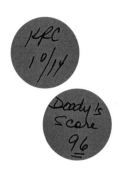

DIAGNOSTIC AND SURGICAL
IMAGING ANATOMY
ULTRASOUND

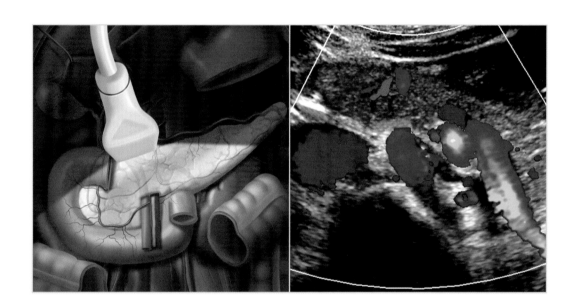

DIAGNOSTIC AND SURGICAL
IMAGING ANATOMY
ULTRASOUND

Anil T. Ahuja, MD, FRCR
Professor
Department of Diagnostic Radiology and Organ Imaging
The Chinese University of Hong Kong
Hong Kong, China

Gregory E. Antonio, MD, FRANZCR
Professor
Department of Diagnostic Radiology and Organ Imaging
The Chinese University of Hong Kong
Hong Kong, China

James F. Griffith, MBBCh, FRCR
Professor
Department of Diagnostic Radiology and Organ Imaging
The Chinese University of Hong Kong
Hong Kong, China

Simon S.M. Ho, MBBS, FRCR
Assistant Professor
Department of Diagnostic Radiology and Organ Imaging
The Chinese University of Hong Kong
Hong Kong, China

K.T. Wong, MBChB, FRCR
Honorary Clinical Associate Professor
Department of Diagnostic Radiology and Organ Imaging
The Chinese University of Hong Kong
Hong Kong, China

Winnie C.W. Chu, MBChB, FRCR
Professor
Department of Diagnostic Radiology and Organ Imaging
The Chinese University of Hong Kong
Hong Kong, China

Stella S.Y. Ho, PhD, RDMS
Adjunct Assistant Professor
Department of Diagnostic Radiology and Organ Imaging
The Chinese University of Hong Kong
Hong Kong, China

Yolanda Y.P. Lee, MBChB, FRCR
Honorary Clinical Tutor
Department of Diagnostic Radiology and Organ Imaging
The Chinese University of Hong Kong
Hong Kong, China

Jill M. Abrigo, MD, DPBR
Clinical Tutor
Department of Diagnostic Radiology and Organ Imaging
The Chinese University of Hong Kong
Hong Kong, China

Bhawan K. Paunipagar, MD, DNB
Clinical Tutor
Department of Diagnostic Radiology and Organ Imaging
The Chinese University of Hong Kong
Hong Kong, China

Chander Lulla, MD, DMRD
Consultant Sonologist
RIA Clinic
Mumbai, India

Deyond Y.W. Siu, MBChB, FRCR
Honorary Clinical Tutor
Department of Diagnostic Radiology and Organ Imaging
The Chinese University of Hong Kong
Hong Kong, China

Eric K.H. Liu, PhD, RDMS
Adjunct Assistant Professor
Department of Diagnostic Radiology and Organ Imaging
The Chinese University of Hong Kong
Hong Kong, China

Vivian Y.F. Leung, PhD, RDMS
Adjunct Assistant Professor
Department of Diagnostic Radiology and Organ Imaging
The Chinese University of Hong Kong
Hong Kong, China

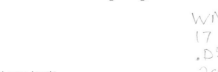

AMIRSYS®
Names you know, content you trust®

WN
17
.D536
2007

AMIRSYS®

Names you know, content you trust®

First Edition

Text and Radiologic Images - Copyright © 2007 Jill M. Abrigo, MD, DPBR, Anil T. Ahuja, MD, FRCR, Gregory E. Antonio, MD, FRANZCR, Winnie C.W. Chu, MBChB, FRCR, James F. Griffith, MBBCh, FRCR, Simon S.M. Ho, MBBS, FRCR, Stella S.Y. Ho, PhD, RDMS, Yolanda Y.P. Lee, MBChB, FRCR, Vivian Y.F. Leung, PhD, RDMS, Eric K.H. Liu, PhD, RDMS, Chander Lulla, MD, DMRD, Bhawan K. Paunipagar, MD, DNB, Deyond Y.W. Siu, MBChB, FRCR, K.T. Wong, MBChB, FRCR

Drawings - Copyright © 2007 Amirsys Inc.

Compilation - Copyright © 2007 Amirsys Inc.

Composition by Amirsys Inc, Salt Lake City, Utah

Printed in Canada by Friesens, Altona, Manitoba, Canada

ISBN-13: 978-1-931884-37-2
ISBN-10: 1-931884-37-4
ISBN-13: 978-1-931884-38-9 (International English Edition)
ISBN-10: 1-931884-38-2 (International English Edition)

Notice and Disclaimer

Library of Congress Cataloging-in-Publication Data

Diagnostic and surgical imaging anatomy. Ultrasound / [edited by] Anil T. Ahuja, Gregory E. Antonio. -- 1st ed.
      p. ; cm.
  Includes index.
  ISBN-13: 978-1-931884-37-2
  ISBN-10: 1-931884-37-4
  ISBN-13: 978-1-931884-38-9 (international English ed.)
  ISBN-10: 1-931884-38-2 (international English ed.)
  1. Human anatomy--Atlases. 2. Ultrasonic imaging--Atlases. I. Ahuja, Anil T. II. Antonio, Gregory E. III. Title: Ultrasound.
  [DNLM: 1. Anatomy, Cross-Sectional--Atlases. 2. Ultrasonography--methods--Atlases. WN 17 D536 2007]
  QM25.D53 2007
  616.07'543--dc22
                    2007038360

This book is dedicated to:

My dear mum, Laj T. Ahuja & dad, Dr. T.S. Ahuja
For your love, and for always being there for the family.

My caring wife, Chu Wai Po, Reann
For your immense patience, support, encouragement & giving
me two beautiful daughters.

My lovely daughters, Sanjali & Tiana
For being a constant source of joy, pride, laughter &
happiness in our lives.

My loving sister, Anita
For all that you do for us.

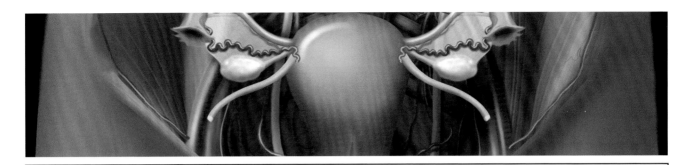

DIAGNOSTIC AND SURGICAL IMAGING ANATOMY: ULTRASOUND

We at Amirsys, together with our distribution colleagues at LWW, are proud to present <u>Diagnostic and Surgical Imaging Anatomy: Ultrasound</u>, the fifth in our brand-new, award-winning series of anatomy reference titles. All books in this exciting series are designed specifically to serve medical imaging specialists as well as clinicians involved in each area's related surgical and allied health subspecialities. Every imaging anatomy textbook contains over 2,500 labeled color graphics and high-resolution radiologic images. The series is designed to give you, the busy medical professional, rapid answers to imaging anatomy questions.

The burgeoning worldwide use of ultrasound in all body parts means today's physicians who utilize this wonderful modality must be intimately familiar with anatomy seen in sometimes-unfamiliar settings. In <u>Diagnostic and Surgical Imaging Anatomy: Ultrasound</u>, Anil Ahuja and colleagues delineate anatomy that is generally visible on ultrasound, presenting bulleted brief introductory text descriptions along with a glorious, rich offering of color normal anatomy graphics together with beautiful multiplanar high-resolution ultrasound images. Both multiplanar grayscale and power Doppler studies are presented. "Mini-graphic" localizers that show probe position accompany each image. Where appropriate, other cross-sectional modalities such as CT and MR are shown side-by-side with their corresponding US images for ease of reference.

For easy reference, <u>Diagnostic and Surgical Imaging Anatomy: Ultrasound</u> is subdivided into separate sections that cover detailed normal anatomy of the brain and spine, neck, thorax, abdomen, pelvis, upper and lower limbs.

In summary, <u>Diagnostic and Surgical Imaging Anatomy: Ultrasound</u> is a product designed with you, the reader, in mind. Today's busy radiologists and clinicians demand both accuracy and efficiency in image interpretation for rapid, accurate decision-making. We think you'll find this new approach to anatomy a highly efficient and wonderfully rich resource that will be the core of your reference collection. Other books in our series that you may find useful are <u>Diagnostic and Surgical Imaging Anatomy: Brain, Spine, Head and Neck</u>, <u>Diagnostic and Surgical Imaging Anatomy: Musculoskeletal</u>, <u>Diagnostic and Surgical Imaging Anatomy: Chest, Abdomen and Pelvis</u> and <u>Diagnostic and Surgical Imaging Anatomy: Knee, Ankle, Foot</u>.

We hope that you will sit back, dig in, and enjoy seeing anatomy and imaging with a whole different eye.

Anne G. Osborn, MD
Executive Vice President and Editor-in-Chief, Amirsys Inc.

H. Ric Harnsberger, MD
CEO & Chairman, Amirsys Inc.

B.J. Manaster, MD
Vice President & Associate Medical Director, Amirsys Inc.

Paula J. Woodward, MD
Senior Vice President & Medical Director, Amirsys Inc.

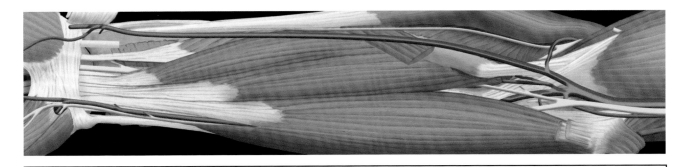

FOREWORD

This book from the team led by Anil Ahuja is a remarkable anatomical text book. Although billed as an ultrasound anatomy book it is a marvellous revision guide for any student in anatomy and anyone using any imaging technique! It will certainly help the inexperienced (and experienced) ultrasonographer avoid pitfalls. The book will also help those more senior radiologists who are extending their ultrasound repertoire into less familiar parts of the body. The graphics which accompany the ultrasound images are extremely informative allowing the reader to see exactly where the probe has been placed in order to obtain the individual ultrasound images. Furthermore schematic anatomical diagrams at the beginning of each section would also be invaluable for people interpreting other imaging investigations (CT, MR, etc). Thus this book should become a classical "bench" book appropriately located in many parts of radiology departments. As ultrasound is, rightly or wrongly, increasingly being used by people with relatively little formal training in imaging, I imagine that such users will come to regard this very welcome addition to the radiology literature with much affection.

Once again, I congratulate Professor Ahuja on overseeing the development of a remarkable text book. The publishers have also done an excellent job in making it so user friendly. I only wish that I had been able to have access to this book when I started my ultrasound training three decades ago. I gave up ultrasound fifteen years later because it became too difficult. With this book I might have been able to keep going a bit longer!

Adrian K. Dixon, MD, FRCR, FRCP, FRCS, FMedSci
Professor of Radiology
University of Cambridge
Honorary Consultant Radiologist
Addenbrooke's Hospital
Cambridge, United Kingdom

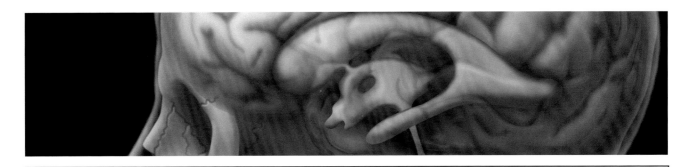

PREFACE

My dad used to have a plaque on his desk which said "hard work is good for health, why not improve yours". My health certainly got a lot better while I worked on this book. All of us involved with this had to go back and relearn anatomy, try and put it into clinical context and marry it with relevant sonograms. Easier said then done, considering ultrasound equipment has significantly improved and now demonstrates structures that were previously invisible.

During routine ultrasound examination, all our attention is focused on areas, structures, and pathology that is relevant to the patient's clinical condition. Instinctively, all other anatomical structures that are seen on the examination, become selectively "invisible", or of doubtful clinical significance. None of us compile images of normal structures or minor anatomical variants. In this book we have concentrated on normal anatomy, examined subjects to demonstrate normal structures routinely seen during sonography, and tried to accurately identify and annotate all visible structures. Graphics alongside sonograms show the approximate location and alignment of the transducer on the skin surface, relevant underlying anatomy and the direction of the scanning beam. These are a general guide. Bear in mind that ultrasound is a real-time examination, and during sonography, the transducer is angulated, rotated, moved side to side to evaluate structures in multiple planes.

I have been fortunate to work with friends who share a unique curiosity. All were interested in identifying anatomy normally visible on ultrasound, and went to great lengths to try and accurately annotate these structures. This book would not have been possible without contribution from all members of the department. I thank them for their patience, help, hard work and generosity in sharing their images, expertise, knowledge and time. On behalf of all the authors, I would particularly like to thank the sonographers for their due diligence and attention to detail, in producing superb quality examinations on a daily basis.

The team from AMIRSYS has been great. They have helped, gently prodded and patiently guided us along the entire process. I am privileged to be associated with Drs. Ric Harnsberger & Anne Osborn. Their support, enthusiasm and friendship have helped me immensely, and I remain grateful for the opportunity.

This book has been hard work, but fun. I have enjoyed the company of friends involved in this venture and remain forever indebted. I learnt a lot during the process and pray you find the book useful.

Anil T. Ahuja, MD, FRCR
Professor
Department of Diagnostic Radiology and Organ Imaging
The Chinese University of Hong Kong
Hong Kong, China

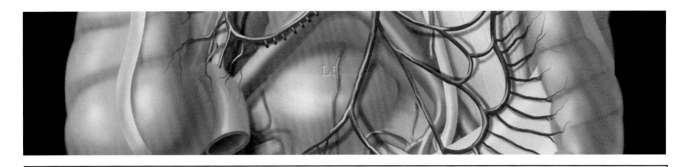

ACKNOWLEDGMENTS

Illustrations
Lane R. Bennion, MS
Richard Coombs, MS

Image/Text Editing
Amanda Hurtado
Melissa A. Hoopes
Kaerli Main
Kevin K.W. Leung
Abby Y.T. Tong

Medical Text Editing
Paula J. Woodward, MD
B.J. Manaster, MD
Daniel N. Sommers, MD
Marta E. Heilbrun, MD

Case Management
Christopher Odekirk

Contributors
Varsha Hardas, MD
Sharad Kondekar, MD
Aniruddha Kulkarni, MD
Pramod Lonikar, MD
Prasanna Mishrikotkar, MD
Asif Momin, MD
Sanjay Surana, MD
Sanjay Vaid, MD
Ki Wang, FRCR

Project Lead
Douglas Grant Jackson

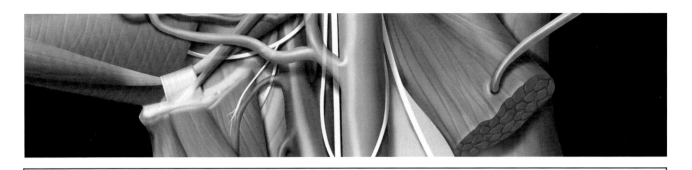

SECTIONS

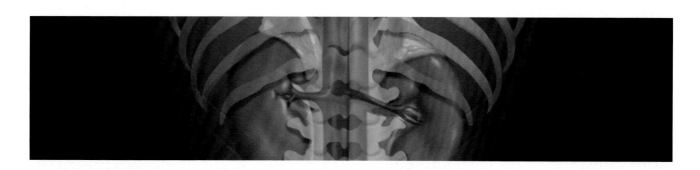

TABLE OF CONTENTS

Section VI
Upper Limb

Section VII
Lower Limb

DIAGNOSTIC AND SURGICAL
IMAGING ANATOMY
ULTRASOUND

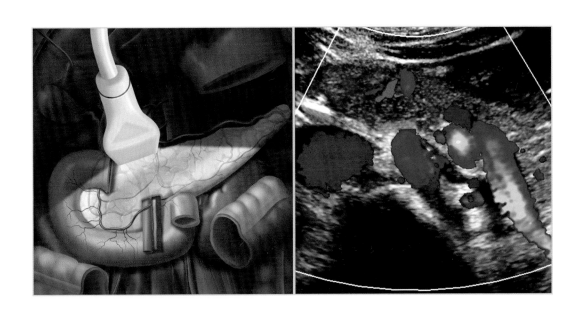

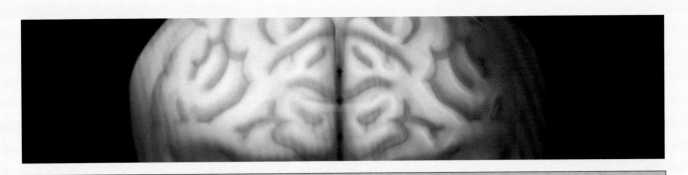

SECTION I: Brain and Spine

SCALP AND CALVARIAL VAULT

Terminology

Definitions
- Fontanelle: Broad areas of connective tissue at the junction of major sutures

Gross Anatomy

Overview
- **Scalp**
  - Scalp has five layers
    - Skin (epidermis, dermis, hair, sebaceous glands)
    - Subcutaneous tissue (very vascular fibro-adipose tissue)
    - Epicranial tissue (scalp muscles, galea aponeurotica)
    - Subaponeurotic tissue (loose areolar connective tissue)
    - Pericranium (periosteum of skull)
- Skull (28 separate bones, mostly connected by fibrous sutures)
  - Cranium has several parts
    - Calvarial vault
    - Cranial base
    - Facial skeleton
  - Calvarial vault composed of several bones
    - 2 frontal bones separated by metopic suture
    - Paired parietal bones
    - Squamous occipital bone
    - Paired squamous temporal bones
  - Three major serrated fibrous joints (sutures) connect bones of vault
    - Coronal suture
    - Sagittal suture
    - Lambdoid suture
  - Outer, inner tables
    - Two thin plates of compact cortical bone
    - Separated by diploic space (cancellous bone containing marrow)
  - Endocranial surface
    - Lined by outer (periosteal) layer of dura
    - Grooved by vascular furrows
    - May have areas of focal thinning (arachnoid granulations), foramina (emissary veins)

Imaging Anatomy

Overview
- Scalp: Hypoechoic, the 5 layers cannot be further separately resolved
- Calvarium echogenic outer/inner tables; diploic space filled with fatty marrow and appears hypoechoic, suture appears as a gap between echogenic calvarium
- Frontal bones
  - Frontal sinuses show wide variation in aeration
  - Frontal bones often appear thickened, hyperostotic (especially in older females)
- Parietal bones
  - Areas of parietal thinning, granular foveolae (for arachnoid granulations) common adjacent to sagittal suture

- Inner tables often slightly irregular (convolutional markings caused by gyri), grooved by paired middle meningeal arteries + vein
- Occipital bone
  - Deeply grooved by superior sagittal, transverse sinuses
  - Internal occipital protuberance marks sinus confluence (torcular Herophili)
- Temporal bones
  - Thin, inner surface grooved by middle meningeal vessels
  - Outer surface grooved by superficial temporal artery
- Fontanelle: Provide acoustic window for US examination of underlying brain parenchyma
  - **Anterior fontanelle**
  - Between 2 frontal and 2 parietal bones, usually disappears by age of 2
  - When fused, corresponds to bregma: Meeting of sagittal, coronal sutures
  - **Posterior fontanelle**
  - Small, usually closes 3-6 month
  - When fused, corresponds to lambda: Meeting of sagittal, lambdoid sutures
  - Pterion
    - Anterolateral fontanelle; closes 3-6 month
    - "H-shaped" junction between frontal, parietal bones plus greater sphenoid wing, squamous temporal bone
  - Asterion
    - Posterolateral fontanelle, persists until 2 years
  - **Mastoid fontanelle**
  - Located at junction of temporosquamous & lambdoid sutures
  - Persists until two years

Anatomy-Based Imaging Issues

Imaging Recommendations
- High frequency, linear array transducers provide superb resolution of near field structures
- Good skin-to-transducer coupling achieved by copious use of acoustic coupling gel
- Superficial standoff pad can be used to increase the depth of focal zone
- US can be used to evaluate cranial sutures and assists diagnosis of craniosynostosis (premature fusion of sutures)

Embryology

Embryologic Events
- Skull base formed from endochondral ossification
- Calvarial vault forms via membranous ossification
  - Curved mesenchymal plates appear at day 30
  - Extend towards each other, skull base
  - As paired bones meet in midline, metopic and sagittal sutures are induced (coronal suture is present from onset of ossification)
  - Unossified centers at edges of parietal bone form fontanelles
  - Vault grows rapidly in first postnatal year

SCALP & CALVARIAL VAULT

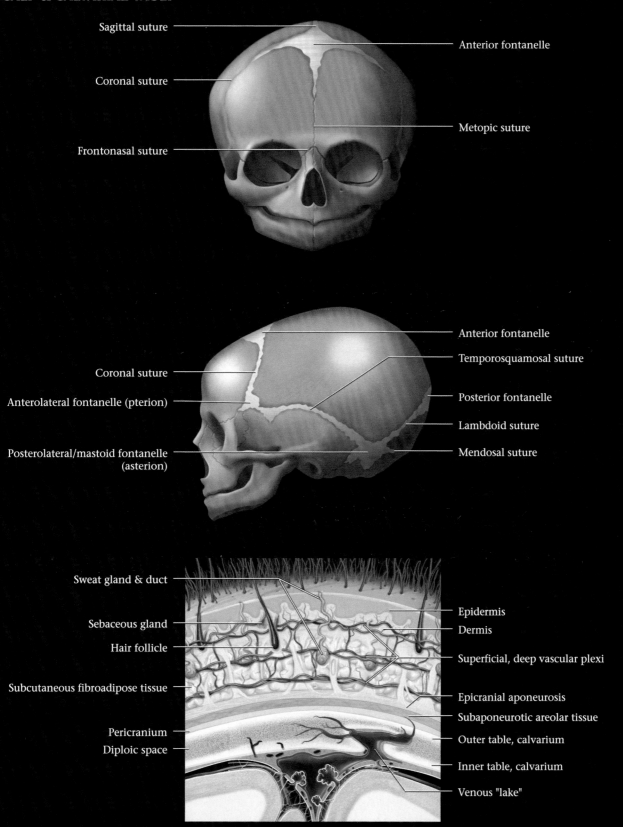

Sagittal suture

Anterior fontanelle

Coronal suture

Metopic suture

Frontonasal suture

Anterior fontanelle

Temporosquamosal suture

Coronal suture

Anterolateral fontanelle (pterion)

Posterior fontanelle

Lambdoid suture

Posterolateral/mastoid fontanelle (asterion)

Mendosal suture

Sweat gland & duct

Epidermis

Sebaceous gland

Dermis

Hair follicle

Superficial, deep vascular plexi

Subcutaneous fibroadipose tissue

Epicranial aponeurosis

Subaponeurotic areolar tissue

Pericranium

Outer table, calvarium

Diploic space

Inner table, calvarium

Venous "lake"

(Top) Graphic depiction of an infant cranium, frontal view. The anterior fontanelle is present between 2 frontal & 2 parietal bones, which usually close by the age of 2. When fused, this site corresponds to bregma: Meeting point of sagittal & coronal sutures. (Middle) Lateral view of an infant calvarial vault. The posterior fontanelle is small and usually closes by 3-6 months. When fused, this corresponds to lambda: Meeting of sagittal & lambdoid sutures. The anterolateral fontanelle (pterion) closes at about 3 months. The posterolateral fontanelle (asterion) often persists until 2 years of age. (Bottom) Scalp and calvarium are depicted in cross section. The five scalp layers are depicted. Skin consists of epidermis and dermis. Hair follicles and a sebaceous gland, the subcutaneous fibro-adipose tissue, sweat glands and ducts, as well as superficial and deep cutaneous vascular plexi are shown.

Brain and Spine

I

SCALP AND CALVARIAL VAULT

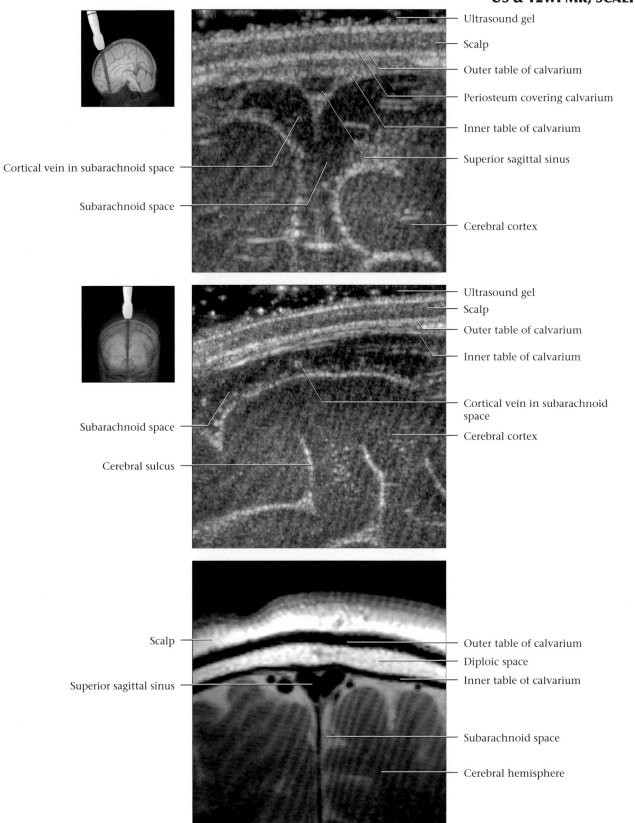

Cortical vein in subarachnoid space

Subarachnoid space

Ultrasound gel

Scalp

Outer table of calvarium

Periosteum covering calvarium

Inner table of calvarium

Superior sagittal sinus

Cerebral cortex

Subarachnoid space

Cerebral sulcus

Ultrasound gel

Scalp

Outer table of calvarium

Inner table of calvarium

Cortical vein in subarachnoid space

Cerebral cortex

Scalp

Superior sagittal sinus

Outer table of calvarium

Diploic space

Inner table of calvarium

Subarachnoid space

Cerebral hemisphere

(Top) Anterior coronal US scan through anterior fontanelle shows the scalp covering the frontal bone of the calvarial vault. The five layers of the scalp are: Skin, connective tissue consisting of lobules of fat, artery and emissary vein, aponeurosis, loose connective tissue which accounts for mobility of the scalp on the underlying bone & periosteum adhering to the outer table of skull. These five layers, however cannot be resolved by ultrasound. **(Middle)** Mid sagittal scan through anterior fontanelle shows the scalp covering the frontal bone of the calvarial vault. Beneath the inner table of the calvarial vault is the anechoic subarachnoid space. **(Bottom)** Coronal T2 MR image shows hypointense outer & inner table of calvarium. The scalp & diploic space are hyperintense. The superior sagittal sinus, appears as signal void structure, below the inner table of calvarium.

SCALP AND CALVARIAL VAULT

US & T2WI MR CALVARIUM

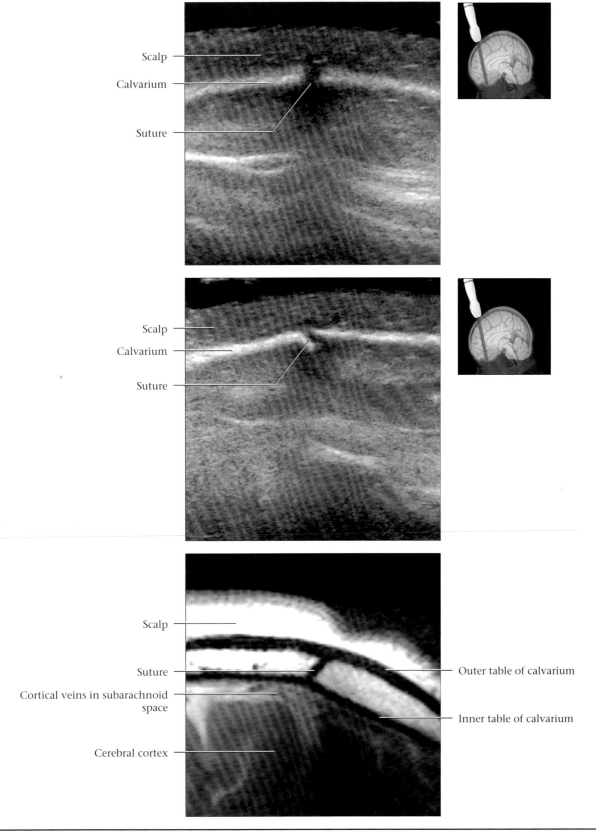

Scalp

Calvarium

Suture

Scalp

Calvarium

Suture

Scalp

Suture

Cortical veins in subarachnoid space

Cerebral cortex

Outer table of calvarium

Inner table of calvarium

(Top) Coronal US scan through the anterior fontanelle shows scalp and calvarium. There is discontinuity: A hypoechoic band extending from the outer to inner table of the calvarial vault. This represents a normal suture. The scalp appears hypoechoic compared to the echogenic outer and inner tables of the calvarium. The five layers of the scalp cannot be resolved by ultrasound. **(Middle)** Coronal US scan through anterior fontanelle shows another suture of the calvarial vault. The width and curvature of sutures is variable and should not be mistaken for a bony fracture. **(Bottom)** T2 MR sagittal image of the scalp and calvarium. The suture line appears as the same signal intensity as the outer and inner table of calvarium. Cortical veins can be seen within hyperintense subarachnoid space, which is immediately under the inner table.

CRANIAL MENINGES

Terminology

Abbreviations
- Extradural space (EDS)
- Subdural space (SDS)
- Subarachnoid space (SAS)
- Subpial space (SPS)
- Perivascular space (PVS)
- Interstitial fluid (ISF)
- Cerebrospinal fluid (CSF)
- Internal carotid artery (ICA)
- External carotid artery (ECA)

Definitions
- Pachymeninges: Dura
- Leptomeninges: Arachnoid, pia
- EDS: Potential space between dura, skull; seen only in pathologic conditions (infection, hematoma, etc.)
- SDS: Potential space between inner dura, arachnoid; seen only in pathologic conditions
- SAS: Normal CSF-filled space between arachnoid, pial-covered brain
- SPS: Potential space between pia, glia limitans of cortex
- PVS: Pial-lined, ISF-filled invagination along penetrating arteries

Gross Anatomy

Overview
- Brain encased by three meninges
  - **Dura**
    - Dense fibrocollagenous sheet
    - Two layers (outer/periosteal, inner/meningeal)
    - Closely adherent except where separate to enclose venous sinus
    - Outer layer forms periosteum of inner calvarium
    - Inner layer folds inward (forming falx cerebri, tentorium cerebelli, etc.) also continues extracranially (into orbit, through foramen magnum into spinal canal)
    - At other foramina, meningeal dura fuses with epineurium of cranial/peripheral nerves, adventitia of carotid/vertebral arteries
    - Blood supply from numerous dural vessels (middle, accessory meningeal arteries; cavernous/tentorial branches of ICA; posterior meningeal branches of vertebral artery; transosseous meningeal branches of ECA, etc.) many with extensive extra/intracranial anastomoses
    - Dura tightly adherent to skull at sutural attachments
  - **Arachnoid**
    - Thin, nearly transparent
    - Outer surface loosely adherent to dura; easily separated
    - Arachnoid follows dura, does **not** invaginate into sulci
    - SAS lies between arachnoid, pia and is traversed by sheet-like bridging trabeculae
    - Arachnoid villi/granulations = endothelial-lined extensions of arachnoid + SAS into dural sinus
  - **Pia**
    - Innermost layer of leptomeninges
    - Covers brain; invaginates into sulci
    - Follows penetrating cortical arteries into brain, forming **PVSs (Virchow-Robin spaces)**

Imaging Anatomy

Overview
- **Dura**
  - Echogenic outer and inner layers enclosing the superior sagittal sinus
  - Best seen on coronal and sagittal scans through anterior fontanelle
  - Superior sagittal sinus: Anechoic with pulsatile flow on color Doppler
    - Echogenicity and lack of flow are suggestive of thrombosis
- **Arachnoid**
  - Normally not seen
  - Pathologic processes typically affect both dura, arachnoid which become involved/thickened and are indistinguishable
  - Pia-arachnoid contains superficial cortical blood vessels visualized by color Doppler
  - Displacement of cortical vessels indicate presence of fluid collection in extra-axial space
- **Extra-axial fluid spaces**
  - Midline space more commonly seen than those over anterior, posterior or lateral surfaces
  - Normal interhemispheric width (widest horizontal distance between the hemispheres at the level of foramen of Monro on coronal plane) ranges from 0.5-8.2 mm

Anatomy-Based Imaging Issues

Imaging Recommendations
- Use high frequency linear transducer
- Color Doppler US helps differentiate fluid in subarachnoid space and subdural space based on displacement of vessels
- Fluid in subarachnoid space
  - Displaces cortical vessels away from brain surface towards cranial vault
  - Cortical vein and branches are seen within fluid collection
- Fluid in subdural space
  - Displaces cortical vessels towards surface of brain

Imaging Pitfalls
- US is relatively insensitive in the detection of small amounts of fluid in extra-axial space
- Differentiation between subdural and epidural fluid is difficult by US

CRANIAL MENINGES

CRANIAL MENINGES

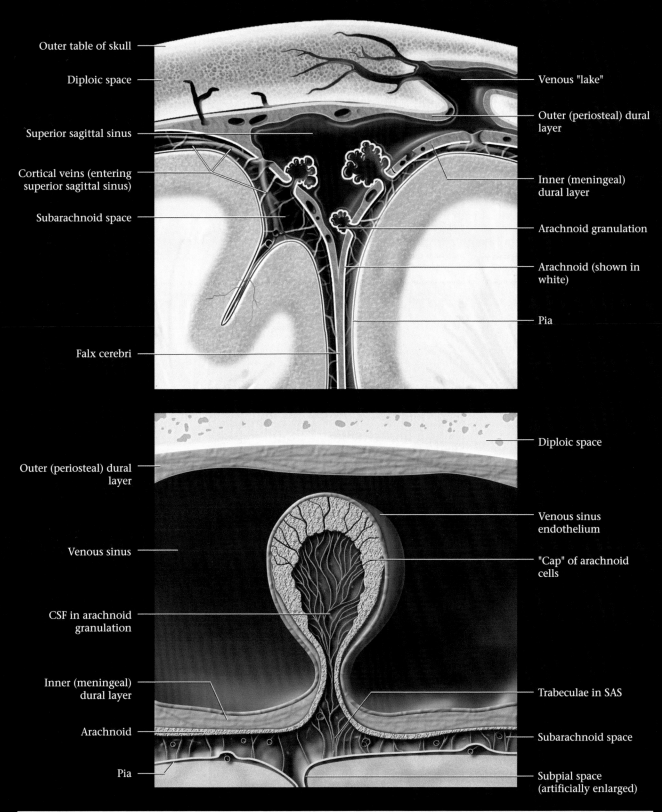

(Top) Close-up coronal view shows the superior sagittal sinus as it is enclosed between the outer and inner dural layers. Note the CSF-containing projections (arachnoid granulations) that extend from the subarachnoid space into the superior sagittal sinuses. (Bottom) Graphic depiction of an arachnoid granulation projecting into a dural venous sinus. A core of CSF extends from the SAS into the granulation and is covered by an apical cap of arachnoid cells. Channels extend through the cap to the sinus endothelium and drain CSF into the venous circulation. Note numerous trabeculae as well as small arteries and veins within the SAS over the brain.

Brain and Spine

I

COLOR DOPPLER US THROUGH ANTERIOR FONTANELLE

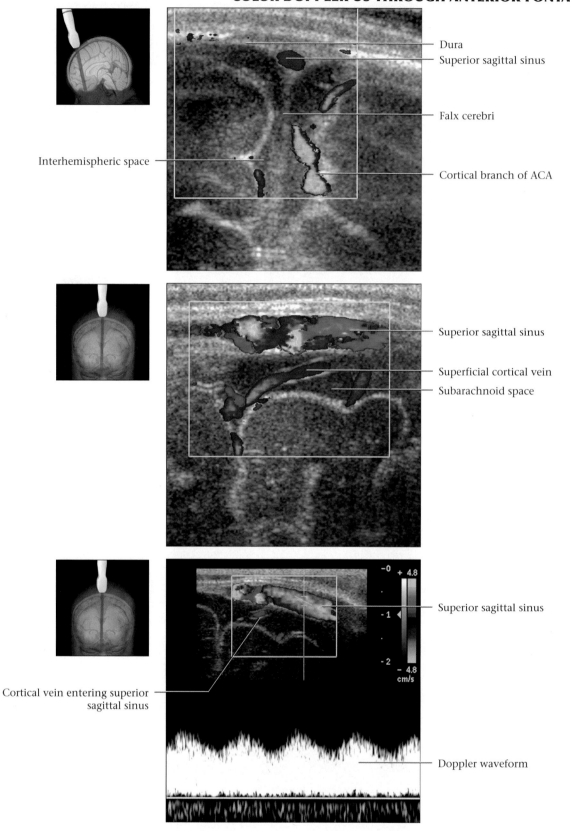

Dura

Superior sagittal sinus

Falx cerebri

Interhemispheric space

Cortical branch of ACA

Superior sagittal sinus

Superficial cortical vein

Subarachnoid space

Superior sagittal sinus

Cortical vein entering superior sagittal sinus

Doppler waveform

(Top) Coronal color Doppler scan through the anterior fontanelle shows transverse section of the superior sagittal sinus, which is enclosed by the dura of the inner table of calvarium. Color signal is seen within the superior sagittal sinus as well as cortical veins traversing the subarachnoid space in the interhemispheric fissure. If flow is absent in the sinus, venous thrombosis should be suspected. In the setting of acute thrombosis, the sinus may also appear echogenic on grayscale ultrasound. (Middle) Sagittal color Doppler scan through the anterior fontanelle shows a superficial cortical vein traversing the subarachnoid space and draining into the superior sagittal sinus. (Bottom) Spectral Doppler waveform of the superior sagittal sinus shows the waveform of the sinus to be pulsatile, under the effect of cardiac pulsation.

COLOR DOPPLER US THROUGH ANTERIOR FONTANELLE

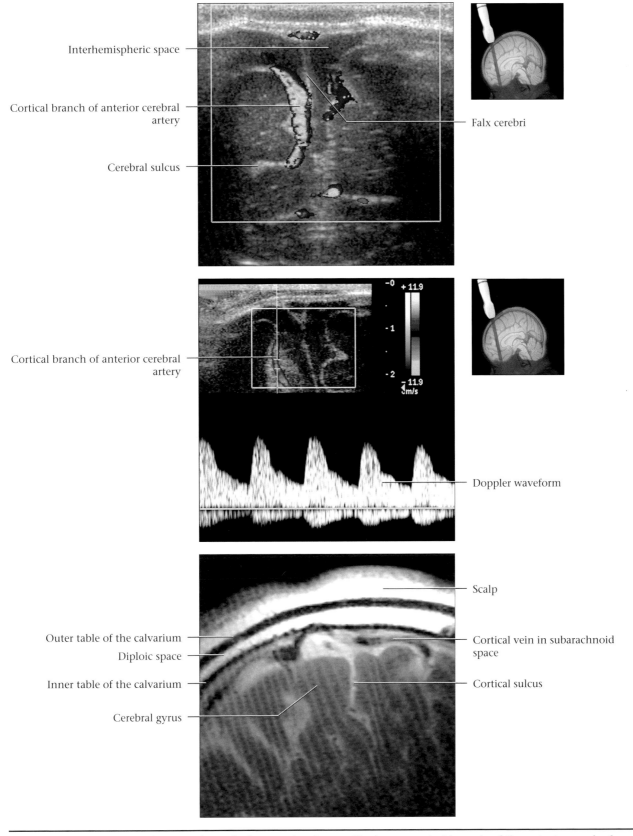

Interhemispheric space

Cortical branch of anterior cerebral artery

Cerebral sulcus

Falx cerebri

Cortical branch of anterior cerebral artery

Doppler waveform

Scalp

Outer table of the calvarium

Diploic space

Inner table of the calvarium

Cerebral gyrus

Cortical vein in subarachnoid space

Cortical sulcus

(Top) Coronal color Doppler scan through the anterior fontanelle shows cortical branch of the anterior cerebral artery (ACA) in the interhemispheric fissure. The falx cerebri is an echogenic midline structure formed by inner, or meningeal, layers of dura. It inserts on the crista galli anteriorly and sweeps backwards in the midline to the straight sinus becoming taller as it passes posteriorly between cerebral hemispheres. **(Middle)** Spectral Doppler waveform of the cortical branch of ACA shows low resistance with abundant antegrade flow throughout diastole. **(Bottom)** T2WI MR coronal image shows a cortical vein within the subarachnoid space. The cortical veins appear as signal void serpiginous structures within the hyperintense CSF space. The meninges cannot be separately resolved on MR. Dura enhances smoothly on post contrast scans while arachnoid and pia are normally not seen on imaging.

CEREBRAL HEMISPHERES OVERVIEW

Terminology

Definitions
- Gyri: Complex convolutions of brain cortex: Hypoechoic on ultrasound (US)
- Sulci (fissure): CSF-filled grooves or clefts that separate gyri; echogenic on ultrasound

Imaging Anatomy

Overview
- **Frontal lobe**
  - Central sulcus separates frontal, parietal lobes
  - Precentral gyrus contains primary motor cortex
    - Detailed topographically-organized map ("motor homunculus") of contralateral body
    - Head/face lateral, legs/feet along medial surface
  - Premotor cortex: Within gyrus just anterior to precentral gyrus (motor cortex)
  - Three additional major gyri: Superior frontal gyrus, middle frontal gyrus & inferior frontal gyrus separated by superior & inferior frontal sulci
- **Parietal lobe**
  - Posterior to central sulcus
  - Separated from occipital lobe by parietooccipital sulcus (medial surface)
  - Postcentral gyrus: Primary somatosensory cortex
    - Contains topographical map of contralateral body
    - Face, tongue, lips are inferior; trunk, upper limb superolateral; lower limb on medial aspect
  - Superior & inferior parietal lobules lie posterior to postcentral gyrus
  - Supramarginal gyrus lies at end of sylvian fissure
  - Angular gyrus lies ventral to supramarginal gyrus
  - Medial surface of parietal lobe is precuneus
- **Occipital lobe**
  - Posterior to parietooccipital sulcus
  - Primary visual cortex on medial occipital lobe
  - Cuneus on medial surface
- **Temporal lobe**
  - Inferior to sylvian fissure
  - Superior temporal gyrus: Contains primary auditory cortex
  - Middle temporal gyrus: Connects with auditory, somatosensory, visual association pathways
  - Inferior temporal gyrus: Higher visual association area
  - Includes major subdivisions of limbic system
    - Parahippocampal gyrus on medial surface, merges into uncus
- **Insula**
  - Lies deep in floor of sylvian fissure, overlapped by frontal, temporal, parietal operculae
- **Limbic system**
  - Subcallosal, cingulate, parahippocampal gyri
  - Cingulate gyrus extends around corpus callosum; tapers rostrally (anteriorly) into paraterminal gyrus, subcallosal area
  - Hippocampus including dentate gyrus, Ammon horn (cornu ammonis)
- **Base of brain**

  - Orbital gyri cover base of frontal lobe: Gyrus rectus medially
- **White matter tracts**: Three major types of fibers
  - Association fibers: Interconnect different cortical regions in same hemisphere including centrum semiovale
    - Cingulum is a long association fiber which lies beneath cingulate gyrus
  - Commissural fibers: Interconnect similar cortical regions of opposite hemispheres
    - Corpus callosum is largest commissural fiber, links cerebral hemispheres
  - Projection fibers: Connect cerebral cortex with deep nuclei, brainstem, cerebellum, spinal cord
    - Internal capsule is a major projection fiber
- **Basal ganglia**
  - Paired deep gray nuclei
  - Caudate nucleus, lentiform nucleus (including putamen, globus pallidus)
- **Thalamus**: Paired nuclear complexes, serve as relay station for most sensory pathways

Anatomy-Based Imaging Issues

Imaging Approaches
- Anterior fontanelle (AF)
  - Sagittal scans
    - Midline scan: Best view for corpus callosum (CC), cerebellar vermis
    - Parasagittal view: To assess degree of sulcal development, size of lateral ventricle
    - Best view for caudothalamic groove: Most common site of germinal matrix hemorrhage in subependymal region of ventricle
  - Coronal scans
    - Important to maintain symmetrical imaging of each half of brain
    - Symmetrical structures (from anterior to posterior) include: Frontal horns, bodies & trigones of lateral ventricles; caudate nuclei, putamen, internal capsule & thalami
    - Midline structures (from anterior to posterior) include: Interhemispheric fissure, genu and anterior body of corpus callosum, septum pellucidum, third ventricle, brainstem
- Posterior fontanelle (PF)
  - Useful to evaluate occipital horns for intraventricular hemorrhage (IVH)
  - Best view for detection of layering clot attached to choroid plexus
- Mastoid fontanelle (MF)
  - Located at junction of squamosal, lambdoidal, occipital sutures
  - Transducer placed about 1 cm behind helix of ear and 1 cm above tragus
  - Allows assessment of brainstem and posterior fossa
  - Best view for fourth ventricle, posterior cerebellar vermis, cerebellar hemispheres and cisterna magna
- Transtemporal (TT)
  - Temporal bone anterior to ear is thin, allowing imaging of brainstem even after sutural closure
  - Best view for cerebral peduncles and third ventricle

CEREBRAL HEMISPHERES OVERVIEW

OVERVIEW

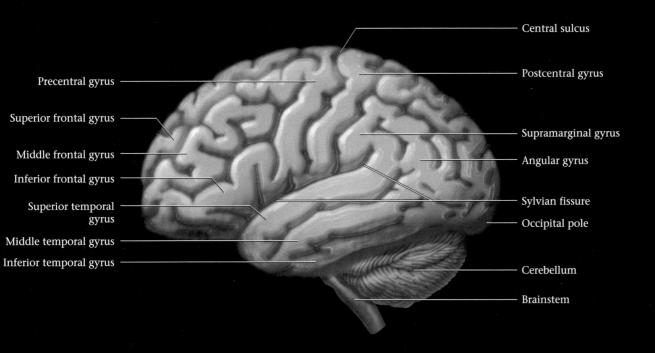

Central sulcus

Precentral gyrus

Postcentral gyrus

Superior frontal gyrus

Supramarginal gyrus

Middle frontal gyrus

Angular gyrus

Inferior frontal gyrus

Superior temporal gyrus

Sylvian fissure

Occipital pole

Middle temporal gyrus

Inferior temporal gyrus

Cerebellum

Brainstem

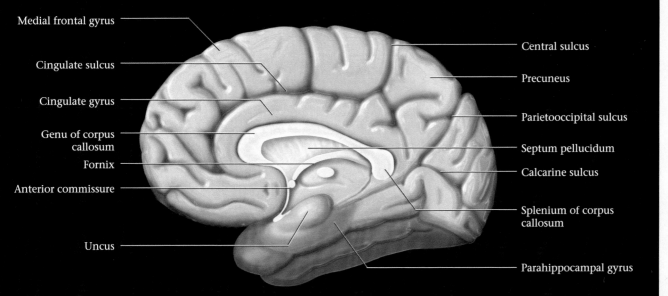

Medial frontal gyrus

Central sulcus

Cingulate sulcus

Precuneus

Cingulate gyrus

Parietooccipital sulcus

Genu of corpus callosum

Septum pellucidum

Fornix

Calcarine sulcus

Anterior commissure

Splenium of corpus callosum

Uncus

Parahippocampal gyrus

(Top) Lateral surface of brain depicts major gyri and sulci. Frontal lobe extends from frontal pole to central sulcus. Supramarginal & angular gyri are part of the parietal lobe. Supramarginal gyrus has somatosensory function while angular gyrus is important in auditory & visual hinput, language comprehension. Superior temporal gyrus contains primary auditory cortex, also forms temporal operculum. Insular cortex lies within sylvian fissure beneath frontal, temporal & parietal opercula. (Bottom) Sagittal graphic shows medial view of cerebral hemisphere. Corpus callosum represents major commissural fiber. Fornix & cingulate gyrus are important in limbic system. Fornix extends from fimbria of hippocampus posteriorly to anterior thalamus, mamillary body and septal region. Cingulate gyrus is involved with emotion formation & processing, learning & memory.

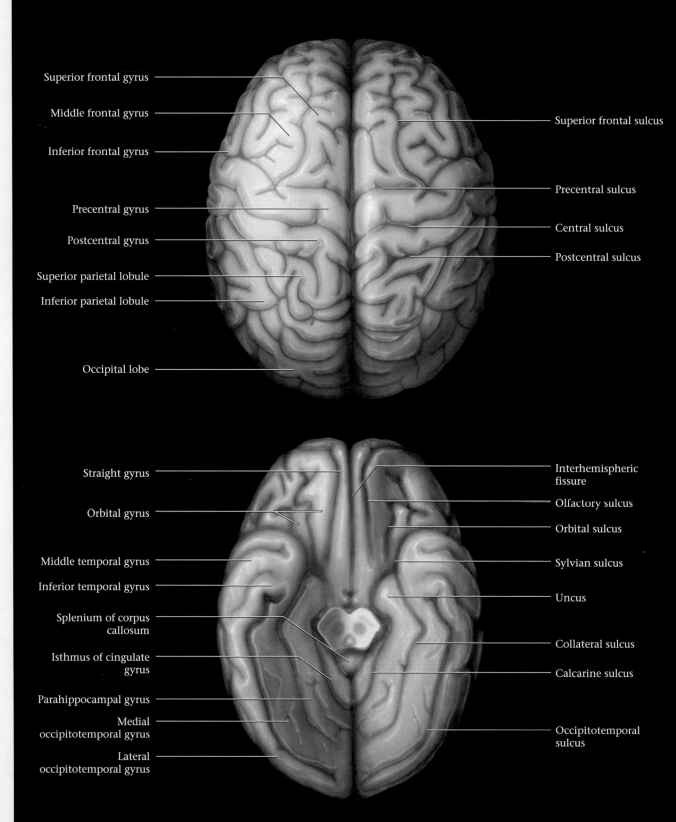

Superior frontal gyrus

Middle frontal gyrus

Inferior frontal gyrus

Precentral gyrus

Postcentral gyrus

Superior parietal lobule

Inferior parietal lobule

Occipital lobe

Superior frontal sulcus

Precentral sulcus

Central sulcus

Postcentral sulcus

Straight gyrus

Orbital gyrus

Middle temporal gyrus

Inferior temporal gyrus

Splenium of corpus callosum

Isthmus of cingulate gyrus

Parahippocampal gyrus

Medial occipitotemporal gyrus

Lateral occipitotemporal gyrus

Interhemispheric fissure

Olfactory sulcus

Orbital sulcus

Sylvian sulcus

Uncus

Collateral sulcus

Calcarine sulcus

Occipitotemporal sulcus

(Top) Surface anatomy of cerebral hemisphere, seen from above. Gyri and lobules shown on left, sulci on right. Central (Rolandic) sulcus separates anterior frontal lobe from posterior parietal lobe. Precentral gyrus of frontal lobe is primary motor cortex while postcentral gyrus of parietal lobe is primary sensory cortex. On ultrasound, the sulci appear echogenic while the adjacent gyri are hypoechoic. **(Bottom)** Inferior view with major sulci, gyri depicted. Orbital gyri cover base of frontal lobe. Gyrus rectus (straight gyrus) is most medial. Olfactory bulb/tract (not shown) lie within olfactory sulcus. Sylvian fissure separates frontal lobe from inferior temporal lobe. Uncus forms medial border of temporal lobe, merges with parahippocampal gyrus. Collateral sulcus separates parahippocampal gyrus from medial occipitotemporal (fusiform or lingual) gyrus.

STANDARD US PLANES VIA ANTERIOR FONTANELLE

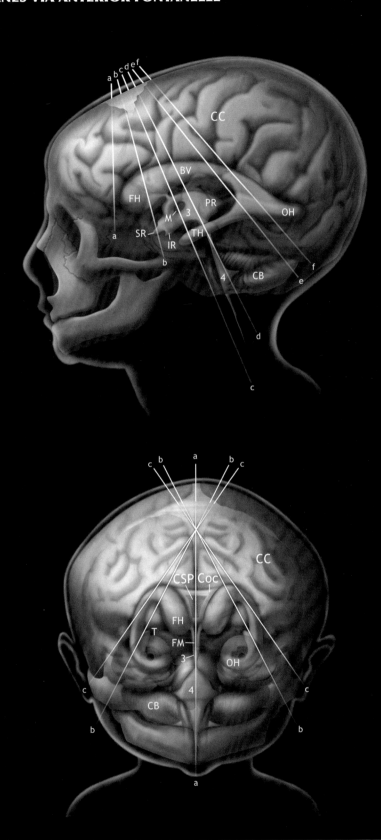

(Top) Graphic shows common coronal planes used in US brain scanning. Plane A to F from front to back. Cerebral cortex (CC); body of lateral ventricle (BV); frontal horn (FH); occipital horn (OH); massa intermedia (M); pineal recess (PR); third ventricle (3); temporal horn (TH); supraoptic recess (SR); infundibular recess (IR); fourth ventricle (4); cerebellum (CB). **(Bottom)** Graphic shows common sagittal planes used in US brain scanning. Plane A to C from midline to lateral. Cerebellum (CB); cerebral cortex (CC); corpus callosum (Coc); cavum septi pellucidi (CSP); frontal horn (FH); foramen of Monro (FM); occipital horn (OH); temporal horn (T); third ventricle (3); fourth ventricle (4). (Both figures are modified from Rumack CM, Johnson ML: Perinatal and Infant Brain Imaging. St. Louis, Mosby- Year Book, 1984).

CEREBRAL HEMISPHERES OVERVIEW

CORONAL US VIA ANTERIOR FONTANELLE

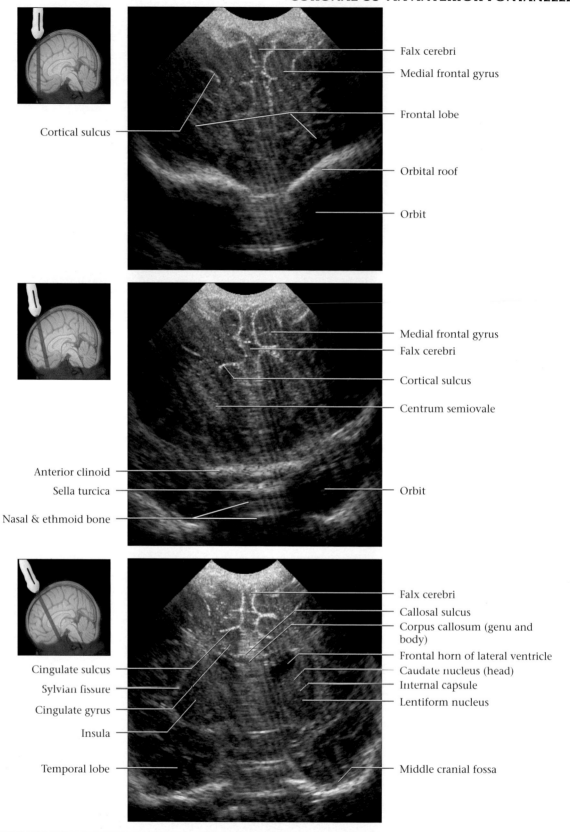

Cortical sulcus

Falx cerebri
Medial frontal gyrus
Frontal lobe
Orbital roof
Orbit

Medial frontal gyrus
Falx cerebri
Cortical sulcus
Centrum semiovale

Anterior clinoid
Sella turcica
Nasal & ethmoid bone

Orbit

Falx cerebri
Callosal sulcus
Corpus callosum (genu and body)
Frontal horn of lateral ventricle
Caudate nucleus (head)
Internal capsule
Lentiform nucleus

Cingulate sulcus
Sylvian fissure
Cingulate gyrus
Insula
Temporal lobe

Middle cranial fossa

(Top) First of nine coronal ultrasound images of the brain through the anterior fontanelle in a term infant. In this image, frontal lobes lie in the anterior cranial fossa with orbital cavities deep to the floor of the skull base. (Middle) Image centered more posteriorly demonstrates slightly more echogenic white matter region of the brain parenchyma known as the centrum semiovale. The bony parts of the skull base that can be seen are the floor of the sella turcica with the anterior clinoid superiorly and the nasal and ethmoid bones inferiorly. (Bottom) Image acquired just anterior to the foramen of Monro. Frontal horns of lateral ventricles are seen. No choroid plexus should be present in the frontal horns. Any intraventricular echogenic material seen at this level should raise the suspicion of blood clot. The head of the caudate nucleus is separated from the lentiform nucleus by the internal capsule.

CEREBRAL HEMISPHERES OVERVIEW

CORONAL T1 MR

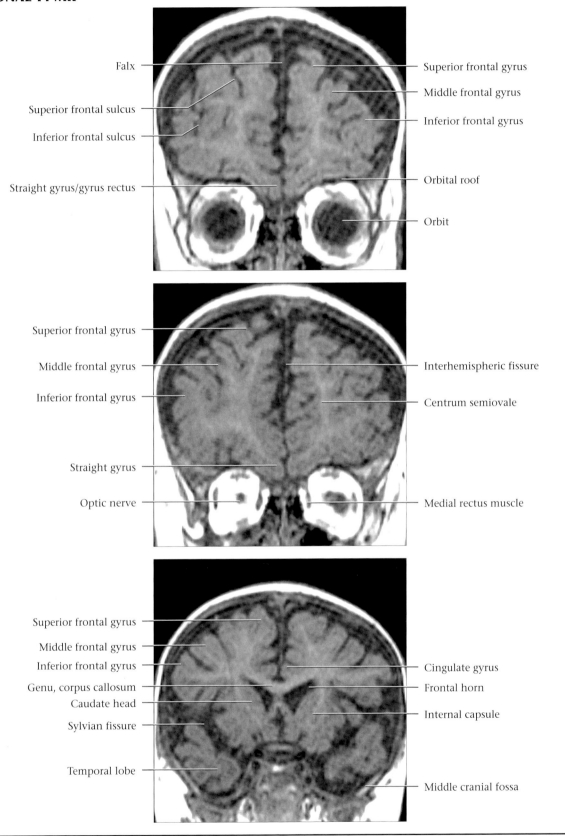

Falx — Superior frontal gyrus

Superior frontal sulcus — Middle frontal gyrus

Inferior frontal sulcus — Inferior frontal gyrus

Straight gyrus/gyrus rectus — Orbital roof

Orbit

Superior frontal gyrus — Interhemispheric fissure

Middle frontal gyrus — Centrum semiovale

Inferior frontal gyrus

Straight gyrus

Optic nerve — Medial rectus muscle

Superior frontal gyrus — Cingulate gyrus

Middle frontal gyrus — Frontal horn

Inferior frontal gyrus — Internal capsule

Genu, corpus callosum

Caudate head

Sylvian fissure

Temporal lobe — Middle cranial fossa

(Top) First of nine coronal T1 MR images through cerebral hemispheres from anterior to posterior. Images are taken through planes/levels corresponding to those commonly used for US scan through the anterior fontanelle. The three major frontal gyri are shown: Superior frontal gyrus, middle frontal gyrus & inferior frontal gyrus, separated by superior & inferior frontal sulci. Straight gyrus (gyrus rectus) is the most medial covering the base of the frontal lobe. (Middle) Slightly more posterior image where superior frontal, middle frontal and inferior frontal gyri are more clearly delineated. Centrum semiovale is the white matter core of cerebral hemispheres containing radiating nerve fibers from the corpus callosum. (Bottom) This image shows the frontal horns. Immediately below each frontal horn is caudate head, separated from the lentiform nucleus by internal capsule.

CEREBRAL HEMISPHERES OVERVIEW

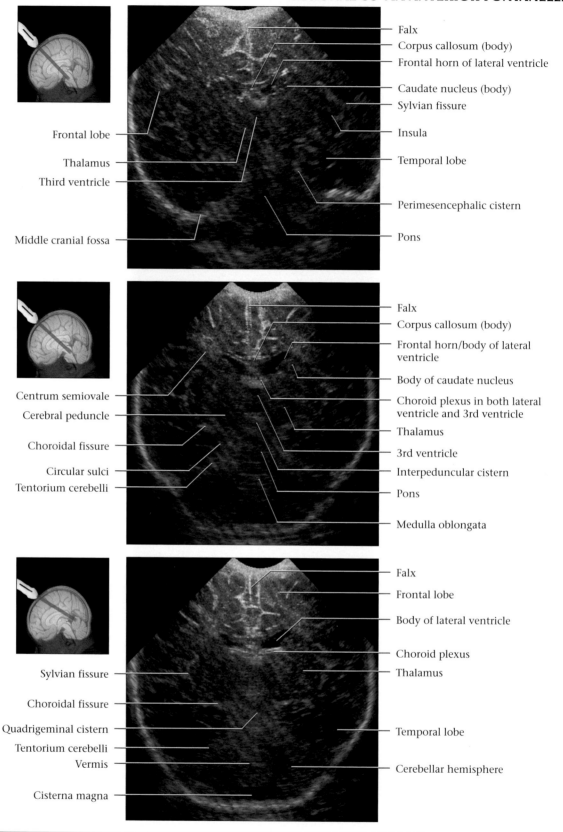

Top image labels:
- Falx
- Corpus callosum (body)
- Frontal horn of lateral ventricle
- Caudate nucleus (body)
- Sylvian fissure
- Insula
- Temporal lobe
- Perimesencephalic cistern
- Pons
- Frontal lobe
- Thalamus
- Third ventricle
- Middle cranial fossa

Middle image labels:
- Falx
- Corpus callosum (body)
- Frontal horn/body of lateral ventricle
- Body of caudate nucleus
- Choroid plexus in both lateral ventricle and 3rd ventricle
- Thalamus
- 3rd ventricle
- Interpeduncular cistern
- Pons
- Medulla oblongata
- Centrum semiovale
- Cerebral peduncle
- Choroidal fissure
- Circular sulci
- Tentorium cerebelli

Bottom image labels:
- Falx
- Frontal lobe
- Body of lateral ventricle
- Choroid plexus
- Thalamus
- Temporal lobe
- Cerebellar hemisphere
- Sylvian fissure
- Choroidal fissure
- Quadrigeminal cistern
- Tentorium cerebelli
- Vermis
- Cisterna magna

(Top) Four of nine coronal US images through AF in term infant. This image is taken at the level of the foramen of Monro. The frontal horns are seen with the body of the caudate nucleus and anterior portions of the thalami below. **(Middle)** Image at the level of the interpeduncular cistern. The choroid plexus is present on the floor of the lateral ventricles and roof of the third ventricle. The three echogenic foci of the choroid plexus, one on the roof of the third ventricle and two located bilaterally on the floor of the lateral ventricles, are known as the "three-dot sign". **(Bottom)** More posterior coronal image at the level of the quadrigeminal cistern. Another US landmark known as the echogenic star is seen which comprises the choroidal fissures as the upper limbs and tentorium cerebelli as the lower limbs. Inferiorly, the vermis appears echogenic while the cerebellar hemispheres on both sides are hypoechoic.

CEREBRAL HEMISPHERES OVERVIEW

CORONAL T1 MR

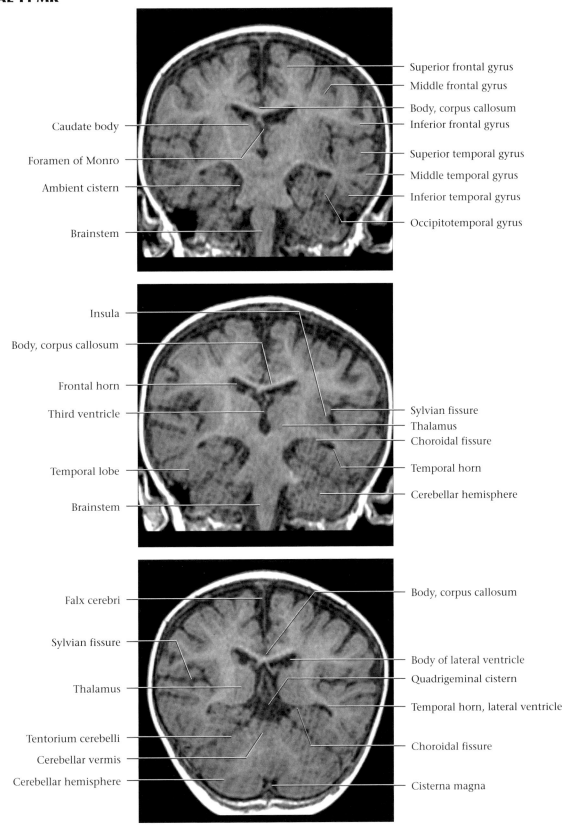

Caudate body

Foramen of Monro

Ambient cistern

Brainstem

Superior frontal gyrus
Middle frontal gyrus
Body, corpus callosum
Inferior frontal gyrus
Superior temporal gyrus
Middle temporal gyrus
Inferior temporal gyrus
Occipitotemporal gyrus

Insula

Body, corpus callosum

Frontal horn

Third ventricle

Temporal lobe

Brainstem

Sylvian fissure
Thalamus
Choroidal fissure
Temporal horn
Cerebellar hemisphere

Falx cerebri

Sylvian fissure

Thalamus

Tentorium cerebelli
Cerebellar vermis
Cerebellar hemisphere

Body, corpus callosum

Body of lateral ventricle
Quadrigeminal cistern
Temporal horn, lateral ventricle
Choroidal fissure
Cisterna magna

(Top) Fourth of nine coronal T1 MR images through the cerebral hemispheres from anterior to posterior. Images are taken through planes/levels corresponding to those commonly used for US scan through AF. This image is taken at the level of the foramen of Monro where both lateral ventricles unite becoming the 3rd ventricle in midline. **(Middle)** This image shows the relationship of the interpeduncular cistern which is in midline, and 2 choroidal fissures which are located in between the temporal horns of the lateral ventricles and perimesencephalic cisterns. These structures are not impressive on MR but give rise to echogenic "3-dot" sign on coronal US scanning. **(Bottom)** This image slightly more posterior shows the quadrigeminal cistern in midline, together with choroidal fissures and tentorium cerebelli on both sides, give rise to the characteristic "echogenic star" appearance on coronal US scanning.

CEREBRAL HEMISPHERES OVERVIEW

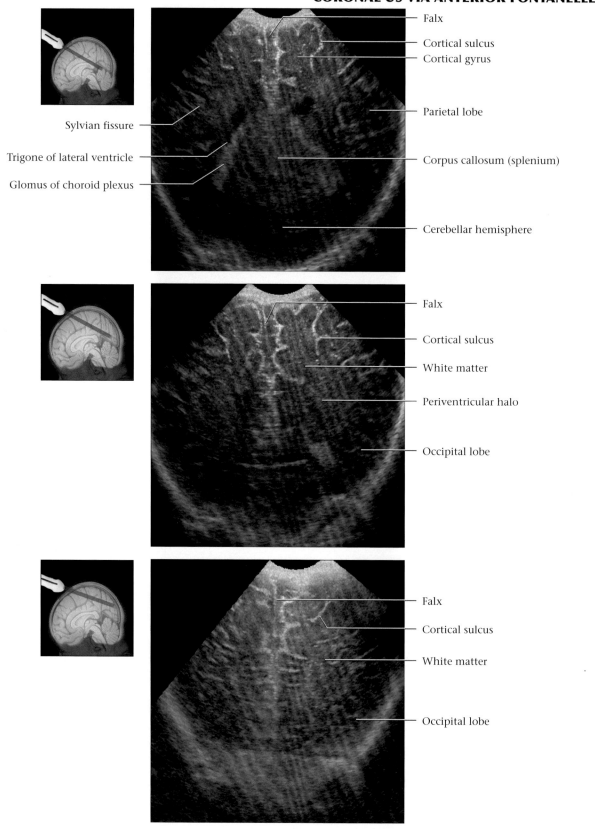

Falx

Cortical sulcus

Cortical gyrus

Parietal lobe

Sylvian fissure

Corpus callosum (splenium)

Trigone of lateral ventricle

Glomus of choroid plexus

Cerebellar hemisphere

Falx

Cortical sulcus

White matter

Periventricular halo

Occipital lobe

Falx

Cortical sulcus

White matter

Occipital lobe

(Top) Seventh of nine coronal US images obtained through the AF in term infant. This image is taken at the trigone of the lateral ventricles. The glomus of the choroid plexus appears highly echogenic nearly occupying the whole trigone. At the midline are the splenium of the corpus callosum and part of the cerebellum. **(Middle)** This image, slightly posterior to the trigone, shows mild echogenic white matter regions, lateral & parallel to both trigones of the lateral ventricles. These regions are known as the periventricular halo, a normal finding, present in almost all normal mature and premature neonates. The echogenicity of the halo should be less than that of the choroid plexus & symmetrical in appearance. **(Bottom)** Most posterior coronal image shows the cortex of the occipital lobe with multiple echogenic sulci extending medially from the lateral margin of the brain. Falx is in midline.

CEREBRAL HEMISPHERES OVERVIEW

CORONAL T1 MR

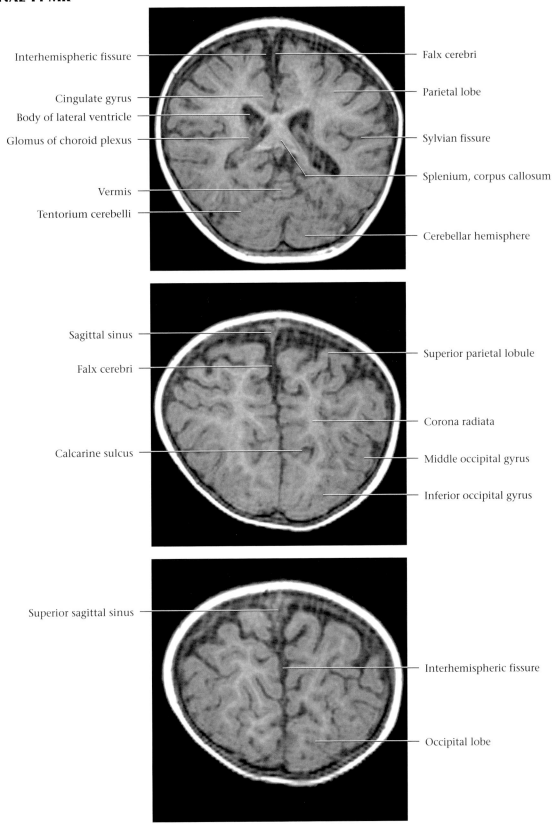

Interhemispheric fissure — Falx cerebri

Cingulate gyrus — Parietal lobe

Body of lateral ventricle

Glomus of choroid plexus — Sylvian fissure

Vermis — Splenium, corpus callosum

Tentorium cerebelli — Cerebellar hemisphere

Sagittal sinus — Superior parietal lobule

Falx cerebri — Corona radiata

Calcarine sulcus — Middle occipital gyrus

Inferior occipital gyrus

Superior sagittal sinus — Interhemispheric fissure

Occipital lobe

(Top) Seven of nine coronal T1 MR images through the cerebral hemispheres from anterior to posterior. Images are taken through planes/levels corresponding to those commonly used for US scan through the anterior fontanelle. The glomus of the choroid plexus is prominent within the trigones of the lateral ventricles. **(Middle)** More posterior image shows the posterior parietal lobes and occipital lobes. Cerebral hemispheres are separated by the interhemispheric fissure which contains the falx cerebri. The ventricular system and cerebellum are no longer seen at this level. Primary visual cortex is on the medial aspect of the occipital lobe. **(Bottom)** Most posterior image shows gyri in the parietal and occipital lobe.

CEREBRAL HEMISPHERES OVERVIEW

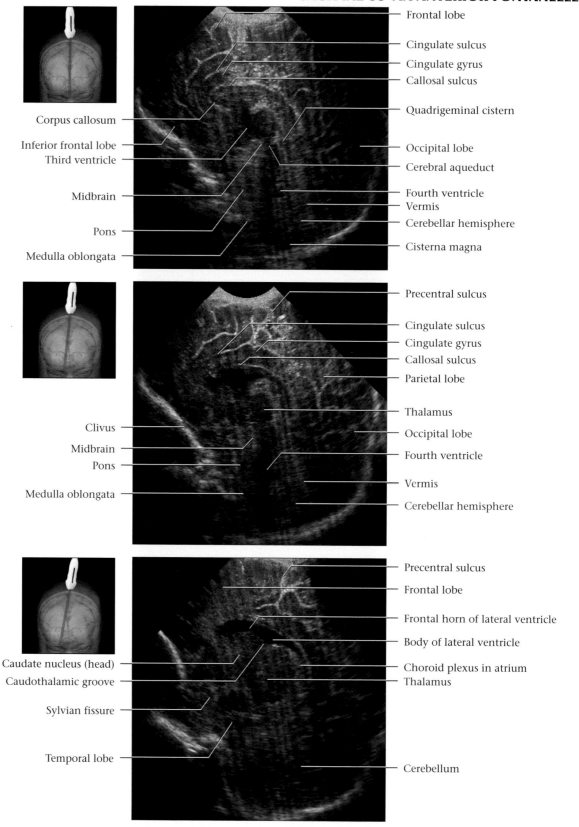

Top image labels:
- Frontal lobe
- Cingulate sulcus
- Cingulate gyrus
- Callosal sulcus
- Quadrigeminal cistern
- Occipital lobe
- Cerebral aqueduct
- Fourth ventricle
- Vermis
- Cerebellar hemisphere
- Cisterna magna
- Corpus callosum
- Inferior frontal lobe
- Third ventricle
- Midbrain
- Pons
- Medulla oblongata

Middle image labels:
- Precentral sulcus
- Cingulate sulcus
- Cingulate gyrus
- Callosal sulcus
- Parietal lobe
- Thalamus
- Occipital lobe
- Fourth ventricle
- Vermis
- Cerebellar hemisphere
- Clivus
- Midbrain
- Pons
- Medulla oblongata

Bottom image labels:
- Precentral sulcus
- Frontal lobe
- Frontal horn of lateral ventricle
- Body of lateral ventricle
- Choroid plexus in atrium
- Thalamus
- Caudate nucleus (head)
- Caudothalamic groove
- Sylvian fissure
- Temporal lobe
- Cerebellum

(**Top**) First of nine sagittal US images of the brain through the anterior fontanelle in term infant. This image obtained in the midline shows the corpus callosum as a hypoechoic curving line. Callosal and cingulate sulci are parallel to & above corpus callosum. From superior to inferior, third ventricle, cerebral aqueduct & fourth ventricle appear hypoechoic while cerebellar vermis appears hyperechoic. (**Middle**) Parasagittal image obtained angling slightly lateral to midline. The thalamus and echogenic sulci can now be seen more clearly. (**Bottom**) Parasagittal image obtained by angling more laterally reaching the level of the caudothalamic groove, the junction between the caudate nucleus and the thalamus. The caudate nucleus is slightly more echogenic than the thalamus. The entire body of the lateral ventricle with part of the choroid plexus within can be seen.

CEREBRAL HEMISPHERES OVERVIEW

SAGITTAL T1 MR

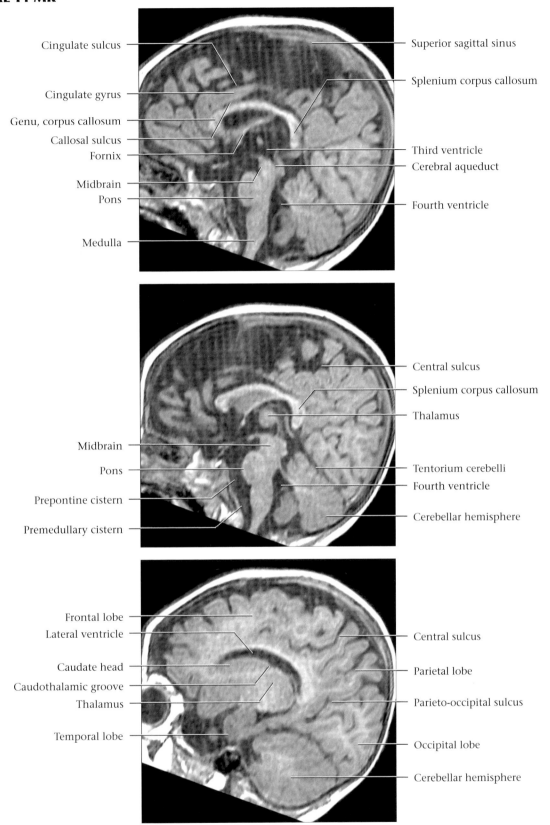

Cingulate sulcus

Cingulate gyrus

Genu, corpus callosum

Callosal sulcus

Fornix

Midbrain

Pons

Medulla

Superior sagittal sinus

Splenium corpus callosum

Third ventricle

Cerebral aqueduct

Fourth ventricle

Central sulcus

Splenium corpus callosum

Thalamus

Midbrain

Pons

Prepontine cistern

Premedullary cistern

Tentorium cerebelli

Fourth ventricle

Cerebellar hemisphere

Frontal lobe

Lateral ventricle

Caudate head

Caudothalamic groove

Thalamus

Temporal lobe

Central sulcus

Parietal lobe

Parieto-occipital sulcus

Occipital lobe

Cerebellar hemisphere

(Top) First of nine sagittal T1 MR images through the cerebral hemispheres from midline to lateral. Images are taken through planes/levels corresponding to those commonly used for US scan through the anterior fontanelle. The midline sagittal image shows the corpus callosum, largest commissural fiber connecting both cerebral hemispheres. More inferiorly is the fornix which is appreciated on MR but not resolved by US. **(Middle)** Parasagittal image just off midline. The tentorium cerebelli is a dural fold separating the brain into supratentorial and infratentorial compartments. When compared with MR, details of the infratentorial compartment are poorly defined by US when scanning through the anterior fontanelle. **(Bottom)** More lateral image shows the caudothalamic groove between the caudate head and thalamus. This is where the vascular germinal matrix is located in premature infants.

CEREBRAL HEMISPHERES OVERVIEW

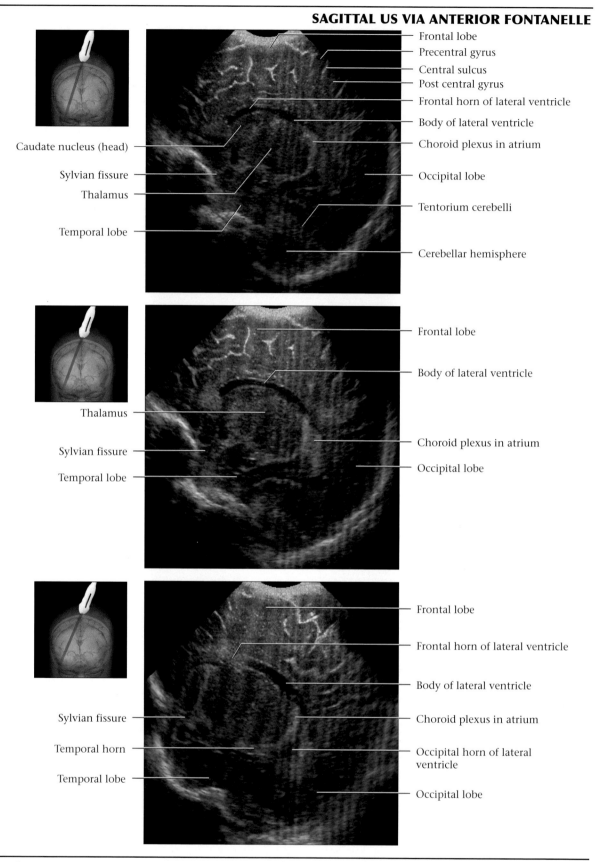

(Top) Fourth image in a series of nine sagittal US images of the brain through the AF in term infant, from medial to lateral. This parasagittal image is obtained slightly more lateral to the caudothalamic groove. The groove is now less distinct but the choroid plexus within the atrium is more clearly demonstrated with extension into the temporal horn of the lateral ventricle. (Middle) This parasagittal image shows the glomus of the choroid plexus in the trigone. Glomus tapers anteriorly as it courses along the floor of the lateral ventricle to the foramen of Monro and continues along the roof of the third ventricle. It also tapers posteriorly from the trigone into the temporal horn of each lateral ventricle. Glomus may appear bulbous and irregular at the trigone and should not be mistaken as a blood clot. (Bottom) This more laterally angled image shows occipital and temporal horns of the lateral ventricle.

CEREBRAL HEMISPHERES OVERVIEW

SAGITTAL T1 MR

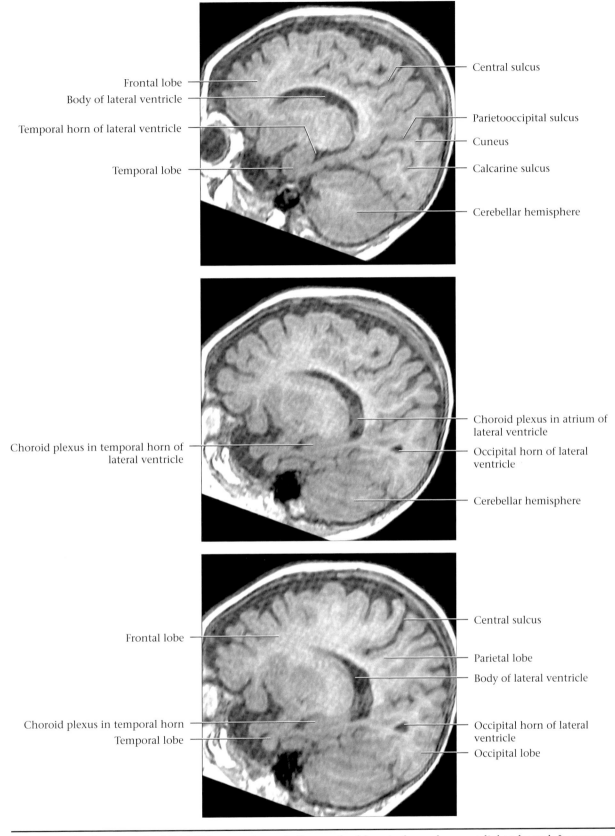

Frontal lobe — (Top image)
Body of lateral ventricle
Temporal horn of lateral ventricle
Temporal lobe

Central sulcus
Parietooccipital sulcus
Cuneus
Calcarine sulcus
Cerebellar hemisphere

Choroid plexus in temporal horn of lateral ventricle

Choroid plexus in atrium of lateral ventricle
Occipital horn of lateral ventricle
Cerebellar hemisphere

Frontal lobe
Choroid plexus in temporal horn
Temporal lobe

Central sulcus
Parietal lobe
Body of lateral ventricle
Occipital horn of lateral ventricle
Occipital lobe

(**Top**) Fourth of nine sagittal T1 MR images through the cerebral hemispheres from medial to lateral. Images are taken through planes/levels corresponding to those commonly used for US scan through the anterior fontanelle. This image shows the central sulcus, bordered anteriorly by the precentral gyrus (motor cortex) and posteriorly by the postcentral gyrus (sensory cortex). Calcarine sulcus and parietooccipital sulcus defines the cuneus of the occipital lobe. (**Middle**) This image shows a prominent choroid plexus within the atrium of the lateral ventricle, which tapers posteriorly and extends into the temporal horn. (**Bottom**) In this image, the occipital horn is more clearly seen. Note the choroid plexus is not present in the occipital horn. Presence of echogenicity in the occipital horn on US in a preterm baby is highly suggestive of intraventricular hemorrhage.

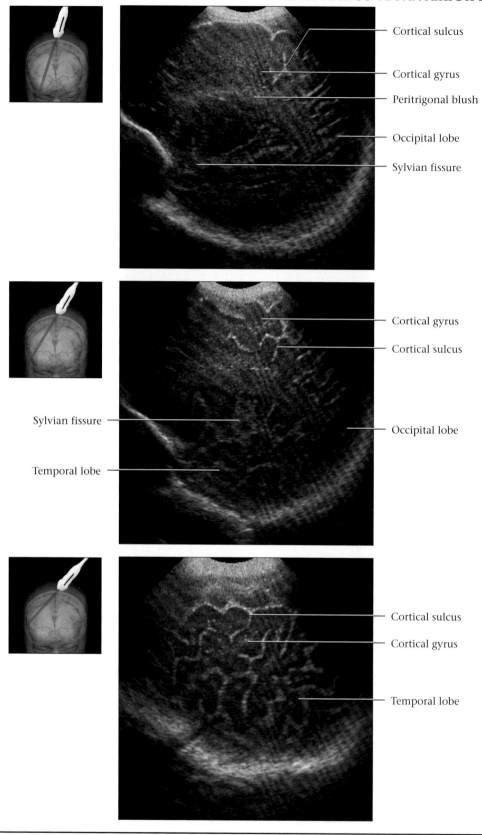

Cortical sulcus

Cortical gyrus

Peritrigonal blush

Occipital lobe

Sylvian fissure

Cortical gyrus

Cortical sulcus

Sylvian fissure

Temporal lobe

Occipital lobe

Cortical sulcus

Cortical gyrus

Temporal lobe

(Top) Seven of nine sagittal ultrasound images of the brain through the anterior fontanelle in term infant from medial to lateral. This parasagittal image is obtained just lateral to the lateral ventricle. The echogenic white matter of the brain just posterior and superior to the ventricular trigone is known as the peritrigonal blush or halo, probably representing radiating white fiber tracts. The peritrigonal blush is more prominent in premature than in term neonates. (Middle) Parasagittal image obtained more laterally. Only the occipital lobe and Sylvian fissure are seen. Cerebral sulci appear as linear or curvilinear echoes scattered throughout the cerebral cortex. The number of sulci increases with brain maturation. (Bottom) This is the last and most lateral sagittal image obtained, and shows the mature sulcal pattern of the occipital lobe in a term infant.

CEREBRAL HEMISPHERES OVERVIEW

SAGITTAL T1 MR

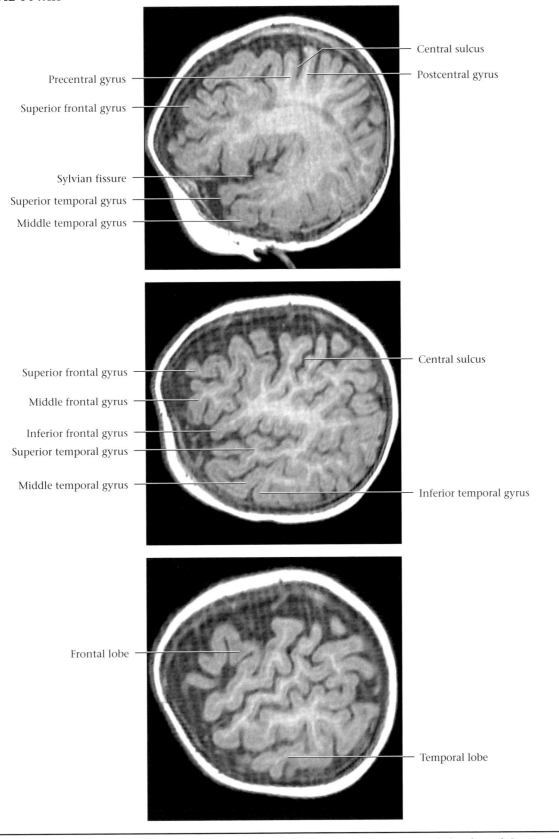

Top image labels:
- Central sulcus
- Postcentral gyrus
- Precentral gyrus
- Superior frontal gyrus
- Sylvian fissure
- Superior temporal gyrus
- Middle temporal gyrus

Middle image labels:
- Central sulcus
- Superior frontal gyrus
- Middle frontal gyrus
- Inferior frontal gyrus
- Superior temporal gyrus
- Middle temporal gyrus
- Inferior temporal gyrus

Bottom image labels:
- Frontal lobe
- Temporal lobe

(Top) Seventh of nine sagittal T1 MR images through the cerebral hemispheres from medial to lateral. Images are through planes/levels corresponding to those commonly used for US scan through AF. Image shows the lateral aspect of the sylvian fissure bound superiorly by the frontal operculum & inferiorly by the temporal operculum. Central sulcus separates the frontal lobe anteriorly from the parietal lobe posteriorly. **(Middle)** Image shows most lateral portion of Sylvian fissure, which contains insular (M2) and opercular (M3) segments of MCA. The temporal lobe is inferior to the Sylvian fissure. The superior temporal gyrus contains the primary auditory cortex. Middle temporal gyrus connects auditory, somatosensory & visual association pathways. The inferior temporal gyrus is the higher visual association area. **(Bottom)** This most lateral image shows only gyri within the frontal and temporal lobes.

CEREBRAL HEMISPHERES OVERVIEW

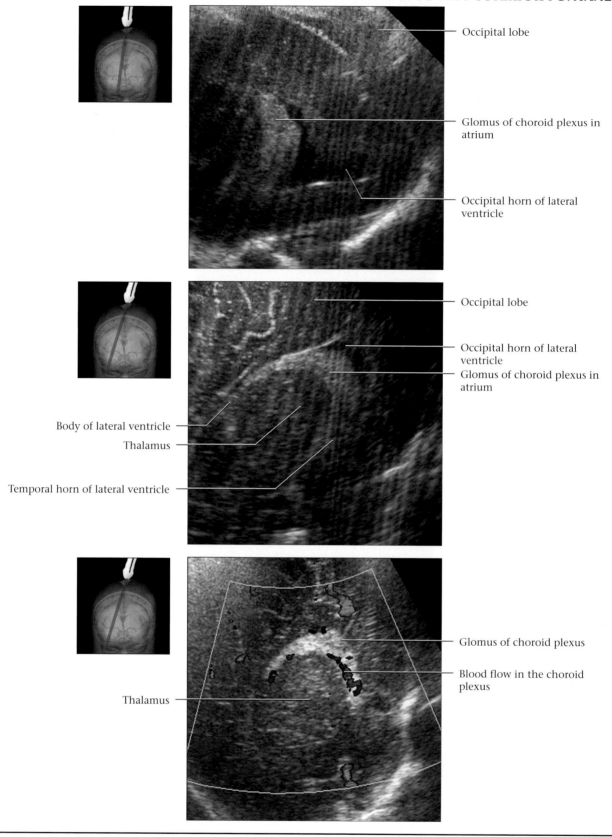

Occipital lobe

Glomus of choroid plexus in atrium

Occipital horn of lateral ventricle

Occipital lobe

Occipital horn of lateral ventricle

Glomus of choroid plexus in atrium

Body of lateral ventricle

Thalamus

Temporal horn of lateral ventricle

Glomus of choroid plexus

Blood flow in the choroid plexus

Thalamus

(Top) First of three sagittal US image of the brain through the posterior fontanelle in term infant. This is the most medial image, best for showing the atrium of the lateral ventricle with occipital horn in the near field. Occipital horn should contain no choroid plexus. Any echogenic material in the occipital horn should raise the suspicion of a blood clot from a intraventricular hemorrhage. (Middle) Parasagittal image obtained at a slightly more lateral view where the occipital horn is less distinct but the glomus of the choroid plexus appears more pronounced. The choroid plexus extends into the body and temporal horn of the lateral ventricle. The thalamus is partially enveloped by the body of the lateral ventricle. (Bottom) Color Doppler image of the choroid plexus within the glomus. The choroid plexus is vascular, which distinguishes it from a blood clot adherent to the choroid plexus. The latter is avascular.

CEREBRAL HEMISPHERES OVERVIEW

CORONAL US VIA POSTERIOR FONTANELLE

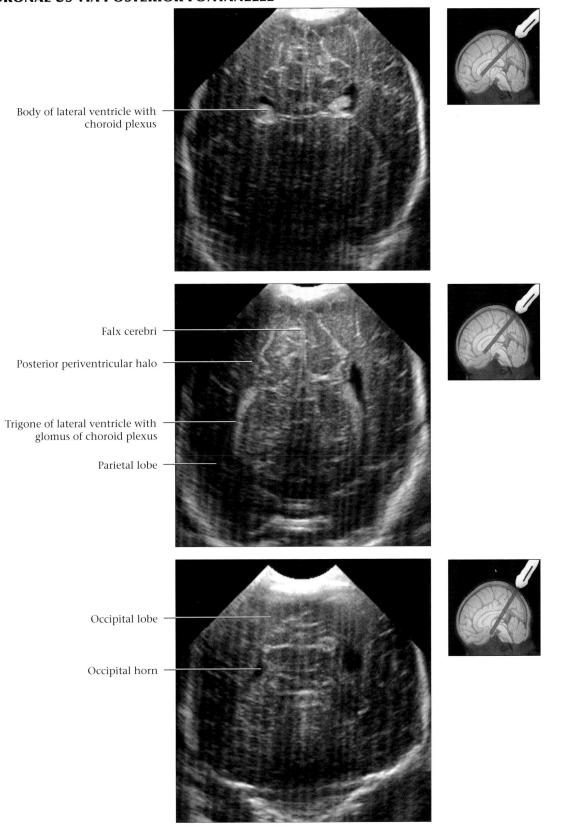

Body of lateral ventricle with choroid plexus

Falx cerebri

Posterior periventricular halo

Trigone of lateral ventricle with glomus of choroid plexus

Parietal lobe

Occipital lobe

Occipital horn

(Top) First of three coronal US images through the posterior fontanelle. This image shows the bodies of the lateral ventricles with echogenic choroid plexus within. (Middle) Slightly inferior image shows the glomus of the choroid plexus in the trigones of the lateral ventricles. Scans through the posterior fontanelle visualize the trigones and posterior periventricular halo much better than the anterior approach. Periventricular halo is a normal finding, more prominent in premature than term infants. (Bottom) Most inferior coronal image shows the occipital horns of the lateral ventricles. The occipital horns should be completely anechoic without the choroid plexus. Any echogenic material within should raise the suspicion of a blood clot resulting from intraventricular hemorrhage. Asymmetry of the occipital horns is common. The left side is usually slightly larger than the right side as in this image.

Brain and Spine

I

27

CEREBRAL HEMISPHERES OVERVIEW

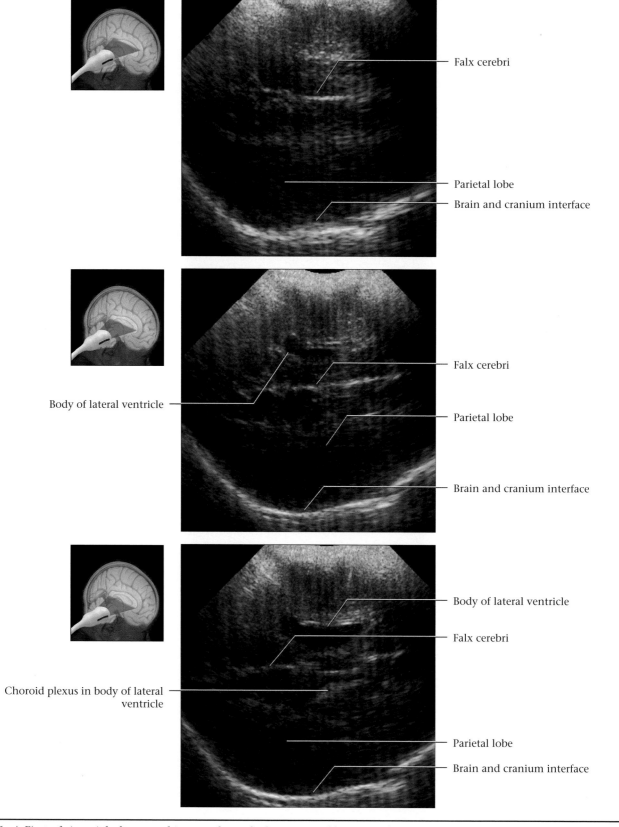

Falx cerebri

Parietal lobe

Brain and cranium interface

Body of lateral ventricle

Falx cerebri

Parietal lobe

Brain and cranium interface

Choroid plexus in body of lateral ventricle

Body of lateral ventricle

Falx cerebri

Parietal lobe

Brain and cranium interface

(Top) First of six axial ultrasound images through the temporal bone. In the most superior image, the falx cerebri is seen as an echogenic midline structure. Only white matter of the frontal, parietal and occipital lobes is seen. This is the view for detection of any extra-axial fluid collection in the far field between the brain and cranium interface and for any gross abnormality in the cerebral cortex. **(Middle)** Axial image obtained at a more inferior level where the body of the lateral ventricle in near field is the first to be seen. **(Bottom)** Axial scan at the level where the bodies of the lateral ventricles are present on either side of the falx. The choroid plexus can be seen in the lateral ventricle in the far field. The ventricular size is well-demonstrated in this view but this is not a common imaging plane used for measuring ventricular size in neonate.

Brain and Spine

I

28

CEREBRAL HEMISPHERES OVERVIEW

AXIAL US THROUGH TEMPORAL BONE

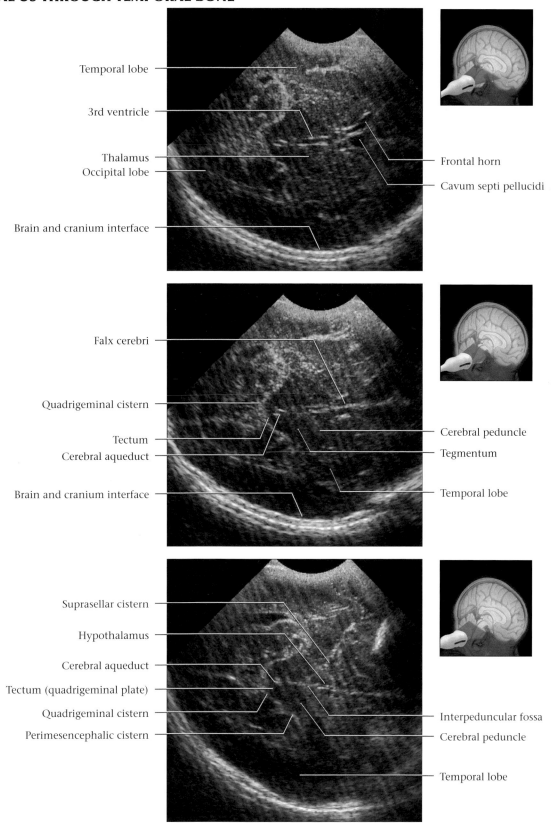

Temporal lobe

3rd ventricle

Thalamus
Occipital lobe

Brain and cranium interface

Frontal horn

Cavum septi pellucidi

Falx cerebri

Quadrigeminal cistern

Tectum
Cerebral aqueduct

Brain and cranium interface

Cerebral peduncle

Tegmentum

Temporal lobe

Suprasellar cistern

Hypothalamus

Cerebral aqueduct

Tectum (quadrigeminal plate)

Quadrigeminal cistern

Perimesencephalic cistern

Interpeduncular fossa

Cerebral peduncle

Temporal lobe

(Top) Fourth of six axial ultrasound images through the temporal bone. In this image, the third ventricle appears slit-like in midline with two thalami lying on either side. The frontal horns of the lateral ventricles & cavum septi pellucidi are seen anteriorly. This is similar to the plane for measuring biparietal diameter in a fetus. **(Middle)** This image shows the midbrain. The cerebral peduncles are butterfly-shaped structures on the ventral surface. In between the cerebral peduncles and echogenic aqueduct is the tegmentum of the midbrain. The tectum is posterior to the aqueduct. **(Bottom)** In this image, the suprasellar cistern appears as an echogenic 5-point star with the hypothalamus within the echogenic cistern. Surrounding the midbrain are the perimesencephalic cisterns bilaterally and quadrigeminal cistern posteriorly. This is the best plane for color Doppler study of the circle of Willis.

COLOR DOPPLER US VIA ANTERIOR FONTANELLE

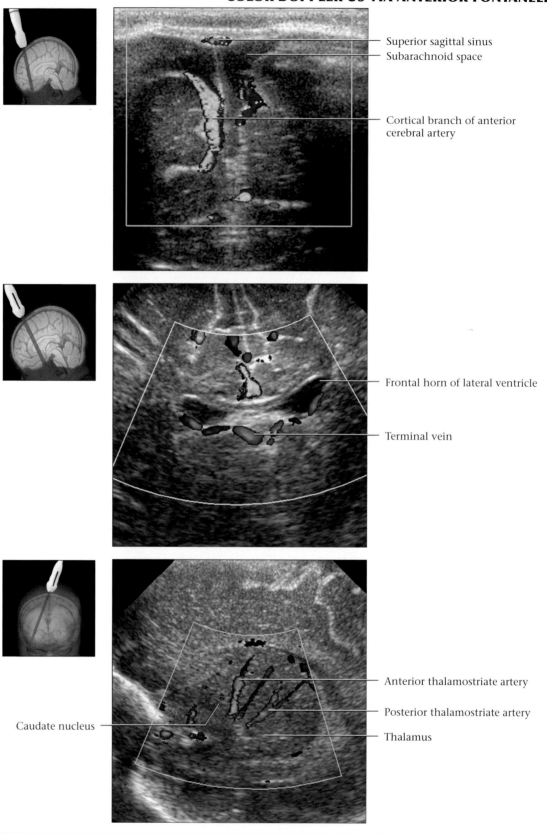

Superior sagittal sinus
Subarachnoid space

Cortical branch of anterior cerebral artery

Frontal horn of lateral ventricle

Terminal vein

Anterior thalamostriate artery

Posterior thalamostriate artery

Caudate nucleus

Thalamus

(Top) Series of three color Doppler US via the anterior fontanelle. Coronal image shows the cortical branch of the anterior cerebral artery in the frontal lobe. (Middle) Coronal color Doppler image through the anterior fontanelle shows the paired terminal veins. At the level of the caudate nucleus, the terminal veins lie closely underneath the frontal horns of the lateral ventricles. Large subependymal hemorrhage may displace terminal veins from the floor of the lateral ventricles, leaving a gap in between the above structures. (Bottom) Color Doppler image obtained by parasagittal scan through the anterior fontanelle shows the thalamostriate arteries. Anteriorly, the caudate nucleus is supplied by the anterior thalamostriate artery while the thalamus posteriorly is supplied by the posterior thalamostriate artery. The thalamostriate arteries arise from the middle cerebral artery.

DOPPLER WAVEFORMS

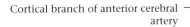

Cortical branch of anterior cerebral artery

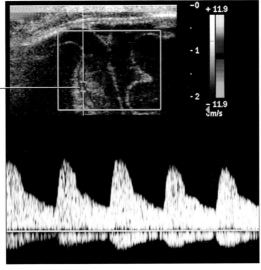

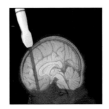

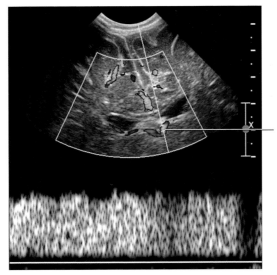

Terminal vein

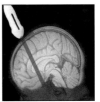

Posterior thalamostriate artery

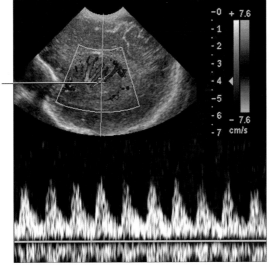

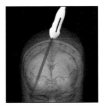

(Top) Doppler waveform of the cortical branch of the anterior cerebral artery which is of low resistance type. There is abundant diastolic flow. Velocity of the cerebral artery is a reliable reflection of intracranial pressure. (Middle) This is the Doppler waveform of the terminal vein. The flow is continuous in this small intracerebral vein. If there is presence of large subependymal hemorrhage and/or associated intraventricular hemorrhage, the terminal veins may be obstructed or compressed leading to periventricular hemorrhagic infarction. (Bottom) This is the Doppler waveform of the posterior thalamostriate artery which shows higher resistance, i.e., less diastolic flow than the large intracerebral arteries. Visualization of these vessels is essential since thromboses in this territory are frequent.

Brain and Spine

I

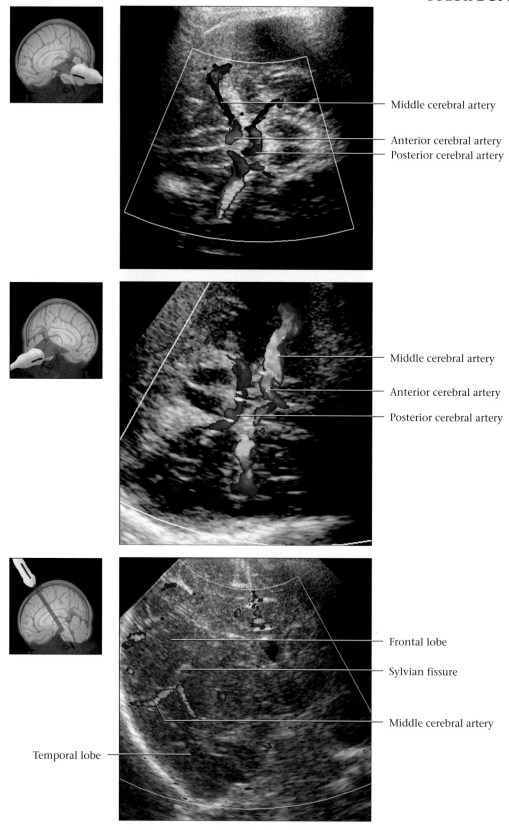

Middle cerebral artery

Anterior cerebral artery
Posterior cerebral artery

Middle cerebral artery

Anterior cerebral artery
Posterior cerebral artery

Frontal lobe

Sylvian fissure

Middle cerebral artery

Temporal lobe

(Top) Axial color Doppler of the circle of Willis, obtained via the transtemporal approach. Major branches of the circle of Willis include middle cerebral (MCA), anterior cerebral (ACA) and posterior cerebral (PCA) arteries. The transtemporal approach provides the best insonation angle between the artery and Doppler beam, thus gives the best estimation of the true blood flow velocity. **(Middle)** Magnified color Doppler image of circle of Willis. The flow direction of the vessels in the near field is opposite to the corresponding one in the far field and hence shows different colors. **(Bottom)** Coronal color Doppler image through the anterior fontanelle. The Sylvian fissure appears as Y-shaped echogenic line with frontal and temporal lobes on either side. The pulsating artery in this fissure is the middle cerebral artery.

CEREBRAL HEMISPHERES OVERVIEW

DOPPLER WAVEFORMS

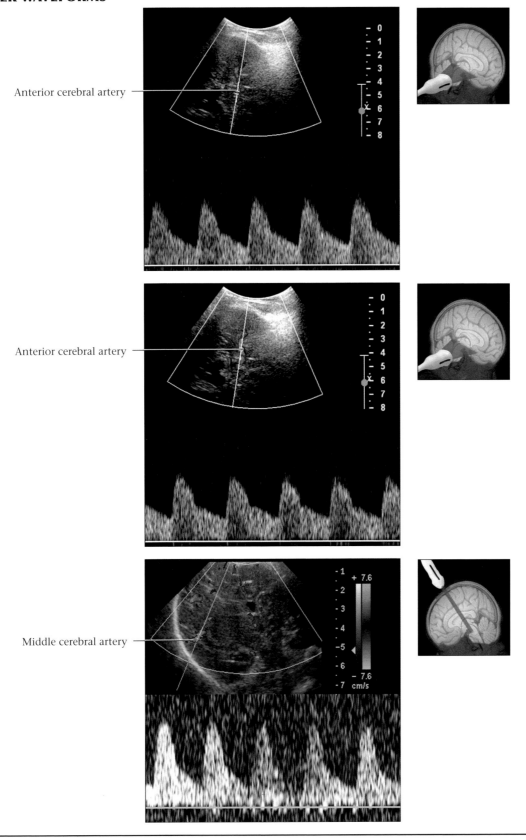

(Top) Doppler waveform of the anterior cerebral artery, which has a low resistance type of flow and hence abundant diastolic flow, i.e., antegrade flow is present throughout diastole. The velocity of the main cerebral arteries in the circle of Willis increase as the gestational age and infant age increases. (**Middle**) Doppler waveform of the middle cerebral artery. Again low resistance with abundant diastolic flow is evident in this vessel. Velocity of flow is more important than the resistive index (RI) since it can be used for both prediction and prognosis of vascular disease. Low blood flow velocity may suggest risk of hypoxic-ischemic injury. High blood flow velocity is associated with increased mean arterial blood pressure. (**Bottom**) Doppler waveform of middle cerebral artery obtained within the Sylvian fissure. Low resistance arterial waveform is again noted.

Brain and Spine

I

33

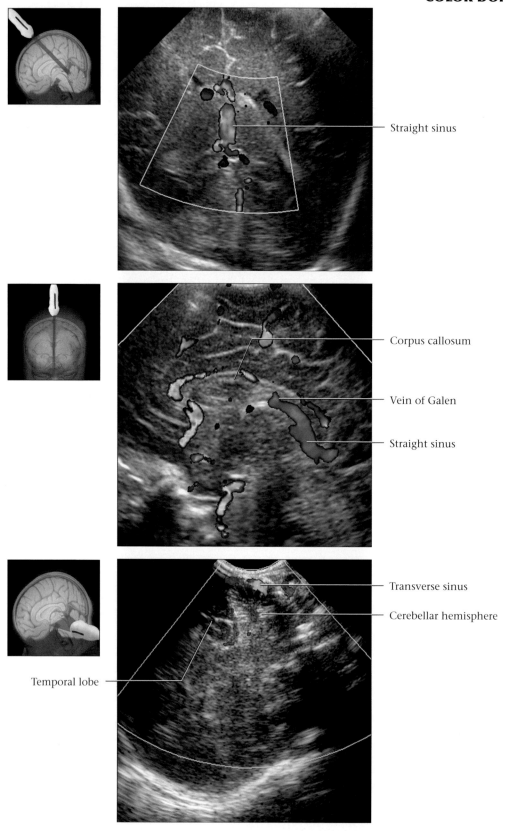

Straight sinus

Corpus callosum

Vein of Galen

Straight sinus

Transverse sinus

Cerebellar hemisphere

Temporal lobe

(Top) Color Doppler image of the straight sinus obtained by coronal scan through AF. The straight sinus runs from falcotentorial apex posteroinferiorly to the sinus confluence (torcular Herophili). It receives tributaries from falx cerebri, tentorium cerebelli and cerebral hemispheres. **(Middle)** Color Doppler image obtained by midline sagittal scan through the anterior fontanelle shows the relationship of the vein of Galen and straight sinus. Vein of Galen is present under the splenium of the corpus callosum. It receives drainage from the paired internal cerebral veins and basal veins of Rosenthal. The vein of Galen continues inferiorly as the straight sinus, which forms torcular Herophili with the two transverse sinuses. **(Bottom)** Axial color Doppler image obtained through the mastoid fontanelle, shows the transverse sinus between the attachment of the tentorial leaves to the calvarium in near field.

DOPPLER WAVEFORMS

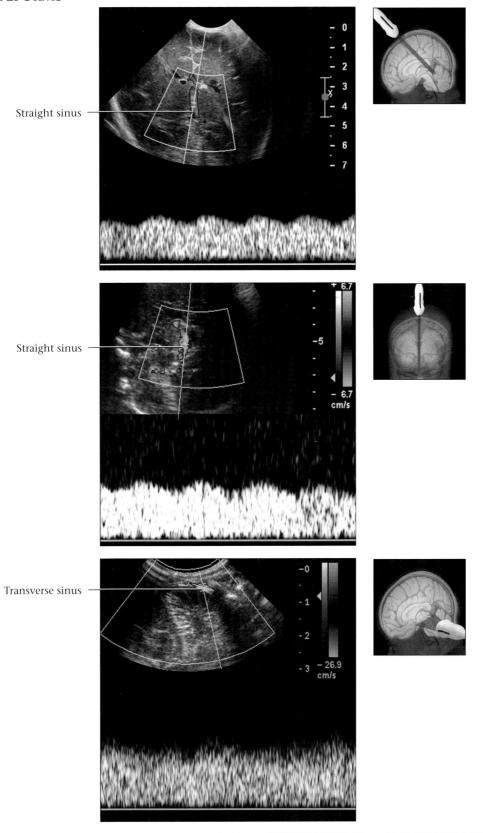

Straight sinus

Straight sinus

Transverse sinus

(Top) Doppler waveform of the straight sinus obtained by coronal scan through the anterior fontanelle. Low amplitude pulsatility is demonstrated relating to cardiac pulsation. Low-amplitude pulsation occurs in the large central venous structures such as straight sinus while continuous flow is present in small terminal veins. There is wide fluctuation in venous flow velocity during forceful crying in infants. (Middle) Doppler waveform of the straight sinus obtained by a sagittal scan through the anterior fontanelle shows low amplitude pulsatility. Abnormal high amplitude waveform is seen when there is elevated right heart pressure and tricuspid regurgitation. (Bottom) Doppler waveform of transverse sinus obtained from axial scan through the mastoid fontanelle, shows continuous flow pattern. Mean blood flow velocity is lower than that in the straight sinus due to its smaller size.

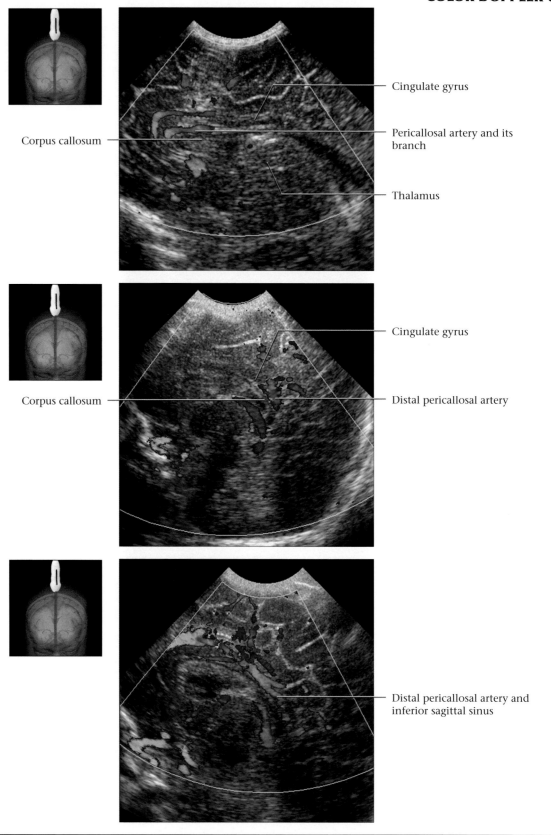

Cingulate gyrus

Pericallosal artery and its branch

Corpus callosum

Thalamus

Cingulate gyrus

Corpus callosum

Distal pericallosal artery

Distal pericallosal artery and inferior sagittal sinus

(Top) Sagittal color Doppler image of the pericallosal artery in the callosal sulcus obtained via anterior fontanelle. In a normal newborn, the pericallosal artery should be close to the surface of the corpus callosum. While in callosal agenesis, this artery remains far from the third ventricle and takes an upward oblique direction. **(Middle)** Sagittal color Doppler image of the distal pericallosal artery obtained via anterior fontanelle. Pericallosal artery arises from A2 near the corpus callosum genu. It courses posterosuperiorly above the corpus callosum and below the cingulate gyrus. **(Bottom)** Sagittal color Doppler image of the distal pericallosal artery obtained in midline through the anterior fontanelle in another newborn. The inferior sagittal sinus and distal pericallosal artery are in close proximity to each other and sometimes cannot be separated by color Doppler.

DOPPLER WAVEFORMS

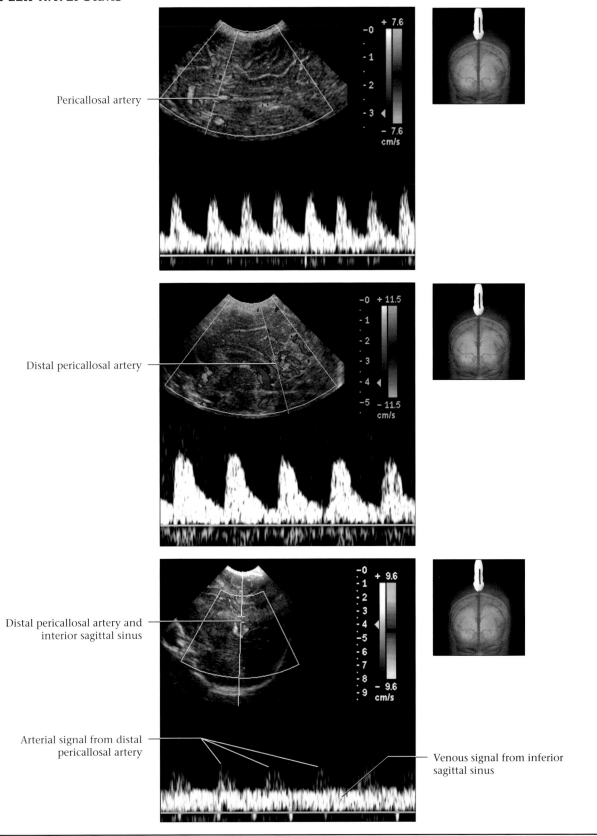

Pericallosal artery

Distal pericallosal artery

Distal pericallosal artery and interior sagittal sinus

Arterial signal from distal pericallosal artery

Venous signal from inferior sagittal sinus

(Top) Doppler waveform of the pericallosal artery obtained by sagittal midline scan through the anterior fontanelle. The flow is of low resistance with abundant antegrade flow throughout diastole. Any abnormalities of flow in the pericallosal arteries may be a result of ischemic change and subsequent hypoplasia of the corpus callosum. (Middle) Doppler waveform of the distal pericallosal artery in the midline sagittal scan through the anterior fontanelle. The arterial waveform should be the same as that in the more proximal segment. (Bottom) Doppler waveform obtained from midline sagittal view of the distal pericallosal artery. Due to the close proximity between distal pericallosal artery and inferior sagittal sinus, the venous signal from the inferior sagittal sinus is superimposed on the arterial signal. This is a common finding.

Brain and Spine

I

37

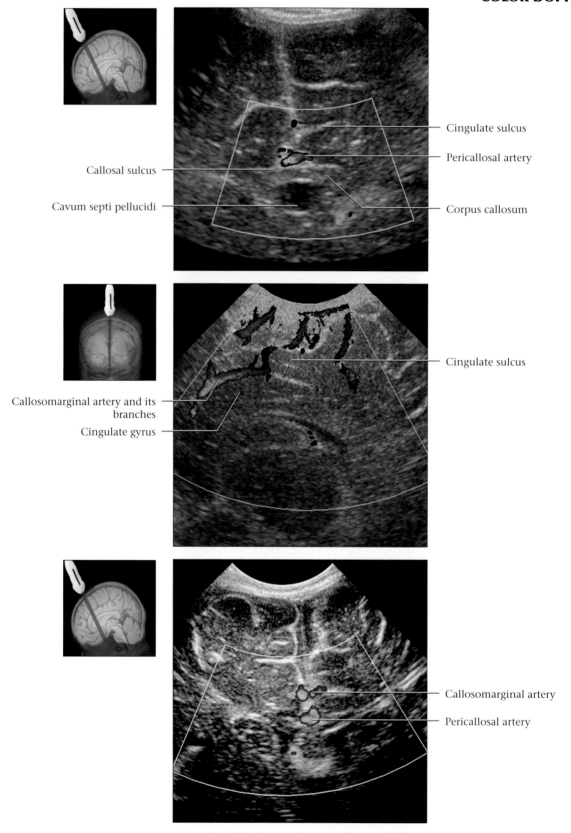

Cingulate sulcus

Pericallosal artery

Callosal sulcus

Corpus callosum

Cavum septi pellucidi

Cingulate sulcus

Callosomarginal artery and its branches

Cingulate gyrus

Callosomarginal artery

Pericallosal artery

(Top) Coronal color Doppler image obtained through anterior fontanelle shows the pericallosal artery within the callosal sulcus above genu of corpus callosum & cavum septi pellucidi in midline. **(Middle)** Sagittal color Doppler image of the callosomarginal artery & its branches obtained through the anterior fontanelle. Callosomarginal artery lies within the echogenic cingulate sulcus above the cingulate gyrus. **(Bottom)** Coronal color Doppler image obtained through the anterior fontanelle shows the relationship between the pericallosal artery & callosomarginal artery. Vascular pulsation of both arteries are noted within the interhemispheric fissure. Callosomarginal artery courses posterosuperiorly in the cingulate sulcus above the cingulate gyrus while the pericallosal artery courses in the callosal sulcus below the cingulate gyrus. Both arteries are major distal ACA branches.

Brain and Spine

I

38

DOPPLER WAVEFORMS

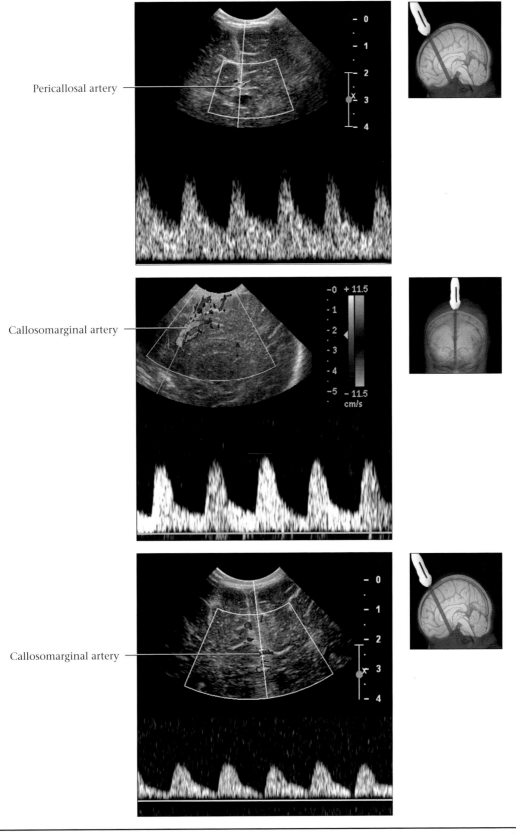

(Top) Doppler waveform of the pericallosal artery, which has a low-resistance waveform with antegrade flow throughout diastole. Systolic & diastolic flow velocities increase as gestational age of infants increases. Resistive index (RI) decreases with increasing gestational age. Mean RI of all intracranial arteries in term infants is 0.726 with a standard deviation (SD) of 0.057. (Middle) Doppler waveform of the callosomarginal artery, sagittal view. The callosomarginal artery has less diastolic flow when compared with the pericallosal artery due to a slightly higher intraarterial resistance when compared with the latter artery; but its waveform remains a low-resistance type. (Bottom) Doppler waveform of the callosomarginal artery, coronal view. Similar waveforms are seen in both the callosomarginal & pericallosal arteries, which are distal branches of the ACA.

Brain and Spine

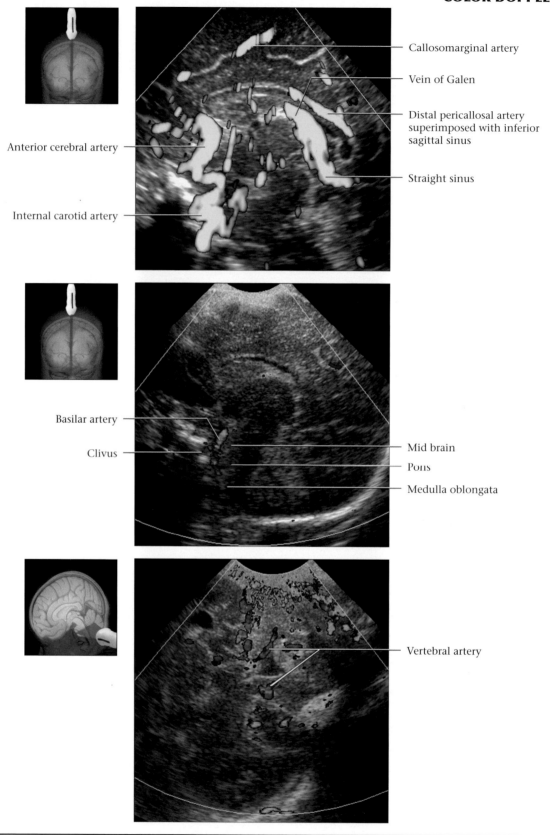

Callosomarginal artery

Vein of Galen

Distal pericallosal artery superimposed with inferior sagittal sinus

Anterior cerebral artery

Straight sinus

Internal carotid artery

Basilar artery

Mid brain

Clivus

Pons

Medulla oblongata

Vertebral artery

(Top) Mid sagittal power Doppler US through the anterior fontanelle shows the internal carotid artery (ICA), anterior cerebral artery (ACA) and its two main distal branches: The larger pericallosal artery & smaller callosomarginal artery. The distal pericallosal artery is superimposed on the inferior sagittal sinus. Other important venous structures seen in the midline are the vein of Galen, which continues inferiorly as the straight sinus. **(Middle)** Mid sagittal color Doppler US through the anterior fontanelle shows the basilar artery lying within the prepontine cistern, in front of the pons & behind the clivus. The basilar artery bifurcates into its terminal branches, PCAs in the interpeduncular or suprasellar cistern at the dorsum sellae. **(Bottom)** Color Doppler US through the mastoid fontanelle shows bilateral vertebral arteries.

DOPPLER WAVEFORMS

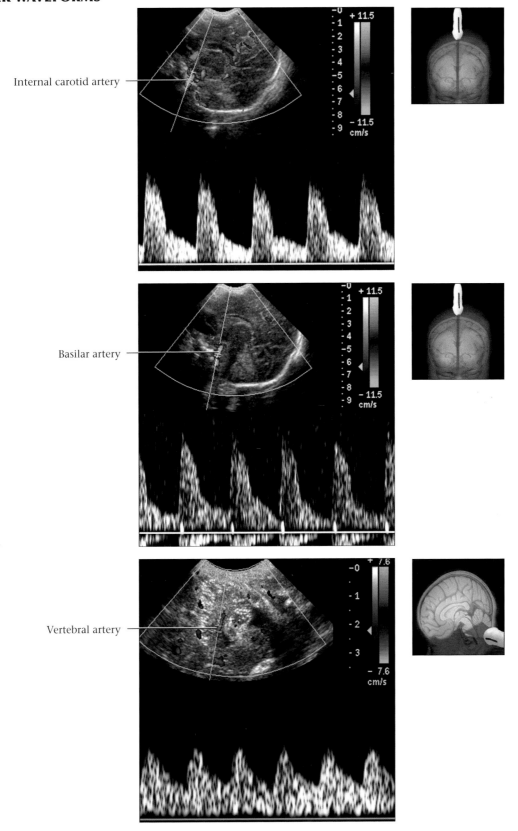

(**Top**) Doppler waveform of the internal carotid artery. Antegrade flow is always present during systole and diastole. In premature infants diastolic flow may be absent due to diastolic steal (shunting of blood from brain during diastole) secondary to a patent ductus arteriosus. (**Middle**) Doppler waveform of the basilar artery. Various factors can cause an increase in the resistive index (RI) or reduced flow during diastole such as hemorrhage, brain edema, subdural effusion, periventricular leukomalacia, hydrocephalus, patent ductus arteriosus, or transiently increased intracranial pressure as the result of pressure on the anterior fontanelle induced by US transducer. Abnormally low RI occurs in intrauterine asphyxia and growth retardation. (**Bottom**) Doppler waveform of the vertebral artery. Again the arterial waveform is of low resistance with abundant diastolic flow.

Brain and Spine

I

CEREBRAL HEMISPHERES OVERVIEW

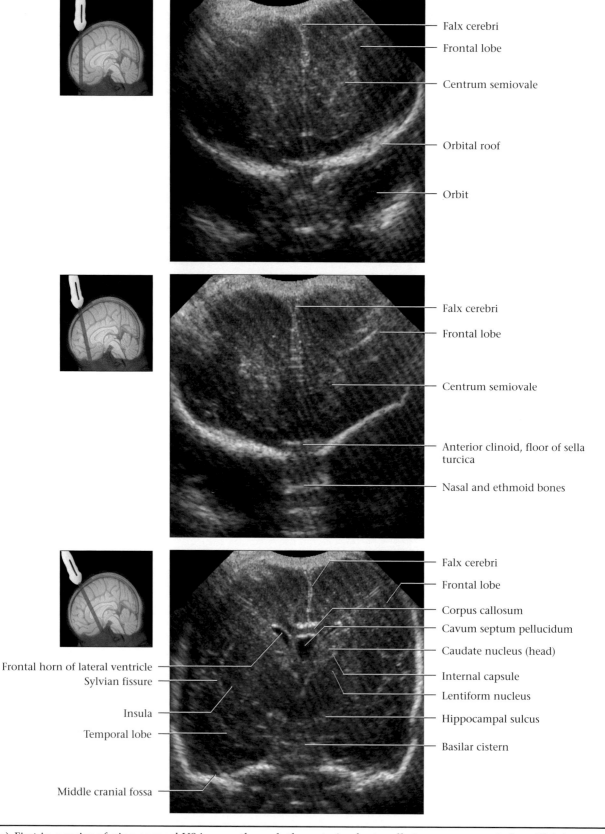

Falx cerebri

Frontal lobe

Centrum semiovale

Orbital roof

Orbit

Falx cerebri

Frontal lobe

Centrum semiovale

Anterior clinoid, floor of sella turcica

Nasal and ethmoid bones

Falx cerebri

Frontal lobe

Corpus callosum

Cavum septum pellucidum

Caudate nucleus (head)

Internal capsule

Lentiform nucleus

Hippocampal sulcus

Basilar cistern

Frontal horn of lateral ventricle

Sylvian fissure

Insula

Temporal lobe

Middle cranial fossa

(Top) First in a series of nine coronal US images through the anterior fontanelle in a premature infant. This image shows the frontal lobe lying in the anterior cranial fossa with orbital cavities below. Premature infants have fewer sulci resulting in smooth & less mature sulcal pattern when compared with mature infants. (Middle) This slightly more posterior image shows the frontal lobe with higher echogenicity in the centrum semiovale than mature infants. The prominent centrum semiovale should not be mistaken for periventricular hemorrhagic infarction associated with large intraventricular hemorrhage. (Bottom) This image is at the level just anterior to the foramen of Monro. The cavum septum pellucidum forms the medial wall of the frontal horns. The cavum septum pellucidum is seen in 50% of term infants and 60% of premature infants. The extraaxial CSF spaces may also be enlarged in preterm neonates.

Brain and Spine

I

CEREBRAL HEMISPHERES OVERVIEW

CORONAL US IN PRETERM BABY

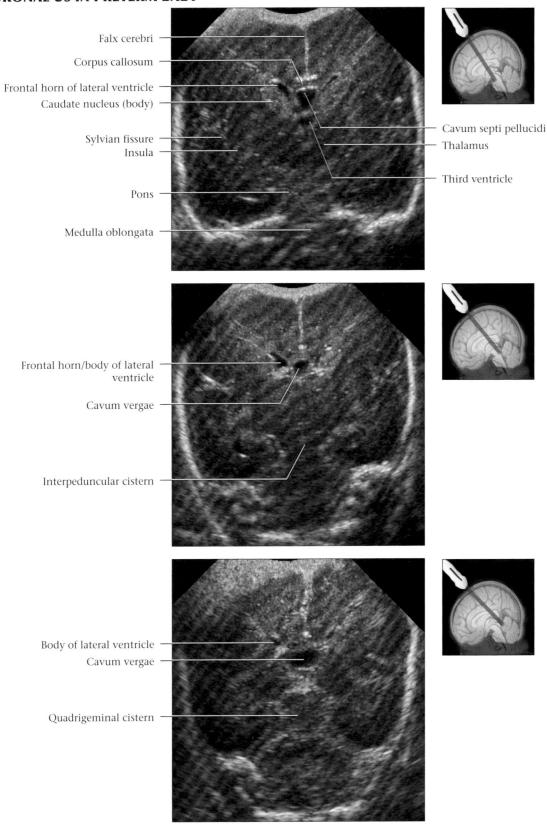

Falx cerebri
Corpus callosum
Frontal horn of lateral ventricle
Caudate nucleus (body)
Sylvian fissure
Insula
Pons
Medulla oblongata

Cavum septi pellucidi
Thalamus
Third ventricle

Frontal horn/body of lateral ventricle
Cavum vergae
Interpeduncular cistern

Body of lateral ventricle
Cavum vergae
Quadrigeminal cistern

(Top) Four of nine coronal US images through the anterior fontanelle in a premature infant. This image is taken at the level of the foramen of Monro, where the cavum septi pellucidi extends back to become the cavum vergae & cavum velum interpositum. Just before term, the cavum septum pellucidum begins to close & is completed by 2 to 6 months of postnatal life. Sometimes linear echoes may be seen in the cavum which represent septal veins. (Middle) Image at the level of the interpeduncular cistern. The ventricles are slightly more prominent in a premature brain. The cavum vergae is the posterior extension of the cavum septi pellucidi, lying between the bodies of the lateral ventricles. (Bottom) Image at the level of the quadrigeminal cistern. The cavum vergae is present, which begins to close from posterior to anterior from gestational age of 6 months and is usually not seen in term infants.

CORONAL US IN PRETERM BABY

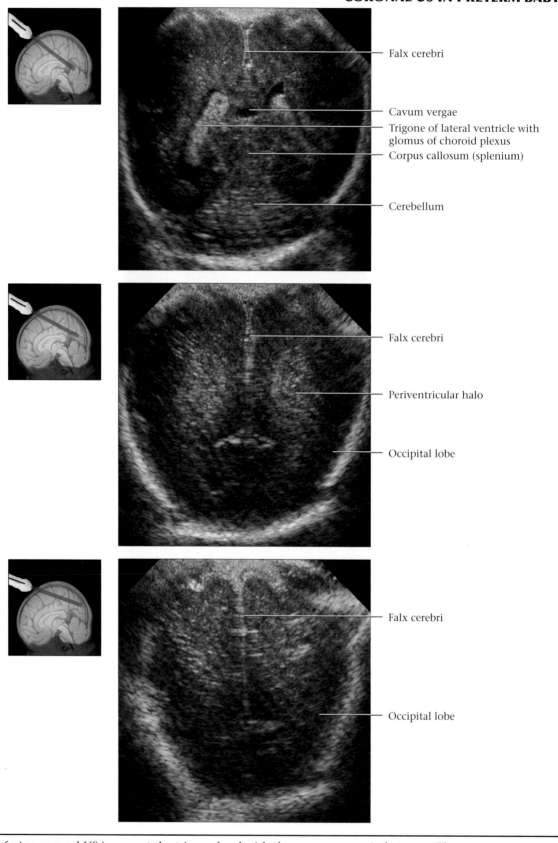

Falx cerebri

Cavum vergae

Trigone of lateral ventricle with glomus of choroid plexus

Corpus callosum (splenium)

Cerebellum

Falx cerebri

Periventricular halo

Occipital lobe

Falx cerebri

Occipital lobe

(Top) Seven of nine coronal US images at the trigone level with the cavum vergae in between. The cavum vergae may extend posteriorly beyond the bodies of the lateral ventricle and become the cavum velum interpositum, projecting behind the quadrigeminal cistern. (Middle) More posterior image shows the periventricular halo in the occipital lobes. The periventricular halo should be symmetrical, homogeneous and brush-like. Its echogenicity is brighter in a premature brain than in a mature brain, and should not be mistaken as periventricular leukomalacia resulting from intraventricular hemorrhage. However, cerebral hemorrhage or periventricular leukomalacia should be suspected if the halo appears coarse or inhomogeneous. (Bottom) Most posterior view shows the occipital lobes. The sulcal pattern appears smooth in the preterm brain with only a few echogenic sulci present.

CEREBRAL HEMISPHERES OVERVIEW

SAGITTAL US IN PRETERM BABY

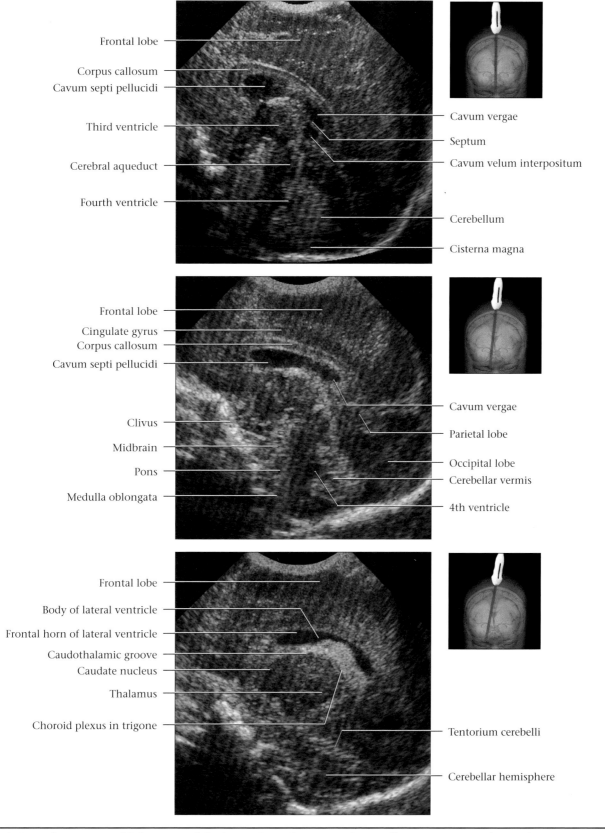

Frontal lobe

Corpus callosum
Cavum septi pellucidi

Third ventricle

Cerebral aqueduct

Fourth ventricle

Cavum vergae
Septum
Cavum velum interpositum

Cerebellum

Cisterna magna

Frontal lobe
Cingulate gyrus
Corpus callosum
Cavum septi pellucidi

Clivus

Midbrain

Pons

Medulla oblongata

Cavum vergae

Parietal lobe

Occipital lobe
Cerebellar vermis

4th ventricle

Frontal lobe

Body of lateral ventricle

Frontal horn of lateral ventricle

Caudothalamic groove
Caudate nucleus

Thalamus

Choroid plexus in trigone

Tentorium cerebelli

Cerebellar hemisphere

(Top) First of nine sagittal US images of the brain through anterior fontanelle in a premature brain. Cavi septi pellucidi & vergae are seen in midline below the curving line of corpus callosum. They appear as a coma-shaped, fluid-filled structure. Cavum septi pellucidi is anterior to foramen of Monro. Most posterior and inferior is the cavum velum interpositum & usually there is a thin septum separating it from the cavum vergae. Cavum does not communicate with the ventricles or subarachnoid space. (Middle) This image is taken just lateral to midline. Sulcal pattern is premature with only a few branches from cingulate sulcus. (Bottom) This image shows the caudothalamic groove. In the preterm brain, the vascular germinal matrix is located anterosuperior to the caudothalamic groove. Echogenicity anterior to the caudothalamic groove should raise suspicions for grade 1 hemorrhage.

Brain and Spine

45

Frontal lobe

Frontal horn of lateral ventricle

Parietal lobe
Body of lateral ventricle

Caudate nucleus

Choroid plexus in trigone

Thalamus

Sylvian fissure

Tentorium cerebelli

Temporal lobe

Cerebellar hemisphere

Frontal lobe
Parietal lobe

Frontal horn of lateral ventricle

Body of lateral ventricle

Choroid plexus in trigone

Sylvian fissure

Occipital horn of lateral ventricle

Temporal lobe

Occipital lobe

Frontal lobe

Body of lateral ventricle

Glomus of choroid plexus in atrium

Sylvian fissure

Temporal horn of lateral ventricle

Temporal lobe

Occipital lobe

(Top) Four of nine sagittal US images of the brain through the anterior fontanelle in a premature brain from medial to lateral. This parasagittal image is obtained by angling slightly more lateral to the caudothalamic groove, which is now less distinct but the choroid plexus of the trigone appears more prominent. (Middle) This parasagittal image at the body of the lateral ventricle clearly shows the glomus of the choroid plexus in the trigone. The occipital horn is more prominent in preterm infants than in mature infants. Note choroid plexus does not extend into the occipital horn. Detection of echogenic material within the occipital horn implies presence of intraventricular hemorrhage in preterm infant, which is best appreciated by US scans through the posterior fontanelle. (Bottom) Parasagittal image obtained more laterally shows glomus of the choroid plexus extending into the temporal horn.

CEREBRAL HEMISPHERES OVERVIEW

SAGITTAL US IN PRETERM BABY

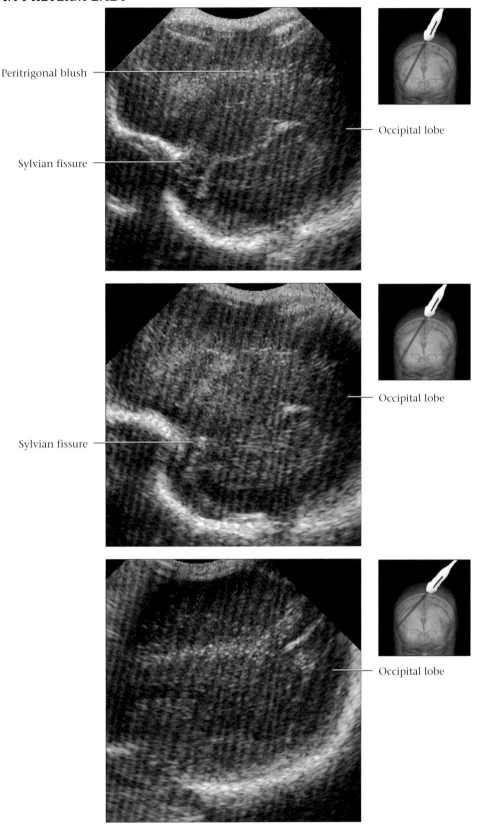

Peritrigonal blush

Occipital lobe

Sylvian fissure

Sylvian fissure

Occipital lobe

Occipital lobe

(Top) Seven of nine sagittal US images of the brain through the anterior fontanelle in a premature brain from medial to lateral. This parasagittal image is just lateral to the lateral ventricle. The echogenic white matter is known as the peritrigonal blush or halo which is more prominent in premature infants than in term infants. The echogenicity probably represents radiating white matter fibers and vascular plexus. (Middle) This more lateral parasagittal image shows the occipital lobe and Sylvian fissure. Compared to term baby, there are far less linear or curvilinear echoes scattered throughout the cerebral cortex compatible with scanty sulcal formation in premature brain. Echogenic sulci become more serpiginous in configuration as the brain matures. (Bottom) The most lateral image shows the premature sulcal pattern with scanty cortical sulci seen.

CEREBRAL HEMISPHERES OVERVIEW

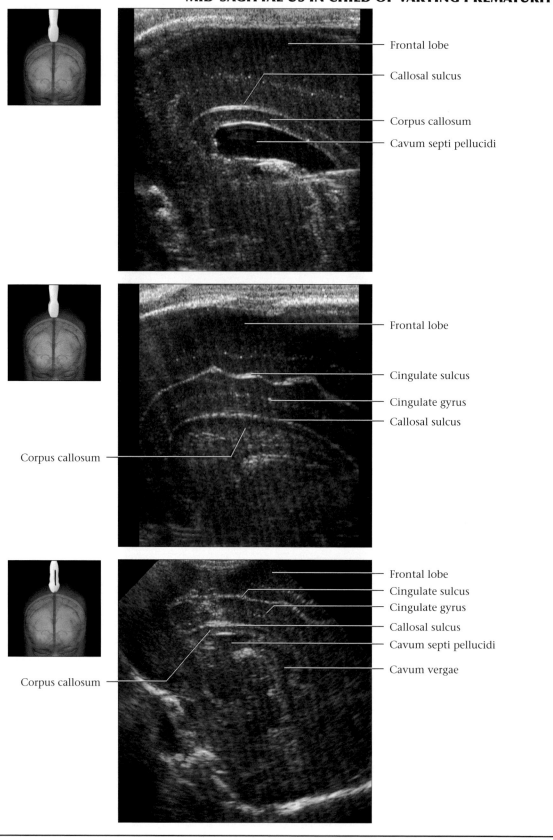

Frontal lobe

Callosal sulcus

Corpus callosum

Cavum septi pellucidi

Frontal lobe

Cingulate sulcus

Cingulate gyrus

Callosal sulcus

Corpus callosum

Frontal lobe

Cingulate sulcus

Cingulate gyrus

Callosal sulcus

Cavum septi pellucidi

Cavum vergae

Corpus callosum

(Top) Midline sagittal image of the brain through the anterior fontanelle in a neonate at 25 weeks of gestation at birth. This is the best view for assessing the sulcal pattern which reflects the degree of gyral maturity of the brain in infants. The brain sulci are not fully developed and appear quite smooth. (Middle) Sulcal pattern of a newborn at 29 weeks of gestation at birth. The brain sulci are still not fully developed and appear quite smooth. The callosal sulcus develops over the corpus callosum and a simple linear cingulate sulcus appears superior and parallel to the corpus callosum without branching. (Bottom) Sulcal pattern of a newborn at 31 weeks of gestation at birth. The cingulate sulcus still appears quite smooth with no branches. The cavum septi pellucidi and the cavum vergae remain completely cystic.

CEREBRAL HEMISPHERES OVERVIEW

MID-SAGITTAL US IN CHILD OF VARYING PREMATURITY

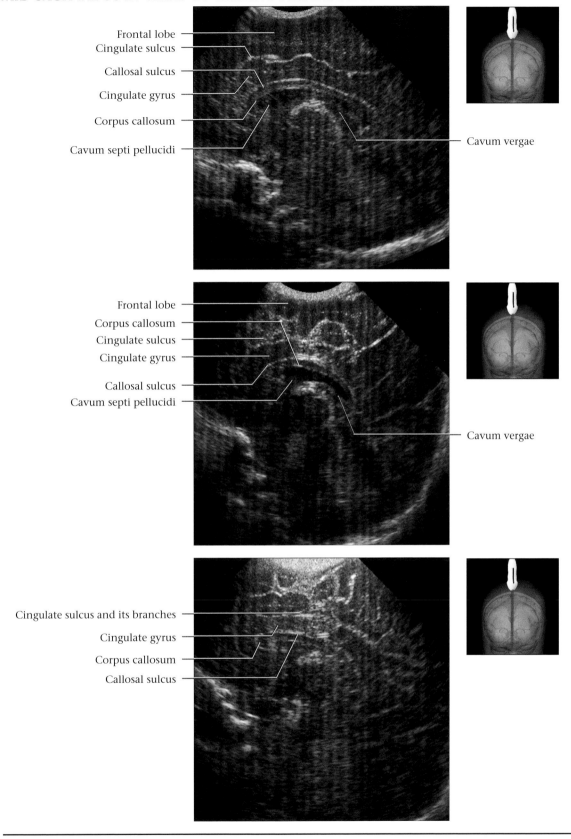

Frontal lobe

Cingulate sulcus

Callosal sulcus

Cingulate gyrus

Corpus callosum

Cavum septi pellucidi

Cavum vergae

Frontal lobe

Corpus callosum

Cingulate sulcus

Cingulate gyrus

Callosal sulcus

Cavum septi pellucidi

Cavum vergae

Cingulate sulcus and its branches

Cingulate gyrus

Corpus callosum

Callosal sulcus

(Top) Sulcal pattern of a newborn at 33 weeks of gestation at birth. The cingulate sulcus has few branches. **(Middle)** Sulcal pattern of a newborn at 35 weeks of gestation at birth. The cingulate sulcus bends, branches and anastomoses with development of many peripheral branches over the brain surface. **(Bottom)** Sulcal pattern of a newborn at 40 weeks of gestation at birth. A full-term infant brain pattern has developed. The sulcal pattern becomes more mature between 33 and 40 weeks of gestation. The number of gyri and sulci increase with increasing gestational age of the infant. Within the cerebral sulci are branches of the anterior cerebral artery and pulsation from these vessels can be seen on real-time examination. The cavum septi pellucidi and cavum vergae are closed.

BRAINSTEM AND CEREBELLUM

Terminology

Abbreviations
- Cranial nerves (CN): Oculomotor nerve (CN3), trochlear nerve (CN4), trigeminal nerve (CN5), abducens nerve (CN6), facial nerve (CN7), vestibulocochlear nerve (CN8), glossopharyngeal nerve (CN9), vagus nerve (CN10), accessory nerve (CN11), hypoglossal nerve (CN12)

Synonyms
- Classical nomenclature (simplified nomenclature)
  - Superior (tentorial), inferior (suboccipital), anterior (petrosal) cerebellar surfaces
  - Primary (tentorial), horizontal (petrosal), prebiventral/prepyramidal (suboccipital) cerebellar fissures

Definitions
- Posterior fossa: Houses brainstem and cerebellum, below tentorium cerebelli (infratentorial)
- Brainstem: Composed of midbrain (mesencephalon), pons and medulla oblongata
- Cerebellum: Largest part of hindbrain, integrates coordinations & fine-tuning of movement & regulation of muscle tone

Gross Anatomy

Overview
- **Posterior fossa**: Infratentorial contents
  - Protected space surrounded by calvarium, contains
    - Brainstem anteriorly, cerebellum posteriorly
    - Cerebral aqueduct and fourth ventricle
    - CSF cisterns containing CNs, vertebrobasilar arterial system and veins
  - CSF cisterns suspend & cushion brainstem and cerebellum
- **Brainstem**
  - Anatomic divisions
    - **Midbrain (mesencephalon)**: Upper brainstem, connects pons and cerebellum with forebrain
    - **Pons**: Mid portion of brainstem, relays information from brain to cerebellum
    - **Medulla**: Caudal (inferior) brainstem, relays information from spinal cord to brain
  - Functional divisions
    - Ventral part contains large descending white matter tracts: Midbrain cerebral peduncles, pontine bulb, medullary pyramids
    - Dorsal part: Tegmentum, common to midbrain, pons and medulla; contains CN nuclei and reticular formation
- **Cerebellum**
  - Two hemispheres & midline vermis, three surfaces
  - Connected to brainstem by three paired peduncles
  - Cortical gray matter, central white matter & four paired deep gray nuclei

Anatomy Relationships
- **Posterior fossa** boundaries
  - Tentorium cerebelli superiorly
  - Bony clivus anteriorly
  - Temporal bones and calvarium laterally
  - Foramen magnum and calvarium inferiorly
- **Midbrain**
  - Ventral: Cerebral peduncles (crus cerebri) containing corticospinal, corticobulbar and corticopontine tracts
  - **Dorsal tegmentum**: Ventral to cerebral aqueduct
    - White matter tracts: Medial longitudinal fasciculus, medial lemniscus, lateral lemniscus, spinothalamic tract, central tegmental tract
    - Gray matter: Substantia nigra and red nucleus
    - Upper midbrain: Contains CN3 nucleus, at superior colliculus level
    - Lower midbrain: Contains CN4 nucleus, at inferior colliculus level
  - **Tectum (quadrigeminal plate)**: Dorsal to cerebral aqueduct
    - Superior & inferior colliculi, periaqueductal gray matter
- **Pons**
  - Ventral: Longitudinal fibers primarily from corticospinal, corticobulbar & corticopontine tracts
  - Dorsal tegmentum: White matter tracts & CN nuclei
    - White matter tracts: Medial longitudinal fasciculus, medial lemniscus, lateral lemniscus, trapezoid body, spinothalamic tract, central tegmental tract
    - Upper pons: Contains main nuclei of CN5
    - Lower pons: Contains nuclei of CN6, 7 & 8
- **Medulla**
  - Ventral: Olives & pyramids
  - Dorsal tegmentum: White matter tracts & CN nuclei
    - White matter tracts: Medial longitudinal fasciculus, medial lemniscus, spinothalamic tract, central tegmental tract, spinocerebellar tract
    - CN nuclei: CN9, 10 & 11 (bulbar portion) in upper & mid medulla; CN12 nuclei in mid medulla
- **Cerebellum**
  - Three surfaces: Superior (tentorial), inferior (suboccipital), anterior (petrosal)
  - Two hemispheres and a midline vermis
    - Divided into lobes & lobules by transverse fissures
    - Major fissures: Primary (tentorial), horizontal (petrosal), prebiventral/prepyramidal (suboccipital) cerebellar fissures
  - Three paired peduncles
    - Superior cerebellar peduncle (brachium conjunctivum) connects cerebellum to cerebrum via midbrain
    - Middle cerebellar peduncle (brachium pontis) connects to pons
    - Inferior cerebellar peduncle (restiform body) connects to medulla

Anatomy-Based Imaging Issues

Imaging Recommendations
- Brainstem and cerebellum not well-demonstrated in standard planes through anterior fontanelle
- Best assessed by transmastoid or transtemporal approach, can be performed in children with closed fontanelles & sutures

BRAINSTEM AND CEREBELLUM

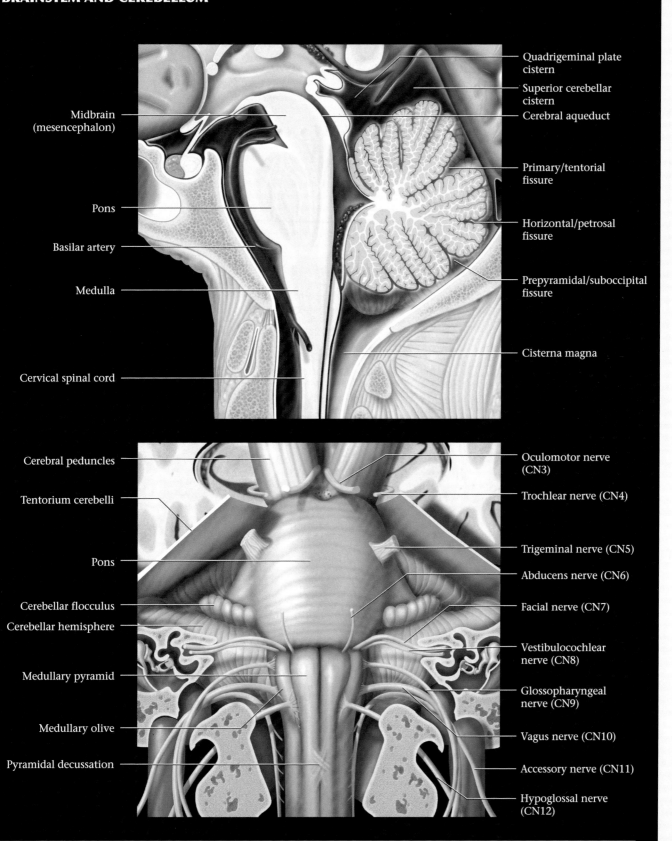

Quadrigeminal plate cistern

Superior cerebellar cistern

Cerebral aqueduct

Midbrain (mesencephalon)

Primary/tentorial fissure

Pons

Horizontal/petrosal fissure

Basilar artery

Medulla

Prepyramidal/suboccipital fissure

Cisterna magna

Cervical spinal cord

Cerebral peduncles

Oculomotor nerve (CN3)

Tentorium cerebelli

Trochlear nerve (CN4)

Trigeminal nerve (CN5)

Pons

Abducens nerve (CN6)

Cerebellar flocculus

Facial nerve (CN7)

Cerebellar hemisphere

Vestibulocochlear nerve (CN8)

Medullary pyramid

Glossopharyngeal nerve (CN9)

Medullary olive

Vagus nerve (CN10)

Pyramidal decussation

Accessory nerve (CN11)

Hypoglossal nerve (CN12)

(Top) Sagittal midline graphic of the posterior fossa shows the anterior brainstem & posterior cerebellum separated by the fourth ventricle. Brainstem consists of midbrain (mesencephalon), pons & medulla. Cerebellum has superior (tentorial), inferior (suboccipital) & anterior (petrosal) surfaces. Primary (tentorial) fissure & horizontal (petrosal) fissures divide vermis & cerebellar hemispheres into lobules. Horizontal fissure is the most prominent fissure on the anterior (petrosal) surface & curves posteriorly onto the inferior (suboccipital) surface. **(Bottom)** Coronal graphic of the anterior brainstem and exiting cranial nerves. CN3 through CN12 nuclei are located within the brainstem. CN3 & 4 nuclei are within the midbrain. CN5 through CN8 nuclei are within the pons. CN9 through CN12 nuclei are within the medulla. CN4 is the only dorsally exiting CN & wraps around the lateral midbrain in the tentorial margin.

Brain and Spine

I

51

TRANSMASTOID & TRANSTEMPORAL US APPROACH

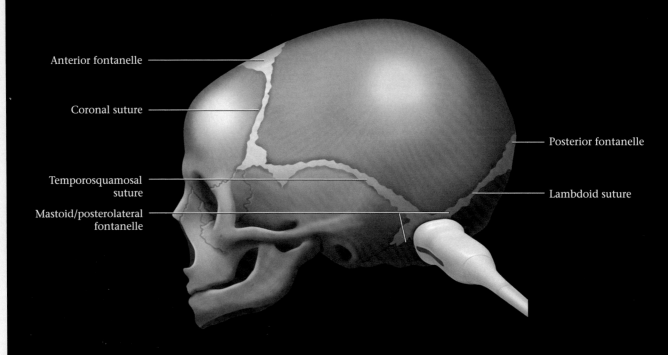

Anterior fontanelle

Coronal suture

Temporosquamosal suture

Mastoid/posterolateral fontanelle

Posterior fontanelle

Lambdoid suture

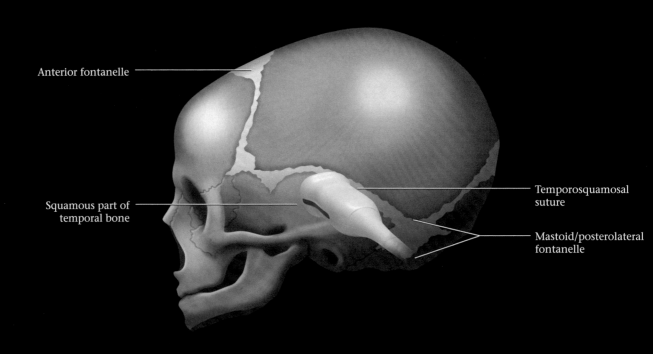

Anterior fontanelle

Squamous part of temporal bone

Temporosquamosal suture

Mastoid/posterolateral fontanelle

(Top) Graphic of the mastoid acoustic window. Mastoid/posterolateral fontanelle is located at the junction of temporosquamosal, lambdoidal & occipital sutures. It allows assessment of brainstem & posterior fossa structures, which are not well-demonstrated in the standard planes through the anterior fontanelle. US probe is placed ~ 1 cm behind the helix of ear and 1 cm above the tragus. This acoustic window allows best visualization of 4th ventricle, posterior cerebellar vermis, cerebellar hemispheres & cisterna magna. **(Bottom)** Graphic of the transtemporal acoustic window. US probe is placed more anterior and superior than mastoid fontanelle approach. Temporal bone anterior to the ear is thin enough to allow imaging of the brainstem even after closure of the temporosquamosal suture. This acoustic window allows the best assessment of cerebral peduncles and the 3rd ventricle.

BRAINSTEM AND CEREBELLUM

SAGITTAL US THROUGH ANTERIOR FONTANELLE

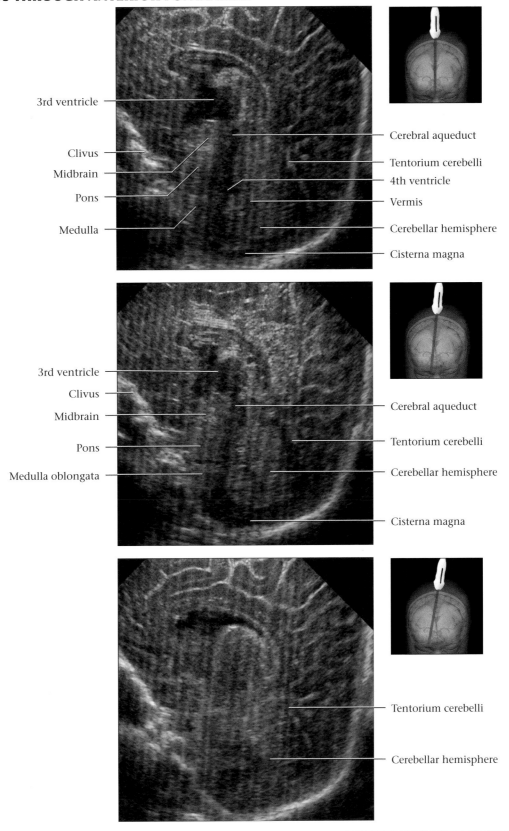

3rd ventricle — Cerebral aqueduct

Clivus — Tentorium cerebelli

Midbrain — 4th ventricle

Pons — Vermis

Medulla — Cerebellar hemisphere

Cisterna magna

3rd ventricle — Cerebral aqueduct

Clivus — Tentorium cerebelli

Midbrain — Cerebellar hemisphere

Pons

Medulla oblongata — Cisterna magna

Tentorium cerebelli

Cerebellar hemisphere

(Top) First of three sagittal US scans through the anterior fontanelle from medial to lateral showing the brainstem. The midline sagittal view shows midbrain, pons and medulla oblongata just behind the clivus of skull base. The cerebral aqueduct is seen within the midbrain communicating with the third ventricle superiorly. The fourth ventricle is triangular in shape just in front of cerebellar vermis. The echogenic vermis and its adjacent cerebellar hemispheres are separated from the occipital lobe by the tentorium cerebelli. Cisterna magna is below the cerebellum and above the foramen magnum. (Middle) Slightly more lateral parasagittal image shows similar structures of the brainstem & cerebellum in the posterior fossa. The cisterna magna is more clearly depicted. (Bottom) Most lateral parasagittal image shows the cerebellar hemisphere, which is less echogenic than the vermis in midline.

BRAINSTEM AND CEREBELLUM

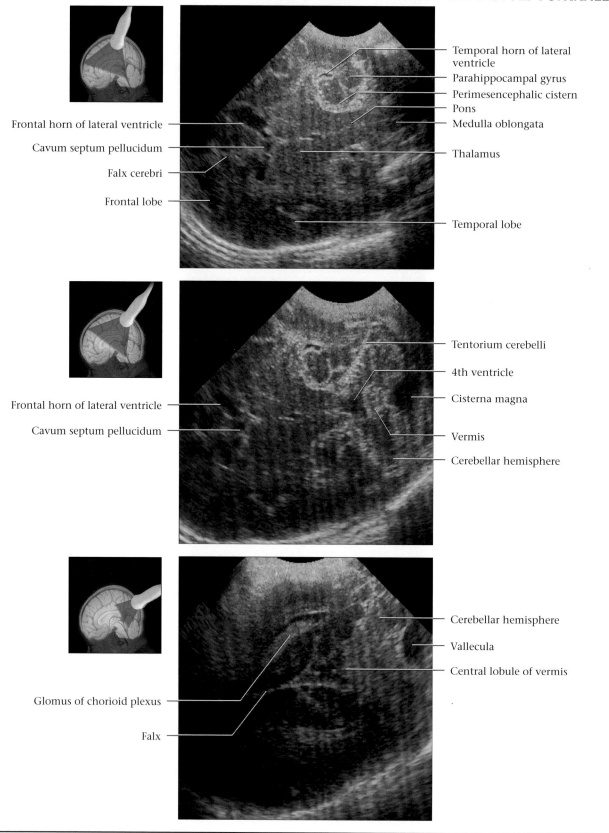

Frontal horn of lateral ventricle

Cavum septum pellucidum

Falx cerebri

Frontal lobe

Temporal horn of lateral ventricle

Parahippocampal gyrus

Perimesencephalic cistern

Pons

Medulla oblongata

Thalamus

Temporal lobe

Frontal horn of lateral ventricle

Cavum septum pellucidum

Tentorium cerebelli

4th ventricle

Cisterna magna

Vermis

Cerebellar hemisphere

Cerebellar hemisphere

Vallecula

Central lobule of vermis

Glomus of chorioid plexus

Falx

(Top) First of three longitudinal US images of the brainstem through mastoid fontanelle. The most anterior view shows frontal horns & cavum septum pellucidum superiorly. The falx cerebri & third ventricle are in midline. Thalami are seen as hypoechoic, inverted heart-shaped structures on both sides of the third ventricle. Inferiorly are two echogenic arcs of perimesencephalic cisterns. Between the two echogenic arcs are pons & medulla oblongata in midline. (Middle) More posterior image shows the fourth ventricle in midline. The cerebellar hemispheres are separated from supratentorial structures by the echogenic tentorium cerebelli. The radiating echogenic folia of the cerebellum are best seen in this view. (Bottom) The most posterior image shows glomus of choroid plexus within trigones of lateral ventricles. Vallecula is seen between cerebellar hemispheres.

BRAINSTEM AND CEREBELLUM

OBLIQUE CORONAL T1 MR

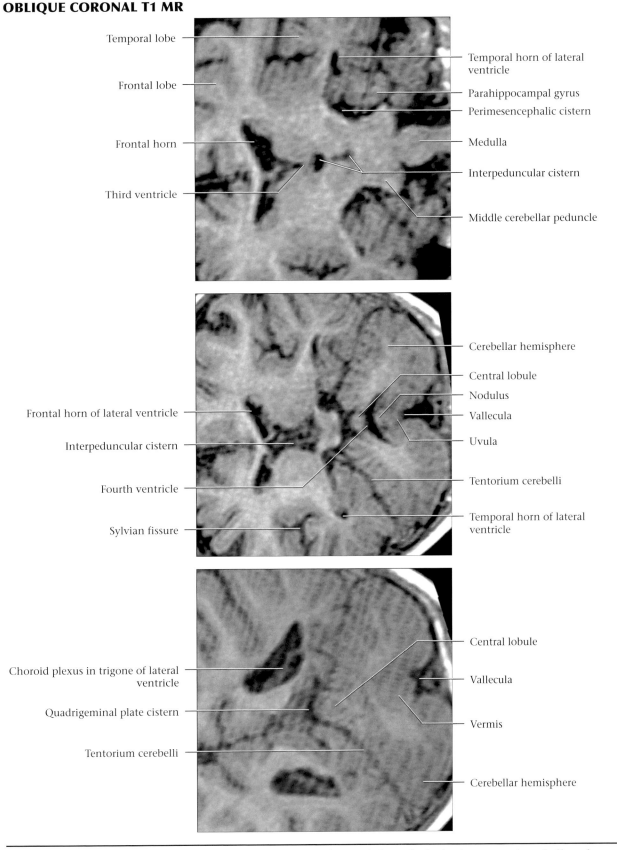

Temporal lobe

Frontal lobe

Frontal horn

Third ventricle

Temporal horn of lateral ventricle

Parahippocampal gyrus

Perimesencephalic cistern

Medulla

Interpeduncular cistern

Middle cerebellar peduncle

Frontal horn of lateral ventricle

Interpeduncular cistern

Fourth ventricle

Sylvian fissure

Cerebellar hemisphere

Central lobule

Nodulus

Vallecula

Uvula

Tentorium cerebelli

Temporal horn of lateral ventricle

Choroid plexus in trigone of lateral ventricle

Quadrigeminal plate cistern

Tentorium cerebelli

Central lobule

Vallecula

Vermis

Cerebellar hemisphere

(Top) First of three rotated oblique coronal T1 MR images obtained through the brainstem and cerebellum from anterior to posterior. Images correspond to scan plane and images obtained by scanning through the mastoid fontanelle. At this level, the brainstem is seen while the cerebellum is out of plane. Note the perimesencephalic cisterns on both sides of the midbrain, which form the "echogenic arcs", a characteristic landmark on US. (Middle) Slightly more posterior image shows the anterior cerebellum, fourth ventricle and cisterna magna. Some of the vermian lobules including central lobule, uvula and nodulus are depicted. (Bottom) More posteriorly, the fourth ventricle is out of plane. The glomus of choroid plexus is seen within the trigones of lateral ventricles. The vallecula is between the two cerebellar tonsils.

BRAINSTEM AND CEREBELLUM

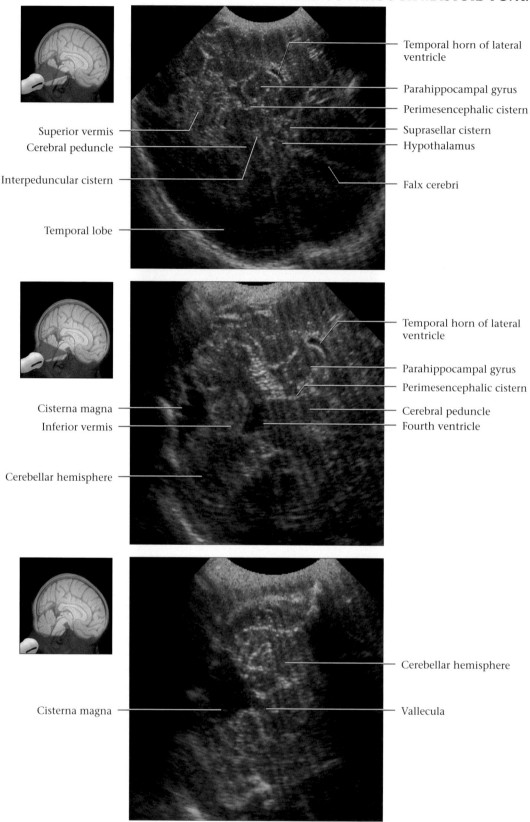

Temporal horn of lateral ventricle

Parahippocampal gyrus

Perimesencephalic cistern

Suprasellar cistern

Hypothalamus

Falx cerebri

Superior vermis

Cerebral peduncle

Interpeduncular cistern

Temporal lobe

Temporal horn of lateral ventricle

Parahippocampal gyrus

Perimesencephalic cistern

Cerebral peduncle

Fourth ventricle

Cisterna magna

Inferior vermis

Cerebellar hemisphere

Cerebellar hemisphere

Cisterna magna

Vallecula

(Top) First of three axial US images of the brainstem and cerebellum through the mastoid fontanelle. In the most superior view, the suprasellar cistern is seen as an echogenic five-point star with hypoechoic hypothalamus present in center. Posterior to this echogenic star are the cerebral peduncles with interpeduncular cistern in between. The midbrain is surrounded by echogenic perimesencephalic cisterns bilaterally. The most posterior structure is the highly echogenic superior vermis. **(Middle)** More inferior axial image shows the fourth ventricle in midline with echogenic vermis and cisterna magna present more posteriorly. The cerebellar hemispheres are on both sides of the vermis. **(Bottom)** Most inferior axial image shows the two cerebellar hemispheres with the vallecula in between. The radiating echogenic folia over the cerebellar surface can be clearly seen.

AXIAL T1 MR

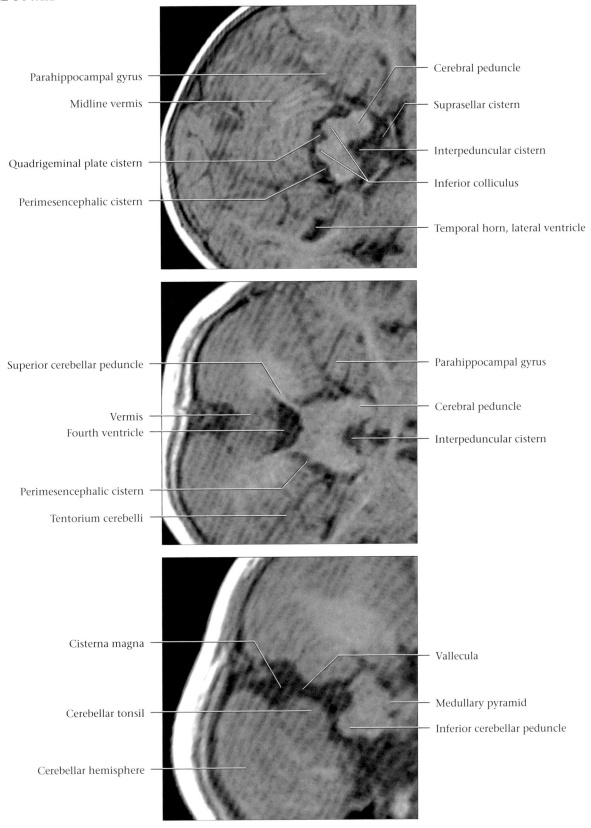

Parahippocampal gyrus

Midline vermis

Quadrigeminal plate cistern

Perimesencephalic cistern

Cerebral peduncle

Suprasellar cistern

Interpeduncular cistern

Inferior colliculus

Temporal horn, lateral ventricle

Superior cerebellar peduncle

Vermis

Fourth ventricle

Perimesencephalic cistern

Tentorium cerebelli

Parahippocampal gyrus

Cerebral peduncle

Interpeduncular cistern

Cisterna magna

Cerebellar tonsil

Cerebellar hemisphere

Vallecula

Medullary pyramid

Inferior cerebellar peduncle

(Top) First of three rotated axial T1 MR images of the brainstem and cerebellum from superior to inferior. Images correspond to scan plane and US images obtained through the mastoid fontanelle. The midbrain is surrounded by CSF-filled cisterns. Anteriorly is the suprasellar cistern. Interpeduncular cistern is between two cerebral peduncles. On both lateral sides of the midbrain are perimesencephalic (ambient) cisterns. The quadrigeminal plate cistern is posterior. Cisterns appear hypointense on T1WI & hyperintense on T2WI MR. They appear echogenic on US. **(Middle)** Image more inferiorly at level of superior cerebellar peduncle. Fourth ventricle & cerebellar hemispheres can be seen in this level. **(Bottom)** Image through inferior cerebellum showing both tonsils, cisterna magna and vallecula.

Brain and Spine   I

MIDBRAIN

Terminology

Abbreviations
- Cerebrospinal fluid (CSF)
- Cranial nerves (CN): Oculomotor nerve (CN3), trochlear nerve (CN4)

Synonyms
- Midbrain, mesencephalon

Definitions
- Midbrain: Portion of brainstem which connects pons and cerebellum with forebrain

Gross Anatomy

Overview
- "Butterfly-shaped" upper brainstem which passes through hiatus in tentorium cerebelli
- Composed of gray matter formations, CN nuclei (CN3-4) and white matter tracts
- Three main parts
  - **Cerebral peduncles**: White matter tracts
    - Continuous with pontine bulb and medullary pyramids
  - **Tegmentum**: CN nuclei, gray matter nuclei, white matter tracts
    - Continuous with pontine tegmentum
    - Ventral to cerebral aqueduct
  - **Tectum (quadrigeminal plate)**: Superior and inferior colliculi
    - Dorsal to cerebral aqueduct
- Midbrain connections
  - Rostral (superior): Cerebral hemispheres, basal ganglia and thalami
  - Dorsal (posterior): Cerebellum
  - Caudal (inferior): Pons
- Cerebral aqueduct passes through dorsal midbrain between tectum posteriorly and tegmentum anteriorly, connecting third and fourth ventricles
- Adjacent CSF cisterns
  - Interpeduncular: Anterior, contains CN3
  - Ambient (perimesencephalic): Lateral, contains CN4
  - Quadrigeminal plate: Posterior, contains CN4
- Blood supply by vertebrobasilar circulation
  - Small perforating branches from basilar, superior cerebellar and posterior cerebral arteries

Cerebral Peduncles (Crus Cerebri)
- Corticospinal, corticobulbar & corticopontine fibers
- Cerebral peduncles separated in midline by interpeduncular fossa

Mesencephalic Tegmentum
- Directly continuous with pontine tegmentum, contains same tracts
- Multiple white matter tracts (not resolved on conventional imaging)
  - Medial longitudinal fasciculus: Oculomotor-vestibular
  - Medial lemniscus: Somatosensory
  - Lateral lemniscus: Auditory
  - Spinothalamic tract: Somatosensory
  - Central tegmental tract: Motor
- **Gray matter formations**
  - **Substantia nigra**: Pigmented nucleus, extends through midbrain from pons to subthalamic region, important in movement
    - Pars compacta: Contains dopaminergic cells (atrophied in Parkinson disease)
    - Pars reticularis: Contains GABAergic cells
  - **Red nucleus**: Relay and control station for cerebellar, globus pallidus and corticomotor impulses
    - Important for muscle tone, posture, locomotion
  - **Periaqueductal grey**: Surrounds cerebral aqueduct
    - Important in modulation of pain and defensive behavior
- **Cranial nerve nuclei**
  - CN3 nuclei at superior colliculus level
    - Paramedian, anterior to cerebral aqueduct
    - Motor nuclei consists of five individual motor subnuclei that supply individual extraocular muscles
    - Edinger-Westphal parasympathetic nuclei: Dorsal to CN3 nucleus in periaquaductal grey
    - CN3 fibers course anteriorly through midbrain to exit at interpeduncular fossa
  - CN4 nuclei at inferior colliculus level
    - Paramedian, anterior to cerebral aqueduct
    - Dorsal to medial longitudinal fasciculus
    - CN4 fibers course posteriorly around cerebral aqueduct, decussate in superior medullary velum
    - CN4 exits dorsal midbrain just inferior to inferior colliculus
- **Reticular formation**: Expands from medulla to rostral midbrain
  - Occupies central tegmentum
  - Afferent and efferent connections
  - Important in consciousness, motor function, respiration and cardiovascular control

Tectum (Quadrigeminal Plate)
- Superior colliculi: Visual pathway
- Inferior colliculi: Auditory pathway

Imaging Anatomy

Overview
- Aqueduct appears as echogenic dot on axial US and as thin line on mid-sagittal plane
- Cerebral peduncles, superior & inferior colliculi best seen on axial image through mastoid fontanelle
- Suprasellar cistern, interpeduncular cistern, perimesencephalic cisterns appear echogenic, best seen on axial planes around midbrain

Anatomy-Based Imaging Issues

Imaging Pitfalls
- Pigmented nuclei: Substantia nigra & red nucleus are not resolved by US, best seen on T2 MR image
- CN nuclei and white matter tracts can be identified by typical location, but are not resolved on imaging

Brain and Spine

I

58

MIDBRAIN

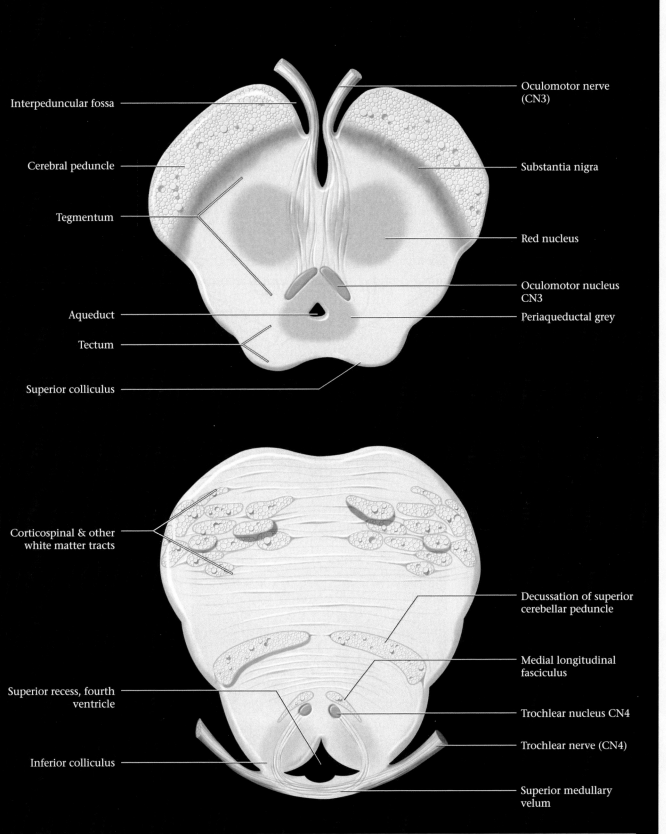

Interpeduncular fossa

Cerebral peduncle

Tegmentum

Aqueduct

Tectum

Superior colliculus

Oculomotor nerve (CN3)

Substantia nigra

Red nucleus

Oculomotor nucleus CN3

Periaqueductal grey

Corticospinal & other white matter tracts

Superior recess, fourth ventricle

Inferior colliculus

Decussation of superior cerebellar peduncle

Medial longitudinal fasciculus

Trochlear nucleus CN4

Trochlear nerve (CN4)

Superior medullary velum

(Top) Axial graphic through level of the superior colliculus shows oculomotor nucleus (CN3) just anterior to the cerebral aqueduct. CN3 exits into the interpeduncular fossa. Cerebral peduncles are anterior & contain corticospinal & other white matter tracts. The tegmentum is anterior & tectum is posterior to the cerebral aqueduct. The substantia nigra consists of two layers of cells: Pars compacta posteriorly & pars reticulata anteriorly, which plays a vital role in Parkinson disease. **(Bottom)** Axial graphic of the midbrain at level of the inferior colliculi shows the trochlear nucleus (CN4) & nerve fibers as they decussate in the superior medullary velum which forms the roof of the fourth ventricle. Each superior oblique muscle is innervated by contralateral trochlear nucleus. CN4 exits dorsally, just inferior to the inferior colliculus & is the only cranial nerve to exit the dorsal brainstem.

Brain and Spine

I

59

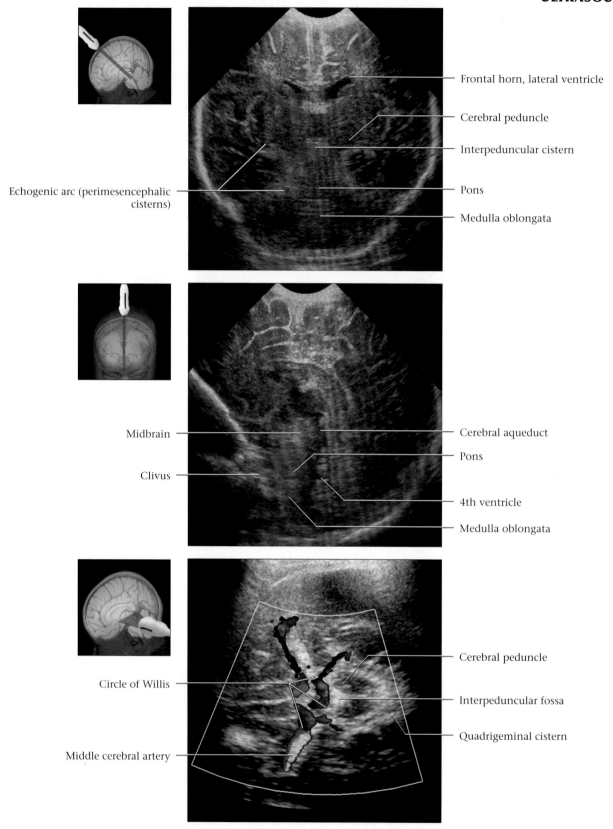

Frontal horn, lateral ventricle

Cerebral peduncle

Interpeduncular cistern

Pons

Medulla oblongata

Echogenic arc (perimesencephalic cisterns)

Midbrain

Clivus

Cerebral aqueduct

Pons

4th ventricle

Medulla oblongata

Circle of Willis

Middle cerebral artery

Cerebral peduncle

Interpeduncular fossa

Quadrigeminal cistern

(Top) Anterior coronal image obtained through the anterior fontanelle at level of the interpeduncular cistern. Structures between the two echogenic arcs are (from top to bottom) as follows: Right & left cerebral peduncles of midbrain, midline echogenic interpeduncular cistern, pons & medulla oblongata. **(Middle)** Midsagittal image obtained through the anterior fontanelle shows the midbrain, pons & medulla oblongata. Echogenic clivus is present anteriorly while the fourth ventricle & cerebellum are seen posteriorly. **(Bottom)** Color Doppler axial image obtained through the temporal bone. The midbrain is the heart-shaped, hypoechoic structure with interpeduncular fossa in between two cerebral peduncles. Anteriorly is the suprasellar cistern which contains the circle of Willis. This is the best view for detecting pathology in the midbrain & circle of Willis.

MIDBRAIN

T1 MR

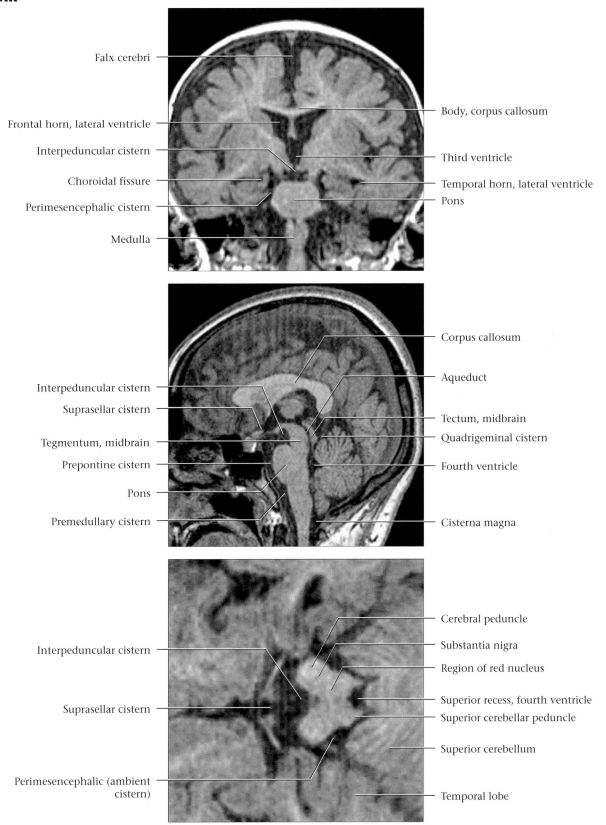

Falx cerebri

Frontal horn, lateral ventricle

Interpeduncular cistern

Choroidal fissure

Perimesencephalic cistern

Medulla

Body, corpus callosum

Third ventricle

Temporal horn, lateral ventricle

Pons

Interpeduncular cistern

Suprasellar cistern

Tegmentum, midbrain

Prepontine cistern

Pons

Premedullary cistern

Corpus callosum

Aqueduct

Tectum, midbrain

Quadrigeminal cistern

Fourth ventricle

Cisterna magna

Interpeduncular cistern

Suprasellar cistern

Perimesencephalic (ambient cistern)

Cerebral peduncle

Substantia nigra

Region of red nucleus

Superior recess, fourth ventricle

Superior cerebellar peduncle

Superior cerebellum

Temporal lobe

(Top) Coronal T1 MR image of the midbrain shows the interpeduncular cistern, perimesencephalic cisterns and choroidal fissures are on same coronal plane. These structures appear echogenic on US and form characteristic landmarks of "three-dot sign" & "echogenic arch" during coronal scans. (Middle) Midsagittal T1 MR image shows the course of the aqueduct. Cerebral peduncles are better visualized on axial images. Ventral to the aqueduct is the tegmentum which consists of CN nuclei, gray matter nuclei & white matter tracts. Dorsal to the aqueduct is the tectum (quadrigeminal plate) which contains superior & inferior colliculi. Colliculi are also better visualized on axial images. (Bottom) Rotated axial T1 MR image of the midbrain, corresponding to scan plane and image obtained on axial ultrasound scan through the temporal bone.

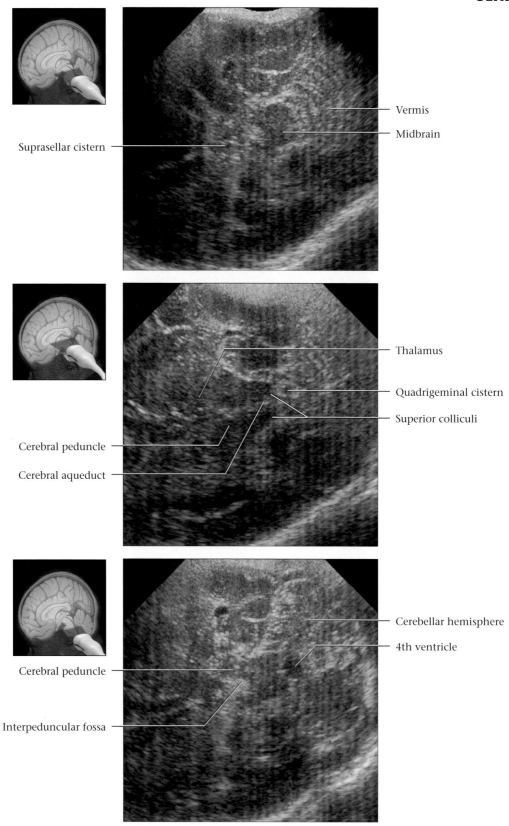

Vermis

Midbrain

Suprasellar cistern

Thalamus

Quadrigeminal cistern

Superior colliculi

Cerebral peduncle

Cerebral aqueduct

Cerebellar hemisphere

4th ventricle

Cerebral peduncle

Interpeduncular fossa

(Top) First of three axial images obtained through the mastoid fontanelle. This image is obtained at the level of the suprasellar cistern, which appears as an echogenic 5-point star and is present most anteriorly. **(Middle)** This image of the midbrain shows both cerebral peduncles & superior colliculi. The aqueduct appears as an echogenic dot on axial US image. On sagittal image, the aqueduct appears as a thin line or occasionally as a thin slit. The quadrigeminal cistern is echogenic, which is present posterior to the superior colliculi, part of the quadrigeminal plate. **(Bottom)** This is the most inferior axial image. The echogenic space between the two cerebral peduncles is known as the interpeduncular fossa which is occupied by the interpeduncular cistern. CN3 exits the midbrain at the level of the superior colliculus and can be seen within the interpeduncular fossa on MR imaging.

MIDBRAIN

T1 MR

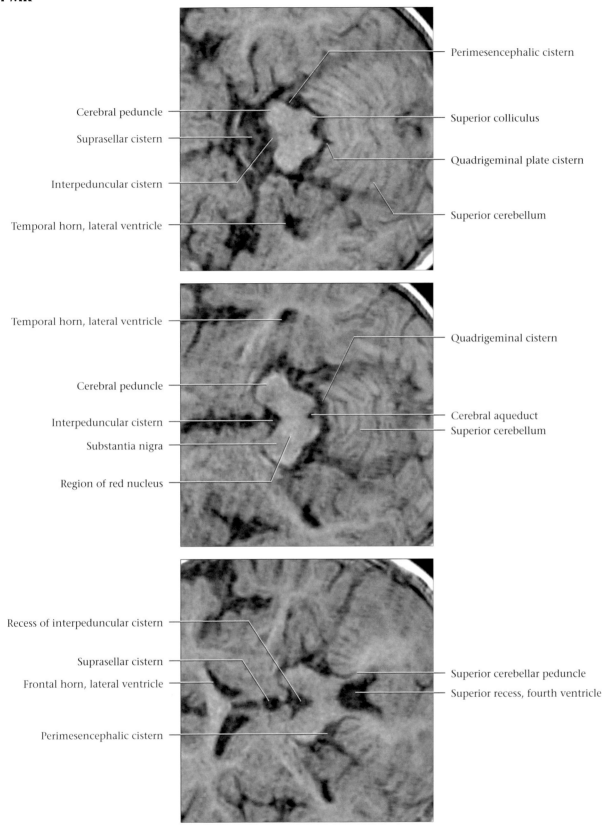

Perimesencephalic cistern

Cerebral peduncle

Superior colliculus

Suprasellar cistern

Quadrigeminal plate cistern

Interpeduncular cistern

Temporal horn, lateral ventricle

Superior cerebellum

Temporal horn, lateral ventricle

Quadrigeminal cistern

Cerebral peduncle

Interpeduncular cistern

Cerebral aqueduct

Substantia nigra

Superior cerebellum

Region of red nucleus

Recess of interpeduncular cistern

Suprasellar cistern

Frontal horn, lateral ventricle

Superior cerebellar peduncle

Superior recess, fourth ventricle

Perimesencephalic cistern

(Top) A set of three rotated T1 MR images, corresponding to scan plane and US image obtained by scanning through the mastoid fontanelle. The relationship of the midbrain with the adjacent cisterns is depicted: The interpeduncular cistern & suprasellar cistern are anterior. The quadrigeminal plate cistern is posterior and the perimesencephalic (ambient) cisterns are located bilaterally. **(Middle)** In this image, the interpeduncular cistern is clearly seen. The pigmented nuclei, substantia nigra and red nucleus are also seen at this level. These nuclei cannot be resolved by US. **(Bottom)** This is the most inferior image of the midbrain. Superior cerebellar peduncles connect the cerebellum to the cerebrum via the midbrain. The superior recess of the fourth ventricle is also seen in this level.

VENTRICLES AND CHOROID PLEXUS

Gross Anatomy

Overview
- **Cerebral ventricles**
  - Paired lateral, midline third and fourth ventricles
  - Communicate with each other as well as central canal of spinal cord, subarachnoid space (SAS)
- **Choroid plexus**
  - CSF flows from lateral ventricles through foramen of Monro into third ventricle, through cerebral aqueduct into fourth ventricle; exits through foramina of Luschka & Magendie to SAS
  - Bulk of CSF resorption through arachnoid granulations in region of superior sagittal sinus

Anatomy Relationships
- **Lateral ventricles**
  - Each has body, atrium, three horns
  - **Frontal horn** formed by
    - Roof: Corpus callosum
    - Lateral wall, floor: Caudate nucleus
    - Medial wall: Septum pellucidum (thin midline structure that separates right, left frontal horns)
  - **Body** formed by
    - Roof: Corpus callosum
    - Floor: Dorsal surface of thalamus
    - Medial wall, floor: Fornix
    - Lateral wall, floor: Body, tail of caudate nucleus
  - **Temporal horn** formed by
    - Roof: Tail of caudate nucleus
    - Medial wall, floor: Hippocampus
    - Lateral wall: Geniculocalcarine tract, arcuate fasciculus
  - **Occipital horn**: Surrounded by white matter (forceps major of corpus callosum, geniculocalcarine tract)
  - **Atrium/trigone**: Confluence of horns; contains glomi of choroid plexus
  - Lateral ventricles communicate with each other, third ventricle via "Y-shaped" foramen of Monro
- **Third ventricle**
  - Midline, slit-like vertical cavity between right, left diencephalon that contains interthalamic adhesion (not a true commissure)
  - Borders
    - Anterior: Lamina terminalis, anterior commissure
    - Lateral: Thalami
    - Roof: Tela choroidea, choroid plexus
    - Floor: Optic chiasm, infundibulum & tuber cinereum, mammillary bodies, posterior perforated substance, tegmentum of midbrain
    - Posterior: Pineal gland, habenular & posterior commissures
  - Recesses
    - Inferior: Optic, infundibular
    - Posterior: Suprapineal, pineal
  - Communicates with fourth ventricle via cerebral aqueduct
- **Fourth ventricle**
  - Diamond-shaped cavity (rhomboid fossa) along dorsal pons & upper medulla
  - Borders
    - Roof/floor: Tent-shaped, covered by anterior (superior) medullary velum above & inferior medullary velum below
    - Walls: Dorsal surface of pons & medulla, cerebral peduncles (superior/middle/inferior)
  - Five recesses
    - Paired posterior-superior: Thin, flat pouch capping tonsils
    - Paired lateral: Curve anteriorly under brachium pontis, contain choroid plexus, communicate with SAS via foramina of Luschka
    - Fastigium: Blind-ending, dorsally pointed midline outpouching from body of fourth ventricle
  - Communicates with SAS via foramina of Magendie and Luschka, with central canal of cord via obex

Imaging Anatomy

Overview
- Lateral ventricles: Paired, "C-shaped", curve posteriorly from temporal horns, arch around/above thalami
  - Asymmetry is common, often L > R, occipital horn > frontal horn
  - Sizes change with maturity, more prominent in preterm infants
- Third ventricle: Thin, usually slit-like; 80% have central adhesion between thalami (massa intermedia)
- Fourth ventricle: Diamond-shaped midline infratentorial ventricle
- Choroid plexus
  - Glomus partially/completely fills trigones
  - Tapers and extends anteriorly to foramen of Monro & roof of third ventricle
  - Tapers laterally to temporal horns
  - Present in roof of fourth ventricle but never extends into frontal or occipital horns

Normal Variants
- Midline cystic structures
  - **Cavum septi pellucidi**: Anterior to foramen of Monro, between anterior horns of lateral ventricles
    - 85% infants completely closed by 3-6 month after birth, some remain open into adulthood
  - **Cavum vergae**: Posterior to foramen of Monro, interposed between bodies of lateral ventricles
    - Begins to close from posterior to anterior from 6 month gestation, 97% infants closed by full-term
  - **Cavum velum interpositum**: Potential space above choroid in roof of third ventricle and below fornices, inferior & posterior to splenium in pineal region
    - Anechoic extension from cavum vergae to quadrigeminal cistern, seen in very premature infants

Anatomy-Based Imaging Issues

Imaging Pitfalls
- Slit-like lateral ventricles common in infants, not to be mistaken for cerebral edema
- Glomus of choroid plexus can be bulbous & irregular, not to be mistaken for blood clot

VENTRICLES AND CHOROID PLEXUS

GRAPHICS

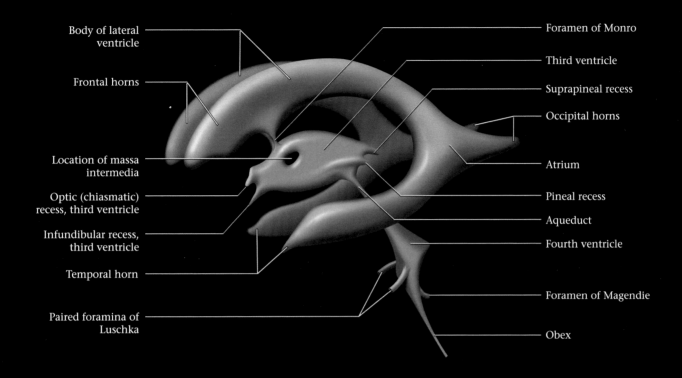

Body of lateral ventricle

Frontal horns

Location of massa intermedia

Optic (chiasmatic) recess, third ventricle

Infundibular recess, third ventricle

Temporal horn

Paired foramina of Luschka

Foramen of Monro

Third ventricle

Suprapineal recess

Occipital horns

Atrium

Pineal recess

Aqueduct

Fourth ventricle

Foramen of Magendie

Obex

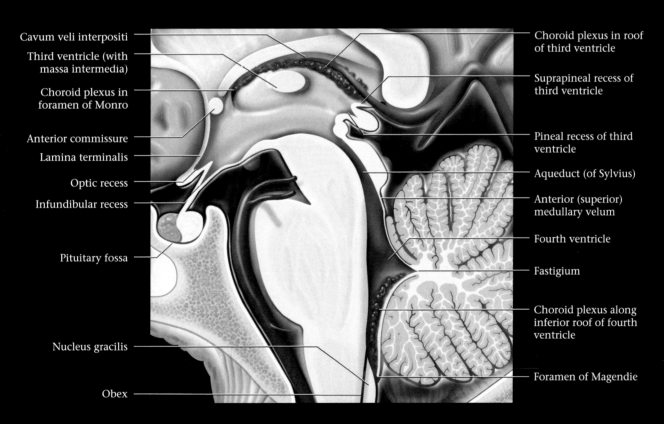

Cavum veli interpositi

Third ventricle (with massa intermedia)

Choroid plexus in foramen of Monro

Anterior commissure

Lamina terminalis

Optic recess

Infundibular recess

Pituitary fossa

Nucleus gracilis

Obex

Choroid plexus in roof of third ventricle

Suprapineal recess of third ventricle

Pineal recess of third ventricle

Aqueduct (of Sylvius)

Anterior (superior) medullary velum

Fourth ventricle

Fastigium

Choroid plexus along inferior roof of fourth ventricle

Foramen of Magendie

(Top) Schematic 3D representation of the ventricular system, viewed in the sagittal plane, demonstrates the normal appearance and communicating pathways of the cerebral ventricles. **(Bottom)** Sagittal midline graphic of normal midline ventricular anatomy. Choroid plexus from the lateral ventricles (not shown) extends through the foramina of Monro and curves dorsally and posteriorly along the roof of the third ventricle. Choroid plexus is not found in the frontal or occipital horns of the lateral ventricles, the cerebral aqueduct or foramen of Magendie. The foramen of Magendie is a slit-like median aperture which allows posterior communication of the fourth ventricle with the cisterna magna. The obex is the inferior terminus of the fourth ventricle in the upper cord.

Brain and Spine

I

65

VENTRICLES AND CHOROID PLEXUS

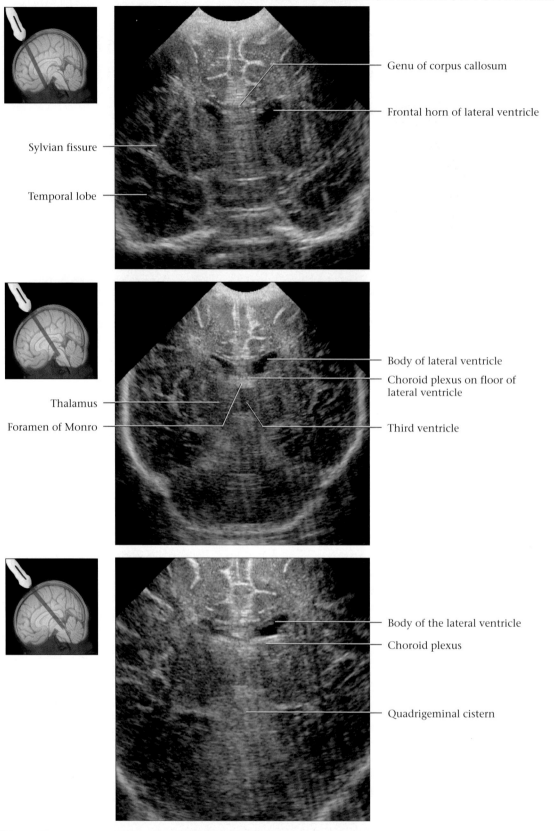

Genu of corpus callosum

Frontal horn of lateral ventricle

Sylvian fissure

Temporal lobe

Body of lateral ventricle

Choroid plexus on floor of lateral ventricle

Thalamus

Foramen of Monro

Third ventricle

Body of the lateral ventricle

Choroid plexus

Quadrigeminal cistern

(Top) First image in a series of six coronal ultrasound images of the ventricular system through the anterior fontanelle. This most anterior image is at the level just anterior to the foramen of Monro. No choroid plexus should be present in the frontal horns. Frontal horns appear as anechoic, fluid-filled spaces with triangular or roundish configuration. In about 60% of term infants, frontal horns appear slit-like, measuring less than 2-3 mm in diameter. **(Middle)** Image at the level of the foramen of Monro shows the choroid plexus on the floor of the lateral ventricles and roof of third ventricle. This is known as the 3-dot sign. The third ventricle may not be visualized on the coronal scan in some infants due to its small transverse diameter. **(Bottom)** Image at the level of the quadrigeminal cistern shows the choroid plexus on the floor of the body of the lateral ventricle.

VENTRICLES AND CHOROID PLEXUS

CORONAL US THROUGH ANTERIOR FONTANELLE

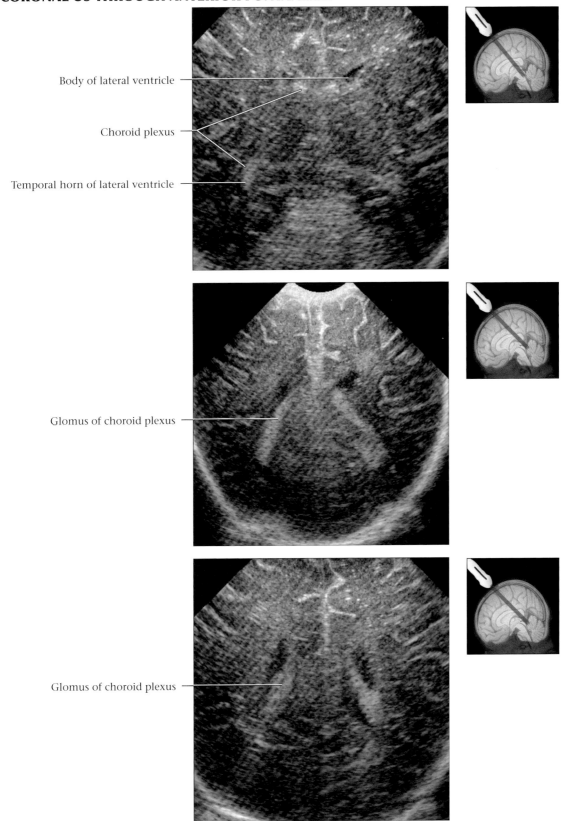

Body of lateral ventricle

Choroid plexus

Temporal horn of lateral ventricle

Glomus of choroid plexus

Glomus of choroid plexus

(Top) Coronal US image at the level just anterior to the trigone of the lateral ventricle shows the temporal horns inferiorly with the choroid plexus within. Asymmetry of lateral ventricles is not uncommon. Most often L > R, and occipital horns are larger than the frontal horns. Ventricular size is more prominent in premature infants than term infants. (Middle) Image at the level of the trigones of the lateral ventricles. Glomus of the choroid plexus can partially or completely fill trigones and appear highly echogenic. The outline of the glomus may be lobulated simulating a blood clot. (Bottom) Most posterior coronal image just posterior to the trigone. The choroid plexus is responsible for the production of CSF in the ventricles. The amount of CSF ranges from tiny anechoic collection to a larger crescentic or C-shaped collection filling the ventricles.

SAGITTAL US THROUGH ANTERIOR FONTANELLE

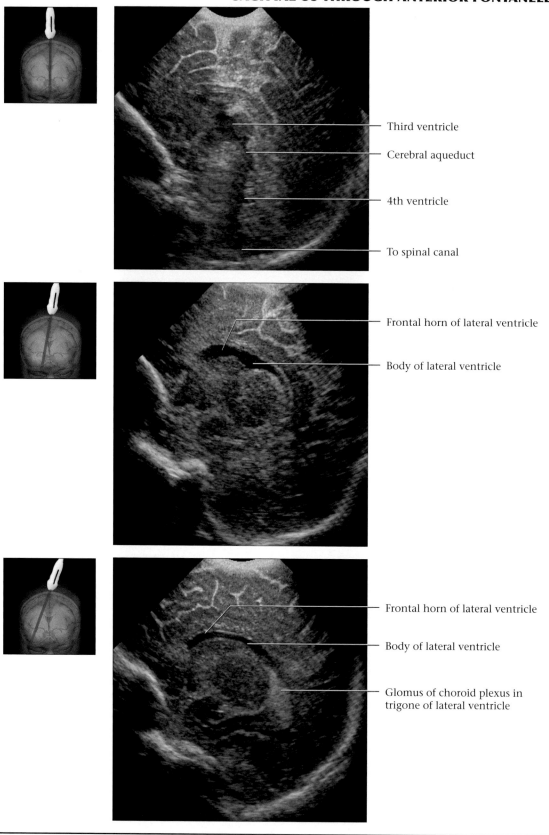

Third ventricle

Cerebral aqueduct

4th ventricle

To spinal canal

Frontal horn of lateral ventricle

Body of lateral ventricle

Frontal horn of lateral ventricle

Body of lateral ventricle

Glomus of choroid plexus in trigone of lateral ventricle

(Top) First of three sagittal US images through the anterior fontanelle. Midline view shows the third ventricle, cerebral aqueduct & triangular-shaped fourth ventricle. Lateral ventricles should not be seen on this view but cavum septum pellucidum & corpus callosum in the midline are seen. Sometimes the choroid plexus may be seen on the roof of the third ventricle but the choroid plexus is rarely seen in the fourth ventricle on this view. (Middle) Parasagittal image at the level of the caudothalamic groove where the germinal matrix is present. Echogenicity anterior to this junction raises the suspicion of hemorrhage in premature infants. (Bottom) Parasagittal fomage at the level of the glomus of the choroid plexus. Choroid plexus tapers & extends anteriorly to the foramen of Monro & along the roof of the third ventricle. Posteriorly the choroid plexus tapers & extends into the temporal horns.

VENTRICLES AND CHOROID PLEXUS

LONGITUDINAL US THROUGH MASTOID FONTANELLE

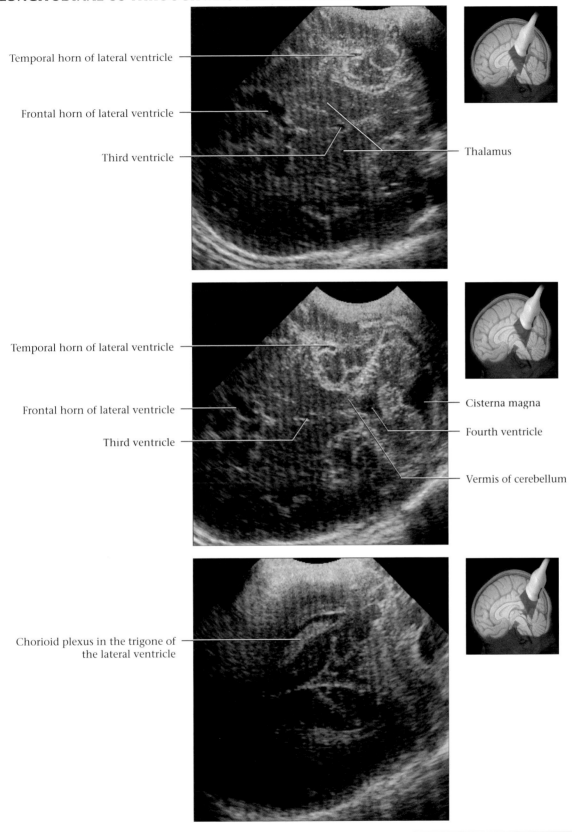

Temporal horn of lateral ventricle

Frontal horn of lateral ventricle

Third ventricle

Thalamus

Temporal horn of lateral ventricle

Frontal horn of lateral ventricle

Third ventricle

Cisterna magna

Fourth ventricle

Vermis of cerebellum

Chorioid plexus in the trigone of the lateral ventricle

(Top) First of three longitudinal ultrasound images through the mastoid fontanelle. The most anterior view shows frontal horns of the lateral ventricles superiorly. The third ventricle is in the middle, between two thalami. Sometimes the temporal horn may also be seen in the near field. Note that asymmetry of ventricular size is common, especially in preterm infants. (Middle) In this slightly more posterior image, frontal horns of the lateral ventricles & third ventricle can still be seen. The fourth ventricle can now be seen in the midline between the vermis superiorly and cisterna magna inferiorly. (Bottom) This is the most posterior longitudinal view through the mastoid fontanelle. The glomus of the choroid plexus is present in the trigones of the lateral ventricles. Usually the glomus is prominent and echogenic, almost completely filling the trigones.

VENTRICLES AND CHOROID PLEXUS

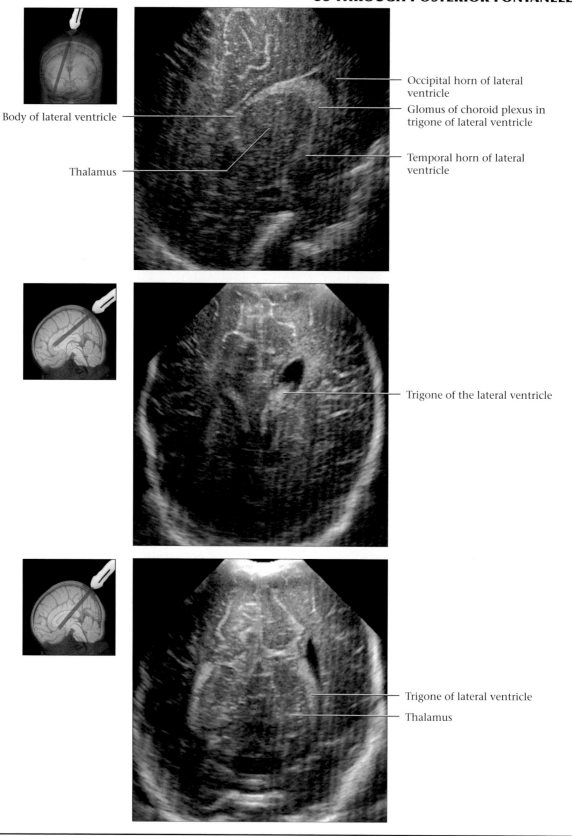

Body of lateral ventricle

Thalamus

Occipital horn of lateral ventricle

Glomus of choroid plexus in trigone of lateral ventricle

Temporal horn of lateral ventricle

Trigone of the lateral ventricle

Trigone of lateral ventricle

Thalamus

(Top) Parasagittal ultrasound image through the posterior fontanelle, shows both occipital horn and body of the lateral ventricle wrapping around the thalamus. The glomus of the choroid plexus is present within the trigone. Chorioid plexus can also be seen extending into the body & temporal horn of the lateral ventricle but no choroid plexus is present in the occipital horn, which should be completely anechoic. This is the best view for detection of intraventricular hemorrhage in occipital horns. (Middle) First of two coronal US images through the posterior fontanelle. This image at a more superior level shows the choroid plexus on the floor of bodies of lateral fontenticles. There is often asymmetry of lateral ventricles with left side larger than right side. (Bottom) More inferior coronal image showing the glomus within the lateral ventricles & thalami in between.

VENTRICLES AND CHOROID PLEXUS

US THROUGH TEMPORAL BONE

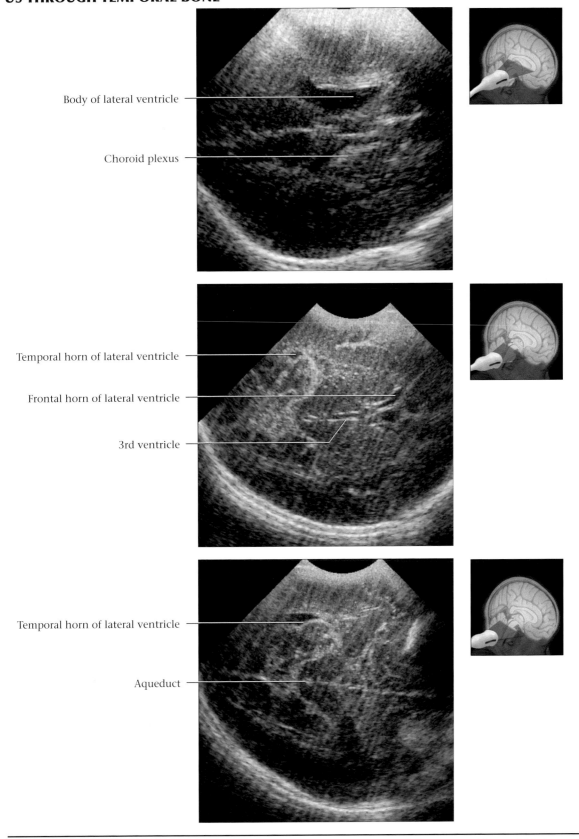

Body of lateral ventricle

Choroid plexus

Temporal horn of lateral ventricle

Frontal horn of lateral ventricle

3rd ventricle

Temporal horn of lateral ventricle

Aqueduct

(Top) First of three axial ultrasound images through the squamous part of the temporal bone. This image at the most superior level shows bodies of the lateral ventricles. Choroid plexus can be seen within the lateral ventricle of the far field. This view was once used to measure the size of the ventricle but is seldom used now. **(Middle)** This mid axial ultrasound image shows the frontal horns of the lateral ventricles and the third ventricle in between the two thalami. In some infants, temporal horn of the lateral ventricle can also be visualized. This image corresponds to the US plane used for measuring biparietal diameter in a fetus. **(Bottom)** This most inferior image shows temporal horns of the lateral ventricles in near field. Choroid plexus in temporal horns is usually thin with smooth contour, compared to bulbous appearance of glomus.

Brain and Spine

I

SUBARACHNOID SPACE/CISTERNS

Terminology

Abbreviations
- SASs: Subarachnoid spaces

Definitions
- SASs: Cerebrospinal fluid-filled spaces between pia, arachnoid; expand at base of brain, around brainstem, tentorial incisura
- Liliequist membrane: Thin arachnoid membrane separates suprasellar, interpeduncular & prepontine cisterns
- Velum interpositum: Double layer of pia (tela choroidea), the result of folding of brain where hemispheres overgrow diencephalon, forms velum interpositum which may remain open & communicate posteriorly with quadrigeminal cistern (cavum veli interpositi)
- Choroidal fissure: Narrow, pial-lined channel between SAS & ventricles; site of attachment of choroid plexus in lateral ventricles

Gross Anatomy

Overview
- Numerous trabeculae, septae, membranes cross SAS → create smaller compartments termed cisterns
  - Liliequist membrane separates suprasellar, interpeduncular & prepontine cisterns
  - Anterior/lateral pontine, medial/lateral pontomedullary membranes separate posterior fossa cisterns
- All cranial nerves, major arteries/veins traverse cisterns
- All structures within cisterns invested with thin pial-like layer of cells
- All SAS cisterns communicate with each other and with ventricular system (through foramina of Magendie and Luschka)
- Cisterns provide natural pathways for disease spread as well as surgical approaches
- SAS cisterns divided into supra- and peritentorial, infratentorial groups
- Sulci separate gyri, fissures separate hemispheres/lobes

Imaging Anatomy

Overview
- Supratentorial/peritentorial cisterns
  - Suprasellar cistern: Superior to pituitary gland
  - Interpeduncular cistern: Between cerebral peduncles, Liliequist membrane
  - Ambient (perimesencephalic) cisterns: Wrap around midbrain, connect suprasellar, quadrigeminal cisterns
  - Quadrigeminal cistern: Under corpus callosum splenium, behind pineal gland, tectum; continuous anteriorly with velum interpositum
  - Cistern of velum interpositum: Formed by double layers of tela choroidea (pia), lies above third ventricle; communicates posteriorly with quadrigeminal cistern

- Infratentorial (posterior fossa) cisterns
  - Midline (unpaired)
    - **Prepontine cistern**: Between upper clivus, anterior pons
    - **Premedullary cistern**: From pontomedullary junction above to foramen magnum below; between lower clivus and medulla
    - **Superior cerebellar cistern**: Between upper vermis, straight sinus
    - **Cisterna magna**: Between medulla (anterior) and occiput (posterior), below/behind inferior vermis
  - Lateral (paired)
    - **Cerebellopontine cistern**: Between anterolateral pons/cerebellum, petrous temporal bone
    - **Cerebellomedullary cistern** (sometimes included as lower cerebellopontine cistern): From dorsal margin of inferior olive laterally around medulla
- Fissures
  - **Interhemispheric fissure**: Longitudinal cerebral fissure separates hemispheres
    - Inferior part contains cistern of the lamina terminalis; upper part contains pericallosal cistern
  - **Sylvian (lateral) fissure**: Separates frontal, temporal lobes anteriorly, courses laterally to cover insula

Internal Structures-Critical Contents
- **Supratentorial/peritentorial cisterns**
  - **Suprasellar cistern**: Infundibulum, optic chiasm, circle of Willis
  - **Interpeduncular cistern**: Oculomotor nerves (CN3), basilar artery (BA) bifurcation, posterior thalamoperforating arteries
  - **Ambient cisterns**: Trochlear nerves (CN4), P2 posterior cerebral artery (PCA) segments and branches, superior cerebellar arteries (SCAs), basal veins of Rosenthal
  - **Quadrigeminal cistern**: Pineal gland, trochlear nerves (CN4), P3 PCA segments, medial & lateral posterior choroidal arteries, vein of Galen (VofG) + tributaries
  - **Cistern of velum interpositum**: Internal cerebral veins (ICVs), medial posterior choroidal artery (MPChAs)
- **Infratentorial cisterns**
  - **Prepontine cistern**: BA, anterior inferior cerebellar artery (AICA), CN5 and 6
  - **Premedullary cistern**: Vertebral arteries (VAs), anterior spinal artery, posterior inferior cerebellar artery (PICAs), CN12
  - **Superior cerebellar cistern**: SCA branches, superior vermian and precentral cerebellar veins
  - **Cisterna magna**: Cerebellar tonsils (often have dense trabecular attachments), tonsillohemispheric PICA branches
  - **Cerebellopontine cistern**: CN5, 7 & 8; AICA; petrosal vein
  - **Cerebellomedullary cistern**: CN9, 10 & 11
- **Fissures**
  - **Interhemispheric fissure**: Falx cerebri with inferior sagittal sinus, anterior cerebral artery (ACA) and branches
  - **Lateral fissure**: Middle cerebral artery (M1-3 segments) & vein

SUBARACHNOID SPACE/CISTERNS

GRAPHICS

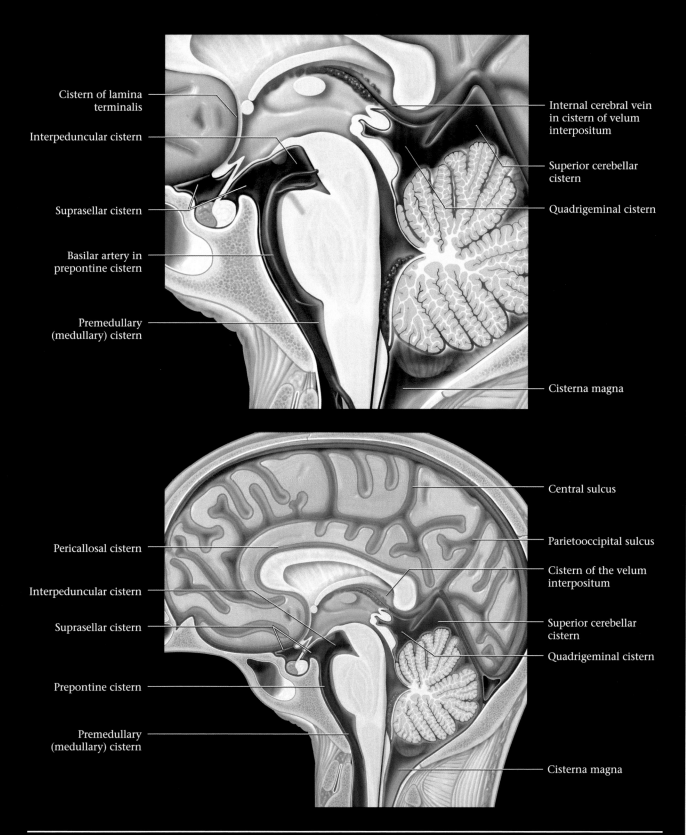

Cistern of lamina terminalis

Interpeduncular cistern

Suprasellar cistern

Basilar artery in prepontine cistern

Premedullary (medullary) cistern

Internal cerebral vein in cistern of velum interpositum

Superior cerebellar cistern

Quadrigeminal cistern

Cisterna magna

Pericallosal cistern

Interpeduncular cistern

Suprasellar cistern

Prepontine cistern

Premedullary (medullary) cistern

Central sulcus

Parietooccipital sulcus

Cistern of the velum interpositum

Superior cerebellar cistern

Quadrigeminal cistern

Cisterna magna

(Top) Sagittal midline graphic demonstrates normal cisternal, regional anatomy. The anterior circulation (anterior cerebral arteries, posterior communicating arteries) have been removed to illustrate some of the major structures in the suprasellar cistern. **(Bottom)** Sagittal midline graphic through interhemispheric fissure depicts SASs with CSF (blue) between arachnoid (purple) and pia (orange). The central sulcus separates frontal lobe (anterior) from parietal lobe (posterior). The pia mater is closely applied to the brain surface whereas the arachnoid is adherent to the dura. The ventricles communicate with the cisterns and subarachnoid space via the foramina of Luschka and Magendie. The cisterns normally communicate freely with each other.

CORONAL US THROUGH ANTERIOR FONTANELLE

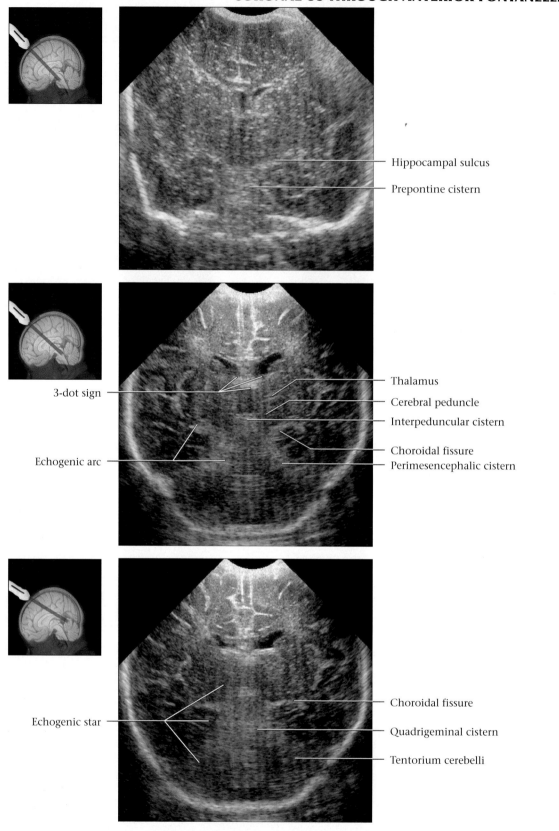

Hippocampal sulcus

Prepontine cistern

3-dot sign

Echogenic arc

Thalamus

Cerebral peduncle

Interpeduncular cistern

Choroidal fissure

Perimesencephalic cistern

Echogenic star

Choroidal fissure

Quadrigeminal cistern

Tentorium cerebelli

(Top) First of three coronal US images obtained through the anterior fontanelle. This is the most anterior view at the level just anterior to the foramen of Monro. The prepontine cistern appears as an echogenic area between the temporal lobes. The echogenic appearance of the cistern on US is due to the presence of arachnoid septation which create multiple interfaces. **(Middle)** Coronal image taken at the level of the 3-dot sign (choroid plexus in frontal horns & third ventricle) & echogenic arcs showing the interpeduncular cistern in midline, which is located between two cerebral peduncles. The echogenic arcs consist of choroidal fissures & perimesencephalic cisterns. **(Bottom)** Image at the level of the echogenic star with quadrigeminal cistern in the center with choroidal fissures as upper limbs and tentorium cerebelli as lower limbs of the star respectively.

SUBARACHNOID SPACE/CISTERNS

US THROUGH MASTOID FONTANELLE

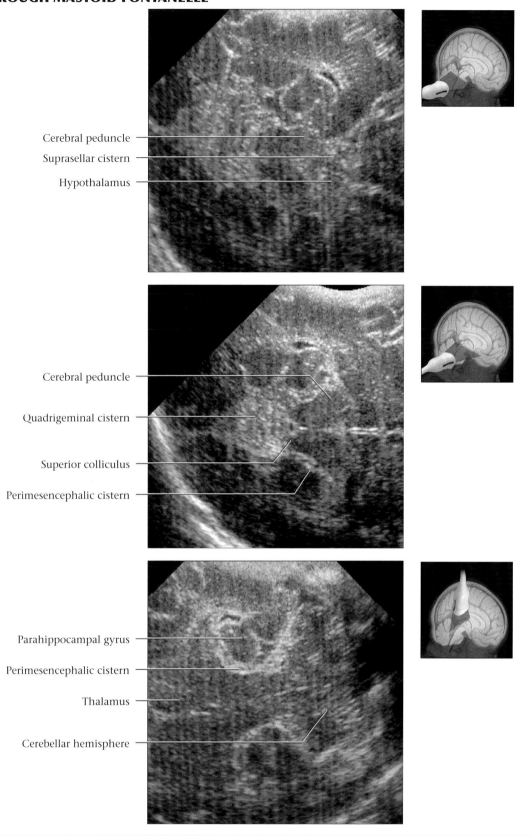

Cerebral peduncle
Suprasellar cistern
Hypothalamus

Cerebral peduncle
Quadrigeminal cistern
Superior colliculus
Perimesencephalic cistern

Parahippocampal gyrus
Perimesencephalic cistern
Thalamus
Cerebellar hemisphere

(Top) First of two axial US images through the mastoid fontanelle shows the suprasellar cistern. The cistern is anterior to the cerebral peduncles and has a five-point star shape with the hypoechoic hypothalamus in its center. The circle of Willis can be seen within the suprasellar cistern on color Doppler. Other important structures within the cistern include infundibulum & optic chiasm. (Middle) Axial image at a more superior level shows the quadrigeminal cistern posterior to the midbrain. Important structures within this cistern include trochlear nerves (CN4) & P3 PCA segments. The perimesencephalic cisterns are on both sides of the midbrain. (Bottom) Anterior longitudinal scan through the mastoid fontanelle shows both perimesencephalic cisterns forming echogenic arcs. Inferior to each arc is a cerebellar hemisphere and laterally is the parahippocampal gyrus.

Brain and Spine I

75

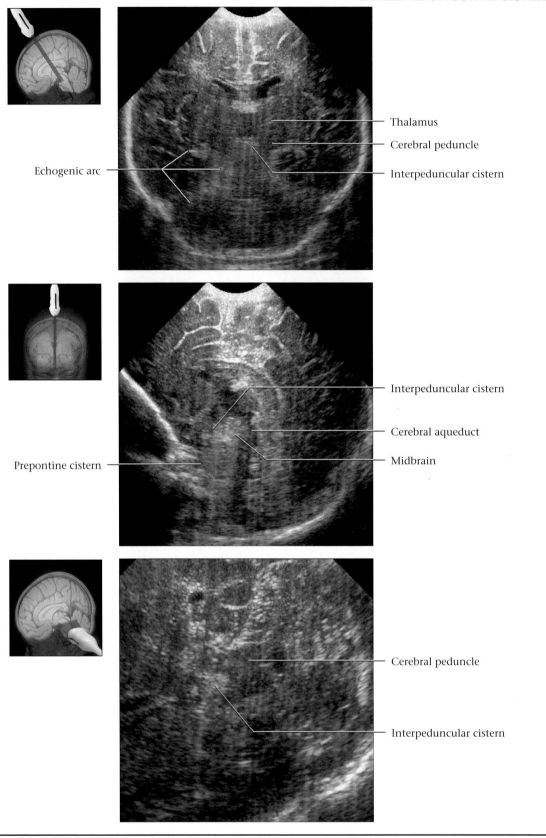

Thalamus

Cerebral peduncle

Interpeduncular cistern

Echogenic arc

Interpeduncular cistern

Cerebral aqueduct

Midbrain

Prepontine cistern

Cerebral peduncle

Interpeduncular cistern

(Top) Anterior coronal US scan through anterior fontanelle shows the interpeduncular cistern at the level of the 3-dot sign & echogenic arcs. The interpeduncular cistern is located between two cerebral peduncles. The choroid on the floor of the lateral ventricles & roof of the third ventricle forms the 3-dot sign. Echogenic arcs consist of choroidal fissures & perimesencephalic cisterns. (Middle) Midsagittal image obtained through anterior fontanelle shows interpeduncular cistern at level of midbrain. The prepontine cistern is more inferior and anterior to pons. (Bottom) Inferior axial US image through mastoid fontanelle shows echogenic interpeduncular cistern in interpeduncular fossa between the two cerebral peduncles. Important structures within interpeduncular cistern include oculomotor nerves (CN3), basilar artery (BA) bifurcation & posterior thalamoperforating arteries.

SUBARACHNOID SPACE/CISTERNS

QUADRIGEMINAL CISTERNS

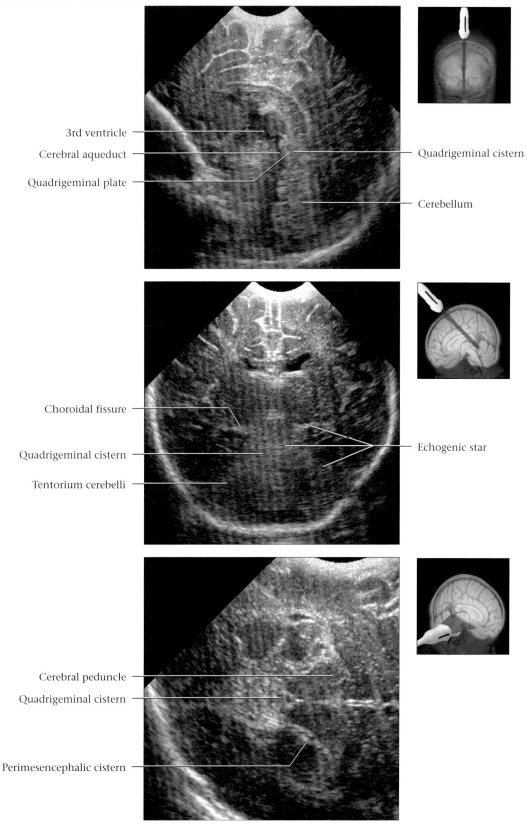

3rd ventricle

Cerebral aqueduct

Quadrigeminal plate

Quadrigeminal cistern

Cerebellum

Choroidal fissure

Quadrigeminal cistern

Tentorium cerebelli

Echogenic star

Cerebral peduncle

Quadrigeminal cistern

Perimesencephalic cistern

(Top) Midsagittal US image through anterior fontanelle shows the quadrigeminal cistern, which is posterior to the cerebral aqueduct & quadrigeminal plate (tectum) of the midbrain. (Middle) Anterior coronal US image through anterior fontanelle shows the quadrigeminal cistern. The quadrigeminal cistern is the center of the echogenic star with choroidal fissures as upper limbs and tentorium cerebelli as lower limbs of the star. (Bottom) Axial US image through mastoid fontanelle shows the quadrigeminal cistern. This cistern is posterior to the midbrain. Important structures within this cistern include the pineal gland, trochlear nerves (CN4), P3 PCA segments, medial & lateral posterior choroidal arteries, vein of Galen (VofG) + tributaries. The perimesencephalic cisterns are on both sides of midbrain, which contain trochlear nerves (CN4) & P2 posterior cerebral artery (PCA) segments.

Brain and Spine   I

77

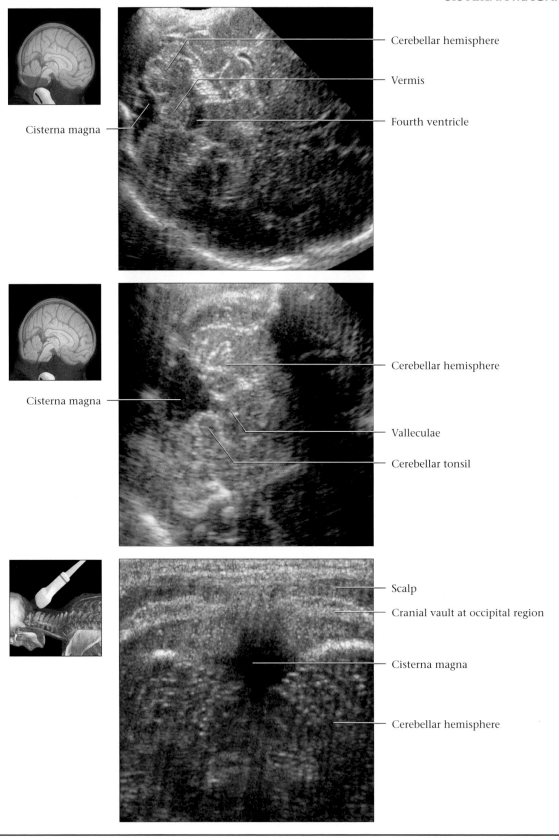

Cerebellar hemisphere

Vermis

Fourth ventricle

Cisterna magna

Cerebellar hemisphere

Cisterna magna

Valleculae

Cerebellar tonsil

Scalp

Cranial vault at occipital region

Cisterna magna

Cerebellar hemisphere

(Top) First of two axial US images through the mastoid fontanelle. This more superior image shows the cisterna magna posterior and inferior to the cerebellar hemispheres & midline echogenic vermis. The cisterna magna is separated from the fourth sventricle by vermis. Free communication between the above two structures is seen in Dandy Walker syndrome. The size of the cisterna magna is variable in normal infants but is markedly reduced in infants with Arnold-Chiari malformation, associated with caudal displacement of cerebellum, tonsils, medulla and fourth ventricle. **(Middle)** More inferior axial US image through mastoid fontanelle shows the cisterna magna between two cerebellar hemispheres & tonsils. **(Bottom)** Axial US image through foramen magnum. Cisterna magna is in midline underneath the cranial vault. Radiating echogenic folia of cerebellar hemisphere can be clearly seen.

SUBARACHNOID SPACE

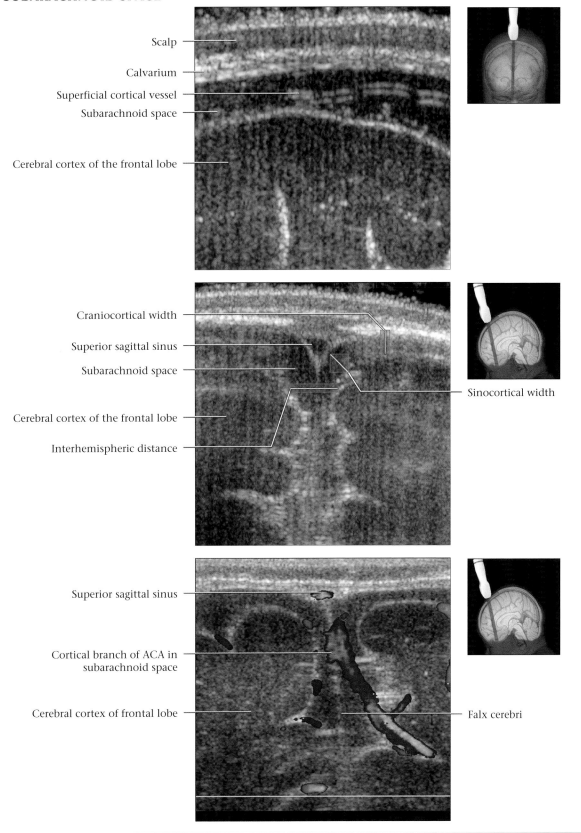

Scalp

Calvarium

Superficial cortical vessel

Subarachnoid space

Cerebral cortex of the frontal lobe

Craniocortical width

Superior sagittal sinus

Subarachnoid space

Cerebral cortex of the frontal lobe

Interhemispheric distance

Sinocortical width

Superior sagittal sinus

Cortical branch of ACA in subarachnoid space

Cerebral cortex of frontal lobe

Falx cerebri

(Top) Sagittal US image through anterior fontanelle shows the superficial cortical vessels running through subarachnoid space. The midline subarachnoid space is more easily seen by US than those located over anterior, posterior or lateral surface of the cerebral hemispheres. (Middle) Coronal US image through anterior fontanelle shows interhemispheric subarachnoid space. This space is usually measured at the level of foramen of Monro. The sinocortical width (shortest distance between lateral wall of superior sagittal sinus to surface of cerebral cortex) < 3 mm. The craniocortical width (vertical distance between calvarium & surface of cerebral cortex) < 4 mm. The widest interhemispheric distance < 6 mm. (Bottom) Coronal color Doppler image through anterior fontanelle shows cortical vessels traversing subarachnoid space & signal within superior sagittal sinus.

Brain and Spine

I

ORBIT

Terminology

Abbreviations
- Ophthalmic artery (OA); lacrimal artery (LA); central retinal artery (CRA); posterior ciliary arteries (PCA)
- Superior & inferior ophthalmic vein (SOV & IOV); central retinal vein (CRV); vortex veins (VV)

Gross Anatomy

Overview
- Bony orbital socket contains eyeball
- Eyeball is embedded in ocular fat, protected and moved by ocular muscles
- Eyeball consists of
  - Cornea: Transparent; covers iris & pupil
  - Anterior chamber: Directly behind cornea; filled with aqueous fluid for maintaining ocular pressure
  - Iris: Colored diaphragm in anterior chamber
  - Pupil: Opening in the center of the iris
  - Lens: Behind the pupil; capable of image focusing
  - Retina: inner wall membrane of eyeball; receives image and converts it into nerve impulses
  - Vitreous body: Clear, jelly-like substance in posterior chamber
  - Macula: Center of retina; > 5% of total retinal layer
  - Sclera: Dense, fibrous outer coating of the eyeball
  - Optic nerve (ON): Transmits nerve impulses from retina to brain

Imaging Anatomy

Internal Structures-Critical Contents
- Ocular structures
  - Anterior chamber difficult to examine
  - Optic nerve
    - Useful landmark for location of ocular vessels
    - Depicted as hypoechoic linear structure exiting eyeball posteromedially
  - Macula: Appears as short bright reflector
  - Retina: Only vitreous body - retinal interface seen normally on ultrasound
  - Sclera: Highly reflective; thickness ↑ with ↓ eye size (anterior 0.6 mm & posterior 1.0 mm)
  - Choroid: Normally indistinguishable from overlying retina and underlying sclera on ultrasound
  - Lens: Well-defined, oval, echolucent structure; visualization: Posterior capsule > anterior capsule
  - Vitreous cavity: Echolucent posterior compartment
- Extraocular muscles
  - Rectus muscles: Periglobal, hypoechoic structures
    - Medial rectus: Thickest of the four recti and is the easiest to examine
    - Lateral rectus: Patient's nose may interfere with transducer movement during examination
    - Inferior rectus: Difficult to examine
    - Superior rectus and levator muscles: Usually depicted as one complex
- Arteries and veins
  - OA
    - Largest ocular artery + fastest Doppler velocity

- Enters the orbital cavity through optic foramen, below and lateral to ON
- Crosses over ON to nasal side of orbit
- Its straight portion is easily seen in the nasal orbit
- Often tortuous in the posterior orbit
- Blood velocities vary with age, systemic blood pressure, smoking and posture
- Waveform: High resistance & resembles that of external carotid artery
- Dicrotic notch is usually present
  - Lacrimal artery
    - One of the large branches of OA
    - Runs along the upper border of lateral rectus
    - Often originates before entering the orbit
    - Sometimes derived from anterior branches of the middle meningeal artery
  - SOV
    - Largest vein detected in center of retrobulbar orbit
    - Runs obliquely and superior to ON
    - Ends in cavernous sinus via superior orbital fissure
    - Enhance visualization by Valsalva maneuver
  - IOV
    - Runs in inferior orbit and has two branches
    - One joins pterygoid venous plexus via inferior orbital fissure
    - Another frequently drains into SOV to end in cavernous sinus via superior orbital fissure
  - VV
    - Located either above/below ON
    - Difficult to detect in normal subjects
  - CRA & CRV
    - Most readily detectable orbital vessels
    - Run parallel to each other within ON
    - Artery on nasal side & vein on temporal side
    - Flow unaffected by blood pressure and postural changes but affected by ↑ intraocular pressure
  - PCA
    - Seen on the nasal and temporal side of ON

Anatomy-Based Imaging Issues

Imaging Recommendations
- Insonation power maintained at a level of low mechanical index (MI) < 0.23
- Avoid prolonged scanning to ↓ chance of lens damage
- Minimal acoustic jelly and gentle transducer pressure applied on closed eyelid during scanning to minimize eye movement due to patient discomfort
- Measurement of PCA should be done in retrobulbar portion about 10-20 mm away from eyeball in order to avoid wrongly measuring choroidal arteries

Clinical Implications

Clinical Importance
- Assessment of OA: Potential for collateral flow in proximal carotid occlusion
- Evaluation of extraocular muscle thickening
- Investigation of CRA/V occlusion; cranial arteritis; nonarteritic ischemic optic neuropathy; diabetic retinopathy; retinal detachment; ocular metastasis

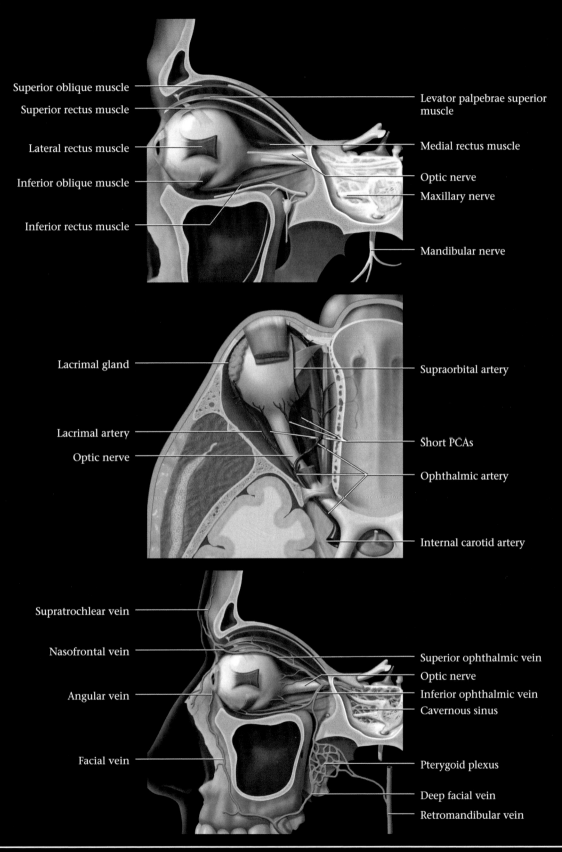

(Top) Lateral graphic illustrates the extraocular muscles of the left orbit. The levator palpebrae lies in front & above ON, separated from it by the superior rectus. Four recti arise posteriorly from a common tendinous ring of ON to attach anteriorly into the sclera. The superior oblique muscle attaches to the sclera by a round ligament & the inferior oblique muscle ends in the inferolateral part of the sclera. **(Middle)** Axial graphic (superior view) shows the relationship of the left OA & its branches. Note OA crosses ON superiorly from temporal side to nasal side in the posterior orbit. **(Bottom)** Lateral graphic shows veins of the left orbit. The SOV begins at the nasofrontal vein ending in the cavernous sinus. The IOV begins at the forepart of the orbital floor & medial orbital wall, joining the pterygoid venous plexus & draining into the cavernous sinus either individually or more frequently in common with SOV.

EXTRAOCULAR MUSCLES, ULTRASOUND

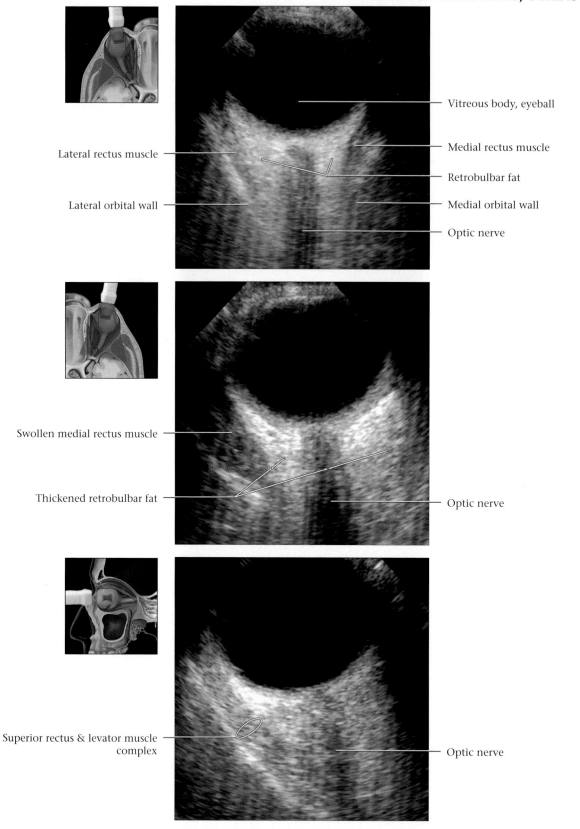

Vitreous body, eyeball

Lateral rectus muscle

Medial rectus muscle

Retrobulbar fat

Lateral orbital wall

Medial orbital wall

Optic nerve

Swollen medial rectus muscle

Thickened retrobulbar fat

Optic nerve

Superior rectus & levator muscle complex

Optic nerve

(Top) Axial grayscale ultrasound of the right orbit at the level of the equator. The transonic eyeball is seen embedded anteriorly within the orbital cavity. Note hypoechoic medial and lateral recti running from posterior to anterior orbit. In the central portion, echogenic retrobulbar fat demonstrates a W-shaped pattern with the ON located within. (Middle) Axial grayscale ultrasound of the left orbit in a patient with thyroid ophthalmopathy. Note retrobulbar fat is hyperechoic suggestive of edema and obliterates lateral rectus. The medial rectus is also swollen. (Bottom) Sagittal grayscale ultrasound of the right orbit shows the superior rectus and levator muscle complex. Although the superior rectus and levator muscles sometimes can be imaged as distinct structures with contact scan, these two muscles are usually displayed as one complex with conventional technique.

ORBIT

3D ULTRASOUND, RIGHT ORBIT

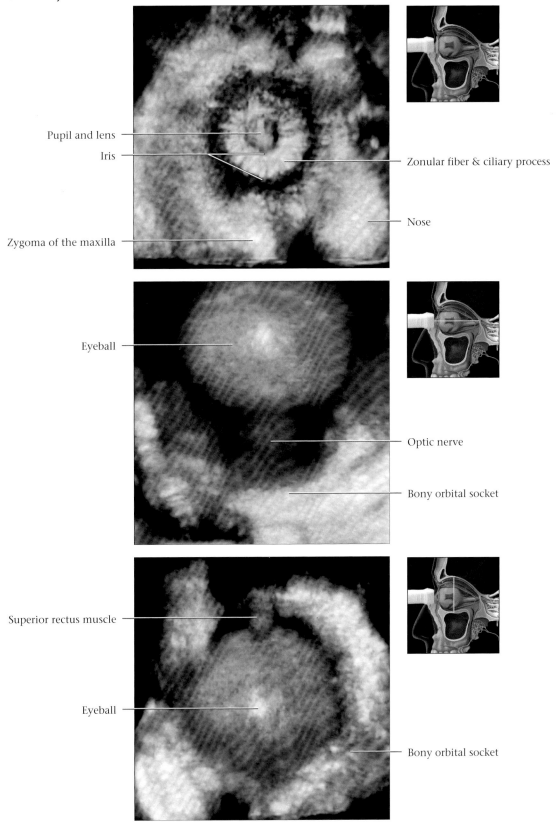

Pupil and lens

Iris

Zonular fiber & ciliary process

Nose

Zygoma of the maxilla

Eyeball

Optic nerve

Bony orbital socket

Superior rectus muscle

Eyeball

Bony orbital socket

(Top) 3D ultrasound of the right orbit (frontal view) using a high-resolution 12 MHz linear 3D transducer demonstrates the anterior chamber of the eyeball. The pupil and lens are seen surrounded by the highly reflective iris, zonular fibers & ciliary processes. (Middle) 3D ultrasound of the right orbit (axial view) shows ON exiting from the posterior aspect of the eyeball. This view is useful in the investigation of retrobulbar abnormality of the orbit. (Bottom) 3D ultrasound of the right orbit (coronal view) shows the attachment of the superior rectus muscle to the eyeball. With proper manipulation of 3D rendered images in three orthogonal planes, different extraocular muscle attachments to the eyeball can be demonstrated.

ORBIT

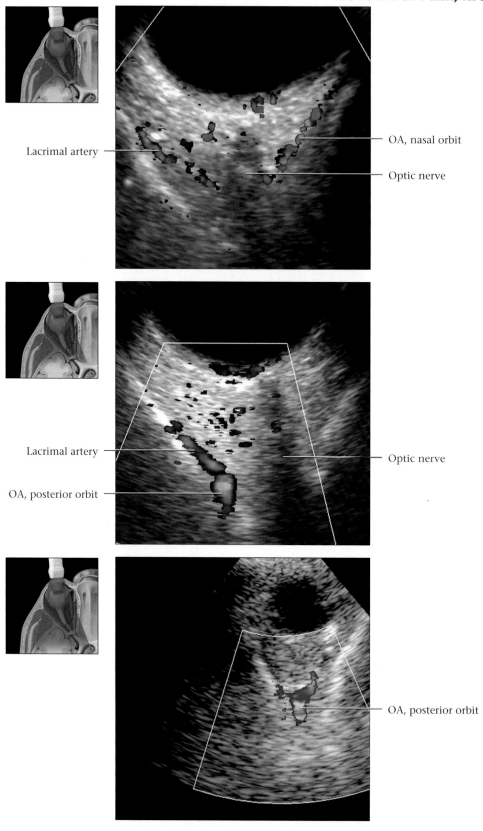

Lacrimal artery — OA, nasal orbit

Optic nerve

Lacrimal artery — Optic nerve

OA, posterior orbit

OA, posterior orbit

(Top) Axial color Doppler ultrasound of the right orbit demonstrates OA on the nasal side and the lacrimal artery on the temporal side. The OA is the largest artery in the orbit with the fastest blood flow and is readily detectable on color Doppler examination. It is more tortuous in the posterior orbit but is relatively straight in the nasal orbit. Normal flow direction is directed toward the transducer. **(Middle)** Axial color Doppler ultrasound of the posterior right orbit demonstrates the LA after branching off from the OA taking a temporal route to supply the lacrimal gland in the superotemporal orbital rim. Its flow direction is toward the transducer. **(Bottom)** Axial color Doppler ultrasound of the right orbit demonstrates the OA as collateral in a patient with proximal internal carotid artery occlusion. Note the blue color coding of the OA indicates abnormal retrograde flow.

ORBIT

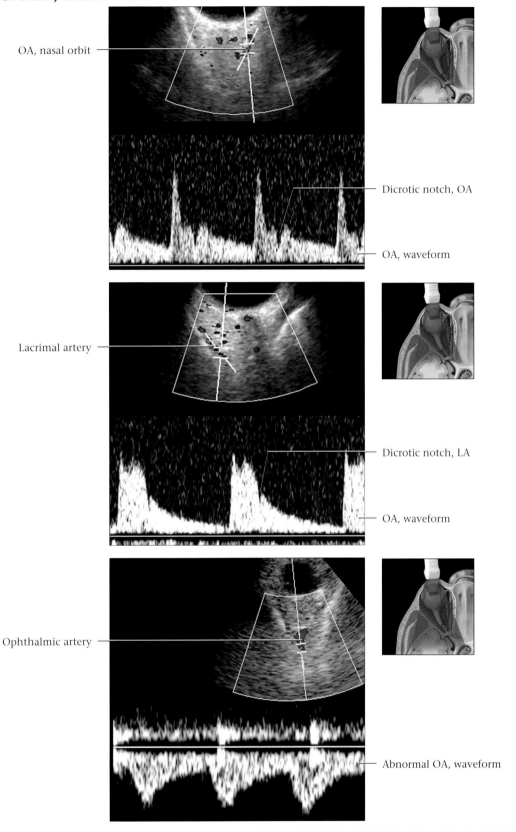

OA, nasal orbit

Dicrotic notch, OA

OA, waveform

Lacrimal artery

Dicrotic notch, LA

OA, waveform

Ophthalmic artery

Abnormal OA, waveform

(Top) Axial spectral Doppler ultrasound of normal right OA. The characteristic waveform is antegrade and of high-resistance with a dicrotic notch. Note the waveform resembles that of the external carotid artery. (Middle) Axial spectral Doppler ultrasound of normal right LA. The waveform of the LA is also antegrade and of high-resistance but the dicrotic notch is less obvious than that of the OA. Note flow resistance in the LA is variable with resistivity index (RI) ranging from 0.63 to 0.81. (Bottom) Axial spectral Doppler ultrasound of the right OA as a collateral. Note the waveform is inverted indicating retrograde flow. In addition, the flow resistance is lowered with absent dicrotic notch. The resulting waveform is similar to that of the normal internal carotid artery.

Brain and Spine

I

ORBIT

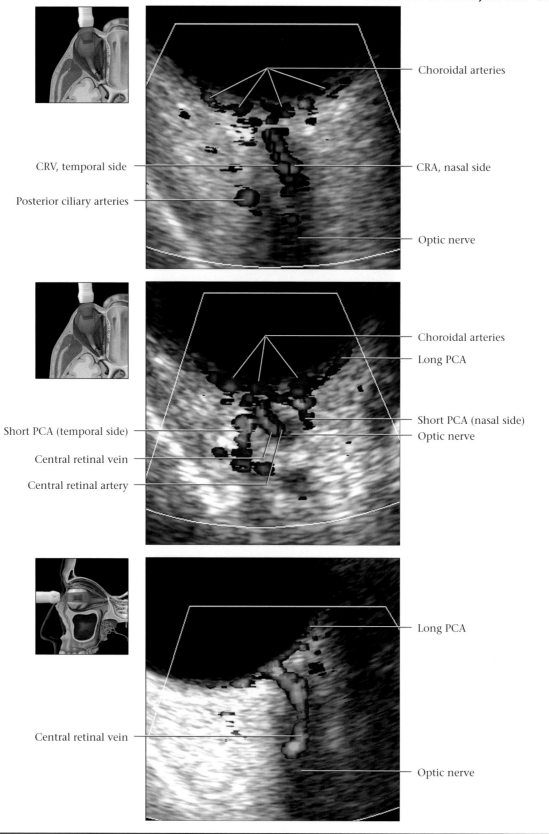

Choroidal arteries

CRV, temporal side

CRA, nasal side

Posterior ciliary arteries

Optic nerve

Choroidal arteries

Long PCA

Short PCA (temporal side)

Short PCA (nasal side)

Central retinal vein

Optic nerve

Central retinal artery

Long PCA

Central retinal vein

Optic nerve

(Top) Axial color Doppler ultrasound of the right orbit shows CRA & CRV. The vessels run parallel to each other within the ON in its retrolaminar portion for a length of approximately 10 mm. The normal orientation of the vessels is CRA on the nasal side and CRV on the temporal side. **(Middle)** Axial color Doppler ultrasound of the right orbit shows the PCA. The short PCAs are seen commencing as trunks approximately 10-20 mm behind the eyeball before forming numerous choroidal branches surrounding the ON in its retrobulbar portion. Care must be taken not to confuse choroidal arteries with the PCA. **(Bottom)** Axial color Doppler ultrasound of the right orbit shows the CRV. The vein is a small vessel seen passing through the ON on the temporal side adjacent to the CRA. Due to its low velocity, false interpretation of absent flow is possible.

Brain and Spine

I

ORBIT

SPECTRAL DOPPLER, RIGHT ORBIT II

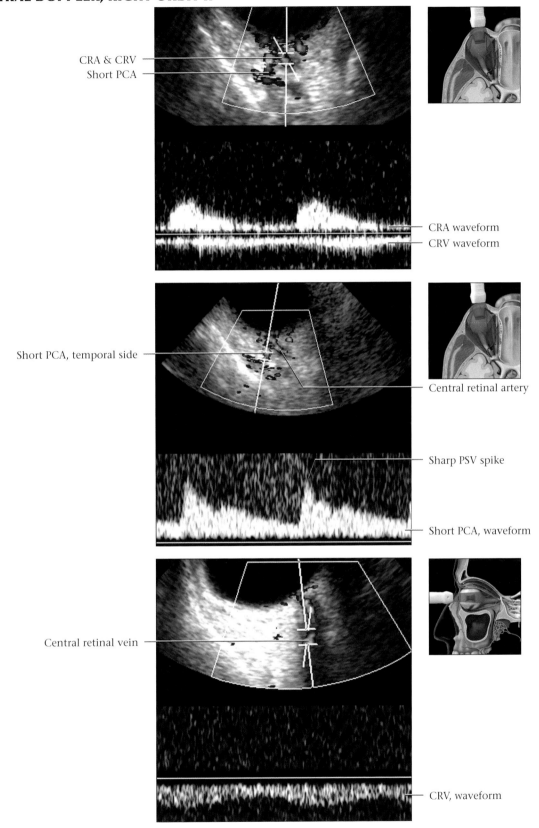

CRA & CRV

Short PCA

CRA waveform

CRV waveform

Short PCA, temporal side

Central retinal artery

Sharp PSV spike

Short PCA, waveform

Central retinal vein

CRV, waveform

(Top) Axial spectral Doppler ultrasound of the right orbit shows CRA & CRV waveforms. Due to the close vicinity of the two vessels, their velocity waveforms are usually inseparable on spectral Doppler trace. Furthermore, arterial waveform normally possesses a flow pattern similar to "tardus parvus waveform" of dampened intrarenal flow. (Middle) Axial spectral Doppler ultrasound of the right orbit shows PCA waveform which normally has velocity values similar to the CRA, but often with a sharper peak systolic velocity (PSV) spike. The PCAs can be assessed either on nasal or temporal sides of the ON. (Bottom) Axial spectral Doppler ultrasound of the right orbit shows a CRV waveform which is of low-velocity with respiratory phasicity. CRV velocities may be better measures of retinal perfusion than CRA velocities because of less flow variations during the cardiac cycle.

Brain and Spine

I

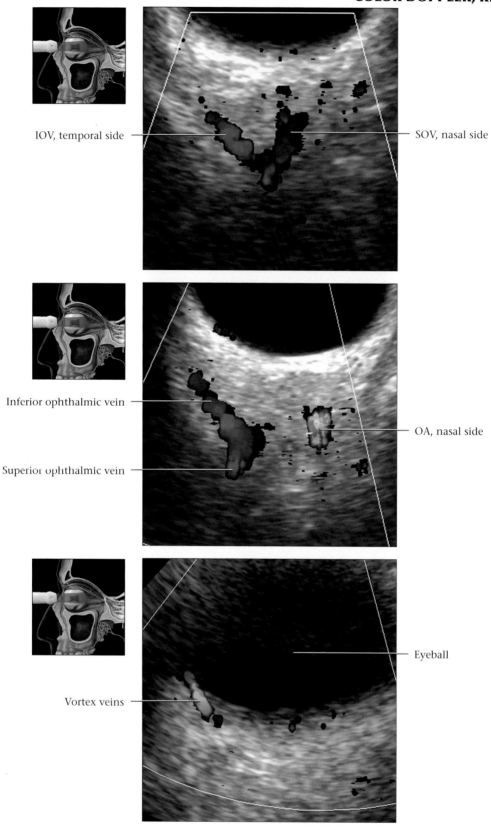

IOV, temporal side ———— SOV, nasal side

Inferior ophthalmic vein ————

———— OA, nasal side

Superior ophthalmic vein ————

———— Eyeball

Vortex veins ————

(Top) Axial color Doppler ultrasound of the right orbit above the ON shows the junction of the SOV and IOV. The SOV runs obliquely in the center of the retrobulbar orbit receiving a branch of the IOV before it ends in the cavernous sinus via the superior orbital fissure. Note the flow direction of both SOV and IOV is away from the transducer. **(Middle)** Axial color Doppler ultrasound of the right orbit shows the IOV with one of its branches coursing temporally to drain into the SOV. The OA with opposite flow direction also appears on the nasal side of the orbit. **(Bottom)** Axial color Doppler ultrasound of the right orbit shows the VV. It is a small vein carrying blood flow away from the transducer as it exits the sclera just posterior to the equator of the eye.

ORBIT

SPECTRAL DOPPLER, RIGHT ORBIT III

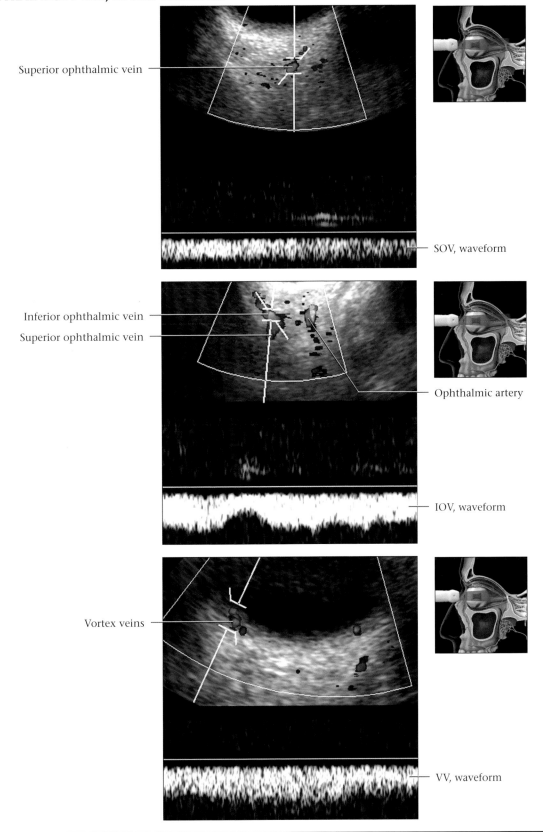

Superior ophthalmic vein

SOV, waveform

Inferior ophthalmic vein

Superior ophthalmic vein

Ophthalmic artery

IOV, waveform

Vortex veins

VV, waveform

(Top) Axial spectral Doppler ultrasound shows a right SOV waveform which is continuous and constant on the negative side of the trace. The flow pattern in this vessel is variable, it may be constant or phasic. In addition, the SOV flow direction may be reversed in Valsalva maneuver. (Middle) Axial spectral Doppler ultrasound of the right IOV with waveform on the negative side of the trace. The waveform of IOV is usually constant but may be enhanced with patient performing Valsalva maneuver. (Bottom) Axial spectral Doppler ultrasound of the right orbit shows the waveform of a VV with respiratory phasicity on the negative side of the trace.

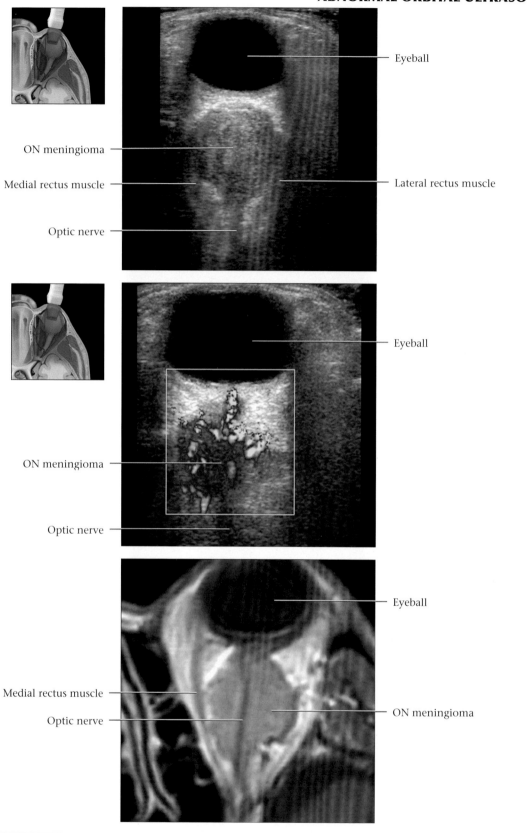

(Top) Axial grayscale ultrasound of the left eye shows histologically proven ON sheath meningioma. The mass is large and moderately echogenic encasing retrobulbar ON and abutting medial and lateral rectus muscles. Although the mass is identified by ultrasound, MR is the examination of choice to evaluate such lesions. **(Middle)** Corresponding axial color Doppler ultrasound of the left eye shows increased vascularity within ON sheath meningioma. **(Bottom)** Corresponding axial post-contrast T1WI MR of the left eye shows a soft tissue mass encasing a normal looking ON with homogeneous contrast-enhancement. Features are consistent with ON meningioma. Note the excellent detail & global anatomical delineation of the mass and its relations to adjacent structures.

ORBIT

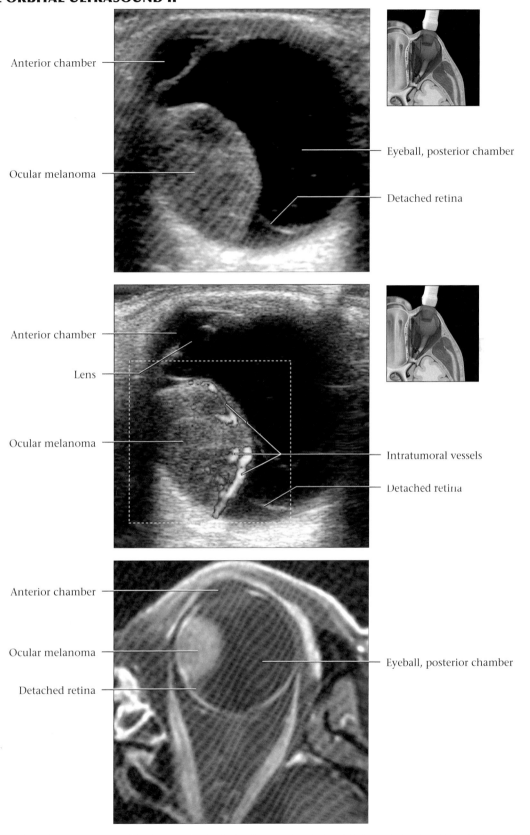

Anterior chamber

Ocular melanoma

Eyeball, posterior chamber

Detached retina

Anterior chamber

Lens

Ocular melanoma

Intratumoral vessels

Detached retina

Anterior chamber

Ocular melanoma

Detached retina

Eyeball, posterior chamber

(Top) Axial grayscale ultrasound of the left eye shows histologically proven ocular melanoma. It arises from the medial wall of the posterior chamber of the eyeball behind the lens and is heterogeneous. The mass is large, occupying nearly 1/3 of the posterior chamber with part of the retina "peeled" off from the underlying sclera. (Middle) Corresponding axial color Doppler ultrasound of the left eye shows multiple small vessels within the ocular melanoma. (Bottom) Corresponding axial post-contrast T1W MR of the left eye with saturation of fat signal shows the ocular melanoma arising from the sclera of the medial wall of the posterior chamber. The mass shows homogeneous enhancement and lifts off part of the retina from the underlying sclera.

Brain and Spine

I

TRANS-CRANIAL COLOR DOPPLER OVERVIEW

Terminology

Abbreviations
- Common carotid arteries (CCA); internal carotid arteries (ICA)
- Anterior, middle, posterior cerebral, posterior communicating arteries (ACA, MCA, PCA, PCoA)
- Vertebral, basilar arteries, ophthalmic (VA, BA, OA)
- Basal, Galen, deep middle cerebral, anterior cerebral, internal cerebral veins (BV, GV, dMCV, ACV, ICV)
- Straight, transverse sinuses (SS, TS)

Anatomy-Based Imaging Issues

Imaging Recommendations
- Performed using low-frequency transducer (1.8-3.6 MHz)
- Grayscale ultrasound: Identify main anatomical structures in correct plane, followed by color Doppler ultrasound
- Unless specified, color coding conventionally displayed on color Doppler ultrasound is
  - Red color: Flow towards transducer
  - Blue color: Flow away from transducer
- Vessel identification depends on window used, beam angulation, insonation depth and flow direction
- Basal skull arteries are extremely variable in size, development and course, supplementary CTA/MRA is useful to enhance its diagnostic accuracy
- For difficult cases, compression test is helpful for arterial identification and assessment of collaterals
  - Must be performed by experienced investigator
  - Exclude risk of embolism in extracranial arteries prior to compression
  - For anterior circulation, compress CCA in lower neck by 2 fingers
  - For vertebrobasilar system, compress VA at mastoid slope
- Normal adults: Highest velocities in MCA or ACA
- Flow velocities in basal cerebral arteries show consistent decrease with increasing age

Imaging Approaches
- Transtemporal approach (commonest approach)
  - Transducer placed on temporal bone superior to zygomatic arch
  - Axial mesencephalic plane
    - Identify the hypoechoic, butterfly-shaped mesencephalon as landmark
    - Assess C5-C7 segments, A1 segment, M1 & M2 segments, P1 & P2 segments, PCoA
    - Also assess dMCV, BV, GV, SS and contralateral TS
  - Axial ventricular plane
    - Tilting of transducer 10 degrees upwards from mesencephalic plane
    - Identify hypoechoic 3rd ventricle, echogenic pineal gland and choroid plexus of trigone
    - Assess A2 segment, M2 & M3 segments and P3
    - Assess midline shift due to MCA infarction
  - Anterior/posterior coronal planes
    - Assess C4 to C7 segments, A1 segment, M1-M3 segments, PCA and distal BA

- Normal mean velocities & depth of insonation
  - Terminal ICA: 39 ± 9 cm/s (60-67 mm)
  - MCA: 62 ± 12 cm/s (30-67 mm)
  - ACA: 50 ± 11 cm/s (60-80 mm)
  - PCA: 39 ± 10 cm/s (55-80 mm)
- Transfrontal approach
  - Insonation depth of 10-16 cm
  - Paramedian frontal bone window
    - Slightly lateral to the midline of forehead
    - Identify echogenic orbital roof, hypoechoic 3rd ventricle & corpus callosum
  - Lateral frontal bone window
    - Just above the lateral aspect of eyebrow
    - Identify echogenic falx cerebri, sylvian fissure and hypoechoic mesencephalon
  - Assess A1 & A2 segments, M1 segment, PCA, PCoA, pericallosal artery
  - Also assess ICV, GV, SS
- Transforaminal/suboccipital approach
  - Transducer placed between squama occipitalis and spinous process of 1st cervical vertebra
  - Ultrasound beam aimed at nasal bridge
  - Identify echogenic processus transversus and clivus
  - Assess VAs and BA which are visualized as "Y"
  - Normal mean velocities & depth of insonation
    - VA: 38 ± 10 cm/s (40-85 mm)
    - BA: 41 ± 10 cm/s (> 80 mm)
- Transorbital approach
  - Problem of insonation of orbital lens
  - Low mechanical index < 0.23 highly recommended
  - Assess intraocular vessels, C4-C6 segments
  - Normal mean velocities & depth of insonation
    - OA: 21 ± 5 cm/s (40-60 mm)
    - Carotid siphon: 47 ± 10 cm/s (60-80 mm)
- Submandibular approach
  - Assess distal C1 & C2 segments
  - Normal mean velocities & depth of insonation
    - Cervical ICA: 37 ± 9 cm/s (35-70 mm)

Imaging Pitfalls
- Extensive variations; incomplete circle of Willis
- Variable probe-to-vessel angle
- Misdiagnosis: Hyperdynamic collaterals → stenosis
- Misdiagnosis: Vasospasm → stenosis
- Misdiagnosis: Displacement of basal vessels by mass lesion → occlusion

Clinical Implications

Clinical Importance
- Diagnosis and assessment of intracranial stenosis
  - Mild stenosis - mild ↑ peak velocity; waveform unchanged
  - Moderate/severe stenosis - greater ↑ in peak velocity, ↑ diastolic velocity ± turbulent flow
  - Near occlusion - damped waveform, pre-occlusive thump, post-stenotic drop in peak velocity
- Diagnosis of intracranial occlusive disease, monitor recanalization after thrombolysis and collateral formation
- Pre-operative compression test to evaluate collateralizing capacity of circle of Willis

INTRACRANIAL ARTERIES & VEINS

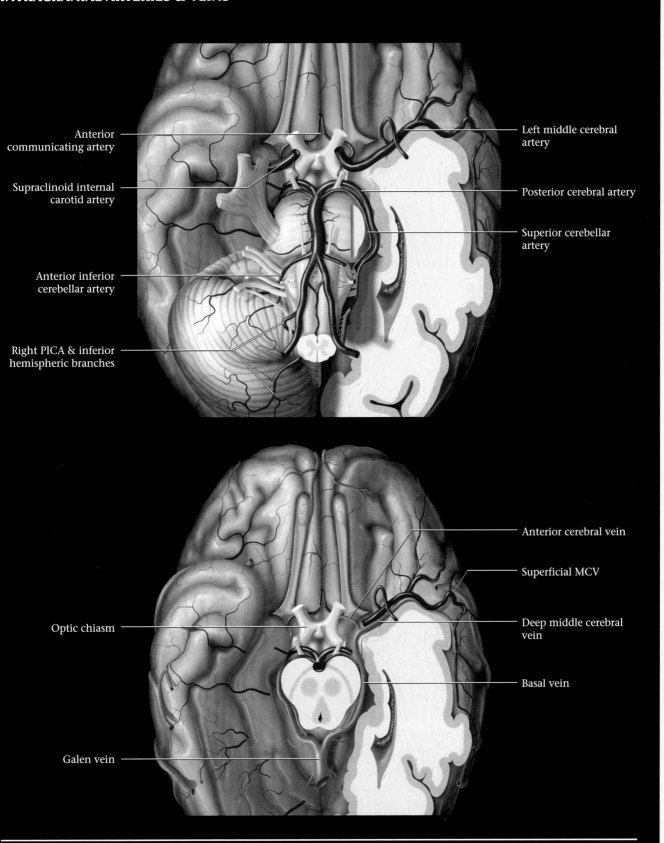

Anterior communicating artery

Supraclinoid internal carotid artery

Anterior inferior cerebellar artery

Right PICA & inferior hemispheric branches

Left middle cerebral artery

Posterior cerebral artery

Superior cerebellar artery

Optic chiasm

Galen vein

Anterior cerebral vein

Superficial MCV

Deep middle cerebral vein

Basal vein

(Top) Graphic shows the brain vascular system and its relationship to the base of the brain. The ACAs course cephalad in the interhemispheric fissure from their junction at the ACoA. They supply most of the medial brain surface except for the posterior third, which is supplied by the MCA. The MCA supplies most of the lateral surface of the hemispheres. The PCA supplies most of the undersurface of the temporal lobe except for its most anterior tip. The right anterior and posterior inferior cerebellar arteries are shown on the right. **(Bottom)** Graphic shows an inferior intracranial view of the deep venous structures. Intracranial veins are valveless veins which pierce the arachnoid membrane and meningeal layer of dura mater. They include external cerebral veins, ICV, ACV, dMCV, BV, GV and cerebellar veins and drain into the cranial venous sinuses.

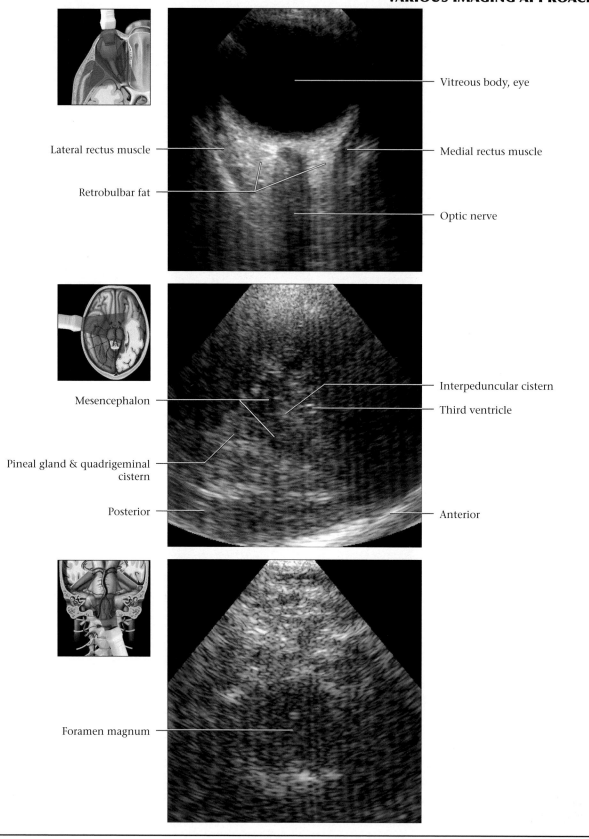

Vitreous body, eye

Lateral rectus muscle

Medial rectus muscle

Retrobulbar fat

Optic nerve

Mesencephalon

Interpeduncular cistern

Third ventricle

Pineal gland & quadrigeminal cistern

Posterior

Anterior

Foramen magnum

(Top) Axial grayscale US of the right orbit (transorbital scan) demonstrates the transonic vitreous body of the eye occupying the anterior part of the orbital socket with the hypoechoic optic nerve behind it. The optic nerve is an important landmark for identification of intraocular vessels. **(Middle)** Grayscale US of the axial mesencephalic plane (transtemporal approach) shows hypoechoic, butterfly-shaped mesencephalon. Anterior to it is the 3rd ventricle surrounded by bright margins and posterior to it is the hyperechoic triangular region of the pineal gland and quadrigeminal cistern. Intracerebral vessels demonstrated on this plane include M1 & M2 of MCA, A1of ACA, C6 & C7 of ICA and P1 & P2 of PCA, and in about 75% of PCoA. **(Bottom)** Axial, suboccipital, grayscale ultrasound shows hypoechoic circular foramen magnum where intradural VAs and BA can be identified.

TRANS-CRANIAL COLOR DOPPLER OVERVIEW

VARIOUS IMAGING APPROACHES

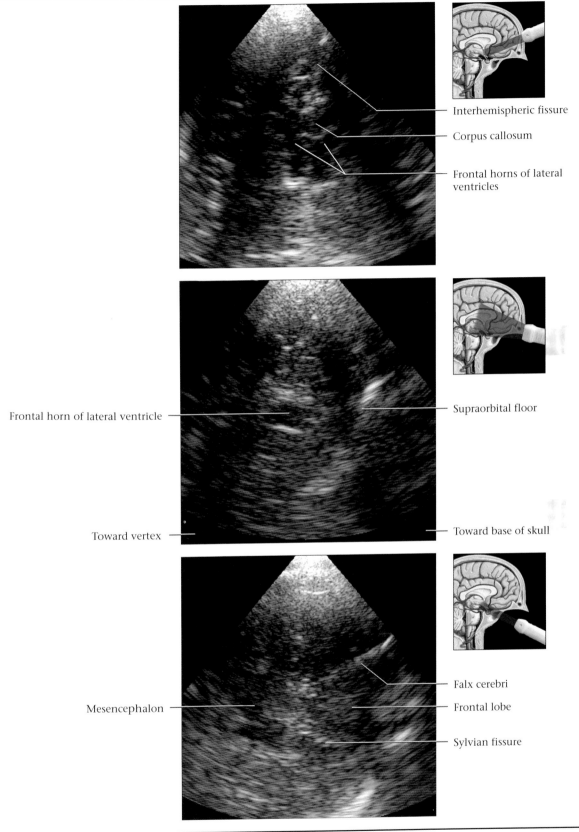

Interhemispheric fissure

Corpus callosum

Frontal horns of lateral ventricles

Frontal horn of lateral ventricle

Supraorbital floor

Toward vertex

Toward base of skull

Mesencephalon

Falx cerebri

Frontal lobe

Sylvian fissure

(Top) Axial grayscale ultrasound (paramedian frontal approach) shows symmetrical anechoic/hypoechoic frontal horns of the lateral ventricles and both frontal lobes separated by the interhemispheric fissure. The hypoechoic corpus callosum forms the roof of the frontal horns of the lateral ventricles. (Middle) Sagittal grayscale ultrasound (paramedian frontal approach) identifies echogenic supraorbital floor, hypoechoic lateral ventricles (frontal horns) and corpus callosum. (Bottom) Axial grayscale ultrasound (lateral frontal approach) identifies echogenic falx cerebri, sylvian fissure and hypoechoic mesencephalon. Intracerebral vessels assessed using transfrontal approach include A1 & A2 segments of ACA, M1 segment of MCA, PCA, PCoA, pericallosal artery, ICV, GV and SS.

Brain and Spine

I

95

DISTAL INTERNAL CAROTID ARTERY

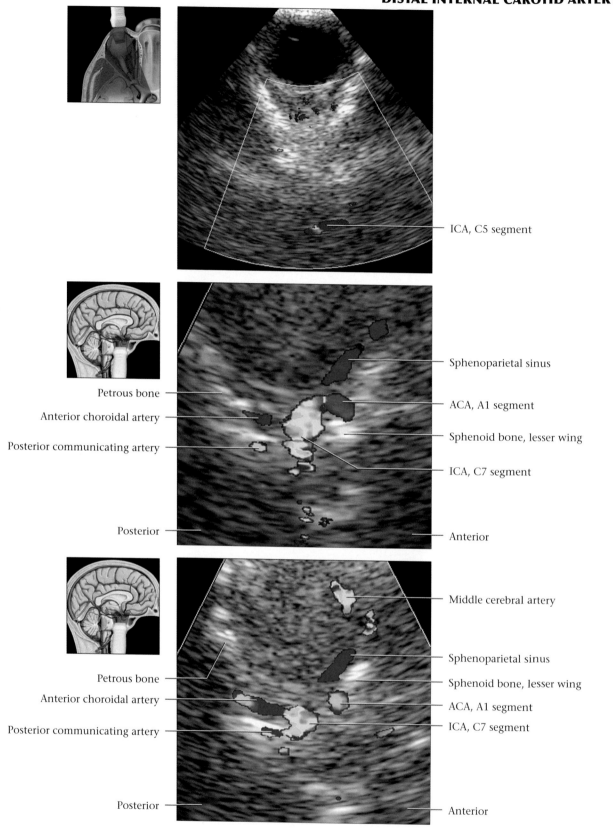

(Top) Axial color Doppler ultrasound (transorbital approach) shows C5 segment of the ICA with flow toward the transducer. Note that C4 to C6 segments can be assessed by transorbital approach where C4, C5 and C6 segments typically show forward, alternating and backward flow respectively. (Middle) Axial color Doppler ultrasound (transtemporal approach) at a plane slightly caudad to the standard mesencephalic plane shows the C7 segment of the ICA, ACA and sphenoparietal sinus. (Bottom) Axial oblique color Doppler ultrasound (transtemporal approach) with slight caudad tilting from the standard axial mesencephalic plane shows the anterior choroidal artery and PCoA branching out from the communicating segment of the ICA.

ANTERIOR CEREBRAL ARTERY

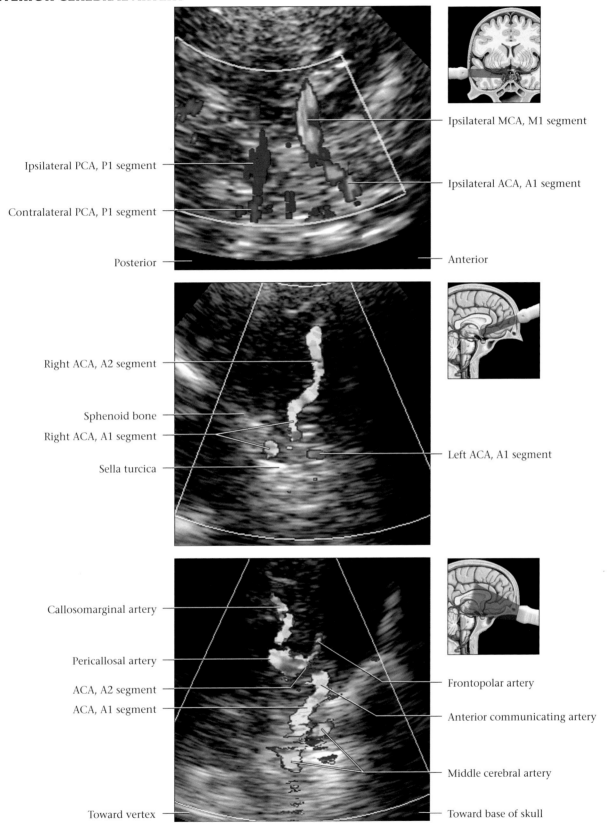

Ipsilateral PCA, P1 segment

Contralateral PCA, P1 segment

Posterior

Ipsilateral MCA, M1 segment

Ipsilateral ACA, A1 segment

Anterior

Right ACA, A2 segment

Sphenoid bone

Right ACA, A1 segment

Sella turcica

Left ACA, A1 segment

Callosomarginal artery

Pericallosal artery

ACA, A2 segment

ACA, A1 segment

Toward vertex

Frontopolar artery

Anterior communicating artery

Middle cerebral artery

Toward base of skull

(Top) Axial color Doppler ultrasound (transtemporal approach) shows the MCA/ACA junction on the mesencephalic plane which is the most useful plane for showing the circle of Willis. However, it is limited in depicting more distal segments of the ACA which can be visualized using a transfrontal approach. (Middle) Axial color Doppler US (paramedian frontal approach) shows the right A2 segment running along the interhemispheric fissure. Echogenic sphenoid bone and sella turcica provide important landmarks for identification of the A2 segment which starts close to the sella turcica and tip of arte sphenoid bone. (Bottom) Sagittal color Doppler US (paramedian frontal approach) shows the frontopolar artery arising anteriorly from the mid A2 segment and the callosomarginal artery branching out from the distal A2 segment. Note the pericallosal artery (A3 segment) can be seen by this approach.

Brain and Spine

I

MCA, M2 segment

MCA, M1 segment

Posterior cerebral artery

Anterior cerebral artery

Anterior communicating artery

Posterior

Anterior

Posterior cerebral artery

MCA, M1 segment

ICA, C7 segment

Posterior communicating artery

Posterior

Anterior

MCA, M1 segment

MCA, M2 segment

Posterior

Anterior

(Top) Axial color Doppler ultrasound (transtemporal approach) on the mesencephalic plane illustrates the MCA appearing in the anterior aspect of the circle of Willis. The origin of the M1 segment can be determined accurately with identification of the MCA/ACA junction. **(Middle)** Axial color Doppler ultrasound (transtemporal approach) on the standard mesencephalic plane depicts the M1 segment arising from the communicating segment of the ICA with flow direction toward the transducer. **(Bottom)** Oblique coronal color Doppler ultrasound (transtemporal approach) shows that the MCA curves and enters the Sylvian fissure where the M2 segment starts. Note the flow direction in the M2 segment is directed away from the transducer as it ascends within the Sylvian fissure.

Brain and Spine

I

TRANS-CRANIAL COLOR DOPPLER OVERVIEW

POSTERIOR CEREBRAL ARTERY

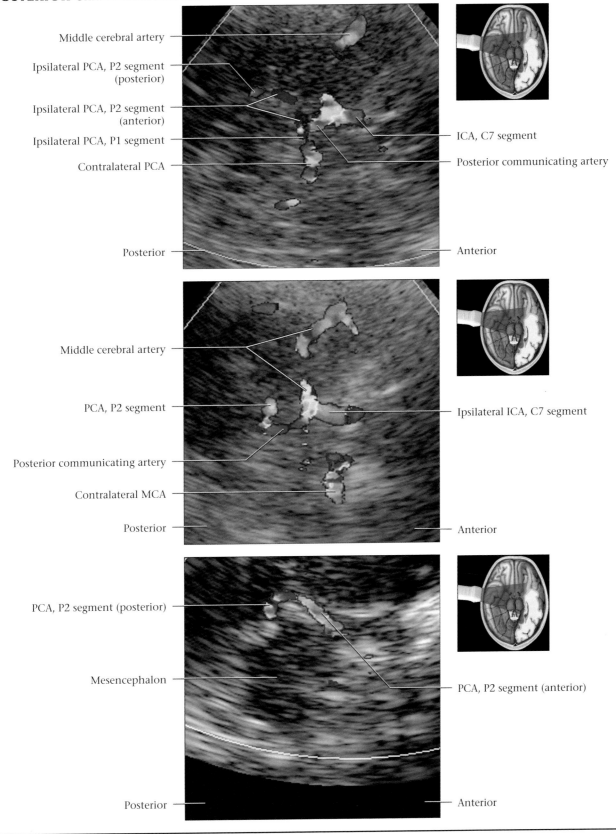

Middle cerebral artery

Ipsilateral PCA, P2 segment (posterior)

Ipsilateral PCA, P2 segment (anterior)

Ipsilateral PCA, P1 segment

Contralateral PCA

ICA, C7 segment

Posterior communicating artery

Posterior — Anterior

Middle cerebral artery

PCA, P2 segment

Posterior communicating artery

Contralateral MCA

Ipsilateral ICA, C7 segment

Posterior — Anterior

PCA, P2 segment (posterior)

Mesencephalon

PCA, P2 segment (anterior)

Posterior — Anterior

(**Top**) Axial color Doppler ultrasound (transtemporal approach) on the mesencephalic plane shows the P1 segment extending laterally from BA to its junction with PCoA and continuing as P2 segment around mesencephalon. The flow direction of P1 and anterior P2 segments is toward the transducer whereas the posterior P2 segment is away from the transducer. (**Middle**) Axial color Doppler ultrasound (transtemporal approach). PCoA is identified as a vascular structure connecting ICA C7 segment to PCA with flow away from the transducer. The clinical importance of investigation of PCoA is due to the prevalence of aneurysm formation and effectiveness of collateralization. (**Bottom**) Axial color Doppler ultrasound (transtemporal approach) shows the P2 segment curving posteriorly around mesencephalon with change in flow direction around the curvature.

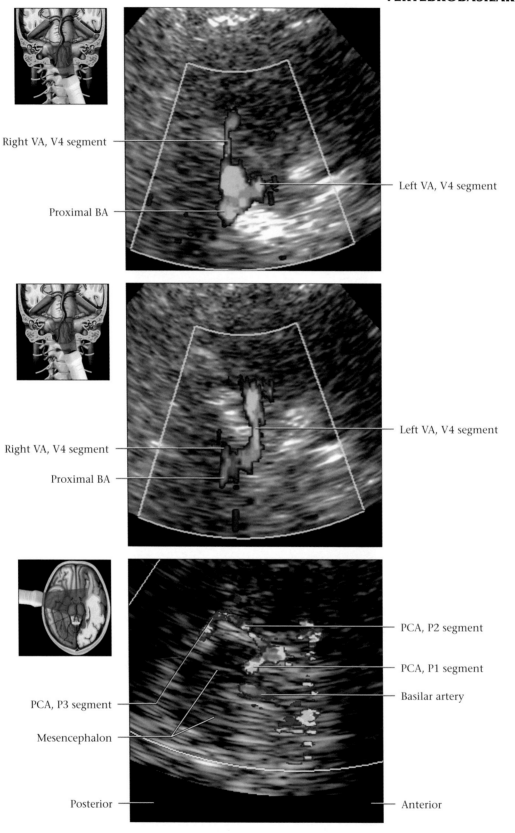

Right VA, V4 segment

Left VA, V4 segment

Proximal BA

Right VA, V4 segment

Left VA, V4 segment

Proximal BA

PCA, P2 segment

PCA, P1 segment

PCA, P3 segment

Basilar artery

Mesencephalon

Posterior

Anterior

(Top) Axial color Doppler ultrasound (suboccipital approach) through the foramen magnum shows the right V4 segment of VA and proximal BA with flow directed away from the transducer. Note that reversed BA flow toward the transducer would signify severe intracranial subclavian steal. **(Middle)** Axial color Doppler ultrasound (suboccipital approach) through the foramen magnum shows the left V4 segment of VA with flow directed away from the transducer. The convergence of two V4 segments forming BA should give rise to a "Y" configuration. However, the "Y" configuration may not be always obtainable because the three vessels are not always on the same plane. **(Bottom)** Axial color Doppler ultrasound (transtemporal approach) on standard mesencephalic plane shows the distal portion of BA which terminates into PCAs in interpeduncular/suprasellar cistern.

INTRACRANIAL VEINS

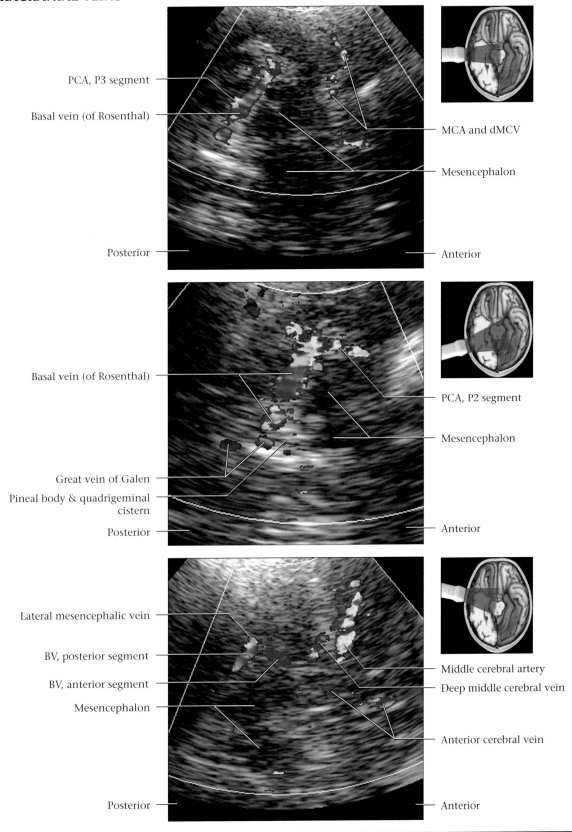

(Top) Axial color Doppler ultrasound (transtemporal approach) illustrates BV running posteriorly along mesencephalon with flow signal away from the transducer. The ipsilateral PCA is often seen closely related to it with opposite flow direction. (Middle) Axial color Doppler ultrasound (transtemporal approach) demonstrates GV. The vein is identified in the midline posterior to mesencephalon in the hyperechoic triangular region of the pineal body and quadrigeminal cistern. (Bottom) Axial color Doppler ultrasound (transtemporal approach) shows the two tributaries of BV: ACV and dMCV. ACV courses posteriorly along the base of the brain and joins dMCV which runs in the Sylvian fissure to form BV just anterior to the mesencephalon. Note both ACV and MCV are accompanied by their respective arteries.

Brain and Spine

I

ANTERIOR CEREBRAL ARTERY

Terminology

Abbreviations
- Anterior, middle & posterior cerebral artery (ACA, MCA, PCA); anterior communicating, internal carotid artery (ACoA, ICA); anterior cerebral vein (ACV)

Gross Anatomy

Overview
- Smaller, more medial terminal branch of communicating segment of ICA
- Three segments
  - Horizontal or precommunicating (A1) segment
  - Vertical or postcommunicating (A2) segment
  - Distal (A3) segment
- ACoA connects left & right A1 segments

Imaging Anatomy

Anatomy Relationships
- ACA runs parallel to ACV
- A1: Extends anteromedially above optic nerve & chiasm, below medial olfactory stria
- A2: From ACoA junction, ascends in interhemispheric fissure, anterior to corpus callosum rostrum
- A3: Pericallosal artery; begins distal to origin of callosomarginal artery
  - Pericallosal, callosomarginal arteries course within interhemispheric fissure, under falx cerebri
- ACoA
  - Communicates both A1 segments in interhemispheric fissure
  - Completes anterior portion of circle of Willis
  - Usually single, may be duplicated/triplicated/hypoplastic
  - Supplies infundibulum, optic chiasm and preoptic areas of hypothalamus

Branches
- Cortical branches
  - Medial orbitofrontal artery (1st cortical branch)
    - Arises from proximal A2/from pericallosal artery
    - Ramifies over inferior surface of frontal lobe
  - Frontopolar artery
    - Arises from mid-A2
    - Extends anteriorly along medial surface of hemisphere to frontal pole
  - Pericallosal artery
    - Begins distal to origin of callosomarginal artery
    - Larger of two major distal ACA branches
    - Courses posterosuperiorly above corpus callosum, below cingulate gyrus
  - Callosomarginal artery
    - Smaller of two distal ACA branches
    - Courses posterosuperiorly in cingulate sulcus, above cingulate gyrus
- Perforating branches
  - Medial lenticulostriate arteries
    - Arise from A1, ACoA; course superiorly through anterior perforated substance
  - Recurrent artery of Heubner
    - Arises from distal A1/proximal A2; curves back parallel to A1 in anterior perforated substance

Vascular Territory
- Cortical branches supply anterior 2/3 of medial hemispheres
- Penetrating branches supply medial basal ganglia, corpus callosum genu, internal capsule anterior limb

Normal Variants, Anomalies
- Normal variants (common)
  - Hypoplastic/absent A1
  - Bihemispheric ACA - distal ACA branches supply part of contralateral hemisphere
  - ACoA: Absent/fenestrated/duplicated/triplicated
- Anomalies (rare)
  - "Azygous" ACA
    - Typically associated with holoprosencephaly
    - Single ACA arises from junction of both A1s
    - Absent ACoA
  - Infraoptic ACA
    - A1 passes underneath optic nerve
    - High prevalence of intracranial aneurysms

Anatomy-Based Imaging Issues

Imaging Recommendations
- Performed using low-frequency transducer (1.8-3.6 MHz)
- Assess flow direction, velocity and patency of vessel
- A1 & A2 segments are amenable for USG assessment
- Normal mean blood velocity for adult A1: 50 ± 11 cm/s
- Transtemporal approach - insonated depth 60-80 mm
  - Axial mesencephalic plane
    - Scans A1 segment: Flow away from transducer
    - Difficult to scan ACoA due to small caliber and unfavorable insonation angle
  - Axial ventricular plane
    - Scans A2 segment: Flow toward transducer
    - Also used to assess severity of midline shift
- Paramedian frontal approach
  - Axial: Scans A1 & A2 segments
  - A1 & A2 segment: Flow direction towards transducer
  - A2 segment: Most prominent vascular structure
  - Sagittal: Scans A1, A2 & A2 branches
    - Frontopolar artery: Flow toward transducer
    - Pericallosal artery: Flow away from transducer
- Lateral frontal approach
  - Axial: Scans A2 segment

Clinical Implications

Clinical Importance
- ACoA is common site for aneurysm formation
- ACoA is common collateral pathway for significant proximal carotid occlusive disease
- Arterial occlusion: MCA, PCA > ACA
  - Peak systolic velocity of ≥ 50% stenosis: ≥ 155 cm/s
- Distal ACA occlusion may occur with severe subfalcine herniation of cingulate gyrus

ANTERIOR CEREBRAL ARTERY

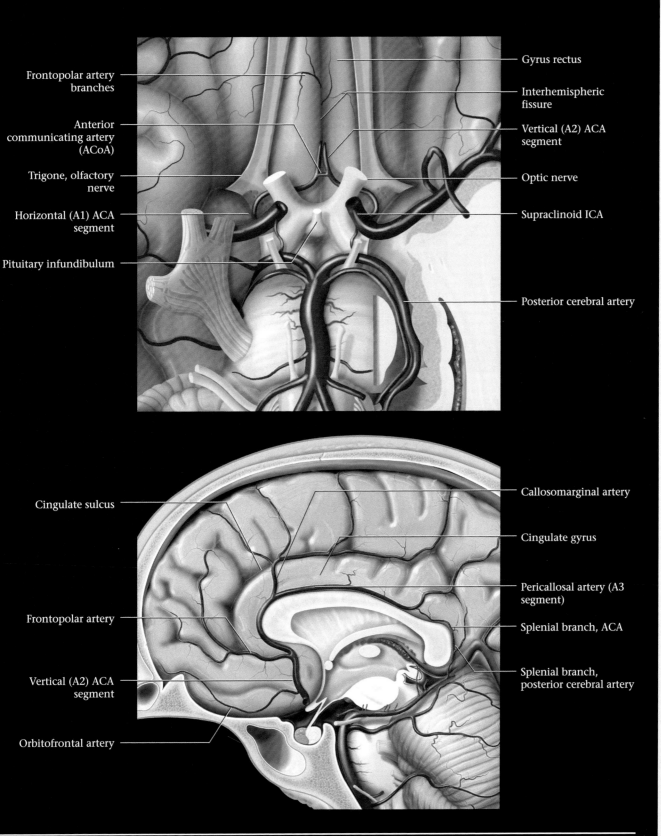

Frontopolar artery branches

Anterior communicating artery (ACoA)

Trigone, olfactory nerve

Horizontal (A1) ACA segment

Pituitary infundibulum

Gyrus rectus

Interhemispheric fissure

Vertical (A2) ACA segment

Optic nerve

Supraclinoid ICA

Posterior cerebral artery

Cingulate sulcus

Frontopolar artery

Vertical (A2) ACA segment

Orbitofrontal artery

Callosomarginal artery

Cingulate gyrus

Pericallosal artery (A3 segment)

Splenial branch, ACA

Splenial branch, posterior cerebral artery

(Top) Submentovertex graphic shows the relationship of the circle of Willis and its components to the cranial nerves. Note that the normal course of the horizontal (A1) segment is over the optic nerves. **(Bottom)** Sagittal (midline) graphic through the interhemispheric fissure shows the relationship of the ACA and its branches to the underlying brain parenchyma. The A2 segment ascends in front of the third ventricle within the cistern of the lamina terminalis. The A3 segment curves around the corpus callosum genu. The branch point of the distal ACA into the pericallosal and callosomarginal arteries varies. Almost the entire anterior 2/3 of the medial hemisphere surface is supplied by the ACA and its branches. Branches of the posterior and anterior cerebral arteries anastomose around the corpus callosum genu.

A1 SEGMENT, TRANSTEMPORAL APPROACH

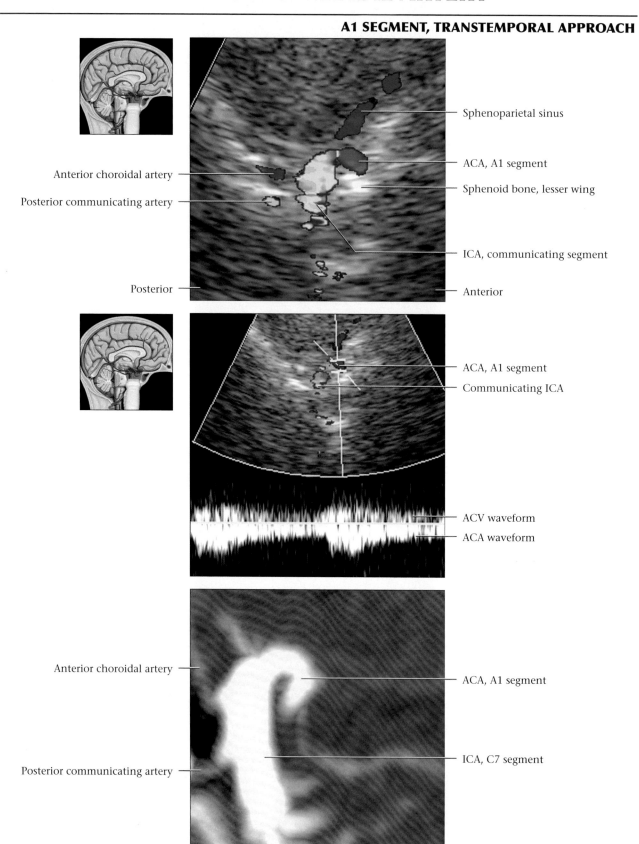

Sphenoparietal sinus

ACA, A1 segment

Sphenoid bone, lesser wing

Anterior choroidal artery

Posterior communicating artery

ICA, communicating segment

Posterior

Anterior

ACA, A1 segment

Communicating ICA

ACV waveform

ACA waveform

Anterior choroidal artery

ACA, A1 segment

Posterior communicating artery

ICA, C7 segment

(Top) Axial color Doppler ultrasound (transtemporal approach) with slight caudad tilting shows the communicating ICA giving off the ACA which extends forward and upward above the optic chiasm. In this precommunicating A1 segment, the flow is directed away from the transducer. (Middle) Axial spectral Doppler ultrasound (transtemporal approach) shows normal arterial waveform of ACA (A1 segment) appearing on the negative scale of the tracing. Although the waveform of ACV (positive scale) is often detected at the same time with ACA, the vein may not be evident on color Doppler imaging. (Bottom) Oblique, axial, reformatted CT arteriogram at the level of the sphenoid bone shows the C7 segment of ICA terminating into the A1 segment of ACA. It gives off the PCoA and anterior choroidal artery before its termination into ACA and MCA.

ANTERIOR CEREBRAL ARTERY

A1 SEGMENT, TRANSTEMPORAL APPROACH

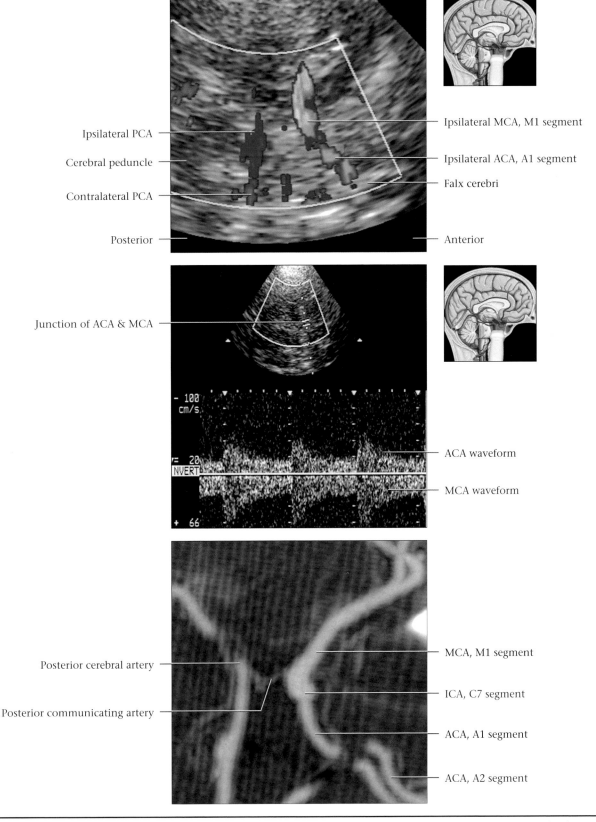

Ipsilateral PCA

Cerebral peduncle

Contralateral PCA

Posterior

Ipsilateral MCA, M1 segment

Ipsilateral ACA, A1 segment

Falx cerebri

Anterior

Junction of ACA & MCA

ACA waveform

MCA waveform

Posterior cerebral artery

Posterior communicating artery

MCA, M1 segment

ICA, C7 segment

ACA, A1 segment

ACA, A2 segment

(Top) Axial color Doppler US shows MCA/ACA junction on the mesencephalic plane. Although the standard mesencephalic plane is the most useful plane for demonstration of circle of Willis, it is limited in depicting more distal segments of the ACA (e.g., A2 & A3 segments) which are best visualized with transfrontal scan. **(Middle)** Axial spectral Doppler US (transtemporal approach) shows typical bidirectional waveform at ACA/MCA junction. The negative waveform denotes flow within the A1 segment whereas positive waveform represents MCA flow. Note flow velocity of the A1 segment is normally lower than that of the MCA. **(Bottom)** Corresponding, oblique, axial, reformatted CT arteriogram shows the distal ICA terminating into the ACA, A1 segment & MCA. A1 segment runs anteromedially to reach the interhemispheric fissure & turns superiorly to become the A2 segment.

Brain and Spine

I

A2 SEGMENT, LATERAL FRONTAL SCAN

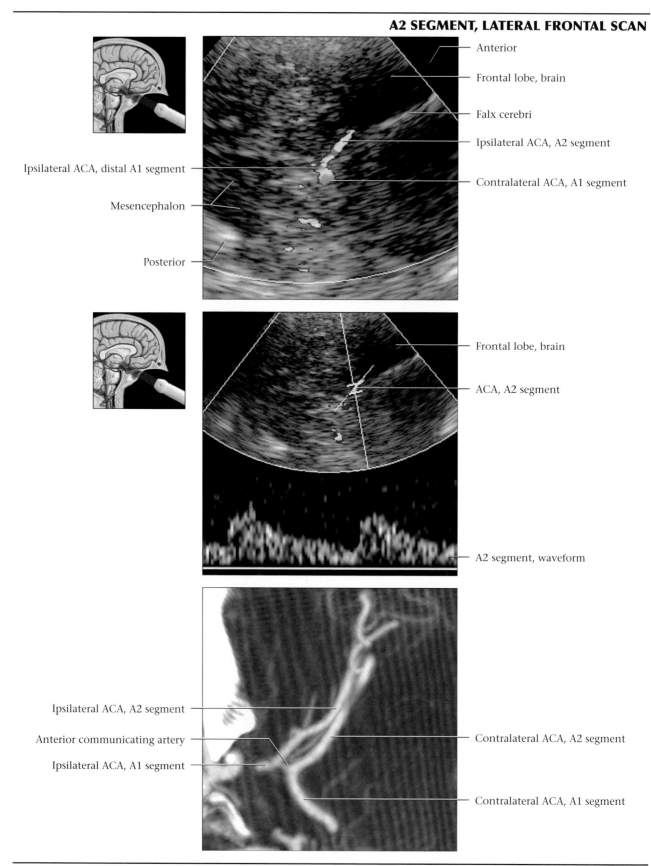

Anterior

Frontal lobe, brain

Falx cerebri

Ipsilateral ACA, A2 segment

Contralateral ACA, A1 segment

Ipsilateral ACA, distal A1 segment

Mesencephalon

Posterior

Frontal lobe, brain

ACA, A2 segment

A2 segment, waveform

Ipsilateral ACA, A2 segment

Anterior communicating artery

Ipsilateral ACA, A1 segment

Contralateral ACA, A2 segment

Contralateral ACA, A1 segment

(Top) Axial color Doppler ultrasound (lateral frontal approach) shows A2 segment seen through the frontal bone at the lateral eyebrow. The ipsilateral A2 segment is often seen as a prominent vessel running along the hyperechoic falx cerebri with flow toward the transducer. Sometimes the contralateral distal A1 or proximal A2 segment can be depicted coursing obliquely toward the ipsilateral A2 segment mimicking ACoA which is infrequently discernible in normal subjects. (Middle) Axial spectral Doppler ultrasound (lateral frontal approach) of A2 segment shows the typical low-resistance waveform with forward flow. (Bottom) Corresponding, oblique, axial, reformatted CT arteriogram shows A1 segments becoming A2 segments after ACoA junction. They then ascend parallel in the interhemispheric fissure.

ANTERIOR CEREBRAL ARTERY

A2 SEGMENT, PARAMEDIAN FRONTAL SCAN

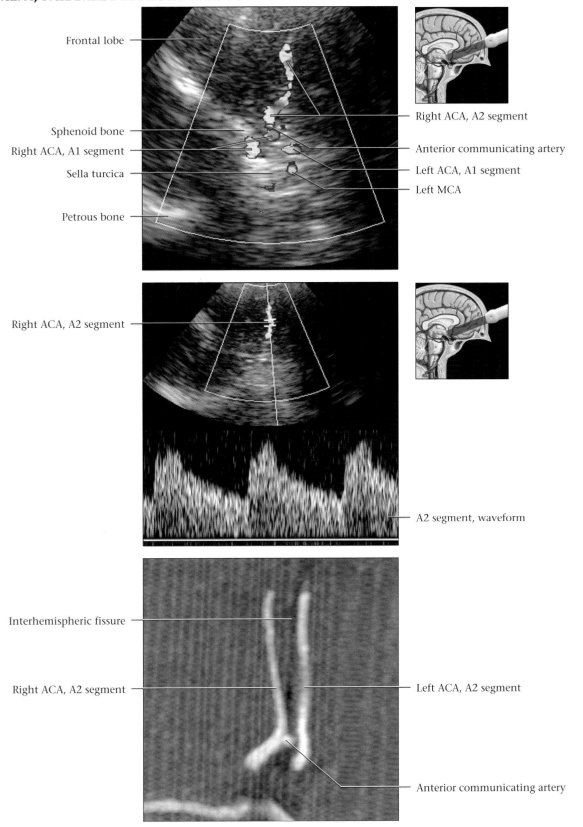

Frontal lobe

Right ACA, A2 segment

Sphenoid bone

Anterior communicating artery

Right ACA, A1 segment

Left ACA, A1 segment

Sella turcica

Left MCA

Petrous bone

Right ACA, A2 segment

A2 segment, waveform

Interhemispheric fissure

Right ACA, A2 segment

Left ACA, A2 segment

Anterior communicating artery

(Top) Oblique, coronal, color Doppler ultrasound (paramedian frontal approach) shows the right A2 segment of the ACA in the interhemispheric fissure. The entry of the small ACoA seen as a "blue" dot defines the origin of the A2 segments. Adjacent, the hyperechoic bony structures such as the sphenoid bone and sella turcica provide important landmarks for identification of the A2 segment because it normally starts close to the anterior aspect of the sella turcica and tip of the sphenoid bone. (Middle) Oblique, coronal, spectral Doppler ultrasound (paramedian frontal approach) of the A2 segment of ACA shows the typical low-resistance forward flow toward the transducer. (Bottom) Oblique, coronal, reformatted MR arteriogram shows the A2 segments ascending parallel in the interhemispheric fissure interconnected by the ACoA.

ANTERIOR CEREBRAL ARTERY

ACA, PARAMEDIAN FRONTAL SCAN

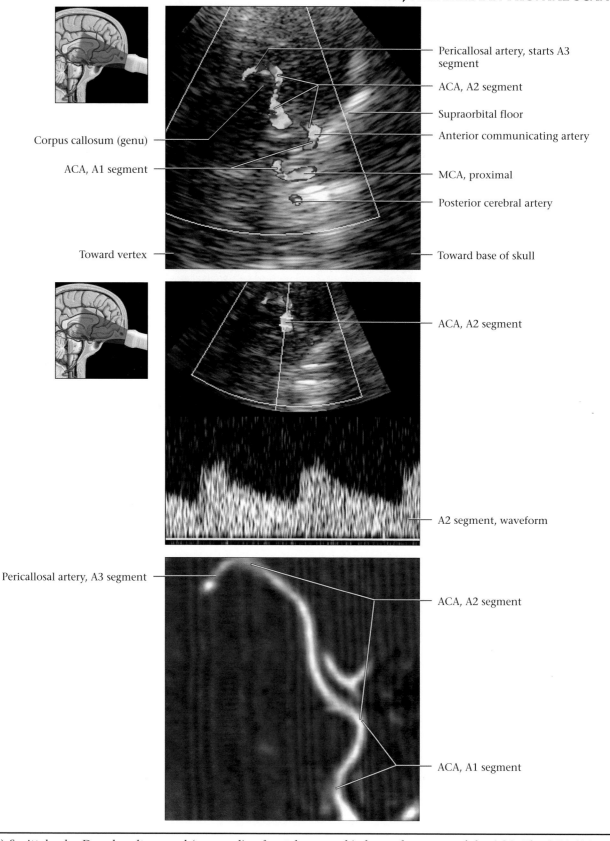

Pericallosal artery, starts A3 segment

ACA, A2 segment

Supraorbital floor

Corpus callosum (genu)

Anterior communicating artery

ACA, A1 segment

MCA, proximal

Posterior cerebral artery

Toward vertex

Toward base of skull

ACA, A2 segment

A2 segment, waveform

Pericallosal artery, A3 segment

ACA, A2 segment

ACA, A1 segment

(Top) Sagittal color Doppler ultrasound (paramedian frontal approach) shows the course of the ACA. The ACA (A1 segment) is shown coursing anteriorly along the base of the brain to its most anterior point, then (A2 segment) turning anterosuperiorly to enter the interhemispheric fissure, and (A3 segment) arching backward along the superior surface of the hypoechoic corpus callosum. Note the ACA is best illustrated by this approach because most of its course can be demonstrated on this plane. **(Middle)** Sagittal spectral Doppler ultrasound (paramedian frontal approach) illustrates the normal waveform of the A2 segment which is antegrade and of low-resistance. **(Bottom)** Corresponding, oblique, sagittal, reformatted CT arteriogram shows the course of the ACA after branching off from the ICA bifurcation.

Brain and Spine

I

ANTERIOR CEREBRAL ARTERY

ACA, FRONTOPOLAR ARTERY

Callosomarginal artery

Frontal horn, right lateral ventricle

ACA, A2 segment

Anterior communicating artery

ACA, A1 segment

Toward vertex

Frontopolar artery

Supraorbital floor

Middle cerebral artery

Toward base of skull

Frontal horn, right lateral ventricle

ACA, A2 segment

Frontopolar artery

Frontopolar artery, waveform

Frontal horn of lateral ventricle

Ipsilateral ACA, A2 segment

Contralateral ACA, A1 segment

Ipsilateral frontopolar artery

Contralateral ACA, A2 segment

Ipsilateral ACA, A1 segment

(Top) Sagittal color Doppler ultrasound (paramedian frontal approach) shows the small frontopolar artery arising from the A2 segment and running anteriorly. It is usually given off in the mid-A2 segment. **(Middle)** Sagittal spectral Doppler ultrasound (paramedian frontal approach) shows the normal waveform of the frontopolar artery. It is antegrade toward the transducer and is of low-resistance but with a much lower velocity than ACA main trunk. **(Bottom)** Corresponding oblique sagittal reformatted MR arteriogram demonstrates the frontopolar artery branching anteriorly from the mid-A2 segment of the ACA.

ACA, CALLOSOMARGINAL ARTERY

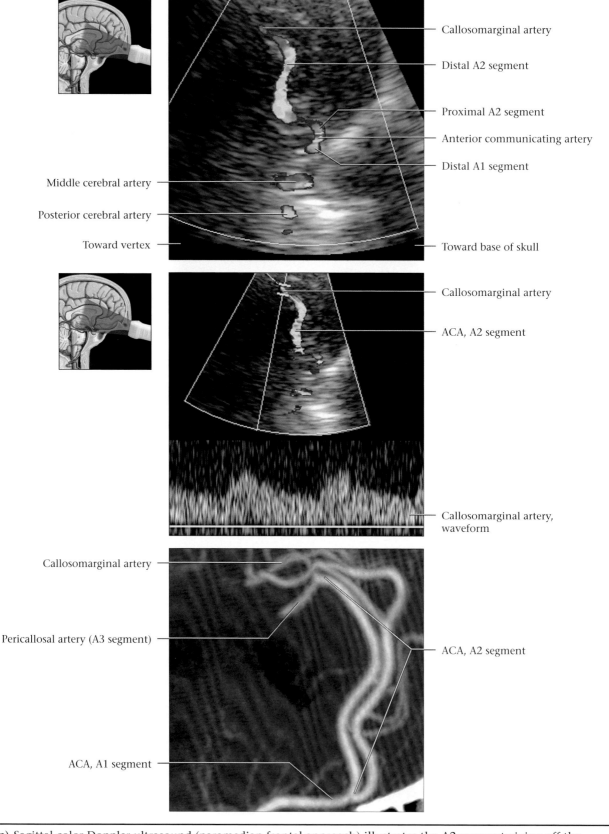

Callosomarginal artery

Distal A2 segment

Proximal A2 segment

Anterior communicating artery

Distal A1 segment

Middle cerebral artery

Posterior cerebral artery

Toward vertex

Toward base of skull

Callosomarginal artery

ACA, A2 segment

Callosomarginal artery, waveform

Callosomarginal artery

Pericallosal artery (A3 segment)

ACA, A2 segment

ACA, A1 segment

(Top) Sagittal color Doppler ultrasound (paramedian frontal approach) illustrates the A2 segment giving off the callosomarginal artery which is the smaller branch of the distal ACA. It runs posterosuperiorly in cingulate sulcus and on the superior surface of the cingulate gyrus. Its flow is directed toward the transducer. (Middle) Sagittal spectral Doppler ultrasound (paramedian frontal approach) shows the antegrade, low-resistance waveform of callosomarginal artery of the A2 segment. (Bottom) Corresponding oblique sagittal reformatted CT arteriogram shows the A2 segment giving off the callosomarginal artery and becoming the A3 segment (pericallosal artery).

ANTERIOR CEREBRAL ARTERY

ACA, PERICALLOSAL ARTERY

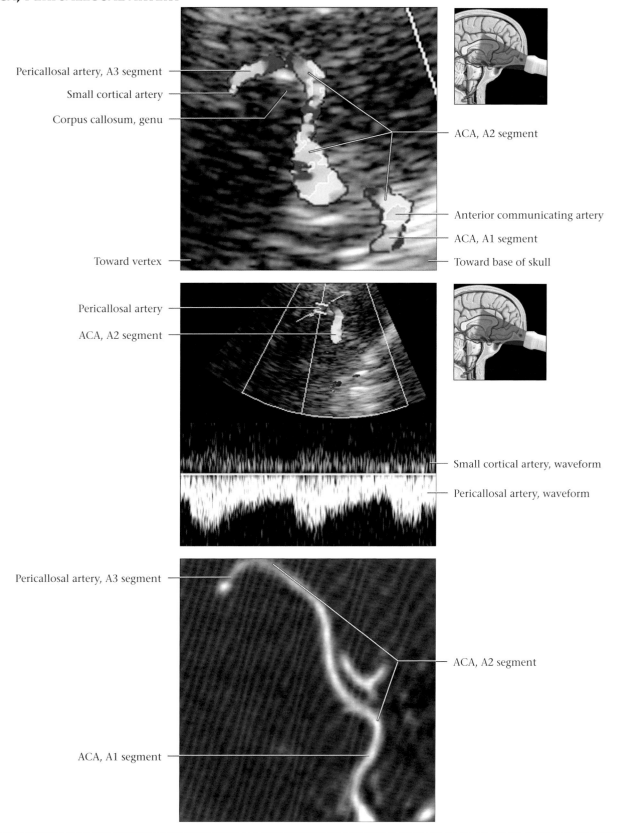

Pericallosal artery, A3 segment

Small cortical artery

Corpus callosum, genu

ACA, A2 segment

Anterior communicating artery

ACA, A1 segment

Toward vertex

Toward base of skull

Pericallosal artery

ACA, A2 segment

Small cortical artery, waveform

Pericallosal artery, waveform

Pericallosal artery, A3 segment

ACA, A2 segment

ACA, A1 segment

(Top) Sagittal color Doppler ultrasound (paramedian frontal approach) illustrates the pericallosal artery (A3 segment) arising as the larger branch from the distal A2 segment near the corpus callosum genu. Its normal flow is directed away from the transducer. (Middle) Sagittal spectral Doppler ultrasound (paramedian frontal approach) shows the low-resistance waveform of the pericallosal artery on the negative scale indicating flow away from the transducer. The waveform is inseparable from that of a small neighboring cortical artery carrying flow toward the transducer. (Bottom) Corresponding, oblique, sagittal, reformatted CT arteriogram shows the A2 segment continuing as the pericallosal artery (larger branch). The pericallosal artery (A3 segment) then curves posteroinferiorly around the corpus callosum genu underneath the falx cerebri.

Brain and Spine

I

111

MIDDLE CEREBRAL ARTERY

Terminology

Abbreviations
- Middle cerebral artery (MCA), anterior cerebral artery (ACA), internal carotid artery (ICA)
- Transcranial color Doppler sonography (TCCD)

Gross Anatomy

Overview
- Larger, lateral terminal branch of supraclinoid ICA
- MCA origin near medial aspect of lesser wing sphenoid
- Four main segments
  - Horizontal (M1) segment
    - From terminal ICA bifurcation to MCA bifurcation
    - Usually bi- or trifurcates just before sylvian fissure
    - Lies lateral to optic chiasm, behind olfactory trigone
    - Courses laterally under anterior perforated substance
    - Young adult: Runs laterally/rostrally; bows dorsally
    - Elderly: Usually straight or tortuous; may bow ventrally coursing closer to sphenoid wing
  - Insular (M2) segments: Superior & inferior trunks
    - Extend from MCA bifurcation to peri-insular sulci
    - Enter sylvian fissure; course superiorly within it
    - Six to eight stem arteries arise from M2 segments
    - M2 segments end at top of sylvian fissure
    - Bifurcate into superior and inferior trunks
  - Superior trunk of M2 segment
    - Prefrontal arteries
    - Precentral (prerolandic) artery
    - Central sulcus (rolandic) artery
    - Anterior parietal artery
    - Orbitofrontal artery may arise from M1 segment
  - Inferior trunk of M2 segment
    - Posterior parietal artery
    - Middle temporal artery
    - Posterior temporal artery
    - Occipital temporal artery
    - Angular (terminal) artery
    - Anterior temporal artery may arise from M1 segment
  - Opercular (M3) segments
    - Begins at top of sylvian fissure, course inferolaterally through sylvian fissure
  - Cortical branches (M4) segments
    - Exit sylvian fissure; ramify over cerebral convexity
    - Origins at insular M2 segments

Imaging Anatomy

Vascular Territory
- Cortical branches
  - Most common pattern - supply most of lateral surface of cerebral hemispheres except for convexity and inferior temporal gyrus
  - Anterior tip of temporal lobe (variable)
- Penetrating branches
  - Lenticulostriate arteries - arise from M1 segment

- Basal ganglia, internal & external capsules

Normal Variants, Anomalies
- High variability in branching patterns
  - Usually bifurcates, ~ 25% trifurcates with individual anterior temporal branch
  - "Early" MCA bifurcation (within 1 cm of origin)
- True anomalies (hypoplasia, aplasia) rare
  - MCA duplication seen in 1-3% of cases
    - Large branch arises from distal ICA just prior to terminal bifurcation, parallels main M1
  - Accessory MCA (rare)
    - Arises from ACA
    - High association with saccular aneurysm
  - Fenestrated MCA (rare)

Anatomy-Based Imaging Issues

Imaging Recommendations
- Performed using 1.8-3.6 MHz transducer
- M1 & M2 segments are amenable for US assessment, M3 may occasionally be seen
- Normal mean velocity and depth of insonation: 62 ± 12 cm/s (30-67 mm)
- Transtemporal approach
  - Axial mesencephalic plane
    - Identify origin of MCA near medial aspect of lesser wing of sphenoid bone
    - M1 & M2 segments - flow towards transducer
    - M2 branches: Usually flow toward transducer but may curve with flow away from transducer
  - Axial ventricular plane
    - Assesses M2 & M3 segments
    - Determine degree of midline shift (MLS) in space-occupying MCA infarct
  - Anterior coronal plane
    - Assesses M1 segment
  - Posterior coronal plane
    - Assesses M2 & M3 segments
- Transfrontal approach (alternative)
  - Lateral frontal bone window better than paramedian window due to insonation angle
  - Identify MCA as echogenic double reflex
  - M1 segment: Flow direction toward transducer

Imaging Pitfalls
- Impenetrable temporal bone (F > M)
- Vessel tortuosity → erroneous velocity measurements
- High anatomical MCA variations leading to misinterpretation

Clinical Implications

Clinical Importance
- Peak systolic velocity ≥ 50% stenosis: ≥ 220 cm/s
- TCCD is useful in acute MCA stroke/occlusion
  - Assess recanalization after thrombolysis therapy
  - Monitoring of midline shift - shown to be of prognostic value
    - Measure distance to center of 3rd ventricle in infarcted (I) & normal (N) sides
    - $MLS = (I-N)/2$

MIDDLE CEREBRAL ARTERY

MIDDLE CEREBRAL ARTERY

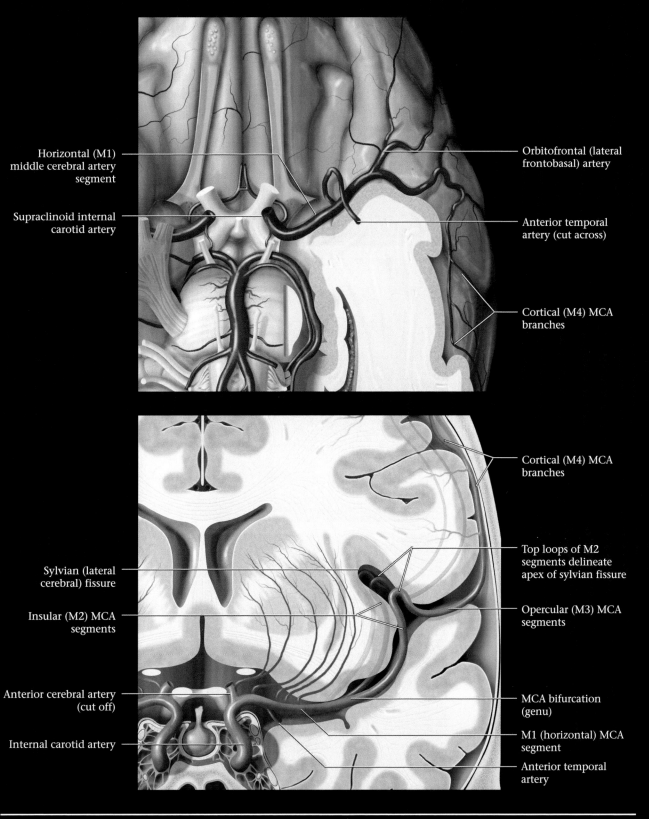

Horizontal (M1) middle cerebral artery segment

Supraclinoid internal carotid artery

Orbitofrontal (lateral frontobasal) artery

Anterior temporal artery (cut across)

Cortical (M4) MCA branches

Cortical (M4) MCA branches

Sylvian (lateral cerebral) fissure

Insular (M2) MCA segments

Top loops of M2 segments delineate apex of sylvian fissure

Opercular (M3) MCA segments

Anterior cerebral artery (cut off)

Internal carotid artery

MCA bifurcation (genu)

M1 (horizontal) MCA segment

Anterior temporal artery

(Top) The middle cerebral artery (MCA) and its relationship to adjacent structures is depicted on these graphics. Submentovertex graphic shows the left temporal lobe sectioned through the temporal horn of the lateral ventricle. The MCA supplies much of the lateral surface of the brain and is the larger of the two terminal branches of the internal carotid artery. **(Bottom)** AP graphic shows the MCA and its relationship to the adjacent brain. The MCA course through the Sylvian fissure and the M1-M4 segments are well-delineated. A few medial and numerous lateral lenticulostriate arteries arise from the top of the horizontal (M1) MCA segment, course superiorly through the anterior perforated substance, and supply the lateral basal ganglia and external capsule.

MCA, COLOR DOPPLER

Ipsilateral MCA, M2 segment (superior trunk)

Ipsilateral MCA, M2 segment (inferior trunk)

Ipsilateral MCA, horizontal M1 segment

Ipsilateral ACA, A1 segment

Contralateral ACA, A1 segment

Mesencephalon

Posterior

Anterior

Small cortical branch

MCA, M2 (insular) segment

MCA, distal M1 segment

Posterior

Anterior

Ipsilateral M2 insula segment

Ipsilateral MCA, M1 segment

Sphenoid bone, lesser wing

Ipsilateral ICA, C7 segment

Posterior communicating artery

Contralateral ICA, C7 segment

Posterior cerebral artery

Mesencephalon

Posterior

Anterior

(Top) Axial color Doppler US (transtemporal approach) of a young adult shows the M1 segment of the MCA on standard mesencephalic plane where it starts from the ICA termination to MCA bi-/trifurcations. In young adults, M1 usually bows dorsally. (Middle) Oblique coronal color Doppler US (transtemporal approach) of the same adult shows the M2 segment in the insula. Note that the flow direction in the M2 segment is directed toward the transducer in the proximal segment and away from the transducer as it ascends within the Sylvian fissure. (Bottom) Axial color Doppler US (transtemporal approach) of the MCA in an elderly patient shows a tortuous M1 segment. Its distal portion bows ventrally bringing the entire segment closer to sphenoid bone. The M1 segment originates near the medial aspect of the lesser wing of the sphenoid & traverses laterally & horizontally to end in the limen insulae.

Brain and Spine

MIDDLE CEREBRAL ARTERY

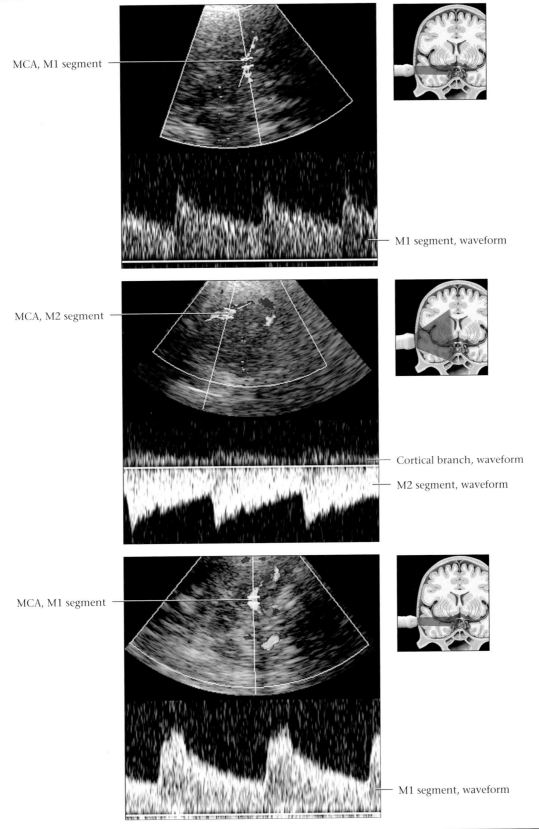

MCA, M1 segment

M1 segment, waveform

MCA, M2 segment

Cortical branch, waveform

M2 segment, waveform

MCA, M1 segment

M1 segment, waveform

(Top) Axial spectral Doppler ultrasound (transtemporal approach) of the MCA in a young adult shows that the waveform pattern is of low-resistance and the mean velocity is within normal range of 62 ± 12 cm/s. The clinical importance of assessing the MCA is its high association with stroke in diseased arteries. (Middle) Oblique, coronal, spectral Doppler ultrasound (transtemporal approach) of a young adult shows waveform of the M2 segment which is away from the transducer. The waveform is inseparable from that of a small neighboring cortical branch with flow toward the transducer. (Bottom) Axial spectral Doppler ultrasound (transtemporal approach) of an elderly patient shows Doppler waveform of the M1 segment. Note accurate flow velocity measurement in an elderly patient may be difficult due to uncertainty in angle correction in a tortuous vessel.

Brain and Spine

I

MCA BRANCHES, COLOR DOPPLER

M2 segment, superior trunk

MCA, M1 segment

Posterior

Prefrontal artery

M2 segment, inferior trunk

Lateral orbitofrontal artery

Anterior

M2 segment, superior trunk

Mesencephalon

Posterior

Prefrontal artery

Lateral orbitofrontal artery

Falx cerebri

Anterior

MCA, M2 segment

M2 segment, superior trunk

MCA bifurcation

Posterior

Anterior temporal artery

M2 segment, inferior trunk

Anterior

(Top) Axial, oblique, color Doppler ultrasound of the MCA bifurcation (transtemporal approach) shows the superior and inferior trunks of the M2 segments. Note the MCA bifurcates in about 75% of normal subjects and the rest trifurcate with an individual anterior temporal artery. (Middle) Axial, oblique, color Doppler ultrasound (transtemporal approach) of the superior trunk of the M2 segments shows the proximal two branches, namely lateral orbitofrontal (LOA) and prefrontal artery (PA). The LOA runs in the cortex of the lateral inferior part of the frontal lobe while the PA is located in the region of the anterior insular point. (Bottom) Axial, oblique, color Doppler ultrasound (transtemporal approach) shows the anterior temporal artery arising from the inferior trunk of the M2 segments. This branch may be given off by the M1 segment in an individual vessel as a normal variant.

Brain and Spine

I

MIDDLE CEREBRAL ARTERY

MCA BRANCHES, SPECTRAL DOPPLER

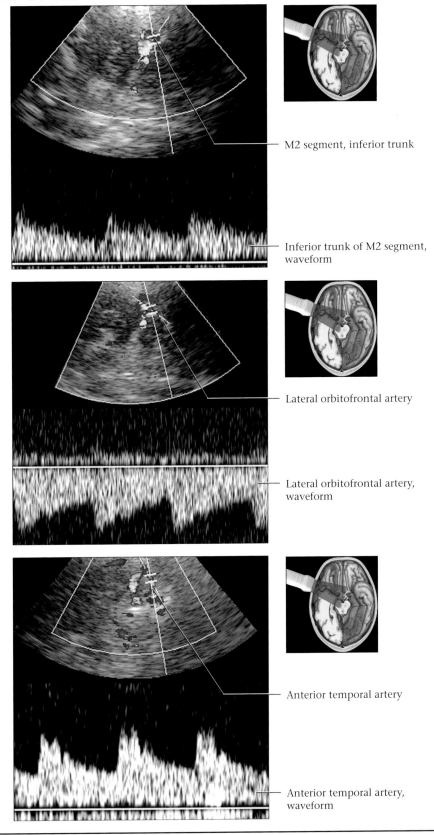

M2 segment, inferior trunk

Inferior trunk of M2 segment, waveform

Lateral orbitofrontal artery

Lateral orbitofrontal artery, waveform

Anterior temporal artery

Anterior temporal artery, waveform

(Top) Axial, oblique, spectral Doppler ultrasound of the MCA bifurcation (transtemporal approach) shows the Doppler waveform of the inferior trunk of the M2 segments. The flow is of low velocity and low resistance with flow direction toward the transducer. (Middle) Axial, oblique, spectral Doppler ultrasound (transtemporal approach) of the first branch, LOA of superior trunk (M2 segments). The waveform is reversed indicating flow away from the transducer. Usually flow in branches from the M2 segment is directed toward the transducer but flow in the opposite direction may be detected in arteries which curve. (Bottom) Axial, oblique, spectral Doppler ultrasound (transtemporal approach) shows the first branch, anterior temporal artery arising from the inferior trunk of the M2 segments. The waveform is typically of low resistance and directed toward the transducer.

Brain and Spine   I

117

POSTERIOR CEREBRAL ARTERY

Gross Anatomy

Overview
- Basilar artery (BA) terminates into two posterior cerebral arteries (PCA)
- Four segments
  - Precommunicating (P1) or mesencephalic segment
  - Ambient (P2) segment
  - Quadrigeminal (P3) segment
  - Calcarine (P4) segment
- Posterior communicating arteries (PCoA) connect PCA to internal carotid artery (ICA) at P1/P2 junction

Imaging Anatomy

Anatomy Relationships
- P1 (precommunicating) segment
  - Extends laterally from BA to junction with PCoA
  - Closely related to anteromedial mesencephalon
  - Courses above cisternal segment of CN3
  - Usually with horizontal course but exact course depends on the length of BA
  - Asymmetry (> 50%) and frequently hypoplastic
- P2 (ambient) segment
  - Extends from P1/PCoA junction
  - Encircles mesencephalon within ambient cistern
  - Lies above tentorium, cisternal segment of CN4
  - Parallels optic tract, basal vein of Rosenthal
- P3 (quadrigeminal) segment
  - Short segment within lateral aspect of quadrigeminal cistern
  - Extends behind mesencephalon, beneath the splenium of corpus callosum
- P4 (calcarine) segment
  - PCA terminates above tentorium in calcarine fissure

Branches
- Perforating (central) branches
  - Thalamoperforating arteries - arise from P1, pass posterosuperiorly in interpeduncular fossa
  - Thalamogeniculate arteries - arise from P2, pass posteromedially into mesencephalon
  - Peduncular perforating arteries arise from P2, pass directly into cerebral peduncles
- Ventricular/choroidal branches (arise from P2)
  - Medial posterior choroidal artery - runs parallel to PCA, enters tela choroidea and runs anteriorly along roof of 3rd ventricle
  - Lateral posterior choroidal arteries - curve anteriorly around thalamus
- Cortical branches
  - Anterior temporal artery - arises from P2, courses anterolaterally under parahippocampal gyrus; anastomoses with MCA branches
  - Posterior temporal artery - arises from P2, courses posterolaterally along hippocampal gyrus
  - Medial & lateral terminal trunks - major branches include parieto-occipital and calcarine arteries

Vascular Territory
- Penetrating branches: Mesencephalon, thalami, posterior limb of internal capsule, optic tract
- Ventricular/choroidal branches: Choroid plexus of 3rd/lateral ventricles, thalami, posterior commissure, cerebral peduncles
- Splenial branches: Posterior body and splenium of corpus callosum
- Cortical branches: Posterior 1/3 of medial hemisphere surface; inferior temporal lobe, occipital lobe (including visual cortex)

Normal Variants, Anomalies
- "Fetal" origin of PCA
  - More common on right side, ~ 8% bilateral
  - PCA has direct supply from anterior circulation with large PCoA giving direct origin to PCA
  - Hypoplastic/absent P1 segment
- Persistent carotid-basilar anastomoses
  - PCAs supplied by persistent trigeminal artery, persistent hypoglossal artery or proatlantal intersegmental artery

Anatomy-Based Imaging Issues

Imaging Recommendations
- Performed using 1.8-3.6 MHz transducer
- Better to begin artery identification from P2 segment
- Normal mean velocity and depth of insonation: 39 ± 10 cm/s (55-80 mm)
- Transtemporal approach (commonly used)
  - Axial mesencephalic plane
    - P1 segment: Flow toward transducer
    - Anterior P2 segment: Flow toward transducer
    - Posterior P2 segment: Flow away from transducer
    - P3 segment: Flow away from transducer
    - PCoA: Flow away from transducer
  - Axial ventricular plane
    - 10 degree upward tilting of mesencephalic plane
    - P3 segment: Flow away from transducer
  - Coronal plane
    - Scans P1, P2 segments and PCoA
- Transforaminal approach
  - Axial plane through foramen magnum, scan cranially from BA
  - Scans P1 segment for short BA and low bifurcation
- Transfrontal approach
  - Paramedian frontal bone window
    - Vertical plane, slightly lateral to forehead midline
  - Lateral frontal bone window
    - Axial plane just above lateral aspect of eyebrow
  - Scans P1, P2 segments and PCoA

Imaging Pitfalls
- Absent P1 segment on transforaminal approach usually due to "fetal" origin, not occlusion

Clinical Implications

Clinical Importance
- Identification of intracranial arterial stenosis or occlusion in posterior circulation
- PCoA is common site for aneurysm formation
- Reversed flow in PCoA indicative of collateral circulation

POSTERIOR ARTERIAL CIRCULATION

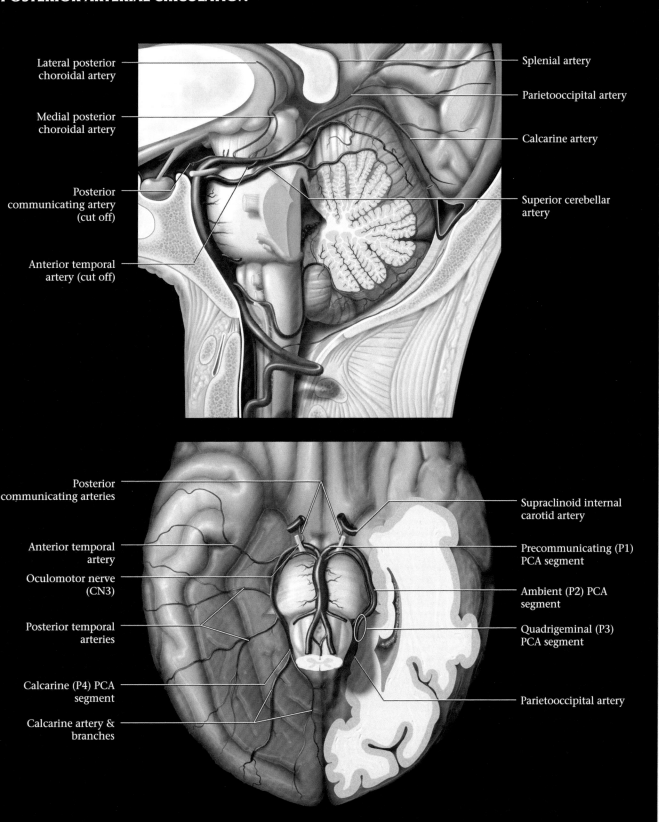

Lateral posterior choroidal artery

Medial posterior choroidal artery

Posterior communicating artery (cut off)

Anterior temporal artery (cut off)

Splenial artery

Parietooccipital artery

Calcarine artery

Superior cerebellar artery

Posterior communicating arteries

Anterior temporal artery

Oculomotor nerve (CN3)

Posterior temporal arteries

Calcarine (P4) PCA segment

Calcarine artery & branches

Supraclinoid internal carotid artery

Precommunicating (P1) PCA segment

Ambient (P2) PCA segment

Quadrigeminal (P3) PCA segment

Parietooccipital artery

(Top) Lateral graphic shows the posterior cerebral artery and its branches. The PCA has central (perforating), choroidal, and cortical branches as well as a small branch to the corpus callosum splenium. The tentorium and CN3 lie between the PCA above and the superior cerebellar artery below. (Bottom) Submentovertex graphic shows the PCA and the relationship of its segments to the midbrain. The PCA supplies the occipital lobe and almost all of the inferior surface of the temporal lobe (except for its tip). The precommunicating (P1) PCA segment extends from the basilar bifurcation to the PCoA junction. The ambient (P2) segment swings posterolaterally around the midbrain. The quadrigeminal segment (P3) lies behind the midbrain. The PCA terminal segment is the calcarine (P4) segment.

Brain and Spine

I

MCA, M2 segment

Ipsilateral PCA, P2 segment (posterior)

MCA, M1 segment

Ipsilateral PCA, P2 segment (anterior)

Ipsilateral ICA, communicating segment

Ipsilateral PCA, P1 segment

Posterior communicating artery

Mesencephalon

Contralateral ICA

Contralateral P1 segment

Posterior

Anterior

MCA, M1 segment

Ipsilateral ICA, communicating segment

Ipsilateral PCA, P2 segment

Ipsilateral PCoA

Ipsilateral PCA, P1 segment

Contralateral PCoA

Distal BA

Contralateral PCA, P1 segment

Contralateral ICA

Ipsilateral PCA, P3 segment

Contralateral PCA, P2 segment

Internal carotid artery

Posterior communicating artery

Posterior cerebral artery

Posterior communicating artery waveform

(Top) Axial color Doppler ultrasound (transtemporal approach) on mesencephalic plane shows the P1 segment emerging in the interpeduncular cistern with P2 segment encircling the mesencephalon with flow toward transducer in P1 and P2 segments. A short P3 segment is also noted with flow away from transducer. With adequate acoustic penetration, the contralateral arterial segments can be visualized with flow direction opposite to ipsilateral arteries. (Middle) Corresponding MR arteriogram in a similar projection plane shows bilateral PCAs and PCoAs in circle of Willis. (Bottom) Axial spectral Doppler ultrasound (transtemporal approach) of PCoA on standard mesencephalic plane shows normal backward flow from ICA to PCA in this artery. Note only 75% of PCoA is discernible transcranially.

Brain and Spine

I

POSTERIOR CEREBRAL ARTERY

POSTERIOR CEREBRAL ARTERY

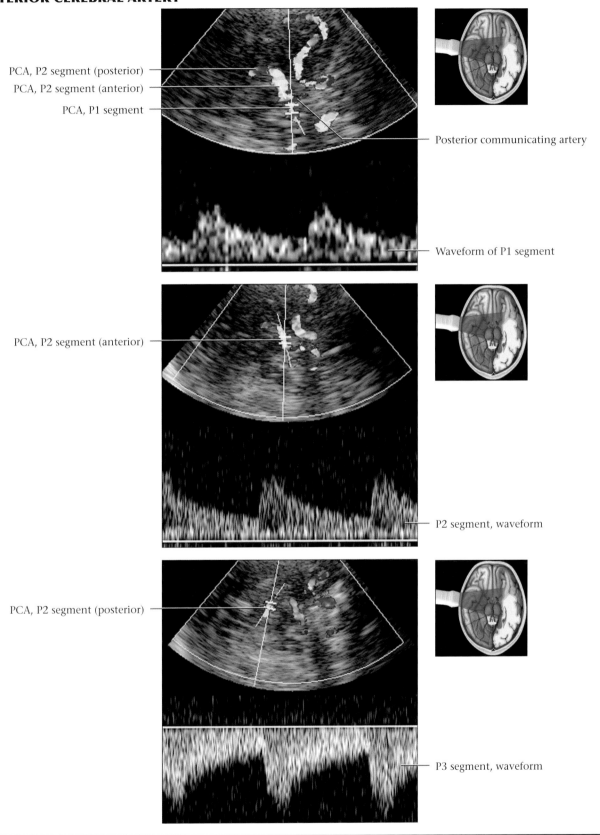

PCA, P2 segment (posterior)

PCA, P2 segment (anterior)

PCA, P1 segment

Posterior communicating artery

Waveform of P1 segment

PCA, P2 segment (anterior)

P2 segment, waveform

PCA, P2 segment (posterior)

P3 segment, waveform

(Top) Axial spectral Doppler ultrasound (transtemporal approach) of P1 segment shows the waveform of P1 flow is of low-resistance and on the positive side of the trace. Note P1 segment is short, often hypoplastic or absent making its visualization difficult. **(Middle)** Axial spectral Doppler ultrasound (transtemporal approach) of anterior P2 segment on axial mesencephalic plane shows normal antegrade low-resistance flow with a waveform pattern similar to P1 segment. **(Bottom)** Axial spectral Doppler ultrasound (transtemporal approach) of posterior P2 segment on axial ventricular plane shows the waveform of this segment is of low-resistance and on the negative side of the trace denoting flow away from transducer.

DISTAL INTERNAL CAROTID ARTERY

Gross Anatomy

Overview
- Internal carotid artery (ICA) is one of the terminal branches of the common carotid artery (CCA)
- ICA has 7 segments, 6 of which are intracranial
- Precavernous: Petrous (C2), lacerum (C3)
- Cavernous: Cavernous (C4), clinoid (C5)
- Supraclinoid: Ophthalmic (C6)
- Terminal: Communicating (C7)

Imaging Anatomy

Petrous (C2) Segment
- Contained within carotid canal of temporal bone
- Two subsegments joined at genu
  - Short vertical segment: ~ 1 cm, passes inside petrous bone anterior to internal jugular vein (IJV)
  - Longer horizontal segment: Passes anteromedial in front of cochlea, emerges near petrous apex
- Branches
  - Vidian artery (artery of pterygoid canal) anastomoses with external carotid artery (ECA)
  - Mandibular artery (arises in foramen lacerum/horizontal portion at carotid canal)
  - Caroticotympanic artery (arises from vertical petrous segment, supplies middle ear)

Lacerum (C3) Segment
- Extends anteromedially from petrous apex to foramen lacerum, curving upwards to posteroinferior aspect of sella turcica
- Also called ganglionar segment as it is in contact with gasserian ganglion located lateral to ICA

Cavernous (C4) Segment
- Lies within cavernous sinus (CS)
- Ascends lateral to inferolateral aspect of sella, passes anteriorly at carotid sulcus then curves upward medial to lower anterior clinoid process
- In contact with abducens nerve (CN6)
- Major branches
  - Meningohypophyseal trunk (arises from posterior genu, supplies pituitary, tentorium and clival dura)
    - Basal tentorial enters tentorium anterior to petrous apex, supplies adjacent tentorium
    - Clivus supply dura of dorsum sellae & clivus
    - Inferior hypophyseal artery supplies posterior pituitary gland
  - Inferolateral trunk (arises from horizontal segment, passes inferolaterally over the lateral aspect of CN6)
    - Supplies gasserian ganglion, CNs in CS, dura of CS and floor of middle fossa
    - Anastomoses with branches of middle & accessory meningeal arteries in the floor of middle fossa and branches of OA near superior orbital fissure

Clinoid (C5) Segment
- Between proximal, distal dural rings of CS
- Ends as ICA enters subarachnoid space near anterior clinoid process
- No important branches unless ophthalmic artery (OA) arises within CS

Ophthalmic (C6) Segment
- Extends from distal dural ring of CS to just below posterior communicating artery (PCoA) origin
- Two important branches
  - OA (runs through optic canal to orbit)
    - 1st supraclinoid branch from anterosuperior ICA
    - Extensive anastomoses with ECA branches
  - Superior hypophyseal artery (can arise from supraclinoid segment or from PCoA)

Communicating (C7) Segment
- Extends from below PCoA to terminate into anterior cerebral artery (ACA) & middle cerebral artery (MCA)
- Passes between optic (CN2), oculomotor (CN3) nerves
- Other branches
  - PCoA
  - Anterior choroidal artery (courses posteromedial, then turns superolateral in suprasellar cistern; enters temporal horn at choroidal fissure)

Common Normal Variants, Anomalies
- Aberrant ICA (aICA)
  - Presents as retrotympanic pulsatile mass; should not be mistaken for glomus tympanicum tumor
  - Absent vertical course of C2; aICA courses more posterolaterally in hypotympanum
- Persistent trigeminal artery
  - Most common carotid-basilar anastomosis
  - Connects cavernous segment of ICA and basilar artery, forms "trident-shape" on lateral DSA
  - Parallels course of CN5, passes posterolaterally around (or through) dorsum sellae

Anatomy-Based Imaging Issues

Imaging Recommendations
- Performed using 1.5-3.5 MHz transducer
- Assess flow direction, velocity and patency of vessel with color Doppler imaging
- Normal mean velocities & depth of insonation: 39 ± 9 cm/s (60-67 mm)
- Different ICA segments are amenable for ultrasound assessment with different windows & approaches
  - Retromandibular approach
    - Examination of distal C1
    - Identify the segment at the retrostyloid region
  - Transorbital approach
    - Examination of carotid siphon (C4 to C6)
    - C4 segment: Flow toward transducer
    - C5 segment: Bidirectional flow
    - C6 segment: Flow away from transducer
  - Transtemporal approach
    - Examination of C7 segment
    - Bifurcation into MCA and ACA: Identify axial mesencephalic plane by depicting hypoechoic butterfly-shaped mesencephalon
    - Bifurcation into other branches: Slight caudad tilting from standard axial mesencephalic plane
- Normal spectral waveform of intracranial ICA
  - Low-resistance flow
  - Similar waveform to CCA but with lower amplitude

DISTAL INTERNAL CAROTID ARTERY

DISTAL INTERNAL CAROTID ARTERY

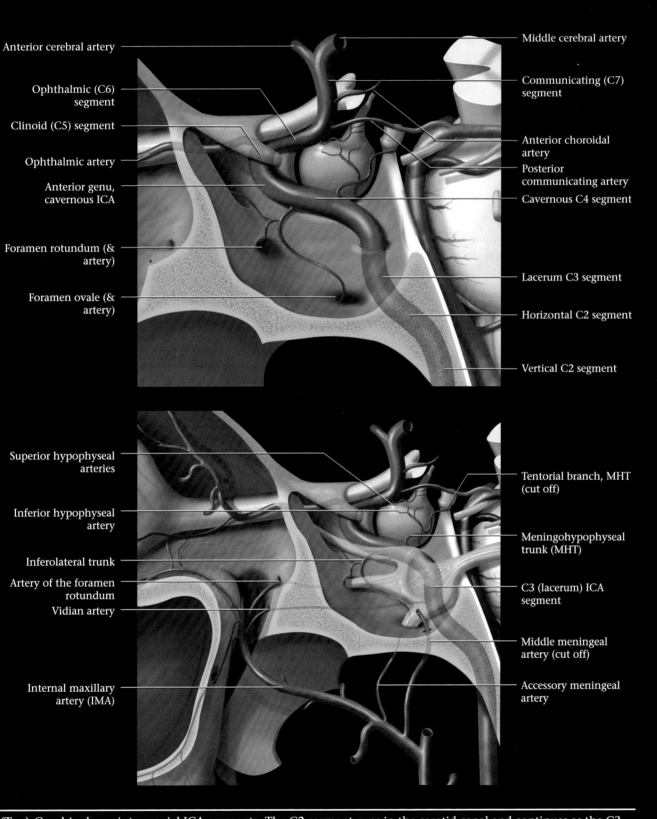

Anterior cerebral artery

Ophthalmic (C6) segment

Clinoid (C5) segment

Ophthalmic artery

Anterior genu, cavernous ICA

Foramen rotundum (& artery)

Foramen ovale (& artery)

Middle cerebral artery

Communicating (C7) segment

Anterior choroidal artery

Posterior communicating artery

Cavernous C4 segment

Lacerum C3 segment

Horizontal C2 segment

Vertical C2 segment

Superior hypophyseal arteries

Inferior hypophyseal artery

Inferolateral trunk

Artery of the foramen rotundum

Vidian artery

Internal maxillary artery (IMA)

Tentorial branch, MHT (cut off)

Meningohypophyseal trunk (MHT)

C3 (lacerum) ICA segment

Middle meningeal artery (cut off)

Accessory meningeal artery

(Top) Graphic shows intracranial ICA segments. The C2 segment runs in the carotid canal and continues as the C3 segment after leaving the canal. The C4 segment as an extension of C3 is depicted with its branches anastomosing extensively with ECA branches. The C5 segment ends near anterior clinoid process and the C6 segment extends to just below PCoA. The C7 segment after giving rise to PCoA branches into ACA and MCA. **(Bottom)** Graphic shows numerous ICA to ECA anastomoses through cavernous and deep facial branches of the two arteries, respectively. These include numerous anastomoses in and around the orbit; small vidian artery anastomosing between IMA and petrous C2 segment and the accessory meningeal artery, an important branch that may supply part of the trigeminal ganglion, anastomosing with the inferolateral trunk of the cavernous ICA.

I

123

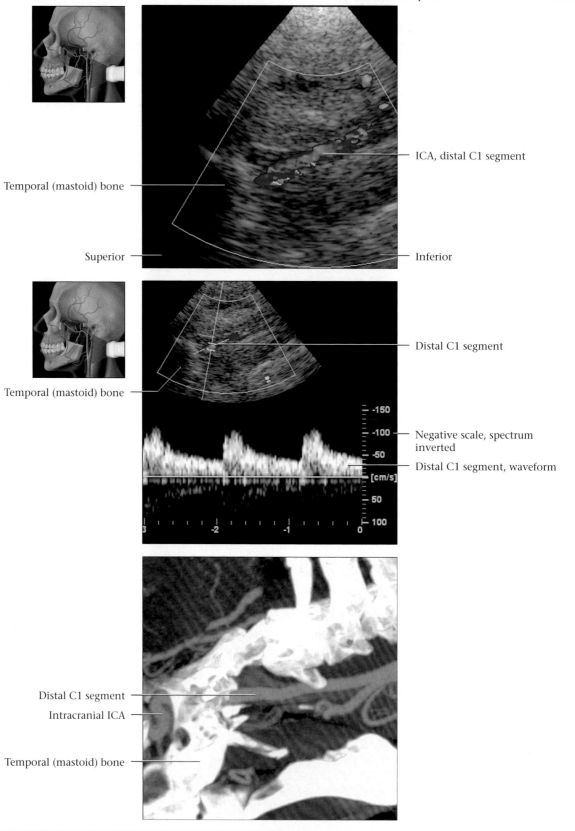

Temporal (mastoid) bone — ICA, distal C1 segment

Superior — Inferior

Temporal (mastoid) bone — Distal C1 segment

Negative scale, spectrum inverted

Distal C1 segment, waveform

Distal C1 segment

Intracranial ICA

Temporal (mastoid) bone

(Top) Longitudinal color Doppler ultrasound (submandibular approach) shows the distal C1 segment at the retromandibular region before it enters the skull via the carotid canal. Normally, there is no branch in this segment. **(Middle)** Corresponding spectral Doppler ultrasound shows typical low-resistance waveform of C1 segment of ICA. Note the flow direction of C1 obtained from this approach is away from the transducer as denoted by the waveform on the negative scale. **(Bottom)** Corresponding, sagittal, reformatted CT angiogram (CTA), displayed in the same orientation as the US, shows the distal C1 segment before ending the carotid canal of the temporal bone.

CAROTID SIPHON, TRANSORBITAL SCAN

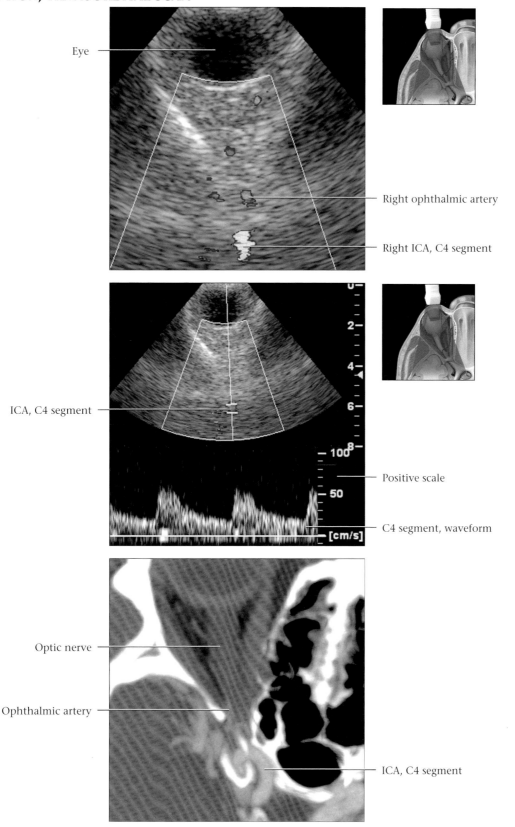

Eye

Right ophthalmic artery

Right ICA, C4 segment

ICA, C4 segment

Positive scale

C4 segment, waveform

Optic nerve

Ophthalmic artery

ICA, C4 segment

(Top) Axial color Doppler ultrasound (transorbital approach) shows the carotid siphon of ICA with its flow direction towards the transducer. Note the flow direction of the carotid siphon varies depending on which segment of the carotid siphon is insonated. Blood flow is toward the transducer in the cavernous C4 segment, bidirectional in clinoid C5 segment and away from the transducer in ophthalmic C6 segment. (Middle) Corresponding spectral Doppler waveform of the carotid siphon (C4 segment) which is usually found at a depth of 6-8 cm from the eyelids. The flow direction is toward the transducer as evidenced by the waveform shown on the positive scale. (Bottom) Corresponding, oblique, axial, reformatted CT arteriogram shows the ophthalmic artery arising from the ophthalmic segment of ICA, running through the optic canal to orbit.

Brain and Spine

I

125

DISTAL INTERNAL CAROTID ARTERY

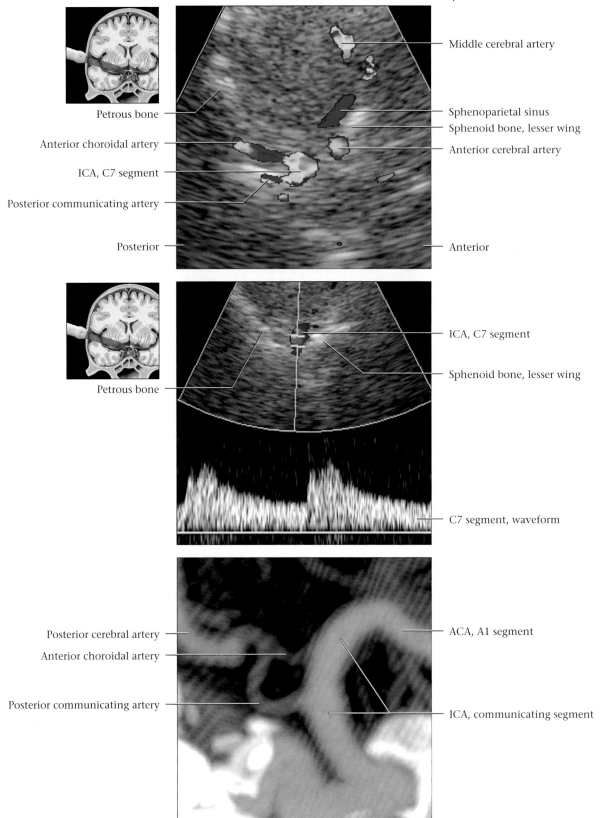

Middle cerebral artery

Sphenoparietal sinus
Sphenoid bone, lesser wing

Anterior cerebral artery

Petrous bone

Anterior choroidal artery

ICA, C7 segment

Posterior communicating artery

Posterior — — Anterior

Petrous bone

ICA, C7 segment

Sphenoid bone, lesser wing

C7 segment, waveform

Posterior cerebral artery

Anterior choroidal artery

Posterior communicating artery

ACA, A1 segment

ICA, communicating segment

(Top) Axial color Doppler ultrasound on a plane slightly caudad to the standard mesencephalic plane shows the communicating C7 segment of the ICA. This segment starts from below the PCoA and terminates into the ACA and MCA, between which the anterior choroidal artery may be identified just distal to the PCoA. **(Middle)** Corresponding spectral Doppler ultrasound of the C7 segment shows the waveform pattern is of low resistance with flow toward the transducer. This segment is easily detected on transtemporal axial scan with caudad tilting of the transducer from the standard mesencephalic plane with identification of the segment between the petrous bone and lesser wing of the sphenoid bone. **(Bottom)** Oblique, sagittal, reformatted MR arteriogram shows the communicating segment of the ICA and its two branches, PCoA proximally and anterior choroidal artery distally.

DISTAL INTERNAL CAROTID ARTERY

C7 SEGMENT, TRANSTEMPORAL SCAN

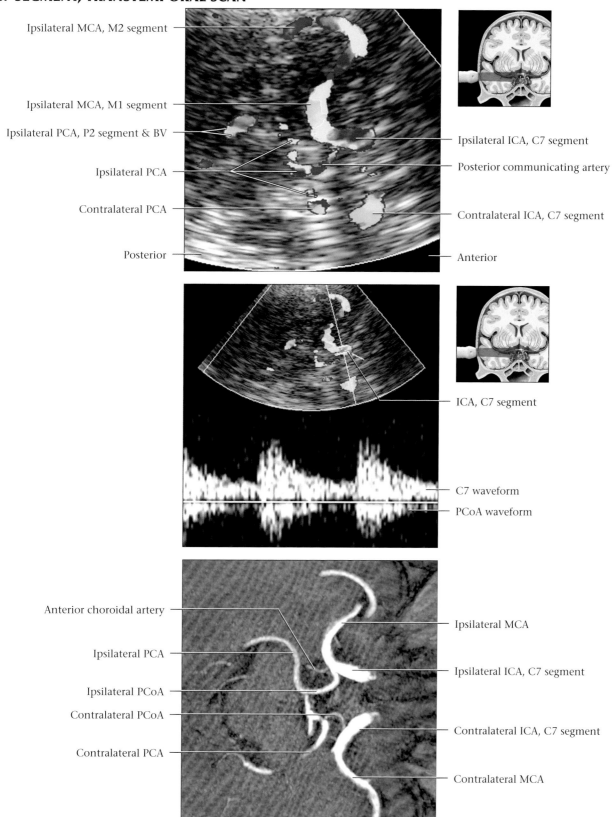

Ipsilateral MCA, M2 segment

Ipsilateral MCA, M1 segment

Ipsilateral PCA, P2 segment & BV

Ipsilateral PCA

Contralateral PCA

Posterior

Ipsilateral ICA, C7 segment

Posterior communicating artery

Contralateral ICA, C7 segment

Anterior

ICA, C7 segment

C7 waveform

PCoA waveform

Anterior choroidal artery

Ipsilateral PCA

Ipsilateral PCoA

Contralateral PCoA

Contralateral PCA

Ipsilateral MCA

Ipsilateral ICA, C7 segment

Contralateral ICA, C7 segment

Contralateral MCA

(Top) Axial color Doppler ultrasound (transtemporal approach) on standard mesencephalic plane shows the C7 segment of ICA branching into the MCA (ACA not shown). The PCoA arising from the C7 segment is demonstrated, with flow directed toward the PCA. (Middle) Corresponding spectral Doppler ultrasound of the C7 segment near the bifurcation shows bidirectional flow on the waveform representing forward flow of the C7 segment and backward flow of the PCoA. (Bottom) Corresponding MRA shows the C7 segment of the ICA terminating into the MCA and ACA (not shown on this plane). The two branches, PCoA and anterior choroidal artery, are consistently identified.

VERTEBROBASILAR SYSTEM

Terminology

Abbreviations
- Vertebral artery (VA); basilar artery (BA)
- Superior cerebellar arteries (SCAs); posterior inferior cerebellar artery (PICA); anterior inferior cerebellar artery (AICA); posterior cerebral artery (PCA)
- Anterior, posterior spinal arteries (ASA, PSA)
- Cranial nerve (CN); internal auditory canal (IAC)

Gross Anatomy

Overview
- V3 segment of VA (Atlas loop)
  - Extracranial/extraspinal
  - From exit at transverse foramen (atlas) to enter into foramen magnum
  - Curves behind superior articular process (atlas)
  - Rest on groove of posterior arch (atlas)
- V4 segment of VA
  - Intradural/intracranial
  - Perforates dura, enters skull through foramen magnum, courses superomedially behind clivus
  - Anterior to medulla oblongata
  - Unites with contralateral VA at/near pontomedullary junction to form BA
  - Branches
    - ASA, PSA
    - Meningeal branches
    - Perforating branches to medulla
    - PICA: Arises from distal VA, curves around/over cerebellar tonsil, gives off perforating medullary, choroid, tonsillar, cerebellar branches
- Basilar artery
  - Large median artery formed by union of two VAs at mid-medullary level
  - Courses superiorly in prepontine cistern (in front of pons, behind clivus)
  - Bifurcates into its terminal branches, PCAs, in interpeduncular or suprasellar cistern behind dorsum sellae
  - Branches
    - Pontine, midbrain perforating branches
    - AICA: Courses inferolaterally, lies ventromedial to CN7 & 8; often loops into IAC; its size is inversely proportional to the size of PICA
    - SCAs: Arise from distal BA, course posterolaterally around mesencephalon below CN3, tentorium; lie above CN5, often in contact with it
    - PCAs (terminal BA branches)

Imaging Anatomy

V3 Segment (Atlas Loop)
- Extracranial approach
  - Insonate posterolaterally from mastoid process
  - Demonstrates segment looping round superior articular process (atlas)
  - Proximal loop exiting from transverse foramen (atlas): Flow toward transducer
  - Distal loop resting on groove of posterior arch (atlas): Flow away from transducer
- Suboccipital approach
  - Insonate slightly off midline
  - Proximal loops: Flow toward transducer

V4 Segment
- Suboccipital approach
  - Insonate through foramen magnum
  - Transducer placed more inferiorly on neck and angled superiorly to obtain V4 segments and BA
  - Vertebrobasilar system typically appears as a "Y" with flow away from transducer
  - Due to vessel tortuosity or normal variation, "Y" configuration may not be seen

Basilar Artery
- Suboccipital approach
  - Proximal segment visualized by tracing up to junction of V4 segments
  - Flow away from transducer
- Transtemporal approach
  - Distal segment identified caudal to PCA origins
  - Flow toward transducer
- Flow is of low-resistance as VA but has higher velocity

Normal Variants, Anomalies
- Normal variants
  - Ectasia, tortuosity, off-midline course, variations in configuration/branching patterns common
  - VA: R/L variation in size, dominance common
    - VA terminates to PICA directly in 0.2%
    - Aortic arch origin ~ 5%
  - BA: Variation in course, branching patterns common; AICA/PICA may share common trunk
- Anomalies
  - Fenestration or duplication (↑ risk of aneurysm)
  - Embryonic carotid-basilar anastomoses; persistent trigeminal artery

Anatomy-Based Imaging Issues

Imaging Recommendations
- Performed using low-frequency transducer (1.8-3.6 MHz)
- For V4 segment
  - Normal adult mean flow velocity: 38 ± 10 cm/s
  - Insonation depth (transoccipital scan): 40-85 mm
- For BA trunk
  - Normal adult mean flow velocity: 41 ± 10 cm/s
  - Insonation depth (transoccipital scan): > 80 mm
  - Insonation depth (transtemporal scan): 75 mm

Clinical Implications

Clinical Importance
- Intracranial subclavian steal: Reversed BA/VA flow
- Intracranial stenosis: Abnormal ↑ flow velocity
- Postocclusive recanalization and collateral formation
- BA vasospasm - 100% sensitivity
  - Mean flow velocity ratio for BA/extracranial VA > 2

VERTEBROBASILAR SYSTEM

VERTEBROBASILAR SYSTEM

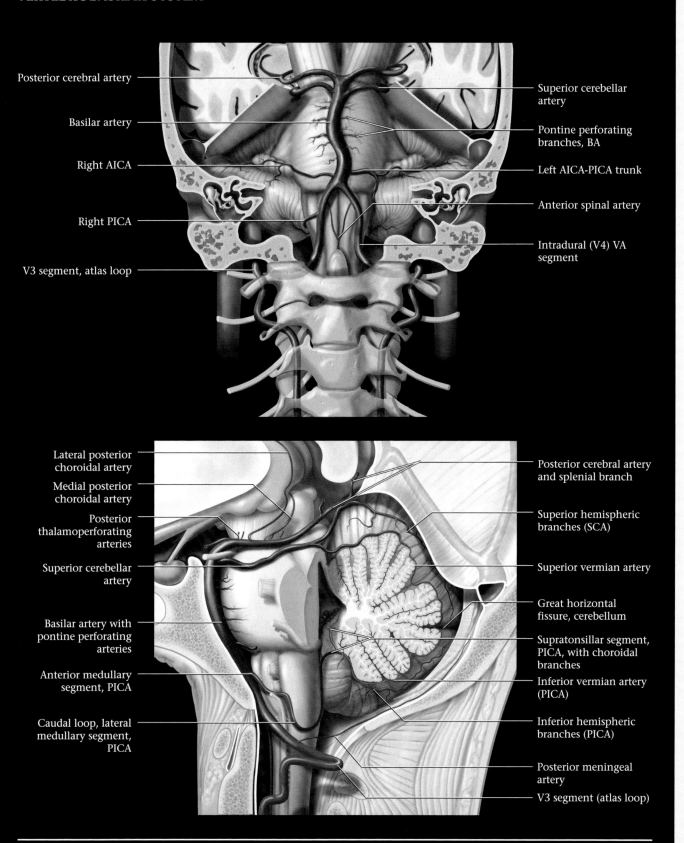

Posterior cerebral artery

Basilar artery

Right AICA

Right PICA

V3 segment, atlas loop

Superior cerebellar artery

Pontine perforating branches, BA

Left AICA-PICA trunk

Anterior spinal artery

Intradural (V4) VA segment

Lateral posterior choroidal artery

Medial posterior choroidal artery

Posterior thalamoperforating arteries

Superior cerebellar artery

Basilar artery with pontine perforating arteries

Anterior medullary segment, PICA

Caudal loop, lateral medullary segment, PICA

Posterior cerebral artery and splenial branch

Superior hemispheric branches (SCA)

Superior vermian artery

Great horizontal fissure, cerebellum

Supratonsillar segment, PICA, with choroidal branches

Inferior vermian artery (PICA)

Inferior hemispheric branches (PICA)

Posterior meningeal artery

V3 segment (atlas loop)

(Top) Frontal graphic depicts the vertebrobasilar system. V3 is the short extraspinal VA segment that extends from the top of C1 to the foramen magnum. V4 is the intradural (intracranial) segment. A right PICA originates from the VA. A combined AICA-PICA trunk is a common normal variant and is shown on the left. **(Bottom)** Lateral graphic depicts the vertebrobasilar system. Note the relationship of the PICA loops to the medulla, cerebellar tonsil. Watershed between SCA, PICA is often near the great horizontal fissure of the cerebellum.

VERTEBRAL ARTERY V3 SEGMENT

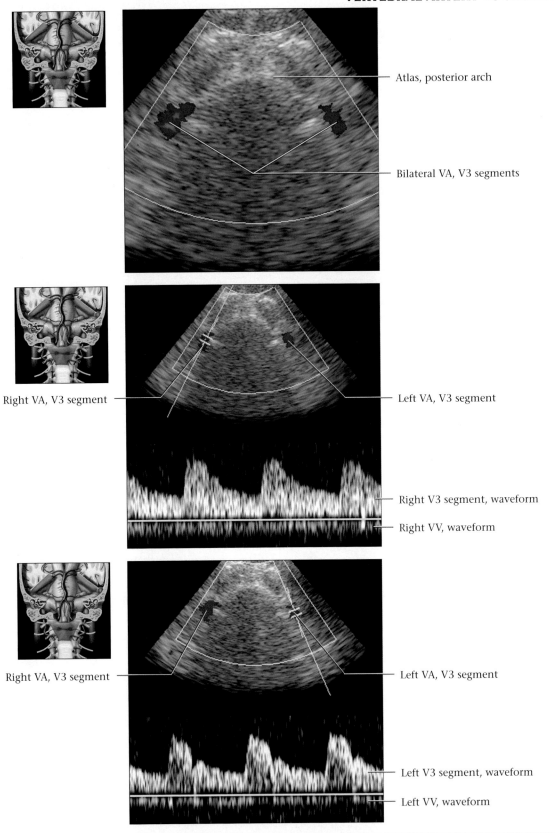

Atlas, posterior arch

Bilateral VA, V3 segments

Right VA, V3 segment — — Left VA, V3 segment

Right V3 segment, waveform

Right VV, waveform

Right VA, V3 segment — — Left VA, V3 segment

Left V3 segment, waveform

Left VV, waveform

(Top) Axial color Doppler ultrasound (suboccipital approach) at a level just above the atlas shows the two short extraspinal V3 segments exiting from the transverse foramina of the atlas and running posteromedially at the horizontal groove on the posterior arch (atlas). The flow direction of these vessels is toward the transducer. **(Middle)** Corresponding spectral Doppler ultrasound of the right V3 segment demonstrates the characteristic antegrade low-resistance flow pattern of this vessel. Note Doppler signal from the ipsilateral vertebral vein is frequently inseparable from the arterial signal and is detected on the opposite side of the trace. **(Bottom)** Corresponding spectral Doppler ultrasound of the left V3 segment shows similar waveform as the contralateral artery.

VERTEBROBASILAR SYSTEM

VERTEBRAL ARTERY V4 SEGMENT

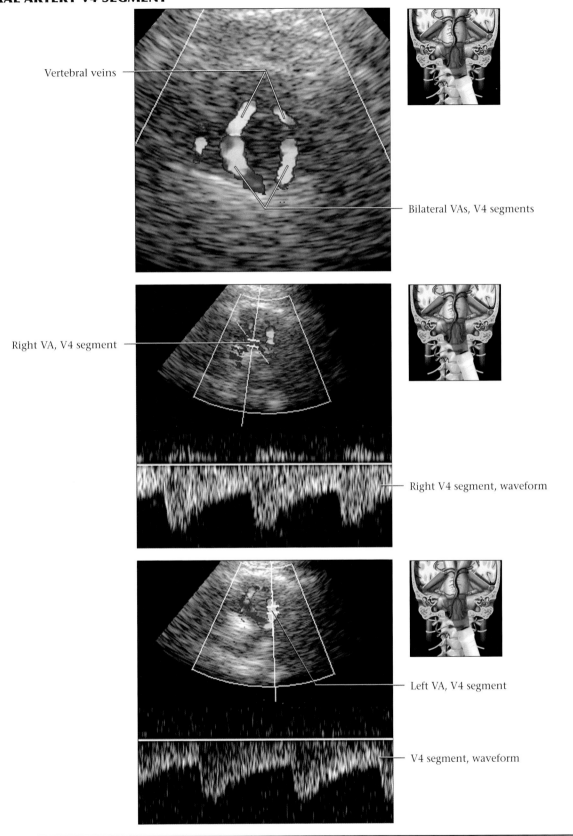

Vertebral veins

Bilateral VAs, V4 segments

Right VA, V4 segment

Right V4 segment, waveform

Left VA, V4 segment

V4 segment, waveform

(Top) Axial color Doppler ultrasound (suboccipital approach) through foramen magnum shows the two intradural V4 segments of VA with flow directed away from the transducer. The two vertebral veins formed in the suboccipital triangle from numerous small tributaries are also visualized with flow toward the transducer. **(Middle)** Corresponding spectral Doppler waveform of the right V4 segment shows the normal antegrade low-resistance flow pattern similar to V3 segment, but with opposite flow direction, as evident by the negative tracing. **(Bottom)** Corresponding spectral Doppler waveform of the left V4 segment shows similar findings as the contralateral artery.

VERTEBROBASILAR ARTERY, COLOR DOPPLER

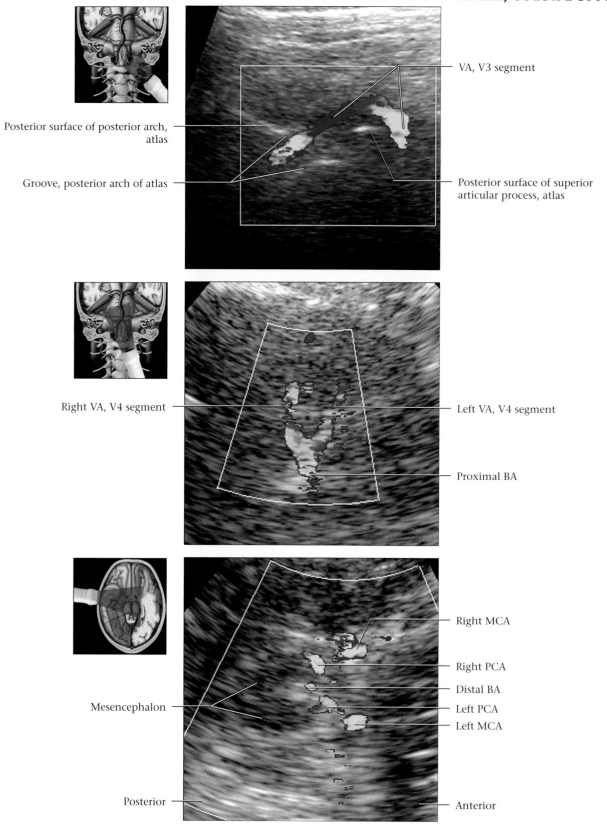

VA, V3 segment

Posterior surface of posterior arch, atlas

Groove, posterior arch of atlas

Posterior surface of superior articular process, atlas

Right VA, V4 segment

Left VA, V4 segment

Proximal BA

Right MCA

Right PCA

Distal BA

Left PCA

Left MCA

Mesencephalon

Posterior

Anterior

(Top) Axial color Doppler ultrasound (extracranial posterolateral approach) shows the V3 segment of VA looping around the superior articular process of atlas after exiting the transverse foramen of the atlas and lying on the groove of the posterior arch (atlas). Flow direction in the proximal loop is toward the transducer (blue color) while it is away in the distal loop (red color). (Middle) Axial color Doppler ultrasound (suboccipital approach) through the foramen magnum shows the convergence of the two V4 segments to form the BA giving rise to a "Y" configuration. The AICA occasionally can be seen branching off from this segment in a posterolateral manner. (Bottom) Axial color Doppler ultrasound (transtemporal approach) of distal BA. The artery is seen terminating into two PCAs in the interpeduncular cistern, just anterior to the cerebral peduncles.

VERTEBROBASILAR SYSTEM

VERTEBROBASILAR ARTERY, SPECTRAL DOPPLER

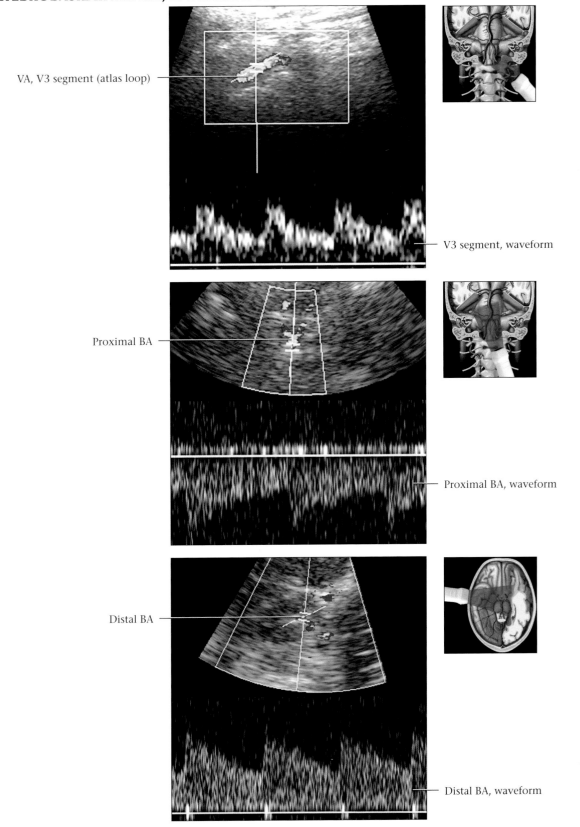

VA, V3 segment (atlas loop)

V3 segment, waveform

Proximal BA

Proximal BA, waveform

Distal BA

Distal BA, waveform

(Top) Axial spectral Doppler ultrasound of the V3 segment (atlas loop) using extracranial posterolateral approach. The flow is of low resistance and directed away from the transducer as shown by the inverted waveform of the trace. Note V3 segment is a common site for extracranial VA stenosis. **(Middle)** Axial spectral Doppler ultrasound of the proximal BA (suboccipital approach). The flow direction of the BA is the same as the V4 that is directed away from the transducer but the magnitude of BA velocity is higher than that of VA. Note flow in the BA may be reversed or alternating in severe subclavian steal. **(Bottom)** Axial spectral Doppler ultrasound (transtemporal approach) shows the antegrade waveform of the distal BA, which is different to the proximal BA assessed by suboccipital approach. Note flow direction of the vessel is dependent on the scanning approach used.

INTRACRANIAL VEINS

Terminology

Abbreviations

- Superior sagittal sinus (SSS); sphenoparietal sinus (SPS); straight sinus (SS); transverse sinus (TS); cavernous sinus (CS); cerebral vein (CV)

Definitions

- Dural venous sinuses
  - Venous channels which drain intracranial veins
  - Lie between two layers of dura mater
  - Postero-superior sinuses: SSS, inferior sagittal, two TS, SS and occipital
  - Antero-inferior sinuses: Two CS, two superior petrosal, two inter-CS, two inferior petrosal and basilar plexus
- Intracranial veins: Cerebral and cerebellar veins
  - Valveless veins which pierce arachnoid membrane and meningeal layer of dura mater
  - Open into the cranial venous sinuses
  - External cerebral veins
    - Superior CV: 8-12 in number; mainly lodged in sulci between gyri; open into SSS
    - Middle CV: Runs along lateral cerebral fissure; ends in CS or SPS; connected with SSS by vein of Trolard or with TS by vein of Labbé
    - Inferior CV: Small; join superior CVs and open into SSS or anastomose with middle CV and basal veins and empty into CS, SPS and superior petrosal sinuses
  - Internal cerebral veins (ICV)
    - Drain deep parts of the hemisphere and are in pair
    - Each formed near the interventricular foramen by the union of the terminal and choroid veins
    - Run parallel with each other posteriorly beneath splenium of the corpus callosum
    - Each receives corresponding basal vein of Rosenthal (BV) before uniting to form great vein of Galen (GV)
  - Basal vein of Rosenthal
    - Formed in lateral cerebral fissures (medial portion)
    - Courses posteriorly around mesencephalon
    - Receives anterior cerebral vein (ACV), deep middle cerebral vein (dMCV), inferior striate veins
    - Also receives tributaries from interpeduncular fossa, inferior horn of the lateral ventricle, hippocampal gyrus and mesencephalon
    - Each ends in its ICV which drains in the GV
    - Many variations: May drain in SPS, lateral mesencephalic vein, contralateral BV
  - Great vein of Galen
    - Receives ICVs, BV, pericallosal veins, and veins draining superior aspect of posterior fossa
    - Curves backward and upward around splenium of corpus callosum
    - Finally drains into SS
  - Cerebellar veins
    - Located on cerebellar surface: Superior and inferior
    - Superior cerebellar veins run anteromedially across the superior vermis to end in SS and ICVs
    - Inferior cerebellar veins (larger) end in TS, superior petrosal, and occipital sinuses

Imaging Anatomy

Overview

- Intracranial venous structures can be insonated through transtemporal window
- Detection rate decreases with advancing age
- Basal vein of Rosenthal
  - Divided into 2 segments
    - Anterior (striate or prepeduncular) segment: From union of inferior striate vein, ACV & dMCV to anterior mesencephalon; flow toward transducer
    - Posterior segment: From lateral mesencephalic vein to point of entrance to GV or inferior CV; flow away from transducer
  - Easily accessible near P2 segments of posterior cerebral artery (PCA)
  - Lateral mesencephalic vein enters BV at the lateral margin of mesencephalon
  - About 90% of BV drain into GV but anastomoses between anterior and posterior segments highly variable
- Great cerebral vein of Galen
  - Located by following BV posteriorly to its point of entrance to GV
  - Identified in midline posterior to pineal region, appears as highly echogenic structure rostral to 3rd ventricle
  - Flow directed away from transducer
  - Common site for congenital arteriovenous malformation
- Deep middle cerebral vein (dMCV)
  - Runs parallel and posterior to middle cerebral artery (MCA)
  - Flow directed away from transducer
  - Venous signal usually contaminated with adjacent arterial signal
- Anterior cerebral vein (ACV)
  - Runs parallel to anterior cerebral artery
  - Drains into 1st segment of BV
  - Flow directed toward transducer
- Sphenoparietal sinus (SPS)
  - Seen along under surface of sphenoid (lesser wing)
  - Flow directed away from transducer

Anatomy-Based Imaging Issues

Imaging Recommendations

- Lowest possible pulse repetition frequency used to detect low-velocity venous flow
- Color gain optimized to reduce color noise
- Enhanced venous flow with patient performing Valsalva maneuver

Clinical Implications

Clinical Importance

- For diagnosis and monitoring of cerebral venous thrombosis
- For evaluation of venous hemodynamics in patients with supratentorial stroke and head injuries
- For pre-operative assessment of skull base surgery

INTRACRANIAL VEINS

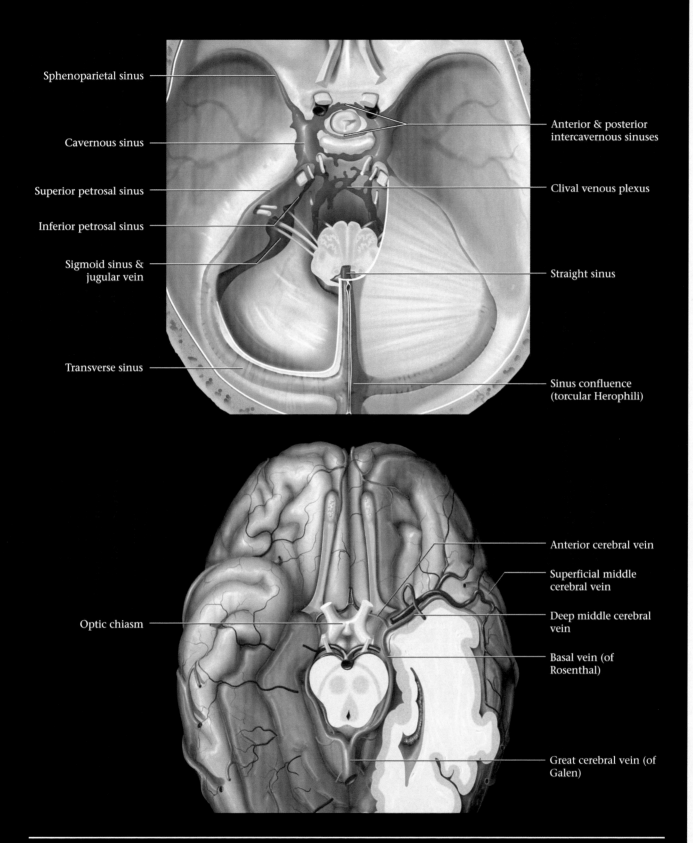

Sphenoparietal sinus

Cavernous sinus

Superior petrosal sinus

Inferior petrosal sinus

Sigmoid sinus & jugular vein

Transverse sinus

Anterior & posterior intercavernous sinuses

Clival venous plexus

Straight sinus

Sinus confluence (torcular Herophili)

Optic chiasm

Anterior cerebral vein

Superficial middle cerebral vein

Deep middle cerebral vein

Basal vein (of Rosenthal)

Great cerebral vein (of Galen)

(Top) Graphic shows the superior intracranial view of the dural venous sinuses. The cerebral hemispheres, midbrain and pons as well as the left half of the tentorium cerebelli have been removed. Note the numerous interconnections between both halves of the cavernous sinus, the clival venous plexus, and the petrosal sinuses. **(Bottom)** Graphic shows the inferior intracranial view of the deep venous structures. Intracranial veins are valveless veins which pierce the arachnoid membrane and meningeal layer of the dura mater. They include the external cerebral veins, internal cerebral veins, anterior cerebral vein, deep middle cerebral vein, basal vein of Rosenthal, great cerebral vein and cerebellar veins. They drain into the cranial venous sinuses.

Brain and Spine

I

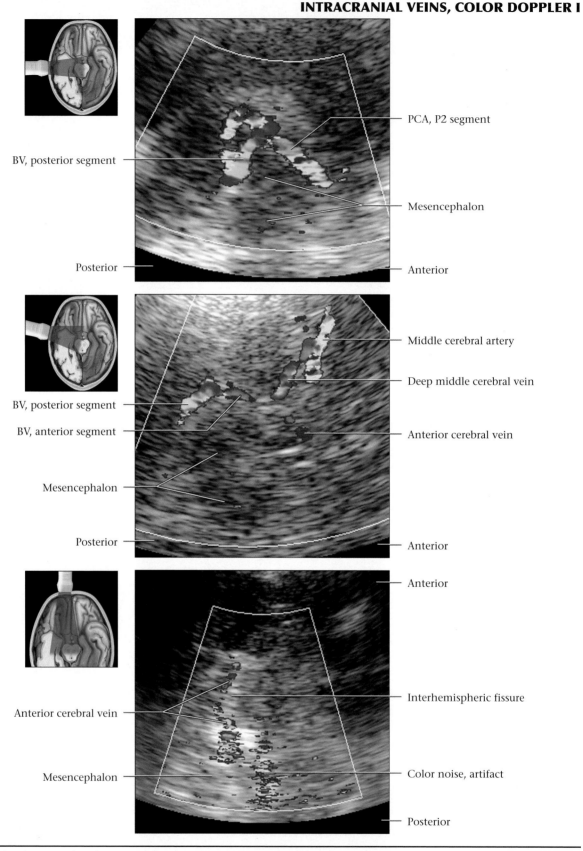

BV, posterior segment

PCA, P2 segment

Mesencephalon

Posterior

Anterior

BV, posterior segment

Middle cerebral artery

BV, anterior segment

Deep middle cerebral vein

Anterior cerebral vein

Mesencephalon

Posterior

Anterior

Anterior

Anterior cerebral vein

Interhemispheric fissure

Mesencephalon

Color noise, artifact

Posterior

(Top) Axial color Doppler ultrasound (transtemporal approach) shows the posterior segment of BV. The vein is seen surrounding the mesencephalon and runs almost parallel to PCA. The blue color coding of the vessel indicates flow directed away from the transducer. **(Middle)** Axial color Doppler ultrasound (transtemporal approach) with more anterior tilting from the plane of the previous image shows the ACV. The ACV is seen running posteriorly to join the dMCV before draining into the anterior segment of BV. The flow in the ACV and anterior segment of BV is directed toward the transducer as denoted by the red color coding. **(Bottom)** Axial color Doppler ultrasound (paramedian frontal approach) shows the ACV which courses posteriorly within the interhemispheric fissure. This small vein after joining the dMCV forms the BV. Identification of this vessel is difficult due to its slow flow.

Brain and Spine

I

INTRACRANIAL VEINS

INTRACRANIAL VEINS, SPECTRAL DOPPLER I

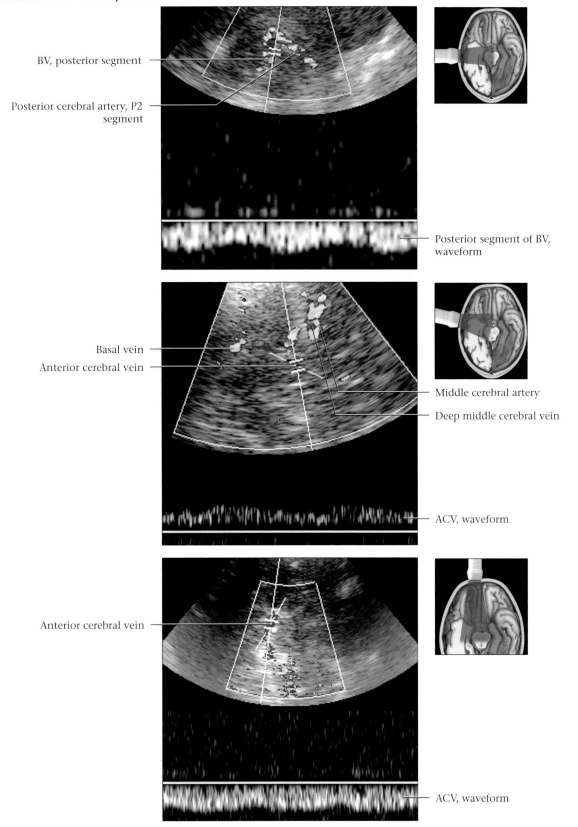

BV, posterior segment

Posterior cerebral artery, P2 segment

Posterior segment of BV, waveform

Basal vein
Anterior cerebral vein

Middle cerebral artery

Deep middle cerebral vein

ACV, waveform

Anterior cerebral vein

ACV, waveform

(Top) Axial spectral Doppler ultrasound (transtemporal approach) shows waveform of the BV (posterior segment) with typical respiratory phasicity. (Middle) Axial spectral Doppler ultrasound (transtemporal approach) shows Doppler waveform of the ACV. Note the waveform is on the positive scale representing flow toward the transducer. (Bottom) Axial spectral Doppler ultrasound shows waveform of the ACV obtained from the paramedian frontal approach shows the flow away from the transducer. Note flow direction of a vessel depends on the scanning approach used and the ACV flow is toward the transducer using transtemporal approach but away from the transducer using transfrontal approach.

INTRACRANIAL VEINS

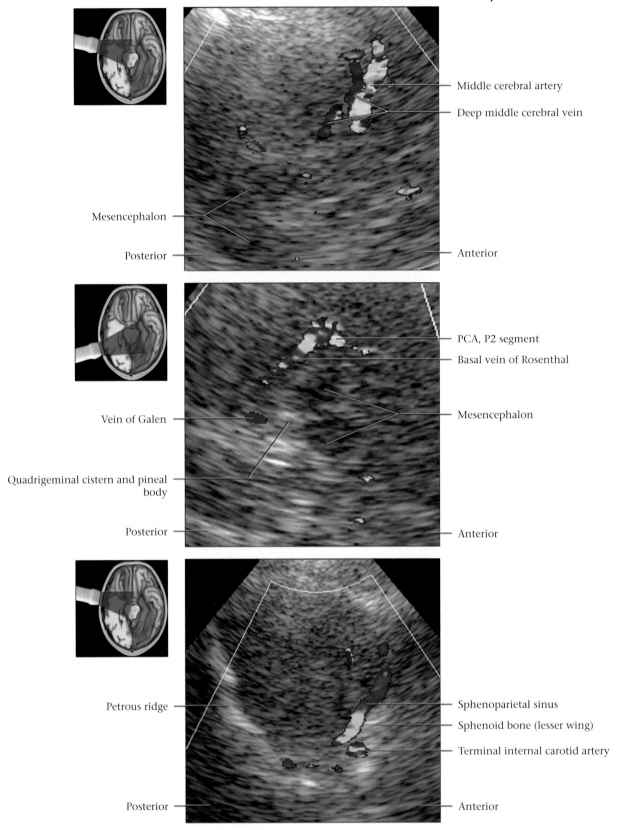

Middle cerebral artery

Deep middle cerebral vein

Mesencephalon

Posterior

Anterior

PCA, P2 segment

Basal vein of Rosenthal

Mesencephalon

Vein of Galen

Quadrigeminal cistern and pineal body

Posterior

Anterior

Petrous ridge

Sphenoparietal sinus

Sphenoid bone (lesser wing)

Terminal internal carotid artery

Posterior

Anterior

(Top) Axial color Doppler ultrasound (transtemporal approach) shows the dMCV, which normally appears dorsal and parallel to the MCA. Note separation of the dMCV signal from the adjacent arterial signal may not be possible. (Middle) Axial color Doppler ultrasound (transtemporal approach) on standard mesencephalic plane shows GV. It is identified in the midline, posterior to the echogenic triangular quadrigeminal cistern and pineal body, with flow directed away from the transducer. (Bottom) Axial color Doppler ultrasound (transtemporal approach) shows the SPS running along the lesser wing of the sphenoid bone with flow directed away from the transducer. The SPS is a venous sinus draining into the cavernous sinus and may receive venous drainage from the BV as a normal variant.

INTRACRANIAL VEINS, SPECTRAL DOPPLER II

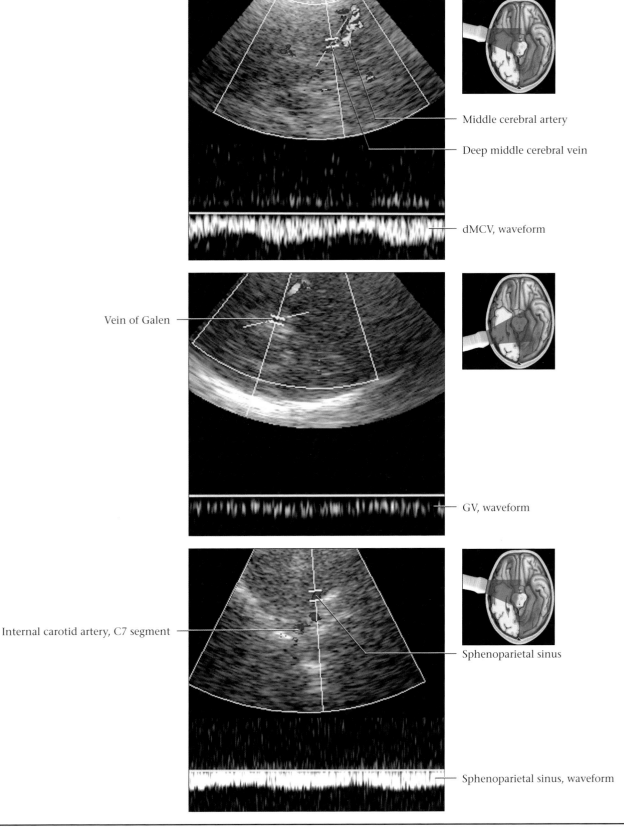

Middle cerebral artery

Deep middle cerebral vein

dMCV, waveform

Vein of Galen

GV, waveform

Internal carotid artery, C7 segment

Sphenoparietal sinus

Sphenoparietal sinus, waveform

(Top) Axial spectral Doppler ultrasound (transtemporal approach) shows waveform of the dMCV with typical respiratory phasicity on the negative trace signifying flow away from the transducer. (Middle) Axial spectral Doppler ultrasound (transtemporal approach) shows GV with constant waveform on the negative trace signifying flow away from the transducer. (Bottom) Axial spectral Doppler ultrasound (transtemporal approach) shows SPS waveform on the negative trace signifying flow away from the transducer.

Brain and Spine

I

VERTEBRAL BODIES, SPINAL CORD & CAUDA EQUINA

Gross Anatomy

Overview
- **Vertebral body**
  - Varies in size, shape depending on region
- **Cervical:** Upper 7 vertebrae
  - **C1 (atlas):** No body, spinous process; circular shape
    - Anterior, posterior arches; 2 lateral masses; transverse processes
  - **C2 (axis):** Body with bony peg (dens/odontoid process)
    - Large, flat ovoid articular facets, broad pedicles, thick laminae
    - Transverse processes contain L-shaped foramina for vertebral artery
  - **C3-6** similar in size, shape
    - Bodies small, thin relative to size of arch, uncinate processes superolaterally
    - Lateral masses rhomboid-shaped with slanted superior/inferior articular surfaces
  - **C7** marked by longest spinous process
- **Thoracic**
  - Bodies heart-shaped, central canal round, short pedicles, broad laminae
  - Costal articular facets on body/transverse processes
- **Lumbar**
  - Body large, wide, thick
  - Pedicles strong, thick, directed posteriorly
  - Laminae strong, broad
- **Sacrum:** Fusion of 5 segments
  - Large triangular shaped bone with base, apex, 3 surfaces (pelvic, dorsal, lateral), 2 alae
  - Base: Round/ovoid; articulates with L5
- **Coccyx:** Fusion of 3-5 segments
  - Apex round, directed caudally, may be bifid
- **Spinal Cord**
  - Suspended within thecal sac
  - Anchored to dura by denticulate ligaments
  - Two enlargements: Cervical enlargement (C3-T2) and lumbar enlargement (T9-12)
  - Cord tapers to diamond-shaped point (conus medullaris), normally ends at T12 to L2-3, most common at T12-L1
- **Filum terminale**
  - Strands of connective tissue extending inferiorly from conus
  - Fuse distally into dura, attaches to dorsal coccyx
- **Cauda equina**
  - "Horse's tail" of lumbar, sacral, coccygeal nerve roots below conus

Imaging Anatomy

Overview
- **Cord:** Relatively hypoechoic
  - Central echogenic complex in center of cord: Interface between myelinated ventral white commissure and central end of anterior median fissure
  - Central spinal canal: Column of fluid within center of central echo complex, seen using high frequency transducer
- Conus medullaris: Terminal part of cord, should taper gradually
- **Filum terminale:** Relatively hypoechoic center with more echogenic outer margin
  - Mobile with CSF pulsation on real time US
  - Should be less than 2 mm in diameter
- **Cauda equina:** Echogenic interface created by divergent nerve rootlets
  - Drape dependently within thecal sac, undulate with each CSF pulsation
- **Vertebral body:** Ossified vertebral body appears echogenic
  - Cartilaginous tip at spinous process appears hypoechoic
- **Cartilaginous coccyx:** Hypoechoic
  - Variable ossification patterns
    - Ossified coccygeal vertebral bodies have rounded central nucleus rather than square contour as in sacrum

Anatomy-Based Imaging Issues

Imaging Recommendations
- Non-ossified state of posterior-median intraneural synchondrosis provides ample acoustic window in newborns
- Spinal cord is best visualized by US within the first month after birth for term infants
- Transverse scan of spinal cord is possible in older infant as cartilaginous gap in vertebral ring allows penetration of US beam
- Determination of position of tip of conus medullaris should always be included in neonatal spine US
  - Conus located over upper third of L3 vertebral body with normal nerve-root pulsation requires no further imaging
  - Conus tip at L3-proper requires follow-up imaging
  - Conus tip at L3/4 disc space is abnormal and requires further MR evaluation

Imaging Approaches
- Infants are preferably scanned in prone position
- Decubitus position is adopted to calm a struggling baby by bottle or breast feeding
- High frequency linear US transducer is used to scan the back both longitudinally and transversely
- Ways to define vertebral levels where conus ends
  - Count downwards from 12th rib
  - Count upwards after defining lumbosacral junction by accentuating lumbar lordosis by elevation of shoulders
- Craniocervical junction can be assessed by scanning base of skull through foramen magnum

Imaging Pitfalls
- Counting of vertebral level upwards from the last ossified vertebral body can be misleading due to variability in ossification of coccygeal vertebral bodies
- Visualization of spinal canal and its content is difficult in older infants due to acoustic shadowing from ossified laminae and loss of acoustic window from intraneural synchondrosis

VERTEBRAL COLUMN & SPINAL CORD

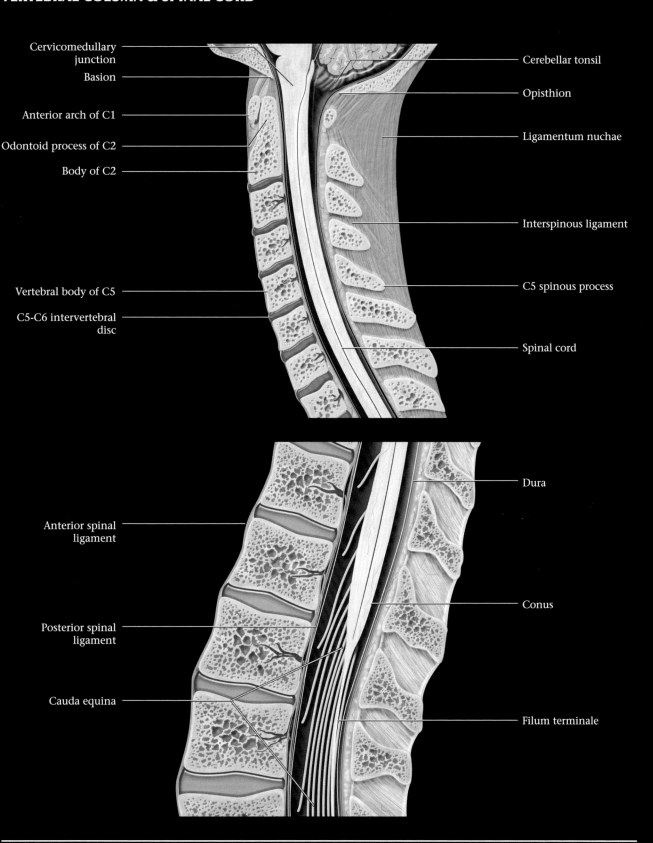

Cervicomedullary junction

Basion

Anterior arch of C1

Odontoid process of C2

Body of C2

Vertebral body of C5

C5-C6 intervertebral disc

Cerebellar tonsil

Opisthion

Ligamentum nuchae

Interspinous ligament

C5 spinous process

Spinal cord

Anterior spinal ligament

Posterior spinal ligament

Cauda equina

Dura

Conus

Filum terminale

(Top) Sagittal midline graphic of the cervical spine and cord showing gentle lordotic curve and smooth alignment of the adjacent vertebrae. The cerebellar tonsils are normally above the line between the basion and opisthion. There is smooth transit of the cervicomedullary junction without kinking. **(Bottom)** Sagittal graphic of the thoracolumbar junction demonstrates normal conus and cauda equina anatomy. The filum terminale lies among the cauda equina roots and affixes the conus to the terminal thecal sac.

Brain and Spine

I

141

VERTEBRAL BODIES, SPINAL CORD & CAUDA EQUINA

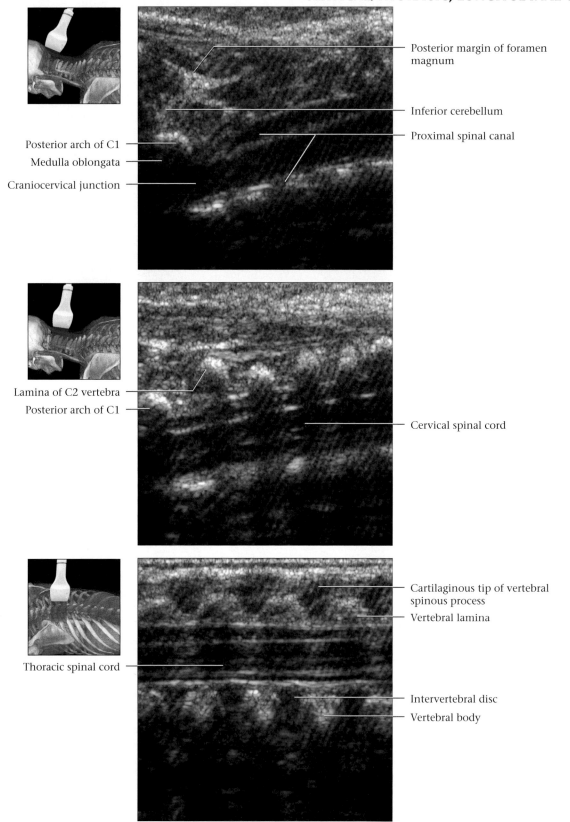

Posterior arch of C1

Medulla oblongata

Craniocervical junction

Posterior margin of foramen magnum

Inferior cerebellum

Proximal spinal canal

Lamina of C2 vertebra

Posterior arch of C1

Cervical spinal cord

Cartilaginous tip of vertebral spinous process

Vertebral lamina

Thoracic spinal cord

Intervertebral disc

Vertebral body

(Top) Longitudinal ultrasound at the craniocervical junction, the spinal cord starts just below the foramen magnum. The inferior cerebellum and medulla oblongata can also be seen. **(Middle)** Longitudinal ultrasound at the cervical portion of the spinal cord. Note the prominent lamina at C2 vertebral level. **(Bottom)** Longitudinal ultrasound at the mid thoracic level of the spinal cord. The diameter of the thoracic spinal cord is the narrowest. There is normal cord enlargement more superiorly (C3 to T2) and inferiorly (T9 to T12).

Brain and Spine

I

142

VERTEBRAL BODIES, SPINAL CORD & CAUDA EQUINA

CERVICAL/THORACIC, SAGITTAL T2 MR

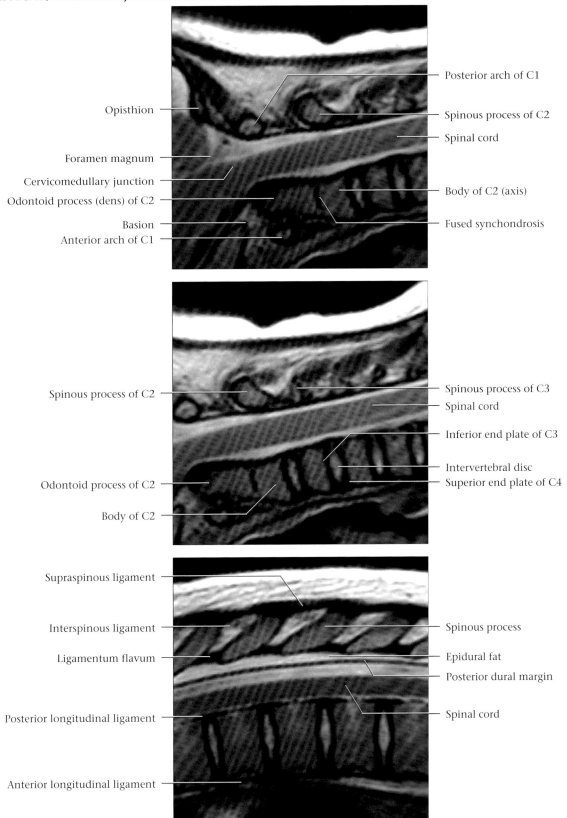

Opisthion

Posterior arch of C1

Spinous process of C2

Spinal cord

Foramen magnum

Cervicomedullary junction

Odontoid process (dens) of C2

Body of C2 (axis)

Basion

Fused synchondrosis

Anterior arch of C1

Spinous process of C2

Spinous process of C3

Spinal cord

Inferior end plate of C3

Intervertebral disc

Superior end plate of C4

Odontoid process of C2

Body of C2

Supraspinous ligament

Interspinous ligament

Spinous process

Ligamentum flavum

Epidural fat

Posterior dural margin

Posterior longitudinal ligament

Spinal cord

Anterior longitudinal ligament

(Top) First of three sagittal T2 MR images of the cervical and thoracic spine presented from superior to inferior. Images are taken through planes/levels corresponding to those commonly used for US scan. Images are presented in prone position. Image at the craniocervical junction shows spacious CSF signal at the foramen magnum. There is smooth transition of the cervicomedullary junction. The cerebellar tonsils should be normally above the line between basion and opisthion. **(Middle)** This image at the cervical junction shows the cervical enlargement of the spinal cord from C3 downwards. **(Bottom)** This image at mid thoracic level shows this segment of the spinal cord is more narrow when compared with the higher level (C3 to T2) and lower level (T9 to T12).

VERTEBRAL BODIES, SPINAL CORD & CAUDA EQUINA

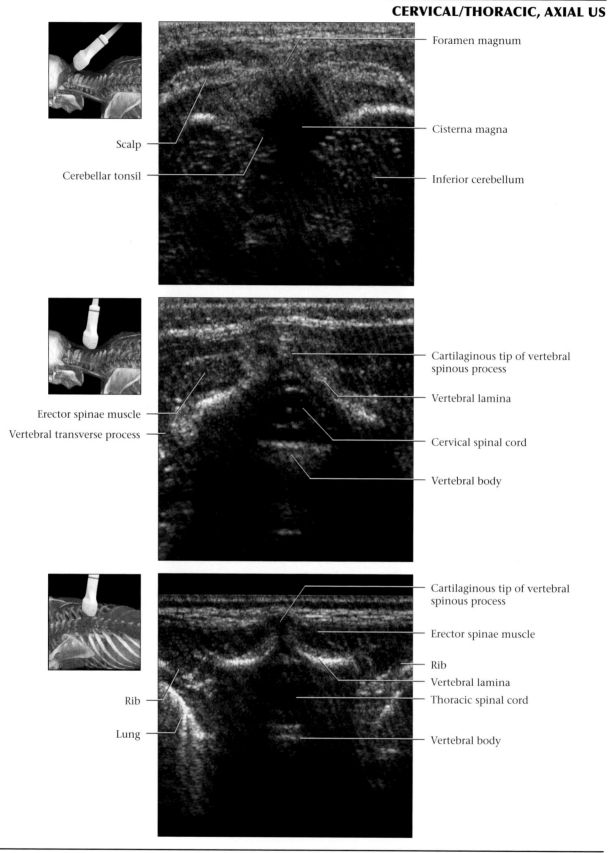

Foramen magnum

Cisterna magna

Inferior cerebellum

Scalp

Cerebellar tonsil

Cartilaginous tip of vertebral spinous process

Vertebral lamina

Cervical spinal cord

Vertebral body

Erector spinae muscle

Vertebral transverse process

Cartilaginous tip of vertebral spinous process

Erector spinae muscle

Rib

Vertebral lamina

Thoracic spinal cord

Vertebral body

Rib

Lung

(Top) Transverse ultrasound image at the foramen magnum level. The cisterna magna is seen between two echogenic inferior cerebellar hemispheres. Below this level begins the cervical spinal cord. This is the most useful view for evaluating the upper spinal canal. (Middle) Transverse ultrasound of the mid cervical spine. The vertebral body is small compared with the transverse processes and neural arch. The spinous process appears hypoechoic in the midline since it is still cartilaginous. Both the lamina and the vertebral body appear highly echogenic. The erector spinae muscle has intermediate echogenicity, and is directly above the lamina. (Bottom) Transverse ultrasound of the mid thoracic spine with echogenic ribs on both sides. Air inside the lungs appears echogenic with ring down artifact.

VERTEBRAL BODIES, SPINAL CORD & CAUDA EQUINA

CERVICAL/THORACIC, AXIAL T2 MR

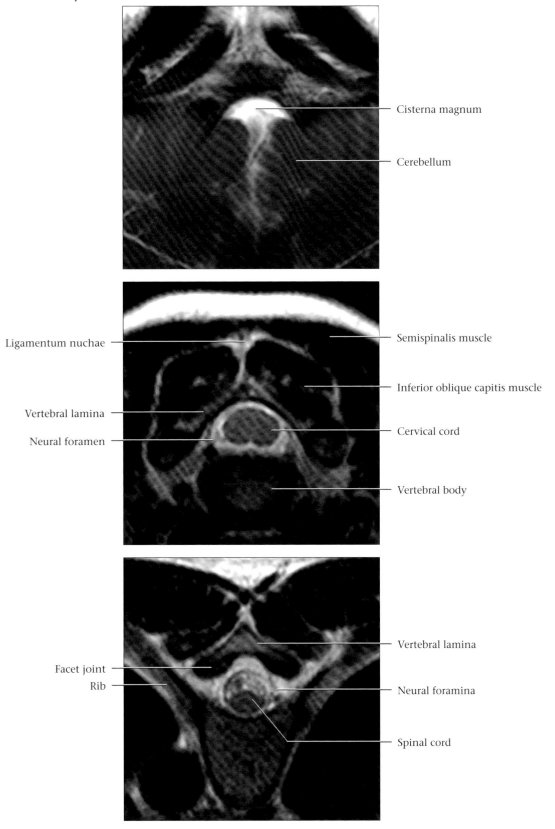

Cisterna magnum

Cerebellum

Ligamentum nuchae

Semispinalis muscle

Inferior oblique capitis muscle

Vertebral lamina

Cervical cord

Neural foramen

Vertebral body

Vertebral lamina

Facet joint

Rib

Neural foramina

Spinal cord

(Top) A set of three axial T2 MR image of lumbar, sacral and coccygeal spine from superior to inferior. Images are taken through planes/levels corresponding to those commonly used for US scan. Images are presented in prone position. This image at the level of the foramen magnum shows the relationship of the cisterna magnum and cerebellar hemispheres. (Middle) Axial image through the neural foramina of C3 shows the neural foraminae are orientated approximately 45 degrees anterolaterally. The cord is enlarged at this level, related to the abundant innervation for the upper limbs. (Bottom) Axial image through foraminal level of the mid thoracic spine shows the neural foraminae are directed laterally. The transverse processes extend out dorsolaterally to articulate with medial ribs. Note the cord is smaller in cross-sectional area and the CSF space around the cord is more capacious.

Brain and Spine

I

Spinal cord

Dorsal cauda equina

Conus

Central echogenic complex

Ventral cauda equina

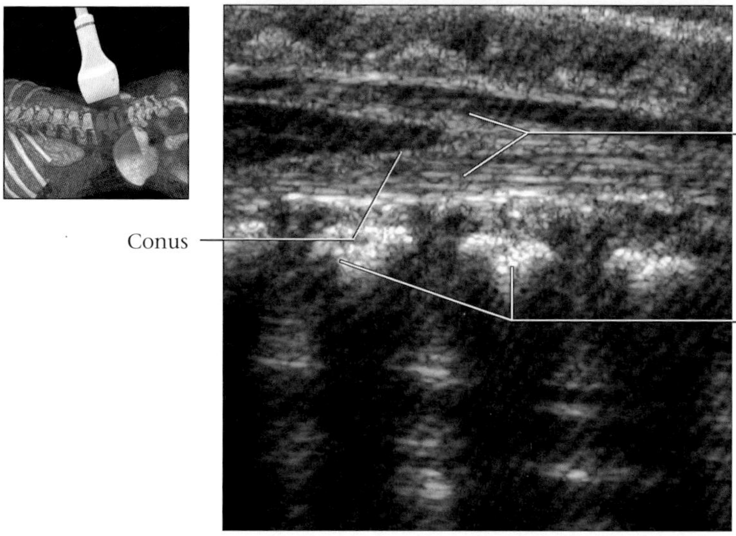

Cauda equina

Conus

Vertebral body

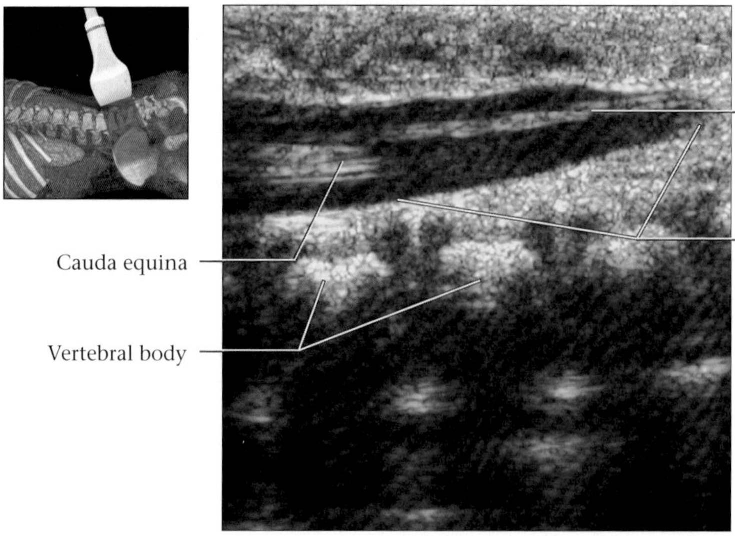

Filum terminale

Terminal theca sac

Cauda equina

Vertebral body

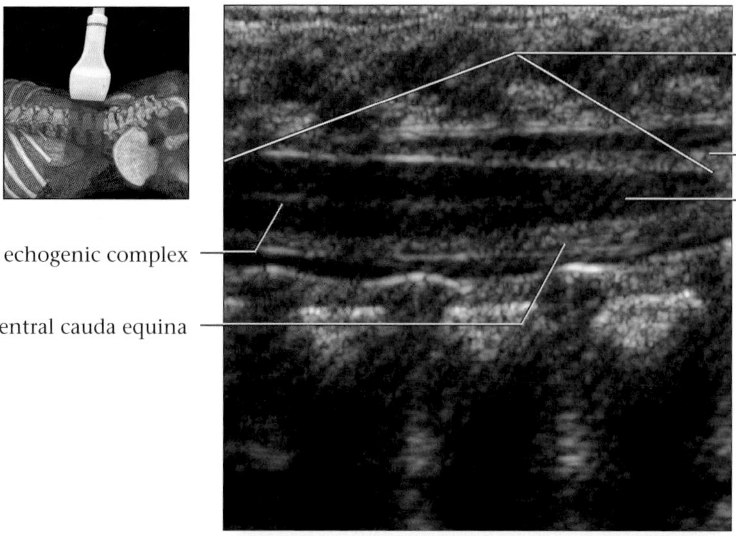

(Top) This is the most cranial longitudinal ultrasound image showing the normal hypoechoic spinal cord with hyperechoic central echo complex. The latter is a reflection of echoes from the interface between the ventral white commissure and CSF within the ventral median fissure. This should not be mistaken for the central canal. **(Middle)** This image centered more caudally demonstrates the hypoechoic spinal cord terminating at the conus. The hyperechoic cauda equina drapes around the conus and undulates with each CSF pulsation during real-time ultrasound. **(Bottom)** This image is acquired at the end of the thecal sac. The mildly hyperechoic filum terminale anchors the spinal cord to the terminal thecal sac. The cauda equina nerve roots drape dependently within the thecal sac.

VERTEBRAL BODIES, SPINAL CORD & CAUDA EQUINA

CONUS, SAGITTAL T2 MR

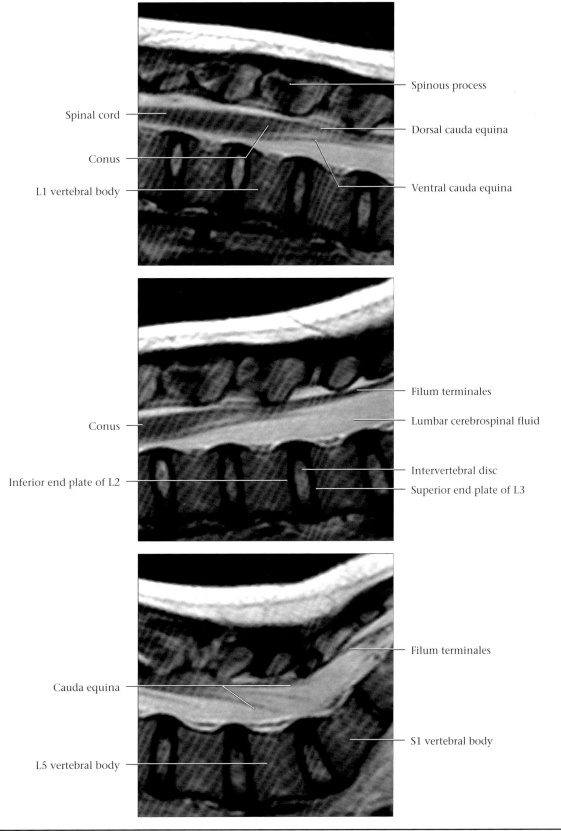

Spinous process

Spinal cord

Dorsal cauda equina

Conus

L1 vertebral body

Ventral cauda equina

Conus

Filum terminales

Lumbar cerebrospinal fluid

Inferior end plate of L2

Intervertebral disc

Superior end plate of L3

Filum terminales

Cauda equina

S1 vertebral body

L5 vertebral body

(Top) First in a series of three sagittal T2 MR images at the lumbosacral region. Images are taken through planes/levels corresponding to those commonly used for US scan. First image shows the position of the conus medullaris which terminates at the normal level of L1. The spinal cord & cauda equina are well-delineated & appear hypointense in contrast to hyperintense CSF. **(Middle)** Sagittal T2 MR image through the lumbar region shows that the prominent filum terminale anchors the spinal cord to the terminal thecal sac. The cauda equina nerve roots are present on both ventral & dorsal side of the conus & float freely in the distal thecal sac. **(Bottom)** Sagittal T2 MR image through the lumbosacral junction shows the filum terminale extends to the distal thecal sac, fuses into dura & is attached to the dorsal coccyx. The nerve roots of cauda equina have the classical "horse's tail" appearance.

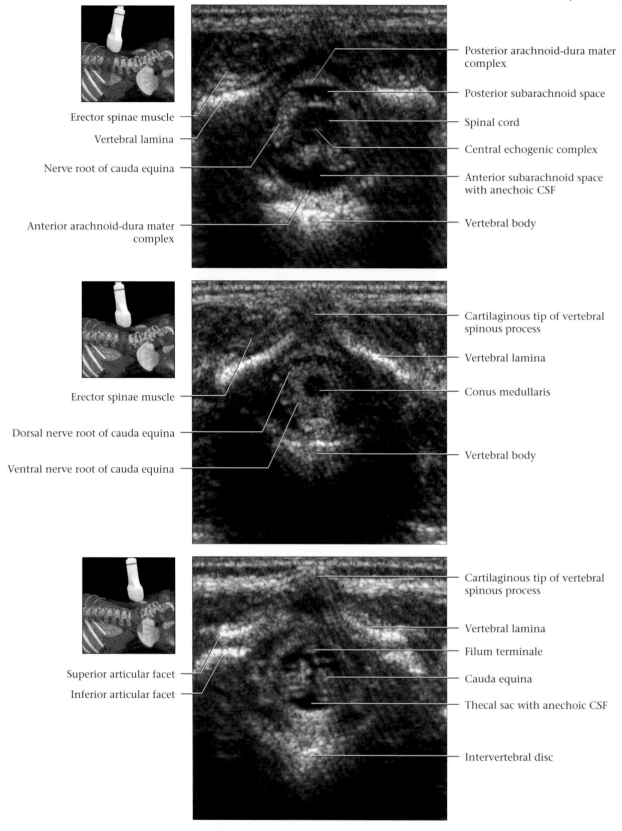

Erector spinae muscle

Vertebral lamina

Nerve root of cauda equina

Anterior arachnoid-dura mater complex

Posterior arachnoid-dura mater complex

Posterior subarachnoid space

Spinal cord

Central echogenic complex

Anterior subarachnoid space with anechoic CSF

Vertebral body

Erector spinae muscle

Dorsal nerve root of cauda equina

Ventral nerve root of cauda equina

Cartilaginous tip of vertebral spinous process

Vertebral lamina

Conus medullaris

Vertebral body

Superior articular facet

Inferior articular facet

Cartilaginous tip of vertebral spinous process

Vertebral lamina

Filum terminale

Cauda equina

Thecal sac with anechoic CSF

Intervertebral disc

(Top) Axial ultrasound at lumbar level shows the normal hypoechoic cord with central echogenic complex. The spinal cord floats freely in the subarachnoid space, which is bound by the dura mater and filled with CSF. The spinal cord is draped around by the echogenic nerve rootlets. (Middle) Axial ultrasound at lower lumbar level shows the conus is draped around by free floating nerve rootlets collectively known as cauda equina. The conus normally should be above L3 level. (Bottom) Axial ultrasound at S2 level shows the filum terminale and nerve rootlets of cauda equina float freely within the thecal sac. The filum terminale is the prolongation of the pia mater and attached to the first coccygeal segment. The filum terminale can be clearly distinguished from the nerve rootlets of the cauda equina and should be less than 2 mm in diameter.

VERTEBRAL BODIES, SPINAL CORD & CAUDA EQUINA

CONUS, AXIAL T2 MR

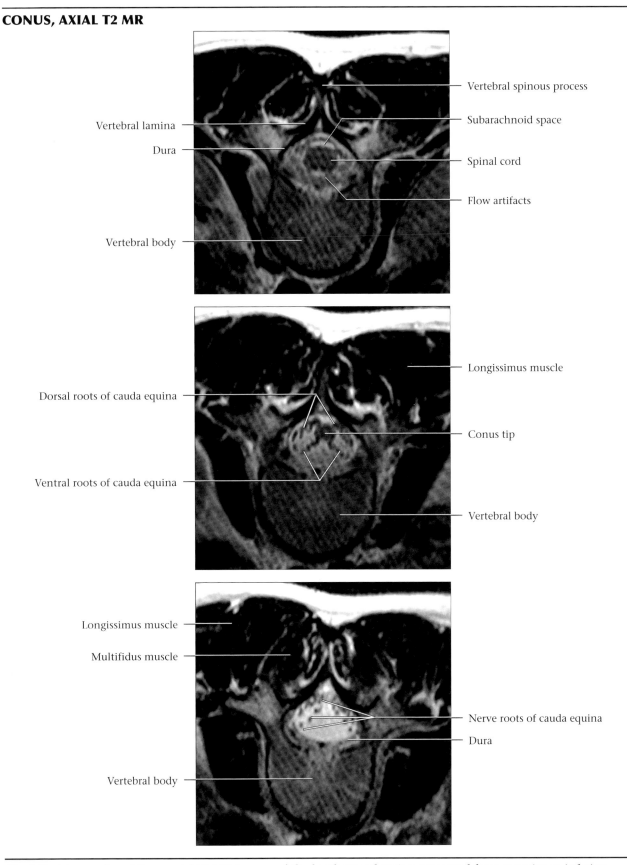

Vertebral spinous process

Subarachnoid space

Spinal cord

Flow artifacts

Vertebral lamina

Dura

Vertebral body

Longissimus muscle

Dorsal roots of cauda equina

Conus tip

Ventral roots of cauda equina

Vertebral body

Longissimus muscle

Multifidus muscle

Nerve roots of cauda equina

Dura

Vertebral body

(Top) First in a series of three axial T2 MR images of the lumbosacral region presented from superior to inferior. Images are taken through planes/levels corresponding to those commonly used for US scan. Images are presented in prone position. This image of the lower thoracic spine demonstrates hypointense dura delineating the thecal sac and its bright CSF contents. Flow artifacts are common around the cord and should not be mistaken for a lesion. (Middle) This image at conus tip, shows the ventral and dorsal nerve roots of the cauda equina are separately positioned xentrally and dorsally respectively within the thecal sac. (Bottom) This image at L4 level shows the nerve roots start losing their ventral/dorsal orientation. The roots assume an inverted "U" shaped configuration around the margin of the thecal sac as the image is in prone position.

LUMBOSACRAL, LONGITUDINAL US

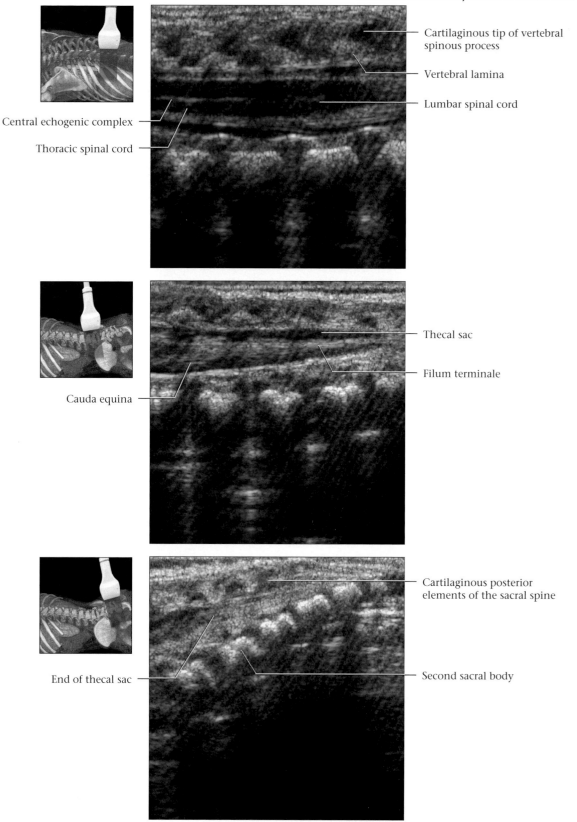

Cartilaginous tip of vertebral spinous process

Vertebral lamina

Lumbar spinal cord

Central echogenic complex

Thoracic spinal cord

Thecal sac

Filum terminale

Cauda equina

Cartilaginous posterior elements of the sacral spine

End of thecal sac

Second sacral body

(Top) Longitudinal ultrasound at the thoraco-lumbar level shows transition in diameter of the spinal cord, from a narrower thoracic to a wider lumbar portion. (Middle) Longitudinal ultrasound at the lower lumbar level showing the thecal sac. The conus terminates at the upper lumbar level. Cauda equina and filum terminale float freely in CSF within the thecal sac. (Bottom) This is the most caudal longitudinal ultrasound showing the five sacral bodies. The hypoechoic area in the posterior part of the sacrum is the cartilaginous element of the sacrum. The thecal sac usually ends at the level of S2 while the filum terminale is continuous down to the first coccygeal segment.

VERTEBRAL BODIES, SPINAL CORD & CAUDA EQUINA

LUMBOSACRAL, SAGITTAL T2 MR

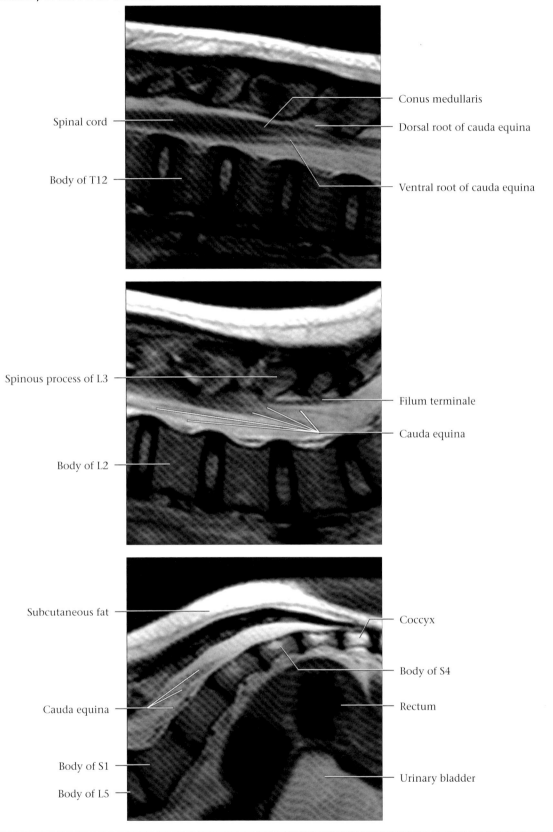

Spinal cord

Body of T12

Conus medullaris

Dorsal root of cauda equina

Ventral root of cauda equina

Spinous process of L3

Body of L2

Filum terminale

Cauda equina

Subcutaneous fat

Cauda equina

Body of S1

Body of L5

Coccyx

Body of S4

Rectum

Urinary bladder

(Top) First of three sagittal T2 MR images of the lower thoracic and lumbosacral spine from superior to inferior. Images are taken through planes/levels corresponding to those commonly used for ultrasound scan. Images are presented in prone positions. In this image, the spinal cord tapers to a diamond-shaped conus medullaris. The cord normally ends between T12 to L2-3, most commonly at level of T12-L1. **(Middle)** This image obtained at the lower lumbar level shows typical "horse-tail" appearance of cauda equina. The filum terminale lies among the cauda equina roots and fixes the conus to the terminal thecal sac. **(Bottom)** This image obtained at the sacral level shows terminal portion of the thecal sac. The lumbosacral junction can be recognized by the transition of sacral kyphosis to lumbar lordosis.

VERTEBRAL BODIES, SPINAL CORD & CAUDA EQUINA

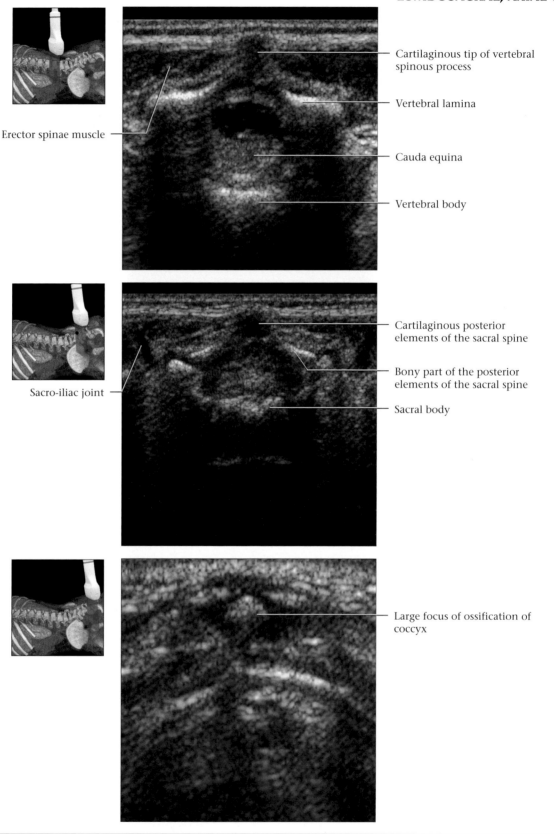

Erector spinae muscle —

— Cartilaginous tip of vertebral spinous process

— Vertebral lamina

— Cauda equina

— Vertebral body

Sacro-iliac joint —

— Cartilaginous posterior elements of the sacral spine

— Bony part of the posterior elements of the sacral spine

— Sacral body

— Large focus of ossification of coccyx

(Top) Transverse ultrasound at the lower lumbar level shows the hypoechoic cartilaginous tip of the spinous process. Within the spinal canal, the echogenic cauda equina lies in the dependent portion of the thecal sac. (Middle) Transverse ultrasound at the sacrum level with the sacro-iliac joints on either side. The posterior elements of the sacrum are divided into two parts: The cartilaginous part in the midline appears hypoechoic while the bony part at the periphery appears echogenic. (Bottom) Transverse ultrasound at the coccyx level. The coccyx appears echogenic due to large focus of ossification nucleus in the first coccygeal segment. The ossified coccygeal vertebral body has a rounded central nucleus rather than a more square contour in the sacral ossification centers.

VERTEBRAL BODIES, SPINAL CORD & CAUDA EQUINA

LUMBOSACRAL, AXIAL T2 MR

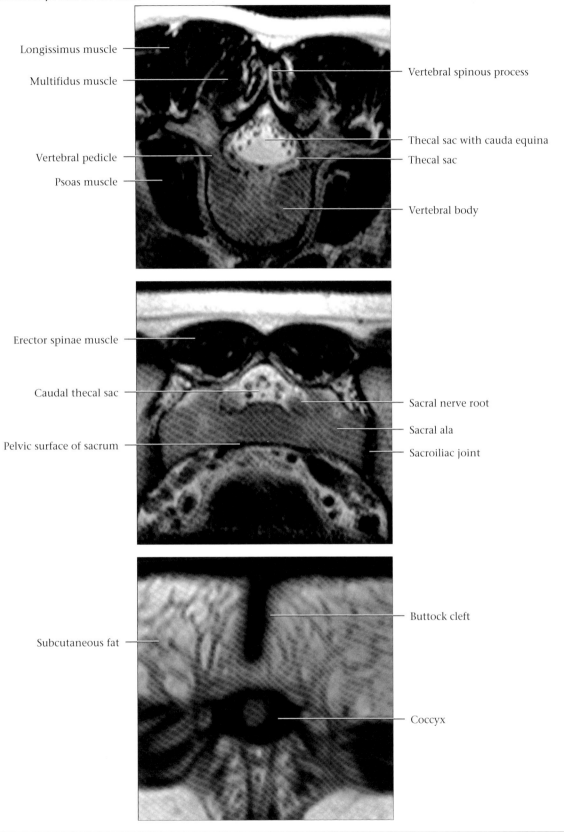

Longissimus muscle

Multifidus muscle

Vertebral pedicle

Psoas muscle

Vertebral spinous process

Thecal sac with cauda equina

Thecal sac

Vertebral body

Erector spinae muscle

Caudal thecal sac

Pelvic surface of sacrum

Sacral nerve root

Sacral ala

Sacroiliac joint

Subcutaneous fat

Buttock cleft

Coccyx

(Top) Series of three axial T2 MR images of the lumbar, sacral and coccygeal spine presented from superior to inferior. Images are taken through planes/levels corresponding to those commonly used for ultrasound scan. Images are presented in prone position. This image at the slumbar level shows the nerve roots of the cauda equina assume an "inverted U" shape configuration at this level. **(Middle)** This image at the mid sacral level shows the sacral body and sacral ala as one large bony mass extending between the lateral sacroiliac joints. The exiting ventral and dorsal nerve roots pass through the ventral and dorsal foramina respectively. **(Bottom)** This image at the coccyx below the termination of the caudal thecal sac, shows the signal of the coccyx is variable depending on the degree of its ossification.

Brain and Spine

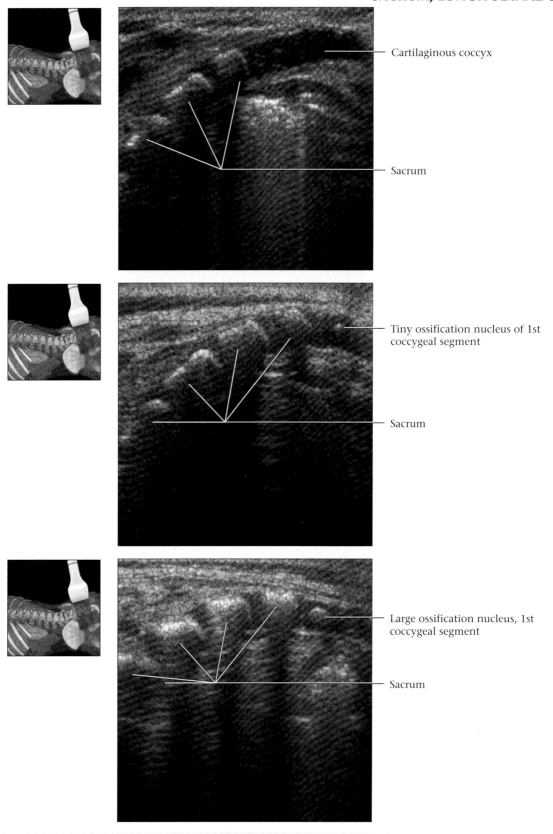

Cartilaginous coccyx

Sacrum

Tiny ossification nucleus of 1st coccygeal segment

Sacrum

Large ossification nucleus, 1st coccygeal segment

Sacrum

(Top) There is wide variability of sonographic appearance of the coccyx on US due to its variable ossification pattern. This longitudinal ultrasound of the sacrococcygeal segment shows ossification is present in the sacral segments, and appears square in configuration. The cartilaginous coccyx appears completely hypoechoic with a smooth classic curve. **(Middle)** This longitudinal ultrasound of sacrococcygeal segment shows a tiny ossification nucleus in the first coccygeal segment, which appears as a round central echogenic focus. **(Bottom)** Longitudinal ultrasound of the sacrococcygeal segment showing a large rounded central focus of ossification nucleus in the first coccygeal segment.

SACRUM, AXIAL & LONGITUDINAL US

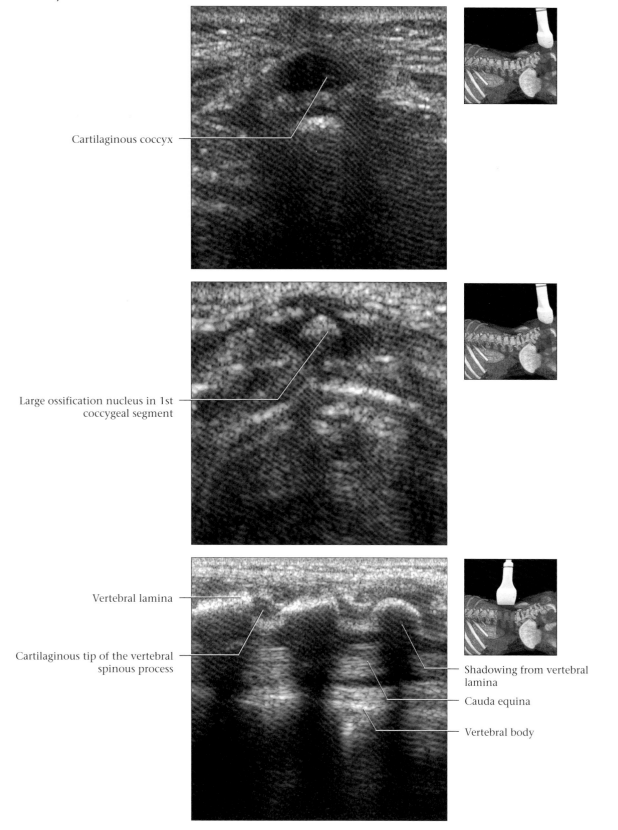

Cartilaginous coccyx

Large ossification nucleus in 1st coccygeal segment

Vertebral lamina

Cartilaginous tip of the vertebral spinous process

Shadowing from vertebral lamina

Cauda equina

Vertebral body

(Top) Transverse ultrasound image of the cartilaginous coccyx which appears completely hypoechoic. (Middle) Transverse ultrasound image of the coccyx with a large focus of ossification nucleus in the first coccygeal segment. (Bottom) Longitudinal ultrasound of the lumbar spine in a mature baby showing marked acoustic shadowing from the lamina of the bony spine. This artifact impairs the visualization of the spinal canal.

Brain and Spine

I

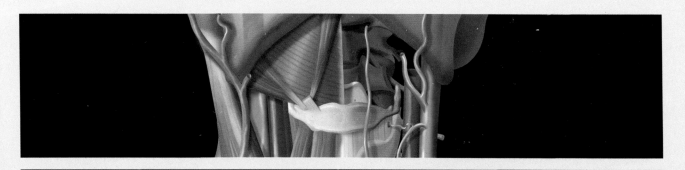

SECTION II: Neck

NECK OVERVIEW

Terminology

Abbreviations
- Suprahyoid neck (SHN)
- Infrahyoid neck (IHN)

Definitions
- SHN: Spaces from skull base to hyoid bone (excluding orbits, paranasal sinuses and oral cavity) including parapharyngeal (PPS), pharyngeal mucosal (PMS), masticator (MS), parotid (PS), carotid (CS), buccal (BS), retropharyngeal (RPS) and perivertebral (PVS) spaces
- IHN: Spaces below hyoid bone to thoracic inlet, including visceral space (VS), posterior cervical space (PCS), anterior cervical space (ACS), CS, RPS, PVS

Imaging Anatomy

Overview
- Fascial spaces of SHN and IHN are key for cross-sectional imaging
  - Concept is difficult to apply for ultrasound
- Ultrasound anatomy is based on division of neck into anterior and posterior triangles
  - Anterior triangle: Bound anteriorly by midline and posteriorly by posterior margin of sternomastoid muscle
    - Further divided into suprahyoid and infrahyoid portions
    - Suprahyoid portion: Divided by anterior belly of digastric muscle into submental and submandibular triangles
    - Infrahyoid portion: Divided by superior belly omohyoid muscle into muscular and carotid triangles
  - Posterior triangle: Bound anteriorly by posterior margin of sternomastoid muscle and posteriorly by anterior border of trapezius muscle
    - Apex formed by the mastoid process, base of the triangle formed by the clavicle
    - Subdivided by posterior belly of omohyoid muscle into occipital triangle (superior) and supraclavicular triangle (inferior)
- Submental region
  - Key structures to identify include anterior belly of digastric, mylohyoid, genioglossus and geniohyoid muscles, sublingual glands, lingual artery
- Submandibular region
  - Key structures to identify are submandibular gland, mylohyoid muscle, hyoglossus muscle, anterior and posterior bellies of digastric, facial vein and anterior division of retromandibular vein (RMV)
- Parotid region
  - Key structures include parotid gland, masseter and buccinator muscles, RMV, external carotid artery (ECA)
- Cervical region
  - Upper cervical region: Skull base to hyoid bone/carotid bifurcation
    - Key structures to identify are internal jugular vein (IJV), carotid bifurcation, jugulodigastric node and posterior belly of digastric

  - Mid cervical region: Hyoid bone to cricoid cartilage
    - Key structures are IJV, common carotid artery (CCA), vagus nerve and lymph nodes
  - Lower cervical region: Cricoid cartilage to clavicle
    - Key structures include: IJV, CCA, superior belly of omohyoid, lymph nodes
- Supraclavicular fossa
  - Key structures include trapezius, sternomastoid, omohyoid muscles, brachial plexus elements, transverse cervical nodes
- Posterior triangle
  - Bordered anteriorly by sternomastoid muscle and posteriorly by trapezius muscle
  - Floor formed by scalene muscles, levator scapulae and splenius capitis muscles
- Midline
  - Key structures are hyoid bone, strap muscles, thyroid, larynx, tracheal rings

Anatomy-Based Imaging Issues

Imaging Recommendations
- Use of high-resolution transducers is essential (> 7.5 MHz)
- Color/power Doppler examination provide useful supplementary information to grayscale US
- US is readily combined with guided fine needle aspiration cytology (FNAC) or biopsy to further enhance its diagnostic accuracy

Imaging Approaches
- Ultrasound imaging protocol
  - Start in the submental region by scanning in the transverse plane
  - Next proceed to submandibular region which is scanned in transverse and longitudinal/oblique planes
  - Then scan the parotid region in transverse and longitudinal planes
  - Next examine the upper cervical region in transverse plane
  - Now proceed to scan mid cervical region in transverse plane
  - Next evaluate lower cervical region in transverse plane
  - Then examine the supraclavicular fossa with transducer held transversely
  - Now scan the posterior triangle transversely along a line drawn from mastoid process to ipsilateral acromion
  - Finally scan the midline including thyroid gland in both transverse and longitudinal planes
- Above protocol is robust and can be tailored to suit individual clinical conditions
- In restless children, it may not be possible to follow the above protocol
  - It is therefore best to evaluate primary area of interest first before child becomes uncooperative

GRAPHICS

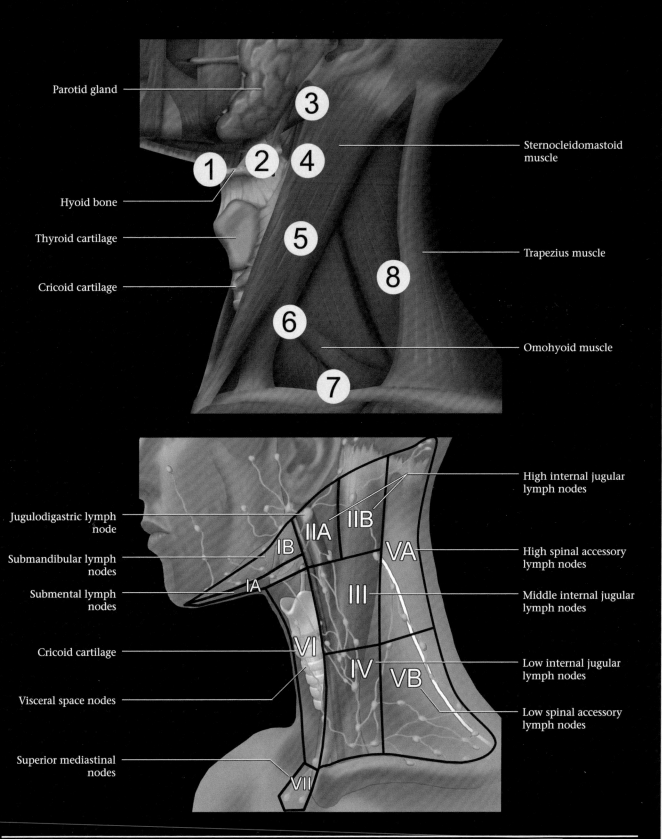

Parotid gland

Sternocleidomastoid muscle

Hyoid bone

Thyroid cartilage

Trapezius muscle

Cricoid cartilage

Omohyoid muscle

Jugulodigastric lymph node

High internal jugular lymph nodes

Submandibular lymph nodes

High spinal accessory lymph nodes

Submental lymph nodes

Middle internal jugular lymph nodes

Cricoid cartilage

Low internal jugular lymph nodes

Visceral space nodes

Low spinal accessory lymph nodes

Superior mediastinal nodes

(Top) Schematic diagram shows the protocol for ultrasound examination of the neck with eight regions scanned in order: Region 1 - submental region; region 2 - submandibular region; region 3 - parotid region; region 4 - upper cervical region; region 5 - mid cervical region; region 6 - lower cervical region; region 7 - supraclavicular fossa; region 8 - posterior triangle. The above protocol is robust and helps to adequately evaluate the neck for common clinical conditions. Note, deep structures cannot be adequately assessed by ultrasound. **(Bottom)** Lateral oblique graphic of the neck shows the anatomic locations for the major nodal groups of the neck. Division of the internal jugular nodal chain into high, middle and low regions is defined by the level of the hyoid bone and cricoid cartilage. Similarly, the spinal accessory nodal chain is divided into high & low regions by the level of the cricoid cartilage.

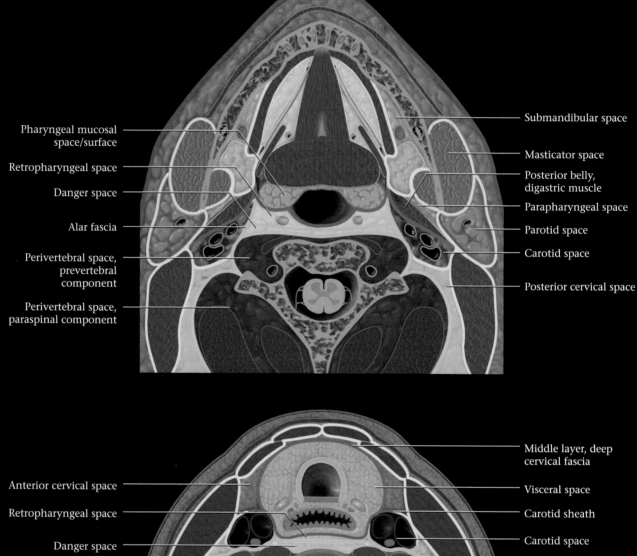

Pharyngeal mucosal space/surface

Retropharyngeal space

Danger space

Alar fascia

Perivertebral space, prevertebral component

Perivertebral space, paraspinal component

Submandibular space

Masticator space

Posterior belly, digastric muscle

Parapharyngeal space

Parotid space

Carotid space

Posterior cervical space

Anterior cervical space

Retropharyngeal space

Danger space

Perivertebral space, prevertebral component

Deep layer, deep cervical fascia touches transverse process

Perivertebral space, paraspinal component

Middle layer, deep cervical fascia

Visceral space

Carotid sheath

Carotid space

Superficial layer, deep cervical fascia

Posterior cervical space

Deep layer, deep cervical fascia

(Top) Axial graphic of the suprahyoid neck spaces at the level of the oropharynx. The superficial (yellow line), middle (pink line) and deep (turquoise line) layers of deep cervical fascia (DCF) outline the suprahyoid neck spaces. Notice the lateral borders of the retropharyngeal & danger spaces are called the alar fascia and represent a slip of the deep layer of DCF. **(Bottom)** Axial graphic depicting the fascia and spaces of the infrahyoid neck. The three layers of DCF are present in the suprahyoid and infrahyoid neck. The carotid sheath is made up of all 3 layers of DCF (tri-color line around carotid space). Notice the deep layer completely circles the perivertebral space, diving in laterally to divide it into prevertebral and a paraspinal components. Although the spaces are not adequately demonstrated by US it is important to be familiar with the concept in order to understand neck anatomy.

NECK OVERVIEW

TRANSVERSE ULTRASOUND

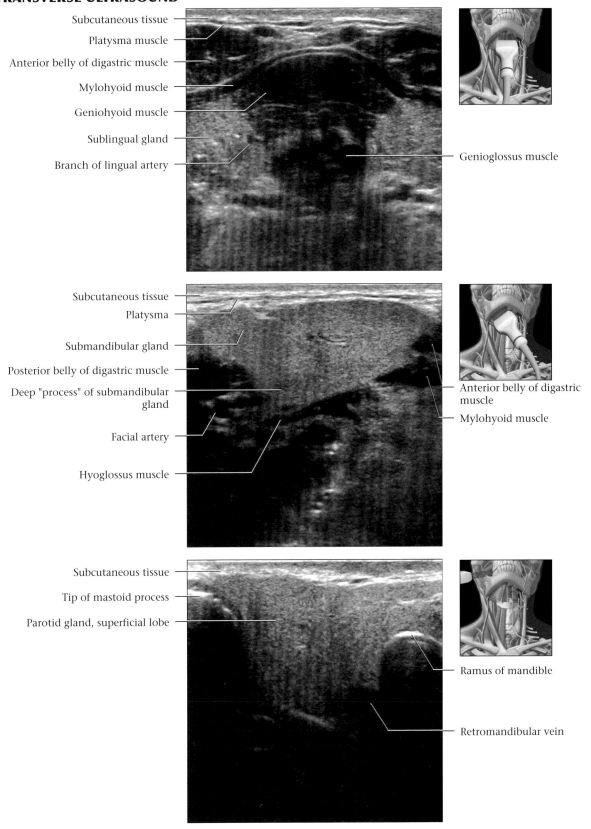

Subcutaneous tissue
Platysma muscle
Anterior belly of digastric muscle
Mylohyoid muscle
Geniohyoid muscle
Sublingual gland
Branch of lingual artery
Genioglossus muscle

Subcutaneous tissue
Platysma
Submandibular gland
Posterior belly of digastric muscle
Deep "process" of submandibular gland
Facial artery
Hyoglossus muscle
Anterior belly of digastric muscle
Mylohyoid muscle

Subcutaneous tissue
Tip of mastoid process
Parotid gland, superficial lobe
Ramus of mandible
Retromandibular vein

(Top) Standard transverse grayscale ultrasound image of the submental region. The mylohyoid muscle is an important landmark for the division of the sublingual (deep to mylohyoid muscle) and submandibular (superficial to mylohyoid muscle) spaces. Part of the extrinsic muscles of the tongue including the geniohyoid and genioglossus are visualized. (Middle) Standard transverse grayscale ultrasound image of the submandibular region. The submandibular gland is the key structure with its homogeneous echotexture. The gland sits astride the mylohyoid and posterior belly of the digastric muscles. (Bottom) Standard transverse grayscale ultrasound image of the parotid region. Note that the deep lobe is obscured by shadowing from the mandible and cannot be evaluated. The retromandibular vein serves as a landmark for the intra-parotid facial nerve.

Subcutaneous tissue

Submandibular gland

Jugulodigastric lymph node

Facial vein

Branches of external carotid artery

External carotid artery

Sternocleidomastoid muscle

Internal jugular vein

Internal carotid artery

Sternohyoid muscle

Sternothyroid muscle

Common carotid artery

Thyroid gland

Longus coli

Sternocleidomastoid muscle

Internal jugular vein

Vagus nerve

Scalenus anterior muscle

Vertebral vessel

Subcutaneous tissue

Sternocleidomastoid muscle

Sternohyoid muscle

Sternothyroid muscle

Thyroid gland

Common carotid artery

Esophagus

Internal jugular vein

Superior belly of omohyoid muscle

Longus coli

(Top) Standard transverse grayscale ultrasound image of the upper cervical level. Key structures include the internal jugular vein, the proximal internal and external carotid arteries and the jugular chain lymph nodes. The jugulodigastric node is the most prominent neck consistently seen on US. **(Middle)** Standard grayscale ultrasound image of the mid cervical level. Note the vagus nerve is clearly seen on US. **(Bottom)** Standard grayscale ultrasound image of the lower cervical level. The thyroid gland is related to the common carotid and internal jugular vein laterally. The anterior strap muscles (including the sternohyoid and sternothyroid muscles) and the superior belly of the omohyoid are clearly visualized.

TRANSVERSE ULTRASOUND

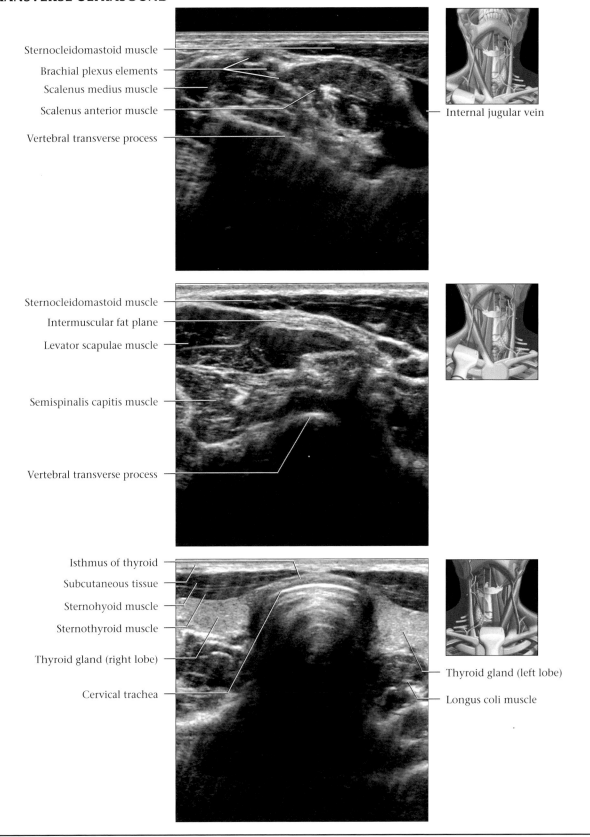

Sternocleidomastoid muscle
Brachial plexus elements
Scalenus medius muscle
Scalenus anterior muscle
Vertebral transverse process

Internal jugular vein

Sternocleidomastoid muscle
Intermuscular fat plane
Levator scapulae muscle

Semispinalis capitis muscle

Vertebral transverse process

Isthmus of thyroid
Subcutaneous tissue
Sternohyoid muscle
Sternothyroid muscle
Thyroid gland (right lobe)
Cervical trachea

Thyroid gland (left lobe)
Longus coli muscle

(Top) Standard grayscale ultrasound image of the supraclavicular fossa. Note that the trunks of the brachial plexus are consistently seen on high resolution US at this site. **(Middle)** Standard transverse grayscale ultrasound image of the posterior triangle. Note that the intermuscular fat plane is visible. The spinal accessory nerve and lymph nodes are important contents of the posterior triangle. **(Bottom)** Standard transverse grayscale ultrasound image of the midline of the lower anterior neck. The isthmus of the thyroid gland, the trachea and the longus colli muscles are key structures to be identified.

SUBLINGUAL/SUBMENTAL REGION

Terminology

Abbreviations
- Submental triangle

Definitions
- Sublingual space (SLS): Paired non-fascial lined spaces of oral cavity in deep oral tongue above floor of mouth superomedial to mylohyoid muscle

Imaging Anatomy

Overview
- Borders of submental triangle are readily defined on ultrasound
  - Floor is formed by mylohyoid muscle
  - Apex is limited anteriorly by symphysis menti
  - Base is bound posteriorly by hyoid bone
  - Anterior belly of digastric muscle represents sides of triangle
- SLS is deep space of oral cavity superomedial to mylohyoid muscles
  - Contains key neurovascular structures of oral cavity
  - Includes glossopharyngeal nerve (CN9), hypoglossal nerve (CN12), lingual nerve (branch of V3), lingual artery and vein

Anatomy Relationships
- Sublingual space relationships
  - SLS in deep oral tongue superomedial to mylohyoid muscle and lateral to genioglossus-geniohyoid muscles
  - Communication between sublingual spaces occurs in midline anteriorly as a narrow isthmus beneath frenulum
  - SLS communicates with submandibular space (SMS) and inferior parapharyngeal space (PPS) at posterior margin of mylohyoid muscle
    - There is no fascia dividing posterior SLS from adjacent SMS
    - Therefore there is direct communication with SMS and PPS in this location

Internal Structures-Critical Contents
- Major muscles forming the borders of submental triangle
  - Anterior belly of digastric muscle
    - It marks the lateral border of the submental triangle
  - Mylohyoid muscle
    - Muscle of the floor of mouth
    - Muscular sling between medial aspect of mandibular bodies
    - Anterior attachment to mandible inferior to origins of genial muscles
    - Differentiating sublingual (deep to mylohyoid muscle plane) and submandibular (superficial to mylohyoid muscle) spaces
  - Genioglossus and geniohyoid muscles
    - Form root of tongue
    - Together with hyoglossus muscle, they make up major extrinsic muscles of tongue

- Posterior aspect of SLS is divided into medial and lateral compartments by hyoglossus muscle
- Lateral compartment contents
  - Hypoglossal nerve
    - Motor to intrinsic and extrinsic muscles of tongue
    - Intrinsic muscles of tongue include inferior lingual, vertical and transverse muscles
  - Lingual nerve: Branch of mandibular division of trigeminal nerve (CN V3) combined with chorda tympani branch of facial nerve
    - Lingual nerve branch of CN V3: Sensation to anterior 2/3 of oral tongue
    - Chorda tympani branch of facial nerve: Anterior 2/3 of tongue taste and parasympathetic secreto-motor fibers to submandibular ganglion/gland
  - Sublingual glands and ducts
    - Lie in anterior SLS bilaterally
    - About 5 small ducts open under oral tongue into oral cavity
    - With age sublingual glands atrophy, becoming difficult to be seen on imaging
  - Submandibular glands and submandibular ducts
    - Submandibular gland deep margin extends into posterior opening of SLS
    - Submandibular duct runs anteriorly to papillae in anteromedial subfrenular mucosa
- Medial compartment contents
  - Glossopharyngeal nerve (CN9)
    - Provides sensation to posterior 1/3 of tongue
    - Carries taste input from posterior 1/3 of tongue
    - Located more cephalad in medial compartment compared to lingual artery and vein
  - Lingual artery and vein
    - Vascular supply to oral tongue
    - Seen running just lateral to genioglossus muscle

Anatomy-Based Imaging Issues

Key Concepts or Questions
- What defines a mass as primary to SLS?
  - Center of lesion is superomedial to mylohyoid muscle and lateral to genioglossus muscle
- Common lesions in submental region include
  - Congenital lesions: Epidermoid cyst
  - Enlarged lymph node: Reactive, inflammatory or neoplastic (metastatic/lymphomatous nodes)
  - Inflammatory conditions: Ranula
  - Sublingual gland lesions: Sialadenitis, calculus, benign/malignant salivary gland tumor

Imaging Recommendations
- High resolution ultrasound is an ideal imaging tool for evaluating submental masses
- Major structures are best seen on transverse scans with patient's neck in slight hyperextension
- For more deep-seated lesions (e.g., deep to root of tongue), MR is necessary for better anatomical assessment
  - Ultrasound may help in directing a needle for guided biopsy of such lesions

SUBLINGUAL/SUBMENTAL REGION

GRAPHICS

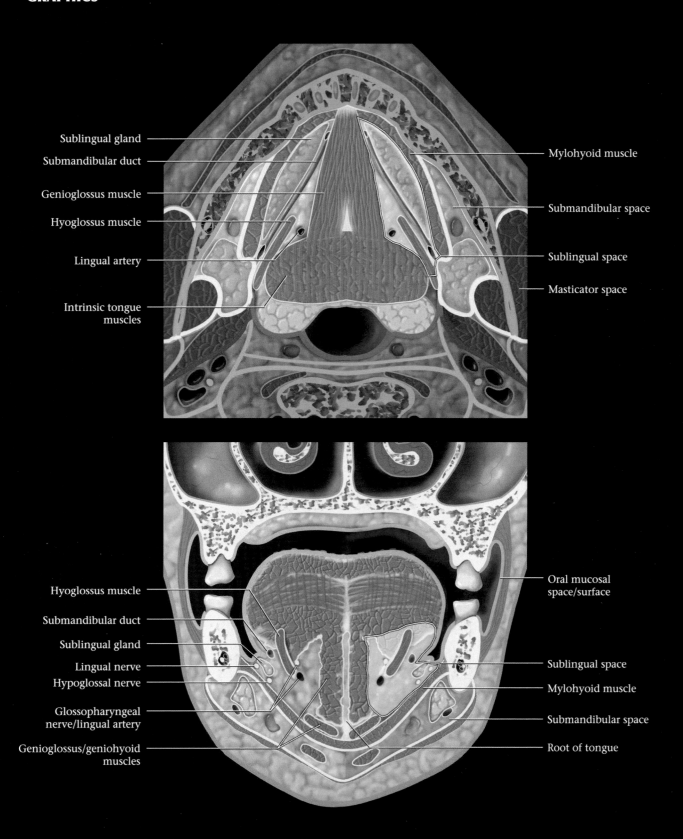

Sublingual gland

Submandibular duct

Genioglossus muscle

Hyoglossus muscle

Lingual artery

Intrinsic tongue muscles

Mylohyoid muscle

Submandibular space

Sublingual space

Masticator space

Hyoglossus muscle

Submandibular duct

Sublingual gland

Lingual nerve

Hypoglossal nerve

Glossopharyngeal nerve/lingual artery

Genioglossus/geniohyoid muscles

Oral mucosal space/surface

Sublingual space

Mylohyoid muscle

Submandibular space

Root of tongue

(Top) Axial graphic through the body of the mandible shows the sublingual space (on patient's left, shaded in green) situated superomedial to the mylohyoid muscle and lateral to the genioglossus muscle. Notice the absence of fascia surrounding the sublingual space. The yellow line represents the superficial layer of deep cervical fascia. **(Bottom)** Coronal graphic through the oral cavity. Note the position of the mylohyoid muscle which is the landmark in this area. The SLS is shaded in green. The SLS medial compartment contents include the glossopharyngeal nerve (CN9) and lingual artery/vein. Lateral SLS compartment contents include the submandibular duct, sublingual gland, lingual nerve and hypoglossal nerve (CN12). The fascia-lined (yellow line) submandibular space is inferolateral to the mylohyoid muscle.

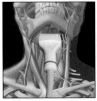
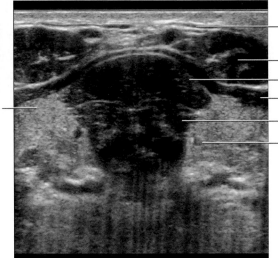
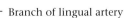

Platysma muscle

Anterior belly of digastric m.

Geniohyoid muscle

Mylohyoid muscle

Genioglossus muscle

Branch of lingual artery

Sublingual gland

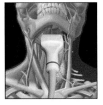
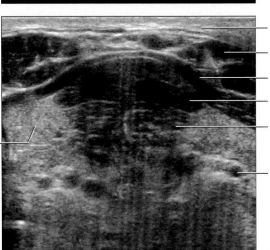

Subcutaneous tissue

Anterior belly of digastric m.

Mylohyoid muscle

Geniohyoid muscle

Genioglossus muscle

Branch of lingual artery

Sublingual gland

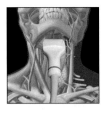
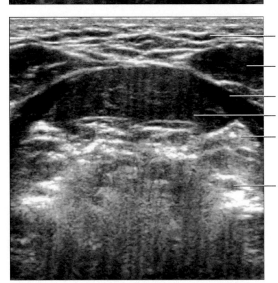

Platysma muscle

Anterior belly of digastric m.

Mylohyoid muscle

Geniohyoid muscle

Sublingual gland

Branch of lingual artery

(Top) The more anterior transverse grayscale ultrasound images of the submental and sublingual region. The mylohyoid muscle is the landmark for division of sublingual space (deep to the mylohyoid plane) and submandibular space (superficial to the muscle plane). The sublingual gland appears as homogeneous, hyperechoic structures lateral to the geniohyoid/genioglossus muscle. Branches of lingual artery can be easily picked up on transverse plane. The submandibular duct sits alongside the lingual vessels and a submandibular calculus may impact at this site. (Middle) The more posterior transverse grayscale ultrasound images allow the clear depiction of extrinsic muscles of the tongue at the root. (Bottom) Transverse grayscale ultrasound of the submental region in a more posterior location.

SUBLINGUAL/SUBMENTAL REGION

POWER DOPPLER ULTRASOUND AND CORONAL MR

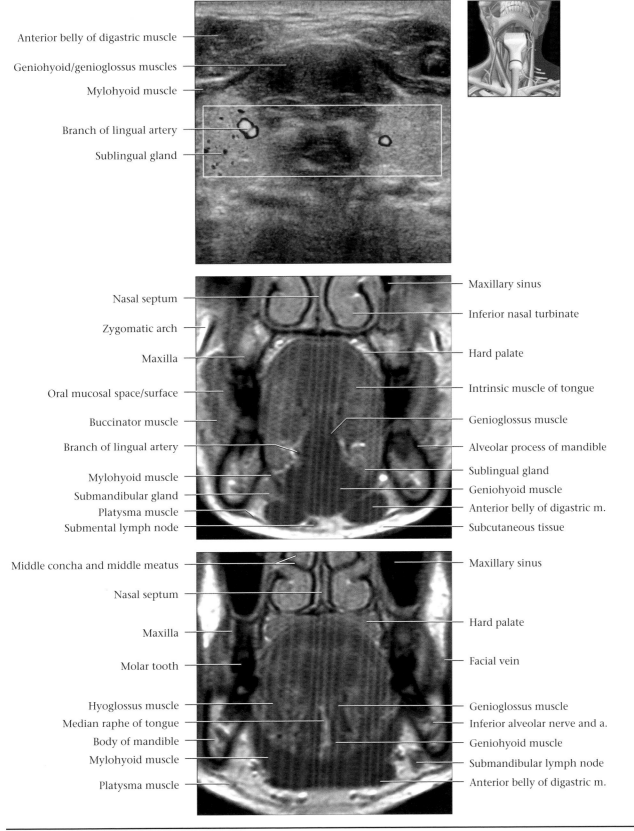

Anterior belly of digastric muscle

Geniohyoid/genioglossus muscles

Mylohyoid muscle

Branch of lingual artery

Sublingual gland

Nasal septum

Zygomatic arch

Maxilla

Oral mucosal space/surface

Buccinator muscle

Branch of lingual artery

Mylohyoid muscle

Submandibular gland

Platysma muscle

Submental lymph node

Maxillary sinus

Inferior nasal turbinate

Hard palate

Intrinsic muscle of tongue

Genioglossus muscle

Alveolar process of mandible

Sublingual gland

Geniohyoid muscle

Anterior belly of digastric m.

Subcutaneous tissue

Middle concha and middle meatus

Nasal septum

Maxilla

Molar tooth

Hyoglossus muscle

Median raphe of tongue

Body of mandible

Mylohyoid muscle

Platysma muscle

Maxillary sinus

Hard palate

Facial vein

Genioglossus muscle

Inferior alveolar nerve and a.

Geniohyoid muscle

Submandibular lymph node

Anterior belly of digastric m.

(**Top**) Power Doppler ultrasound of the submental region shows the presence of color flow within the branches of the lingual artery. The use of Doppler examination aids in differentiation from the dilated submandibular duct. (**Middle**) Correlative coronal T1WI MR image of the floor of the mouth and tongue. The mylohyoid muscle is the landmark to separate the sublingual space and submandibular spaces. (**Bottom**) Correlative coronal T1WI MR image of the floor of the mouth and tongue (in a more posterior location to the middle image). For optimal use of US the operator must also be familiar with the correlative anatomy on other imaging modalities.

LONGITUDINAL ULTRASOUND AND PATHOLOGY

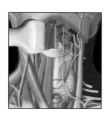
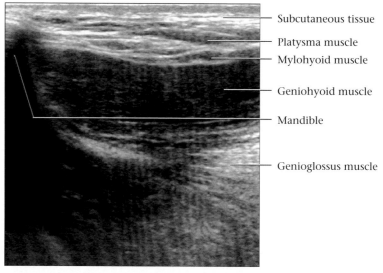

— Subcutaneous tissue
— Platysma muscle
— Mylohyoid muscle

— Geniohyoid muscle

— Mandible

— Genioglossus muscle

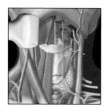
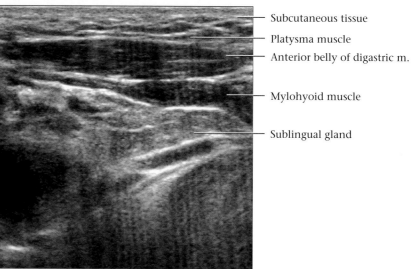

— Subcutaneous tissue

— Platysma muscle
— Anterior belly of digastric m.

— Mylohyoid muscle

— Sublingual gland

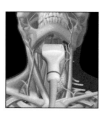
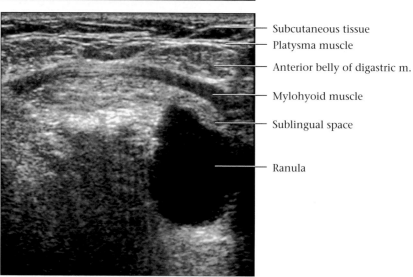

— Subcutaneous tissue
— Platysma muscle

— Anterior belly of digastric m.

— Mylohyoid muscle

— Sublingual space

— Ranula

(Top) Longitudinal grayscale ultrasound of the submental region shows the relationship of the mylohyoid, geniohyoid and genioglossus muscles. Note if you scan just off the midline you will see more of the anterior belly of the digastric rather than the mylohyoid anteriorly. (Middle) Parasagittal longitudinal grayscale ultrasound of the submental region. The sublingual gland is visualized within the sublingual space (deep to the mylohyoid muscle) underneath the anterior belly of the digastric and mylohyoid muscles. (Bottom) Transverse grayscale ultrasound shows a well-circumscribed, anechoic, cystic lesion in the left sublingual space (i.e., deep to the mylohyoid muscle plane), the appearances are suggestive of a ranula. Its relationship to the mylohyoid defines whether it is a simple or diving ranula.

SUBLINGUAL/SUBMENTAL REGION

SAGITTAL MR AND PATHOLOGY

Pituitary gland — Nasal septum — Hard palate — Soft palate — Superior longitudinal muscle — Genioglossus muscle — Geniohyoid muscle — Mylohyoid muscle — Hyoid bone

Medulla oblongata and cerebellum — Sphenoid sinus — Clivus — Anterior arch of atlas and odontoid process — Lingual follicles — Epiglottis — Hypopharynx — Spinal cord — Tracheal ring

Ethmoid air cells — Middle meatus — Inferior nasal concha — Superior longitudinal muscle — Genioglossus muscle — Sublingual gland — Mandible — Anterior belly of digastric muscle

Cavernous portion of internal carotid artery — Longus capitis — Oropharynx — Geniohyoid muscle — Hyoid bone — Piriform fossa — Thyroid cartilage

Anterior belly of digastric muscle — Mylohyoid muscle — Geniohyoid/genioglossus muscles

Epidermoid cyst

(Top) Correlative sagittal T1WI MR image of the floor of the mouth close to the midline. Note the positions of the mylohyoid and geniohyoid muscles between the mandible anteriorly and hyoid bone posteriorly. **(Middle)** T1WI sagittal MR image of the floor of the mouth in the paramedian plane. Note that the anterior belly of the digastric muscle is now seen as it extends anteromedially to insert on the inner cortex of the mandible. **(Bottom)** Transverse grayscale ultrasound of the submental region shows a well-circumscribed, homogeneous, hyperechoic, midline mass deep to the mylohyoid and geniohyoid/genioglossus muscles. The appearances and anatomical location of the lesion are suggestive of an epidermoid cyst. Congenital lesions in the neck are site specific and familiarity with the correlative anatomy is often the best clue to their diagnosis.

SUBMANDIBULAR REGION

Terminology

Abbreviations
- Submandibular space (SMS)

Definitions
- Fascial-lined space inferolateral to mylohyoid muscle containing submandibular gland, lymph nodes and anterior belly of digastric muscles

Imaging Anatomy

Overview
- SMS is one of the distinct locations within oral cavity that may be used to develop location specific differential diagnoses
  - Other locations include oral mucosal space/surface, sublingual space and root of tongue

Anatomy Relationships
- Inferolateral to the mylohyoid muscle
- Deep to the platysma muscle
- Cephalad to the hyoid bone
- Communicates posteriorly with sublingual space and inferior parapharyngeal space at posterior margin of mylohyoid muscle
- Continues inferiorly into infrahyoid neck as anterior cervical space

Internal Structures-Critical Contents
- Submandibular gland
  - One of the three major salivary glands
  - Divided anatomically into superficial and deep lobes by the mylohyoid muscle
  - Superficial lobe is larger and in the SMS itself
    - Superficial layer, deep cervical fascia (SL-DCF) forms the submandibular gland capsule
    - Crossed by facial vein and cervical branches of facial nerve (marginal mandibular branch)
  - Smaller deep lobe, often called deep "process"
    - Tongue-like extension of gland which wraps around behind mylohyoid muscle
    - Projects into posterior aspect of sublingual space
    - Submandibular duct projects off deep lobe into sublingual space
  - Submandibular gland innervation
    - Parasympathetic secretomotor supply from chorda tympani branch of facial nerve
    - Comes via lingual branch of cranial nerve V3
- Submental (level IA) and submandibular (level IB) nodal groups
  - Receive lymphatic drainage from anterior facial region
    - Including oral cavity, anterior sinonasal and orbital areas
  - A few elliptical lymph nodes with preserved internal architecture is a constant normal finding
- Anterior belly of digastric muscle
  - Divide the suprahyoid portion into submental and submandibular triangles
- Hyoglossus muscle
  - Deep to mylohyoid muscle and marks the anterior margin of submandibular gland

- The submandibular duct runs between hyoglossus muscle and mylohyoid muscle
- Facial vein and artery pass through SMS
  - Facial vein courses anteriorly and superiorly to the submandibular gland
- Anterior division of retromandibular vein (RMV)
  - It outlines the posterior border of submandibular gland
- Caudal loop of CN12
  - Passes through SMS on the way before looping anteriorly and cephalad into tongue muscle
- Tail of parotid gland may "hang down" into posterior submandibular space

Anatomy-Based Imaging Issues

Key Concepts or Questions
- Major clinical-radiological question when mass present in SMS: Is lesion nodal or submandibular gland in origin?
  - "Beaking" of submandibular gland tissue around lesion margin and if lesion is completely surrounded by glandular parenchyma, lesion is submandibular gland in origin
  - Fatty cleavage plane between the mass and submandibular gland identifies lesion as nodal in origin
  - Internal architecture (e.g., presence of echogenic hilus) helps to identify lymph node
- Major differential diagnoses for mass in submandibular region
  - Congenital lesion: Epidermoid cyst, cystic hygroma
  - Inflammatory condition: Submandibular gland sialadenitis/abscess, diving ranula, Kuttner tumor, Sjögren syndrome
  - Lymph node enlargement: Reactive, inflammatory or neoplastic (secondary or lymphomatous)
  - Benign salivary gland tumor: Benign mixed tumor, lipoma
  - Malignant salivary gland tumor

Imaging Recommendations
- Scan the submandibular region in transverse and longitudinal/oblique planes as these best demonstrate floor of submandibular region, hyoglossus and mylohyoid muscles
- Always establish origin of mass (i.e., submandibular glandular or extraglandular mass) as this will help to narrow differential diagnosis
- Remember to evaluate glandular/extraglandular ductal dilatation and lymph nodes at this location

Imaging Pitfalls
- Distinction between submandibular glandular mass and enlarged lymph node can be difficult, especially if mass is large
- Lesions of parotid tail may appear in posterior submandibular region clinically
- Coronal MR helps to evaluate and localize large masses at this site

GRAPHICS

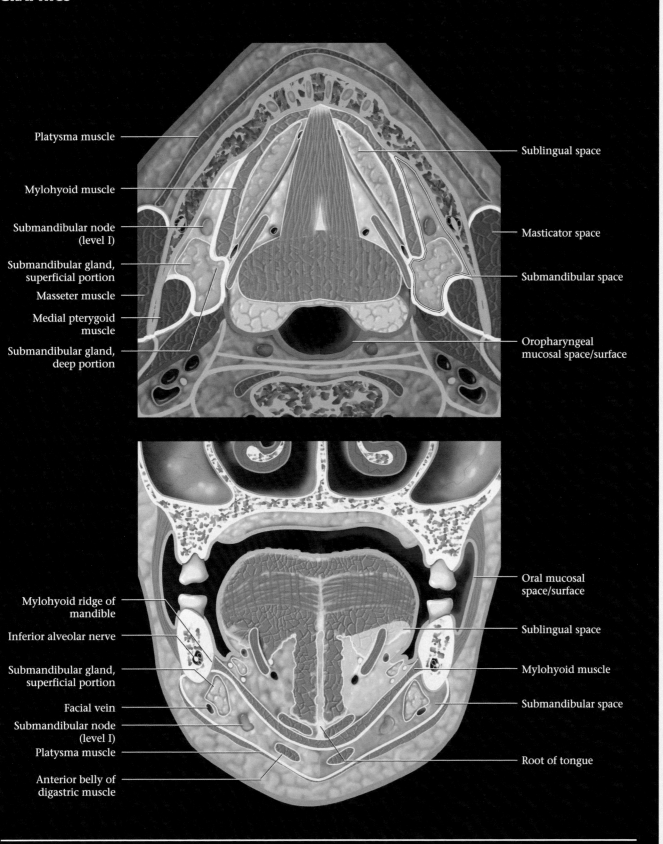

Platysma muscle

Mylohyoid muscle

Submandibular node
(level I)

Submandibular gland,
superficial portion

Masseter muscle

Medial pterygoid
muscle

Submandibular gland,
deep portion

Sublingual space

Masticator space

Submandibular space

Oropharyngeal
mucosal space/surface

Mylohyoid ridge of
mandible

Inferior alveolar nerve

Submandibular gland,
superficial portion

Facial vein

Submandibular node
(level I)

Platysma muscle

Anterior belly of
digastric muscle

Oral mucosal
space/surface

Sublingual space

Mylohyoid muscle

Submandibular space

Root of tongue

(Top) Axial graphic of oral cavity with emphasis on the SMS shaded in light blue on patient's left. The submandibular space is inferolateral to the mylohyoid muscle. Note that the principal structures of the SMS are the submandibular gland and lymph nodes. **(Bottom)** In this coronal graphic through the oral cavity, the submandibular space is shaded in light blue. The superficial layer of the deep cervical fascia (yellow line) is seen lining the "vertical horseshoe-shaped" SMS inferolateral to the mylohyoid muscle. The contents of SMS are the anterior belly of the digastric muscle, submandibular nodes, submandibular gland and facial vein. Notice that the platysma forms the superficial margin of the SMS.

SUBMANDIBULAR REGION

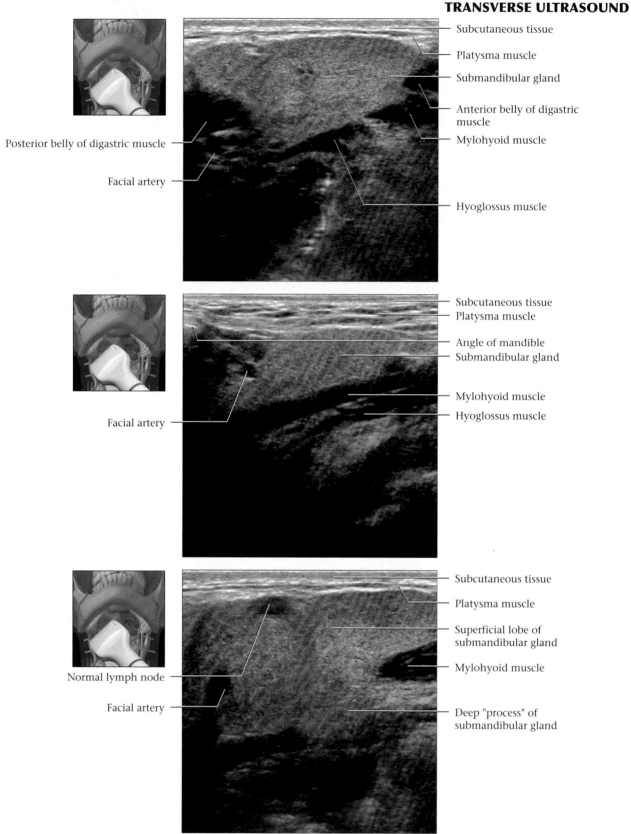

Top image labels:
- Subcutaneous tissue
- Platysma muscle
- Submandibular gland
- Anterior belly of digastric muscle
- Mylohyoid muscle
- Hyoglossus muscle
- Posterior belly of digastric muscle
- Facial artery

Middle image labels:
- Subcutaneous tissue
- Platysma muscle
- Angle of mandible
- Submandibular gland
- Mylohyoid muscle
- Hyoglossus muscle
- Facial artery

Bottom image labels:
- Subcutaneous tissue
- Platysma muscle
- Superficial lobe of submandibular gland
- Mylohyoid muscle
- Deep "process" of submandibular gland
- Normal lymph node
- Facial artery

(Top) Transverse grayscale ultrasound image of the submandibular region. The submandibular gland sits astride the posterior belly of digastric and mylohyoid muscles. The hyoglossus muscle is seen deep to the submandibular gland. **(Middle)** Transverse grayscale ultrasound of the submandibular region (slightly more posterior scan to the top image) shows the consistent relationship of the submandibular gland superficial to the mylohyoid and hyoglossus muscles. The submandibular duct runs between these two muscles. **(Bottom)** Transverse grayscale ultrasound image of the submandibular gland. The gland is divided into superficial and deep lobe, demarcated by the free posterior edge of mylohyoid muscle. Normal lymph nodes are a constant finding in this region.

SUBMANDIBULAR REGION

AXIAL MR AND POWER DOPPLER ULTRASOUND

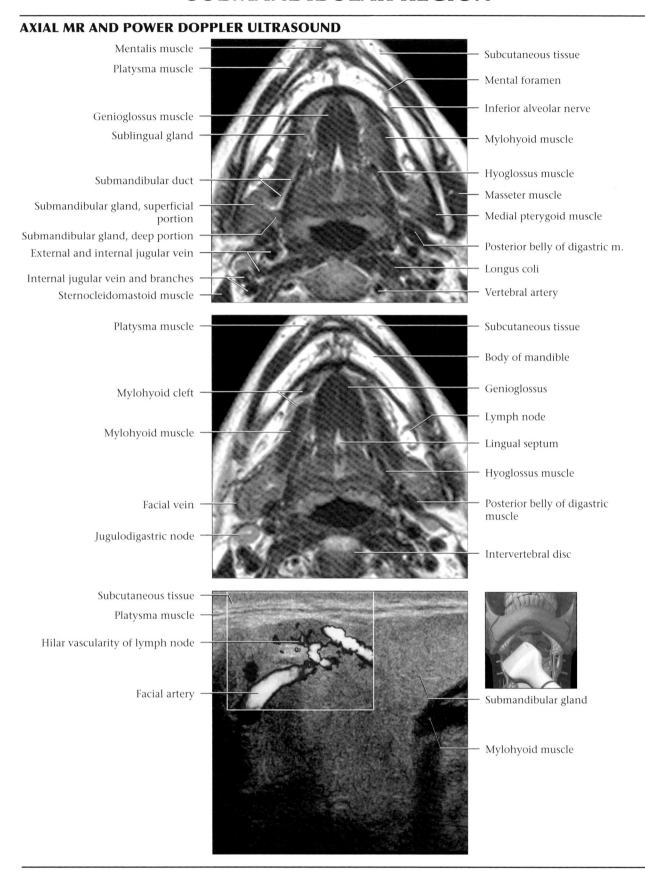

Mentalis muscle
Platysma muscle
Genioglossus muscle
Sublingual gland
Submandibular duct
Submandibular gland, superficial portion
Submandibular gland, deep portion
External and internal jugular vein
Internal jugular vein and branches
Sternocleidomastoid muscle

Subcutaneous tissue
Mental foramen
Inferior alveolar nerve
Mylohyoid muscle
Hyoglossus muscle
Masseter muscle
Medial pterygoid muscle
Posterior belly of digastric m.
Longus coli
Vertebral artery

Platysma muscle
Mylohyoid cleft
Mylohyoid muscle
Facial vein
Jugulodigastric node

Subcutaneous tissue
Body of mandible
Genioglossus
Lymph node
Lingual septum
Hyoglossus muscle
Posterior belly of digastric muscle
Intervertebral disc

Subcutaneous tissue
Platysma muscle
Hilar vascularity of lymph node
Facial artery

Submandibular gland
Mylohyoid muscle

(Top) Axial T2WI MR of the floor of the mouth. The SMS contains submandibular glands, fat and lymph nodes. Notice the high signal submandibular ducts entering the posterior aspect of sublingual spaces bilaterally. **(Middle)** In a more inferior image both submandibular glands are seen wrapping around the posterior margins of the mylohyoid muscles. The neurovascular pedicle to each side of the tongue is closely related to the hyoglossus muscle. **(Bottom)** Transverse power Doppler ultrasound image of submandibular gland shows vascular flow within the facial artery. Note the presence of normal hilar vascularity within lymph node.

GRAYSCALE ULTRASOUND AND PATHOLOGY

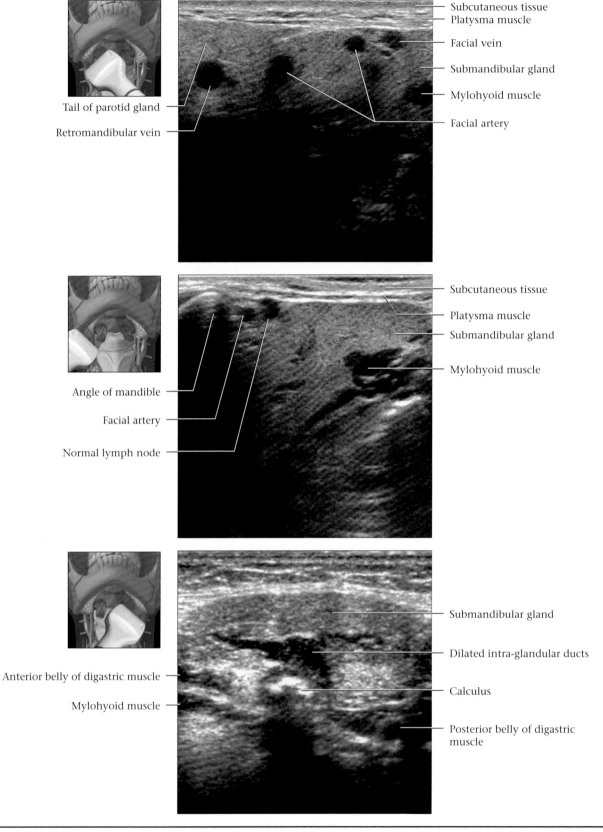

(Top) Transverse grayscale ultrasound image of the posterior submandibular region. Note the close proximity of the submandibular gland to the tail of the parotid gland. On US it may be difficult to localize the origin of large lesions at this site. Displacement of vessels often provides the clue. **(Middle)** Longitudinal grayscale ultrasound image of the submandibular region. The submandibular gland is located inferior and posterior to the mandible and superficial to the mylohyoid muscle. **(Bottom)** Transverse grayscale ultrasound of the left submandibular gland shows a large obstructing calculus with intra-glandular ductal dilatation. Note the glandular parenchyma appears heterogeneous, hypoechoic compatible with sialadenitis secondary to obstruction.

SUBMANDIBULAR REGION

POWER DOPPLER ULTRASOUND AND PATHOLOGY

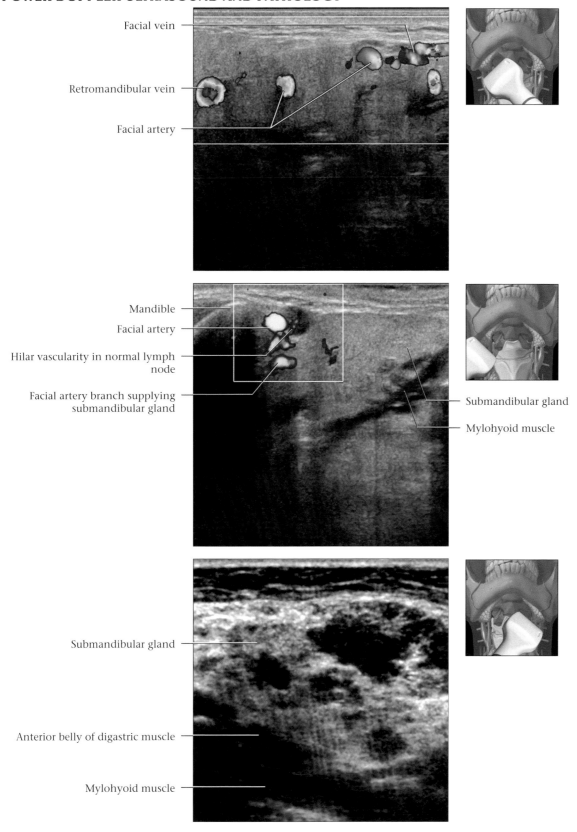

Facial vein

Retromandibular vein

Facial artery

Mandible

Facial artery

Hilar vascularity in normal lymph node

Facial artery branch supplying submandibular gland

Submandibular gland

Mylohyoid muscle

Submandibular gland

Anterior belly of digastric muscle

Mylohyoid muscle

(Top) Transverse color Doppler ultrasound helps to identify and confirm important vascular landmarks in the posterior submandibular region including the retromandibular vein and facial artery. (Middle) Longitudinal power Doppler ultrasound of the submandibular region shows the relationship of facial artery to the superficial portion of submandibular gland. The hilar vascularity of a normal lymph node and the vessels supplying the submandibular gland are seen. (Bottom) Transverse grayscale ultrasound of the left submandibular region shows an enlarged, heterogeneous submandibular gland with patchy hypoechoic areas. No ductal dilatation or calculus is seen. The changes were also seen in the opposite gland (not shown) suggesting chronic sclerosing sialadenitis (Kuttner tumor).

PAROTID REGION

Terminology

Abbreviations
- Parotid space (PS)

Definitions
- PS: Paired lateral suprahyoid neck spaces enclosed by superficial layer deep cervical fascia containing parotid glands, nodes & extracranial facial nerve branches

Imaging Anatomy

Extent
- PS extends from external auditory canal (EAC) & mastoid tip superiorly to below angle of mandible (parotid tail)

Internal Structures-Critical Contents
- Parotid gland
  - Divided anatomically into superficial lobe and deep lobe by extracranial facial nerve
    - Superficial lobe - constitutes ~ 2/3 of parotid glandular parenchyma
    - Deep lobe - smaller component and projects into lateral PPS
- Extracranial facial nerve (CN7)
  - Exits stylomastoid foramen as single trunk; ramifies within PS lateral to retromandibular vein
  - Ramifying intraparotid facial nerve creates surgical plane between superficial & deep lobes
- External carotid artery (ECA)
  - The medial and smaller vessel of the two vessels seen just behind mandibular ramus in PS
- Retromandibular vein (RMV)
  - The lateral and larger of the two vessels seen just behind mandibular ramus in parotid
  - Form by union of superficial temporal vein and maxillary vein
  - Intraparotid facial nerve branches course just lateral to retromandibular vein
- Intraparotid lymph nodes
  - ~ 20 lymph nodes found in each parotid gland
  - Parotid nodes are 1st order drainage for EAC, pinna & surrounding scalp
- Parotid duct
  - Emerges from anterior PS, runs along surface of masseter muscle
  - Duct then arches through buccal space to pierce buccinator muscle at level of upper 2nd molar
- Accessory parotid glands
  - Project over surface of masseter muscles
  - Present in ~ 20% of normal anatomic dissections
- Masseter muscle
  - Muscle of mastication related to the outer surface of mandibular ramus
  - Parotid duct runs anteriorly on its surface
- Buccinator muscle
  - Deep muscle of buccal space, extends anteriorly and just medially to anterior margin of masseter muscle
  - Through which parotid duct pierces to enter buccal mucosa at upper 2nd molar level

Anatomy-Based Imaging Issues

Key Concepts or Questions
- How to determine whether deep lobe of parotid gland is involved?
  - For a parotid mass, it is important to determine location and extent of involvement in relation to extracranial facial nerve (i.e., superficial/deep lobe involvement)
    - Difference in surgical approach and risk of perioperative facial nerve injury
  - Intraparotid facial nerve is not visible with USG, CT or MR except proximally with high-resolution MR
  - On USG, RMV is taken as a marker for division of parotid gland into superficial and deep lobes (due to close proximity to CN7)

Imaging Approaches
- Scan parotid region in both transverse and longitudinal planes
  - Transverse scans help to define anatomic location of salivary gland masses in relation to ECA and RMV
  - Longitudinal scans help in better evaluating lesions in parotid tail and for Doppler examination
- USG does not evaluate deep lobe mass or deep extension of superficial masses
  - Lower frequency transducer (e.g., 5 MHz) with gel block/standoff pad helps to evaluate large parotid mass with suspicious deep lobe extension
  - MR/CT is required for full anatomical delineation
  - US helps direct needle for guided biopsy
- Always remember to evaluate masseter muscle as its lesions will clinically mimic parotid pathology
- Normal intraglandular ducts are seen as echogenic streaks within parotid parenchyma
  - When dilated they are seen as two bright lines separated by fluid within
  - Extraglandular portion of duct is seen on US only if it is dilated

Imaging Pitfalls
- Facial nerve plane in parotid can only be estimated
- Deep lobe cannot be assessed on USG

Clinical Implications

Clinical Importance
- Parotid tumors: Benign mixed tumor (75%), Warthin tumor (5%), adenoid cystic carcinoma (5%), mucoepidermoid carcinoma (5%), other (10%)

Embryology

Embryologic Events
- Parotid space undergoes late encapsulation in embryogenesis

Practical Implications
- Late encapsulation results in intraparotid lymph nodes
- Parotid nodes are 1st-order drainage for malignancies of adjacent scalp, EAC & deep face
- No such nodes in submandibular gland

GRAPHICS

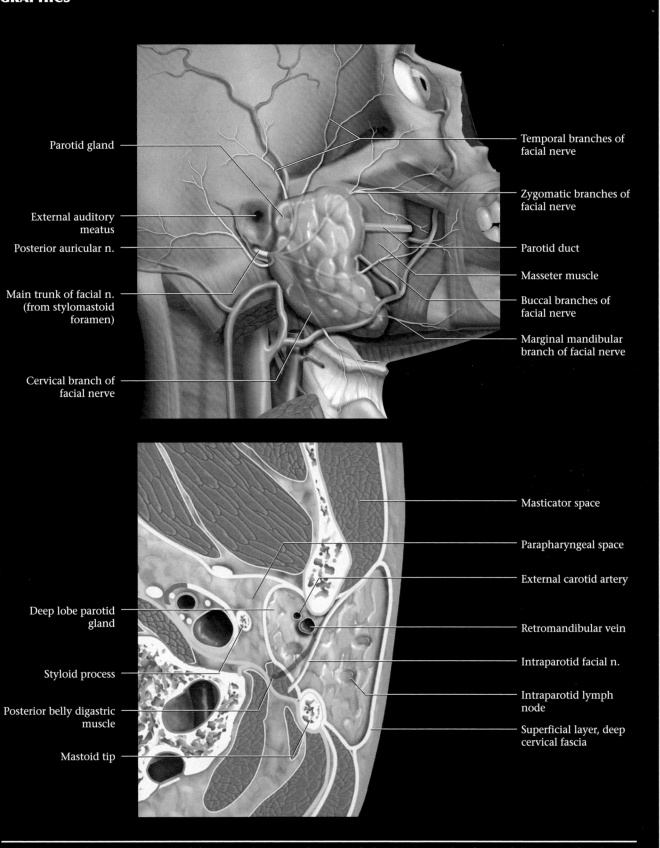

Parotid gland

External auditory meatus

Posterior auricular n.

Main trunk of facial n. (from stylomastoid foramen)

Cervical branch of facial nerve

Temporal branches of facial nerve

Zygomatic branches of facial nerve

Parotid duct

Masseter muscle

Buccal branches of facial nerve

Marginal mandibular branch of facial nerve

Deep lobe parotid gland

Styloid process

Posterior belly digastric muscle

Mastoid tip

Masticator space

Parapharyngeal space

External carotid artery

Retromandibular vein

Intraparotid facial n.

Intraparotid lymph node

Superficial layer, deep cervical fascia

(Top) Lateral schematic diagram of the parotid region. The parotid gland is situated in front of the external auditory meatus and below the zygomatic arch. The parotid duct emerges from the anterior margin and passes superficial to the masseter muscle. The facial nerve, after emerging from the stylomastoid foramen, enters the parotid gland and divides into terminal branches to supply muscles of facial expression. **(Bottom)** Axial graphic of the PS at the level of C1 vertebral body. The intraparotid course of the facial nerve extends from just medial to the mastoid tip to a position just lateral to the retromandibular vein, dividing the parotid gland into superficial and deep lobes.

Neck

II

PAROTID REGION

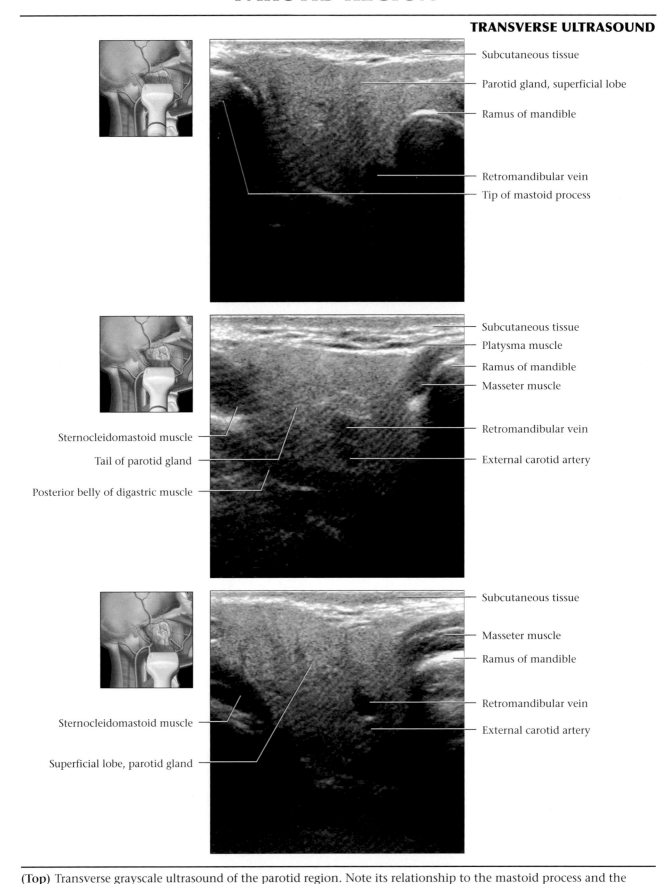

Top image labels:
- Subcutaneous tissue
- Parotid gland, superficial lobe
- Ramus of mandible
- Retromandibular vein
- Tip of mastoid process

Middle image labels:
- Subcutaneous tissue
- Platysma muscle
- Ramus of mandible
- Masseter muscle
- Retromandibular vein
- External carotid artery
- Sternocleidomastoid muscle
- Tail of parotid gland
- Posterior belly of digastric muscle

Bottom image labels:
- Subcutaneous tissue
- Masseter muscle
- Ramus of mandible
- Retromandibular vein
- External carotid artery
- Sternocleidomastoid muscle
- Superficial lobe, parotid gland

(Top) Transverse grayscale ultrasound of the parotid region. Note its relationship to the mastoid process and the mandibular ramus. The glandular parenchyma shows a homogeneous, hyperechoic echo pattern. The retromandibular vein is visualized as a round, anechoic structure within the parotid gland. **(Middle)** Transverse grayscale ultrasound of the parotid tail region. The sternocleidomastoid muscle and the posterior belly of the digastric muscle are related to the posterior margin of parotid tail. The retromandibular vein and external carotid artery serve as markers to infer the location of CN7. **(Bottom)** Transverse grayscale ultrasound of the parotid gland. The retromandibular vein is usually larger and lateral to the external carotid artery within the parotid gland. Note that the deep lobe is obscured by shadowing from the mandibular ramus.

PAROTID REGION

AXIAL T1 MR & POWER DOPPLER ULTRASOUND

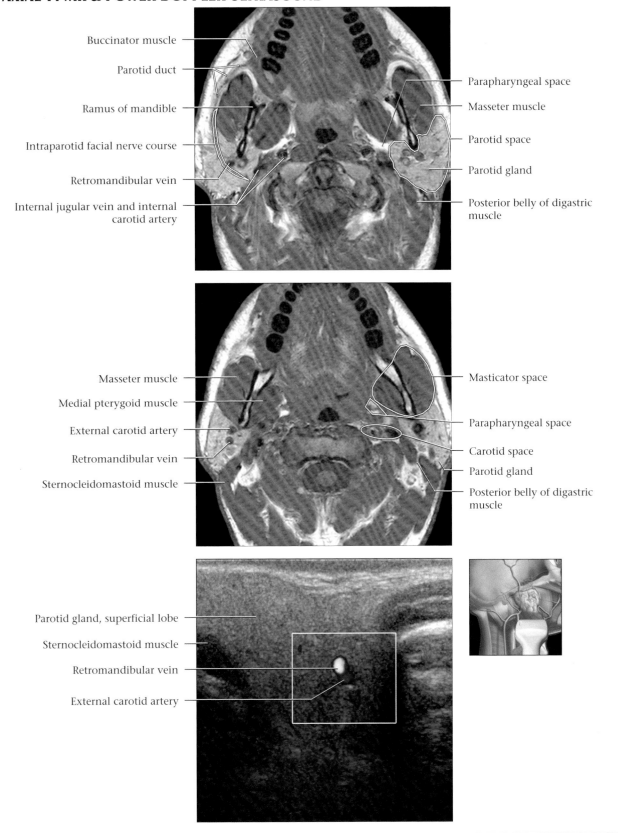

Buccinator muscle

Parotid duct

Ramus of mandible

Intraparotid facial nerve course

Retromandibular vein

Internal jugular vein and internal carotid artery

Parapharyngeal space

Masseter muscle

Parotid space

Parotid gland

Posterior belly of digastric muscle

Masseter muscle

Medial pterygoid muscle

External carotid artery

Retromandibular vein

Sternocleidomastoid muscle

Masticator space

Parapharyngeal space

Carotid space

Parotid gland

Posterior belly of digastric muscle

Parotid gland, superficial lobe

Sternocleidomastoid muscle

Retromandibular vein

External carotid artery

(Top) Axial T1-weighted MR image at the oral pharyngeal level. The parotid gland is seen as a homogeneous T1WI hyperintense structure posterolateral to the mandibular ramus and masseter muscle. Note the projected intraparotid facial nerve course drawn on the right. (Middle) Axial T1-weighted image of a more inferior level of the parotid glands. The parotid space relates anteriorly to the masticator space, medially to the parapharyngeal space and is separated medially by the posterior belly of digastric muscle from the carotid space. (Bottom) Power Doppler ultrasound helps to depict the retromandibular vein and external carotid artery, which are sometimes difficult to see in patients with bright fatty parotid glands. The RMV and ECA help to infer location of CN7.

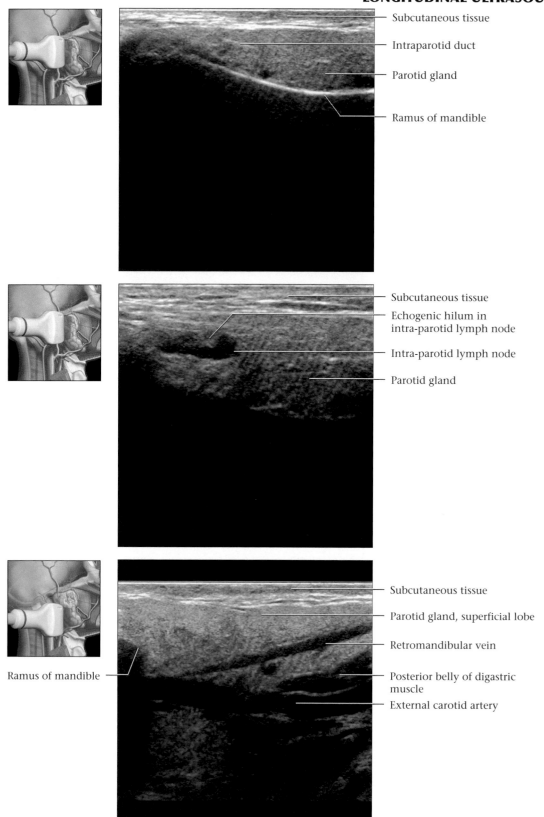

Subcutaneous tissue

Intraparotid duct

Parotid gland

Ramus of mandible

Subcutaneous tissue

Echogenic hilum in intra-parotid lymph node

Intra-parotid lymph node

Parotid gland

Subcutaneous tissue

Parotid gland, superficial lobe

Retromandibular vein

Ramus of mandible

Posterior belly of digastric muscle

External carotid artery

(Top) First image of a series of longitudinal grayscale ultrasound scans of the parotid gland. The parotid gland is superficial to the ramus of mandible. (Middle) Second image shows a normal intra-parotid lymph node in the superficial lobe of parotid gland. On high resolution US normal nodes are invariably seen in the parotid tail and in the pretragal parotid gland. The elliptical shape and normal internal architecture with echogenic hilum suggest its benign nature. (Bottom) Third image at the plane of retromandibular vein. Such anatomy is best seen in children and young adults where there is not much fat deposition in the gland.

PAROTID REGION

CORONAL T1 MR & POWER DOPPLER ULTRASOUND

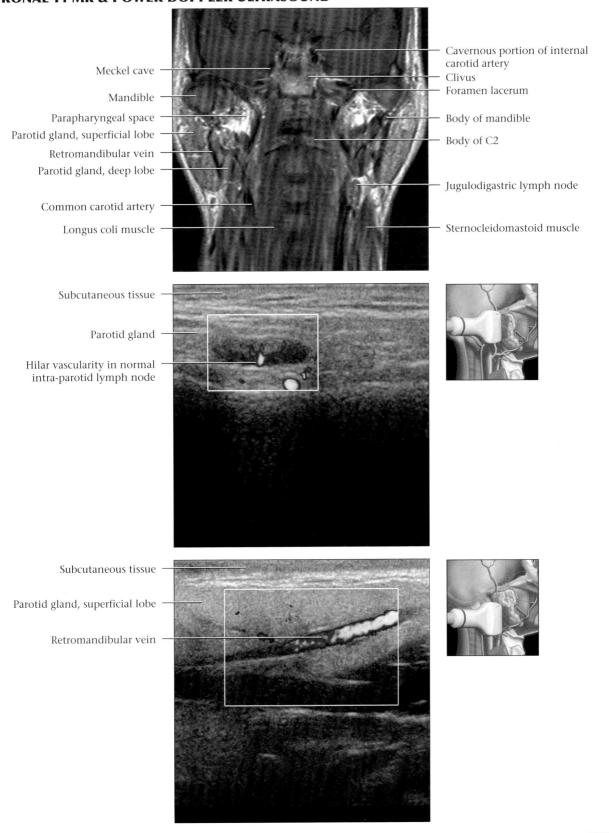

Meckel cave

Mandible

Parapharyngeal space

Parotid gland, superficial lobe

Retromandibular vein

Parotid gland, deep lobe

Common carotid artery

Longus coli muscle

Cavernous portion of internal carotid artery

Clivus

Foramen lacerum

Body of mandible

Body of C2

Jugulodigastric lymph node

Sternocleidomastoid muscle

Subcutaneous tissue

Parotid gland

Hilar vascularity in normal intra-parotid lymph node

Subcutaneous tissue

Parotid gland, superficial lobe

Retromandibular vein

(Top) Coronal T1-weighted MR image of the parotid glands. The retromandibular vein is seen as a signal void tubular structure traversing the parotid gland vertically helping to suggest location of CN7. **(Middle)** Longitudinal power Doppler ultrasound of the parotid gland shows the presence of hilar vascularity within a normal intra-parotid lymph node. On high resolution US more nodes are seen in children compared to adults. **(Bottom)** Longitudinal power Doppler ultrasound of the parotid gland clearly delineating the retromandibular vein.

TRANSVERSE ULTRASOUND & PATHOLOGY

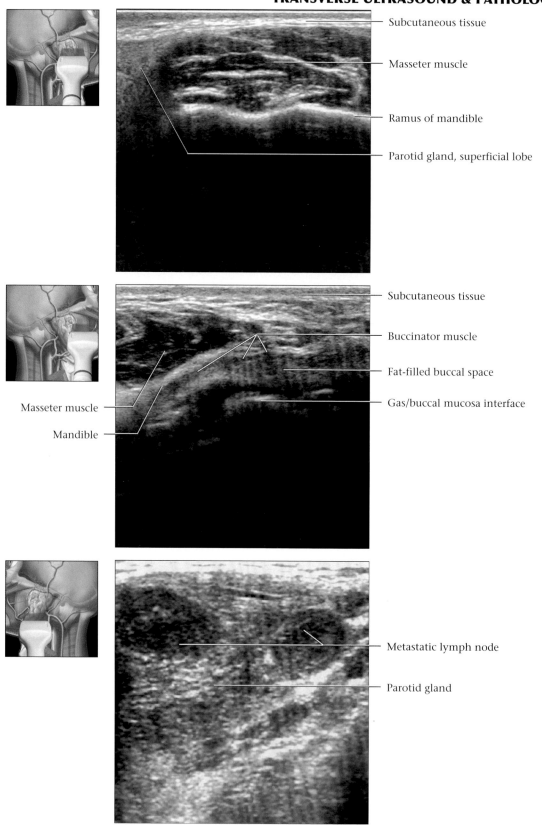

Subcutaneous tissue

Masseter muscle

Ramus of mandible

Parotid gland, superficial lobe

Subcutaneous tissue

Buccinator muscle

Fat-filled buccal space

Gas/buccal mucosa interface

Masseter muscle

Mandible

Metastatic lymph node

Parotid gland

(Top) Transverse grayscale ultrasound of the anterior parotid region. The masseter muscle is superficial to the ramus of mandible and closely related to the parotid gland. Note that masseter muscles lesions will clinically mimic parotid pathology. (Middle) Transverse grayscale ultrasound of the anterior parotid region/facial region. The buccinator muscle appears as a thin hypoechoic structure extending anteriorly and just medial to the anterior margin of the masseter muscle. The buccal space, which lies lateral to the buccinator muscle, is fat-filled and contains the facial nerve, vein, artery and the parotid duct. (Bottom) Transverse grayscale ultrasound of the left parotid gland shows multiple, well-defined, hypoechoic, solid nodules in the superficial lobe. Pathology: Metastatic undifferentiated lymph nodes, from nasopharyngeal carcinoma.

PAROTID REGION

AXIAL T1 MR & PATHOLOGY

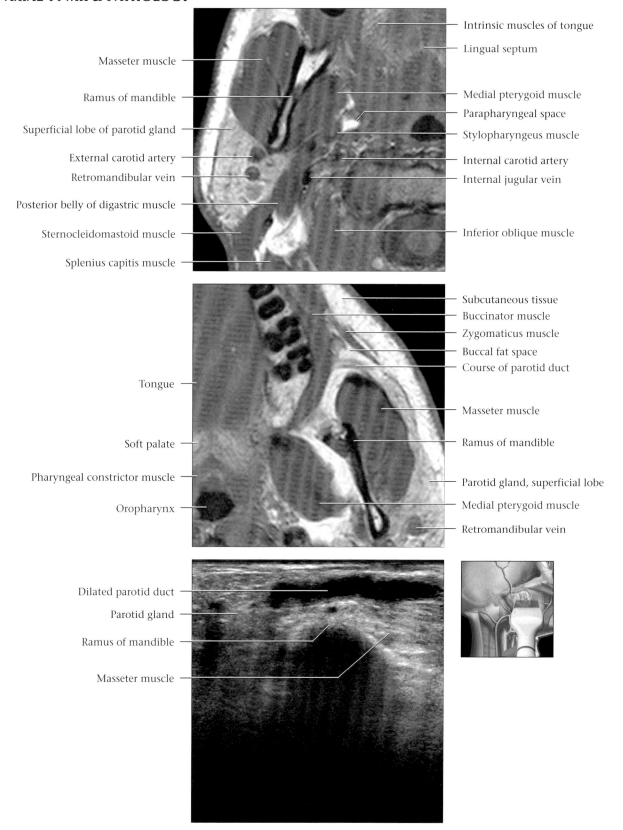

Masseter muscle

Ramus of mandible

Superficial lobe of parotid gland

External carotid artery

Retromandibular vein

Posterior belly of digastric muscle

Sternocleidomastoid muscle

Splenius capitis muscle

Intrinsic muscles of tongue

Lingual septum

Medial pterygoid muscle

Parapharyngeal space

Stylopharyngeus muscle

Internal carotid artery

Internal jugular vein

Inferior oblique muscle

Tongue

Soft palate

Pharyngeal constrictor muscle

Oropharynx

Subcutaneous tissue

Buccinator muscle

Zygomaticus muscle

Buccal fat space

Course of parotid duct

Masseter muscle

Ramus of mandible

Parotid gland, superficial lobe

Medial pterygoid muscle

Retromandibular vein

Dilated parotid duct

Parotid gland

Ramus of mandible

Masseter muscle

(Top) Axial T1WI MR of right parotid region shows the relationship of parotid gland to the masseter muscle, ramus of mandible; parapharyngeal space, posterior belly of digastric muscle; the upper sternocleidomastoid muscle. (Middle) Axial T1WI MR of anterior parotid region. The parotid duct courses anteromedially within the buccal fat space and pierces the buccinator muscle at the level of upper 2nd molar into the buccal mucosa. (Bottom) Transverse grayscale ultrasound of the right parotid gland shows a grossly dilated parotid duct superficial to the ramus of the mandible and masseter muscles. The ductal dilatation is due to distal parotid ductal stricture close to the orificial opening. Note that the parotid gland itself is atrophic and heterogeneous, secondarily to chronic infection.

UPPER CERVICAL LEVEL

Terminology

Abbreviations
- Internal carotid artery (ICA)
- External carotid artery (ECA)
- Internal jugular vein (IJV)
- Jugulodigastric (JD) lymph node

Synonyms
- Carotid triangle
- Suprahyoid anterior triangle

Definitions
- Portion of anterior triangle adjacent to major vessels of carotid sheath
- Extending from skull base superiorly to hyoid bone inferiorly

Imaging Anatomy

Overview
- Cervical region is divided into upper, mid and lower cervical levels in order to identify relevant groups of jugular cervical lymph nodes
- On US upper cervical region is best scanned transversely from submandibular/parotid tail region to the carotid bifurcation
- Major structures of upper cervical level: Cervical portion of ICA, ECA with origins of major branches, carotid bifurcation, IJV, posterior belly of digastric muscle, JD lymph node

Internal Structures-Critical Contents
- Cervical portion of ICA
  - One of two branches from common carotid artery
    - Runs lateral or posterolateral to ECA
    - Usually of larger caliber than ECA
    - Low resistance arterial flow waveform on Doppler ultrasound
  - Supplies anterior part of brain, eye and its appendages
  - Divided into bulbous, cervical, petrous, cavernous and cerebral portions
  - Only first two portions lie extracranially and accessible by ultrasound
  - No branch in extracranial portions
- ECA
  - Runs medial to cervical ICA
  - Smaller than ICA
  - High resistance arterial flow waveform on Doppler ultrasound
  - Plays a pivotal role in collateral circulation if there is arterial occlusion of ICA/vertebral artery
  - First branch: Superior thyroid artery
    - Readily detected by grayscale and Doppler examination
- Carotid bifurcation
  - Approximately at level of hyoid bone (i.e., division between upper and mid cervical levels)
  - Bulbous dilatation of proximal ICA beyond carotid bifurcation: Carotid bulb
  - Carotid body is located at carotid bifurcation
- IJV
  - Inferior continuation of sigmoid sinus from level of jugular foramen at skull base
  - Right usually of larger caliber than left
  - Lateral/posterolateral to internal carotid artery
  - Acts as landmark for jugular cervical lymph nodes
- Posterior belly of digastric muscle
  - Key structure in separating parotid region superiorly from upper cervical level inferiorly
  - Runs anteroinferiorly from mastoid process to hyoid bone
  - Emerges deep to sternocleidomastoid muscle to abut tail of parotid gland
  - Major vessels (from posterior to anterior: Internal jugular vein, internal carotid artery and external carotid artery) run deep to muscle
- JD lymph node
  - Largest and most superior lymph node of deep jugular chain, also known as "sentinel" node of internal jugular chain
  - Resides in close to carotid bifurcation/IJV
  - Orientated along line of digastric muscle
  - Commonly involved in head and neck cancer
- Vagus nerve
  - Descends from skull base within the carotid sheath
  - Sandwiched between ICA medially and IJV
  - More difficult to see than in mid and lower cervical levels

Anatomy-Based Imaging Issues

Key Concepts or Questions
- Common differential diagnoses for a mass in upper cervical level
  - Enlarged lymph nodes: Reactive, inflammatory and neoplasm (metastases/lymphoma)
  - Congenital lesion: Second branchial cleft cyst
  - Vascular lesion: IJV varix, IJV thrombosis
  - Neoplasm: Vagal schwannoma, carotid body tumor
- JD lymph node is common site of nodal metastases from head and neck cancer
  - Common sites of primary include oral cavity (including tonsils and tongue), nasopharyngeal carcinoma
  - JD node also commonly involved in lymphoma
    - Multiple, often bilateral nodal involvement, pseudocystic/reticulated internal architecture on US

Imaging Recommendations
- Scan in transverse plane from submandibular region/parotid tail down to carotid bifurcation
- Color flow imaging helps to identify major vessels and their anatomic relation to node/mass
  - Also provides flow information of cervical masses to characterize their nature
- US provides safe real-time guidance for fine needle aspiration cytology (FNAC)/biopsy to further enhance diagnostic yield
  - FNAC/biopsy is not recommended for suspected carotid body tumor due to risk of uncontrolled bleeding

GRAPHICS

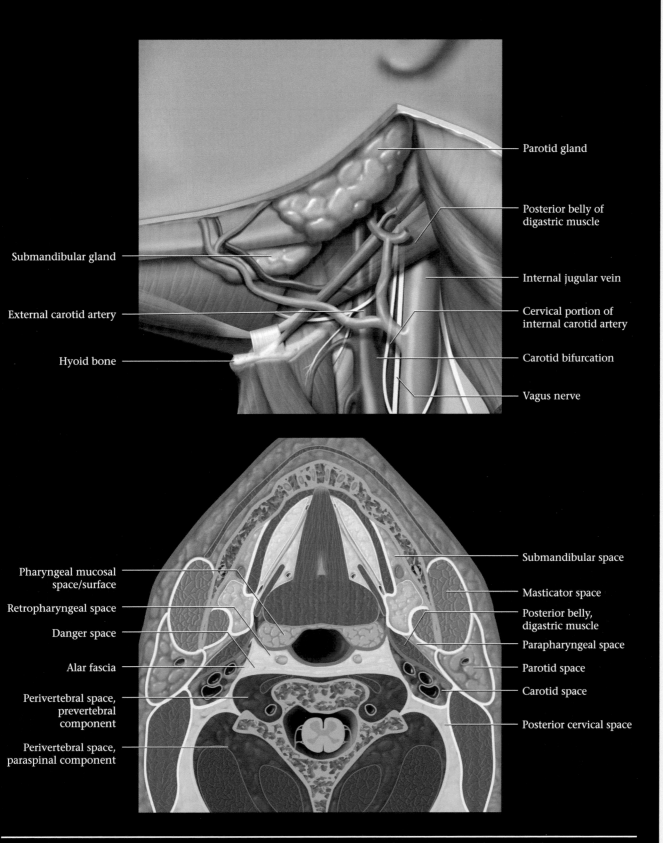

Parotid gland

Posterior belly of digastric muscle

Submandibular gland

Internal jugular vein

External carotid artery

Cervical portion of internal carotid artery

Hyoid bone

Carotid bifurcation

Vagus nerve

Pharyngeal mucosal space/surface

Submandibular space

Retropharyngeal space

Masticator space

Danger space

Posterior belly, digastric muscle

Alar fascia

Parapharyngeal space

Perivertebral space, prevertebral component

Parotid space

Carotid space

Perivertebral space, paraspinal component

Posterior cervical space

(Top) Schematic diagram shows the key structures in the upper cervical level. The hyoid bone and the carotid bifurcation are two anatomical landmarks for the inferior margin of the upper cervical level. Note, with high resolution US, the jugulodigastric lymph node will be consistently seen at this site & should not be mistaken for pathology. Visualization of a similar node on the opposite side helps. **(Bottom)** Axial graphic of the suprahyoid neck spaces at the level of the oropharynx. The superficial (yellow line), middle (pink line) and deep (turquoise line) layers of the deep cervical fascia outline the suprahyoid neck spaces. Ultrasound assessment of the upper cervical level involves scanning transversely along the major vessels of the carotid sheath (i.e., the internal carotid artery and internal jugular vein).

TRANSVERSE ULTRASOUND

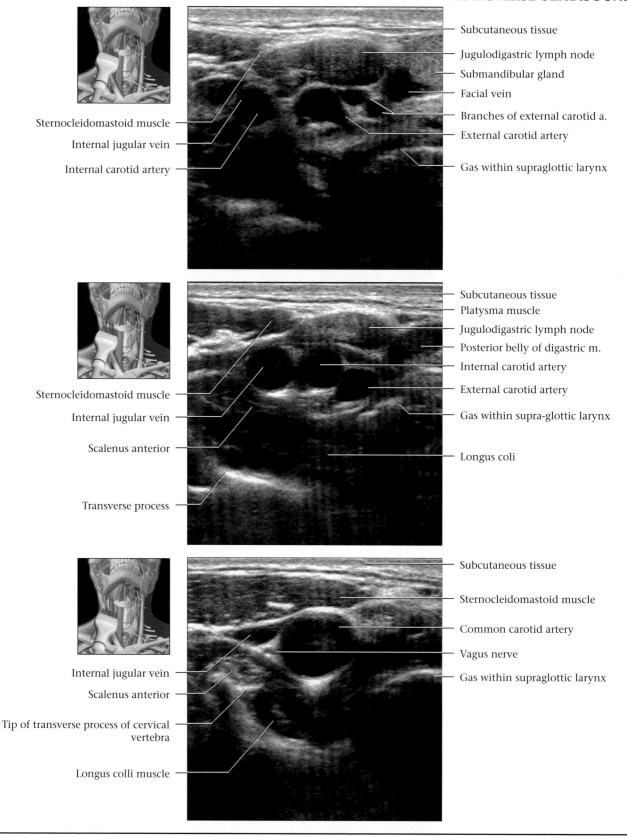

(Top) First image of a series of consecutive transverse grayscale ultrasound images of the upper cervical level. Key vascular landmarks, including the internal and external carotid arteries and the internal jugular vein, are clearly identified. The uppermost and largest deep cervical lymph node (i.e., the jugulodigastric lymph node) is constantly seen on US in the upper cervical level anterior to the carotid arteries. It is usually elliptical, hypoechoic and with echogenic hilum. **(Middle)** Second image shows the carotid bifurcation in the transverse plane. The external carotid artery is usually more medial and smaller than the internal carotid artery. **(Bottom)** The third image is below the level of carotid bifurcation. The common carotid artery, internal jugular vein and vagus nerve are major structures within the carotid sheath and are clearly seen on US.

AXIAL CECT

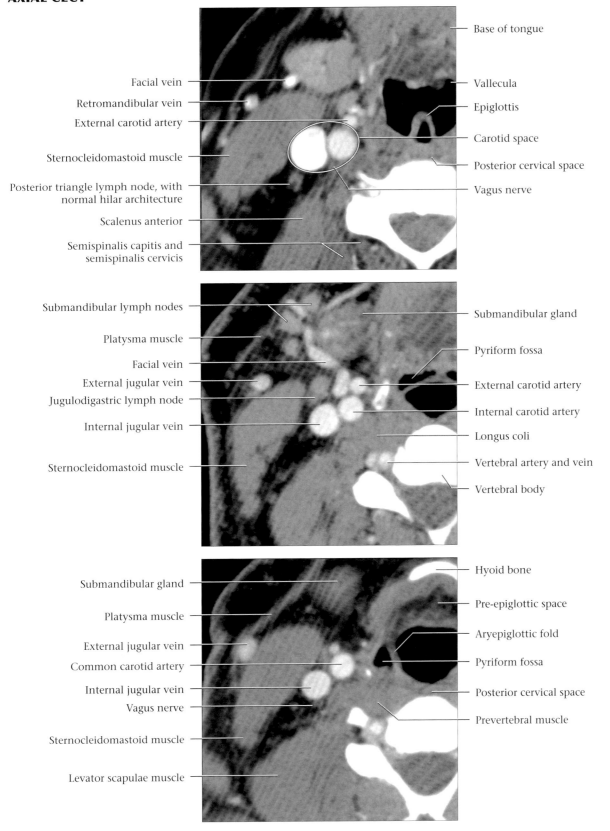

Base of tongue

Facial vein

Retromandibular vein

External carotid artery

Sternocleidomastoid muscle

Posterior triangle lymph node, with normal hilar architecture

Scalenus anterior

Semispinalis capitis and semispinalis cervicis

Vallecula

Epiglottis

Carotid space

Posterior cervical space

Vagus nerve

Submandibular lymph nodes

Platysma muscle

Facial vein

External jugular vein

Jugulodigastric lymph node

Internal jugular vein

Sternocleidomastoid muscle

Submandibular gland

Pyriform fossa

External carotid artery

Internal carotid artery

Longus coli

Vertebral artery and vein

Vertebral body

Submandibular gland

Platysma muscle

External jugular vein

Common carotid artery

Internal jugular vein

Vagus nerve

Sternocleidomastoid muscle

Levator scapulae muscle

Hyoid bone

Pre-epiglottic space

Aryepiglottic fold

Pyriform fossa

Posterior cervical space

Prevertebral muscle

(Top) At the level just above the hyoid bone, the carotid bifurcation can be seen. The vagus nerve is seen within the carotid sheath. (Middle) First image of series of axial CECT of the suprahyoid neck at the level of the free margin of epiglottis. The jugulodigastric lymph node is commonly seen. However the internal architecture is better assessed on ultrasound than CECT. (Bottom) At the level of the hyoid bone, the carotid space now contains the common carotid artery, internal jugular vein and vagus nerve only. The submandibular space is seen anteriorly, predominantly fat-filled at this level. Familiarity with cross-sectional anatomy is key to optimal US examination of the neck, as lesions at this level are site specific.

TRANSVERSE ULTRASOUND AND PATHOLOGY

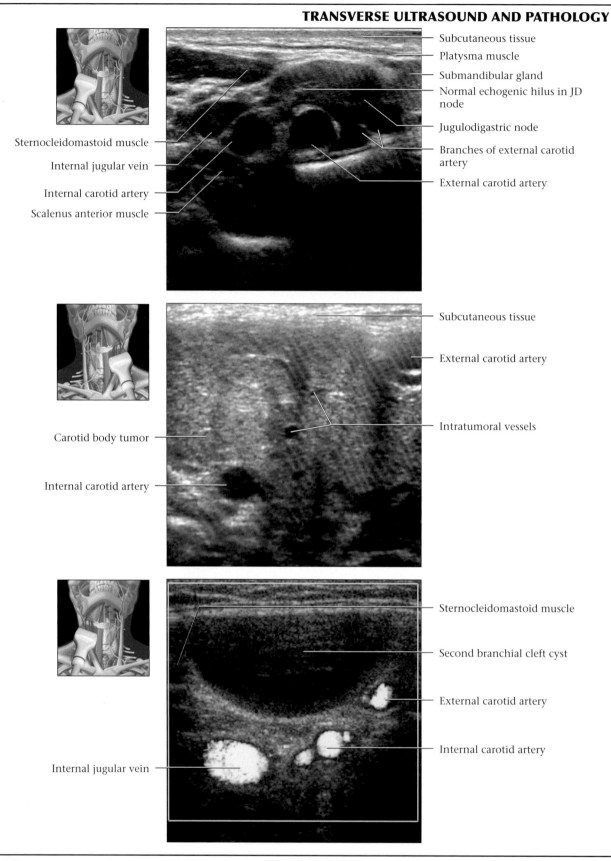

(Top) Transverse grayscale ultrasound of upper cervical level. The normal jugulodigastric lymph node is elliptical in shape with preserved echogenic hilum. Its anatomical relationship with the major neck vessels is better appreciated on power Doppler ultrasound. **(Middle)** Transverse grayscale ultrasound of the left upper cervical level shows a large heterogeneous hypoechoic mass centered at the carotid bifurcation splaying the internal and external carotid arteries. The appearances and location are suggestive of a carotid body tumor. **(Bottom)** Transverse power Doppler ultrasound of the right upper cervical level shows a well-circumscribed cystic mass along the medial edge of the sternomastoid muscle and superficial to the major vessels of the carotid sheath. The location and appearances are suggestive of a second branchial cleft cyst.

POWER DOPPLER ULTRASOUND AND PATHOLOGY

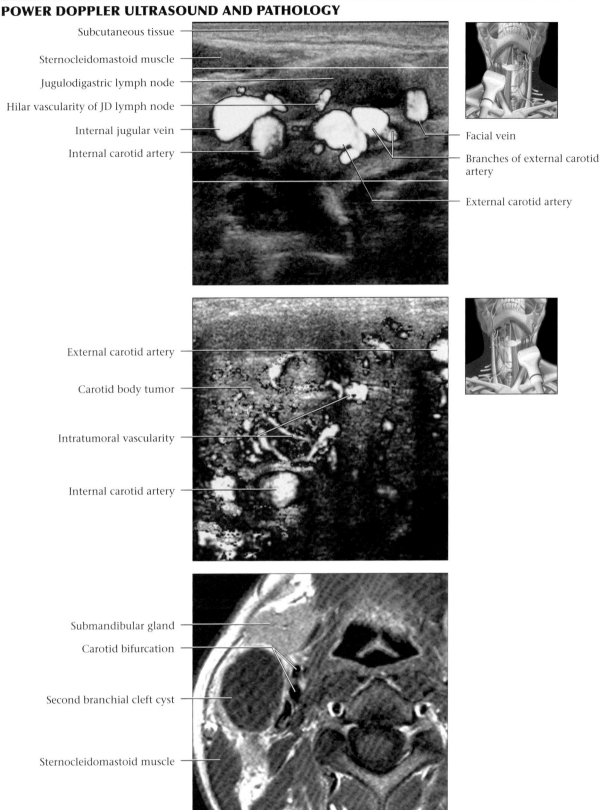

Subcutaneous tissue
Sternocleidomastoid muscle
Jugulodigastric lymph node
Hilar vascularity of JD lymph node
Internal jugular vein
Internal carotid artery

Facial vein
Branches of external carotid artery
External carotid artery

External carotid artery
Carotid body tumor
Intratumoral vascularity
Internal carotid artery

Submandibular gland
Carotid bifurcation
Second branchial cleft cyst
Sternocleidomastoid muscle

(Top) Transverse power Doppler ultrasound of the upper cervical level. The major vessels, including the internal and external carotid arteries and the internal jugular vein, show color flow. Note the presence of normal hilar vascularity within the echogenic hilum of the jugulodigastric lymph node. (Middle) Transverse power Doppler ultrasound shows florid intra-tumoral vessels in a carotid body tumor. Note the splaying of the internal and external carotid arteries. (Bottom) Post-gadolinium axial T1WI MR shows the typical appearances of a second branchial cleft cyst - cystic in signal with no enhancement, well-circumscribed margin, posterior to the submandibular gland and along the medial edge of the sternocleidomastoid muscle.

MID CERVICAL LEVEL

Terminology

Abbreviations
- Common carotid artery (CCA)
- Internal jugular vein (IJV)
- Vagus nerve (CN10)

Definitions
- Portion of anterior triangle adjacent to the major vessels of carotid sheath
- Extends from hyoid bone superiorly to cricoid cartilage inferiorly

Imaging Anatomy

Overview
- Major lymphatic drainage of the head and neck region is via the deep jugular cervical lymph nodes which are distributed along upper, mid and lower cervical levels
- Key structures in mid cervical level include CCA, IJV, vagus nerve, lymph nodes, omohyoid muscle and esophagus

Internal Structures-Critical Contents
- CCA
  - Arises from aortic arch directly on the left, from brachiocephalic trunk on the right
  - Ascends the neck within the carotid sheath
    - Medial to the IJV
    - Vagus nerve sandwiched between CCA and IJV
  - No named branches in mid cervical level
  - Bifurcates into internal carotid artery (ICA) and external carotid artery (ECA) at the level of hyoid bone
  - Low resistance arterial flow pattern
- IJV
  - Inferior continuation of sigmoid sinus from jugular foramen at skull base
  - Major deep venous drainage from brain and neck
  - Descends within the carotid sheath
    - Lateral to CCA at mid cervical level
  - Joins subclavian vein to form brachiocephalic vein
  - During sonography, make sure the IJV is compressible and has respiratory phasicity to rule out presence of thrombus
  - Occasionally presence of slow venous flow may mimic IJV thrombus
    - Real-time visualization of layering and a sharp linear interface help to distinguish it from thrombus
- Vagus nerve/CN10
  - Extracranial segment starts superiorly from jugular foramen at skull base
  - Descends along posterolateral aspect of carotid artery within carotid sheath
    - Passes anterior to aortic arch on the left and subclavian artery on the right
  - Major autonomic nerve supply to visceral organs in thorax and abdomen
  - On transverse sonography it appears as a round, hypoechoic structure with central echogenicity
    - Its close relation to CCA, IJV are clue to its identification
    - On longitudinal scan it is seen as a long tubular hypoechoic structure with fibrillary pattern
- Lymph nodes
  - Numerous lymph nodes are seen along deep jugular chain in mid cervical level
  - Receive lymphatic drainage from upper jugular chain and directly from adjacent structures including larynx, hypopharynx and thyroid gland
    - Commonly involved in nodal metastases from common head and neck cancers
  - Usually located anterior to vessels of carotid sheath
  - Normal ultrasound appearances: Small, elliptical in shape, presence of echogenic hilus, preserved hilar vascularity on Doppler imaging
- Omohyoid muscle
  - Arises from anterior portion of body of hyoid bone
  - Runs obliquely to cross anterior to CCA and deep to sternocleidomastoid muscle
  - Intermediate tendon overlies the IJV
    - Occasionally mistaken for a lymph node
  - Then runs obliquely across the inferior posterior triangle to attach to posterior aspect of lateral clavicle
- Cervical esophagus
  - The junction of cricopharyngeus muscle and proximal cervical esophagus is located in mid cervical level
  - Lies posterior/posterolateral to the trachea and medial to CCA
    - More commonly slightly off midline to the left
    - Asking the patient to swallow during real time sonography helps to accurately identify the esophagus
  - On US, it may be mistaken for parathyroid adenoma or paratracheal lymph node

Anatomy-Based Imaging Issues

Key Concepts or Questions
- Common differential diagnoses for mass in mid cervical level
  - Enlarged lymph nodes - reactive, inflammatory or neoplasm (metastases/lymphoma)
  - Inflammatory - abscess
  - Congenital lesion - lymphangioma, off-midline thyroglossal duct cyst
  - Neoplasm - vagal Schwannoma

Imaging Approaches
- Scan in transverse plane along major vessels of carotid sheath
  - From carotid bifurcation down to level of cricoid cartilage
- Color flow imaging helps to identify major vessels and characterize lesions in this region
- USG also provides safe real-time guidance for fine needle aspiration cytology (FNAC) or biopsy

GRAPHICS

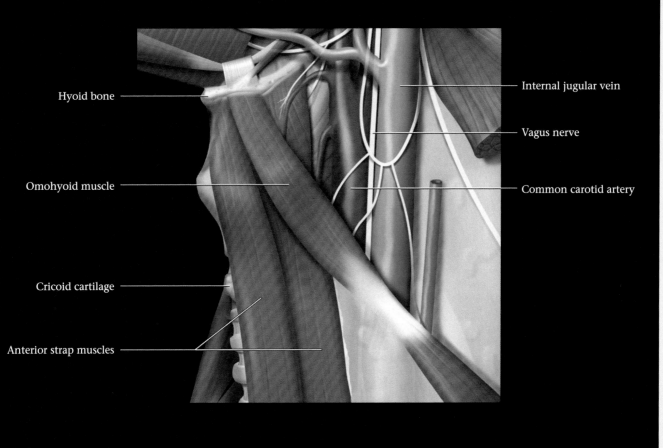

Hyoid bone

Omohyoid muscle

Cricoid cartilage

Anterior strap muscles

Internal jugular vein

Vagus nerve

Common carotid artery

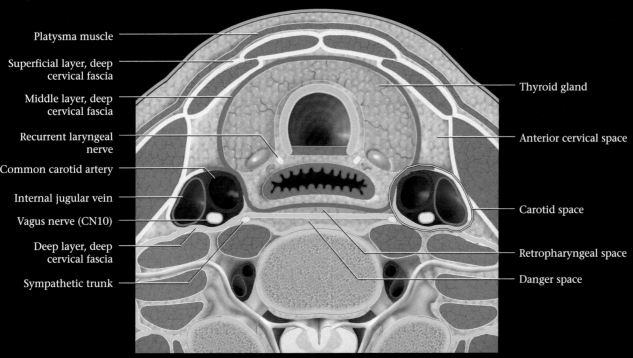

Platysma muscle

Superficial layer, deep cervical fascia

Middle layer, deep cervical fascia

Recurrent laryngeal nerve

Common carotid artery

Internal jugular vein

Vagus nerve (CN10)

Deep layer, deep cervical fascia

Sympathetic trunk

Thyroid gland

Anterior cervical space

Carotid space

Retropharyngeal space

Danger space

(Top) Schematic diagram of the mid cervical level containing key structures including the common carotid artery, the internal jugular vein and the vagus nerve within the carotid sheath. The hyoid bone and the cricoid cartilage are the anatomical landmarks for the superior and inferior borders of the mid cervical level respectively. Note, with high resolution US, normal small jugular chain lymph nodes may be seen at this site & should not be mistaken for pathology. (Bottom) Axial graphic of the middle cervical level in the infrahyoid neck. Note that the carotid sheath contains all 3 layers of the deep cervical fascia (tri-color line). In the infrahyoid neck the carotid sheath is tenacious throughout its length. The infrahyoid carotid space contains the common carotid artery, the internal jugular vein and only the vagus cranial nerve.

TRANSVERSE ULTRASOUND

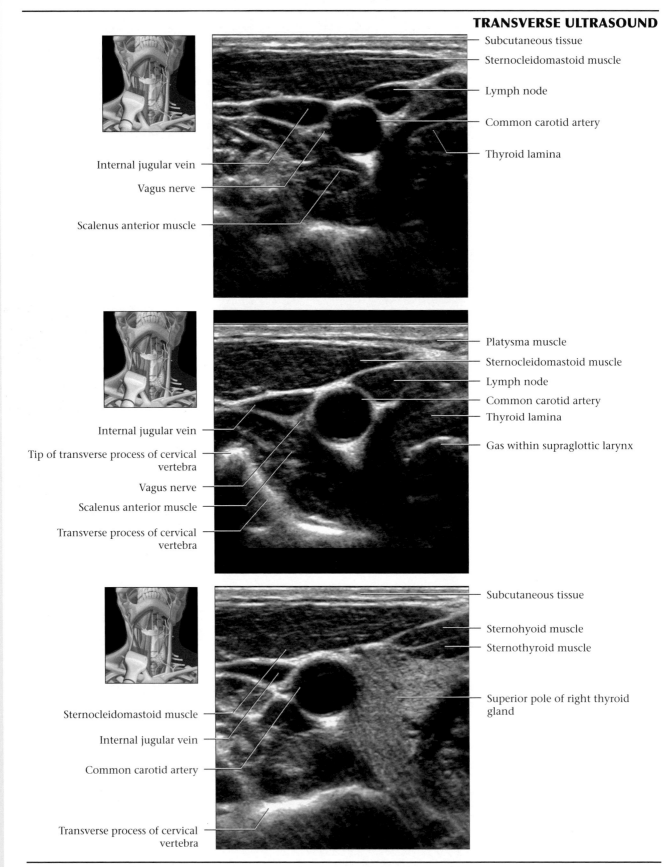

Top image labels:
- Subcutaneous tissue
- Sternocleidomastoid muscle
- Lymph node
- Common carotid artery
- Thyroid lamina
- Internal jugular vein
- Vagus nerve
- Scalenus anterior muscle

Middle image labels:
- Platysma muscle
- Sternocleidomastoid muscle
- Lymph node
- Common carotid artery
- Thyroid lamina
- Gas within supraglottic larynx
- Internal jugular vein
- Tip of transverse process of cervical vertebra
- Vagus nerve
- Scalenus anterior muscle
- Transverse process of cervical vertebra

Bottom image labels:
- Subcutaneous tissue
- Sternohyoid muscle
- Sternothyroid muscle
- Superior pole of right thyroid gland
- Sternocleidomastoid muscle
- Internal jugular vein
- Common carotid artery
- Transverse process of cervical vertebra

(Top) First image of consecutive transverse grayscale ultrasound of mid cervical level. Deep cervical lymph nodes are commonly found along and anterior to major vessels of the carotid sheath. These are commonly hypoechoic and elliptical with a normal echogenic hilum and hilar vascularity. **(Middle)** The second image of mid cervical level in transverse plane. At this level, common carotid artery, internal jugular vein and vagus nerve are the main structures within the carotid sheath. The vagus nerve is usually located between the CCA and the IJV, and appears as a small round hypoechoic round nodule with a central echogenic dot. **(Bottom)** The third image of the mid cervical level. The cricoid cartilage may not be routinely seen on ultrasound and visualization of the superior pole of the thyroid gland approximately coincides with this level.

MID CERVICAL LEVEL

AXIAL CECT

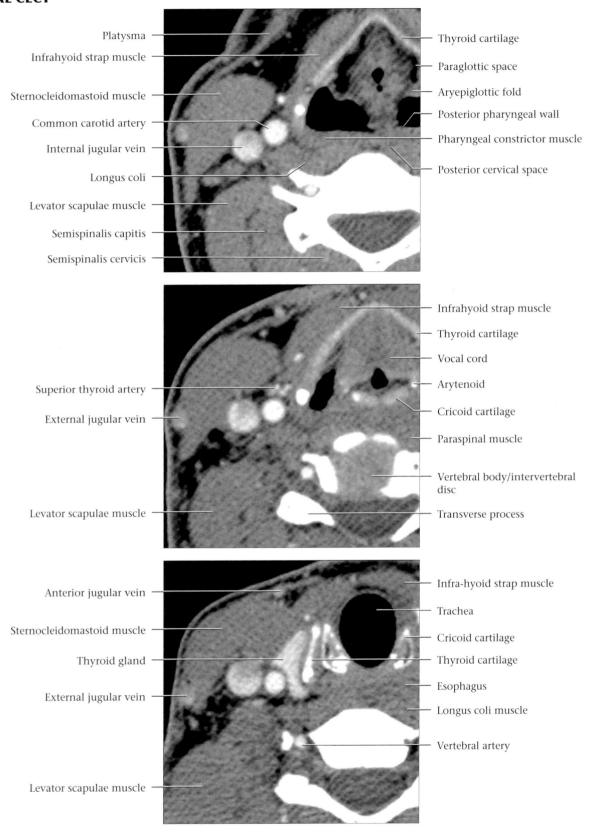

Platysma

Infrahyoid strap muscle

Sternocleidomastoid muscle

Common carotid artery

Internal jugular vein

Longus coli

Levator scapulae muscle

Semispinalis capitis

Semispinalis cervicis

Thyroid cartilage

Paraglottic space

Aryepiglottic fold

Posterior pharyngeal wall

Pharyngeal constrictor muscle

Posterior cervical space

Superior thyroid artery

External jugular vein

Levator scapulae muscle

Infrahyoid strap muscle

Thyroid cartilage

Vocal cord

Arytenoid

Cricoid cartilage

Paraspinal muscle

Vertebral body/intervertebral disc

Transverse process

Anterior jugular vein

Sternocleidomastoid muscle

Thyroid gland

External jugular vein

Levator scapulae muscle

Infra-hyoid strap muscle

Trachea

Cricoid cartilage

Thyroid cartilage

Esophagus

Longus coli muscle

Vertebral artery

(Top) CECT at the upper thyroid cartilage level. Major structures of the mid cervical level including the common carotid artery, the internal jugular vein, and the sternocleidomastoid muscle are well-demonstrated. Small lymph nodes are commonly seen adjacent to major vessels of the carotid sheath. **(Middle)** CECT at the level of the lower thyroid lamina. Apart from the common carotid artery and the internal jugular vein, branches of the external carotid artery such as the superior thyroid artery can be demonstrated. **(Bottom)** CECT at the level of the cricoid cartilage. The upper pole of the thyroid gland begins to be included in cross-section. Note the presence of calcification/ossification in thyroid lamina and cricoid cartilages which is a normal age-related change.

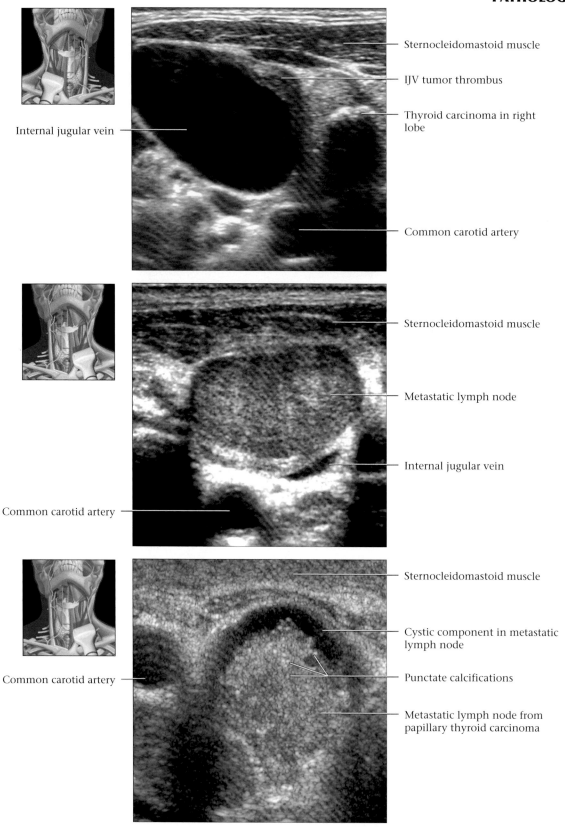

Internal jugular vein

Sternocleidomastoid muscle

IJV tumor thrombus

Thyroid carcinoma in right lobe

Common carotid artery

Common carotid artery

Sternocleidomastoid muscle

Metastatic lymph node

Internal jugular vein

Common carotid artery

Sternocleidomastoid muscle

Cystic component in metastatic lymph node

Punctate calcifications

Metastatic lymph node from papillary thyroid carcinoma

(Top) Transverse grayscale ultrasound of right mid cervical level shows an eccentric hypoechoic thrombus in the anteromedial wall of the right internal jugular vein. Note the presence of an adjacent thyroid carcinoma in right lobe. (Middle) Transverse grayscale ultrasound of the left mid cervical level shows an enlarged, round, solid, hypoechoic, deep cervical lymph node with loss of echogenic hilum. The adjacent left internal jugular vein is compressed. Pathology: Metastatic squamous cell carcinoma. (Bottom) Transverse grayscale ultrasound of left mid cervical level shows an enlarged, round, solid, slightly hyperechoic, internal jugular lymph node with punctate calcifications and cystic changes suggesting a metastatic lymph node from papillary thyroid carcinoma.

PATHOLOGY

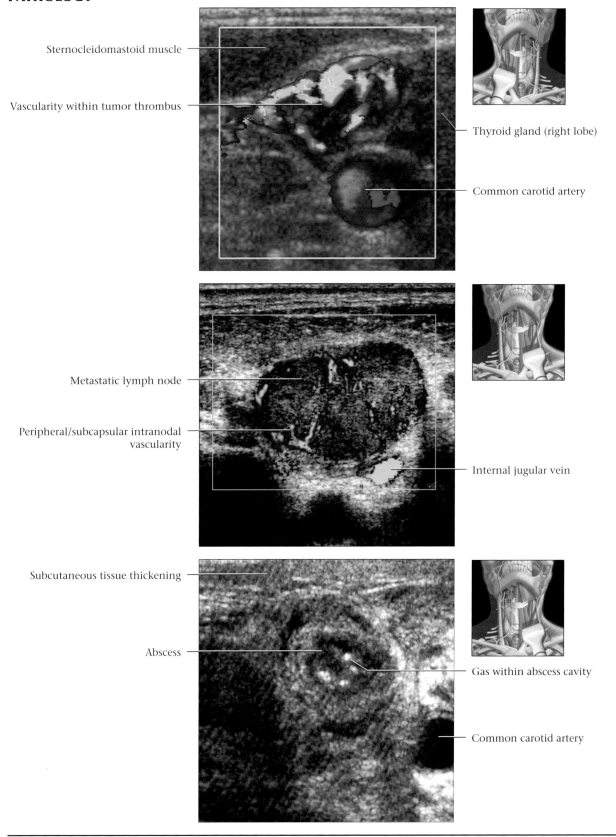

Sternocleidomastoid muscle

Vascularity within tumor thrombus

Thyroid gland (right lobe)

Common carotid artery

Metastatic lymph node

Peripheral/subcapsular intranodal vascularity

Internal jugular vein

Subcutaneous tissue thickening

Abscess

Gas within abscess cavity

Common carotid artery

(Top) Transverse color Doppler ultrasound in a patient with occlusive IJV thrombus. Note the presence of vascularity within the IJV thrombus suggesting it is a tumor thrombus rather than a bland venous thrombus. (Middle) Transverse power Doppler ultrasound shows the presence of peripheral/subcapsular intranodal vessels in a metastatic lymph node from head and neck squamous cell carcinoma. The vascularity is completely different from the hilar pattern of a normal cervical lymph node. (Bottom) Transverse grayscale ultrasound of a neck abscess with fluid and gas within. The adjacent soft tissue is edematous and thickened. Note its close proximity to the CCA putting it at a risk of rupture.

LOWER CERVICAL LEVEL & SUPRACLAVICULAR FOSSA

Terminology

Abbreviations
- Common carotid artery (CCA)
- Internal jugular vein (IJV)

Definitions
- Portion of lower anterior neck adjacent to carotid sheath below the level of cricoid cartilage and above the level of clavicle

Imaging Anatomy

Overview
- Key structures in lower cervical level include CCA, IJV, vagus nerve, subclavian artery, scalenus anterior muscle, lymph nodes
- Important structures in supraclavicular fossa include trapezius muscle, sternocleidomastoid muscle, omohyoid muscle, brachial plexus trunks/divisions, transverse cervical chain lymph nodes

Internal Structures-Critical Contents
- Subclavian artery
  - Arises from brachiocephalic trunk on the right and aortic arch on the left
  - Major arterial supply to upper limb
  - Contributes to arterial supply to neck structures and brain via vertebral artery
  - The junction of subclavian artery and CCA is readily identified on scanning in transverse plane in lower cervical level
    - Location marks root of the neck
  - Origin of the subclavian artery can be seen by angulating the transducer inferiorly behind the medial head of clavicle
- Scalenus anterior muscle
  - Runs inferiorly from transverse processes of cervical spine
  - Passes posterior to IJV to dip behind clavicle
  - Lies between second part of subclavian artery posteriorly and subclavian vein anteriorly
  - Related posteriorly to scalenus medius muscle
    - Brachial plexus elements lie between scalenus anterior muscle and scalenus medius muscle in supraclavicular fossa
    - Scanning inferiorly in transverse plane, brachial plexus elements appear as small, round, hypoechoic structures emerging from behind the lateral border of scalenus anterior muscle
- Brachial plexus (BP)
  - Formed from ventral rami of C5-T1 ± minor branches from C4, T2
  - BP divided into roots/rami, trunks, division, cords and terminal branches
  - Roots/rami: Originate from spinal cord levels C5-T1 enter posterior triangle by emerging between scalenus anterior and medius muscle
  - Trunks: Upper (C5-6), middle (C7), lower (C8-T1)
  - Divisions: Formed by each trunk, dividing into anterior and posterior branches in supraclavicular fossa
  - Cords: Lateral, medial, posterior cords, descend behind clavicle to leave posterior triangle and enter axilla
  - Branches: In axilla
- Trapezius muscle
  - Anterior border marks posterior margin of posterior triangle and supraclavicular fossa and is easily recognized
  - Distal portion is attached to lateral clavicle
- Inferior belly of omohyoid muscle
  - Runs obliquely from intermediate tendon to transverse the inferior portion of supraclavicular fossa
  - It divides the occipital triangle superiorly from supraclavicular triangle inferiorly
- Transverse cervical chain lymph nodes
  - Seen adjacent to transverse cervical artery and vein which arise from thyrocervical trunk and IJV
  - Related to and just superior to inferior belly of omohyoid muscle

Anatomy-Based Imaging Issues

Key Concepts or Questions
- Enlarged lymph node still most common cause of mass in lower cervical level and supraclavicular fossa
  - Terminology
    - Omohyoid node: Deep cervical chain node just superior to omohyoid (where it crosses IJV)
    - Virchow node: Signal node; lowest node of deep cervical chain nodes
    - Troisier node: Most medial node of transverse cervical chain nodes
  - Reactive nodes: Enlarged, cortical hypertrophy, preserved echogenic hilus and hilar vascularity
  - Tuberculous lymphadenitis: Matted, necrotic enlarged nodes with soft tissue edema, hypovascular/displaced hilar vascularity on power Doppler examination
  - Metastatic nodes: Round, hypoechoic nodes with peripheral/subcapsular vascularity
  - Lymphomatous nodes: Large, heterogeneous, reticulated/pseudocystic appearance, increased peripheral and central vascularity, bilateral involvement
- Isolated metastatic lymph node in supraclavicular fossa is unusual from primary in head and neck region
  - Careful search for infraclavicular primary is suggested
- Differential diagnoses
  - Brachial plexus schwannoma
  - Lipoma
  - Venous vascular malformation
  - Lymphangioma

Imaging Approaches
- From mid-cervical level, proceed scan in transverse plane along carotid sheath until the medial head of clavicle
- Then sweep laterally in transverse plane above the mid/lateral portion of clavicle to assess supraclavicular fossa

LOWER CERVICAL LEVEL & SUPRACLAVICULAR FOSSA

GRAPHICS

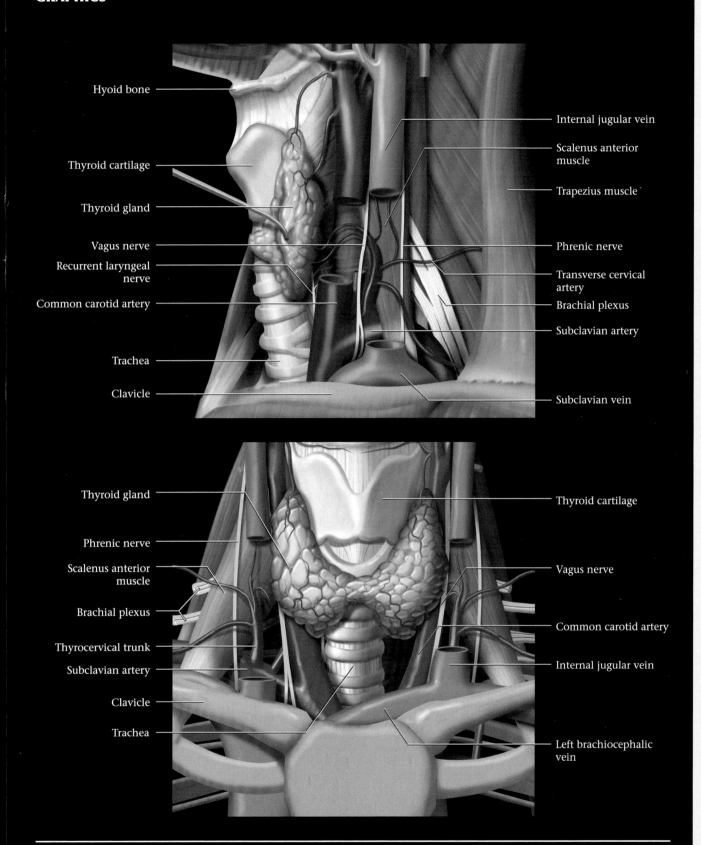

Hyoid bone

Thyroid cartilage

Thyroid gland

Vagus nerve

Recurrent laryngeal nerve

Common carotid artery

Trachea

Clavicle

Internal jugular vein

Scalenus anterior muscle

Trapezius muscle

Phrenic nerve

Transverse cervical artery

Brachial plexus

Subclavian artery

Subclavian vein

Thyroid gland

Phrenic nerve

Scalenus anterior muscle

Brachial plexus

Thyrocervical trunk

Subclavian artery

Clavicle

Trachea

Thyroid cartilage

Vagus nerve

Common carotid artery

Internal jugular vein

Left brachiocephalic vein

(Top) Graphic in lateral projection shows the anatomical relationship of major structures in the lower cervical level and supraclavicular fossa including the common carotid artery, internal jugular vein, subclavian vessels and brachial plexus. In assessing the supraclavicular fossa on ultrasound, adequate visualization is achieved by sweeping the transducer laterally in the transverse plane from the medial head of the clavicle. **(Bottom)** Graphic in frontal projection of the lower cervical level and medial portion of the supraclavicular fossa. The major lymph nodes in these regions are mainly located close to the major vessels of the carotid sheath including the Virchow node and the Troisier node. Presence of isolated malignant nodes at this site usually points towards an infraclavicular primary. Proximity of these nodes to adjacent pulsatile vessels makes Doppler examination at this site suboptimal/difficult.

TRANSVERSE ULTRASOUND

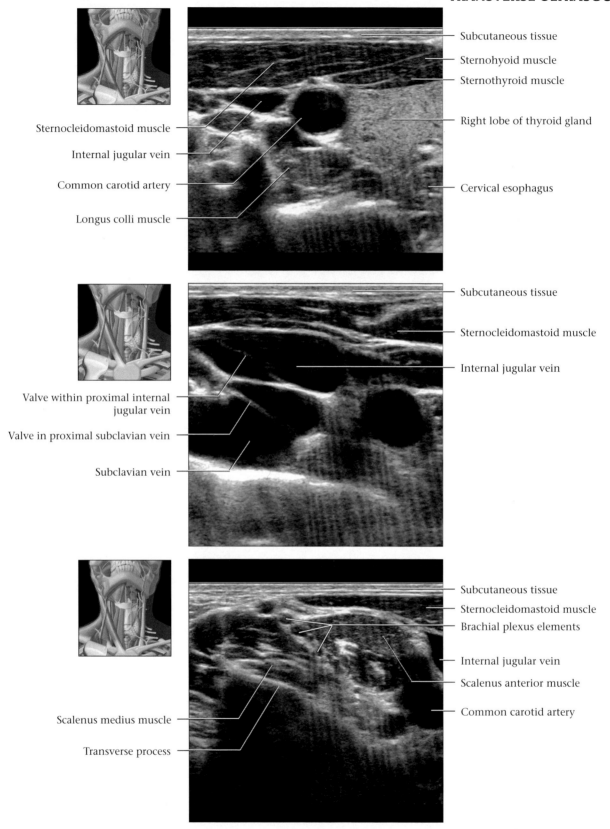

Sternocleidomastoid muscle

Internal jugular vein

Common carotid artery

Longus colli muscle

Subcutaneous tissue

Sternohyoid muscle

Sternothyroid muscle

Right lobe of thyroid gland

Cervical esophagus

Valve within proximal internal jugular vein

Valve in proximal subclavian vein

Subclavian vein

Subcutaneous tissue

Sternocleidomastoid muscle

Internal jugular vein

Scalenus medius muscle

Transverse process

Subcutaneous tissue

Sternocleidomastoid muscle

Brachial plexus elements

Internal jugular vein

Scalenus anterior muscle

Common carotid artery

(**Top**) First image of a series of transverse grayscale ultrasound images of the lower cervical level. Major structures at this level include the common carotid artery, the internal jugular vein, the thyroid gland and the overlying muscles of the anterior neck. (**Middle**) Second image at the level of the medial supraclavicular fossa. Note the close proximity of the proximal internal jugular vein and the subclavian vein at this site which join to form the brachiocephalic vein. Supraclavicular lymph nodes are commonly found adjacent to these major vessels. (**Bottom**) Third image in the lateral supraclavicular fossa. The scalenus anterior and medius muscles are clearly visualized with the trunks of the brachial plexus between them. US is often used to guide brachial plexus blocks. US also helps to exclude brachial plexus involvement by metastases at this site.

LOWER CERVICAL LEVEL & SUPRACLAVICULAR FOSSA

AXIAL CECT AND POWER DOPPLER ULTRASOUND

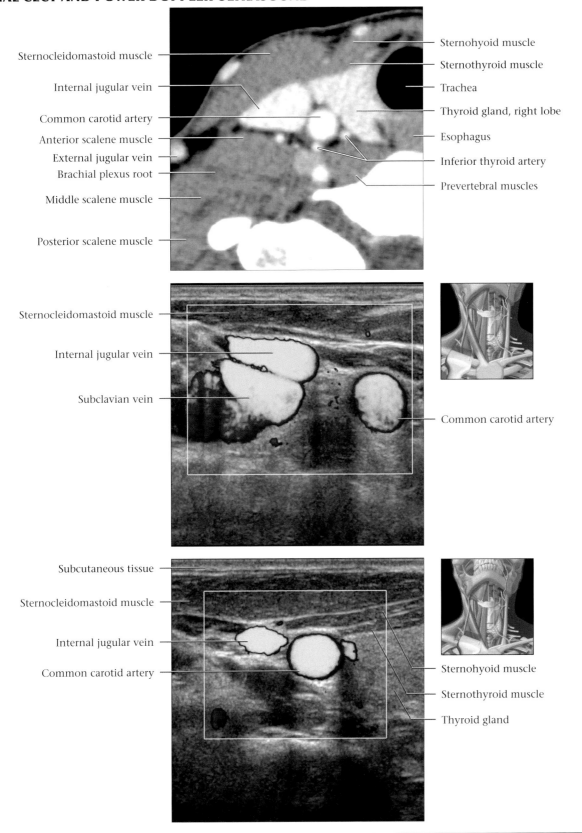

Sternocleidomastoid muscle —

Internal jugular vein —

Common carotid artery —

Anterior scalene muscle —

External jugular vein —

Brachial plexus root —

Middle scalene muscle —

Posterior scalene muscle —

— Sternohyoid muscle

— Sternothyroid muscle

— Trachea

— Thyroid gland, right lobe

— Esophagus

— Inferior thyroid artery

— Prevertebral muscles

Sternocleidomastoid muscle —

Internal jugular vein —

Subclavian vein —

— Common carotid artery

Subcutaneous tissue —

Sternocleidomastoid muscle —

Internal jugular vein —

Common carotid artery —

— Sternohyoid muscle

— Sternothyroid muscle

— Thyroid gland

(Top) Axial CECT image through the lower-cervical level. The relationship of the thyroid gland with the adjacent structures including the carotid sheath, strap muscles, trachea and esophagus is demonstrated. **(Middle)** Transverse power Doppler ultrasound in the supraclavicular fossa helps to delineate vascular structures in this region including the confluence of the internal jugular vein and the subclavian vein. The proximal portion of the common carotid artery from the brachiocephalic trunk is also seen at this level. **(Bottom)** Transverse power Doppler ultrasound of the lower cervical level allows the clear depiction of the color-filled common carotid artery and internal jugular vein. Nodes are often seen at this site and are readily evaluated by US and biopsied/FNAed under guidance.

LONGITUDINAL ULTRASOUND AND PATHOLOGY

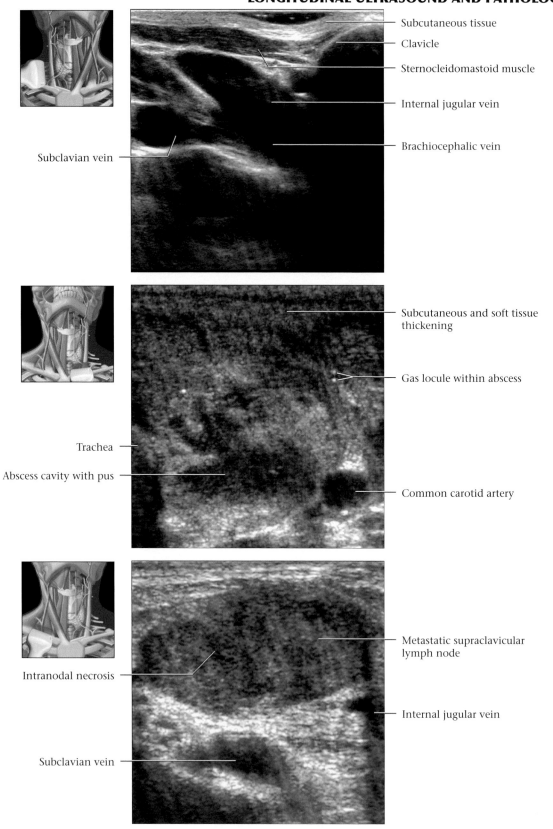

Subcutaneous tissue

Clavicle

Sternocleidomastoid muscle

Internal jugular vein

Brachiocephalic vein

Subclavian vein

Subcutaneous and soft tissue thickening

Gas locule within abscess

Trachea

Abscess cavity with pus

Common carotid artery

Metastatic supraclavicular lymph node

Intranodal necrosis

Internal jugular vein

Subclavian vein

(Top) Longitudinal grayscale ultrasound of the supraclavicular fossa shows the confluence of the internal jugular vein and the subclavian vein to form the brachiocephalic vein just above the medial portion of the clavicle. Nodes often nestle under these vessels making biopsy access difficult. Pulsation from the vessels also makes Doppler evaluation of nodes at this level suboptimal. (Middle) Transverse grayscale ultrasound of the left lower-cervical level shows abscess formation in the left lobe and perithyroidal soft tissue due to acute suppurative thyroiditis. Note the presence of pus and echogenic foci due to gas bubbles. (Bottom) Transverse grayscale ultrasound shows an enlarged, abnormal lymph node in the right supraclavicular fossa. Isolated nodes at this site point to an infraclavicular primary.

LOWER CERVICAL LEVEL & SUPRACLAVICULAR FOSSA

CECT AND PATHOLOGY

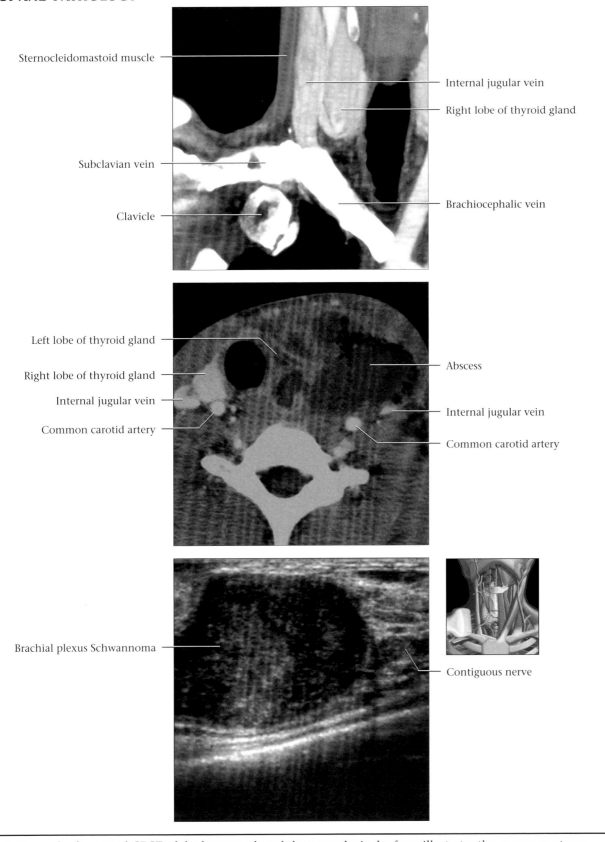

Sternocleidomastoid muscle

Internal jugular vein

Right lobe of thyroid gland

Subclavian vein

Clavicle

Brachiocephalic vein

Left lobe of thyroid gland

Right lobe of thyroid gland

Internal jugular vein

Common carotid artery

Abscess

Internal jugular vein

Common carotid artery

Brachial plexus Schwannoma

Contiguous nerve

(**Top**) Coronal reformatted CECT of the lower neck and the supraclavicular fossa illustrates the venous anatomy. (**Middle**) Axial CECT of acute suppurative thyroiditis shows a large heterogeneous abscess with thick peripheral enhancement involving the left lobe of the thyroid gland and perithyroidal soft tissue. Note the presence of fluid and gas within the abscess cavity and marked subcutaneous thickening in left lower neck. (**Bottom**) Longitudinal grayscale ultrasound of the right supraclavicular fossa shows a solid, hypoechoic lobulated mass contiguous with a thickened nerve. The appearances suggest a brachial plexus schwannoma. The continuation with a nerve is the clue to its diagnosis.

POSTERIOR TRIANGLE

Terminology

Abbreviations
- Posterior cervical space (PCS)

Definitions
- Posterolateral fat-containing space in neck with complex fascial boundaries that extends from posterior mastoid tip to clavicle behind the sternocleidomastoid muscle

Imaging Anatomy

Overview
- Posterolateral fat-filled space just deep & posterior to sternomastoid muscle
- Posterior border bound by anterior edge of trapezius muscle

Extent
- PCS extends from small superior component near mastoid tip to broader base at level of clavicle
- When viewed from side, appears as "tilting tent"

Anatomy Relationships
- Superficial space lies superficial to PCS
- Deep to PCS is perivertebral space
  - Anterior PCS is superficial to prevertebral component of perivertebral space
  - Posterior PCS is superficial to paraspinal component of perivertebral space

Internal Structures-Critical Contents
- Fat is primary occupant of PCS
- Floor is formed by muscles running obliquely: Scalenus muscles, levator scapulae and splenius capitis muscles (from anterior to posterior)
  - Subdivided by inferior belly of omohyoid muscle into occipital & subclavian triangles
- The muscular floor is covered by superficial and deep layers of deep cervical fascia
- Spinal accessory nerve (CN11)
  - Arise from nerve cells in the anterior gray column of upper five segments of spinal cord
  - Ascend alongside the spinal cord and enter the skull through foramen magnum
  - United with cranial root to exit through jugular foramen
  - The spinal portion then separates from the cranial root
  - Motor supply to soft palate, pharynx, larynx, sternocleidomastoid and trapezius muscles
- Spinal accessory lymph node chain
  - Level 5 spinal accessory nodes (SAN) further subdivided into A & B levels at hyoid bone
    - Level 5A: SAN above cricoid cartilage level
    - Level 5B: SAN below cricoid cartilage level
- Pre-axillary brachial plexus
  - Segment of brachial plexus emerging from anterior & middle scalene gap passes through PCS
  - Leaves PCS with axillary artery into axillary fat
- Dorsal scapular nerve
  - Arises from brachial plexus (spinal nerves C4 & C5)
  - Motor innervation to rhomboid & levator scapulae muscles
- Transverse cervical artery and vein
  - Arises from thyrocervical trunk of subclavian artery and IJV respectively
  - Course in inferior posterior triangle and parallel to the clavicle

Anatomy-Based Imaging Issues

Key Concepts or Questions
- Most lesions in posterior triangle arises from spinal accessory chain lymph nodes
  - Reactive lymphadenopathy
  - Infective lymphadenitis such as tuberculous lymphadenitis
    - Enlarged hypoechoic necrotic nodes with matting and soft tissue edema, avascular or displaced hilar vascularity
  - Metastatic lymph nodes
    - Primary from nasopharyngeal carcinoma and squamous cell carcinoma from other H&N sites
    - Enlarged, round, hypoechoic nodes with intranodal necrosis and peripheral vascularity
  - Lymphomatous nodes
    - Usually bilateral neck involvement
    - Enlarged, heterogeneous, reticulated/pseudocystic appearance, increased central and peripheral vascularity
- Other diseases which may occur in posterior triangle include
  - Congenital lesion: Lymphangioma, usually transpatial
  - Benign tumor: Lipoma, nerve sheath tumor

Imaging Approaches
- Scanning is usually undertaken in a transverse plane
- From mastoid tip superiorly to acromion process inferiorly
  - Spinal accessory chain lymph nodes run from a point midway between mastoid process and angle of mandible to outer third of the clavicle

Imaging Pitfalls
- On transverse scan, tips of transverse process of cervical vertebrae may be seen as echogenic structures with posterior acoustic shadowing
  - Do not mistake these for calcified lymph nodes

Clinical Implications

Clinical Importance
- CN11 runs in floor of posterior triangle
  - Accessory cranial neuropathy results when CN11 injured
  - Most commonly injured during neck dissection for malignant SCC nodes
  - Less commonly injured by extranodal spread of squamous cell carcinoma
- Spinal accessory nodes are main normal occupants of posterior cervical space

POSTERIOR TRIANGLE

GRAPHICS

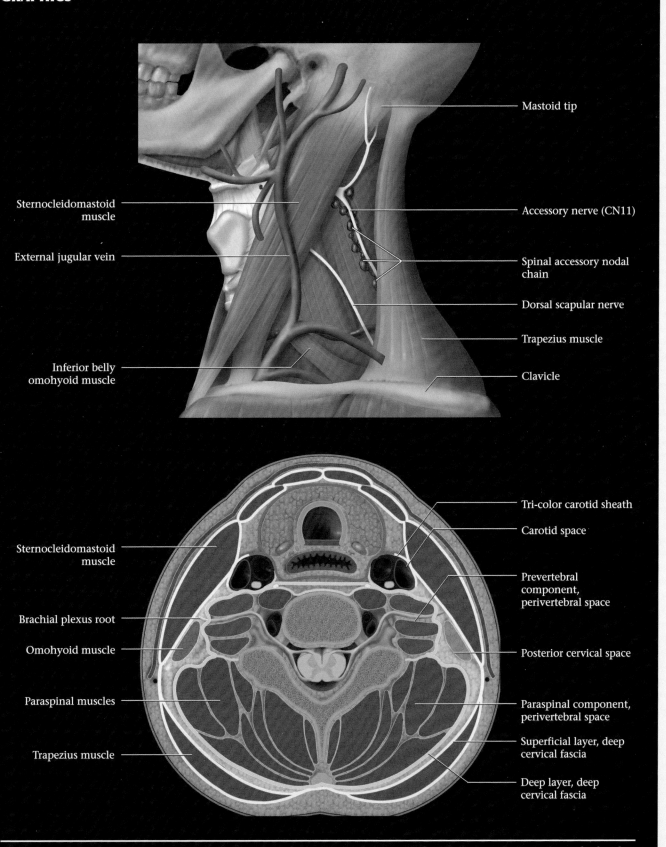

Mastoid tip

Sternocleidomastoid muscle

Accessory nerve (CN11)

External jugular vein

Spinal accessory nodal chain

Dorsal scapular nerve

Trapezius muscle

Inferior belly omohyoid muscle

Clavicle

Sternocleidomastoid muscle

Tri-color carotid sheath

Carotid space

Prevertebral component, perivertebral space

Brachial plexus root

Omohyoid muscle

Posterior cervical space

Paraspinal muscles

Paraspinal component, perivertebral space

Superficial layer, deep cervical fascia

Trapezius muscle

Deep layer, deep cervical fascia

(Top) Lateral graphic of the neck shows the posterior triangle as a "tilting tent" with its superior margin at the level of the mastoid tip and its inferior border at the clavicle. Notice that it has two main nerves in its floor, the accessory nerve (CN11) and the dorsal scapular nerve. The spinal accessory nodal chain is its key occupant with regards to the kind of lesions found in the posterior triangle. **(Bottom)** Axial graphic through the thyroid bed of the infrahyoid neck depicts the posterior cervical space with its complex fascial borders. The superficial layer of the deep cervical fascia is its superficial border while the deep layer of the deep cervical fascia is its deep border. Note the tri-color carotid sheath is its anteromedial border. The brachial plexus roots travel through the PCS on their way to the axillary apex.

POSTERIOR TRIANGLE

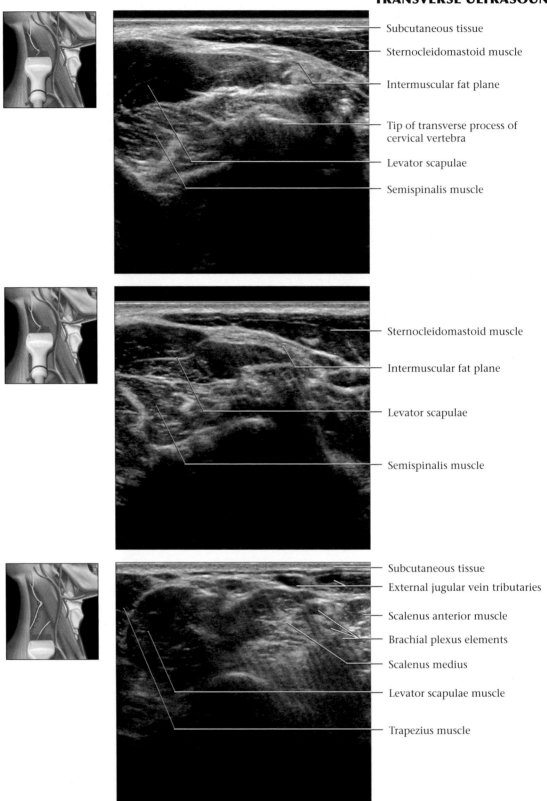

(Top) — Subcutaneous tissue
— Sternocleidomastoid muscle
— Intermuscular fat plane
— Tip of transverse process of cervical vertebra
— Levator scapulae
— Semispinalis muscle

(Middle) — Sternocleidomastoid muscle
— Intermuscular fat plane
— Levator scapulae
— Semispinalis muscle

(Bottom) — Subcutaneous tissue
— External jugular vein tributaries
— Scalenus anterior muscle
— Brachial plexus elements
— Scalenus medius
— Levator scapulae muscle
— Trapezius muscle

(Top) First image of a series of transverse grayscale ultrasound images of the posterior triangle. The sternocleidomastoid muscle marks the anterior border of posterior triangle. Muscles form the floor of the posterior triangle. Note the accessory nerve and nodes lie in the intermuscular fat plane. **(Middle)** Standard transverse grayscale ultrasound image of the posterior triangle. Note the intermuscular fat plane. This fat plane is best screened in the transverse plane. Once pathology is detected further examination, particularly Doppler, is best done longitudinally. **(Bottom)** Third image at the lower level of the posterior triangle. The trapezius muscle marks the posterior margin of the posterior triangle. The main bulk of the levator scapulae muscle forms the muscular floor.

AXIAL MR

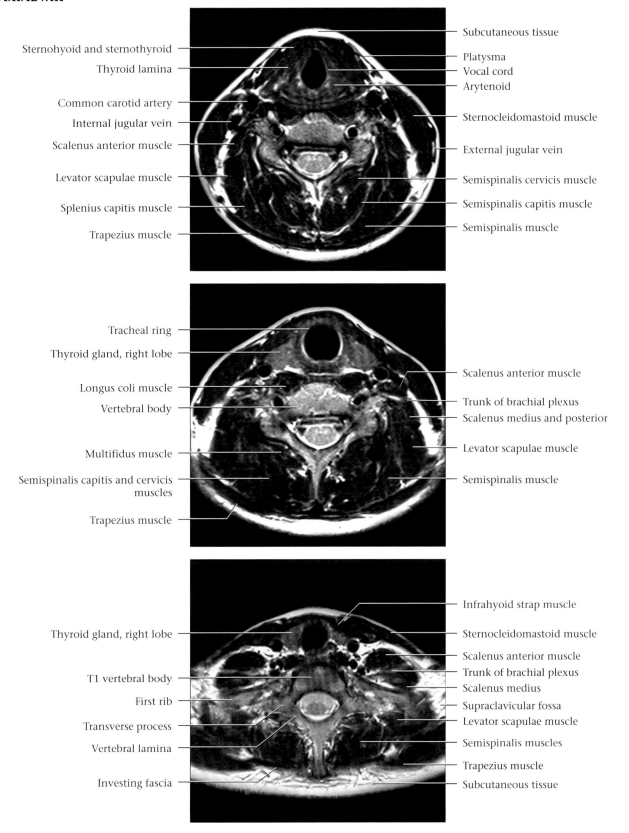

Subcutaneous tissue

Sternohyoid and sternothyroid

Thyroid lamina

Platysma

Vocal cord

Arytenoid

Common carotid artery

Internal jugular vein

Sternocleidomastoid muscle

Scalenus anterior muscle

External jugular vein

Levator scapulae muscle

Semispinalis cervicis muscle

Splenius capitis muscle

Semispinalis capitis muscle

Trapezius muscle

Semispinalis muscle

Tracheal ring

Thyroid gland, right lobe

Longus coli muscle

Scalenus anterior muscle

Vertebral body

Trunk of brachial plexus

Scalenus medius and posterior

Multifidus muscle

Levator scapulae muscle

Semispinalis capitis and cervicis muscles

Semispinalis muscle

Trapezius muscle

Infrahyoid strap muscle

Thyroid gland, right lobe

Sternocleidomastoid muscle

Scalenus anterior muscle

Trunk of brachial plexus

T1 vertebral body

Scalenus medius

First rib

Supraclavicular fossa

Transverse process

Levator scapulae muscle

Vertebral lamina

Semispinalis muscles

Trapezius muscle

Investing fascia

Subcutaneous tissue

(Top) Axial PD MR image of the neck at the level of the vocal cord. Note the largely fat-filled posterior triangle with muscular floor. (Middle) Axial PD MR image of the neck at the level of thyroid gland. Note the scalenus medius muscle begins at the mid cervical level. The nerve roots and the trunk of the brachial plexus is seen emerging between the scalenus anterior and medius muscles. (Bottom) Axial PD MR image of the lower posterior triangle. The trunks of the brachial plexus are seen between the scalenus anterior and the medius muscles and diverge posterior to the clavicle to axillary region. Note the content of the posterior triangle is predominantly fat with large muscles forming its boundaries.

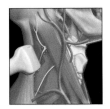

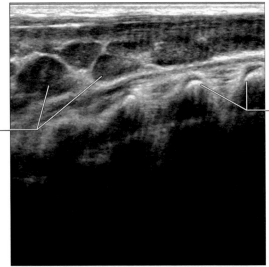

Reactive nodes — Tips of transverse process

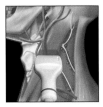

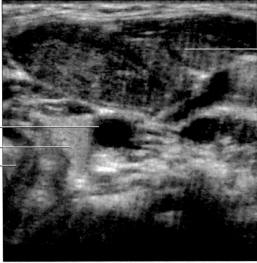

Sternocleidomastoid muscle pseudotumor

Common carotid artery

Left lobe of thyroid gland

Trachea

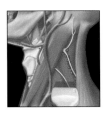

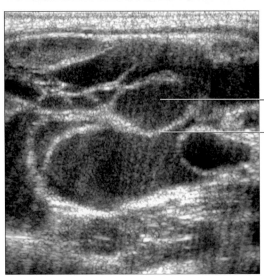

Lymphangioma

Internal septation

(Top) Longitudinal grayscale ultrasound of the posterior triangle shows a chain of reactive accessory nodes. Note their location in the intermuscular fat plane. Do not mistake the tips of the transverse processes with calcified nodes. **(Middle)** Transverse grayscale ultrasound in an infant with torticollis shows a heterogeneously enlarged left sternocleidomastoid muscle. The appearance is compatible with a sternocleidomastoid pseudotumor. **(Bottom)** Transverse grayscale ultrasound shows a large, multiseptated, cystic mass occupying the left posterior triangle in a child. The appearance is suggestive of a lymphangioma (cystic hygroma). These lesions are trans-spatial and frequently extend in to other neck spaces.

PATHOLOGY

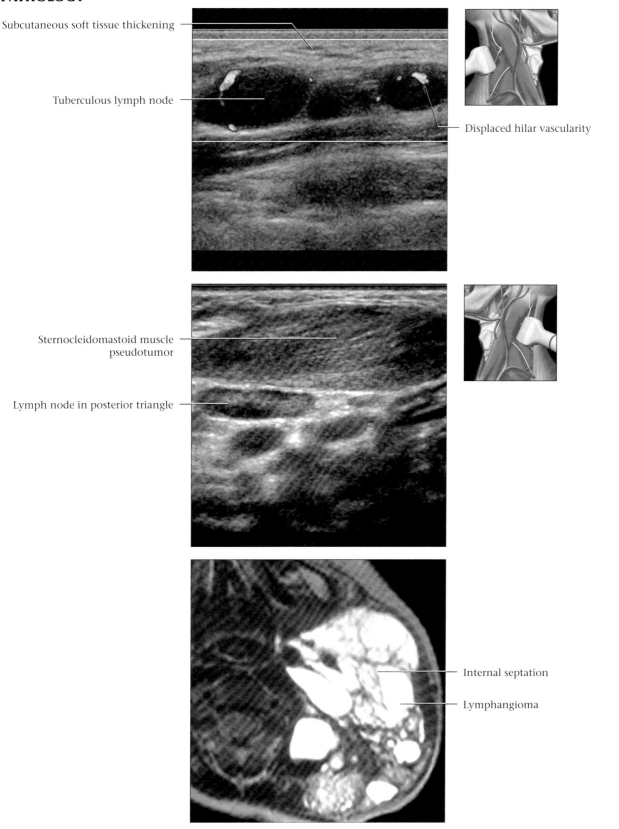

Subcutaneous soft tissue thickening

Tuberculous lymph node

Displaced hilar vascularity

Sternocleidomastoid muscle pseudotumor

Lymph node in posterior triangle

Internal septation

Lymphangioma

(Top) Longitudinal color Doppler ultrasound in the posterior triangle shows multiple, enlarged, hypoechoic lymph nodes with displaced hilar vascularity. Pathology: Tuberculous lymphadenitis. Once pathology is detected in transverse scans, it is better evaluated on a longitudinal scan, particularly if performing a Doppler examination. (Middle) Longitudinal grayscale ultrasound of the left posterior triangle shows the sternocleidomastoid muscle pseudotumor. Part of the normal muscular striations are preserved. (Bottom) Fat-suppressed T2WI MR of the neck shows the large lymphangioma occupying the left posterior triangle. Note the trans-spatial distribution of the lesion is better delineated by MR.

THYROID GLAND

Imaging Anatomy

Overview
- "H" or "U" shaped gland in anterior cervical neck formed from 2 elongated lateral lobes with superior & inferior poles connected by median isthmus
- 40% of people have pyramidal lobe ascending from isthmus area toward hyoid bone

Extent
- Extends from level of 5th cervical vertebra to 1st thoracic vertebra

Anatomy Relationships
- Thyroid gland lies anterior & lateral to trachea in visceral space of infrahyoid neck
- Posteromedially are tracheoesophageal grooves
  - Paratracheal lymph nodes, recurrent laryngeal nerve, parathyroid glands lie within it
- Posterolaterally are carotid spaces
  - Contains common carotid artery, internal jugular vein, vagus nerve
- Anteriorly are infrahyoid strap muscles
- Anterolaterally are sternocleidomastoid muscles

Internal Structures-Critical Contents
- Thyroid gland
  - Two lateral lobes (i.e., right and left lobes)
    - Measures ~ 4 cm in height
    - Each lobe has upper & lower poles
    - Lateral lobes are commonly asymmetric in size
  - Lateral lobes joined by midline isthmus
  - On ultrasound, the thyroid parenchymal echoes are fine, uniform and hyperechoic compared to adjacent muscles
  - The echogenic thyroid capsule is clearly visualized and helps to differentiate thyroid lesions from extrathyroidal masses
- Arterial supply to thyroid gland
  - Superior thyroid arteries
    - First anterior branch of external carotid artery
    - Runs superficially on anterior border of lateral lobe, sending a branch deep into gland before curving toward isthmus where it anastomoses with contralateral artery
    - Proximal course closely associated with superior laryngeal nerve
  - Inferior thyroid arteries
    - Arises from thyrocervical trunk, a branch of subclavian artery
    - Ascends vertically, then curves medially to enter tracheoesophageal groove in plane posterior to carotid space
    - Most of its branches penetrate posterior aspect of lateral thyroid lobe
    - Closely associated with recurrent laryngeal nerve
  - Thyroidea ima occasionally present (3%)
    - Single vessel originating from aortic arch or innominate artery
    - Enters thyroid gland at inferior border of isthmus
- Venous drainage of thyroid gland
  - 3 pairs of veins arise from venous plexus on surface of thyroid gland
    - Superior & middle thyroid veins drain into internal jugular vein
    - Inferior thyroid veins drain into left brachiocephalic vein
- Lymphatic drainage of thyroid gland
  - Lymphatic drainage is extensive & multidirectional
  - Initial lymphatic drainage courses to periglandular nodes
    - Prelaryngeal, pretracheal (Delphian) & paratracheal nodes along recurrent laryngeal nerve
    - Paratracheal nodes drain along recurrent laryngeal nerve into mediastinum
    - Regional drainage occurs laterally into internal jugular chain (level 2-4) & spinal accessory chain (level 5), higher in the neck along internal jugular vein

Anatomy-Based Imaging Issues

Imaging Approaches
- Both longitudinal and transverse scans are required for comprehensive USG assessment of thyroid gland
  - Transverse scan helps to locate thyroid nodules, their relationship to trachea, major vessels in carotid sheath, evaluate internal architecture and extrathyroid extension
  - Longitudinal scan helps to evaluate internal architecture, vascularity on Doppler and extrathyroidal extension
- When evaluating thyroid nodule, the examination is divided into
  - Ultrasound features of the thyroid nodule
  - Assessment of adjacent structures (including trachea, esophagus, strap muscles, carotid artery and internal jugular vein) and cervical lymph nodes

Embryology

Embryologic Events
- Thyroid gland originates from 1st & 2nd pharyngeal pouches (medial anlage)
- Originates as proliferation of endodermal epithelial cells on median surface of developing pharyngeal floor termed foramen cecum
- Bilobed thyroid gland descends anterior to pharyngeal gut along thyroglossal duct
- Inferior descent of thyroid gland carries it anterior to hyoid bone & laryngeal cartilages

Practical Implications
- Thyroglossal duct cyst: Results from failure of involution of portion of thyroglossal duct
- Thyroid tissue remnants: From sequestration of thyroid tissue along thyroglossal duct
  - Seen anywhere along course of thyroglossal duct from foramen cecum to superior mediastinum
- Ectopic thyroid gland: From incomplete descent of thyroid into low neck
  - Seen anywhere along course from foramen cecum in tongue base to superior mediastinum
  - Most common location in neck is just deep to foramen cecum in tongue base = lingual thyroid

GRAPHICS

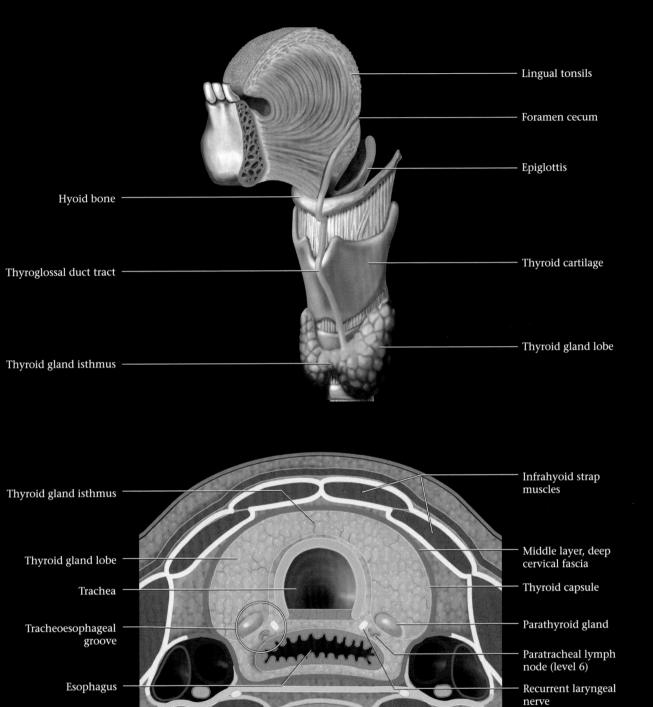

Lingual tonsils

Foramen cecum

Epiglottis

Hyoid bone

Thyroglossal duct tract

Thyroid cartilage

Thyroid gland lobe

Thyroid gland isthmus

Thyroid gland isthmus

Infrahyoid strap muscles

Thyroid gland lobe

Middle layer, deep cervical fascia

Trachea

Thyroid capsule

Tracheoesophageal groove

Parathyroid gland

Paratracheal lymph node (level 6)

Esophagus

Recurrent laryngeal nerve

(Top) Sagittal oblique graphic displays the thyroglossal duct tract as it traverses the cervical neck from its origin at the foramen cecum to its termination in the anterior & lateral visceral space of the infrahyoid neck. The medial thyroid anlage arises from the paramedian aspect of the 1st & 2nd branchial pouches (foramen cecum area), then descends inferiorly through the tongue base, floor of mouth, around and in front of the hyoid bone. **(Bottom)** Axial graphic at thyroid level, depicts the thyroid lobes & isthmus in the anterior visceral space wrapping around the trachea. Notice that there are three key structures found in the area of the tracheoesophageal groove, the recurrent laryngeal nerve, the paratracheal lymph node chain and the parathyroid gland. The parathyroid glands may be inside or outside of the thyroid capsule.

Neck

II

53

THYROID GLAND

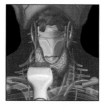

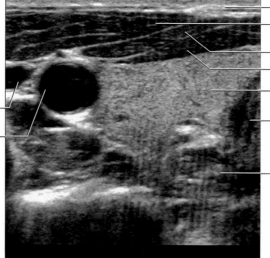

- Subcutaneous tissue
- Sternocleidomastoid muscle
- Sternohyoid muscle
- Sternothyroid muscle
- Right lobe of thyroid gland
- Trachea
- Esophagus

Internal jugular vein —

Common carotid artery —

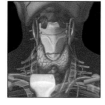

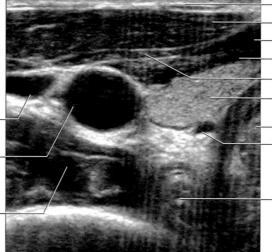

- Subcutaneous tissue
- Sternocleidomastoid muscle
- Sternohyoid muscle
- Sternothyroid muscle
- Omohyoid muscle
- Lower pole of right thyroid gland
- Trachea
- Inferior thyroid artery
- Esophagus

Internal jugular vein —

Common carotid artery —

Longus colli muscle —

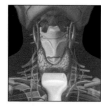

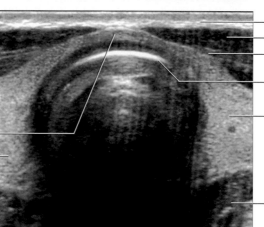

- Subcutaneous tissue
- Strap muscle
- Thyroid capsule
- Tracheal ring
- Left lobe of thyroid gland
- Longus colli muscle

Thyroid isthmus —

Right lobe of thyroid gland —

(Top) Transverse grayscale ultrasound of the right lobe of the thyroid gland shows homogeneous, hyperechoic echo pattern of the glandular parenchyma. Note its close anatomical relationship with the major vessels of the carotid sheath (IJV and CCA) laterally, the trachea medially and the cervical esophagus posteromedially. (Middle) Transverse grayscale ultrasound at the level of inferior pole of thyroid gland. The inferior thyroid artery is a consistent finding related to and supplying the inferior pole. (Bottom) Midline transverse grayscale ultrasound shows the thyroid isthmus connecting the two lobes. The isthmus lies on the anterior surface of the trachea. In view of the intimate anatomical relationship between the thyroid gland and the trachea, local tumor invasion to trachea from malignant thyroid carcinoma is commonly seen, rendering surgical excision more extensive than total thyroidectomy.

THYROID GLAND

AXIAL CECT

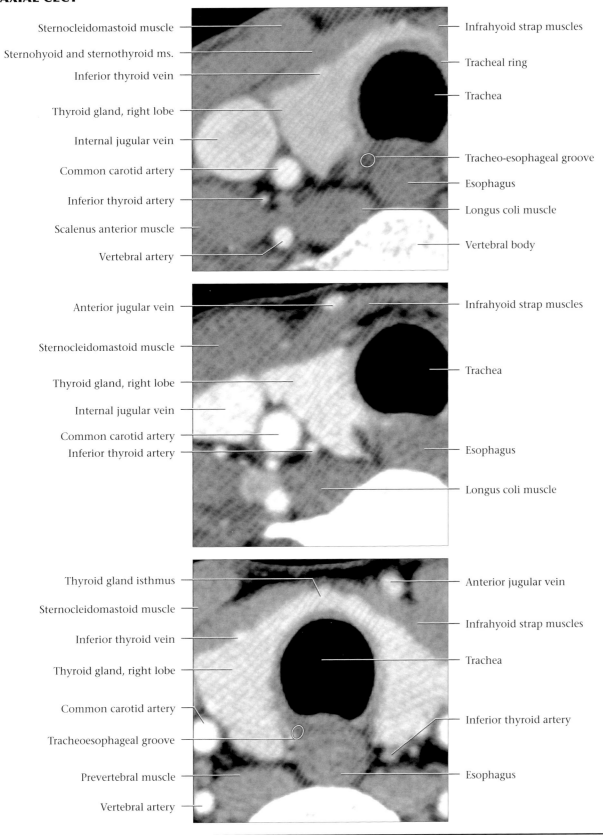

Sternocleidomastoid muscle

Sternohyoid and sternothyroid ms.

Inferior thyroid vein

Thyroid gland, right lobe

Internal jugular vein

Common carotid artery

Inferior thyroid artery

Scalenus anterior muscle

Vertebral artery

Infrahyoid strap muscles

Tracheal ring

Trachea

Tracheo-esophageal groove

Esophagus

Longus coli muscle

Vertebral body

Anterior jugular vein

Sternocleidomastoid muscle

Thyroid gland, right lobe

Internal jugular vein

Common carotid artery

Inferior thyroid artery

Infrahyoid strap muscles

Trachea

Esophagus

Longus coli muscle

Thyroid gland isthmus

Sternocleidomastoid muscle

Inferior thyroid vein

Thyroid gland, right lobe

Common carotid artery

Tracheoesophageal groove

Prevertebral muscle

Vertebral artery

Anterior jugular vein

Infrahyoid strap muscles

Trachea

Inferior thyroid artery

Esophagus

(Top) Correlative CECT image of the right thyroid gland. The thyroid gland is seen as a triangular, homogeneously enhancing structure embracing the anterior aspect of the cervical trachea. The inferior thyroid artery seen on this CT is the main trunk while that seen on the ultrasound image is a branch. **(Middle)** Axial CECT at the lower pole of the thyroid gland. **(Bottom)** Axial CECT of the neck at midline indicating the tracheoesophageal groove. Remember that the recurrent laryngeal nerve, paratracheal nodes and parathyroid glands may be seen on ultrasound in this location but they normally cannot be well-demonstrated on routine CT images. Always evaluate extensions of the tumor into the trachea, tracheoesophageal groove, nodes, strap muscles, CCA and IJV.

THYROID GLAND

Subcutaneous tissue
Anterior portion of sternocleidomastoid muscle
Sternohyoid muscle
Sternothyroid muscle
Inferior pole of thyroid gland
Inferior thyroid artery
Longus colli muscle

Superior pole of thyroid gland

Cervical vertebrae

Subcutaneous tissue
Sternocleidomastoid muscle
Sternohyoid muscle
Sternothyroid muscle
Inferior thyroid artery
Esophagus

Thyroid gland

Cervical vertebra

Subcutaneous tissue
Sternohyoid muscle
Sternothyroid muscle
Thyroid gland

Superior thyroid artery

(Top) Parasagittal longitudinal grayscale ultrasound of thyroid gland. The homogeneous, hyperechoic echo pattern of the glandular parenchyma is better assessed on longitudinal scans. Part of the tortuous course of the inferior thyroid artery is constantly seen in relation to the lower pole. (Middle) Parasagittal longitudinal grayscale ultrasound shows the inferior thyroid artery coursing superiorly from the inferior pole within the glandular parenchyma. (Bottom) Parasagittal longitudinal grayscale ultrasound shows the superior thyroid artery, the first anterior branch of the external carotid artery, running inferiorly within and supplying the upper pole of the thyroid gland. Longitudinal scans best evaluate the glandular parenchyma and vascularity.

THYROID GLAND

CORONAL REFORMATTED CECT AND VARIANT

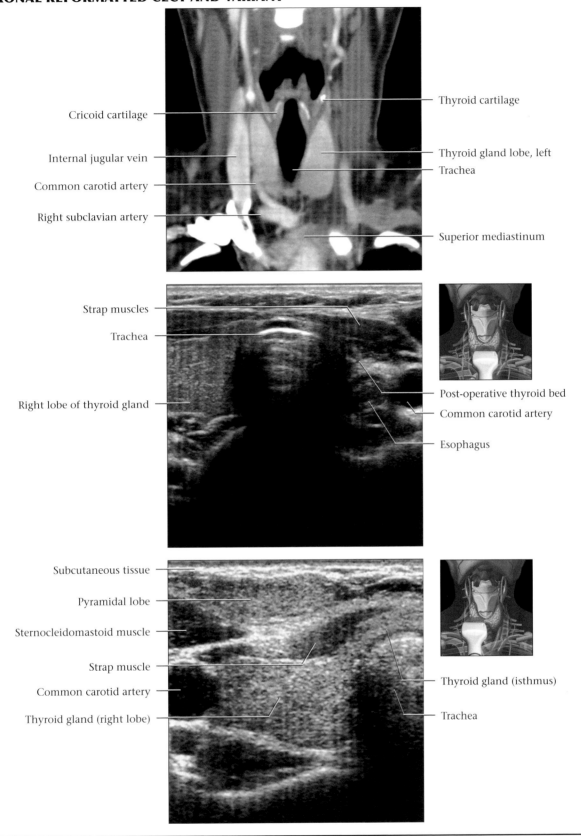

Thyroid cartilage

Cricoid cartilage

Thyroid gland lobe, left

Internal jugular vein

Trachea

Common carotid artery

Right subclavian artery

Superior mediastinum

Strap muscles

Trachea

Right lobe of thyroid gland

Post-operative thyroid bed

Common carotid artery

Esophagus

Subcutaneous tissue

Pyramidal lobe

Sternocleidomastoid muscle

Strap muscle

Thyroid gland (isthmus)

Common carotid artery

Trachea

Thyroid gland (right lobe)

(Top) In this image the "H" or "U" shaped lobes of the thyroid gland are particularly well-seen. Note the intimate relationship between the superomedial thyroid gland and the larynx. Remember that for thyroid malignancies the first order nodes are the paratracheal nodes which drain inferiorly into the superior mediastinum. **(Middle)** Transverse grayscale ultrasound in a patient with a previous history of a left thyroidectomy. Note that the left thyroid bed is devoid of thyroid tissue and is occupied by the cervical portion of the esophagus and connective tissue. **(Bottom)** Transverse grayscale ultrasound shows the pyramidal lobe of the thyroid gland. The echo pattern is identical to the normal right thyroid lobe (i.e., homogeneous, hyperechoic) and is located anterior to the anterior strap muscle and connected to the isthmus.

PARATHYROID GLAND

Terminology

Abbreviations
- Parathyroid gland (PTG)

Definitions
- Posterior visceral space (VS) endocrine glands that control calcium metabolism by producing parathormone

Imaging Anatomy

Anatomy Relationships
- PTG closely applied to posterior surface of thyroid lobes within visceral space
- Extracapsular (outside thyroid capsule) in most cases
- In vicinity of tracheoesophageal groove

Internal Structures-Critical Contents
- Parathyroid glands
  - Small lentiform glands posterior to thyroid glands in visceral space
  - Normal measurements
    - Approximately 6 mm length, 3-4 mm transverse & 1-2 mm in anteroposterior diameter
  - In general, normal glands are not clearly visualized on US/CT/MR
    - Normal PTG may be seen by use of modern US machine and high frequency transducer
    - Appear as small, well-circumscribed, hypoechoic nodules posterior to thyroid gland separated from echogenic thyroid capsule
  - Normal number = 4
    - Two superior & two inferior PTGs
    - May be as many as 12 total PTGs
  - Normal positions of superior PTGs
    - Superior PTGs are more constant in position as compared with lower PTGs
    - Lie on posterior border of middle 1/3 of thyroid 75% of time
    - 25% found behind upper or lower 1/3 of thyroid
    - 7% found below inferior thyroidal artery
    - Rarely found behind pharynx or esophagus
  - Normal positions of inferior PTGs
    - More variable in location
    - Inferior glands lie lateral to lower pole of thyroid gland (50%)
    - 15% lie within 1 cm of inferior thyroid poles
    - 35% position is variable residing anywhere from angle of mandible to lower anterior mediastinum
    - Intrathyroidal PTG are rare
  - Arterial supply of PTGs
    - Superior PTG supplied by superior thyroid artery
    - Inferior PTG supplied by inferior thyroid artery

Anatomy-Based Imaging Issues

Key Concepts or Questions
- Main indication for imaging of the parathyroid glands is localization of parathyroid adenoma causing hyperparathyroidism with hypercalcemia

Imaging Approaches
- Imaging for pre-operative localization of parathyroid adenoma (PTA)
  - Ultrasonography
    - Best first examination for localizing most PTA
    - Use high-resolution linear array transducer (7.5-10 MHz)
    - Identifies 95% of PTA weighing > 1 gram
    - **It is easier to start scanning in transverse plane with the patient's neck hyperextended**
    - Start above the thyroid at the angle of mandible and move downwards scanning through the thyroid to level of clavicle
    - Angulate transducer at clavicle to see any obvious lesion in mediastinum
    - **On color flow imaging most PTAs demonstrate hypervascularity, mainly intraparenchymal and arterial**
    - Color flow imaging is best done in longitudinal plane
  - Nuclear scintigraphy
    - Tc-99m sestamibi concentrates in PTA
    - Useful for detection of ectopic PTA (most common site below inferior thyroid pole)
  - Cross-sectional imaging (CT or MR)
    - Used for anatomic localization of ectopic PTA discovered with radionuclide exam

Imaging Pitfalls
- Parathyroid lesion may be confused with normal anatomical structures such as
  - Longus colli muscle, esophagus, blood vessels
  - Para-tracheal lymph nodes (FNA and internal vascularity help to identify)
  - Thyroid nodules in subcapsular location

Embryology

Embryologic Events
- Superior PTG develop from the 4th branchial pouch along with primordium of thyroid gland
- Inferior PTG develop from the 3rd branchial pouch along with anlage of thymus
  - Descend variable distance with thymic anlage in thymopharyngeal duct tract
  - May descend into anterior mediastinum as far as pericardium

Practical Implications
- Abnormal PTG descent may cause inferior PTG to occupy "ectopic" sites
  - May be of critical importance when searching for parathyroid adenoma
    - In cases where surgical exploration for PTA is done without imaging, no PTA may be found if PTG is ectopic

GRAPHICS

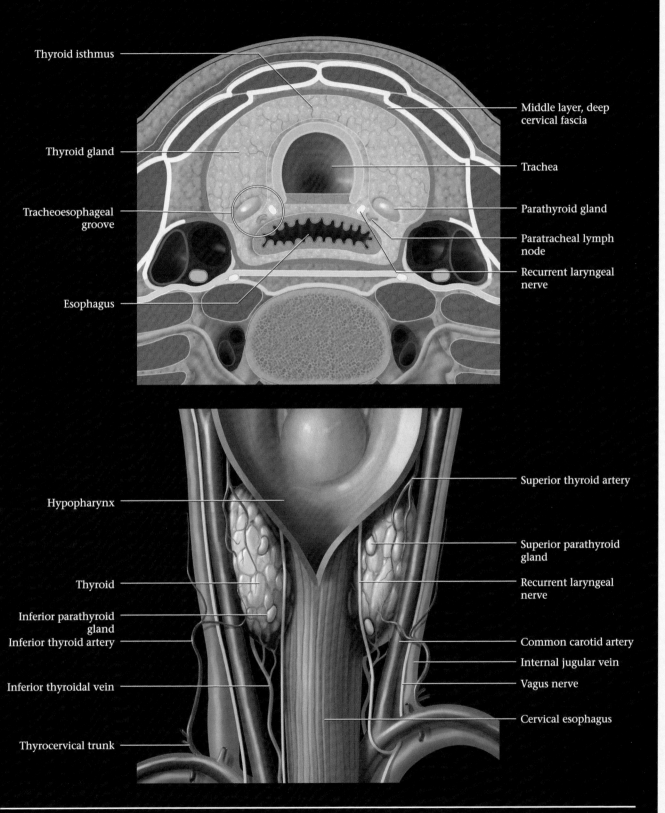

Thyroid isthmus

Thyroid gland

Tracheoesophageal groove

Esophagus

Middle layer, deep cervical fascia

Trachea

Parathyroid gland

Paratracheal lymph node

Recurrent laryngeal nerve

Hypopharynx

Thyroid

Inferior parathyroid gland

Inferior thyroid artery

Inferior thyroidal vein

Thyrocervical trunk

Superior thyroid artery

Superior parathyroid gland

Recurrent laryngeal nerve

Common carotid artery

Internal jugular vein

Vagus nerve

Cervical esophagus

(Top) Axial graphic at thyroid level, depicts the superior parathyroid glands in the visceral space just posterior to the thyroid gland. Notice that there are three key structures found in the area of the tracheoesophageal groove, the recurrent laryngeal nerve, the paratracheal lymph node chain and the parathyroid gland. **(Bottom)** Coronal graphic views the esophagus, parathyroid glands and thyroid gland from behind. The drawing depicts the typical anatomic relationships of the paired superior and inferior parathyroid glands in the visceral space. Note the arterial supply to superior and inferior parathyroid glands, the superior and inferior thyroid arteries respectively.

PARATHYROID GLAND

Sternocleidomastoid muscle

Infrahyoid strap muscle

Trachea

Parathyroid gland

Internal jugular vein

Common carotid artery

Right lobe thyroid gland

Sternocleidomastoid muscle

Infrahyoid strap muscle

Left lobe thyroid gland

Common carotid artery

Trachea

Parathyroid gland

Esophagus

Sternocleidomastoid muscle

Infrahyoid strap muscle

Trachea

Parathyroid gland

Common carotid artery

(Top) First of three transverse, grayscale sonographic images of the right neck shows a well-circumscribed, hypoechoic, right-superior parathyroid gland medial to the common carotid artery and posterior to the superior right thyroid lobe. (Middle) Image of the left neck at the level of the thyroid gland shows the left inferior parathyroid gland as a hypoechoic, ovoid lesion closely applied to the posterior left thyroid lobe. The esophagus is barely visible posterior to the parathyroid gland. (Bottom) Image of right neck, demonstrates a right inferior parathyroid gland medial to the common carotid artery, lateral to the cervical trachea and inferior to the right thyroid lobe. Note, it is not always possible to see normal parathyroid glands even with high resolution ultrasound. Doppler will help in distinguishing it from paratracheal node.

PARATHYROID GLAND

AXIAL CECT

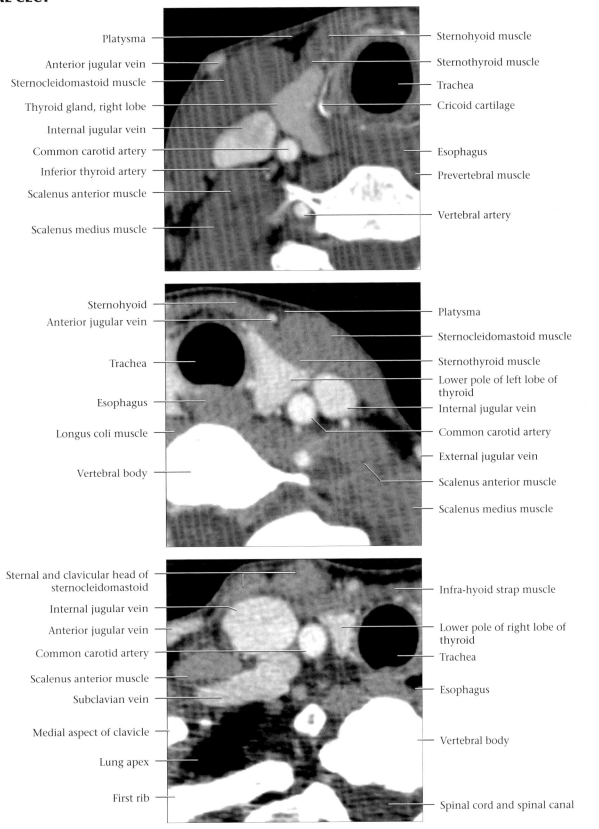

(Top) Axial CECT image of the neck, at the level of the upper pole of the thyroid gland. A normal parathyroid gland is normally not seen. The anatomical location is commonly at the tracheoesophageal groove posterior to the thyroid gland. **(Middle)** Axial CECT image of the neck showing the region of the lower pole of the thyroid's left lobe. **(Bottom)** Axial CECT of the lower cervical level at the region of the lower pole of the right lobe of the thyroid gland. Note the normal parathyroid gland is not seen. Both CT and MR are used for anatomic localization of ectopic PTA discovered with radionuclide scan.

PARATHYROID GLAND

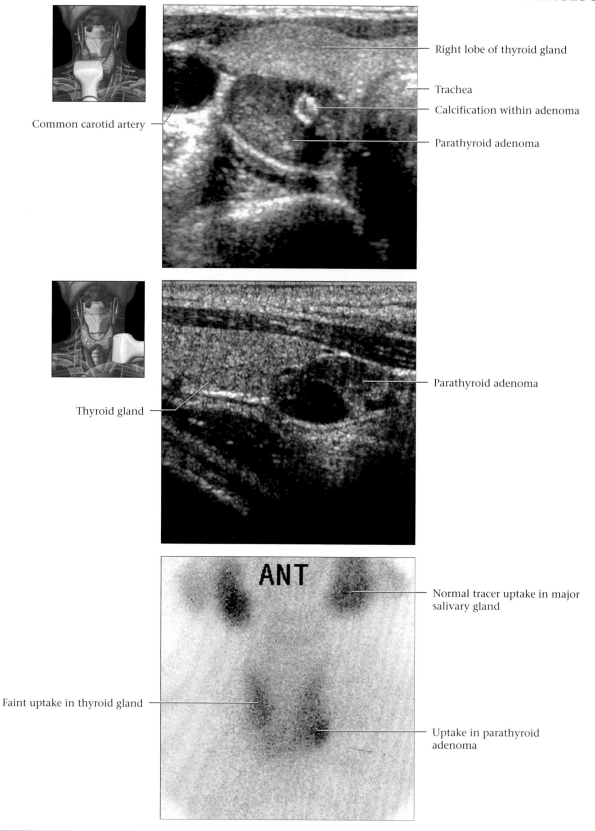

Right lobe of thyroid gland

Trachea

Calcification within adenoma

Parathyroid adenoma

Common carotid artery

Parathyroid adenoma

Thyroid gland

ANT

Normal tracer uptake in major salivary gland

Faint uptake in thyroid gland

Uptake in parathyroid adenoma

(Top) Transverse grayscale ultrasound shows a well-circumscribed, solid, round, hypoechoic PTA posterior to the upper pole of the right thyroid lobe. This patient had biochemical evidence of primary hyperparathyroidism. Note the presence of calcification within adenoma is uncommon, it is more commonly seen with carcinoma. (Middle) Longitudinal grayscale ultrasound shows a well-circumscribed PTA inferoposterior to the lower pole of left lobe of the thyroid gland. The echotexture of the adenoma is heterogeneous. (Bottom) Planar sestamibi scintigraphy shows a solitary focus of increased tracer uptake superimposed on the lower pole of the left thyroid gland. The scintigraphic features are suggestive of solitary hyperfunctioning parathyroid adenoma.

PARATHYROID GLAND

PATHOLOGY

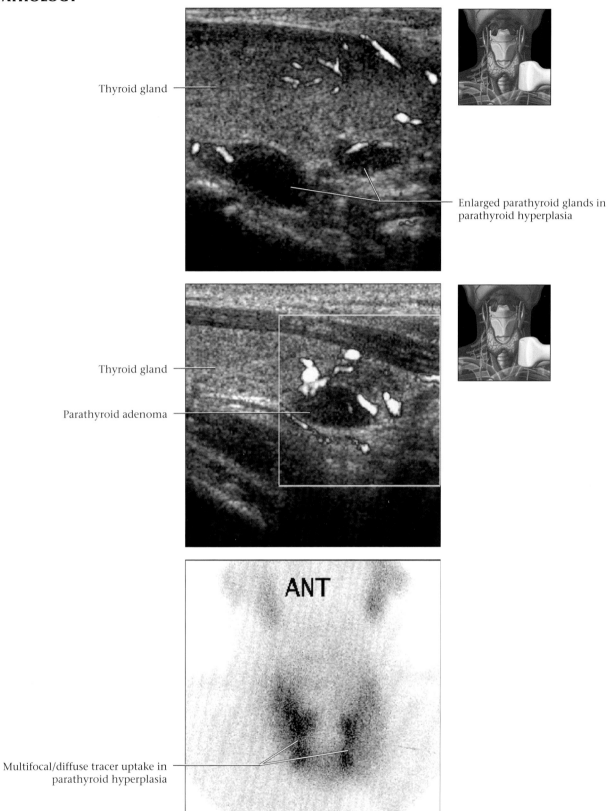

Thyroid gland — Enlarged parathyroid glands in parathyroid hyperplasia

Thyroid gland

Parathyroid adenoma

ANT

Multifocal/diffuse tracer uptake in parathyroid hyperplasia

(Top) Power Doppler ultrasound at the level of the lower pole of the thyroid gland shows two enlarged, hypoechoic parathyroid glands with increased vascularity located posterior to the lower pole of thyroid gland. Multiplicity usually indicates parathyroid hyperplasia rather than double adenoma. **(Middle)** Longitudinal power Doppler ultrasound of a parathyroid adenoma. Note the adenoma is slightly hypervascular in 90% of cases. Vascularity is best examined on longitudinal scans. **(Bottom)** Planar sestamibi scintigraphy reveals multifocal/diffuse tracer uptake superimposed on both sides of thyroid gland. The scintigraphic features are compatible with parathyroid hyperplasia.

LARYNX

Terminology

Abbreviations
- Aryepiglottic fold (AE fold)
- True vocal cord (TVC); false vocal cord (FVC)

Definitions
- Larynx: Cartilaginous skeleton bound by ligaments and muscle at the junction of upper & lower airway
- Hypopharynx: Caudal continuation of pharyngeal mucosal space, between oropharynx & esophagus

Imaging Anatomy

Extent
- Larynx: Cranial margin at level of glossoepiglottic & pharyngoepiglottic folds with caudal margin defined by lower edge of cricoid
  - Superior: Oropharynx
  - Inferior: Trachea
- Hypopharynx: Extends from level of glossoepiglottic & pharyngoepiglottic folds superiorly to inferior cricoid cartilage (cricopharyngeus muscle)
  - Superior: Oropharynx
  - Inferior: Cervical esophagus

Internal Structures-Critical Contents
- Laryngeal cartilages
  - Thyroid cartilage: Largest laryngeal cartilage; "shields" larynx
    - Two anterior laminae meet anteriorly at acute angle
    - Superior thyroid notch at anterosuperior aspect
    - Superior cornua are elongated & narrow, attach to thyrohyoid ligament
    - Inferior cornua are short & thick, articulating medially with sides of cricoid cartilage
  - Cricoid cartilage: Only complete ring in endolarynx, provides structural integrity
    - Two portions, posterior lamina & anterior arch
    - Lower border of cricoid cartilage is junction between larynx above & trachea below
  - Arytenoid cartilage: Paired pyramidal cartilages that sit on the top posterior aspect of cricoid cartilage
    - Vocal & muscular processes are at level of TVC
    - Vocal processes: Anterior projections of arytenoids where posterior margins of TVC attach
  - Corniculate cartilage: Rests on top of superior process of arytenoid cartilage, within AE folds
- Supraglottic larynx
  - Extends from tip of epiglottis above to laryngeal ventricle below
  - Contains vestibule, epiglottis, pre-epiglottic fat, AE folds, FVC, paraglottic space, arytenoid cartilages
  - Epiglottis: Leaf-shaped cartilage, larynx lid with free margin (suprahyoid), fixed portion (infrahyoid)
    - Petiole is "stem" of leaf which attaches epiglottis to thyroid lamina via thyroepiglottic ligament
    - Hyoepiglottic ligament attaches epiglottis to hyoid; glossoepiglottic fold is midline mucous membrane covering hyoepiglottic ligament
  - Pre-epiglottic space: Fat-filled space between hyoid bone anteriorly & epiglottis posteriorly
  - AE folds: Projects from cephalad tip of arytenoid cartilages to inferolateral margin of epiglottis
    - Represents superolateral margin of supraglottis, dividing it from pyriform sinus (hypopharynx)
  - FVC: Mucosal surfaces of laryngeal vestibule of supraglottis
  - Paraglottic spaces: Paired fatty regions beneath false & true vocal cords
    - Superiorly they merge into pre-epiglottic space
    - Terminates inferiorly at under surface of TVC
- Glottic larynx
  - TVC & anterior & posterior commissures
    - Comprised of thyroarytenoid muscle (medial fibers are "vocalis muscle") covered by mucosa
    - Anterior commissure: Midline, anterior meeting point of TVC
- Subglottic larynx
  - Subglottis extends from under surface of TVC to inferior surface of cricoid cartilage
  - Mucosal surface of subglottic area is closely applied to cricoid cartilage
- Hypopharynx: Consists of 3 regions
  - Piriform sinus: Anterolateral recess of hypopharynx
    - Between inner surface of thyrohyoid membrane (above), thyroid cartilage (below) & lateral AE fold
    - Pyriform sinus apex (inferior tip) at level of TVC
    - Anteromedial margin of pyriform sinus is posterolateral wall of AE fold ("marginal supraglottis")
  - Posterior hypopharyngeal wall: Inferior continuation of posterior oropharynx wall
  - Post cricoid region: Anterior wall of lower hypopharynx
    - Interface between hypopharynx & larynx
    - Extends from cricoarytenoid joints to lower edge of cricoid cartilage

Anatomy-Based Imaging Issues

Imaging Recommendations
- Role of ultrasound in laryngeal cancer is limited particularly in the era of MDCT and MR
- US may serve a supplementary role with clinical examination and CT/MRI in assessing superficial extent of laryngeal tumor
- US combined with FNAC is useful for nodal staging of laryngeal tumor
- Although the role of US in imaging the larynx is very limited, sonologist doing neck US should be familiar with its anatomy in order not to mistake its appearances for abnormalities

Imaging Pitfalls
- Presence of motion and calcification/ossification within laryngeal cartilages (common in adult) makes detailed assessment of internal laryngeal structures impossible
- Real time US is well-suited to evaluate vocal cord mobility on children presenting with hoarseness and stridor

GRAPHICS

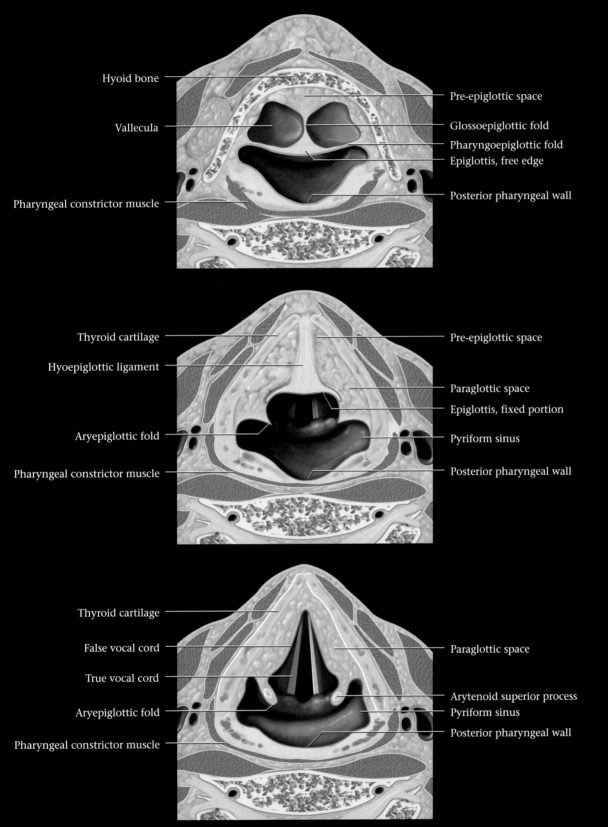

Hyoid bone

Vallecula

Pharyngeal constrictor muscle

Pre-epiglottic space

Glossoepiglottic fold

Pharyngoepiglottic fold

Epiglottis, free edge

Posterior pharyngeal wall

Thyroid cartilage

Hyoepiglottic ligament

Aryepiglottic fold

Pharyngeal constrictor muscle

Pre-epiglottic space

Paraglottic space

Epiglottis, fixed portion

Pyriform sinus

Posterior pharyngeal wall

Thyroid cartilage

False vocal cord

True vocal cord

Aryepiglottic fold

Pharyngeal constrictor muscle

Paraglottic space

Arytenoid superior process

Pyriform sinus

Posterior pharyngeal wall

(Top) First of six axial graphics of the larynx & hypopharynx from superior to inferior shows the roof of hypopharynx at hyoid bone level & the high supraglottic structures. The free edge of the epiglottis is attached to the hyoid bone via the hyoepiglottic ligament which is covered by the glossoepiglottic fold. **(Middle)** Graphic at the mid-supraglottic level shows the hyoepiglottic ligament dividing the lower pre-epiglottic space. No fascia separates the pre-epiglottic space from the paraglottic space. These two endolaryngeal spaces are submucosal locations where tumors hide from clinical detection. The aryepiglottic fold represents junction between larynx & hypopharynx. **(Bottom)** Graphic at low supraglottic level shows false vocal cords (FVC) formed by mucosal surfaces of laryngeal vestibule. Paraglottic space is beneath FVC, a common location for submucosal tumor spread.

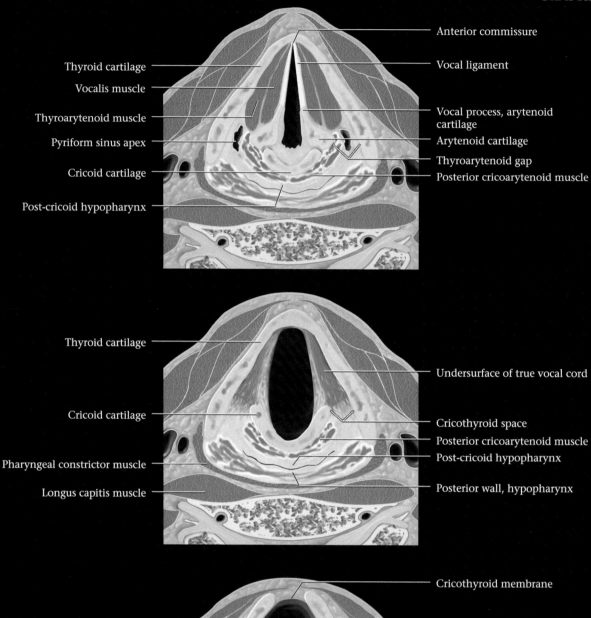

Anterior commissure

Thyroid cartilage

Vocalis muscle

Thyroarytenoid muscle

Pyriform sinus apex

Cricoid cartilage

Post-cricoid hypopharynx

Vocal ligament

Vocal process, arytenoid cartilage

Arytenoid cartilage

Thyroarytenoid gap

Posterior cricoarytenoid muscle

Thyroid cartilage

Cricoid cartilage

Pharyngeal constrictor muscle

Longus capitis muscle

Undersurface of true vocal cord

Cricothyroid space

Posterior cricoarytenoid muscle

Post-cricoid hypopharynx

Posterior wall, hypopharynx

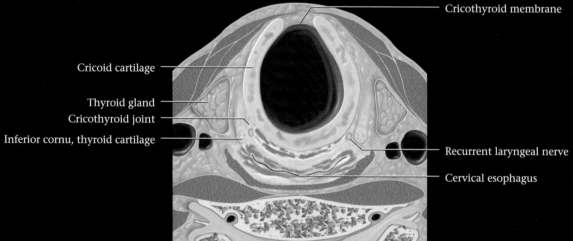

Cricothyroid membrane

Cricoid cartilage

Thyroid gland

Cricothyroid joint

Inferior cornu, thyroid cartilage

Recurrent laryngeal nerve

Cervical esophagus

(Top) Graphic at glottic, true vocal cord level shows thyroarytenoid muscle which makes up bulk of true vocal cord. Medial fibers of thyroarytenoid muscle are known as vocalis muscle. Pyriform sinus apex is seen at glottic level. **(Middle)** Graphic at level of undersurface of true vocal cord shows posterior lamina of cricoid cartilage. Post-cricoid hypopharynx represents anterior wall of lower hypopharynx & extends from cricoarytenoid joints to lower edge of cricoid cartilage at cricopharyngeus muscle. Posterior wall of hypopharynx represents inferior continuation of posterior oropharyngeal wall & extends to cervical esophagus. **(Bottom)** Graphic at subglottic level shows cricothyroid joint immediately adjacent to recurrent laryngeal nerve, located in tracheoesophageal groove.

LARYNX

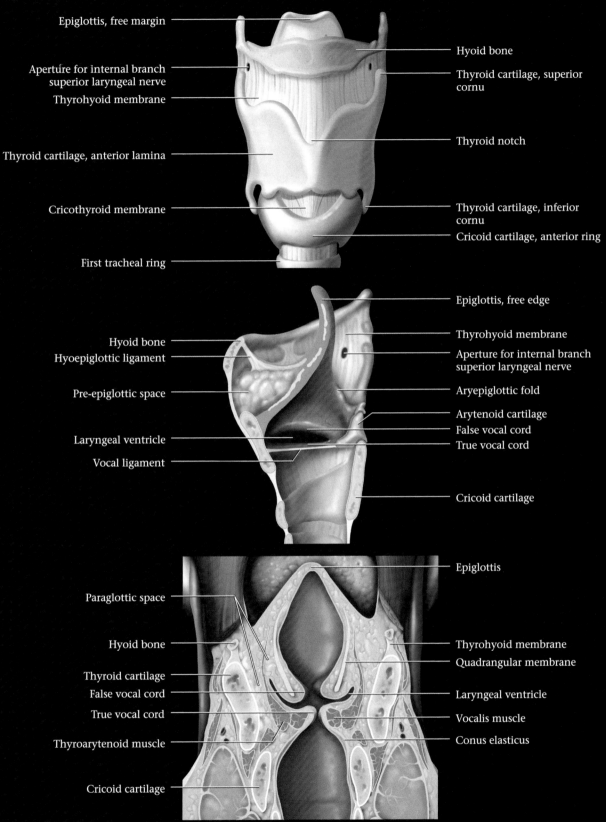

Epiglottis, free margin

Hyoid bone

Aperture for internal branch superior laryngeal nerve

Thyroid cartilage, superior cornu

Thyrohyoid membrane

Thyroid notch

Thyroid cartilage, anterior lamina

Cricothyroid membrane

Thyroid cartilage, inferior cornu

Cricoid cartilage, anterior ring

First tracheal ring

Epiglottis, free edge

Thyrohyoid membrane

Hyoid bone

Hyoepiglottic ligament

Aperture for internal branch superior laryngeal nerve

Pre-epiglottic space

Aryepiglottic fold

Arytenoid cartilage

False vocal cord

Laryngeal ventricle

True vocal cord

Vocal ligament

Cricoid cartilage

Epiglottis

Paraglottic space

Hyoid bone

Thyrohyoid membrane

Quadrangular membrane

Thyroid cartilage

False vocal cord

Laryngeal ventricle

True vocal cord

Vocalis muscle

Thyroarytenoid muscle

Conus elasticus

Cricoid cartilage

(Top) Anterior view of the laryngeal cartilage which provides the structural framework for the soft tissues of the larynx. Note that two large anterior laminae "shield" the larynx. The thyrohyoid membrane contains an aperture through which the internal branch of the superior laryngeal nerve & associated vessels course. (Middle) Sagittal graphic of midline larynx shows laryngeal ventricle air-space, which separates false vocal cords above with true vocal cords below. (Bottom) Coronal graphic posterior view shows the false & true vocal cords separated by the laryngeal ventricle. The quadrangular membrane is a fibrous membrane which extends from the upper arytenoid & corniculate cartilages to the lateral epiglottis. The conus elasticus is a fibroelastic membrane which extends from the vocal ligament of the true vocal cord to the cricoid.

Neck

II

67

LARYNX

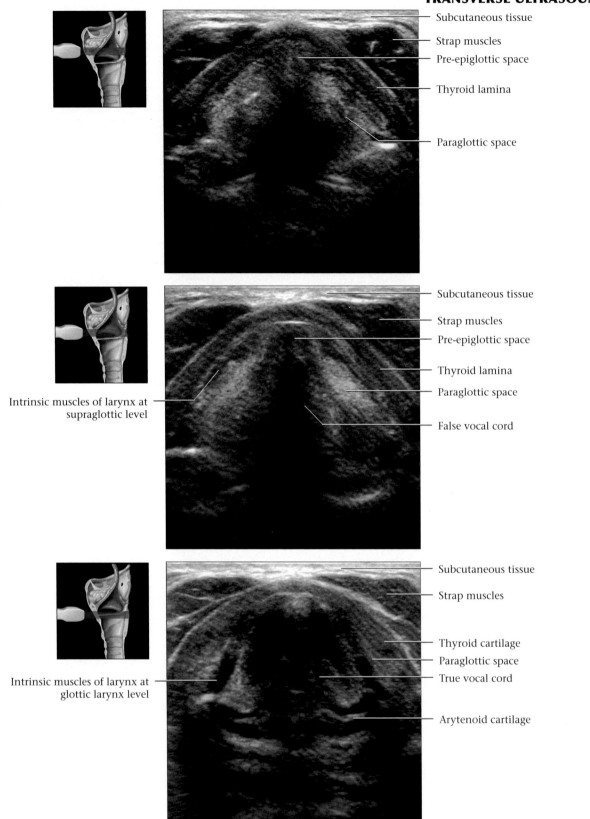

Subcutaneous tissue
Strap muscles
Pre-epiglottic space
Thyroid lamina
Paraglottic space

Subcutaneous tissue
Strap muscles
Pre-epiglottic space
Thyroid lamina
Paraglottic space
False vocal cord

Intrinsic muscles of larynx at supraglottic level

Subcutaneous tissue
Strap muscles
Thyroid cartilage
Paraglottic space
True vocal cord
Arytenoid cartilage

Intrinsic muscles of larynx at glottic larynx level

(Top) First of three consecutive axial grayscale ultrasound images of the larynx (from above downwards) at the supraglottic larynx level. The thyroid laminae are the largest cartilaginous skeleton of the larynx and appear as thin, hypoechoic bands which join at the midline anteriorly. The hyperechoic, fat-filled paraglottic and pre-epiglottic spaces are important surgical landmarks for the staging of laryngeal carcinoma. **(Middle)** Transverse grayscale ultrasound of the larynx at the level of the false vocal cord shows abundant fat in the paraglottic spaces. The echo poor intrinsic muscles of the larynx are embedded within the echogenic paraglottic fat. **(Bottom)** Transverse grayscale ultrasound of the larynx at the level of the true vocal cord. Note that the arytenoid cartilage appears as echogenic foci posteriorly with attachments to the true vocal cords which have distinct echo poor appearances.

LARYNX

AXIAL CECT

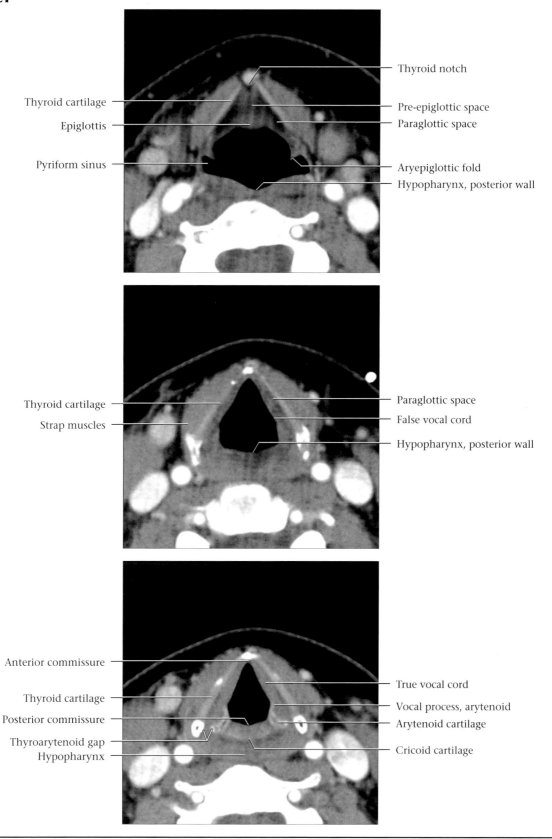

Thyroid cartilage

Epiglottis

Pyriform sinus

Thyroid notch

Pre-epiglottic space

Paraglottic space

Aryepiglottic fold

Hypopharynx, posterior wall

Thyroid cartilage

Strap muscles

Paraglottic space

False vocal cord

Hypopharynx, posterior wall

Anterior commissure

Thyroid cartilage

Posterior commissure

Thyroarytenoid gap

Hypopharynx

True vocal cord

Vocal process, arytenoid

Arytenoid cartilage

Cricoid cartilage

(Top) Image of the high supraglottic level shows that pre-epiglottic & paraglottic spaces are continuous. This allows tumors to spread submucosally in these locations. The aryepiglottic fold, part of the larynx, represents transition between larynx & hypopharynx. **(Middle)** Image of the low supraglottic level at the false vocal cord level. The paraglottic space represents deep fatty space beneath false vocal cords. Tumors that cross the laryngeal ventricle & involve false & true vocal cords are considered transglottic. **(Bottom)** Image at glottic level shows the true vocal cords in abduction in quiet respiration. True vocal cord level is identified on CT when the arytenoid & cricoid cartilages are seen & muscle fills the inferior paraglottic space. The anterior & posterior commissures of the true vocal cords should be less than 1 mm in normal patients. The post-cricoid hypopharynx is typically collapsed.

Medial edge of strap muscle
Subcutaneous tissue
Thyrohyoid ligament
Isthmus of thyroid cartilage
Pre-epiglottic space
Hyoid bone

Subcutaneous tissue
Strap muscle
Thyroid cartilage
Cricoid cartilage
Intrinsic muscles of larynx
Paraglottic space

Subcutaneous tissue
Strap muscle
Cricoid cartilage
Intrinsic muscle of larynx
Thyroid cartilage
Paraglottic space

(Top) Midline sagittal longitudinal grayscale ultrasound of the supraglottic larynx, shows the fat-filled, echogenic, pre-epiglottic space underneath the thyrohyoid membrane. Tumor spread here is readily assessed by US. (Middle) Parasagittal longitudinal grayscale ultrasound of the larynx, shows sonolucent thyroid and cricoid cartilages with no laryngeal calcification/ossification in a young adult. The paraglottic space is fat-filled and appears echogenic. The intrinsic muscles of the larynx are embedded within paraglottic space and are hypoechoic on ultrasound. (Bottom) Parasagittal longitudinal grayscale ultrasound of the larynx further lateral than the previous image. Gas within the laryngeal lumen appears highly echogenic casting posterior acoustic shadowing.

LARYNX

SAGITTAL & CORONAL REFORMATTED CECT

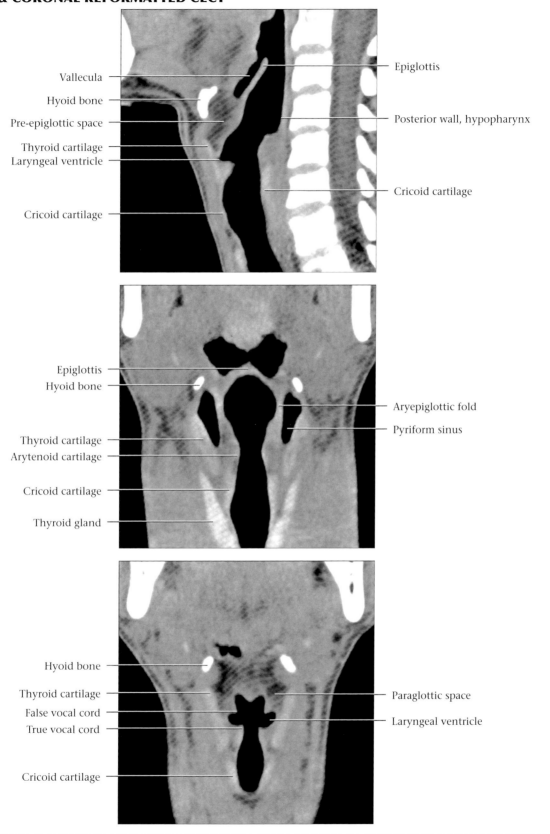

Vallecula
Hyoid bone
Pre-epiglottic space
Thyroid cartilage
Laryngeal ventricle
Cricoid cartilage

Epiglottis
Posterior wall, hypopharynx
Cricoid cartilage

Epiglottis
Hyoid bone
Thyroid cartilage
Arytenoid cartilage
Cricoid cartilage
Thyroid gland

Aryepiglottic fold
Pyriform sinus

Hyoid bone
Thyroid cartilage
False vocal cord
True vocal cord
Cricoid cartilage

Paraglottic space
Laryngeal ventricle

(Top) Parasagittal reformatted NECT shows the laryngeal ventricle, the air space that separates the false vocal cords above from the true vocal cords below. **(Middle)** In this coronal reformatted NECT, aryepiglottic folds are well seen as they extend from the lateral epiglottis to the arytenoid cartilage. The pyriform sinus is the most common location for tumors of the hypopharynx. **(Bottom)** In this coronal reformatted NECT, the laryngeal ventricle is visible as an air space between false vocal cords above, & true vocal cords below. When a tumor crosses the laryngeal ventricle to involve the true & false cords it is transglottic, which has important treatment implications. Coronal imaging is particularly useful for evaluation of transglottic disease. Note that US is unable to demonstrate such detailed anatomy, particularly of deeper structures.

CERVICAL TRACHEA AND ESOPHAGUS

Terminology

Definitions
- Cervical trachea: Air-conveying flexible tube made of cartilage & fibromuscular membrane connecting larynx to lungs
- Cervical esophagus: Muscular food & fluid-conveying tube connecting pharynx to stomach

Imaging Anatomy

Overview
- Trachea
  ○ 10-13 cm tube extending in midline from inferior larynx at ~ 6th cervical vertebral body to carina at upper margin of 5th thoracic vertebral body (carina)
- Esophagus
  ○ 25 cm tube extending in midline from inferior hypopharynx at ~ 6th cervical vertebral body to 11th thoracic vertebral body
  ○ Descends behind trachea & thyroid, lying in front of lower cervical vertebrae
    ▪ Inclines slightly to left in lower cervical neck & upper mediastinum, returning to midline at T5 vertebral body level

Anatomy Relationships
- Cervical trachea
  ○ Anterior structures: Infrahyoid strap muscles; isthmus of thyroid gland
  ○ Lateral structures: Lobes of thyroid gland
    ▪ Tracheoesophageal groove structures: Recurrent laryngeal nerve, paratracheal nodes, parathyroid glands
  ○ Posterior structure: Cervical esophagus
- Cervical esophagus
  ○ Anterior structure: Cervical trachea
  ○ Anterolateral structures: Tracheoesophageal groove structures
  ○ Lateral structures: Common carotid artery, internal jugular vein, vagus nerve
  ○ Posterior structures: Retropharyngeal fascia/muscle

Internal Structures-Critical Contents
- Cervical trachea
  ○ Tracheal cartilages
    ▪ Each cartilage is "imperfect ring" of cartilage surrounding anterior two-thirds of trachea
    ▪ Flat deficient posterior portion is completed with fibromuscular membrane
    ▪ Cross-sectional shape of trachea is that of letter D, with flat side posterior
    ▪ Smooth muscle fibers in posterior membrane (trachealis muscle) attach to free ends of tracheal cartilages & provide alteration in tracheal cross-sectional area
    ▪ Hyaline cartilage calcifies with age
    ▪ Minor salivary glands sporadically distributed in tracheal mucosa
  ○ Blood supply: Inferior thyroid arteries & veins
  ○ Lymphatic drainage: Level VI pretracheal & paratracheal nodes

- Cervical esophagus
  ○ Begins at lower border of cricoid cartilage as continuation of hypopharynx
    ▪ Upper limit is defined by cricopharyngeus muscle, which encircles it from front to back
  ○ Usually in slightly off midline position towards the left in cervical portion
  ○ Long muscular tube consists of longitudinal and circular smooth muscles
  ○ Active peristalsis in antegrade (i.e., downward) direction
  ○ Blood supply: Inferior thyroid arteries & veins
  ○ Lymphatic drainage: Level VI paratracheal nodes

Anatomy-Based Imaging Issues

Imaging Recommendations
- US best done with patient's head slightly hyperextended
- Ask patient not to swallow during ultrasound
- Transverse and longitudinal scans necessary for a comprehensive ultrasound examination
- Always assess adjacent structures and regional neck nodes

Imaging Approaches
- Multislice CT is the imaging modality to assess local tumor extent of cervical esophageal/tracheal cancer
- Tumor extent
  ○ Thyroid cancer: Assessment of tumor invasion to trachea and esophagus, CT and MR better than US
  ○ Esophageal cancer: To determine local tumor extent and invasion to adjacent structures (e.g., thyroid gland/trachea), CT better than US

Imaging Pitfalls
- Tracheal ring calcification and intraluminal air render complete assessment of trachea difficult
- Intraluminal gas due to swallowing obscures posterior esophageal wall
- As the esophagus is a mobile tube, it may slip side to side in the neck depending on direction which the head is turned
  ○ On US you may see the esophagus on the right when the head is turned to the left

Embryology

Embryologic Events
- During 4th gestational week respiratory primordium begins with formation of laryngotracheal groove that extends lengthwise in floor of gut just caudal to pharyngeal pouches
- Groove then deepens into laryngotracheal diverticulum whose ventral ectoderm become larynx & trachea
- Lateral furrows develop on either side of laryngotracheal diverticulum, then deepen to form laryngotracheal tube
- Tracheoesophageal septum then develops caudally to cranially, separating respiratory system from esophagus

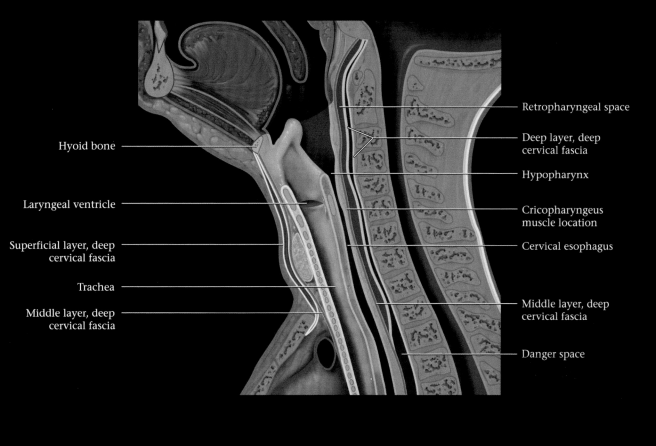

Hyoid bone

Laryngeal ventricle

Superficial layer, deep cervical fascia

Trachea

Middle layer, deep cervical fascia

Retropharyngeal space

Deep layer, deep cervical fascia

Hypopharynx

Cricopharyngeus muscle location

Cervical esophagus

Middle layer, deep cervical fascia

Danger space

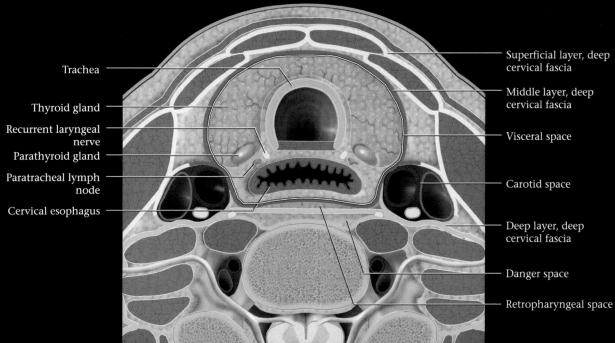

Trachea

Thyroid gland

Recurrent laryngeal nerve

Parathyroid gland

Paratracheal lymph node

Cervical esophagus

Superficial layer, deep cervical fascia

Middle layer, deep cervical fascia

Visceral space

Carotid space

Deep layer, deep cervical fascia

Danger space

Retropharyngeal space

(Top) Sagittal graphic shows the longitudinal relationships of the infrahyoid neck. Note that the middle layer of the deep cervical fascia (pink) encircles the trachea & esophagus as part of the visceral space. The trachea & esophagus are the inferior continuations of the airway & pharynx. **(Bottom)** Axial graphic shows the anteroposterior relationship of the trachea and esophagus in the lower neck. Note that the middle layer of the deep cervical fascia as it surrounds the visceral space. Important components of the tracheoesophageal groove include the recurrent laryngeal nerve, paratracheal nodes & parathyroid glands.

TRANSVERSE ULTRASOUND

Subcutaneous tissue

Sternocleidomastoid muscle

Strap muscles

Internal jugular vein

Common carotid artery

Left lobe of thyroid gland

Trachea

Cervical esophagus

Thyroid isthmus

Subcutaneous tissue

Sternohyoid muscle

Sternothyroid muscle

Trachea

Left lobe of thyroid gland

Tracheal ring cartilage

Right lobe of thyroid gland

Subcutaneous tissue in suprasternal region

Sternocleidomastoid muscle

Sternothyroid muscle

Trachea

Internal jugular vein

(Top) Transverse grayscale ultrasound of left lower cervical level. Note the location of cervical esophagus posterior to the left lobe of thyroid gland and posterolateral to the trachea. The recurrent laryngeal nerve is located in the tracheoesophageal groove (the nerve is not visualized on USG). Note the circular configuration with alternating concentric echogenic/hypoechoic rings of the esophagus in cross section. (Middle) Transverse grayscale ultrasound of the midline anterior neck at the level of thyroid gland. The trachea is a midline structure underneath the isthmus of thyroid gland and related laterally to thyroid lobes. Note the hypoechoic tracheal ring composed of hyaline cartilage which is incomplete posteriorly. (Bottom) Transverse grayscale ultrasound of the suprasternal region shows the lower cervical trachea underneath the insertion sites of the strap muscles.

CERVICAL TRACHEA AND ESOPHAGUS

AXIAL CECT

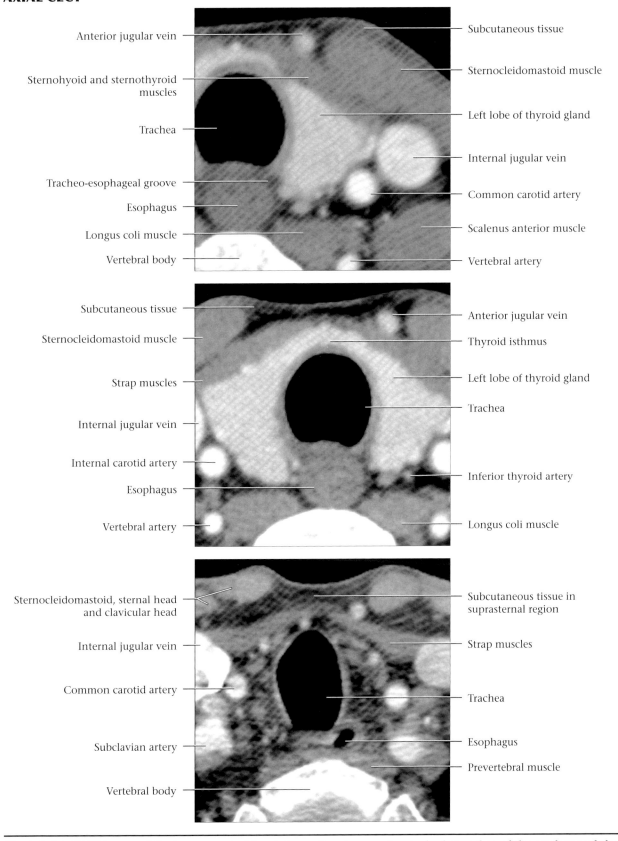

Anterior jugular vein

Sternohyoid and sternothyroid muscles

Trachea

Tracheo-esophageal groove

Esophagus

Longus coli muscle

Vertebral body

Subcutaneous tissue

Sternocleidomastoid muscle

Left lobe of thyroid gland

Internal jugular vein

Common carotid artery

Scalenus anterior muscle

Vertebral artery

Subcutaneous tissue

Sternocleidomastoid muscle

Strap muscles

Internal jugular vein

Internal carotid artery

Esophagus

Vertebral artery

Anterior jugular vein

Thyroid isthmus

Left lobe of thyroid gland

Trachea

Inferior thyroid artery

Longus coli muscle

Sternocleidomastoid, sternal head and clavicular head

Internal jugular vein

Common carotid artery

Subclavian artery

Vertebral body

Subcutaneous tissue in suprasternal region

Strap muscles

Trachea

Esophagus

Prevertebral muscle

(Top) Axial CECT image of the lower cervical level shows the close anatomical relationship of the trachea and the esophagus with adjacent structures such as the thyroid gland. **(Middle)** Axial CECT of the lower cervical level with the trachea surrounded by thyroid lobes and the isthmus and esophagus posterior to the trachea. **(Bottom)** Axial CECT at the level of the suprasternal region. The esophagus at this level is usually slightly off midline towards the left in relation to the trachea. The two structures are surrounded by mediastinal fat and related to the major vessels in the superior mediastinum. Although US is able to detect the spread of a thyroid tumor to the trachea and esophagus (and vice versa), CT and MR delineate the involvement much better.

LONGITUDINAL ULTRASOUND AND PATHOLOGY

Subcutaneous tissue

Strap muscles

Left lobe of thyroid gland

Esophagus

Subcutaneous tissue
Fourth tracheal ring
Third tracheal ring
Second tracheal ring
First tracheal ring

Cricoid cartilage

Artifact from tracheal air and calcification

Strap muscles

Right lobe of thyroid gland

Thyroid carcinoma

Tracheal invasion

(Top) Longitudinal grayscale ultrasound of the lower left neck at the thyroid gland level. The cervical esophagus is seen posterior to the left lobe of the thyroid gland. It is a long tubular structure with alternating echogenic/hypoechoic layers representing the mucosal, submucosal, muscular and serosal layers. (Middle) Longitudinal grayscale ultrasound of the midline anterior neck shows the presence of hypoechoic tracheal rings along the cervical portion of the trachea. Note the hypoechoic, non-calcified, cricoid cartilage above the tracheal rings. (Bottom) Transverse grayscale ultrasound in patient with thyroid carcinoma involving isthmus, adjacent right lobe with local tumor invasion into trachea. Note the loss of definition of the hypoechoic tracheal ring which is replaced by the tumor.

CERVICAL TRACHEA AND ESOPHAGUS

SAGITTAL REFORMATTED CECT AND PATHOLOGY

Vallecula — Retropharyngeal space

Hyoid cartilage — Aryepiglottic fold

Strap muscles — Pyriform fossa

Thyroid cartilage

Cricoid cartilage — Cervical esophagus

Left lobe of thyroid — Vertebral body

Sternocleidomastoid muscle — Spinal canal

Cervical esophagus

Thyroid cartilage — Spinous process

Trachea

Isthmus of thyroid — Spinal cord and spinal canal

Vertebral body

Sternum

Branches from aorta

Common carotid artery

Left lobe of thyroid gland

Metastatic left lower jugular lymph node

Air in esophageal lumen

Esophageal tumor

(Top) Oblique sagittal reformatted CECT image of the neck correlating the image plane on ultrasound. The thyroid lobe is seen superficial to the esophagus. (Middle) Sagittal reformatted CECT of the neck in the midline. The trachea is seen anterior to the cervical esophagus, which is gas-filled and inferior to the pharyngeal constrictor. (Bottom) Transverse grayscale ultrasound of the left lower-cervical level. There is a large heterogeneous mass posterior to and invading the lower pole of the left thyroid gland compatible with known locally extensive esophageal carcinoma. Note the presence of left lower-jugular lymph node metastases.

BRACHIAL PLEXUS

Gross Anatomy

Overview

- Brachial plexus (BP)
  - Major neural supply to upper limbs
  - Formed from ventral rami of C5-T1 ± minor branches from C4, T2
  - Has some proximal branches originating above BP proper
    - Dorsal scapular nerve; long thoracic nerve; nerves to scalene/longus colli muscles; branch to phrenic nerve
  - Remaining minor, all major peripheral branches arise from BP proper
  - BP divided into roots/rami, trunks, divisions, cords, terminal branches
  - Roots/rami
    - Originate from spinal cord levels C5 to T1
    - Enter the posterior triangle by emerging between scalenus anterior and scalenus medius muscles
  - Trunks
    - Upper (C5-6), middle (C7), lower (C8, T1)
    - Lower trunk - lies behind the third part of subclavian artery
    - Minor nerves arising directly from trunks: Suprascapular nerve, nerve to subclavius muscle
  - Divisions
    - Form by each trunk's dividing into anterior and posterior branches in supraclavicular triangle
    - Anterior divisions innervate anterior (flexor) muscles
    - Posterior divisions innervate posterior (extensor) muscles
    - No named minor nerves arising directly from divisions
  - Cords
    - Lateral cord (anterior divisions of superior, middle trunks) innervates anterior (flexor) muscles
    - Medial cord (anterior division of inferior trunk) innervates anterior (flexor) muscles
    - Posterior cord (posterior divisions of all 3 trunks) innervates posterior (extensor) muscles
    - Descend behind the clavicle to leave the posterior triangle and enter the axilla
  - Branches (terminal)
    - Within the axillary content
    - Musculocutaneous nerve (C5-6) arises from lateral cord
    - Ulnar nerve (C8-T1) arises from medial cord
    - Axillary nerve (C5-6), radial nerve (C5-T1), thoracodorsal nerve (C6-8), upper (C6-7) and lower (C5-6) subscapular nerves all arise from posterior cord

Anatomy Relationships

- Close anatomic proximity to subclavian artery and lymphatics
- Subclavian vein courses anterior to anterior scalene muscle, not in direct proximity to brachial plexus
- Enter the axilla behind the clavicle

Imaging Anatomy

Overview

- MR is the best modality for visualization of BP
  - Surrounding perineural fat provides excellent visualization of nerves, and allows them to be distinguished from adjacent soft tissues
- USG is an alternative imaging technique to visualize small component of brachial plexus
  - Excellent spatial resolution provided by high frequency transducer
  - Appear as long, tubular, hypoechoic structures against background hyperechoic fat on longitudinal scan
  - Several small ovoid/round hypoechoic nodules in lower posterior triangle/supraclavicular region between scalenus anterior and scalenus medius muscles on transverse scan
  - Lack of flow distinguish them from vascular structures

Anatomy-Based Imaging Issues

Key Concepts or Questions

- Knowledge of normal brachial plexus anatomy is critical for evaluating clinical abnormalities
- Nerve sheath tumor is one of the differential diagnoses for a mass in lower posterior triangle/supraclavicular region
  - Demonstration of mass being contiguous with brachial plexus elements provides a definite diagnosis
- Sonographic appearances of nerve sheath tumor may overlap with abnormal lymph node
  - Identification of contiguous nerve obviates the need for needle aspiration/biopsy which is particularly painful for nerve sheath tumor

Imaging Recommendations

- USG is ideal for initial investigation of suspected brachial plexus schwannoma in the neck
- USG also helps to evaluate brachial plexus involvement with metastatic nodes in lower posterior triangle/supraclavicular fossa

Imaging Approaches

- On US it is not possible to definitively differentiate between rami, trunks, divisions, cords
  - They are therefore often referred to as brachial plexus elements
- Roots/rami emerging from the spine are better seen on longitudinal scans
- Brachial plexus elements are readily identified on transverse scans between scalenus anterior and medius
- Longitudinal scans help to evaluate along their length
- Color/power Doppler help to distinguish them from vessels

Imaging Pitfalls

- The infraclavicular portion of brachial plexus cannot be well demonstrated on USG

GRAPHICS

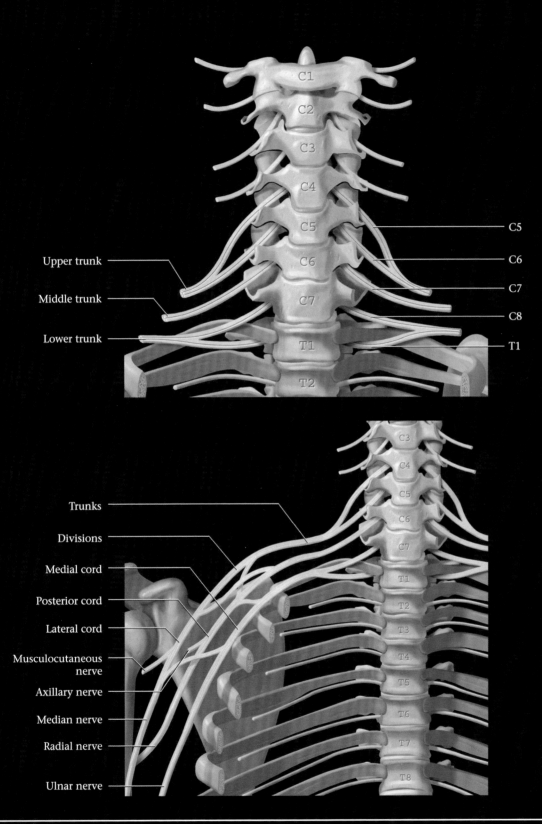

C1
C2
C3
C4
C5 — C5
C6 — C6
C7 — C7
— C8
Upper trunk
Middle trunk
Lower trunk — T1 — T1
T2

Trunks
Divisions
Medial cord
Posterior cord
Lateral cord
Musculocutaneous nerve
Axillary nerve
Median nerve
Radial nerve
Ulnar nerve

C3
C4
C5
C6
C7
T1
T2
T3
T4
T5
T6
T7
T8

(Top) Coronal graphic of the cervical spine and supraclavicular brachial plexus demonstrates the cervical ventral primary rami combining to form the brachial plexus. The C1-7 roots exit above the same numbered pedicle, C8 exits above the T1 pedicle, and more caudal roots exit below their numbered pedicle. The trunks are visualized on ultrasound in the lower posterior triangle and supraclavicular fossa. **(Bottom)** Coronal graphic of the brachial plexus demonstrates the more distal plexus elements extending into the axilla. The trunks recombine into posterior and anterior divisions that form the cords. The posterior cord forms the radial and axillary nerves. The medial cord forms the ulnar nerve, while the lateral cord forms the musculocutaneous nerve. The median nerve is formed from branches of both the lateral and medial cords.

Neck

II

79

BRACHIAL PLEXUS

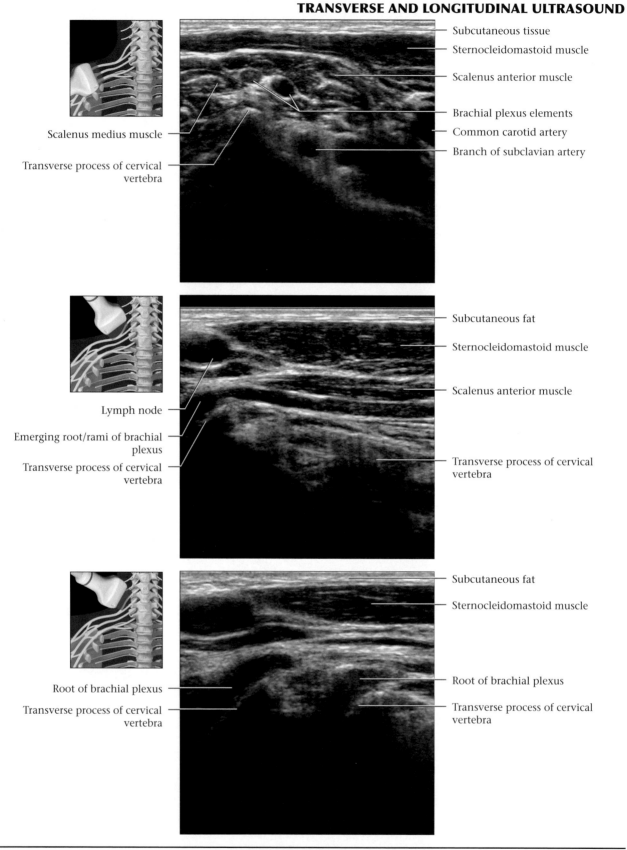

Scalenus medius muscle

Transverse process of cervical vertebra

Subcutaneous tissue

Sternocleidomastoid muscle

Scalenus anterior muscle

Brachial plexus elements

Common carotid artery

Branch of subclavian artery

Lymph node

Emerging root/rami of brachial plexus

Transverse process of cervical vertebra

Subcutaneous fat

Sternocleidomastoid muscle

Scalenus anterior muscle

Transverse process of cervical vertebra

Root of brachial plexus

Transverse process of cervical vertebra

Subcutaneous fat

Sternocleidomastoid muscle

Root of brachial plexus

Transverse process of cervical vertebra

(Top) Short axis view, grayscale ultrasound of lower posterior triangle shows the elements of brachial plexus which appear as round hypoechoic structures between scalenus anterior muscle and scalenus medius muscle. (Middle) Longitudinal grayscale ultrasound of posterior triangle of the neck shows root and trunk of brachial plexus which appears as thin tubular hypoechoic structure related superficially to scalenus anterior muscle and deeply with cervical vertebrae. (Bottom) Longitudinal grayscale ultrasound of the posterior triangle shows the emerging roots of the brachial plexus. Although USG identifies elements of the brachial plexus in the neck, MR delineates entire anatomy better.

BRACHIAL PLEXUS

AXIAL AND CORONAL MR

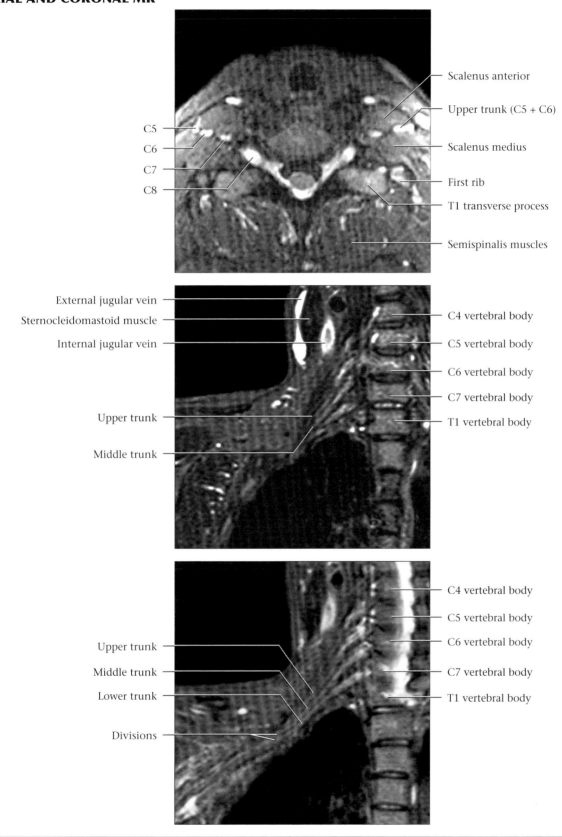

Scalenus anterior

Upper trunk (C5 + C6)

C5

C6

C7

C8

Scalenus medius

First rib

T1 transverse process

Semispinalis muscles

External jugular vein

Sternocleidomastoid muscle

Internal jugular vein

C4 vertebral body

C5 vertebral body

C6 vertebral body

C7 vertebral body

T1 vertebral body

Upper trunk

Middle trunk

Upper trunk

Middle trunk

Lower trunk

Divisions

C4 vertebral body

C5 vertebral body

C6 vertebral body

C7 vertebral body

T1 vertebral body

(Top) Axial STIR MR image at the C7/T1 level depicts the linear alignment of the C5 through C8 ventral primary rami (VPR). C5 and C6 are closely approximated and forming the left upper trunk. (Middle) Coronal T2-weighted image of the brachial plexus showing the proximal cervical roots/VPR combining to form the upper and middle trunks of the brachial plexus. Normal nerve is slightly hyperintense to muscle on STIR and fat-saturated T2-weighted MR. (Bottom) Coronal reformatted oblique coronal T2-weighted image of the brachial plexus. The trunks and divisions of the brachial plexus can be seen continuing from cervical nerve roots to the axilla.

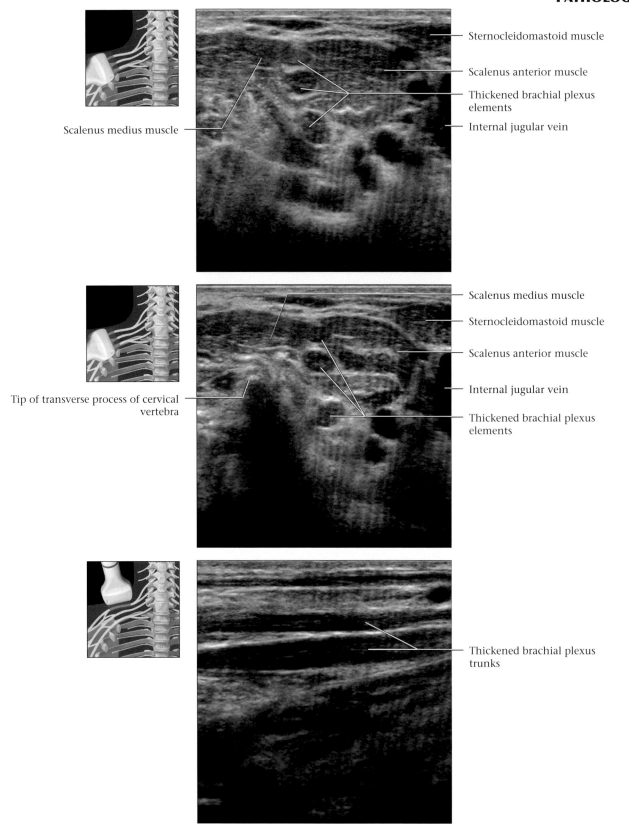

Sternocleidomastoid muscle

Scalenus anterior muscle

Thickened brachial plexus elements

Internal jugular vein

Scalenus medius muscle

Scalenus medius muscle

Sternocleidomastoid muscle

Scalenus anterior muscle

Internal jugular vein

Thickened brachial plexus elements

Tip of transverse process of cervical vertebra

Thickened brachial plexus trunks

(Top) Transverse grayscale ultrasound of right lower posterior triangle/supraclavicular fossa shows round smooth hypoechoic nodules between the scalenus anterior and medius muscles. The anatomical location suggests the possibility of thickened brachial plexus elements. **(Middle)** Transverse grayscale ultrasound at lower level of right posterior triangle/supraclavicular fossa. The hypoechoic nodules persist and diverge. **(Bottom)** Longitudinal grayscale ultrasound of right posterior triangle/supraclavicular fossa confirms the elongated linear hypoechoic thickened elements of the brachial plexus. This patient had past history of neck irradiation for metastatic neck nodal disease, the nerve thickening is likely secondary to post-radiation changes.

PATHOLOGY

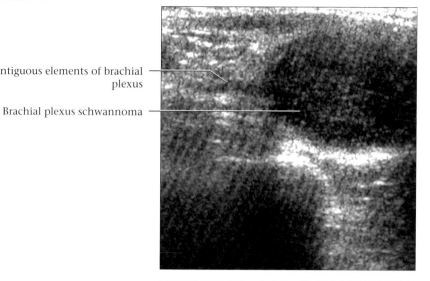
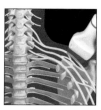

Contiguous elements of brachial plexus

Brachial plexus schwannoma

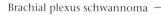
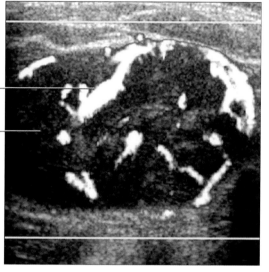
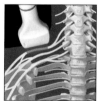

Intratumoral vascularity

Brachial plexus schwannoma

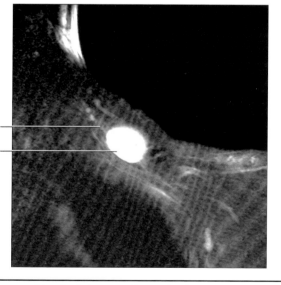

Adjacent trunks of brachial plexus

Brachial plexus schwannoma

(Top) Longitudinal grayscale ultrasound in the left supraclavicular fossa shows a round, solid, heterogeneous hypoechoic mass which continues with brachial plexus elements suggesting a brachial plexus schwannoma. (Middle) Power Doppler ultrasound of a brachial plexus schwannoma demonstrates increased intralesional vascularity. (Bottom) Coronal fat-suppressed T2WI MR of a brachial plexus schwannoma, which shows high signal intensity. The adjacent trunks of brachial plexus also appear mildly hyperintense on T2WI. The lesion is typically hypo/isointense on T1WI and shows marked homogeneous enhancement after intravenous gadolinium (not shown).

VAGUS NERVE

Terminology

Abbreviations
- Vagus nerve (CN10, CN X)

Synonyms
- Tenth cranial nerve

Imaging Anatomy

Overview
- Mixed nerve (sensory, taste, motor, parasympathetic)
  - Parasympathetic nerve supplying regions of head and neck and thoracic and abdominal viscera
  - Additional vagus nerve components
    - Motor to soft palate (except tensor veli palatini muscle), pharyngeal constrictor muscles, larynx and palatoglossus muscle of tongue
    - Visceral sensation from larynx, esophagus, trachea, thoracic and abdominal viscera
    - Sensory nerve to external tympanic membrane, external auditory canal (EAC) and external ear
- Four major segments: Intra-axial, cisternal, skull base and extracranial
- Intra-axial segment
  - Vagal nuclei are in upper and middle medulla
    - Contains motor, sensory (including taste from epiglottis) and parasympathetic fibers
  - Fibers to and from these nuclei exit lateral medulla in postolivary sulcus inferior to CN9 and superior to bulbar portion of CN11
- Cisternal segment
  - Exits lateral medulla in postolivary sulcus between CN9 and bulbar portion of CN11
  - Travel anterolaterally through basal cistern together with CN9 and bulbar portion of CN11
- Skull base segment
  - Passes through posterior pars vascularis portion of jugular foramen (JF)
    - Accompanied by CN11 and jugular bulb
    - Superior vagal ganglion is found within JF
- Extracranial segment
  - Exits JF into nasopharyngeal carotid space
  - Inferior vagal ganglion lies just below skull base
  - Descends along posterolateral aspect of internal carotid artery into thorax
    - Passes anterior to aortic arch on left and subclavian artery on right
  - Forms plexus around esophagus and major blood vessels to heart and lungs
  - Gastric nerves emerge from esophageal plexus and provide parasympathetic innervation to stomach
  - Innervation to intestines and visceral organs follows arterial blood supply to that organ
- Extracranial branches in head and neck
  - Auricular branch (Arnold nerve)
    - Sensation from external surface of tympanic membrane, EAC and external ear
    - Passes through mastoid canaliculus extending from posterolateral JF to mastoid segment CN7 canal
  - Pharyngeal branches

- Pharyngeal plexus exits just below skull base
- Sensory to epiglottis, trachea and esophagus, motor to soft palate and pharyngeal constrictor muscles
  - Superior laryngeal nerve
    - Motor to cricothyroid muscle, sensory to mucosa of supraglottis
- Recurrent laryngeal nerve
  - On right recurs at cervicothoracic junction, passes posteriorly around subclavian artery
  - On left recurs in mediastinum by passing posteriorly under aorta at aortopulmonary window
  - Nerves recur in tracheoesophageal grooves
  - Motor to all laryngeal muscles except cricothyroid muscle
  - Sensory to mucosa of infraglottics

Anatomy-Based Imaging Issues

Imaging Recommendations
- Extracranial segment is only portion accessible for USG evaluation (upper, mid, lower cervical regions)
  - Lies between internal/common carotid artery (ICA/CCA) and internal jugular vein (IJV) on transverse scans
  - Linear hypoechoic structure with central echogenic fibrillary pattern on longitudinal scan
  - On axial scans seen as round, hypoechoic structure with central echogenic focus
  - Best seen from level of carotid bifurcation down to lower cervical region
  - Color/power Doppler helps to distinguish it from small vessels in the vicinity of major vessels of carotid sheath
- USG readily identifies a vagal nerve Schwannoma in upper, mid, lower cervical region
  - Appears as round/ovoid solid hypoechoic mass
  - Related to ICA/CCA and IJV
    - Not causing splaying of carotid bifurcation (carotid body tumor)
  - Vagus nerve contiguous with the mass
  - Increased intranodular vascularity on power Doppler
  - USG features obviate the need for fine needle aspiration/biopsy which is particularly painful
- The recurrent laryngeal nerve cannot be confidently visualized on USG (in our experience)
  - In patient with vocal cord palsy, USG may help to detect abnormality in the tracheoesophageal groove

Clinical Implications

Clinical Importance
- Vagal nerve dysfunction
  - Proximal symptom complex (lesion between medulla and hyoid bone)
    - Multiple cranial nerves involved (CN9-12) with oropharyngeal and laryngeal dysfunction
  - Distal symptom complex (lesion below hyoid bone)
    - Isolated CN10 involvement with laryngeal dysfunction only

VAGUS NERVE

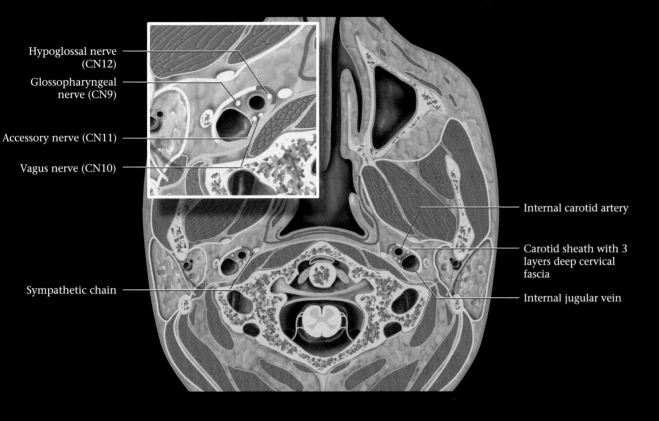

Hypoglossal nerve (CN12)

Glossopharyngeal nerve (CN9)

Accessory nerve (CN11)

Vagus nerve (CN10)

Sympathetic chain

Internal carotid artery

Carotid sheath with 3 layers deep cervical fascia

Internal jugular vein

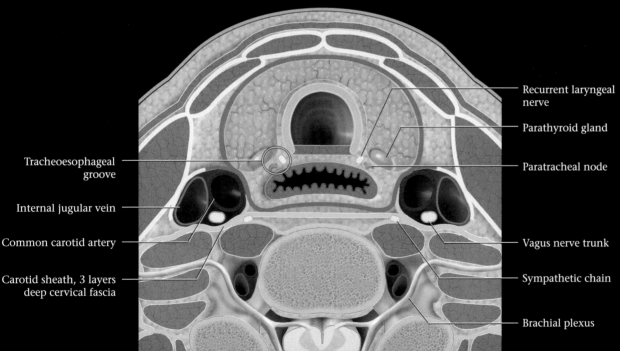

Tracheoesophageal groove

Internal jugular vein

Common carotid artery

Carotid sheath, 3 layers deep cervical fascia

Recurrent laryngeal nerve

Parathyroid gland

Paratracheal node

Vagus nerve trunk

Sympathetic chain

Brachial plexus

(Top) Axial graphic of nasopharyngeal carotid spaces shows the extracranial vagus nerve situated posteriorly in the gap between the internal carotid artery and the internal jugular vein. Notice that at this level, CN9, CN11 and CN12 are all still within the carotid space. This site is not accessible to US. (Bottom) Axial graphic through the infrahyoid carotid spaces at the level of the thyroid gland demonstrates that the vagus trunk is the only remaining cranial nerve within the carotid space. It remains in the posterior gap between the common carotid artery and the internal jugular vein. Note the recurrent laryngeal nerve in the tracheoesophageal groove within the visceral space. Remember that the left recurrent laryngeal nerve turns cephalad in the aortopulmonary window in the mediastinum whereas the right recurrent nerve turns at the cervicothoracic junction around the subclavian artery.

VAGUS NERVE

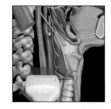
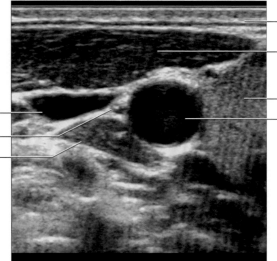

Internal jugular vein

Vagus nerve

Scalenus anterior muscle

Subcutaneous tissue

Sternocleidomastoid muscle

Right lobe of thyroid gland

Common carotid artery

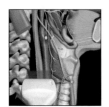
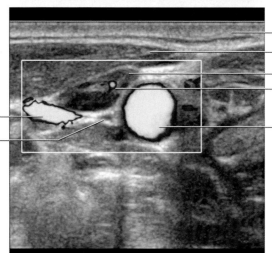

Internal jugular vein

Vagus nerve

Subcutaneous tissue

Sternocleidomastoid muscle

Lymph node

Hilar vascularity in lymph node

Common carotid artery

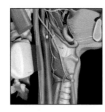
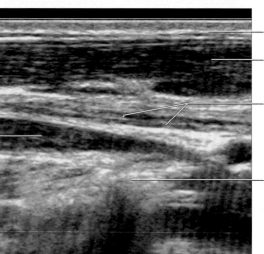

Common carotid artery

Subcutaneous tissue

Sternocleidomastoid muscle

Vagus nerve

Transverse process of cervical vertebra

(Top) Transverse grayscale ultrasound of the lower cervical level at the thyroid gland level. The vagus nerve appears as a small, round, hypoechoic structure with central echogenicity within the carotid sheath and is located between the common carotid artery and the internal jugular vein. (Middle) Power Doppler ultrasound of the mid cervical level in the transverse plane. Note the avascular nature of the vagus nerve adjacent to the common carotid artery and internal jugular vein. Note the presence of hilar vascularity in the adjacent normal deep cervical lymph node. (Bottom) Longitudinal grayscale ultrasound of the vagus nerve which appears as a long, thin, tubular, hypoechoic structure with central echogenic fibrillary pattern within. On US CN10 is readily seen from the carotid bifurcation to the lower cervical region.

VAGUS NERVE

AXIAL AND CORONAL CECT

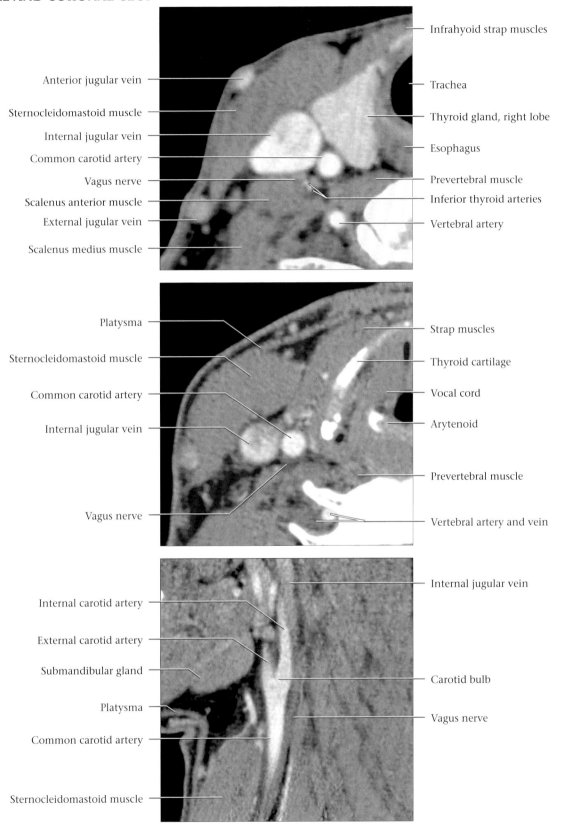

Anterior jugular vein	Infrahyoid strap muscles
Sternocleidomastoid muscle	Trachea
Internal jugular vein	Thyroid gland, right lobe
Common carotid artery	Esophagus
Vagus nerve	Prevertebral muscle
Scalenus anterior muscle	Inferior thyroid arteries
External jugular vein	Vertebral artery
Scalenus medius muscle	

Platysma	Strap muscles
Sternocleidomastoid muscle	Thyroid cartilage
Common carotid artery	Vocal cord
Internal jugular vein	Arytenoid
	Prevertebral muscle
Vagus nerve	Vertebral artery and vein

	Internal jugular vein
Internal carotid artery	
External carotid artery	
Submandibular gland	Carotid bulb
Platysma	Vagus nerve
Common carotid artery	
Sternocleidomastoid muscle	

(Top) Axial CECT of the neck at mid cervical level. The vagus nerve is seen as an isodense dot in the posterior aspect of the carotid sheath. The inferior thyroid arteries are seen as contrast-enhanced dots in it proximity. **(Middle)** Axial CECT image of the neck in a different patient. The vagus nerve is again seen as an isodense dot in the posterior aspect of the carotid space. **(Bottom)** Oblique sagittal reformatted CECT image of the neck, showing the course of the vagus nerve. It is closely related to the posterior aspect of the common carotid artery. Although CT demonstrates CN10 in the neck, high resolution US clearly evaluates its internal architecture.

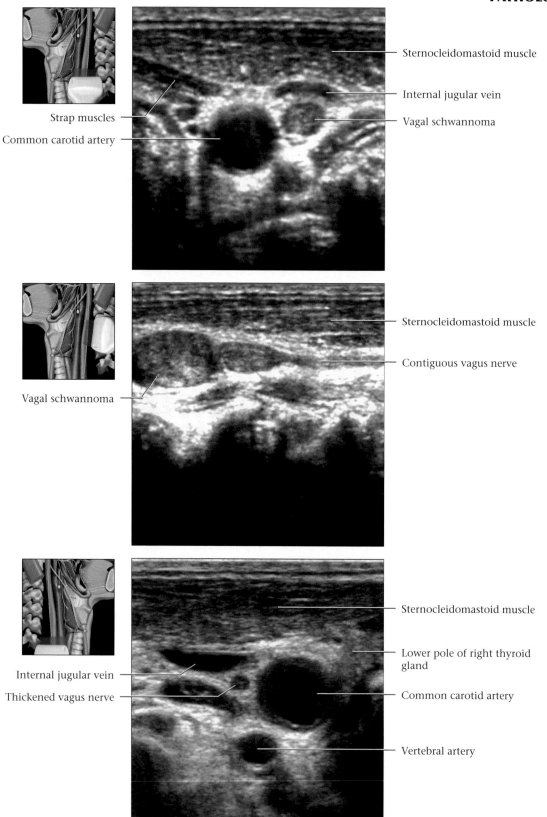

Strap muscles
Common carotid artery

Sternocleidomastoid muscle
Internal jugular vein
Vagal schwannoma

Vagal schwannoma

Sternocleidomastoid muscle
Contiguous vagus nerve

Internal jugular vein
Thickened vagus nerve

Sternocleidomastoid muscle
Lower pole of right thyroid gland
Common carotid artery
Vertebral artery

(Top) Transverse grayscale ultrasound of left mid cervical level shows a well-circumscribed, hypoechoic mass closely related to the left internal jugular vein and common carotid artery. The anatomical location helps to identify the mass originating from the vagus nerve. **(Middle)** Longitudinal grayscale ultrasound shows two well-circumscribed, oblong, solid, hypoechoic masses contiguous with vagus nerve inferiorly. The appearances are of vagal schwannomas. **(Bottom)** Transverse grayscale ultrasound of the lower cervical level in a patient with previous neck irradiation for head and neck cancer. The vagus nerve is diffusely thickened with smooth contour as a result of post-irradiation change.

VAGUS NERVE

PATHOLOGY

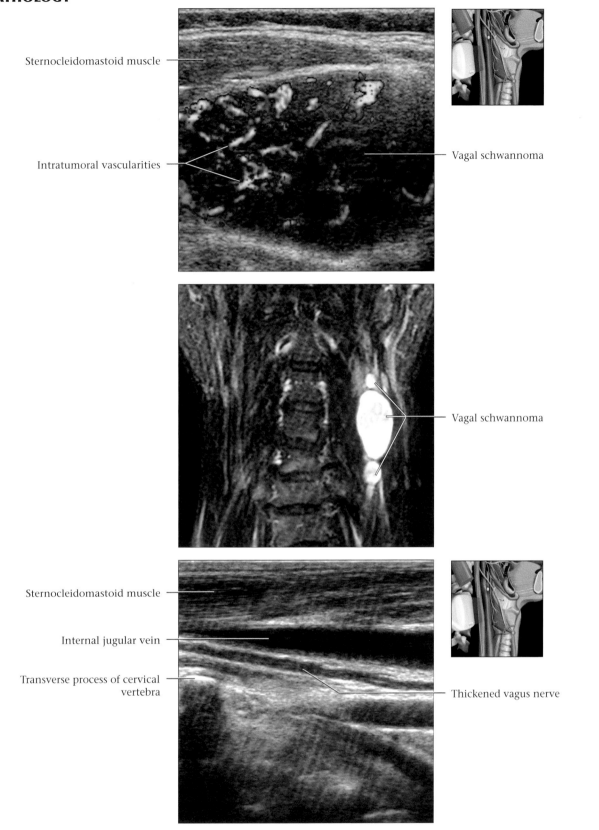

Sternocleidomastoid muscle

Intratumoral vascularities

Vagal schwannoma

Vagal schwannoma

Sternocleidomastoid muscle

Internal jugular vein

Transverse process of cervical vertebra

Thickened vagus nerve

(Top) Longitudinal power Doppler ultrasound of a vagal schwannoma reveals marked increased intratumoral vascularity. US readily identifies a vagal nerve schwannoma and obviates the need for FNAC/biopsy. **(Middle)** Coronal fat-suppressed T2WI MR shows marked T2-hyperintensity of vagal schwannoma. **(Bottom)** Longitudinal grayscale ultrasound shows the diffusely thickened vagus nerve in relation to the IJV.

CERVICAL CAROTID ARTERIES

Terminology

Abbreviations
- Aortic arch (AA); brachiocephalic trunk (BCT)
- Common (CCA), internal (ICA), external (ECA) carotid arteries, vertebral artery (VA)

Gross Anatomy

Overview
- CCA terminates by dividing into ECA and ICA
- ECA is the smaller of the two terminal branches
  - Supplies most of head, neck (except eye, brain)
  - Has numerous anastomoses with ICA and VA (may become important source of collateral blood flow)
- ICA has no normal extracranial branches

Imaging Anatomy

Overview
- CCA
  - Right CCA originates from BCT; left CCA from AA
  - Course superiorly in carotid space, anteromedial to internal jugular vein
  - Divide into ECA, ICA at approximately C3-4 level
- Cervical ICA
  - 90% are posterolateral to ECA
  - Carotid bulb
    - Focal dilatation of ICA at its origin from CCA
    - Flow reversal occurs in carotid bulb
  - Ascending cervical segment
    - Courses superiorly within carotid space
    - Enters carotid canal of skull base (petrous temporal bone)
    - No named branch in neck
- ECA
  - Smaller and medial compared with ICA
  - Has 8 major branches in the neck
  - Superior thyroid artery
    - First ECA branch (may arise from CCA bifurcation)
    - Arises anteriorly, courses inferiorly to apex of thyroid
    - Supplies superior thyroid, larynx
    - Anastomoses with inferior thyroid artery (branch of thyrocervical trunk)
  - Ascending pharyngeal artery
    - Arises from posterior ECA (or CCA bifurcation)
    - Courses superiorly between ECA, ICA
    - Visceral branches, muscular branches and neuromeningeal branches
  - Lingual artery
    - Second anterior ECA branch
    - Loops anteroinferiorly, then superiorly to tongue
    - Major vascular supply to tongue, oral cavity, submandibular gland
  - Facial artery
    - Originates just above lingual artery
    - Curves around mandible, then passes anterosuperiorly across cheek and is closely related to the submandibular gland

- Supplies face, palate, lip, cheek
  - Occipital artery
    - Originates from posterior aspect of ECA
    - Courses posterosuperiorly between occiput and C1
    - Supplies scalp, upper cervical musculature, posterior fossa meninges
  - Posterior auricular artery
    - Arises from posterior ECA above occipital artery
    - Courses superiorly to supply pinna, scalp, external auditory canal, chorda tympani
  - Superficial temporal artery
    - Smaller of two terminal ECA branches
    - Runs superiorly behind mandibular condyle, across zygoma
    - Supplies scalp, gives off transverse facial artery
  - Internal maxillary artery
    - Larger of two terminal ECA branches
    - Arises within parotid gland, behind mandibular neck
    - Gives off middle meningeal artery (supplies cranial meninges)

Anatomy-Based Imaging Issues

Imaging Recommendations
- Normal USG appearances of carotid arteries
  - CCA - diameter: 6.3 +/- 0.9 mm, smooth and thin intima, antegrade low resistance arterial flow
  - ICA - diameter: 4.8 +/- 0.7 mm, smooth and thin intima, antegrade low resistance flow
  - ECA - diameter: 4.1 +/- 0.6 mm, smooth and thin intima, antegrade high resistance flow
- In assessing carotid arteries on USG, the following parameters should be examined
- Intima-media thickness (IMT)
  - Distance between the leading edges of the lumen-intima interface and the media-adventia interface at the far edge
  - Ranges from 0.5 mm to 1 mm in healthy adults
- Presence of atherosclerotic plaques
  - Eccentric/concentric, non-circumferential/circumferential
  - Calcified plaque/soft plaque
- Luminal diameter/area reduction
  - Should be made on the true cross sectional view of affected artery
  - Color flow imaging helps to detect residual lumen in tight stenosis or in assessing an indeterminate total occlusion
- Spectral Doppler analysis
  - Arterial flow pattern: Low resistance/high resistance flow, antegrade/retrograde flow, special waveform - e.g., damped waveform, pre-occlusive "thump"
  - Peak systolic velocity (PSV) measurement
  - Systolic velocity ratio (SVR) measurement

Imaging Pitfalls
- Scanning technique must be meticulous to produce reliable Doppler ultrasound results
- Obliquity of imaging plane in relation to cross-section of artery may wrongly estimate degree of arterial stenosis

CERVICAL CAROTID ARTERIES

GRAPHIC & DIGITAL SUBTRACTION ANGIOGRAM

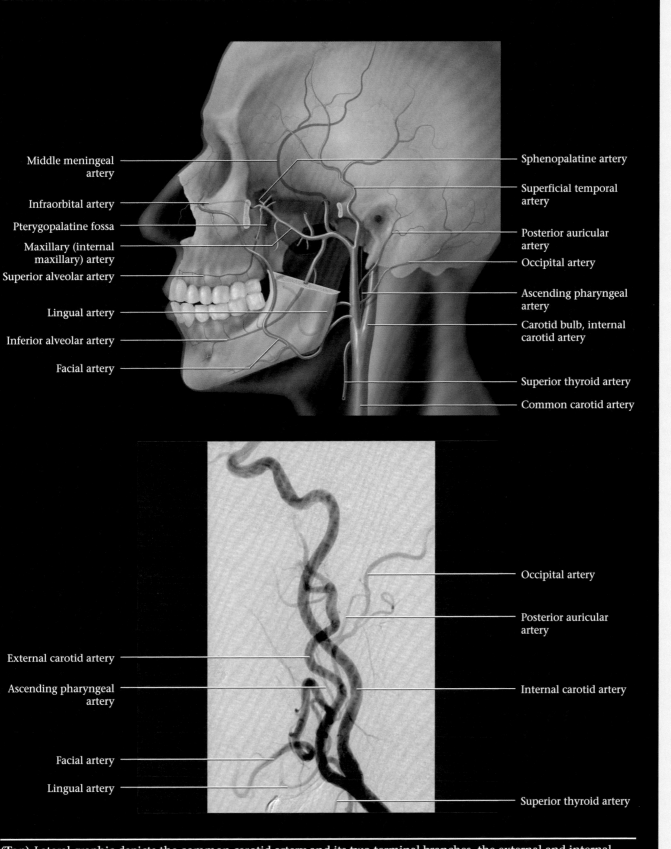

Middle meningeal artery — Infraorbital artery — Pterygopalatine fossa — Maxillary (internal maxillary) artery — Superior alveolar artery — Lingual artery — Inferior alveolar artery — Facial artery — Sphenopalatine artery — Superficial temporal artery — Posterior auricular artery — Occipital artery — Ascending pharyngeal artery — Carotid bulb, internal carotid artery — Superior thyroid artery — Common carotid artery

Occipital artery — Posterior auricular artery — External carotid artery — Ascending pharyngeal artery — Internal carotid artery — Facial artery — Lingual artery — Superior thyroid artery

(Top) Lateral graphic depicts the common carotid artery and its two terminal branches, the external and internal carotid arteries. The scalp and the superficial facial structures are removed to show the deep ECA branches. The ECA terminates by dividing into the superficial temporal and internal maxillary arteries (IMA). Within the pterygopalatine fossa, the IMA divides into numerous deep branches. Its distal termination is the sphenopalatine artery, which passes medially into the nasal cavity. Numerous anastomoses between the ECA branches (e.g., between the facial and maxillary arteries) as well as between the ECA and the orbital and cavernous branches of the ICA provide potential sources for collateral blood flow. **(Bottom)** The early arterial phase of CCA angiogram is shown with bony structures subtracted. The major ECA branches are opacified.

COMMON CAROTID ARTERY

Subcutaneous tissue

Sternocleidomastoid muscle

Sternohyoid muscle

Sternothyroid muscle

Omohyoid muscle

Internal jugular vein

Common carotid artery

Right lobe of thyroid gland

Cervical esophagus

Sternocleidomastoid muscle

Internal jugular vein

Common carotid artery

Thyroid gland

Sternocleidomastoid muscle

Common carotid artery

Brachiocephalic artery

Subclavian artery

(Top) Transverse grayscale ultrasound of the distal common carotid artery at the level of the upper pole of the thyroid gland. Note the wall in a normal individual is smooth with no intimal thickening or atherosclerotic plaque. The lumen is circular in cross-section. There is no major named branch in the neck apart from the termination into external and internal carotid arteries at the level of the hyoid bone. **(Middle)** Longitudinal grayscale ultrasound of the common carotid artery. Note the smooth outline of the intimal layer. **(Bottom)** Color Doppler ultrasound of the proximal common carotid artery at the root of the neck in the longitudinal plane. The normal antegrade arterial flow towards the cranial direction is well demonstrated. Its origin along with the subclavian artery from the right brachiocephalic artery is well demonstrated.

CERVICAL CAROTID ARTERIES

COMMON CAROTID ARTERY

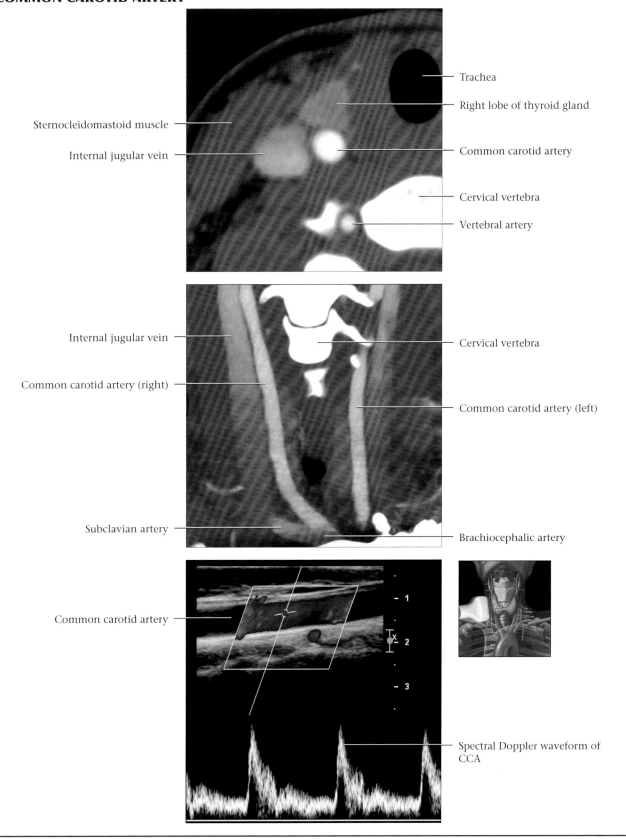

Sternocleidomastoid muscle

Internal jugular vein

Trachea

Right lobe of thyroid gland

Common carotid artery

Cervical vertebra

Vertebral artery

Internal jugular vein

Common carotid artery (right)

Subclavian artery

Cervical vertebra

Common carotid artery (left)

Brachiocephalic artery

Common carotid artery

Spectral Doppler waveform of CCA

(Top) Axial CECT of lower neck shows contrast-filled common carotid artery related anteriorly and medially to the right lobe of the thyroid gland and laterally to the internal jugular vein. **(Middle)** Coronal reformatted CECT shows the normal contour and vertical course of the common carotid artery. It originates from the brachiocephalic artery on the right at the root of the neck with the right subclavian artery. **(Bottom)** Spectral Doppler ultrasound of the common carotid artery is of low resistance arterial flow with a forward diastolic component. The scanning technique has to be meticulous to produce a reliable Doppler assessment.

CAROTID BIFURCATION

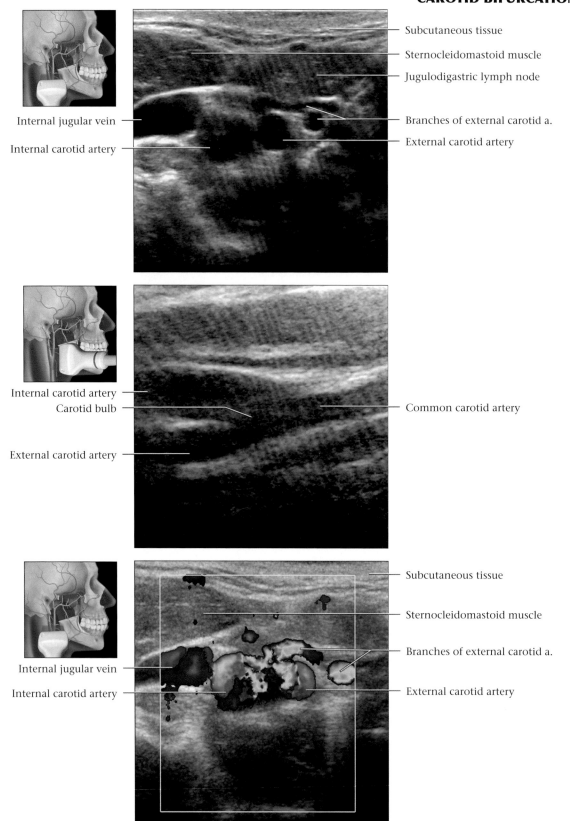

Subcutaneous tissue

Sternocleidomastoid muscle

Jugulodigastric lymph node

Internal jugular vein

Branches of external carotid a.

Internal carotid artery

External carotid artery

Internal carotid artery

Carotid bulb

Common carotid artery

External carotid artery

Subcutaneous tissue

Sternocleidomastoid muscle

Branches of external carotid a.

Internal jugular vein

Internal carotid artery

External carotid artery

(Top) Transverse grayscale ultrasound of upper cervical level at carotid bifurcation. The common carotid artery bifurcates into the internal and external carotid artery. The former is usually of larger caliber, laterally located and has no branches in the neck. (Middle) Longitudinal grayscale ultrasound in coronal orientation demonstrates the carotid bifurcation. The proximal portion of the internal carotid artery is usually mildly dilated and is termed carotid bulb. At this site the color/spectral Doppler study is more complex due to a disturbance of laminar flow and should not be misinterpreted as an abnormality. (Bottom) Color Doppler ultrasound of carotid bifurcation in transverse plane demonstrates turbulent flow in carotid bulb. Branches of external carotid artery are easier to depict than on grayscale examination.

CERVICAL CAROTID ARTERIES

CAROTID BIFURCATION

Hyoid bone — Hypopharynx

Submandibular gland — Aryepiglottic fold

Facial artery

External carotid artery

Internal jugular vein — Internal carotid artery

External jugular vein — Vertebral artery

Sternocleidomastoid muscle

Levator scapulae muscle

Facial artery — Internal carotid artery

External carotid artery — Carotid bulb

Hyoid bone

Superior thyroid artery — Internal jugular vein

Carotid bulb

Spectral Doppler waveform in carotid bulb

Flow reversal in separation zone

(Top) Axial CECT of the upper neck just beyond the carotid bifurcation. The internal carotid artery is larger and more posterolateral in position than the external carotid artery. (Middle) Maximum intensity projection of carotid bifurcation in the sagittal plane demonstrates carotid bifurcation into the external and internal carotid arteries at the level of the hyoid bone. Note the branching nature of the external carotid artery in contrast to the internal carotid artery. (Bottom) Spectral Doppler ultrasound of the carotid bulb which shows a different flow pattern than in the rest of internal carotid artery. In early systole, blood flow is accelerated in a forward direction. As the peak systole is approached, a large separation zone with flow reversal develops. Flow separation should be seen in normal individuals, its absence should raise the suspicion of plaque formation.

CERVICAL CAROTID ARTERIES

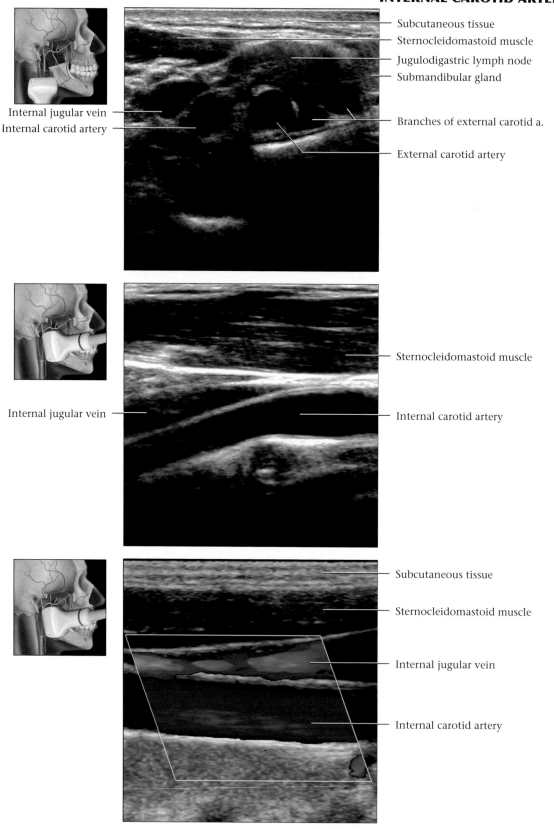

Subcutaneous tissue

Sternocleidomastoid muscle

Jugulodigastric lymph node

Submandibular gland

Internal jugular vein

Internal carotid artery

Branches of external carotid a.

External carotid artery

Sternocleidomastoid muscle

Internal jugular vein

Internal carotid artery

Subcutaneous tissue

Sternocleidomastoid muscle

Internal jugular vein

Internal carotid artery

(Top) Transverse grayscale ultrasound of the upper neck just beyond the carotid bifurcation shows its close anatomical relationship with the internal jugular vein, the external carotid artery and the jugulodigastric lymph node. (Middle) Longitudinal grayscale ultrasound of the internal carotid artery. Note its smooth wall with no intimal thickening and free of atherosclerotic plaque in a normal individual. No branch is seen in the cervical region. (Bottom) Color Doppler ultrasound of the internal carotid artery and the internal jugular vein in the longitudinal plane. Note the normal antegrade flow is towards the cranial direction of the ICA and opposite the caudal direction of flow in the adjacent IJV.

CERVICAL CAROTID ARTERIES

INTERNAL CAROTID ARTERY

Subcutaneous tissue

Platysma

Submandibular gland

Jugulodigastric lymph node

External carotid artery

External jugular vein

Internal jugular vein

Internal carotid artery

Sternocleidomastoid muscle

Levator scapulae muscle

Hypopharynx

Branches of external carotid artery

Vertebral body

Vertebral artery

Transverse process

Internal carotid artery

Facial artery

External carotid artery

Cervical vertebra

Internal jugular vein

Carotid bulb

Internal jugular vein

Internal carotid artery

PSV -75.6 cm/s
EDV -30.3 cm/s
RI   0.60

Spectral Doppler waveform of ICA

(Top) Axial CECT of upper neck shows the anatomical relation of the internal carotid artery with the internal jugular vein and branches of the external carotid artery. (Middle) Maximum intensity projection (MIP) CECT in the sagittal plane shows the normal configuration and contour of the cervical portion of the internal carotid artery. Note the lack of an arterial branch from the cervical ICA in the neck, in contrast to the external carotid artery. Note the mild dilatation of the ICA at its origin - "carotid bulb". (Bottom) Spectral Doppler ultrasound of the cervical portion of the internal carotid artery in the longitudinal plane which is of low resistance flow pattern with antegrade flow in the diastolic phase. The waveform is different from that of carotid bulb.

EXTERNAL CAROTID ARTERY

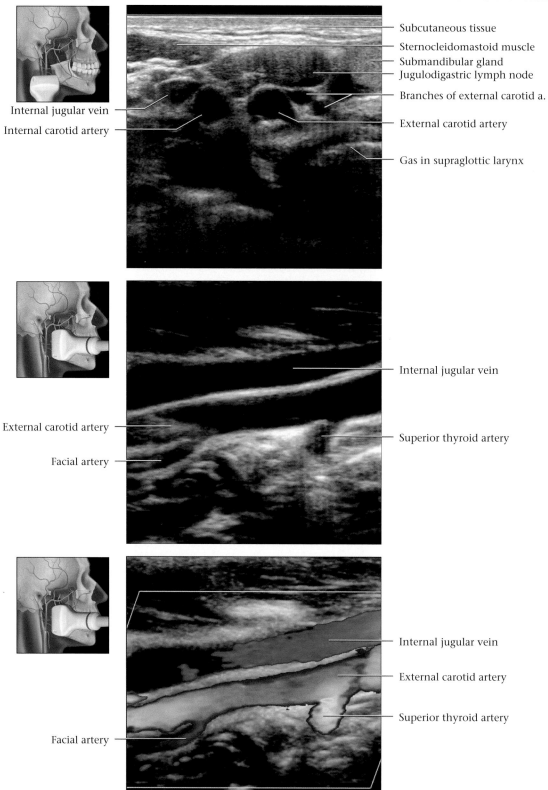

Internal jugular vein

Internal carotid artery

Subcutaneous tissue
Sternocleidomastoid muscle
Submandibular gland
Jugulodigastric lymph node
Branches of external carotid a.
External carotid artery
Gas in supraglottic larynx

Internal jugular vein

External carotid artery
Facial artery

Superior thyroid artery

Internal jugular vein
External carotid artery
Superior thyroid artery

Facial artery

(Top) Transverse grayscale ultrasound of the upper neck above the carotid bifurcation. The position of the external carotid artery medial to the internal carotid artery and internal jugular vein, posterior to the jugulodigastric lymph node, is well demonstrated. (Middle) Longitudinal grayscale ultrasound of the external carotid artery. Two anterior branches: The superior thyroid artery and the facial artery are seen arising from the proximal portion of the external carotid artery. They course inferiorly to the upper pole of the thyroid and superiorly to the facial region. (Bottom) Color Doppler ultrasound of the external carotid artery in the longitudinal plane. The antegrade flow in the cranial direction of the external carotid artery is demonstrated. Note the opposite flow direction of the adjacent internal jugular vein.

CERVICAL CAROTID ARTERIES

EXTERNAL CAROTID ARTERY

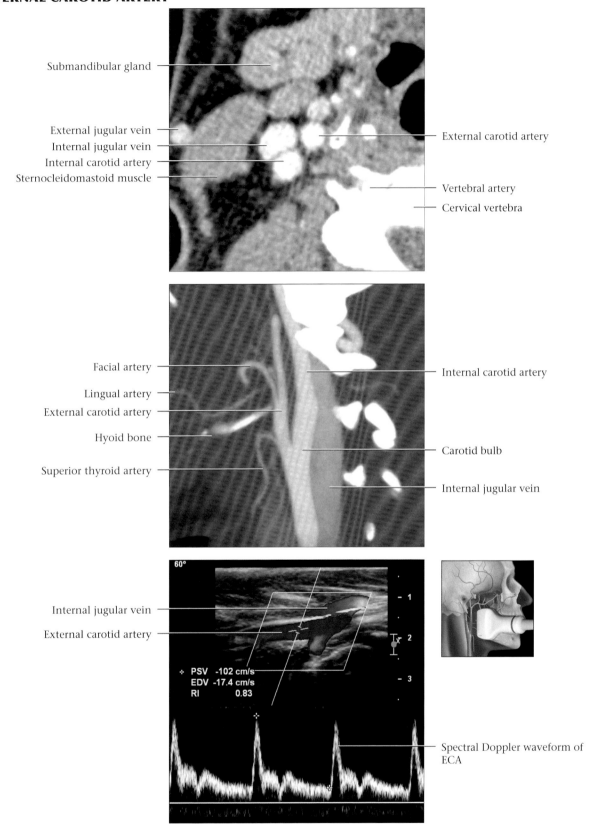

Submandibular gland

External jugular vein
Internal jugular vein
Internal carotid artery
Sternocleidomastoid muscle

External carotid artery

Vertebral artery
Cervical vertebra

Facial artery
Lingual artery
External carotid artery
Hyoid bone
Superior thyroid artery

Internal carotid artery

Carotid bulb

Internal jugular vein

Internal jugular vein
External carotid artery

60°

PSV -102 cm/s
EDV -17.4 cm/s
RI   0.83

- 1

- 2

- 3

Spectral Doppler waveform of ECA

(**Top**) Axial CECT of the upper neck at the hyoid bone level shows the relationship of the external carotid artery with the adjacent internal carotid artery and the internal jugular vein. (**Middle**) Maximum intensity projection (MIP) CECT image in the sagittal plane shows the normal contour and configuration of the external carotid artery. Note some of its major branches including the superior thyroid artery, lingual artery and facial artery in its proximal portion. (**Bottom**) Spectral Doppler ultrasound of the external carotid artery in longitudinal plane shows a high resistance flow pattern with a low diastolic component. This is different to that of the CCA and ICA which are of a low resistance pattern with a high diastolic component.

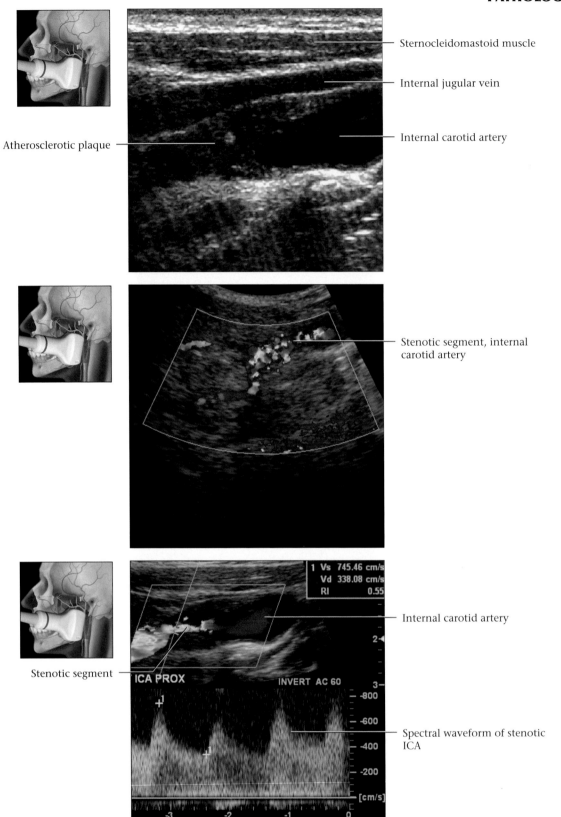

Sternocleidomastoid muscle

Internal jugular vein

Internal carotid artery

Atherosclerotic plaque

Stenotic segment, internal carotid artery

1 Vs 745.46 cm/s
Vd 338.08 cm/s
RI 0.55

Internal carotid artery

Stenotic segment

ICA PROX

INVERT AC 60

Spectral waveform of stenotic ICA

(Top) Longitudinal grayscale ultrasound of the cervical portion of the internal carotid artery shows hypoechoic atherosclerotic plaque with marked luminal narrowing. (Middle) Longitudinal color Doppler ultrasound (same patient as in top image) helps to demonstrate the turbulent arterial flow through the severe stenotic segment in the proximal internal carotid artery. Color flow imaging is a useful tool to distinguish severe stenosis from complete occlusion. (Bottom) Spectral Doppler ultrasound of the proximal internal carotid artery demonstrates markedly elevated peak systolic and peak diastolic velocity indicating severe stenosis.

PATHOLOGY

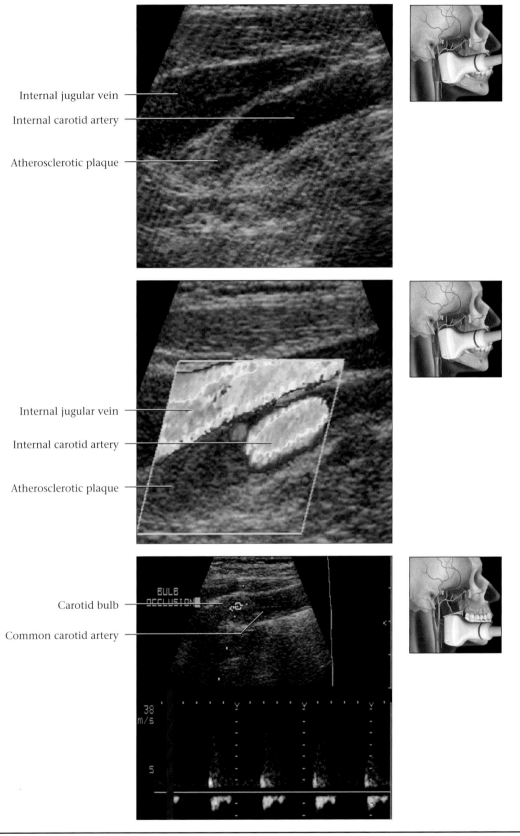

Internal jugular vein

Internal carotid artery

Atherosclerotic plaque

Internal jugular vein

Internal carotid artery

Atherosclerotic plaque

BULB
OCCLUSION

Carotid bulb

Common carotid artery

38
m/s

5

(Top) Longitudinal grayscale ultrasound of the cervical portion of the internal carotid artery. There is slightly hyperechoic atherosclerotic plaque causing complete arterial occlusion. (Middle) Color Doppler ultrasound (same patient as in top image) reveals an absence of arterial flow in the occluded segment of the internal carotid artery. (Bottom) Spectral Doppler ultrasound at the carotid bifurcation shows no detectable signal within the occluded segment and pre-occlusive "thump" proximal to the occluded segment. The carotid bulb was occluded on grayscale imaging (not shown).

VERTEBRAL ARTERIES

Terminology

Abbreviations
- Vertebrobasilar (VB); vertebral artery (VA); basilar artery (BA)
- Superior cerebellar arteries (SCAs); posterior inferior cerebellar artery (PICA); anterior inferior cerebellar artery (AICA)
- Anterior, posterior spinal arteries (ASA, PSA)

Imaging Anatomy

Overview
- VA - four segments
  - V1 segment (extraosseous segment)
    - Arises from first part of subclavian artery
    - Courses posterosuperiorly to enter C6 transverse foramen
    - Branches: Segmental cervical muscular, spinal branches
  - V2 segment (foraminal segment)
    - Ascends through C6-C3 transverse foramina
    - Turns superolaterally through the inverted "L-shaped" transverse foramen of axis (C2)
    - Courses short distance superiorly through C1 transverse foramen
    - Branches: Anterior meningeal artery, unnamed muscular/spinal branches
  - V3 segment (extraspinal segment)
    - Exits top of atlas (C1) transverse foramen
    - Lies on top of C1 ring, curving posteromedially around atlanto-occipital joint
    - As it passes around back of atlanto-occipital joint, turns sharply anterosuperiorly to pierce dura at foramen magnum
    - Branches: Posterior meningeal artery
  - V4 segment (intradural/intracranial segment)
    - After VA enters skull through foramen magnum, courses superomedially behind clivus
    - Unites with contralateral VA at/near pontomedullary junction to form BA
    - Branches: Anterior, posterior spinal arteries, perforating branches to medulla, PICA - arises from distal VA, curves around/over tonsil, gives off perforating medullary, choroid, tonsillar, cerebellar branches
- BA
  - Courses superiorly in prepontine cistern (in front of pons, behind clivus)
  - Bifurcates into its terminal branches, PCAs, in interpeduncular or suprasellar cistern at/slightly above dorsum sellae
  - Branches: Pontine, midbrain perforating branches (numerous), AICA, SCAs, PCAs (terminal branches)

Vascular Territory
- VA
  - ASA: Upper cervical spinal cord, inferior medulla
  - PSA: Dorsal spinal cord to conus medullaris
  - Penetrating branches: Olives, inferior cerebellar peduncle, part of medulla
  - PICA: Lateral medulla, choroid plexus of fourth ventricle, tonsil, inferior vermis/cerebellum
- BA
  - Pontine perforating branches: Central medulla, pons, midbrain
  - AICA: IAC, CN7 and 8, anterolateral cerebellum
  - SCA: Superior vermis, superior cerebellar peduncle, dentate nucleus, brachium pontis, superomedial surface of cerebellum, upper vermis

Normal Variants, Anomalies
- Normal variants
  - VA: R/L variation in size, dominance common; aortic arch origin 5%
- Anomalies
  - VA/BA may be fenestrated, duplicated (may have increased prevalence of aneurysms)
  - Embryonic carotid-basilar anastomoses (e.g., persistent trigeminal artery)

Anatomy-Based Imaging Issues

Imaging Recommendations
- V1 and V2 segments are amenable for USG examination
- Examination usually starts in V2 segment and proceeds downwards to V1 segment, then to its origin
- Examination of V2 segment
  - Transducer orientated longitudinally in mid cervical region between the trachea and sternocleidomastoid muscle
  - Angle transducer laterally from CCA and locate V2 segment posterior to the acoustic shadowing of transverse processes
- Examination of V1 segment
  - Trace caudally from V2 to its origin
  - Left VA more difficult to visualize than right VA
  - Beware not to confuse vertebral vein (VV) lying adjacent to VA which can appear pulsatile
    - Color flow imaging helps to differentiate
- Normal waveform of vertebral artery on spectral Doppler analysis
  - Low resistance flow
  - Similar to that of CCA but with lower amplitude
  - PSV: 59 ± 17 cm/s, EDV: 19 ± 8 cm/s
  - Flow velocity asymmetry is common and related to caliber of VA

Embryology

Embryologic Events
- Plexiform longitudinal anastomoses between cervical intersegmental arteries → VA precursors
- Paired plexiform dorsal longitudinal neural arteries (LNAs) develop, form precursors of BA
- Transient anastomoses between dorsal longitudinal neural arteries, developing ICAs appear (primitive trigeminal/hypoglossal arteries, etc.)
- Definitive VAs arise from 7th cervical intersegmental arteries, anastomose with LNAs
- LNAs fuse as temporary connections with ICAs regress → definitive BA, VB circulation formed

GRAPHICS AND VOLUME RENDERED CTA

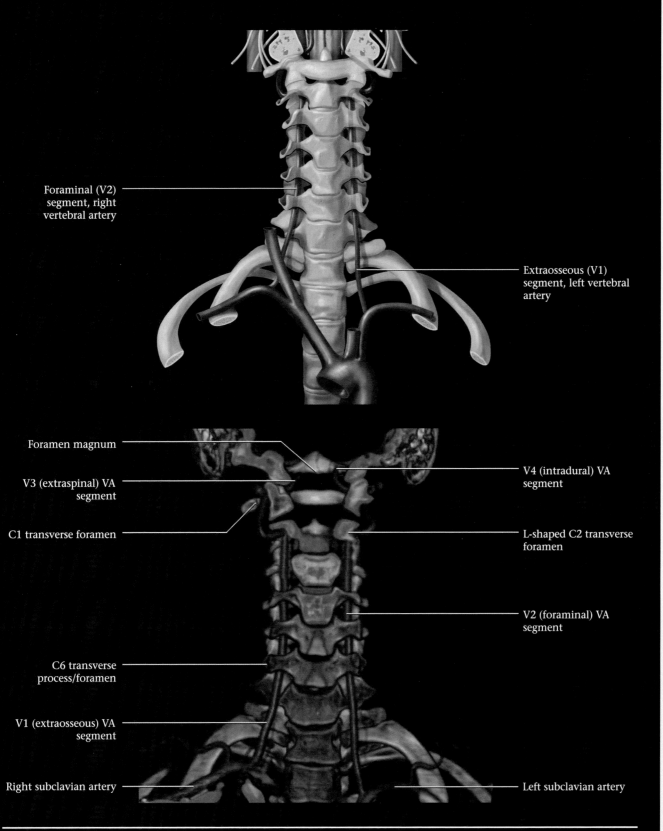

Foraminal (V2) segment, right vertebral artery

Extraosseous (V1) segment, left vertebral artery

Foramen magnum

V4 (intradural) VA segment

V3 (extraspinal) VA segment

C1 transverse foramen

L-shaped C2 transverse foramen

V2 (foraminal) VA segment

C6 transverse process/foramen

V1 (extraosseous) VA segment

Right subclavian artery

Left subclavian artery

(Top) Two of the three extracranial segments of the VAs and their relationship to the cervical spine are shown here in an AP graphic. The extraosseous (V1) VA segments extend from the superior aspect of the subclavian arteries to the C6 transverse foramina. The V2 (foraminal) segment extends afrom C6 to the VA exit from the C1 transverse foramina. (Bottom) A 3D-VRT CTA shows the extracranial VAs. They originate from the superior aspect of the subclavian arteries. The VAs typically enter the transverse foramina of C6 and ascend almost vertically to C2, where they make a 90 degree turn laterally in the L-shaped C2 transverse foramen before ascending vertically again to C1.

VERTEBRAL ARTERIES

TRANSVERSE, LONGITUDINAL AND COLOR DOPPLER

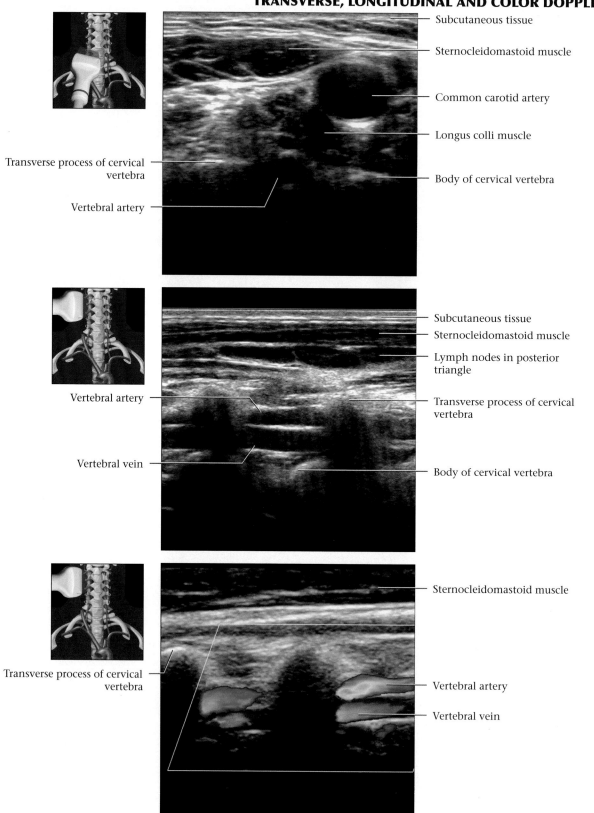

Subcutaneous tissue

Sternocleidomastoid muscle

Common carotid artery

Longus colli muscle

Body of cervical vertebra

Transverse process of cervical vertebra

Vertebral artery

Subcutaneous tissue

Sternocleidomastoid muscle

Lymph nodes in posterior triangle

Transverse process of cervical vertebra

Body of cervical vertebra

Vertebral artery

Vertebral vein

Sternocleidomastoid muscle

Transverse process of cervical vertebra

Vertebral artery

Vertebral vein

(Top) Transverse grayscale ultrasound of the lower neck shows the proximal V1 segment of the vertebral artery which arises from the first part of the subclavian artery and courses superiorly to enter the transverse foramina of the lower cervical vertebra. Note its posterior relationship to the longus colli muscle at this level. (Middle) Longitudinal grayscale ultrasound of the posterior neck demonstrates the V2 segment of the vertebral artery within the transverse foramina of cervical vertebrae. Note the presence of dense posterior acoustic shadowing from the transverse processes obscuring a clear view of the underlying vertebral vessels. (Bottom) Color Doppler ultrasound of the V2 segment of the vertebral artery in the longitudinal plane. Note the opposite flow direction of the vertebral vein (i.e., craniocaudal direction) as compared with that of the vertebral artery (caudocranial direction).

VERTEBRAL ARTERIES

AXIAL AND CORONAL CECT, SPECTRAL DOPPLER

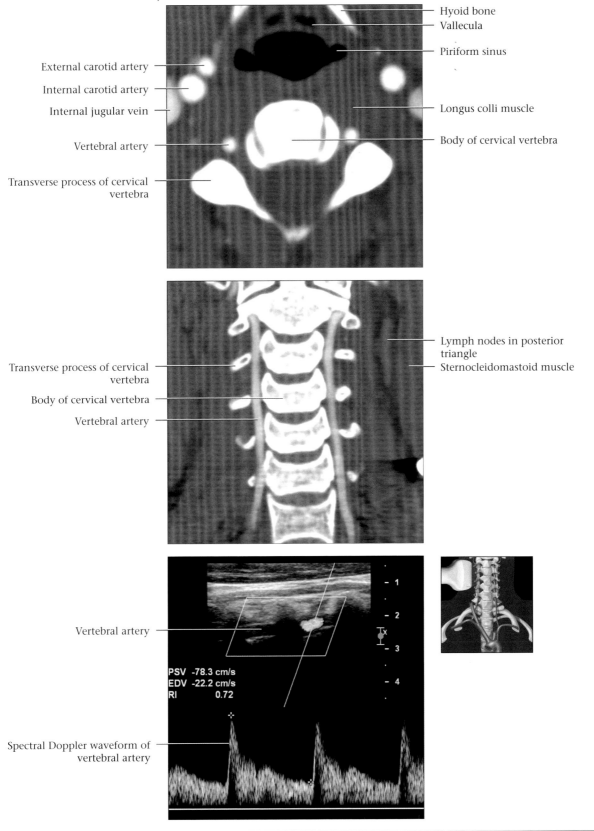

(Top) Axial CECT of the neck at the level of the hyoid bone shows the vertebral artery running in a caudocranial direction within the foramen transversarium of the cervical vertebrae. This portion is amenable for ultrasound examination. **(Middle)** Coronal reformatted CECT of the neck shows the vertical course of the vertebral arteries through the transverse foramina of C6 to C2 vertebrae. Note its close anatomical relationship with the transverse processes and bodies of the cervical vertebrae. **(Bottom)** Spectral Doppler ultrasound of the V2 segment of the vertebral artery is of low resistance, similar to that of the common carotid artery but with lower amplitude. Spectral analysis of the V2 segment provides a clue to stenosis/occlusion proximally and distally. For example, a high resistance flow pattern without a diastolic flow component is often associated with a distal flow obstruction.

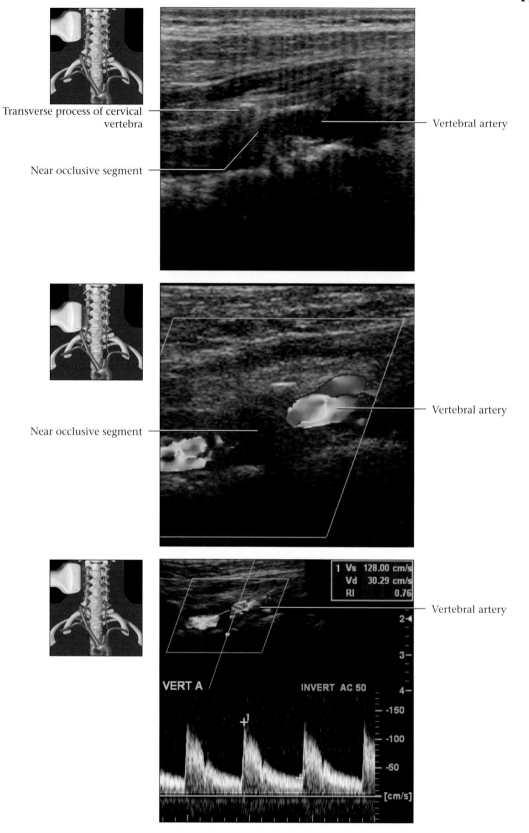

Transverse process of cervical vertebra

Near occlusive segment

Vertebral artery

Near occlusive segment

Vertebral artery

Vertebral artery

(Top) Longitudinal grayscale ultrasound of the V2 segment of the vertebral artery shows the presence of hypoechoic atherosclerotic plaque causing near complete occlusion. **(Middle)** Color Doppler ultrasound of the vertebral artery (same patient as previous image) shows a lack of arterial color flow within the nearly occluded segment. **(Bottom)** Spectral Doppler ultrasound (same patient as previous two images) shows a high resistance flow pattern with elevated peak systolic and diastolic velocities.

PATHOLOGY

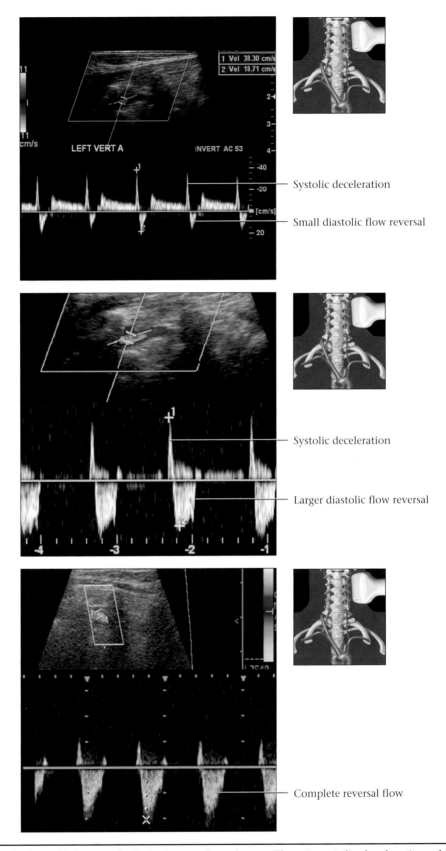

(Top) Spectral Doppler ultrasound of a mild degree of subclavian steal syndrome. There is systolic deceleration of the vertebral flow in an antegrade direction with small diastolic flow reversal. **(Middle)** Spectral Doppler ultrasound of a moderate degree of subclavian steal syndrome. The degree of systolic deceleration and diastolic flow reversal is more pronounced with alternating vertebral flow demonstrated. **(Bottom)** Spectral Doppler ultrasound of severe subclavian steal syndrome. There is near complete reversal of flow in the vertebral artery with relative absent antegrade systolic flow. This pattern is commonly associated with the occurrence of vertebrobasilar symptoms.

Neck

II

NECK VEINS

Terminology

Abbreviations
- Internal jugular vein (IJV)
- External jugular vein (EJV)
- Retromandibular vein (RMV)

Gross Anatomy

Overview
- Major extracranial venous system comprised of facial veins, neck veins, scalp, skull (diploic) and orbital veins
- Facial veins
  - Facial vein
    - Begins at angle between eye, nose
    - Descends across masseter, curves around mandible
    - Joins IJV at hyoid level
    - Tributaries from orbit (supraorbital, superior ophthalmic veins), lips, jaw, facial muscles
  - Deep facial vein
    - Receives tributaries from deep face, connects facial vein with pterygoid plexus
  - Pterygoid plexus
    - Network of vascular channels in masticator space between temporalis/lateral pterygoid muscles
    - Connects cavernous sinuses, clival venous plexus with face/orbit tributaries
    - Drains into maxillary vein
  - RMV
    - Formed from union of maxillary and superficial temporal veins
    - Lies within parotid space
    - Passes between external carotid artery (ECA) and CN7 to empty into IJV
- Neck veins
  - EJV
    - From union of retromandibular and posterior auricular veins
    - Courses inferiorly on the surface of sternocleidomastoid muscle
    - Drain into subclavian vein in supraclavicular fossa
    - Receives tributaries from scalp, ear, face
    - Size, extent highly variable
  - IJV
    - Caudal continuation of sigmoid sinus from jugular foramen at skull base
    - Jugular bulb = dilatation at origin
    - Courses inferiorly in carotid space posterolateral to internal/common carotid arteries underneath the sternocleidomastoid muscle
    - Unites with subclavian vein to form brachiocephalic vein
    - Size highly variable; significant side-to-side asymmetry common, right usually larger than left
  - Subclavian vein
    - Proximal continuation of axillary vein in thoracic inlet
    - EJV drains into subclavian vein
    - Join IJV to form brachiocephalic vein
  - Vertebral venous plexus
    - Suboccipital venous plexus
    - Tributaries from basilar (clival) plexus, cervical musculature
    - Interconnects with sigmoid sinuses, cervical epidural venous plexus
    - Terminates in brachiocephalic vein

Imaging Anatomy

Overview
- Low pressure inside; easily compressible
  - Light probe pressure with good surface contact between the transducer and skin to ensure optimal visualization
  - Use of Valsalva maneuver helps to distend the major neck veins
- IJV
  - Largest vein of the neck
  - Deep cervical chain lymph nodes commonly found along its course
  - Beware of thrombosis in patients with previous central venous catheterization or adjacent tumors
  - Always check for compressibility and phasicity on respiration
  - Presence of vascularity in IJV thrombosis is usually seen with a tumor thrombus rather than bland venous thrombus
- Subclavian vein
  - Accessible on USG by inferior tilting of the transducer in supraclavicular fossa
  - Venous valves are present in most patients
  - Thrombosis/stenosis commonly seen in patients on chronic hemodialysis or previous subclavian venous catheterization
- RMV
  - Serves as landmark on USG to infer position of intra-parotid portion of facial nerve
  - Anterior division of RMV sandwiched between submandibular gland anteriorly and parotid tail posteriorly
    - Its displacement helps to determine origin of a mass in posterior submandibular region

Anatomy-Based Imaging Issues

Imaging Pitfalls
- Neck veins are often overlooked as most sonologist pay more attention to arteries in the neck than veins
- Not all neck veins are readily assessed by ultrasound
  - Only large and superficial veins are clearly seen
- Asymmetric IJVs are common; one IJV may be many times the size of the contralateral IJV
  - IJV venous varix; extreme dilatation of IJV upon Valsalva maneuver with clinically palpable neck lump
- Slow flow within IJV may appears as low level hyperechoic intraluminal "mass"
  - May mimic IJV thrombus
  - Moving nature of the echoes on real time ultrasound and sharp linear near-field interface help to distinguish artifacts from slow flow and IJV thrombus

GRAPHIC

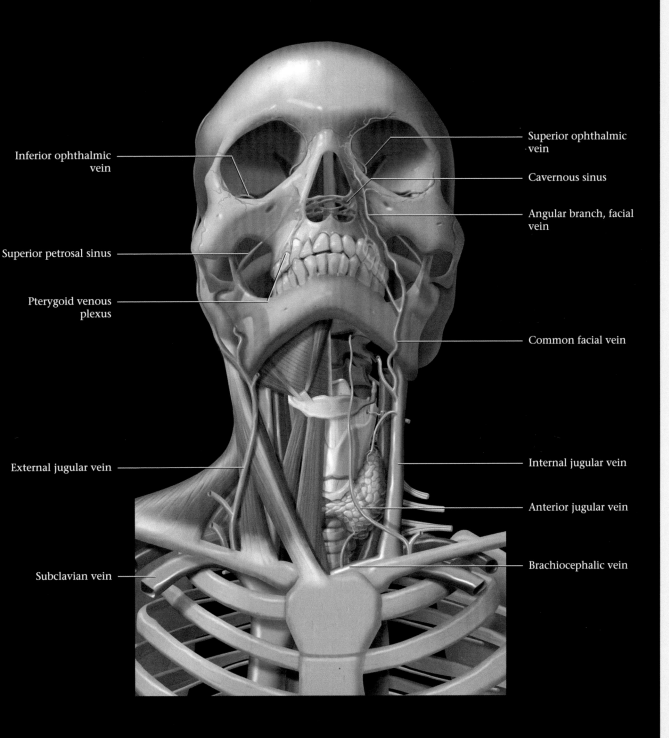

Inferior ophthalmic vein

Superior petrosal sinus

Pterygoid venous plexus

External jugular vein

Subclavian vein

Superior ophthalmic vein

Cavernous sinus

Angular branch, facial vein

Common facial vein

Internal jugular vein

Anterior jugular vein

Brachiocephalic vein

Anteroposterior view of the extracranial venous system depicts the major neck veins, their drainage into the mediastinum, and their numerous interconnections with the intracranial venous system. The pterygoid venous plexus receives tributaries from the cavernous sinus and provides an important potential source of collateral venous drainage if the transverse or sigmoid sinuses become occluded.

GRAYSCALE AND COLOR DOPPLER ULTRASOUND (IJV)

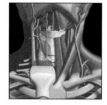

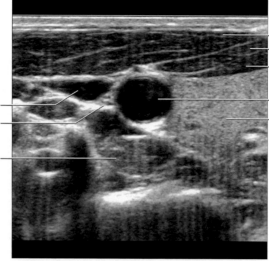

Sternocleidomastoid muscle
Sternohyoid muscle
Sternothyroid muscle

Internal jugular vein

Vagus nerve

Common carotid artery

Right lobe of thyroid gland

Scalenus anterior muscle

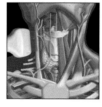

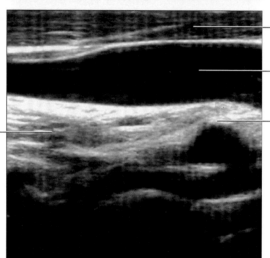

Sternocleidomastoid muscle

Internal jugular vein

Scalenus anterior muscle

Transverse process of cervical vertebra

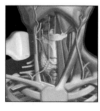

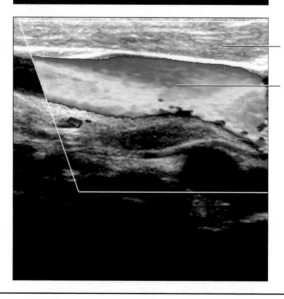

Sternocleidomastoid muscle

Internal jugular vein

(Top) Transverse grayscale ultrasound of the lower cervical level, shows the normal anatomical relationship between the internal jugular vein and the adjacent structures. It is underneath the sternocleidomastoid muscle and lateral to the common carotid artery and vagus nerve within the carotid sheath. (Middle) Longitudinal grayscale ultrasound of the internal jugular vein in the mid cervical level. The internal jugular vein appears as a tubular anechoic structure coursing in a vertical direction. It should be examined with light probe pressure and with compression to exclude a venous thrombosis. (Bottom) Color Doppler ultrasound in the longitudinal plane (corresponding to previous image) shows color flow filling the entire lumen of the internal jugular vein. The use of color Doppler helps to identify and evaluate the presence and nature of an IJV thrombus.

NECK VEINS

CECT AND SPECTRAL DOPPLER ULTRASOUND (IJV)

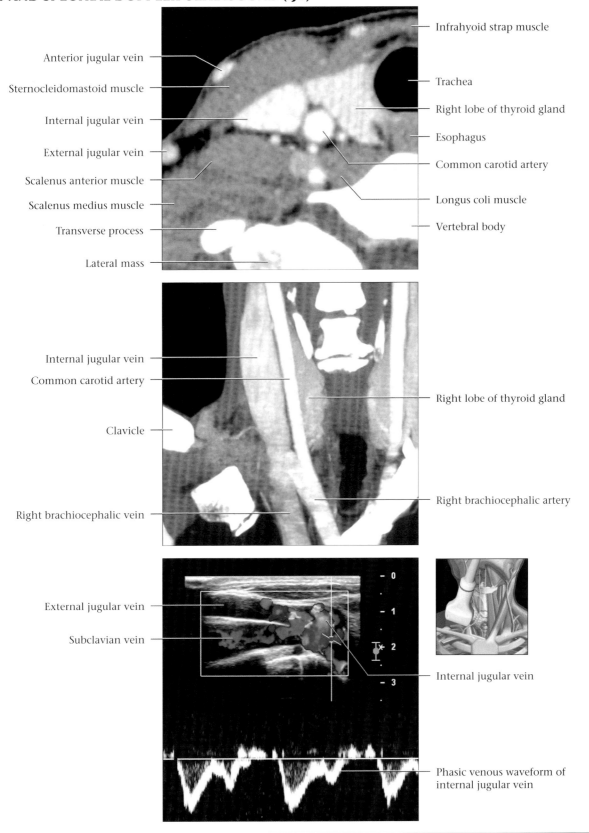

Anterior jugular vein

Sternocleidomastoid muscle

Internal jugular vein

External jugular vein

Scalenus anterior muscle

Scalenus medius muscle

Transverse process

Lateral mass

Infrahyoid strap muscle

Trachea

Right lobe of thyroid gland

Esophagus

Common carotid artery

Longus coli muscle

Vertebral body

Internal jugular vein

Common carotid artery

Clavicle

Right brachiocephalic vein

Right lobe of thyroid gland

Right brachiocephalic artery

External jugular vein

Subclavian vein

Internal jugular vein

Phasic venous waveform of internal jugular vein

(Top) Axial CECT of the lower neck shows the internal jugular vein which is usually larger than and lateral to the common carotid artery. The external jugular vein is subcutaneous layer in location. (Middle) Coronal reformatted CECT of the lower neck shows the close anatomical relationship of the internal jugular vein and common carotid artery within the carotid sheath. The internal jugular vein continues inferiorly below the clavicle to join the subclavian vein to form the brachiocephalic vein. (Bottom) Transverse spectral Doppler ultrasound of the internal jugular vein at spe level of the supraclavicular fossa at the junction with the subclavian vein. The normal biphasic venous waveform which varies with respiratory motion can be easily demonstrated and helps to exclude the presence of obstructing venous thrombus.

NECK VEINS

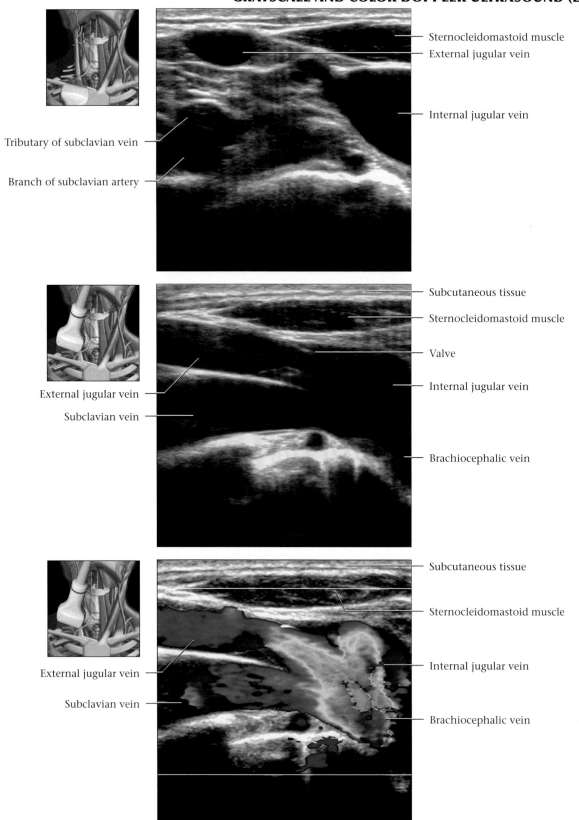

Sternocleidomastoid muscle

External jugular vein

Internal jugular vein

Tributary of subclavian vein

Branch of subclavian artery

Subcutaneous tissue

Sternocleidomastoid muscle

Valve

Internal jugular vein

External jugular vein

Subclavian vein

Brachiocephalic vein

Subcutaneous tissue

Sternocleidomastoid muscle

Internal jugular vein

External jugular vein

Subclavian vein

Brachiocephalic vein

(**Top**) Transverse grayscale ultrasound at right lower neck shows the location of the external jugular vein in relation to the sternocleidomastoid muscle. It appears as a distended, round, anechoic structure on Valsalva maneuver using light transducer pressure. (**Middle**) Transverse grayscale ultrasound of the external jugular vein at the supraclavicular level, at the site of union with the subclavian vein, close to the terminal portion of the internal jugular vein. Valve leaflets are commonly seen within the major veins at the thoracic inlet level. (**Bottom**) Transverse color Doppler ultrasound at the supraclavicular level (corresponding to previous image) helps to depict the venous drainage of the external jugular vein to the subclavian vein. Note that the subclavian vein joins the internal jugular vein to form the brachiocephalic vein.

NECK VEINS

CECT AND SPECTRAL DOPPLER ULTRASOUND (EJV)

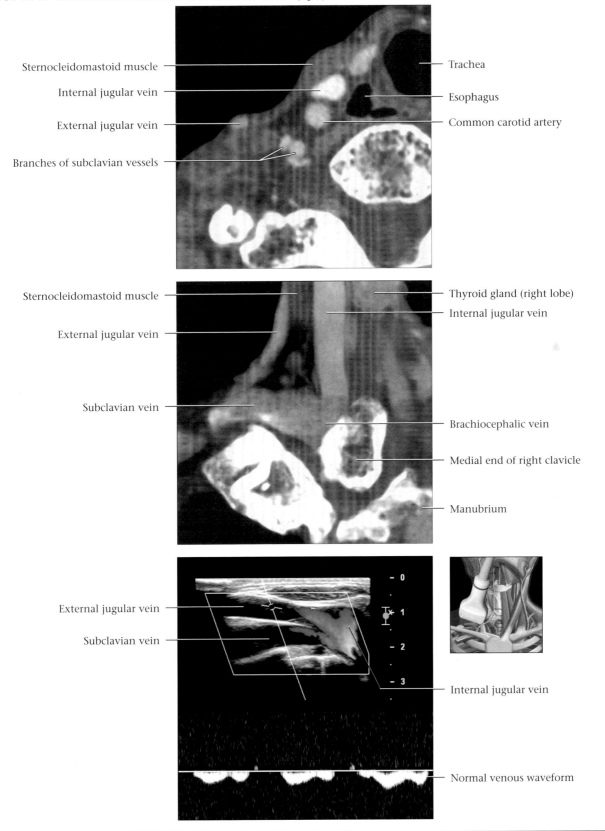

Sternocleidomastoid muscle — Trachea

Internal jugular vein — Esophagus

External jugular vein — Common carotid artery

Branches of subclavian vessels

Sternocleidomastoid muscle — Thyroid gland (right lobe)

— Internal jugular vein

External jugular vein

Subclavian vein — Brachiocephalic vein

— Medial end of right clavicle

— Manubrium

External jugular vein

Subclavian vein — Internal jugular vein

— Normal venous waveform

(Top) Axial CECT of the right lower neck. Note the superficial anatomical location of the external jugular vein. Thus light probe pressure is necessary for the assessment of the external jugular vein on ultrasound as with increasing pressure the vein will be compressed. **(Middle)** Coronal reformatted CECT image of the right lower neck. Note the drainage of the external jugular vein to the subclavian vein which join the IJV to form the brachiocephalic vein at the thoracic inlet level. **(Bottom)** Spectral Doppler ultrasound interrogating the terminal portion of the external jugular vein shows a normal, phasic, low-pressure venous waveform which helps to confirm its patency.

NECK VEINS

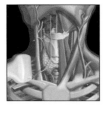
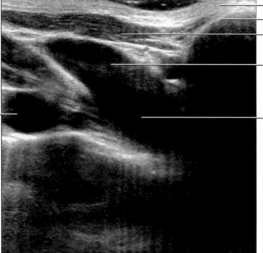

Subcutaneous tissue
Clavicle
Sternocleidomastoid muscle

Internal jugular vein

Subclavian vein

Brachiocephalic vein

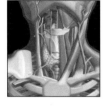
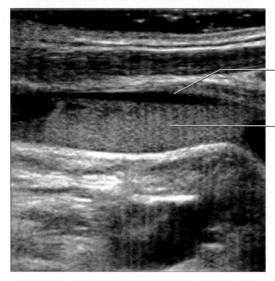

Internal jugular vein

Pseudothrombus from slow venous flow

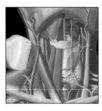
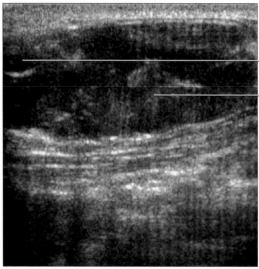

External jugular vein

Venous vascular malformation

(Top) Longitudinal grayscale ultrasound at the supraclavicular level shows the union of internal jugular vein and subclavian vein to form the brachiocephalic vein. The more distal portion of the brachiocephalic vein is obscured by the overlying clavicle, thus not assessed by ultrasound. (Middle) Longitudinal grayscale ultrasound of the right internal jugular vein shows a pseudothrombus phenomenon due to slow venous flow within the internal jugular vein. Note the layering with sharp linear border in the IJV lumen in the near field which is the clue to distinguish it from venous thrombus. (Bottom) Transverse grayscale ultrasound of the right posterior triangle shows a well-defined, hypoechoic mass with multiple internal sinusoidal spaces. The lesion is inseparable from the external jugular vein. Surgery confirmed a venous vascular malformation arising from the external jugular vein.

NECK VEINS

CECT, COLOR AND POWER DOPPLER ULTRASOUND

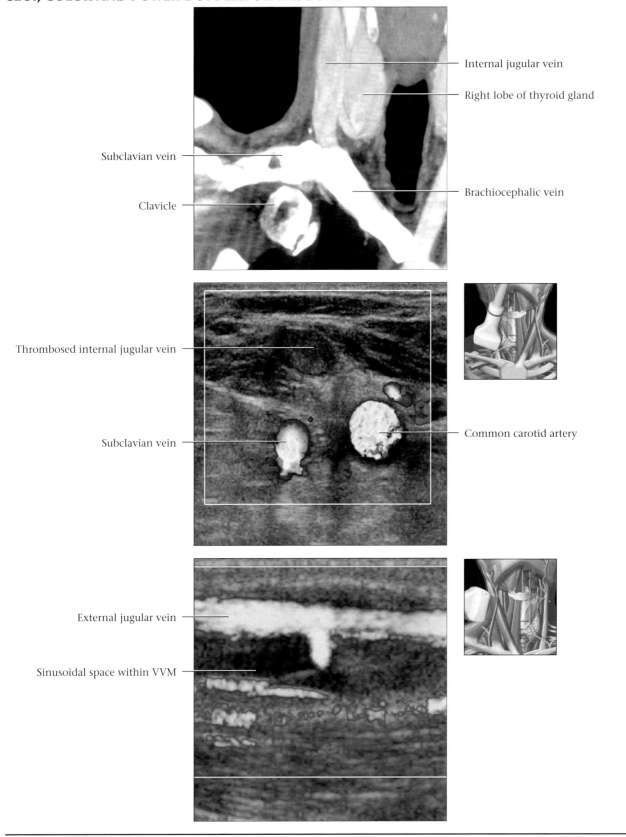

Internal jugular vein

Right lobe of thyroid gland

Subclavian vein

Clavicle

Brachiocephalic vein

Thrombosed internal jugular vein

Subclavian vein

Common carotid artery

External jugular vein

Sinusoidal space within VVM

(**Top**) Coronal reformatted CECT of the right supraclavicular fossa shows the formation of the brachiocephalic vein by union of subclavian vein (dense contrast filling due to injection in ipsilateral anti-cubital fossa) and internal jugular vein. The brachiocephalic vein can be fully assessed on CECT as compared with ultrasound. (**Middle**) Transverse color Doppler ultrasound of the right supraclavicular level reveals intraluminal, hypoechoic, avascular echoes causing occlusion of the internal jugular vein. The appearances are of a bland venous thrombus due to prolonged central venous catheterization. (**Bottom**) Longitudinal power Doppler ultrasound of the external jugular vein venous vascular malformation (VVM). Note the intimate relationship of the VVM and the external jugular vein. Sinusoidal spaces are usually not color-filled due to very slow flow within.

CERVICAL LYMPH NODES

Terminology

Abbreviations
- Internal jugular chain (IJC)

Synonyms
- Internal jugular chain: Deep cervical chain
- Spinal accessory chain (SAC): Posterior triangle chain
- Transverse cervical chain: Supraclavicular chain
- Anterior cervical chain: Prelaryngeal, pretracheal, paratracheal nodes
- Paratracheal node: Recurrent laryngeal node

Definitions
- Jugulodigastric node: "Sentinel" (highest) node, found at apex of IJC at angle of mandible
- Virchow node: "Signal" node, lowest node of deep cervical chain
- Troisier node: Most medial node of transverse cervical chain
- Omohyoid node: Deep cervical chain node superior to omohyoid as it crosses jugular vein
- Delphian node: Pretracheal node

Imaging Anatomy

Overview
- In normal adult neck there may be up to 300 lymph nodes
  - Small, oval/reniform shape
  - Internal structures: Capsule, cortex, medulla, hilum
- USG appearances of normal cervical lymph node
  - Small ovoid shape
  - Well-defined margin
  - Homogeneous hypoechoic cortex with echogenic hilus
  - Hilar vascularity on color/power Doppler examination
- Imaging-based nodal classification
  - Level I: Submental & submandibular nodes
    - Level IA: Submental nodes: Found between anterior bellies of digastric muscles
    - Level IB: Submandibular nodes: Found around submandibular glands in submandibular space
  - Level II: Upper IJC nodes - from posterior belly of digastric muscle to hyoid bone
    - Level IIA: Level II node anterior, medial, lateral or posterior to internal jugular vein (IJV); if posterior to IJV, node must be inseparable from IJV
    - Level IIA contains jugulodigastric nodal group
    - Level IIB: Level II node posterior to IJV with fat plane visible between node & IJV
  - Level III: Mid IJC nodes
    - From hyoid bone to inferior margin of cricoid cartilage
  - Level IV: Lower IJC nodes
    - From inferior cricoid margin to clavicle
  - Level V: Nodes of posterior cervical space/spinal accessory chain
    - SAC nodes lie posterior to back margin of sternocleidomastoid muscle
    - Level VA: Upper SAC nodes from skull base to bottom of cricoid cartilage
    - Level VB: Lower SAC nodes from cricoid to clavicle
  - Level VI: Nodes of visceral space
    - Found from hyoid bone above to top of manubrium below
    - Midline group of cervical lymph nodes
    - Includes prelaryngeal, pretracheal and paratracheal subgroups
  - Level VII: Superior mediastinal nodes
    - Between carotid arteries from top of manubrium above to innominate vein below
- Other nodal groups not included in standard imaging-based nodal classification
  - Parotid nodal group: Intraglandular or extraglandular
  - Retropharyngeal (RPS) nodal group: Medial RPS nodes and lateral RPS nodes (Rouviere node)
  - Facial nodal group

Anatomy-Based Imaging Issues

Key Concepts or Questions
- Useful USG features suspicious of malignancy
  - Shape: Round, long/short axis ratio < 2
  - Loss of echogenic hilus
  - Presence of intranodal necrosis (cystic/coagulation)
  - Presence of extracapsular spread - ill-defined margin
  - Peripheral/subcapsular flow on color/power Doppler ultrasound
  - Increased intranodal intravascular resistance: Resistive index (RI) > 0.8, pulsatility index (PI) > 1.6
  - Internal architecture: Punctate calcifications in metastatic node from papillary thyroid carcinoma, reticulated/pseudocystic appearances of lymphomatous node
- No single finding is sensitive or specific enough, these signs should be used in combination
- FNAC helps to improve diagnostic accuracy

Clinical Implications

Clinical Importance
- Presence of malignant SCCa nodes in staging associated with 50% ↓ in long term survival
  - If extranodal spread present, further 50% ↓
- Location of metastatic nodes in the neck help predict the site of primary tumor
  - When Virchow node found on imaging without upper neck nodes, primary is not in neck
  - Posterior triangle LN raises the suspicion of nasopharyngeal carcinoma in Southern Chinese populations

GRAPHICS

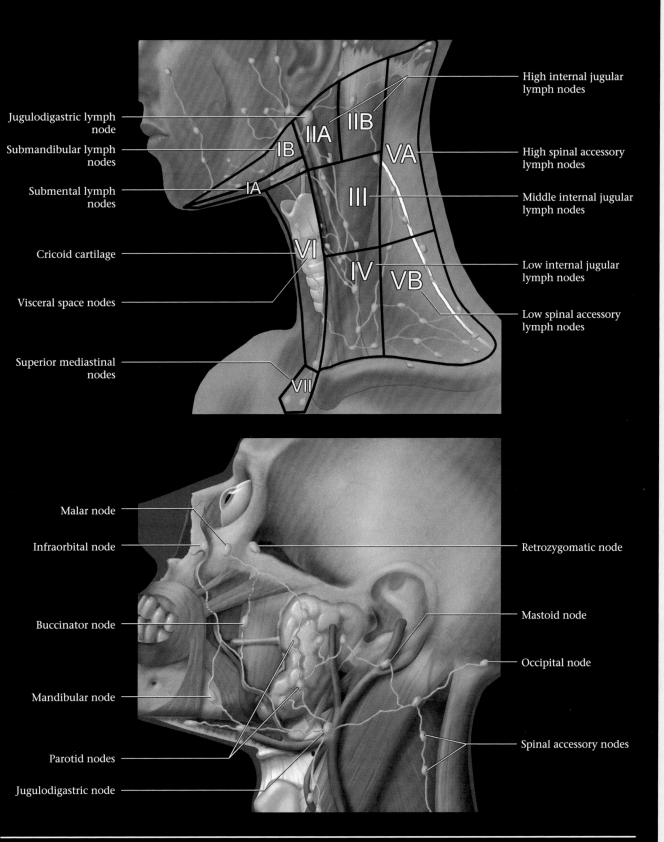

(Top) Lateral oblique graphic of the neck shows the anatomic locations for the major nodal groups of the neck. Division of the internal jugular nodal chain into high, middle and low regions is defined by the level of the hyoid bone and cricoid cartilage. Similarly, cer spinal accessory lyndal chain is divided into high & low regions by the level of the cricoid cartilage. **(Bottom)** Lateral view of facial nodes plus parotid nodes. None of these nodes bear level numbers but instead must be described by their anatomic location. Note that the IJC is the final common pathway for all lymphatics of upper aerodigestive tract and neck.

CERVICAL LYMPH NODES

TRANSVERSE AND LONGITUDINAL ULTRASOUND AND PATHOLOGY

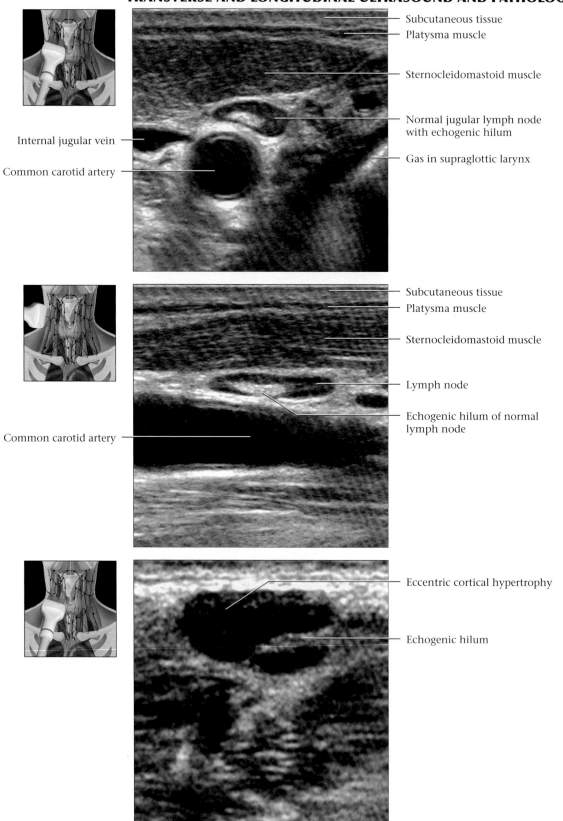

Subcutaneous tissue

Platysma muscle

Sternocleidomastoid muscle

Normal jugular lymph node with echogenic hilum

Gas in supraglottic larynx

Internal jugular vein

Common carotid artery

Subcutaneous tissue

Platysma muscle

Sternocleidomastoid muscle

Lymph node

Echogenic hilum of normal lymph node

Common carotid artery

Eccentric cortical hypertrophy

Echogenic hilum

(Top) Transverse grayscale ultrasound of the mid cervical level shows the normal appearance of a cervical lymph node, i.e., ovoid shape with echogenic hilum. It is commonly found anterior to the carotid artery/internal jugular vein. (Middle) Longitudinal grayscale ultrasound of the mid cervical level shows a normal elliptical hypoechoic lymph node with echogenic hilum anterior to the common carotid artery. (Bottom) Transverse grayscale ultrasound of a reactive lymph node. It is mildly enlarged with cortical hypertrophy and preserved echogenic hilum. Note, with high resolution ultrasound the jugulodigastric node and other nodes in the jugular chain and accessory chain are invariably seen.

CERVICAL LYMPH NODES

POWER DOPPLER ULTRASOUND AND PATHOLOGY

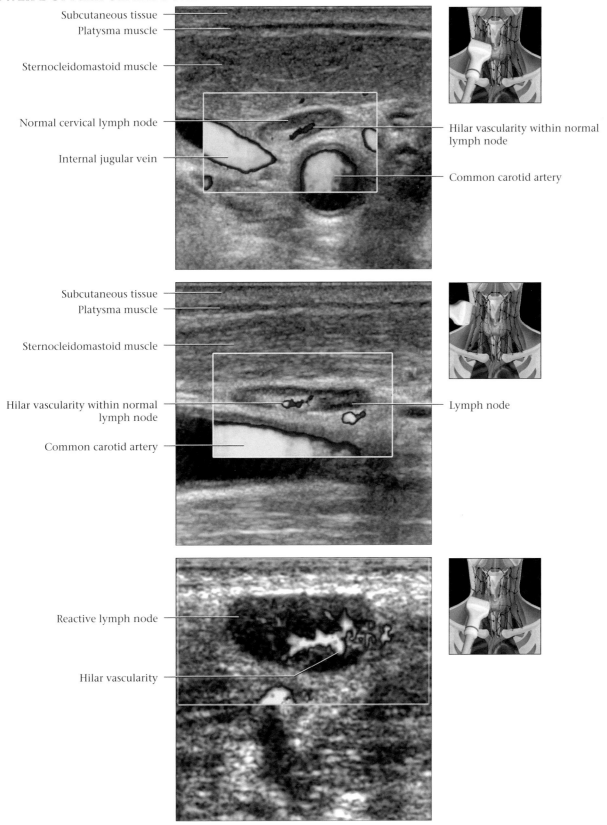

Subcutaneous tissue
Platysma muscle
Sternocleidomastoid muscle
Normal cervical lymph node
Internal jugular vein
Hilar vascularity within normal lymph node
Common carotid artery

Subcutaneous tissue
Platysma muscle
Sternocleidomastoid muscle
Hilar vascularity within normal lymph node
Common carotid artery
Lymph node

Reactive lymph node
Hilar vascularity

(Top) Transverse power Doppler ultrasound shows the presence of hilar vascularity within the echogenic hilum of a normal cervical lymph node. (Middle) Longitudinal power Doppler ultrasound shows hilar vascularity within the echogenic hilum of a normal cervical lymph node. The presence of echogenic hilum and hilar vascularity are good sign of benignity of cervical lymph node. (Bottom) Transverse power Doppler ultrasound shows mild increase but preserved hilar vascularity in a reactive lymph node. Newer high resolution transducers readily demonstrate nodal vascularity, both normal and abnormal.

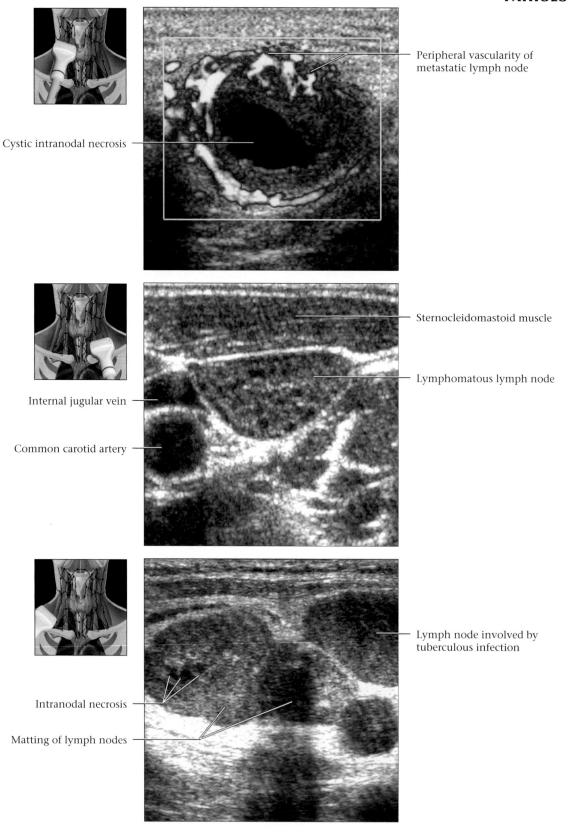

Peripheral vascularity of metastatic lymph node

Cystic intranodal necrosis

Sternocleidomastoid muscle

Lymphomatous lymph node

Internal jugular vein

Common carotid artery

Lymph node involved by tuberculous infection

Intranodal necrosis

Matting of lymph nodes

(Top) Transverse power Doppler ultrasound of a metastatic lymph node from head and neck squamous cell carcinoma. It is round with cystic intranodal necrosis and peripheral vascularity. (Middle) Transverse grayscale ultrasound of a lymphomatous lymph node in mid deep jugular chain which demonstrates the typical reticulated echo pattern. (Bottom) Transverse grayscale ultrasound in right posterior triangle shows multiple, enlarged, round, hypoechoic lymph nodes. Some of them contain intranodal necrosis and are matted. A mild degree of soft tissue edema is also noted. Features are highly suspicious of tuberculous lymphadenitis which was subsequently confirmed.

CERVICAL LYMPH NODES

PATHOLOGY

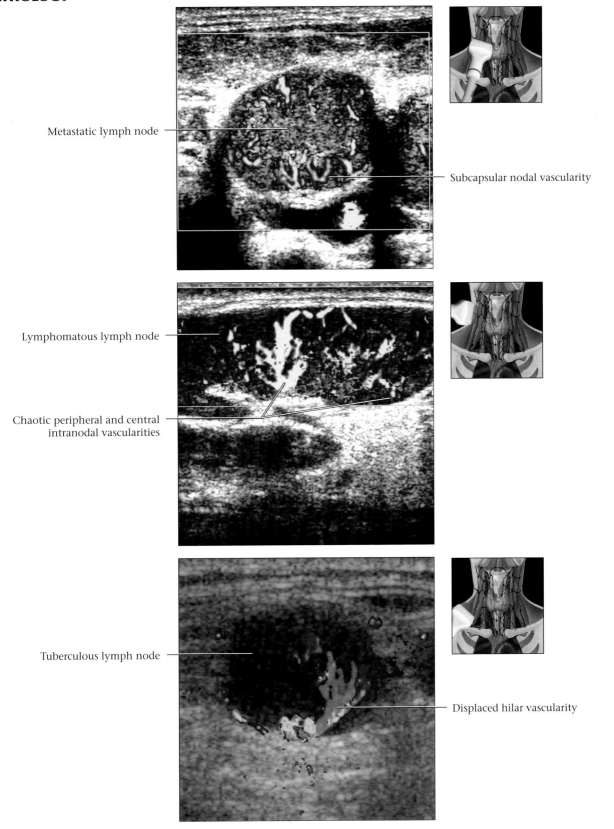

Metastatic lymph node

Subcapsular nodal vascularity

Lymphomatous lymph node

Chaotic peripheral and central intranodal vascularities

Tuberculous lymph node

Displaced hilar vascularity

(Top) Transverse power Doppler ultrasound shows the presence of multiple subcapsular intranodal vessels in a round, hypoechoic, solid lymph node in the upper cervical level. Pathology - metastatic squamous cell carcinoma. **(Middle)** Longitudinal power Doppler ultrasound of a lymphomatous lymph node showing marked increase and chaotic peripheral and central intranodal vessels. **(Bottom)** Transverse color Doppler ultrasound of a tuberculous lymph node in the posterior triangle which is predominantly hypovascular with displaced hilar vascularity. The hypovascular portion corresponds to the portion of tuberculous node with caseating necrosis. The confirmation of shape and abnormal vascularity help to suggest metastatic nodes, in a patient with known head and neck primary.

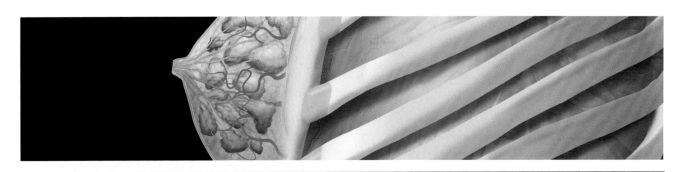

SECTION III: Thorax

PLEURA

General Anatomy

Pleural Structure
- Continuous surface epithelium and underlying connective tissue
- Visceral pleura adheres to pulmonary surfaces
- Parietal pleura is a continuation of visceral pleura; lines corresponding half of thoracic wall, covers ipsilateral diaphragm and ipsilateral mediastinal surface
- Visceral and parietal pleurae form right and left pleural cavities, which are potential spaces containing a small amount of serous pleural fluid
- Combined thickness of visceral and parietal pleurae and fluid-containing pleural space is < 0.5 mm

Pleural Space
- Potential space; normally contains 2-10 mL of fluid
- Fluid production capacity, 100 mL/hr; fluid absorption capacity, 300 mL/hr
- Fluid flux normally from parietal pleura capillaries to pleural space; absorbed by microscopic stomata in parietal pleura

Costodiaphragmatic Recesses
- Pleura extends caudally beyond inferior lung border
- Costal and diaphragmatic pleura separated by narrow slit, the costodiaphragmatic recess
- Extends approximately 5 cm below inferior border of the lung during quiet inspiration; caudal extent at 12th rib posteromedially

Visceral Pleura
- Covers lung parenchyma surfaces
- Blood Supply and Drainage
  ○ Supply by systemic bronchial vessels, drainage by pulmonary and bronchial veins
  ○ Lymphatic drainage to deep pulmonary plexus within interlobar and peribronchial spaces toward hilum
- Histology
  ○ Mesothelial layer, thin connective tissue layer, chief layer of connective tissue, vascular layer, limiting lung membrane (connected to chief layer by collagen and elastic fibers)
  ○ Single layer of flat mesothelial cells separated by basal lamina from underlying lamina propria of loose connective tissue

Parietal Pleura
- Covers non-parenchymal surfaces; forms lining of thoracic cavities
- Blood supply and drainage
  ○ Supply from adjacent chest wall (intercostal, internal mammary, diaphragmatic arteries)
  ○ Drainage to bronchial veins (diaphragmatic pleural drainage to inferior vena cava and brachiocephalic trunk)
- Histology
  ○ Single layer of parietal mesothelial cells over loose, fat-containing areolar connective tissue; bounded externally by endothoracic fascia

Imaging

Ultrasound
- Provides detailed imaging of the costal surfaces of the pleura
- Ribs cause posterior acoustic shadowing
  ○ Scanning in both inspiration and expiration helps examine pleura which may have been obscured by ribs
- Clinical uses
  ○ Differentiation of solid pleural masses from fluid
  ○ Assessment of echogenicity and morphology (may change shape with respiration) of fluid collections
  ○ Guide pleural drainage or biopsy

Imaging Anatomic Correlations

Pleural Effusion
- Categorized as transudates or exudates; based on composition of fluid obtained by thoracentesis
  ○ Transudates not associated with pleural disease; systemic abnormalities (cardiac failure, pericardial disease, cirrhosis, pregnancy, hypoalbuminemia, overhydration, renal failure)
  ○ Exudates indicate presence of pleural disease (pneumonia, empyema, tuberculosis, neoplasm, pulmonary embolism, collagen vascular disease)
- Ultrasound
  ○ Anechoic effusions suggest transudative or exudative
  ○ Septations suggestive exudative effusion

Pleural Thickening
- Focal thickening
  ○ Pleural plaques occur 15-20 years after asbestos exposure; focal collections of acellular collagen on parietal pleura (costal, diaphragmatic and mediastinal pleura)
    ■ Imaging may show discontinuous areas of pleural thickening, predominantly: Along 6th-8th ribs, on parietal pleura at domes of diaphragms, along mediastinal pleura
    ■ They may be non-calcified or calcified
    ■ There is usually sparing apices and costophrenic sulci
  ○ Localized fibrous tumor, solitary lenticular, round, or lobulated neoplasm; benign (80%) or malignant
  ○ Bronchogenic carcinoma may focally invade pleura or produce diffuse pleural thickening
- Diffuse thickening may be benign (fibrothorax) or malignant (metastases, mesothelioma, lymphoma, invasive thymoma)

PLEURA

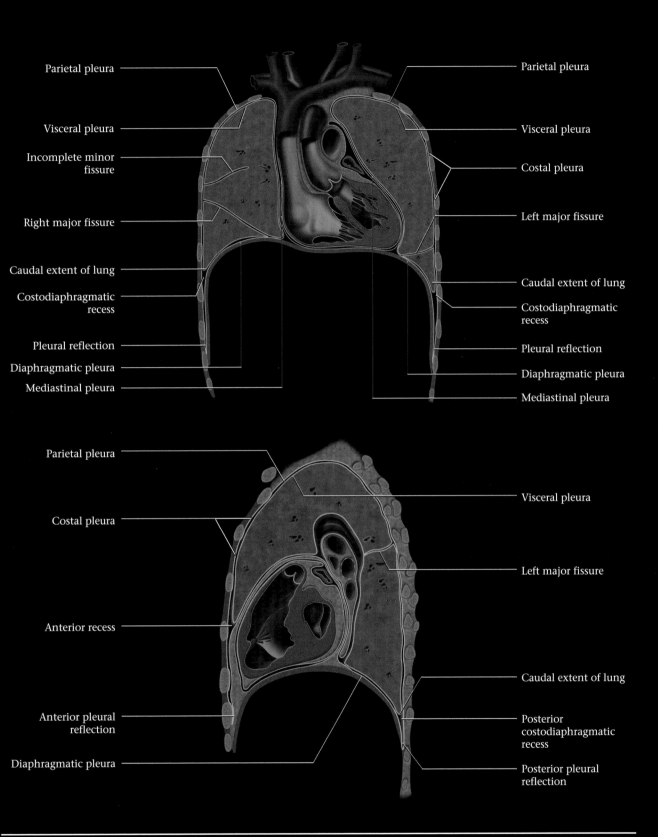

Parietal pleura

Visceral pleura

Incomplete minor fissure

Right major fissure

Caudal extent of lung

Costodiaphragmatic recess

Pleural reflection

Diaphragmatic pleura

Mediastinal pleura

Parietal pleura

Visceral pleura

Costal pleura

Left major fissure

Caudal extent of lung

Costodiaphragmatic recess

Pleural reflection

Diaphragmatic pleura

Mediastinal pleura

Parietal pleura

Costal pleura

Anterior recess

Anterior pleural reflection

Diaphragmatic pleura

Visceral pleura

Left major fissure

Caudal extent of lung

Posterior costodiaphragmatic recess

Posterior pleural reflection

(Top) Graphic shows the extensive distribution of the pleura as visualized in the coronal plane. Visceral pleura covers the surfaces of both lungs and forms interlobar fissures that may be complete or incomplete in their extension to the hila. Parietal pleura lines both thoracic cavities and may be designated by its location as costal, diaphragmatic or mediastinal pleurae. Inferiorly, the parietal pleura extends deep into the costodiaphragmatic recesses where costal and diaphragmatic pleura are in apposition. **(Bottom)** Graphic shows the extent of parietal and visceral pleura as visualized in the sagittal plane in the left mid-clavicular zone. The posterior pleural reflection in the costodiaphragmatic recess extends caudally to the level of the 12th rib.

Thorax III

3

PLEURA

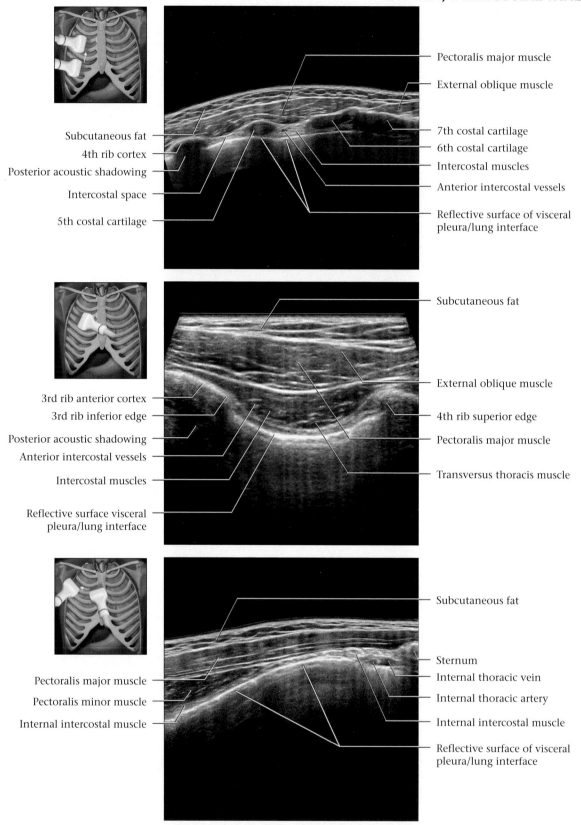

Pectoralis major muscle

External oblique muscle

7th costal cartilage

6th costal cartilage

Intercostal muscles

Anterior intercostal vessels

Reflective surface of visceral pleura/lung interface

Subcutaneous fat

4th rib cortex

Posterior acoustic shadowing

Intercostal space

5th costal cartilage

Subcutaneous fat

3rd rib anterior cortex

3rd rib inferior edge

Posterior acoustic shadowing

Anterior intercostal vessels

Intercostal muscles

Reflective surface visceral pleura/lung interface

External oblique muscle

4th rib superior edge

Pectoralis major muscle

Transversus thoracis muscle

Subcutaneous fat

Pectoralis major muscle

Pectoralis minor muscle

Internal intercostal muscle

Sternum

Internal thoracic vein

Internal thoracic artery

Internal intercostal muscle

Reflective surface of visceral pleura/lung interface

(Top) Panoramic sagittal scan of the lower anterior chest wall and pleura. The cortex of the ribs produce significant posterior acoustic shadowing which obscures the underlying pleura, this is less of an issue with costal cartilage (which is relatively sonolucent). By scanning during respiration (and thus pleural movement), all of the pleura can be evaluated with ultrasound. **(Middle)** Sagittal scan of the anterior pleura. The intercostal muscles run in between the edges of the ribs. The innermost intercostal muscle is separated from the external and internal intercostal muscles by the intercostal vessels and nerve. **(Bottom)** Oblique transverse scan of the anterior pleura just lateral to the sternum using an intercostal window. Uninterrupted strips of pleura can be demonstrated by placing the transducer obliquely along the intercostal space.

PLEURA

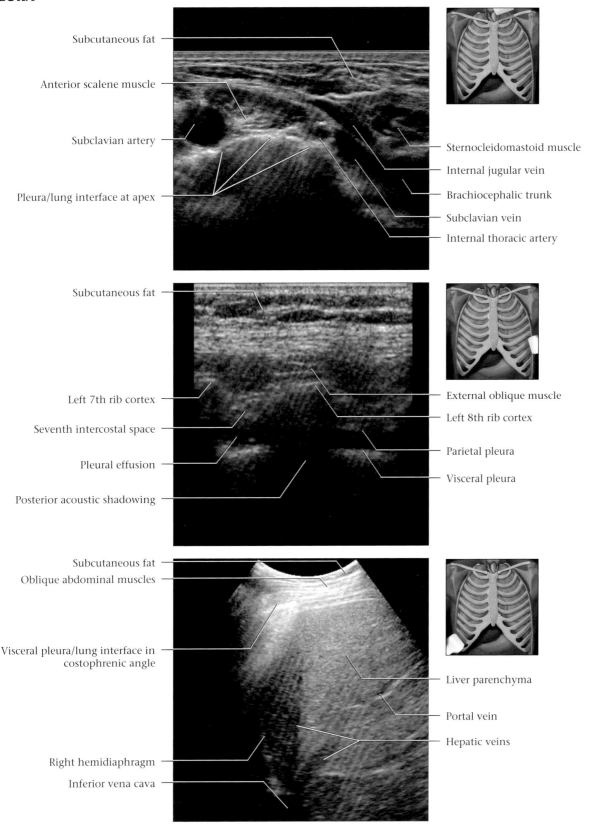

Subcutaneous fat

Anterior scalene muscle

Subclavian artery

Pleura/lung interface at apex

Sternocleidomastoid muscle

Internal jugular vein

Brachiocephalic trunk

Subclavian vein

Internal thoracic artery

Subcutaneous fat

Left 7th rib cortex

Seventh intercostal space

Pleural effusion

Posterior acoustic shadowing

External oblique muscle

Left 8th rib cortex

Parietal pleura

Visceral pleura

Subcutaneous fat

Oblique abdominal muscles

Visceral pleura/lung interface in costophrenic angle

Right hemidiaphragm

Inferior vena cava

Liver parenchyma

Portal vein

Hepatic veins

(Top) Oblique transverse scan of the apical pleura. The apical pleura is adjacent to important cervical structures. Pathology in the lung apex, such as a Pancoast tumor, can therefore extend readily into the neck. **(Middle)** Coronal scan of the lower pleura in a patient with pleural effusion. The pleural effusion allows both pleural layers (parietal and visceral) to be visualized. The high resolution of ultrasound allows even small volumes of pleural fluid to be identified and safely aspirated under ultrasound guidance. **(Bottom)** Oblique coronal scan of the costophrenic angle. A slip of lung, and its pleura, is in the costophrenic angle. One must take this into account when performing a percutaneous biopsy of the liver to avoid puncturing the lung or pleural space.

Thorax

III

DIAPHRAGM

Imaging Anatomy

Overview
- Sheet of central aponeurotic tendon contributed by peripheral muscle fibers
- Separates the thoracic cavity from abdominal cavity

Anatomy Relationships
- Superiorly: Heart, lower lobes of lungs and pleura
- Peripherally: Rib cage
- Inferiorly: Liver, gastric cardia, spleen, colon

Muscular Component
- Costal part
  - Muscle fibers from internal surface of ribs 6-12
  - Forms the left and right hemidiaphragms
- Lumbar part
  - Originates as the diaphragmatic crura and from three arcuate ligaments (see below)
- Sternal part
  - Slips of muscle from the xiphoid process running posteriorly to insert on central tendon
  - Sternocostal hiatus on each side of these central slips of muscle
    - Internal thoracic vessels run through the hiatus to enter the abdomen

Central Tendon
- Aponeurosis with interlacing fibers
- Peripheral muscular component inserts centrally onto this aponeurosis
- Trefoiled appearance due to three parts
  - Central leaf for the heart to rest on
    - Right side of central leaf contains the foramen for the inferior vena cava
  - Left and right leaves represent the domes of the hemidiaphragms

Diaphragmatic Crura
- Left crus
  - Narrower and shorter than right crus
  - Attached to left side of aorta, left anterolateral surfaces of L1 and L2 vertebral bodies and discs
- Right crus
  - Broader and longer than left crus
  - Attached to right side of aorta, right anterolateral surfaces of L1 to L3 vertebral bodies and discs
  - Surrounds the esophageal hiatus

Arcuate Ligaments
- Medial arcuate ligament
  - Fibrous thickening of the thoracolumbar fascia over the proximal aspect of psoas major muscle
  - Runs in an arch from one of the diaphragmatic crura, over ipsilateral psoas major and inserts on L1 transverse process
- Lateral arcuate ligament
  - Fibrous thickening of thoracolumbar fascia over quadratus lumborum muscle
  - Runs in an arch from L1 transverse process to ipsilateral 12th rib
- Median arcuate ligament
  - Joins the medial aspects of both crura
  - Runs over anterior surface of aorta
  - Contributes fibers to right diaphragmatic crus

Diaphragmatic Hiatus
- Vena caval foramen
  - Located in right posterior margin of central leaf of central tendon
  - At T8/9 intervertebral disc level
  - IVC wall adheres to this foramen: Therefore diaphragmatic movement on inspiration dilates IVC lumen and helps increase flow of blood to right atrium
- Esophageal hiatus
  - Located in posterocentral (left of midline) aspect of muscular component of diaphragm
  - At T10 vertebral level
  - Encircled by right crus fibers, which constricts esophagus on inspiration and thus prevents reflux
  - Contains left gastric artery branches, anterior and posterior vagal trunks and esophagus
- Aortic hiatus
  - Located behind median arcuate ligament (thus outside diaphragm) and thus not constricted by respiration
  - At T12 vertebral level
  - Contains azygos vein, thoracic duct and aorta

Phrenic Nerve (C3 to C5 Ventral Rami)
- Right phrenic nerve
  - Runs posterolateral to right brachiocephalic vein and superior vena cava
  - Then between mediastinal pleura and right parietal pericardium, runs anterior to right lung hilum
  - Finally runs on right side of inferior vena cava to enter right hemi-diaphragm lateral to vena caval foramen
- Left phrenic nerve
  - Runs between left common carotid artery and left subclavian artery
  - Passes on left side of aortic arch
  - Runs on left parietal pericardium (over left auricle and left ventricle)
  - Enters left hemidiaphragm lateral to left pericardial margin

Anatomy-Based Imaging Issues

Imaging Recommendations
- Sonographic imaging of the diaphragm is best done using the abdominal contents (liver, spleen) as a window
  - Gas in the lung precludes using a thoracic approach to examine the diaphragm (except when there is a sizable pleural effusion displacing the intervening lung)
- Ultrasound allows real-time evaluation of diaphragmatic movement, which is essential for investigating neurological or muscular diaphragmatic abnormalities

GRAPHIC, DIAPHRAGM

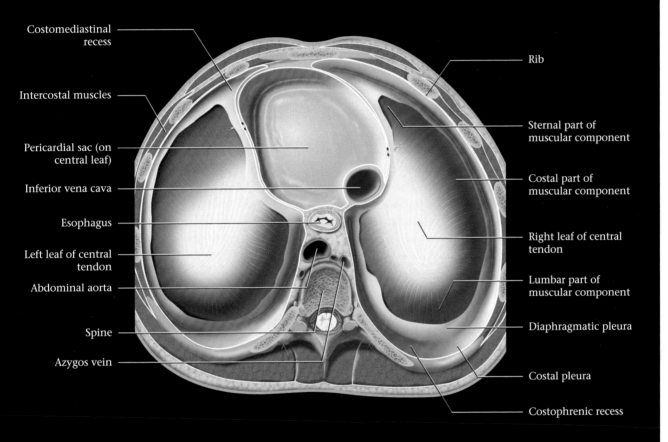

Costomediastinal recess

Intercostal muscles

Pericardial sac (on central leaf)

Inferior vena cava

Esophagus

Left leaf of central tendon

Abdominal aorta

Spine

Azygos vein

Rib

Sternal part of muscular component

Costal part of muscular component

Right leaf of central tendon

Lumbar part of muscular component

Diaphragmatic pleura

Costal pleura

Costophrenic recess

Graphic of the diaphragm looking from above. The diaphragm is composed of a central tendon and a peripheral muscular component. The central tendon is made up of three leaves: Central leaf (on which rests the pericardium); left and right leaves form the dome of each hemidiaphragm. The muscular component is composed of three parts: Costal, lumbar and sternal. The muscular component contracts to lower the diaphragm in inspiration. There are several hiatuses present for conducting structures between the thorax and abdomen. The vena caval foramen is in the right posterior margin of the central leaf. The esophageal hiatus is in the posterocentral aspect of the muscular component. The aortic hiatus is behind the median arcuate ligament and contains the aorta, azygos vein and thoracic duct.

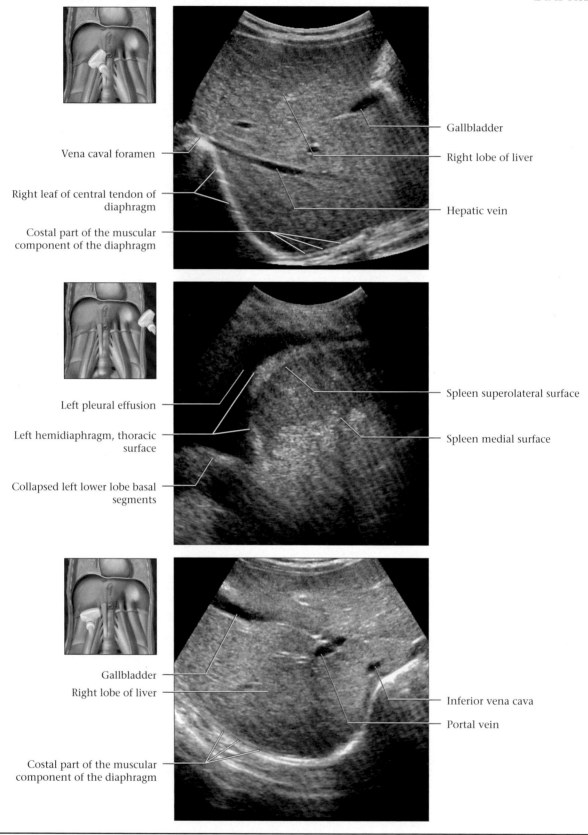

Gallbladder

Vena caval foramen

Right lobe of liver

Right leaf of central tendon of diaphragm

Hepatic vein

Costal part of the muscular component of the diaphragm

Left pleural effusion

Spleen superolateral surface

Left hemidiaphragm, thoracic surface

Spleen medial surface

Collapsed left lower lobe basal segments

Gallbladder

Right lobe of liver

Inferior vena cava

Portal vein

Costal part of the muscular component of the diaphragm

(Top) Oblique sagittal scan of the upper abdomen using subcostal window. The dome of the diaphragm is well-demonstrated with ultrasound due to its strong reflection (a result of the gas-containing lung on the other side of the diaphragm). The vena caval foramen is at the right posterior edge of the middle leaf of the central tendon of diaphragm. **(Middle)** Oblique coronal scan using left lower intercostal window in a patient with left pleural effusion. The thoracic surface of the diaphragm is outlined by the pleural effusion. Without the effusion, this diaphragmatic surface is difficult to visualize. **(Bottom)** Oblique transverse scan of the upper abdomen. The costal part of the muscular portion of the diaphragm arises from the internal surface of the inferior six ribs. The contraction of this muscular component causes depression of the diaphragm on inspiration.

DIAPHRAGM

DIAPHRAGMATIC MOVEMENT

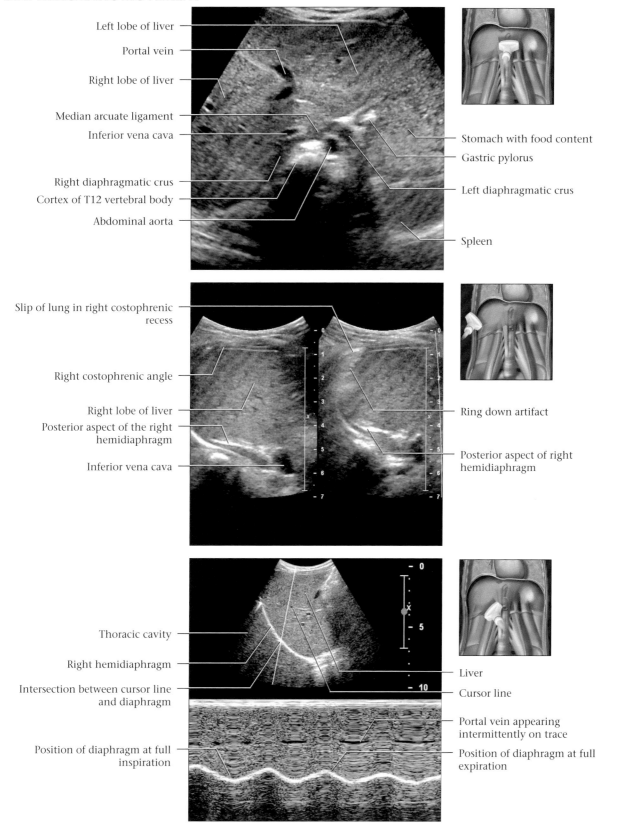

Left lobe of liver

Portal vein

Right lobe of liver

Median arcuate ligament

Inferior vena cava

Right diaphragmatic crus

Cortex of T12 vertebral body

Abdominal aorta

Stomach with food content

Gastric pylorus

Left diaphragmatic crus

Spleen

Slip of lung in right costophrenic recess

Right costophrenic angle

Right lobe of liver

Posterior aspect of the right hemidiaphragm

Inferior vena cava

Ring down artifact

Posterior aspect of right hemidiaphragm

Thoracic cavity

Right hemidiaphragm

Intersection between cursor line and diaphragm

Position of diaphragm at full inspiration

Liver

Cursor line

Portal vein appearing intermittently on trace

Position of diaphragm at full expiration

(Top) Transverse scan at the T12 vertebral body level. The aorta emerges under the median arcuate ligament to enter the abdomen. Thus the aorta is outside the diaphragm & therefore not constricted by it during inspiration. The diaphragmatic crura lie on both sides of the aorta, taking orgin from the cortical surface of the lumbar vertebrae. The crura are hypoechoic and should not be mistaken for lymph nodes. **(Middle)** Oblique transverse scans of the right hemidiaphragm using the same intercostal window during full expiration (left image) & full inspiration (right image). With inspiration, a slip of lung may enter the costophrenic recess & cause posterior acoustic shadowing (gas ring-down). **(Bottom)** Trace obtained in M-mode. The cursor line was placed to cut through the liver and right hemidiaphragm. The respiratory motion of diaphragm (bright line) can thus be traced.

THORACIC OUTLET

Terminology

Synonyms
- Anatomical literature refers to thoracic outlet as inferior thoracic aperture opening into abdominal cavity
  - However, in clinical medicine thoracic outlet usually implies area at and around junction of neck and thorax

Definitions
- Transition area between cervical/brachial spaces and thoracic cavity, extending from cervical spine, mediastinum to lower border of pectoralis minor muscle

Imaging Anatomy

Overview
- Thoracic outlet is clinically divided into three compartments (from medial to lateral): Interscalene triangle, costoclavicular space, retropectoralis minor space

Interscalene Triangle
- Boundaries
  - Anterior scalene (anteriorly)
  - Middle & posterior scalene (posteriorly)
  - First rib (inferiorly)
- Contents
  - Subclavian artery (inferiorly)
  - Three trunks of brachial plexus (upper and middle trunks in superior part of triangle, inferior trunk behind subclavian artery)
- Subclavian vein is anterior to anterior scalene muscle and is thus not within interscalene triangle

Costoclavicular Space
- Boundaries
  - Clavicle (superiorly)
  - Subclavius muscle (anterior)
  - First rib & middle scalene muscle (posterior)
- Contents
  - Subclavian artery and vein
  - 1st part of axillary vein
    - Axillary artery begins at lateral border of first rib as a direct continuation of subclavian artery
    - Axillary artery ends laterally at inferior border of teres major muscle
    - Posterior to axillary vein
  - First part of axillary vein
    - Anterior to axillary artery
  - Two divisions and three cords of brachial plexus form within this space
    - Posterior cord of brachial plexus is formed by posterior division of upper, middle and lower trunks
    - Lateral cord is formed by anterior division of upper and middle trunks
    - Medial cord is formed by anterior division of lower trunk

Retropectoralis Minor Space
- Boundaries
  - Posterior border of pectoralis minor muscle (anteriorly)
  - Subscapularis muscle (posterosuperiorly)
  - Anterior chest wall (posteroinferiorly)
- Contents
  - Second part of axillary vein and artery
  - Three cords of brachial plexus: Posterior, lateral and medial
    - Names of the three cords of brachial plexus indicate their relationship with second part of axillary artery
    - Lateral to pectoralis major muscle, cords divide into five terminal branches

Superior Thoracic Aperture
- Boundaries
  - Manubrium (anteriorly)
  - Medial borders of first ribs and costal cartilages (anterolaterally)
  - First thoracic vertebra (posteriorly)
- Contents
  - Trachea, esophagus, great vessels, nerves, strap muscles of neck

Clinical Significance
- Thoracic outlet syndrome is a compression syndrome of neurovascular structure(s) when arm is abducted
- Neurological compression is common in both costoclavicular space and interscalene triangle
- Arterial compression is most common in costoclavicular space followed by interscalene triangle
- Compression is rare in retropectoralis space

Anatomy-Based Imaging Issues

Imaging Recommendations
- Ultrasound allows simultaneous, real-time grayscale (anatomical) and color Doppler (functional) evaluation of vessels to assess compression and flow restriction
- Ultrasound can be performed with dynamic maneuvers, which exacerbates thoracic outlet syndrome clinically, allowing simultaneous imaging assessment
- Ultrasound allows patients to be scanned in upright position, which frequently exacerbates compression (CT and MR requires patients to be scanned supine)

Imaging Pitfalls
- Ultrasound cannot evaluate the lungs
- Eighth cervical and first thoracic nerve roots are not adequately visualized, especially in patients with short necks

GRAPHICS, THORACIC OUTLET

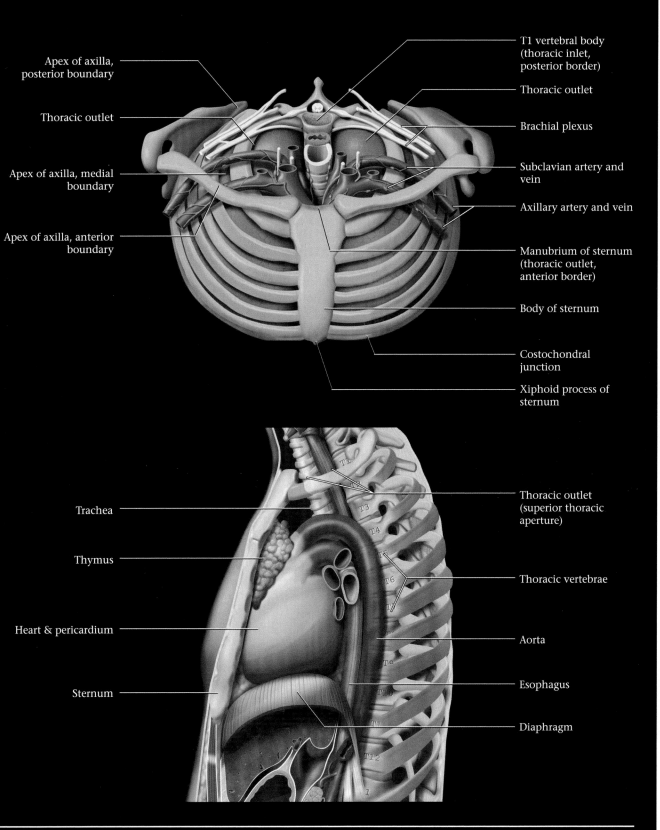

Apex of axilla, posterior boundary

Thoracic outlet

Apex of axilla, medial boundary

Apex of axilla, anterior boundary

T1 vertebral body (thoracic inlet, posterior border)

Thoracic outlet

Brachial plexus

Subclavian artery and vein

Axillary artery and vein

Manubrium of sternum (thoracic outlet, anterior border)

Body of sternum

Costochondral junction

Xiphoid process of sternum

Trachea

Thymus

Heart & pericardium

Sternum

Thoracic outlet (superior thoracic aperture)

Thoracic vertebrae

Aorta

Esophagus

Diaphragm

(Top) Graphic depicts the superior thoracic aperture, supraclavicular structures & axillary regions. The superior thoracic aperture (part of thoracic outlet) is bound by the T1 vertebral body, right & left first ribs & their costal cartilages, & the manubrium of sternum. The apex of the axillary region is bound by the clavicle, scapula, and outer border of the first rib. Vascular structures allow blood flow to enter and exit through the superior thoracic aperture. **(Bottom)** Graphic depicts a sagittal view of the mediastinum and lower neck. The superior thoracic aperture is the junction between the two regions and is part of the thoracic outlet. The aerodigestive tract and the great vessels of the thorax exit via the superior thoracic aperture to enter the neck and upper limbs.

SUPERIOR THORACIC APERTURE

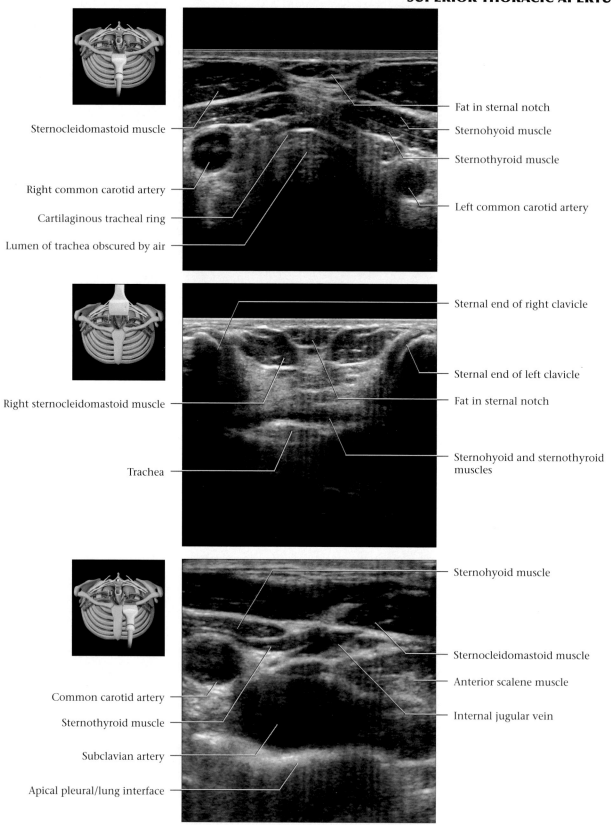

Sternocleidomastoid muscle

Right common carotid artery

Cartilaginous tracheal ring

Lumen of trachea obscured by air

Fat in sternal notch

Sternohyoid muscle

Sternothyroid muscle

Left common carotid artery

Sternal end of right clavicle

Sternal end of left clavicle

Fat in sternal notch

Right sternocleidomastoid muscle

Sternohyoid and sternothyroid muscles

Trachea

Sternohyoid muscle

Sternocleidomastoid muscle

Anterior scalene muscle

Internal jugular vein

Common carotid artery

Sternothyroid muscle

Subclavian artery

Apical pleural/lung interface

(Top) Transverse scan of superior thoracic aperture at the sternal notch. Trachea is located in the center of the image, where its cartilaginous ring is well-visualized but lumen obscured (by gas). Strap muscles of the neck, which are anterior to the trachea, are well-delineated. (Middle) Transverse scan at sternal notch level with caudal tilting of transducer to better demonstrate the thoracic outlet. The strap muscles appear thinner using this scanning plane. A retrosternal extension of goiter can be demonstrated in this view of the superior thoracic aperture. (Bottom) Transverse scan of left supraclavicular fossa. The lung apex is located deep to the vessels and immediately behind the subclavian vein. This view is good for searching for supraclavicular lymphadenopathy.

THORACIC OUTLET

SUPERIOR THORACIC APERTURE

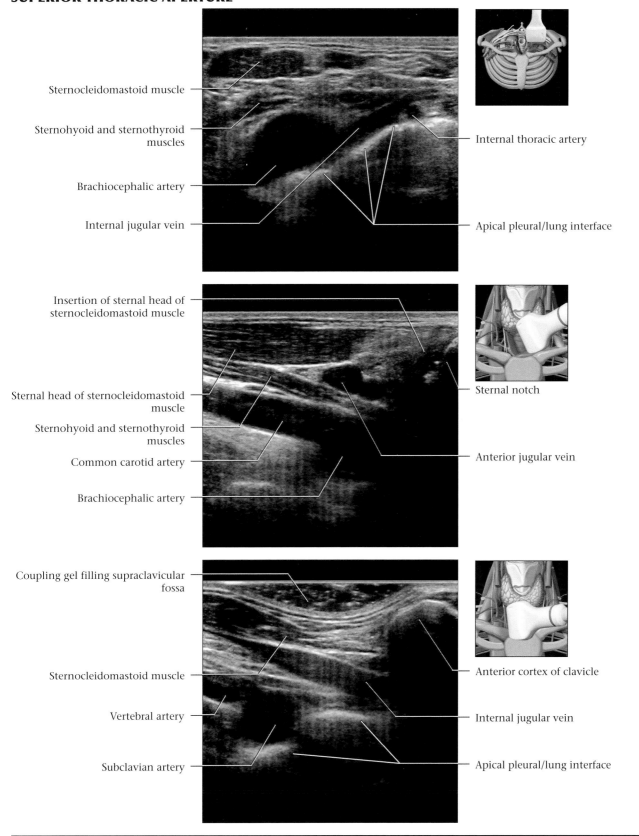

Sternocleidomastoid muscle

Sternohyoid and sternothyroid muscles

Brachiocephalic artery

Internal jugular vein

Internal thoracic artery

Apical pleural/lung interface

Insertion of sternal head of sternocleidomastoid muscle

Sternal head of sternocleidomastoid muscle

Sternohyoid and sternothyroid muscles

Common carotid artery

Brachiocephalic artery

Sternal notch

Anterior jugular vein

Coupling gel filling supraclavicular fossa

Sternocleidomastoid muscle

Vertebral artery

Subclavian artery

Anterior cortex of clavicle

Internal jugular vein

Apical pleural/lung interface

(Top) Transverse scan of left supraclavicular fossa with caudal tilting of the transducer. The apical pleural/lung interface is visualized immediately behind brachiocephalic artery, internal jugular vein and internal thoracic artery. (Middle) Longitudinal scan of superior thoracic aperture at the sternal notch. Insertion of sternocleidomastoid at the sternal notch appears echogenic and tapered compared to the muscle belly. The anterior jugular vein crosses anterior to strap muscles and common carotid artery. (Bottom) Longitudinal scan of supraclavicular fossa along the internal jugular vein. The supraclavicular fossa is filled with coupling gel to provide good transducer contact. The apical pleural/lung interface is visualized immediately behind internal jugular vein and subclavian artery.

Thorax

III

13

THORACIC OUTLET

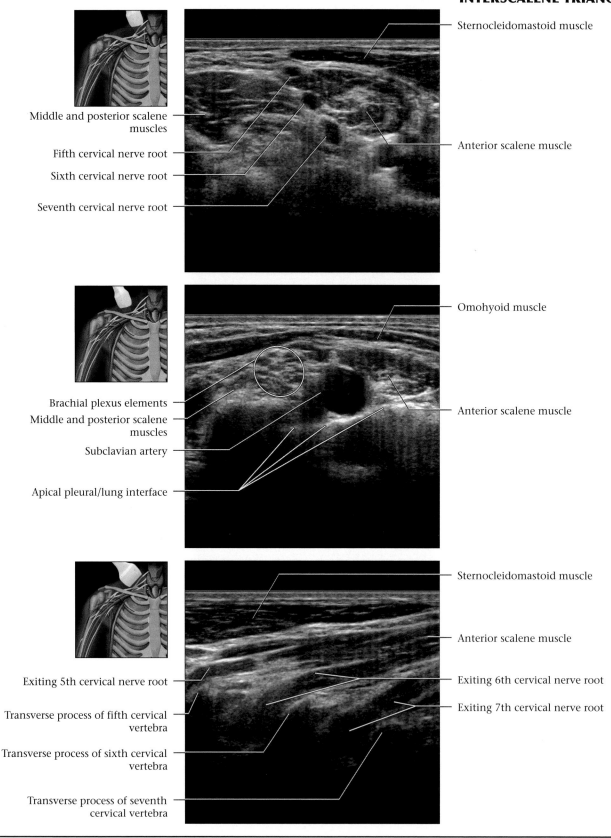

(Top) Sternocleidomastoid muscle

Middle and posterior scalene muscles

Fifth cervical nerve root

Sixth cervical nerve root

Seventh cervical nerve root

Anterior scalene muscle

Omohyoid muscle

Brachial plexus elements

Middle and posterior scalene muscles

Subclavian artery

Apical pleural/lung interface

Anterior scalene muscle

Sternocleidomastoid muscle

Anterior scalene muscle

Exiting 5th cervical nerve root

Transverse process of fifth cervical vertebra

Transverse process of sixth cervical vertebra

Transverse process of seventh cervical vertebra

Exiting 6th cervical nerve root

Exiting 7th cervical nerve root

(Top) Oblique coronal scan of upper interscalene triangle. The fifth, sixth and seventh cervical nerve roots are well-demonstrated in cross-section, lying between anterior and middle scalene muscles. The eighth cervical and first thoracic nerve roots are usually more difficult to visualize on ultrasound because of their deeper location behind subclavian artery. **(Middle)** Oblique coronal scan of lower interscalene triangle. The brachial plexus elements appear as a cluster of well-delineated, round, hypoechoic structures that result from the divisions of the nerve trunks. The subclavian artery is seen posterior and medial to the brachial plexus. **(Bottom)** Oblique coronal scan of interscalene triangle. The extraforaminal parts of fifth, sixth and seventh cervical nerve roots are well-visualized as they exit from the intervertebral foramina in the downward and outward direction.

COSTOCLAVICULAR SPACE

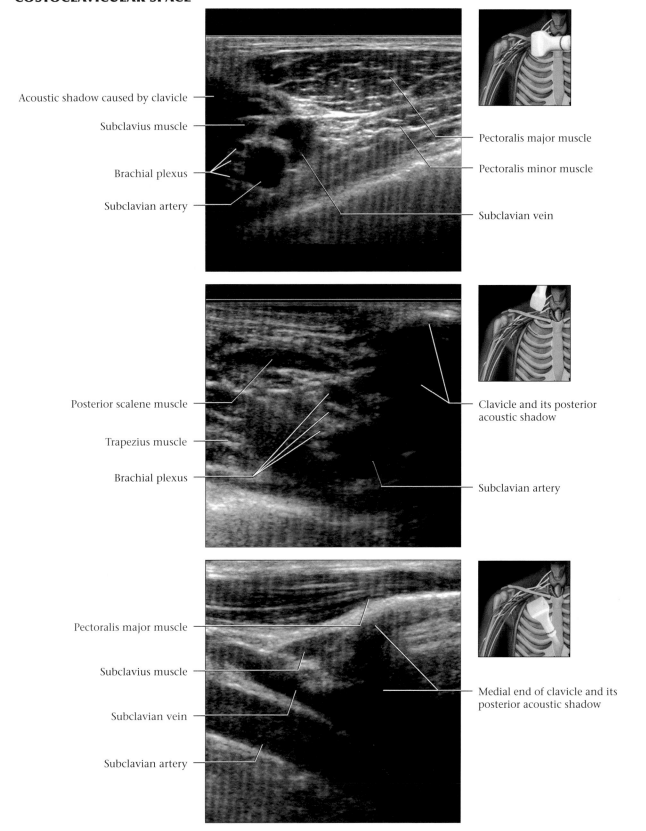

Acoustic shadow caused by clavicle

Subclavius muscle

Brachial plexus

Subclavian artery

Pectoralis major muscle

Pectoralis minor muscle

Subclavian vein

Posterior scalene muscle

Trapezius muscle

Brachial plexus

Clavicle and its posterior acoustic shadow

Subclavian artery

Pectoralis major muscle

Subclavius muscle

Subclavian vein

Subclavian artery

Medial end of clavicle and its posterior acoustic shadow

(Top) Sagittal scan of costoclavicular space using an infra-clavicular approach. This space is limited superiorly by the clavicle and anteriorly by the subclavius muscle, and contains the subclavian vein anteriorly, the subclavian artery immediately posterior to it, and three cords of brachial plexus. (Middle) Sagittal scan of costoclavicular space from supraclavicular approach. The brachial plexus and subclavian artery are demonstrated while the subclavian vein is obscured by the shadowing posterior to the clavicle. (Bottom) Transverse scan of the costoclavicular space. Long axis of subclavian artery and vein are visualized in this view, but the brachial plexus is difficult to visualize because of its proximity to the clavicle.

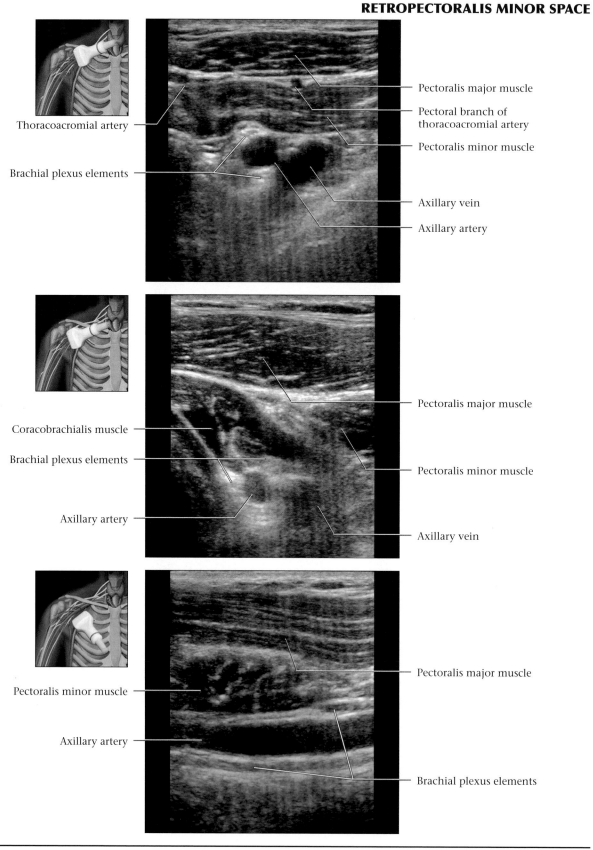

Thoracoacromial artery

Brachial plexus elements

Pectoralis major muscle

Pectoral branch of thoracoacromial artery

Pectoralis minor muscle

Axillary vein

Axillary artery

Coracobrachialis muscle

Brachial plexus elements

Axillary artery

Pectoralis major muscle

Pectoralis minor muscle

Axillary vein

Pectoralis minor muscle

Axillary artery

Pectoralis major muscle

Brachial plexus elements

(Top) Sagittal scan of retropectoralis minor space. This space is bound anteriorly by the pectoralis minor muscle and posteriorly by the anterior chest wall. The axillary artery and vein are well-depicted, and the cords of brachial plexus are visualized above and posterior to the axillary artery. (Middle) Sagittal scan just lateral to the retropectoralis minor space. The brachial plexus, subclavian artery and vein are away from pectoralis minor space, but with similar configuration as seen in retropectoralis minor space. (Bottom) Transverse scan of the retropectoralis minor space. The brachial plexus is seen running parallel to, above and posterior to the axillary artery. On a longitudinal scan the axillary vein cannot be visualized together with axillary artery and brachial plexus in the same image because of their triangular configuration.

DYNAMIC INTERROGATION

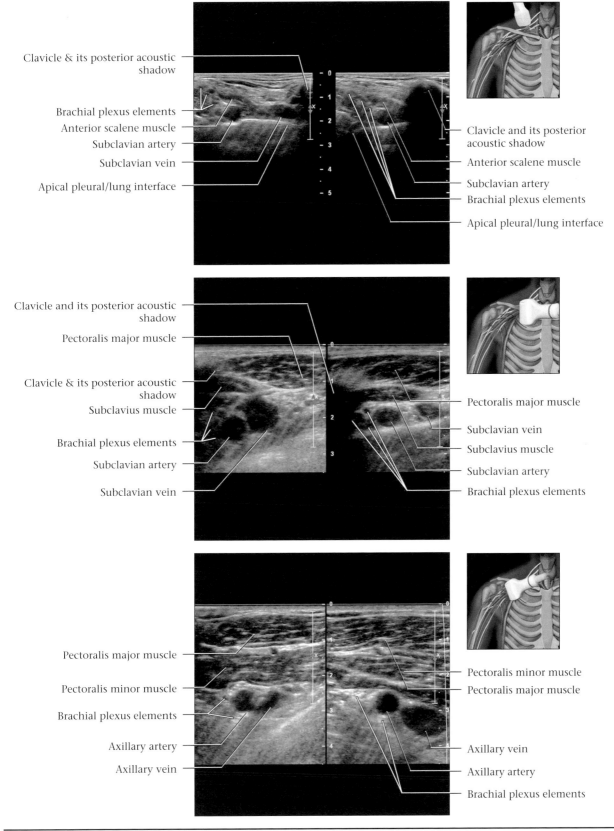

Clavicle & its posterior acoustic shadow
Brachial plexus elements
Anterior scalene muscle
Subclavian artery
Subclavian vein
Apical pleural/lung interface

Clavicle and its posterior acoustic shadow
Anterior scalene muscle
Subclavian artery
Brachial plexus elements
Apical pleural/lung interface

Clavicle and its posterior acoustic shadow
Pectoralis major muscle
Clavicle & its posterior acoustic shadow
Subclavius muscle
Brachial plexus elements
Subclavian artery
Subclavian vein

Pectoralis major muscle
Subclavian vein
Subclavius muscle
Subclavian artery
Brachial plexus elements

Pectoralis major muscle
Pectoralis minor muscle
Brachial plexus elements
Axillary artery
Axillary vein

Pectoralis minor muscle
Pectoralis major muscle
Axillary vein
Axillary artery
Brachial plexus elements

(Top) Dual sagittal image of lower interscalene triangle with arm in neutral position (left image) and 180 degree abduction (right image). The space in the interscalene triangle decreases with the arm abducted. The brachial plexus and subclavian arterial caliber show no significant change. **(Middle)** Dual sagittal image of costoclavicular space (from infraclavicular approach) with arm in neutral position (left image) and arm 180 degree (right image). The subclavian vein appears to be compressed by approximately 50%, which is due to the compressive effect of arm abduction in costoclavicular space. **(Bottom)** Dual sagittal image of retropectoralis minor space with arm in neutral position (left image) and 180 degree abduction (right image). The axillary artery and brachial plexus show no significant change. The axillary vein is more distended with arm abducted.

THORACIC OUTLET

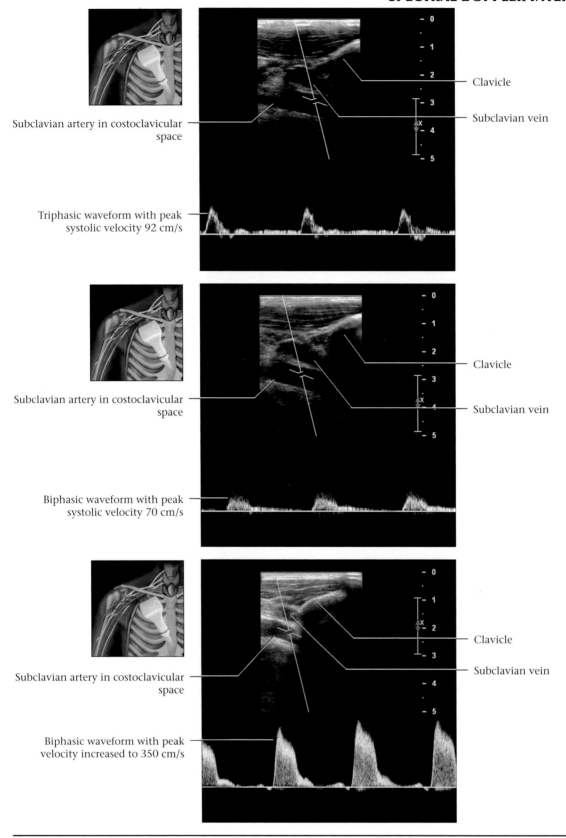

Subclavian artery in costoclavicular space

Clavicle

Subclavian vein

Triphasic waveform with peak systolic velocity 92 cm/s

Subclavian artery in costoclavicular space

Clavicle

Subclavian vein

Biphasic waveform with peak systolic velocity 70 cm/s

Subclavian artery in costoclavicular space

Clavicle

Subclavian vein

Biphasic waveform with peak velocity increased to 350 cm/s

(Top) Doppler spectrum of subclavian artery in costoclavicular space with the arm in neutral position. Normal triphasic waveform is recorded with peak systolic velocity 92 cm/s. **(Middle)** Doppler spectrum of subclavian artery in costoclavicular space with arm in 90 degree abduction (same subject as previous image). The waveform changes from triphasic to biphasic, with no significant change in peak systolic velocity. **(Bottom)** Doppler spectrum of subclavian artery with the arm in 180 degrees abduction (same subject as previous image). Biphasic waveform is still present, with the peak systolic velocity markedly increased to 350 cm/s. Features are indicative of arterial compression in costoclavicular space. The costoclavicular space is the most frequent site of arterial compression.

THORACIC OUTLET

SPECTRAL DOPPLER INTERROGATION

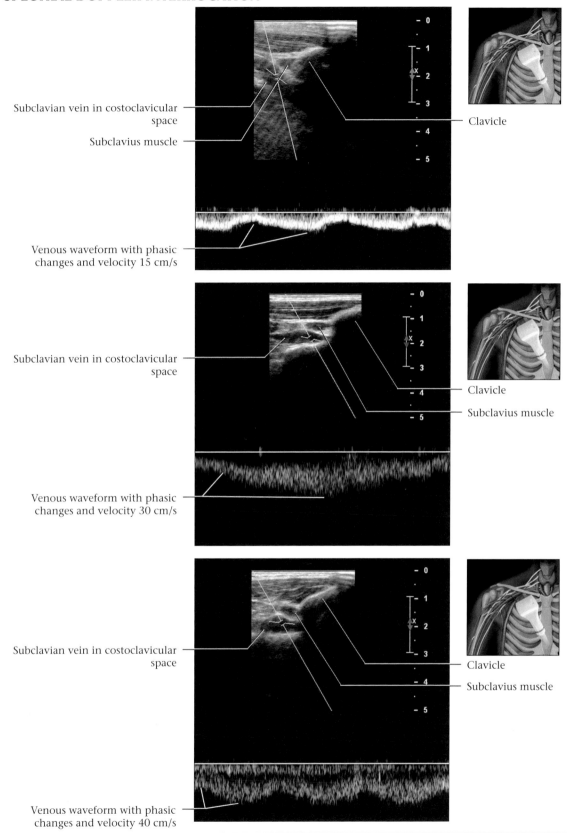

Subclavian vein in costoclavicular space

Subclavius muscle

Clavicle

Venous waveform with phasic changes and velocity 15 cm/s

Subclavian vein in costoclavicular space

Clavicle

Subclavius muscle

Venous waveform with phasic changes and velocity 30 cm/s

Subclavian vein in costoclavicular space

Clavicle

Subclavius muscle

Venous waveform with phasic changes and velocity 40 cm/s

(Top) Doppler spectrum of subclavian vein in costoclavicular space with the arm in neutral position. Normal venous waveform with phasic changes are recorded. **(Middle)** Doppler spectrum of subclavian vein in costoclavicular space (same subject as previous image). Normal venous waveform with phasic changes is again recorded. The velocity increases from 15-30 cm/s. **(Bottom)** Doppler spectrum of subclavian waveform in costoclavicular space with arm 180 degrees abduction (same patient as previous image). The velocity increases to 40 cm/s while normal venous waveform with phasicity is preserved. This indicates a mild compressive effect of arm abduction on subclavian vein.

RIBS AND INTERCOSTAL SPACE

General Anatomy and Function

Chest Wall Anatomy
- Skin, subcutaneous fat
- Blood vessels, lymphatics, nerves
- Bone, cartilage
- Muscles
- Endothoracic fascia, fibroelastic connective tissue between inner aspect of chest wall and costal pleura

Function
- Musculoskeletal cage: Surrounds cardiorespiratory system; effects respiration by expanding and contracting during ventilation

Surface Landmarks
- Suprasternal (jugular) notch: At superior manubrium of sternum; between sternal ends of clavicles
- Sternal angle: Landmark for internal thoracic anatomy; anterior projection at level of costal cartilage of 2nd rib
- Costal margin: Inferior margins of lowest ribs and costal cartilages

Skeletal Structures

Sternum
- Flat, broad bone forms anterior thoracic wall; three parts (manubrium, body, xiphoid process)
- Manubrium forms superior part of sternum
- Body articulates with manubrium superiorly, xiphoid process inferiorly, bilateral costal cartilages of 2nd-7th ribs
- Xiphoid process variable size, shape, ossification; articulates with body of sternum superiorly

Ribs
- 12 pairs, symmetrically arrayed; numbered in accordance with attached vertebral body
- True ribs (1-7) attach to sternum by costal cartilages (synovial joints)
- False ribs (8-10) articulate by costal cartilages with costal cartilage of 7th rib
- Floating ribs (11-12) do not articulate with sternum or rib costal cartilages; short costal cartilages terminate in abdominal wall muscle
- Head articulates with demi-facets of two adjacent vertebral bodies; neck located between head and tubercle of each rib; tubercle articulates with vertebral transverse process
- Body: Longest part of each rib
- Angle: Most posterior part
- Costal groove on inner surface of inferior border; accommodates intercostal neurovascular bundle

Muscles

Pectoral
- Pectoralis major: Largest muscle in breast and pectoral region; originates from anterior chest wall, sternum, and clavicle; adducts, flexes and medially rotates arm

- Pectoralis minor: Deep to pectoralis major; originates from chest wall, inserts onto coracoid process of scapula; stabilizes scapula

Intercostal
- External: Contained within 11 intercostal spaces; extend from tubercle of ribs to costochondral junction
- Internal: Middle layer; occupy 11 intercostal spaces; extend from border of sternum to angle of ribs
- Innermost: Form inner layer of chest wall muscles with subcostales and transversus thoracis muscles

Serratus Anterior
- Thin muscular sheet; overlies lateral thoracic cage and intercostal muscles; arises from upper eight ribs; wraps around rib cage; inserts along medial border of anterior surface of scapula

Vessels and Nerves

Arteries
- Internal thoracic (internal mammary): Branch of subclavian artery; descends posterior to first six costal cartilages; supplies upper anterior chest wall
  - Supplies anterior intercostal arteries to first six intercostal spaces

Veins
- Azygos vein receives drainage from posterior intercostal veins, hemi-azygos and accessory hemi-azygos veins

Nerves
- Anterior rami of thoracic spinal nerves (T1-T11) supply skin, tissues of chest wall; form intercostal nerves
- Intercostal nerves run in costal groove, between internal and innermost intercostal muscles
- Brachial plexus: Branching network of nerve roots, trunks, divisions, cords and branches
  - Spinal roots form three trunks; behind clavicle, each dividing into anterior and posterior divisions

Imaging

Radiography
- Limited capabilities; may detect congenital deformities, soft-tissue masses, bone destruction

Ultrasound
- Allows detailed examination of intercostal spaces and contents
- Intercostal muscles are seen as hypoechoic structures
- Intercostal membrane is seen as hyperechoic layer
  - However, the intercostal structures are often thin, making it difficult to separate them into distinct layers
- Only anterior cortex of ribs evaluated (medulla obscured)

Computed Tomography
- Helical CT and multiplanar reformations optimal for visualization of osseous lesions

RIBS AND INTERCOSTAL SPACE

GRAPHICS, RIBS AND INTERCOSTAL SPACES

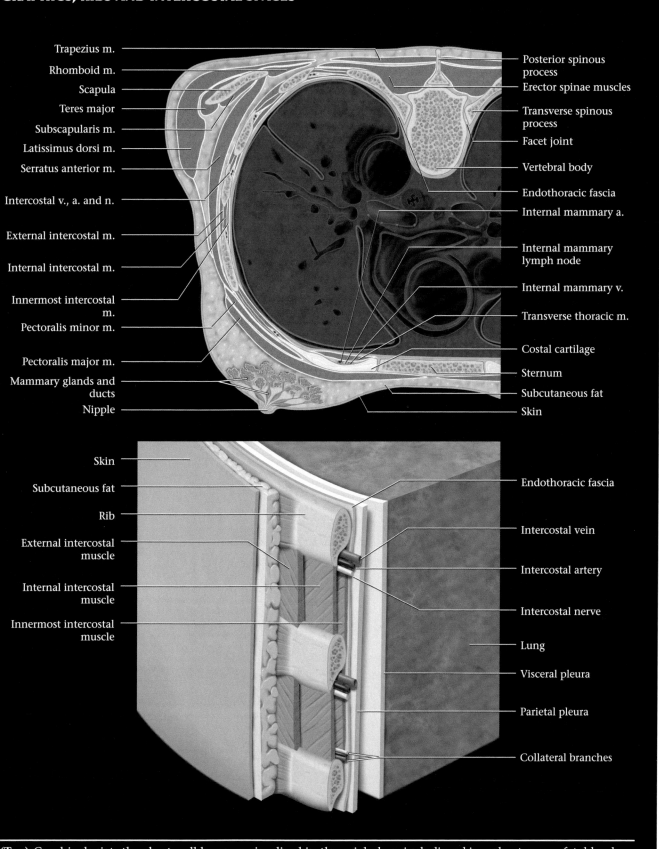

Trapezius m.
Rhomboid m.
Scapula
Teres major
Subscapularis m.
Latissimus dorsi m.
Serratus anterior m.
Intercostal v., a. and n.
External intercostal m.
Internal intercostal m.
Innermost intercostal m.
Pectoralis minor m.
Pectoralis major m.
Mammary glands and ducts
Nipple

Posterior spinous process
Erector spinae muscles
Transverse spinous process
Facet joint
Vertebral body
Endothoracic fascia
Internal mammary a.
Internal mammary lymph node
Internal mammary v.
Transverse thoracic m.
Costal cartilage
Sternum
Subcutaneous fat
Skin

Skin
Subcutaneous fat
Rib
External intercostal muscle
Internal intercostal muscle
Innermost intercostal muscle

Endothoracic fascia
Intercostal vein
Intercostal artery
Intercostal nerve
Lung
Visceral pleura
Parietal pleura
Collateral branches

(Top) Graphic depicts the chest wall layers as visualized in the axial plane including skin, subcutaneous fat, blood vessels, lymphatics, and musculoskeletal structures. The innermost layer, the endothoracic fascia, is a fibroelastic connective tissue layer between the inner aspect of the chest wall and the pleura. (Bottom) Graphic demonstrates details of the intercostal region, showing three layers of intercostal muscles (external, internal and innermost) between the ribs. The costal groove along the inferomedial aspect of each rib accommodates the intercostal neurovascular bundle (vein, artery and nerve). Small collateral branches of the major intercostal vessels and nerves may be present above the body of the subjacent rib. The endothoracic fascia forms a connective tissue layer between the inner aspect of the chest wall and the costal parietal pleura.

Thorax II

21

RIBS AND INTERCOSTAL SPACE

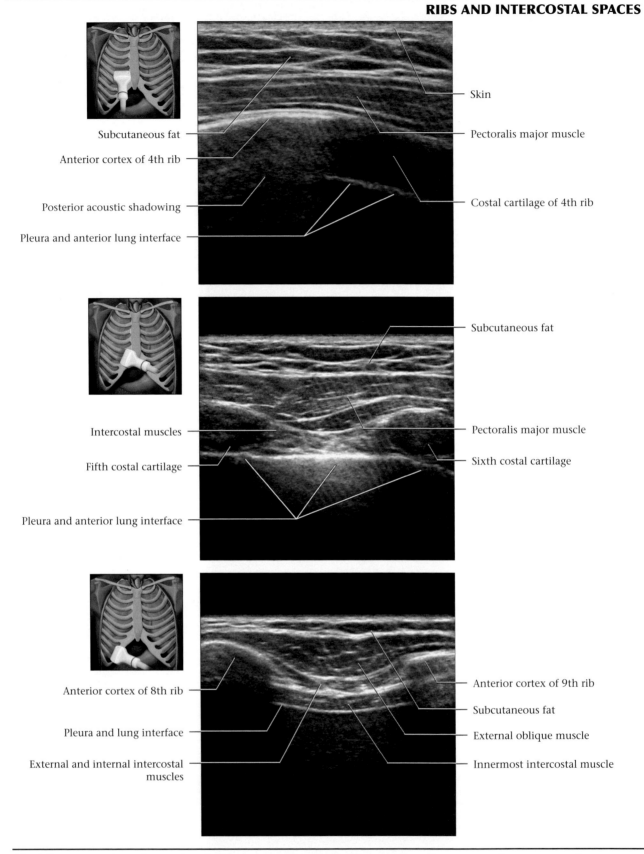

Skin

Subcutaneous fat

Pectoralis major muscle

Anterior cortex of 4th rib

Posterior acoustic shadowing

Costal cartilage of 4th rib

Pleura and anterior lung interface

Subcutaneous fat

Intercostal muscles

Pectoralis major muscle

Fifth costal cartilage

Sixth costal cartilage

Pleura and anterior lung interface

Anterior cortex of 8th rib

Anterior cortex of 9th rib

Subcutaneous fat

Pleura and lung interface

External oblique muscle

External and internal intercostal muscles

Innermost intercostal muscle

(Top) Transverse view of costochondral junction of fourth rib. The costal cartilage appears homogeneously hypoechoic and does not produce significant posterior acoustic shadowing, thus allowing the underlying pleural surface to be seen. The cortex of 4th rib casts a strong posterior shadow, obscuring the underlying pleura. (Middle) Oblique sagittal view of intercostal space between costal cartilages in the anterior chest wall. The costal cartilages are well-defined and oval-shaped on cross-section. Intercostal muscles between costal cartilages and overlying pectoralis muscle can be clearly visualized. (Bottom) More laterally, oblique sagittal view shows intercostal spaces between ribs. Areas behind the ribs are obscured by acoustic shadowing. The intercostal muscles in here are better differentiated compared to more medially.

RIBS AND INTERCOSTAL SPACE

RIBS AND INTERCOSTAL SPACES

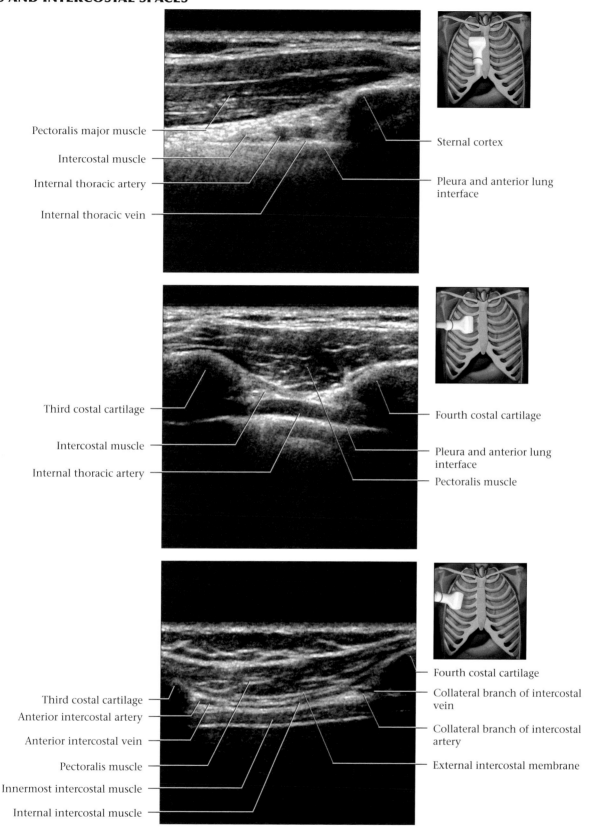

Pectoralis major muscle

Intercostal muscle

Internal thoracic artery

Internal thoracic vein

Sternal cortex

Pleura and anterior lung interface

Third costal cartilage

Intercostal muscle

Internal thoracic artery

Fourth costal cartilage

Pleura and anterior lung interface

Pectoralis muscle

Third costal cartilage

Anterior intercostal artery

Anterior intercostal vein

Pectoralis muscle

Innermost intercostal muscle

Internal intercostal muscle

Fourth costal cartilage

Collateral branch of intercostal vein

Collateral branch of intercostal artery

External intercostal membrane

(Top) Transverse view of the anterior intercostal space just lateral to the sternum. The internal thoracic artery and vein next to the sternum are well-visualized with this approach, as are the overlying pectoralis muscle and underlying pleura. (Middle) Sagittal view of the anterior intercostal space showing internal thoracic artery. Long axis of internal thoracic artery can be well-delineated by scanning along the lateral margin of the sternum. (Bottom) Sagittal view of anterior intercostal space and the anterior intercostal vessels. The anterior intercostal artery and anterior intercostal vein are identified just inferior to rib above. Smaller collateral branches of intercostal artery and vein can be identified just superior to the rib above. At the anterior intercostal space, the external intercostal muscle is seen as a thin membrane.

Thorax

III

23

BREAST

Terminology

Definitions
- Lobe (segment): Drainage territory defined by each major duct
- Terminal duct: Final branch of segmental duct
  - Has two parts: Extralobular terminal duct (ELTD) and intralobular terminal duct (ILTD)
- Lobule: Composed of ILTD and complex system of tiny ducts terminating in blind-ending acini (alveoli)
- Terminal ductal lobular unit (TDLU): Lobule + ELTD
- Cooper ligament: Strands of suspensory ligaments extending from the anterior mammary fascia into the dermis to support the breast

Lobe/Segment

Composition
- Major ducts and branches → ELTDs → ILTDs → acini

Clinical Considerations
- Average of 15-20 lobes per breast
- Lobar volume and anatomy variable
- No discrete histologic or anatomic lobar boundaries
- Most, but not all, lobes drain to corresponding nipple duct orifice (some share common ducts)

Ductal System

Duct Orifices
- Usually 8-12 per nipple
- Arranged radially in nipple crevices
- Some major ducts merge deep to nipple surface
- Quadrant of duct orifice on nipple surface does not always correspond to quadrant of lobe

Lactiferous Sinus (Ampullary Segment)
- Widened duct segment just deep to nipple orifice
- Average diameter = 4-5 mm

Major Ducts
- Average diameter = 1 mm
- Arborize into segmental and subsegmental branches of variable length and number
- Branches may extend into multiple breast quadrants
- Segmental and subsegmental branches give rise to terminal ducts
- Drain 20-40 lobules each containing 10-100 acini

Terminal Duct Lobular Unit (TDLU)

Overview
- Functional, glandular unit of breast
- May arise directly from major ducts or lactiferous sinuses
  - Possible explanation for subareolar invasive malignancies
- Multiple rows of TDLUs arise from distal segmental/subsegmental ducts
  - More numerous anterior rows have longer ELTDs
  - Less numerous posterior rows have shorter ELTDs

- Composition
  - ELTD is extralobar segment of terminal duct
  - ILTD is terminal intralobular segment of terminal duct
  - 10-100 acini drain into each ILTD
  - Loose stromal matrix of collagen and reticular fibers less dense than interlobular stroma

TDLU Proliferation
- Late adolescence
- Pregnancy and lactation
- Exogenous hormones: Birth control pills and hormone replacement therapy (HRT)
- Post-ovulatory (secretory) phase of menstrual cycle

TDLU Regression
- Postpartum and menopause
- May be nonuniform between breasts causing mammographic asymmetries

Zonal Anatomy

Premammary Zone
- Between skin and anterior mammary fascia
- Contains subcutaneous fat, blood vessels and Cooper ligaments

Mammary Zone
- Between anterior and posterior mammary fasciae
- Contains TDLUs and ducts, stromal fat and stromal connective tissue

Retromammary Zone
- Between posterior mammary fascia and chest wall
- Contains fat and posterior suspensory ligaments

Imaging Issues

Ultrasound
- Ducts frequently visible as linear, branching hypo- to isoechoic channels
- Cooper ligaments visible in premammary zone
- TDLUs often visible
- Interlobular stromal fibrous tissue is usually hyperechoic compared to subcutaneous fat and glandular elements are usually iso or slightly hyperechoic to subcutaneous fat

Clinical Implications

Clinical Importance
- Most invasive cancers arise from TDLU
- Ductal carcinoma in situ (DCIS) may extend into segmental and main ducts
- Papillomas and duct ectasia arise from ductal elements
- Duct orifices and subareolar ducts avenues for mastitis

GRAPHICS, BREAST

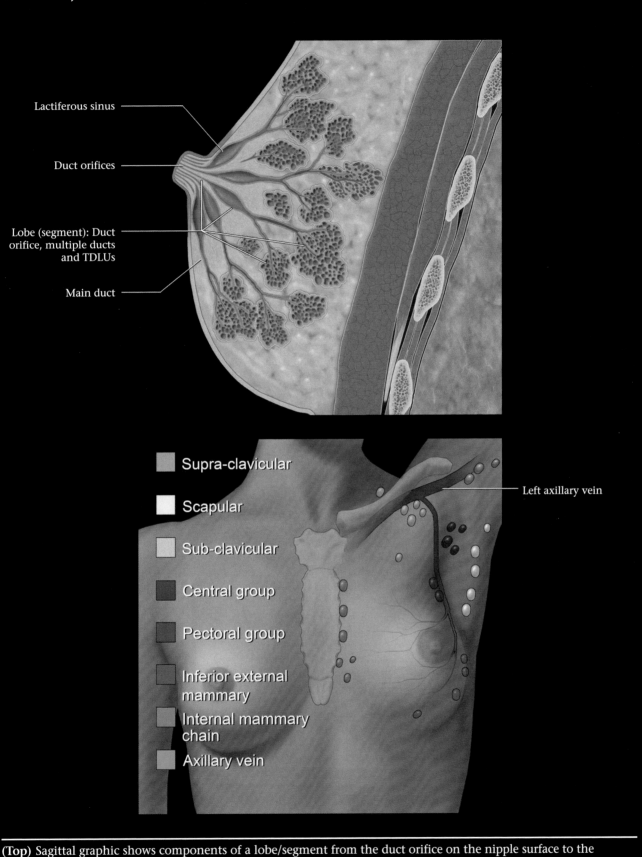

Lactiferous sinus

Duct orifices

Lobe (segment): Duct orifice, multiple ducts and TDLUs

Main duct

Supra-clavicular

Scapular

Sub-clavicular

Central group

Pectoral group

Inferior external mammary

Internal mammary chain

Axillary vein

Left axillary vein

(Top) Sagittal graphic shows components of a lobe/segment from the duct orifice on the nipple surface to the TDLUs. Breasts average 15-20 lobes, draining into 8-12 duct orifices. **(Bottom)** Each major lymph node group has well-defined anatomy. The axillary vein group is medial and posterior to the axillary vein, the pectoral group projects at the lower margin of the pectoral muscle, the scapular group projects at the intersection of posterior axilla & scapula, the central group projects posterior to pectoralis minor muscle into the axillary fat, the interpectoral group (not labeled) projects between pectoralis major and pectoralis minor, the subclavicular group projects at the apex of the axilla, the inferior external mammary group is lateral and inferior to the breast and the internal mammary chain in the parasternal intercostal spaces.

BREAST

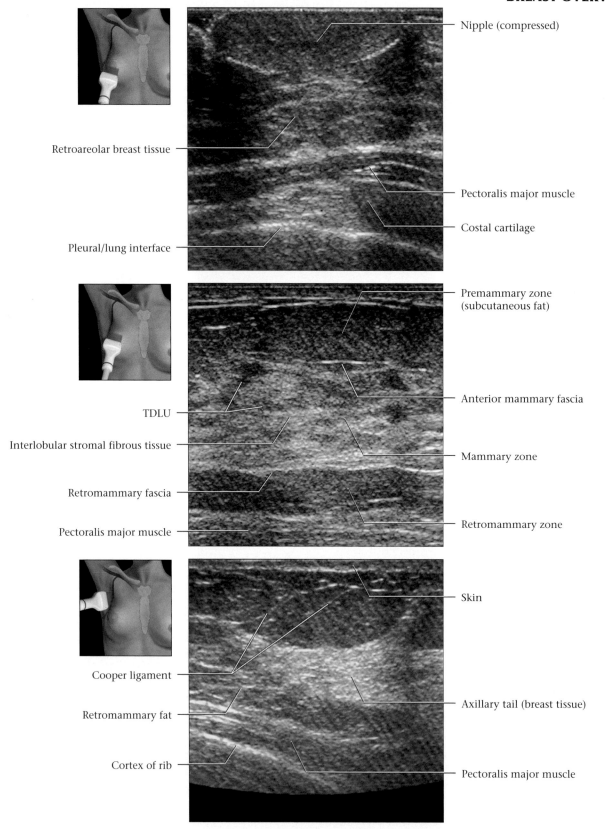

Nipple (compressed)

Retroareolar breast tissue

Pectoralis major muscle

Costal cartilage

Pleural/lung interface

Premammary zone
(subcutaneous fat)

Anterior mammary fascia

TDLU

Interlobular stromal fibrous tissue

Mammary zone

Retromammary fascia

Pectoralis major muscle

Retromammary zone

Skin

Cooper ligament

Axillary tail (breast tissue)

Retromammary fat

Cortex of rib

Pectoralis major muscle

(Top) Transverse view of the nipple. Copious amount of transducer gel should be used to fill in gaps when scanning the nipple. Behind the nipple lies the retroareolar region. (Middle) Transverse view of the breast to illustrate the three mammary zones. The premammary zone is the subcutaneous fat layer and is separated from the mammary zone by the anterior mammary fascia. The mammary zone (contains TDLUs) is separated from the retromammary zone (of fat) by the retromammary fascia. The pectoralis muscle and chest wall lie deep to these mammary zones. (Bottom) Oblique transverse view showing the axillary tail of breast tissue. The breast tissue may extend laterally to form an axillary tail, which must be evaluated before the examination is complete. (Courtesy ALM Pang, MD).

BREAST

BREAST PARENCHYMAL VARIATION

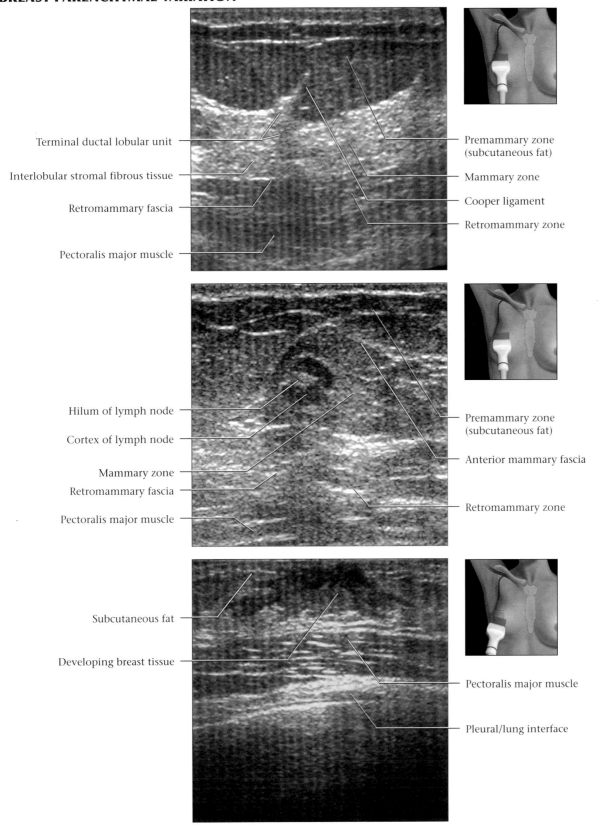

Terminal ductal lobular unit

Interlobular stromal fibrous tissue

Retromammary fascia

Pectoralis major muscle

Premammary zone (subcutaneous fat)

Mammary zone

Cooper ligament

Retromammary zone

Hilum of lymph node

Cortex of lymph node

Mammary zone

Retromammary fascia

Pectoralis major muscle

Premammary zone (subcutaneous fat)

Anterior mammary fascia

Retromammary zone

Subcutaneous fat

Developing breast tissue

Pectoralis major muscle

Pleural/lung interface

(Top) Transverse scan showing Cooper ligament in a breast with a moderate degree of atrophy. With age, the fibroglandular tissue between Cooper ligaments regress. This results in residual fibroglandular elements being trapped within the Cooper ligament. (Courtesy ALM Pang, MD). (Middle) Transverse view of the breast showing an intramammary lymph node. These are frequently found incidentally and usually lie in the upper outer quadrant. They may present as a palpable lump, especially in small-breasted or thin women. (Bottom) Transverse view of the retroareolar area of a 10 year old girl. The developing breast tissue consists of proliferating ducts and periductal stromal fibrous tissue, resulting in a hypo-/iso-echoic mass deep to the nipple. Clinically this is a palpable disc of tissue deep to the nipple. (Courtesy ALM Pang, MD).

BREAST

Premammary zone (subcutaneous fat)

Cooper ligament

Interlobular stromal fibrous tissue

Retromammary fascia

Pectoralis major muscle

Anterior mammary fascia

Mammary zone

Retromammary zone

TDLUs

Interlobular stromal fibrous tissue

Retromammary fascia

Pectoralis major muscle

Premammary zone (subcutaneous fat)

Anterior mammary fascia

Mammary zone

Retromammary zone

Isoechoic glandular tissue

Retromammary fascia

Pectoralis major muscle

Premammary zone (subcutaneous fat)

Anterior mammary fascia

Mammary zone

Retromammary zone

(Top) Transverse view of a breast with atrophy, consisting of hyperechoic interlobular stromal fibrous tissue. No terminal ductal lobular units can be demonstrated. (Middle) Transverse view of a breast with both isoechoic glandular tissue (terminal ductal lobular units) and hyperechoic stomal fibrous tissue. As can be seen in these examples, the echopattern ranges from purely hyperechoic (compared to subcutaneous fat) stomal fibrous tissue to purely isoechoic (compared to subcutaneous fat) glandular tissue. A combination of different types is the most common appearance. (Bottom) Transverse view of a breast with purely isoechoic glandular tissue. This is more likely to be seen in patients in their second or early third decade due to lobule proliferation, or during lactation or pregnancy.

BREAST

BREAST PARENCHYMAL VARIATION

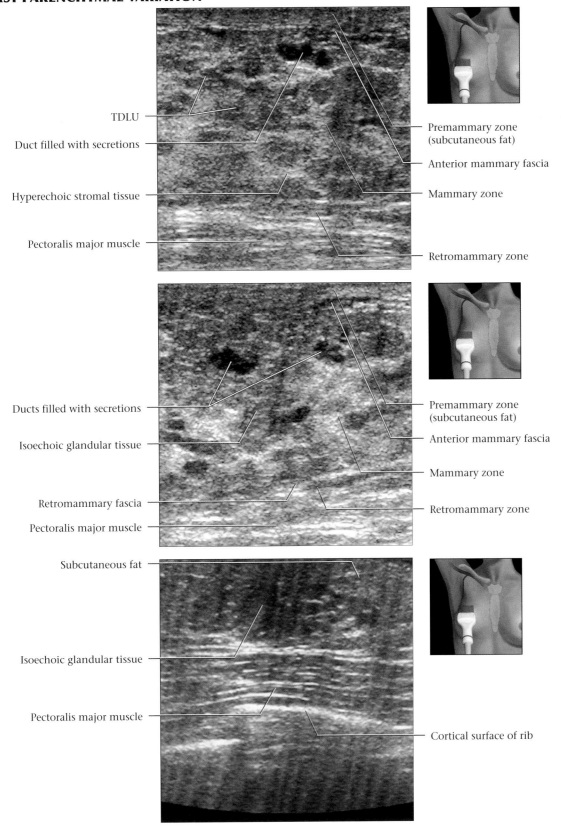

TDLU

Duct filled with secretions

Hyperechoic stromal tissue

Pectoralis major muscle

Premammary zone (subcutaneous fat)

Anterior mammary fascia

Mammary zone

Retromammary zone

Ducts filled with secretions

Isoechoic glandular tissue

Retromammary fascia

Pectoralis major muscle

Premammary zone (subcutaneous fat)

Anterior mammary fascia

Mammary zone

Retromammary zone

Subcutaneous fat

Isoechoic glandular tissue

Pectoralis major muscle

Cortical surface of rib

(Top) Transverse view of the breast during pregnancy shows that the terminal ductal lobular units have hypertrophied and multiplied in number. The hypertrophic glandular tissue tends to be hypoechoic in pregnancy, becoming more hypoechoic during lactation, representing intralobular acini filled with secretions. The hyperechoic stromal fibrous tissue is replaced by glandular tissue. (Middle) Transverse view of a lactating breast. During lactation, glandular tissue tends to be more hypoechoic, with many hypoechoic ducts. (Bottom) Transverse view of breast tissue in a man with gynecomastia. This markedly hypoechoic mass, reflects enlarged subareolar ducts, and is the proliferative phase of gynecomastia. In the mixed phase, hyperechoic fibrous tissue is seen in between hypoechoic ducts. (Courtesy ALM Pang, MD).

Thorax

III

29

BREAST

Premammary zone (subcutaneous fat)

Major lobular duct and tributaries

Interlobular stromal fibrous tissue

Retromammary fascia

Pectoralis major muscle

Anterior mammary fascia

Mammary zone

Retromammary zone

Premammary zone (subcutaneous fat)

Nipple

Pectoralis major muscle

Dilated duct

Mammary zone

Premammary zone (subcutaneous fat)

Ectatic duct

TDLU

Pectoralis major muscle

Anterior mammary fascia

Inflamed periductal tissue

Mammary zone

(Top) Transverse view of breast just inferior to the nipple to illustrate the ductal system. Lobules drain into small branch ducts, which join to form gradually larger ducts. These then drain into a single major lobular duct. Deep to the nipple, major ducts dilate to form lactiferous sinuses for milk storage. (Courtesy ALM Pang, MD). **(Middle)** Oblique scan of the breast demonstrating a prominent retroareolar duct. Despite the dilatation, there is an absence of periductal inflammation, distinguishing this from duct ectasia. Prominent or dilated retroareolar ducts are common especially in women older than 50 years of age. **(Bottom)** Oblique scan of the breast demonstrating duct ectasia. This represents large subareolar and intermediate-sized ducts dilated by thick secretions, with inflammation in and around the duct.

BREAST

AXILLARY LYMPH NODE

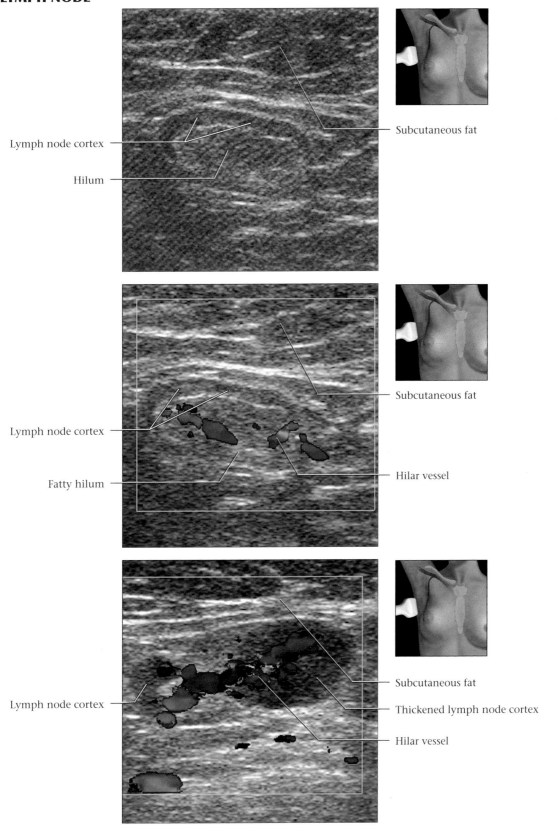

Lymph node cortex

Hilum

Subcutaneous fat

Lymph node cortex

Fatty hilum

Subcutaneous fat

Hilar vessel

Lymph node cortex

Subcutaneous fat

Thickened lymph node cortex

Hilar vessel

(Top) Oblique scan of the axilla showing a normal lymph node. The hilum is similar in appearance to the surrounding axillary fat. The normal lymph node cortex is smooth, hypoechoic and uniform in thickness. (Middle) Oblique color Doppler scan of a normal axillary node showing hilar vessels. These vessels are consistently seen on high resolution sonography. (Bottom) Oblique color Doppler scan of the axilla showing a lymph node with thickened cortex. Here the cortical thickening is uniform, the surface appears smooth and the hilum is preserved. These features suggest that this may be an inflamed or reactive lymph node (this was a reactive node on biopsy).

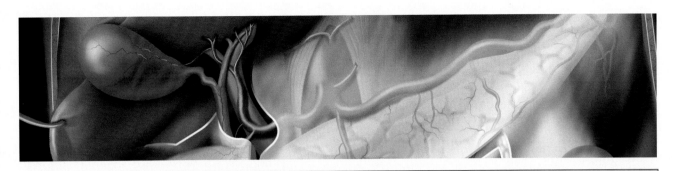

SECTION IV: Abdomen

LIVER

Gross Anatomy

Overview
- Liver is largest gland & largest internal organ (average weight = 1,500 grams)
  - Functions
    - Processes all nutrients (except fats) absorbed from GI tract; conveyed via portal vein
    - Stores glycogen, secretes bile
  - Relations
    - Anterior & superior surfaces are smooth and convex
    - Posterior & inferior surfaces are indented by colon, stomach, right kidney, duodenum, IVC, gallbladder
  - Covered by peritoneum except at gallbladder fossa, porta hepatis and bare area
    - Bare area: Nonperitoneal posterior superior surface where liver abuts diaphragm
  - Porta hepatis: Site of entry/exit of portal vein, hepatic artery and bile duct
  - Falciform ligament: Extends from liver to anterior abdominal wall
    - Separates right & left subphrenic peritoneal recesses (between liver & diaphragm)
    - Marks plane separating medial and lateral segments of left hepatic lobe
    - Carries round ligament (lig. teres), fibrous remnant of umbilical vein
- Vascular anatomy (unique dual afferent blood supply)
  - Portal vein
    - Carries nutrients from gut and hepatotrophic hormones from pancreas to liver along with oxygen (contains 40% more oxygen than systemic venous blood)
    - 75-80% of blood supply to liver
  - Hepatic artery
    - Supplies 20-25% of blood
    - Liver is less dependent than biliary tree on hepatic arterial blood supply
    - Usually arises from celiac artery
    - Variations are common including arteries arising from superior mesenteric artery
  - Hepatic veins
    - Usually 3 (right, middle and left)
    - Many variations & accessory veins
    - Collect blood from liver and return it to IVC at confluence of hepatic veins just below diaphragm and entrance of IVC into right atrium
  - Portal triad
    - At all levels of size and subdivision, branches of hepatic artery, portal vein and bile ducts travel together
    - Blood flows into hepatic sinusoids from interlobular branches of hepatic artery & portal vein → hepatocytes (detoxify blood and produce bile) → bile collects into ducts, blood collects into central veins → hepatic veins
- Segmental anatomy of liver
  - Eight hepatic segments
    - Each receives secondary or tertiary branch of hepatic artery and portal vein

- Each is drained by its own bile duct (intrahepatic) and hepatic vein branch
  - Caudate lobe = segment 1
    - Has independent portal triads and hepatic venous drainage to IVC
  - Left lobe
    - Lateral superior = segment 2
    - Lateral inferior = segment 3
    - Medial superior = segment 4A
    - Medial inferior = segment 4B
  - Right lobe
    - Anterior inferior = segment 5
    - Posterior inferior = segment 6
    - Posterior superior = segment 7
    - Anterior superior = segment 8

Imaging Anatomy

Internal Structures-Critical Contents
- Capsule
  - Reflective capsule making borders of liver well-defined
- Left lobe
  - Contains segments 2, 3, 4A and 4B
  - Longitudinal scan
    - Triangular in shape
    - Rounded upper surface
    - Sharp inferior border
  - Transverse scan
    - Wedge-shaped tapering to left
  - Liver parenchyma echoes are mid gray with a uniform sponge-like pattern interrupted by vessels
- Right lobe
  - Contains segments 5, 6, 7 and 8
  - Liver parenchymal echoes similar to left lobe
  - Sections of right lobe show same basic shape, though right lobe is usually larger than left
- Caudate lobe
  - Longitudinal scan
    - Almond-shaped structure posterior to left lobe
  - Transverse scan
    - Seen as an extension of right lobe
- Portal veins
  - Have thicker reflective walls than hepatic veins - portal veins have fibromuscular walls
  - Wall reflectivity also depends on angle of interrogation - portal vein cut at more oblique angle may have less apparent wall
  - Can be traced back towards porta hepatis
  - Normal portal flow is hepatopetal on color Doppler - absent or reversal of flow may be seen in portal hypertension
  - Mean flow velocity is about 15-18 cm/s with a wide normal range
  - Portal waveform has an undulating appearance due to variations with cardiac activity and respiration
  - Branches run in a transverse plane
  - Hepatic portal vein anatomy is variable
- Hepatic veins
  - Appear as echolucent defects within liver parenchyma with no reflective wall - large sinusoids with thin or absent wall

- o Branches enlarge and can be traced towards inferior vena cava
- o Flow pattern has a chaotic and pulsatile pattern
  - ▪ Resulting from transmission of right atrial pulsations into veins
  - ▪ Doppler spectrum reflects a combination of phasic variations and transmitted pulsation
- o Right hepatic vein
  - ▪ Runs in a coronal plane between anterior and posterior segments of right hepatic lobe
- o Middle hepatic vein
  - ▪ Lies in a sagittal or parasagittal plane between right and left hepatic lobe
- o Left hepatic vein
  - ▪ Runs between medial and lateral segments of left hepatic lobe
  - ▪ Frequently duplicated
- o One of the three major branches of hepatic veins may be absent
  - ▪ Absent right hepatic vein ~ 6%
  - ▪ Less commonly middle and left hepatic vein
- Hepatic artery
  - o Common hepatic artery usually arises from celiac axis
  - o Classic configuration - 72%
    - ▪ Celiac axis → common hepatic artery → gastroduodenal artery and proper hepatic artery → latter gives rise to right and left hepatic artery
  - o Variations from classic configuration
    - ▪ Common hepatic artery arising from SMA - 4%
    - ▪ Right hepatic artery arising from SMA (replaced right hepatic artery) - 11%
    - ▪ Left hepatic artery arising from left gastric artery - 10%
  - o Flow pattern has low resistance characteristics with a large amount of continuous forward flow throughout diastole
- Bile ducts
  - o Normal peripheral intrahepatic bile ducts are too small to be demonstrated
  - o Normal right and left hepatic ducts measuring a few millimeters are usually visible
  - o Normal common duct
    - ▪ Most visible in its proximal portion just caudal to porta hepatis - less than 5 mm
    - ▪ Distal common duct should typically measure < 6 mm
    - ▪ In the elderly, generalized loss of tissue elasticity with advancing age leads to increase in bile duct diameter - < 8 mm (somewhat controversial)
    - ▪ Post cholecystectomy patients - less than 10 mm

Anatomy-Based Imaging Issues

Key Concepts or Questions
- Designating and remembering hepatic segments
  - o Portal triads are intra-segmental, hepatic veins are inter-segmental
  - o Separating right from left lobe
    - ▪ Plane extending vertically through gallbladder fossa & middle hepatic vein
  - o Separating right anterior from posterior segments

- ▪ Vertical plane through right hepatic vein
- o Separating left lateral from medial segments
  - ▪ Plane of falciform ligament
- o Separating superior from inferior segments
  - ▪ Plane of main right & left portal veins
- o Segments are numbered in clockwise order as if looking at anterior surface of liver

Imaging Recommendations
- Transducer
  - o 2-5 MHz curvilinear transducer is generally most suitable
  - o Higher frequency linear transducer (e.g., 7.5 MHz) can be useful for detailed evaluation of contour of liver
- Left lobe
  - o Subcostal window with full inspiration generally most suitable
- Right lobe
  - o Subcostal window
    - ▪ Cranial and right-wards angulation useful for visualization of right lobe below dome of hemidiaphragm
    - ▪ Can sometimes be obscured by bowel gas
  - o Intercostal window
    - ▪ Usually gives better resolution for parenchyma without influence from bowel gas
    - ▪ Right lobe just below hemidiaphragm may not be visible due to obscuration from lung bases
    - ▪ Important to tilt transducer parallel to intercostal space to minimize shadowing from ribs

Imaging Pitfalls
- Because of variations of vascular & biliary branching within liver (common), it is frequently impossible to designate precisely the boundaries between hepatic segments on imaging studies

Clinical Implications

Clinical Importance
- Advances in hepatic surgery (tumor resection, transplantation) make it essential to depict lobar and segmental anatomy, volume, blood supply, biliary drainage as accurately as possible
  - o Combination of axial, coronal, sagittal and 3D imaging by CT, MR and sonography may be needed
  - o "Invasive" imaging studies (catheter angiography and percutaneous transhepatic or endoscopic cholangiography) can be avoided in many cases by CT & MR angiography and cholangiography
- Liver metastases are common
  - o Primary carcinomas of colon, pancreas, & stomach are common
  - o Portal venous drainage usually results in liver being initial site of metastatic spread from these tumors
- Primary hepatocellular carcinoma
  - o Common worldwide, usually result of viral hepatitis B or C, alcoholism

LIVER

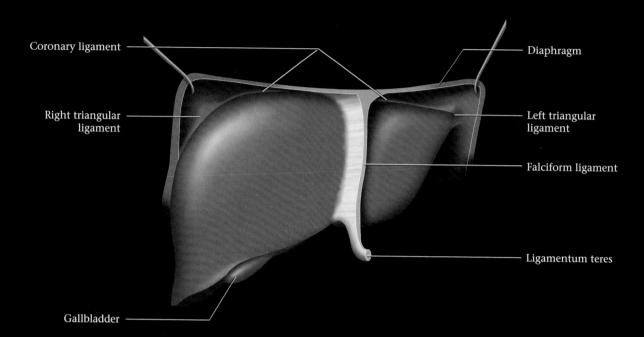

Coronary ligament

Diaphragm

Right triangular ligament

Left triangular ligament

Falciform ligament

Ligamentum teres

Gallbladder

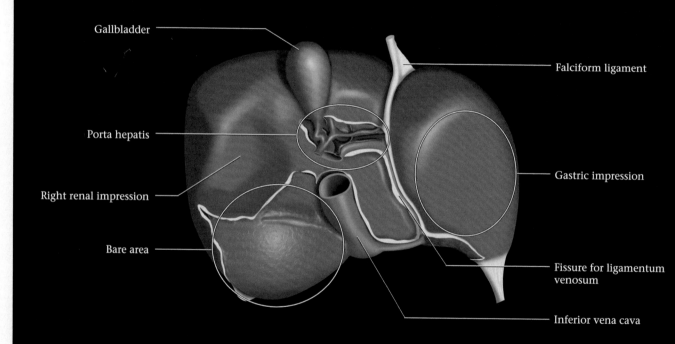

Gallbladder

Falciform ligament

Porta hepatis

Gastric impression

Right renal impression

Bare area

Fissure for ligamentum venosum

Inferior vena cava

(Top) The anterior surface of the liver is smooth and molds to the diaphragm & anterior abdominal wall. Generally, only the anterior/inferior edge of the liver is palpable on physical exam. The liver is covered with peritoneum, except for the gallbladder bed, porta hepatis, and the bare area. Peritoneal reflections form various ligaments that connect the liver to the diaphragm & abdominal wall, including the falciform ligament, the inferior edge of which contains the ligamentum teres, the obliterated remnant of the umbilical vein. **(Bottom)** Graphic shows the liver inverted, somewhat similar to the surgeon's view of the upwardly retracted liver. The structures in the porta hepatis include the portal vein (blue), hepatic artery (red), and the bile ducts (green). The visceral surface of the liver is indented by adjacent viscera. The bare area is not easily accessible.

LIVER

HEPATIC ATTACHMENTS AND RELATIONS

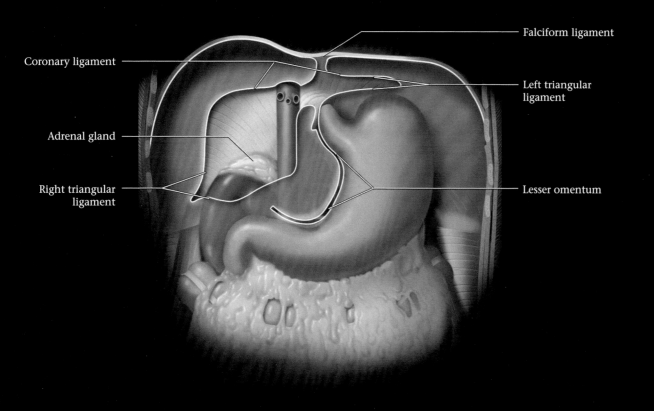

Falciform ligament

Coronary ligament

Left triangular ligament

Adrenal gland

Right triangular ligament

Lesser omentum

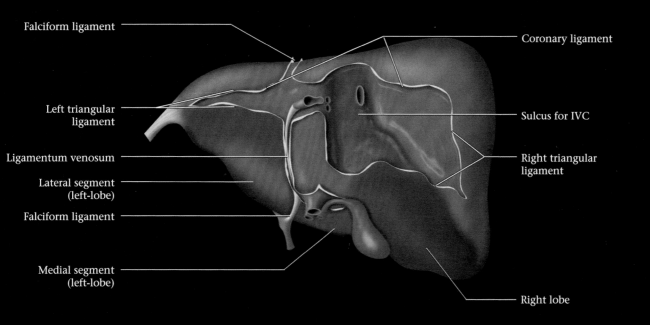

Falciform ligament

Coronary ligament

Left triangular ligament

Sulcus for IVC

Ligamentum venosum

Right triangular ligament

Lateral segment (left-lobe)

Falciform ligament

Medial segment (left-lobe)

Right lobe

(Top) The liver is attached to the posterior abdominal wall and diaphragm by the left & right triangular and coronary ligaments. The falciform ligament attaches the liver to the anterior abdominal wall. The bare area is in direct contact with the right adrenal gland & kidney, and the IVC. (Bottom) Posterior view of the liver shows the ligamentous attachments. While these may help to fix the liver in position, abdominal pressure alone is sufficient, as evidenced by orthotopic liver transplantation, after which the ligamentous attachments are lost without the liver shifting position. The diaphragmatic peritoneal reflection is the coronary ligament whose lateral extensions are the right & left triangular ligaments. The falciform ligament separates the medial & lateral segments of the left lobe.

LIVER

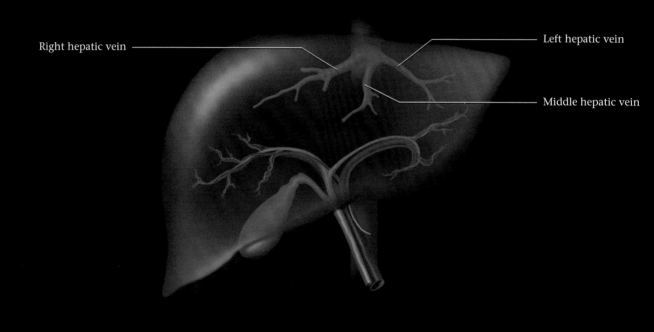

Right hepatic vein

Left hepatic vein

Middle hepatic vein

This graphic emphasizes that, at every level of branching and subdivision, the portal veins, hepatic arteries and bile ducts course together, constituting the "portal triad". Each segment of the liver is supplied by branches of these vessels. Conversely, hepatic venous branches lie between hepatic segments and interdigitate with the portal triads, but never run parallel to them.

LIVER

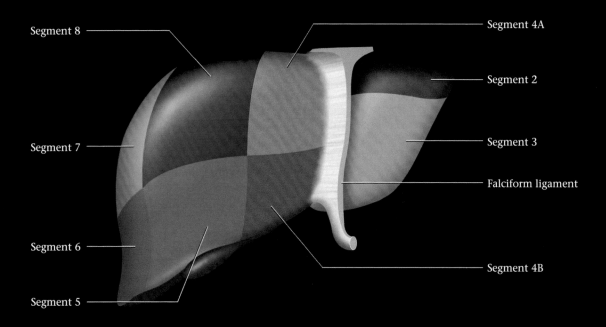

Segment 8

Segment 4A

Segment 2

Segment 7

Segment 3

Falciform ligament

Segment 6

Segment 4B

Segment 5

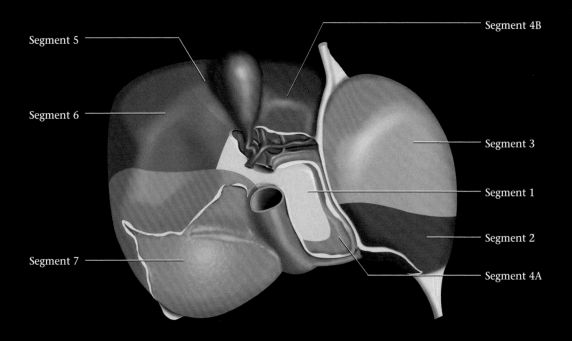

Segment 4B

Segment 5

Segment 6

Segment 3

Segment 1

Segment 2

Segment 7

Segment 4A

(Top) First of two graphics demonstrating the segmental anatomy of the liver in a somewhat idealized fashion. Segments are numbered in a clockwise direction, starting with the caudate lobe (segment 1), which cannot be seen on this frontal view. The falciform ligament divides the lateral (segments 2 & 3) from the medial (segments 4A & 4B) left lobe. The horizontal planes separating the superior from the inferior segments follow the course of the right and left portal veins. An oblique vertical plane through the middle hepatic vein, gallbladder fossa and IVC divides the right & left lobes. (Bottom) Inferior view of the liver shows that the caudate is entirely posterior, abutting the IVC, ligamentum venosum & porta hepatis. In this view, a plane through the IVC and gallbladder approximately divides the left & right lobes.

LIVER

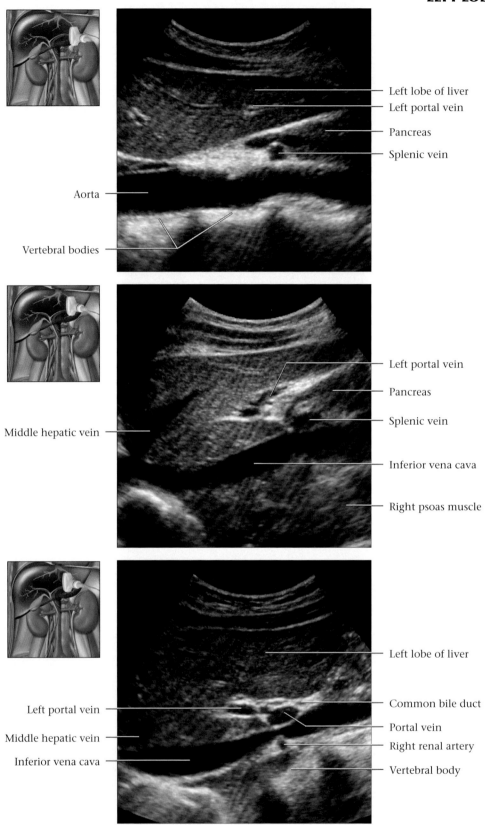

(Top) First of three sagittal ultrasound images of the left lobe of the liver, moving from left to right. (Middle) Sagittal ultrasound of the left lobe cutting through the inferior vena cava and medial aspect of the right psoas muscle. The middle hepatic vein is just coming into view joining the inferior vena cava. Note the triangular shape and sharp borders of the left lobe of the liver on sagittal scans. (Bottom) Sagittal ultrasound of the left lobe of the liver cutting through the common bile duct and portal vein which is seen anterior to the inferior vena cava.

LIVER

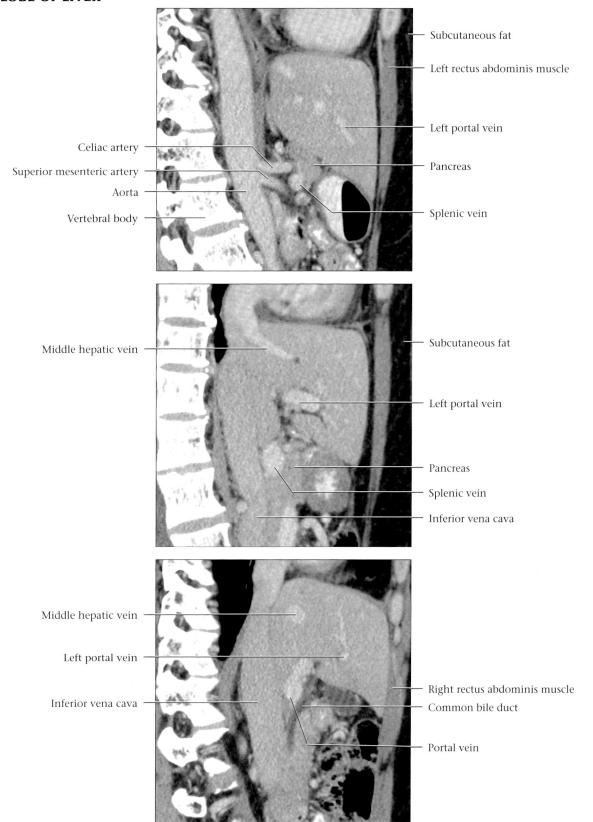

Subcutaneous fat

Left rectus abdominis muscle

Left portal vein

Celiac artery

Pancreas

Superior mesenteric artery

Aorta

Vertebral body

Splenic vein

Middle hepatic vein

Subcutaneous fat

Left portal vein

Pancreas

Splenic vein

Inferior vena cava

Middle hepatic vein

Left portal vein

Inferior vena cava

Right rectus abdominis muscle

Common bile duct

Portal vein

(Top) First of three correlative sagittal CT images. The left lobe of the liver is seen anterior to the aorta. (Middle) Sagittal correlative CT cutting through the inferior vena cava. Note that the middle hepatic vein is just coming into view joining the inferior vena cava. (Bottom) Sagittal CT of the left lobe of the liver, just to the right of midline, showing the common bile duct and the portal vein.

LIVER

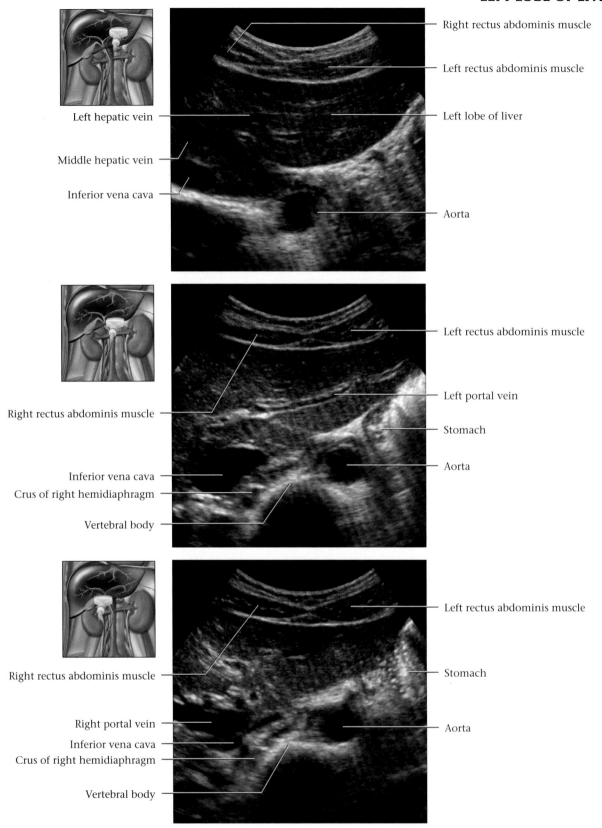

(Top) First of three transverse ultrasound images of the left lobe of the liver, just below the confluence of the hepatic veins, with the left hepatic vein coming into view. **(Middle)** Transverse ultrasound of the left lobe of the liver at the level of the left portal vein. **(Bottom)** Transverse ultrasound of the left lobe of the liver at the level of the right portal vein. Note on transverse scans the left lobe is wedge-shaped, tapering to the left. The hepatic parenchymal echoes are mid-gray, with a sponge-like pattern interrupted by vessels.

LIVER

LEFT LOBE OF LIVER

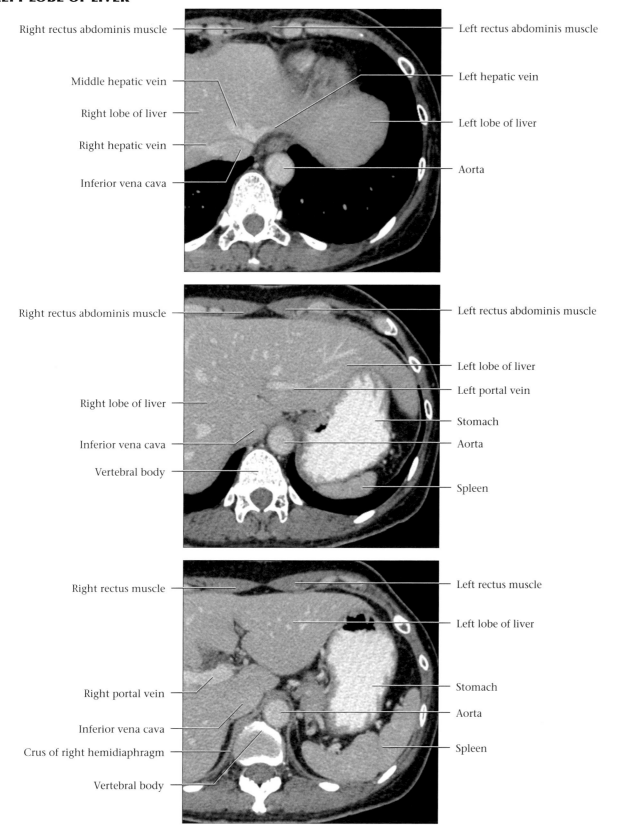

Right rectus abdominis muscle

Middle hepatic vein

Right lobe of liver

Right hepatic vein

Inferior vena cava

Left rectus abdominis muscle

Left hepatic vein

Left lobe of liver

Aorta

Right rectus abdominis muscle

Right lobe of liver

Inferior vena cava

Vertebral body

Left rectus abdominis muscle

Left lobe of liver

Left portal vein

Stomach

Aorta

Spleen

Right rectus muscle

Right portal vein

Inferior vena cava

Crus of right hemidiaphragm

Vertebral body

Left rectus muscle

Left lobe of liver

Stomach

Aorta

Spleen

(Top) Correlative transverse CT of the left lobe of the liver just below the confluence of the hepatic veins with the left hepatic vein coming into view. **(Middle)** Correlative transverse CT of the left lobe of the liver at the level of the left portal vein. **(Bottom)** Correlative transverse CT of the left lobe of the liver at the level of the right portal vein.

LIVER

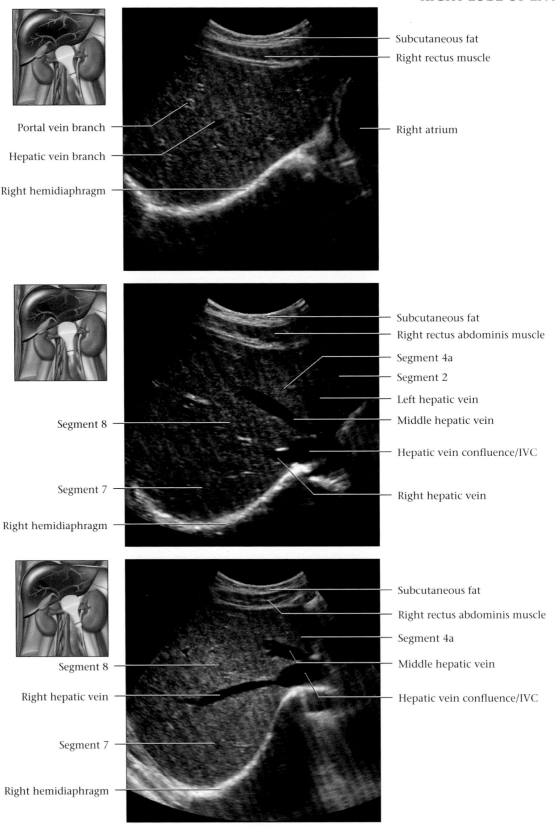

Top image labels:
- Subcutaneous fat
- Right rectus muscle
- Right atrium
- Portal vein branch
- Hepatic vein branch
- Right hemidiaphragm

Middle image labels:
- Subcutaneous fat
- Right rectus abdominis muscle
- Segment 4a
- Segment 2
- Left hepatic vein
- Middle hepatic vein
- Hepatic vein confluence/IVC
- Right hepatic vein
- Segment 8
- Segment 7
- Right hemidiaphragm

Bottom image labels:
- Subcutaneous fat
- Right rectus abdominis muscle
- Segment 4a
- Middle hepatic vein
- Hepatic vein confluence/IVC
- Segment 8
- Right hepatic vein
- Segment 7
- Right hemidiaphragm

(Top) Subcostal, transverse, oblique ultrasound of the right lobe of the liver with cranial angulation. This view is particularly useful for visualization of the subdiaphragmatic portion of the right lobe of the liver. Note the heart (right atrium) coming into view on the left of the image. **(Middle)** Subcostal, transverse, oblique ultrasound of the right lobe of the liver with slight cranial angulation cutting through the hepatic vein confluence. This is a useful view for identifying the plane of the hepatic veins to designate liver segments. **(Bottom)** Subcostal transverse oblique ultrasound view of the right lobe of the liver with slight cranial angulation cutting through the middle and right hepatic veins. This is a useful view for identifying the plane of the hepatic veins to designate liver segments.

LIVER

RIGHT LOBE OF LIVER

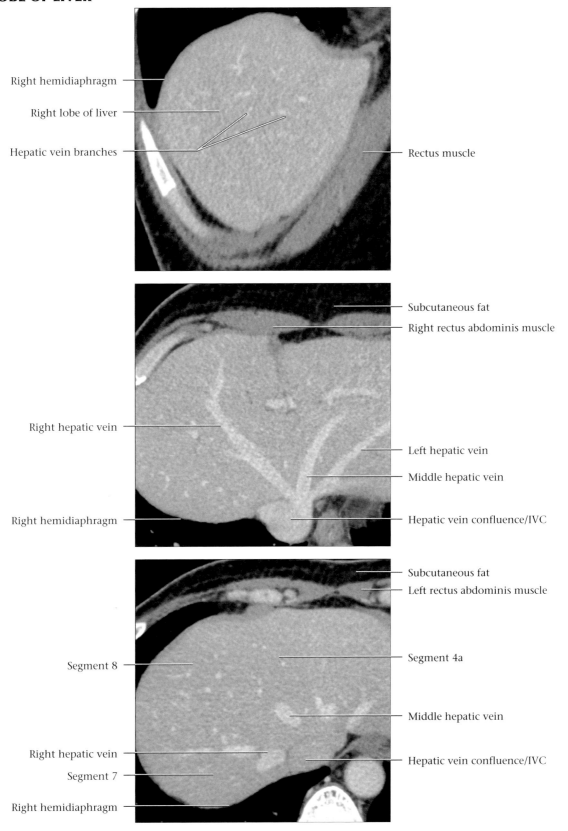

Right hemidiaphragm

Right lobe of liver

Hepatic vein branches

Rectus muscle

Subcutaneous fat

Right rectus abdominis muscle

Right hepatic vein

Left hepatic vein

Middle hepatic vein

Right hemidiaphragm

Hepatic vein confluence/IVC

Subcutaneous fat

Left rectus abdominis muscle

Segment 8

Segment 4a

Middle hepatic vein

Right hepatic vein

Hepatic vein confluence/IVC

Segment 7

Right hemidiaphragm

(Top) Correlative, transverse, oblique CT image showing the subdiaphragmatic portion of the right lobe of the liver. **(Middle)** Correlative, transverse, oblique CT image of the right lobe of the liver cutting through the hepatic vein confluence. Note how hepatic vein branches enlarge towards the confluence. **(Bottom)** Correlative, coronal, oblique CT image of the liver cutting through the middle and right hepatic veins. These planes are useful for identifying the plane of the hepatic veins to designate liver segments.

LIVER

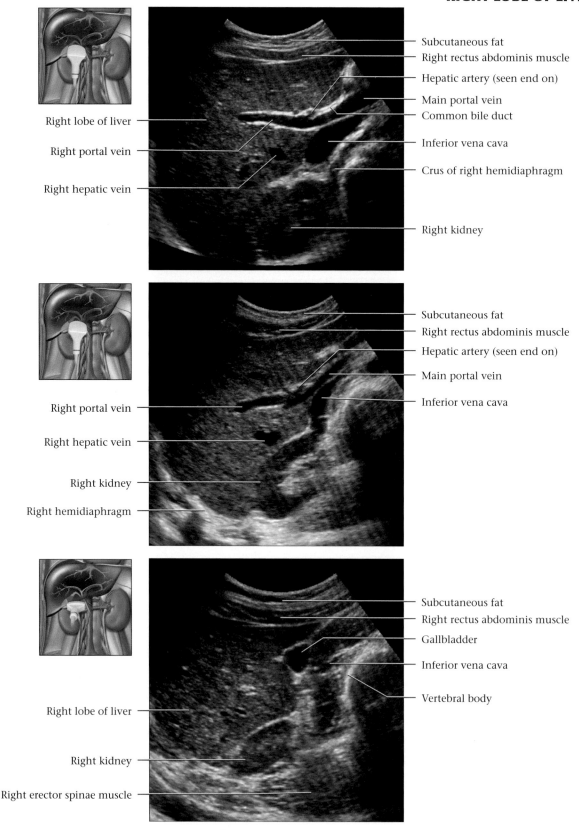

(Top) Subcostal transverse ultrasound of the right lobe of the liver at the level of the right portal vein, main portal vein and common bile duct. **(Middle)** Subcostal transverse ultrasound of the right lobe of the liver at the level of the right portal vein and main portal vein just inferior to the previous image. **(Bottom)** Subcostal transverse ultrasound of the right lobe of the liver at the level of the lower pole of the right kidney and gallbladder. Compare the reflectivity of the walls of the portal vein to hepatic vein walls. Portal veins have fibromuscular walls and hence are more reflective on ultrasound. Reflectivity of walls also depends on the angle of interrogation; a portal vein cut at more oblique angles has a less apparent wall.

LIVER

RIGHT LOBE OF LIVER

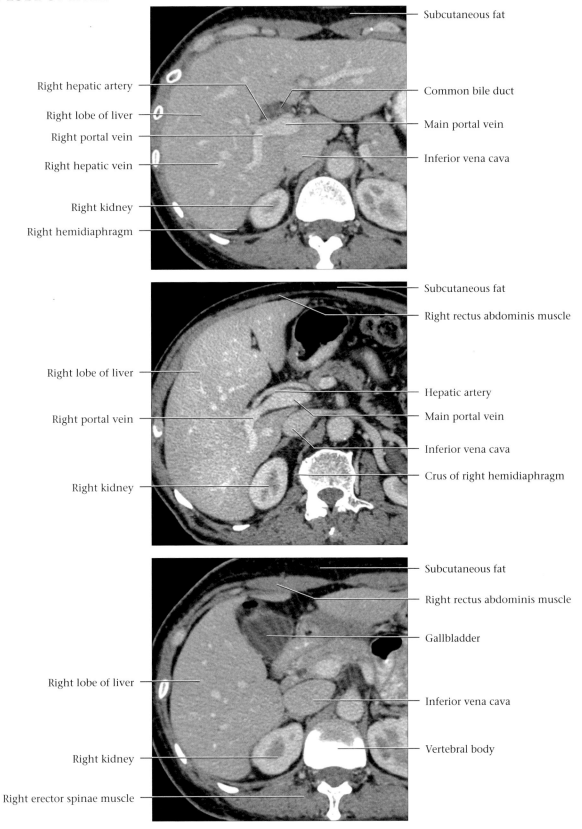

Subcutaneous fat

Right hepatic artery

Right lobe of liver

Right portal vein

Right hepatic vein

Right kidney

Right hemidiaphragm

Common bile duct

Main portal vein

Inferior vena cava

Subcutaneous fat

Right rectus abdominis muscle

Right lobe of liver

Right portal vein

Right kidney

Hepatic artery

Main portal vein

Inferior vena cava

Crus of right hemidiaphragm

Subcutaneous fat

Right rectus abdominis muscle

Gallbladder

Right lobe of liver

Inferior vena cava

Vertebral body

Right kidney

Right erector spinae muscle

(Top) Correlative transverse CT of the right lobe of the liver at the level of the right portal vein, main portal vein and common bile duct. **(Middle)** Correlative transverse CT of the right lobe of the liver at the level of the right portal vein and main portal vein, just inferior to the previous image. Note how branches portal veins diverge from the main portal vein. **(Bottom)** Correlative transverse CT of the right lobe of the liver at the level of the gallbladder.

LIVER

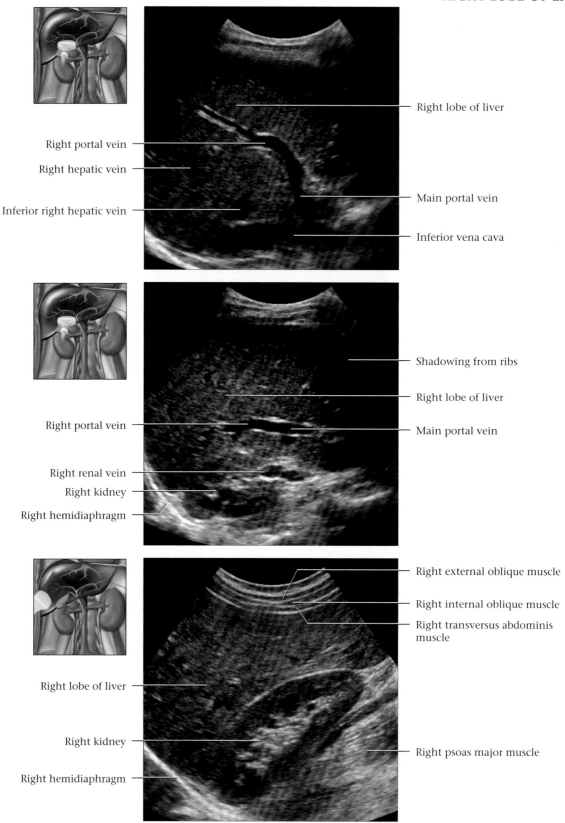

Right lobe of liver

Right portal vein

Right hepatic vein

Inferior right hepatic vein

Main portal vein

Inferior vena cava

Shadowing from ribs

Right lobe of liver

Right portal vein

Main portal vein

Right renal vein

Right kidney

Right hemidiaphragm

Right external oblique muscle

Right internal oblique muscle

Right transversus abdominis muscle

Right lobe of liver

Right kidney

Right psoas major muscle

Right hemidiaphragm

(Top) Intercostal transverse ultrasound of the right lobe of the liver through the intercostal window cutting through the main portal vein. This is a useful method for visualization of the main portal vein especially in patients who have small livers (e.g., in cirrhosis) or in patients with a large amount of bowel gas. **(Middle)** Intercostal transverse ultrasound of the right lobe of the liver through the intercostal window cutting through the main portal vein and right portal vein at a level inferior to the previous image. This is a useful window for assessment of liver parenchymal lesions in the right lobe of the liver. It is important to keep the probe parallel to the intercostal space to avoid shadowing from the ribs. **(Bottom)** Posterolateral intercostal view of the right lobe of the liver angling to achieve a longitudinal view of the right kidney.

LIVER

RIGHT LOBE OF LIVER

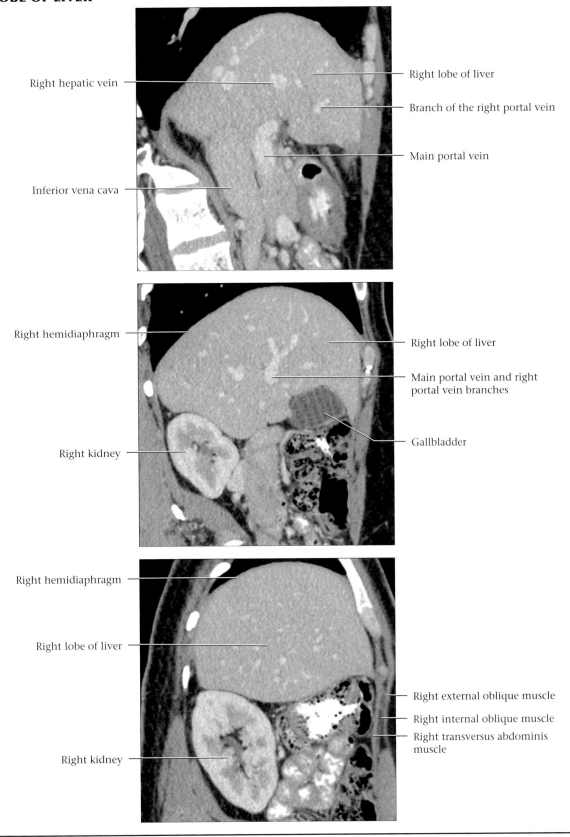

(Top) Correlative oblique CT image from multiplanar reconstruction at a plane showing the inferior vena cava and main portal vein. **(Middle)** Correlative oblique CT image from multiplanar reconstruction at a plane showing the gallbladder and superior pole of the right kidney. Note how branches of the portal vein diverge from the main portal vein. **(Bottom)** Correlative oblique CT image from multiplanar reconstruction at a plane showing most of the right kidney. For hepatic tumor surgery it is essential to accurately depict lobar and segmental anatomy, biliary drainage and blood supply. A combination of axial, sagittal, 3D imaging using multidetector CT, magnetic resonance imaging and ultrasound may be required.

LIVER

Subcutaneous fat

Right rectus abdominis muscle

Left lobe of liver

Middle hepatic vein

Portal vein

Inferior vena cava

Right renal artery

Subcutaneous fat

Right rectus abdominis muscle

Left lobe of liver

Portal vein

Middle hepatic vein

Inferior vena cava

Pulsatile flow in proximal IVC with mixed color signal

Proximal intrahepatic IVC

Pulsatile Doppler waveform reflecting right atrial pulsation

−40
−20
cm/s
−20
−40

(Top) Sagittal, longitudinal, grayscale ultrasound of the intrahepatic inferior vena cava. (Middle) Sagittal, longitudinal, color Doppler ultrasound of the intrahepatic inferior vena cava. Note the pulsatile flow in the proximal inferior vena cava with mixed color signal. (Bottom) Spectral Doppler ultrasound of the intrahepatic inferior vena cava. Note the chaotic, pulsatile waveform in the proximal inferior vena cava reflecting phasic variations and right atrial pulsation.

INFERIOR VENA CAVA

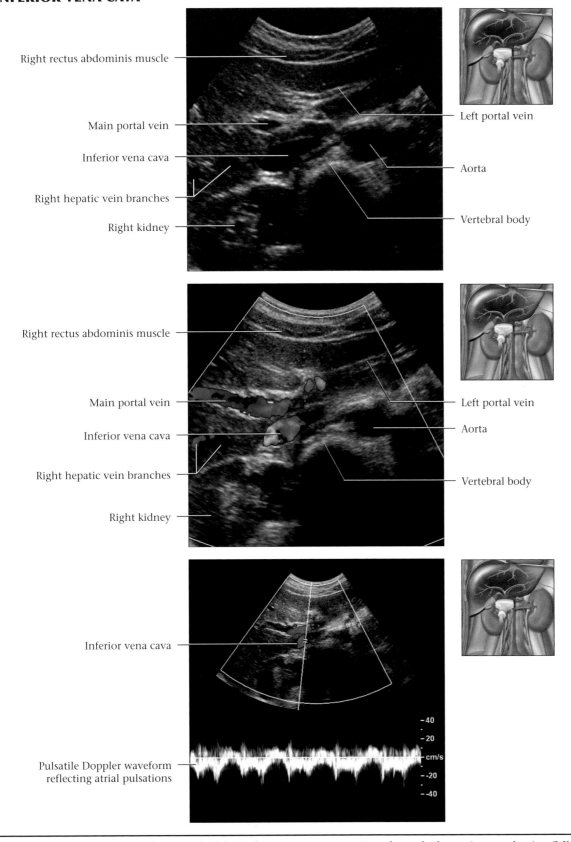

Right rectus abdominis muscle

Main portal vein

Inferior vena cava

Right hepatic vein branches

Right kidney

Left portal vein

Aorta

Vertebral body

Right rectus abdominis muscle

Main portal vein

Inferior vena cava

Right hepatic vein branches

Right kidney

Left portal vein

Aorta

Vertebral body

Inferior vena cava

Pulsatile Doppler waveform reflecting atrial pulsations

-40
-20
cm/s
--20
--40

(Top) Transverse grayscale ultrasound of the inferior vena cava cutting through the main portal vein. **(Middle)** Transverse color Doppler ultrasound of the inferior vena cava cutting through the main portal vein. **(Bottom)** Spectral Doppler image of the intrahepatic inferior vena cava. Note the chaotic, pulsatile waveform in the proximal inferior vena cava reflecting phasic variations and right atrial pulsation.

LIVER

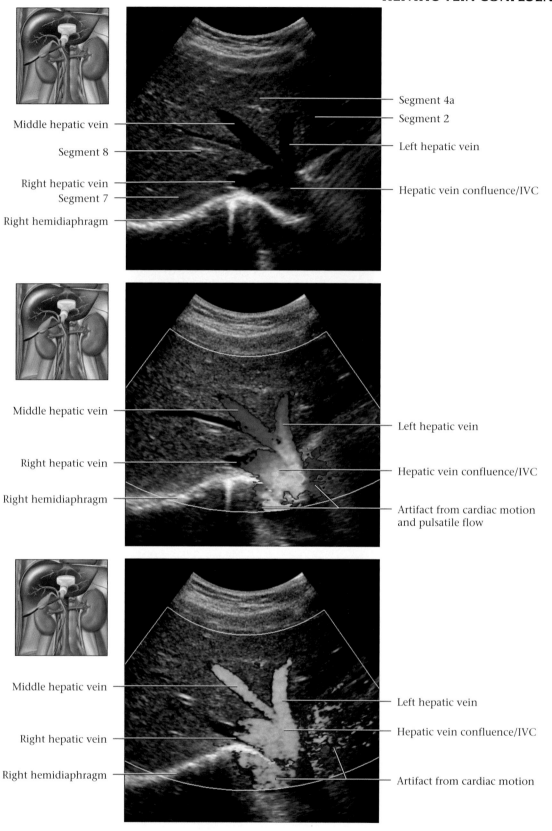

Segment 4a
Segment 2
Middle hepatic vein
Left hepatic vein
Segment 8
Right hepatic vein
Hepatic vein confluence/IVC
Segment 7
Right hemidiaphragm

Middle hepatic vein
Left hepatic vein
Right hepatic vein
Hepatic vein confluence/IVC
Right hemidiaphragm
Artifact from cardiac motion and pulsatile flow

Middle hepatic vein
Left hepatic vein
Right hepatic vein
Hepatic vein confluence/IVC
Right hemidiaphragm
Artifact from cardiac motion

(**Top**) Subcostal, transverse, grayscale ultrasound of the hepatic vein confluence. A degree of cranial angulation of the transducer is generally required to evaluate this part of the liver. Note the increasing size of hepatic veins towards the confluence. (**Middle**) Transverse color Doppler ultrasound of the hepatic vein confluence. Artifact from cardiac motion and pulsatile flow is common at this location. (**Bottom**) Transverse power Doppler ultrasound view of the hepatic vein confluence. Although power Doppler is more sensitive than color Doppler in the detection of flow, unlike color Doppler it is unable to provide information about direction of flow.

LIVER

LEFT HEPATIC VEIN

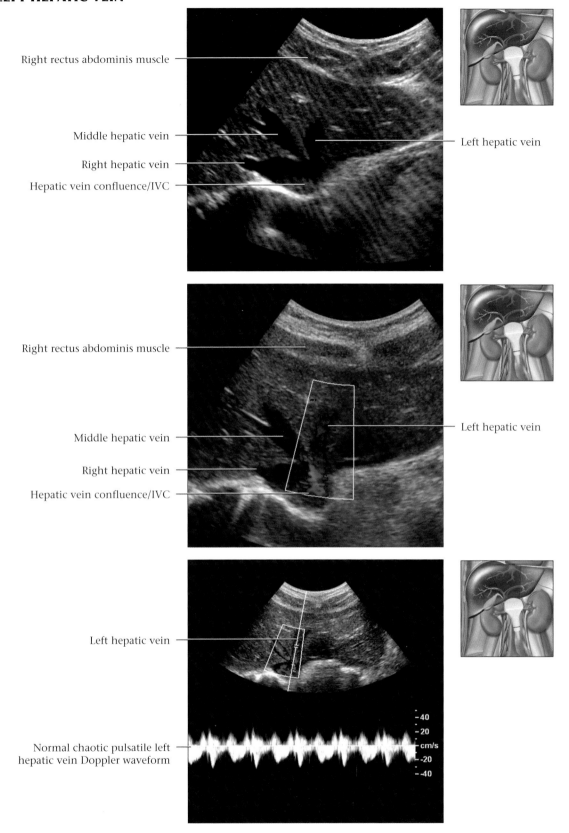

Right rectus abdominis muscle

Middle hepatic vein

Right hepatic vein

Hepatic vein confluence/IVC

Left hepatic vein

Right rectus abdominis muscle

Middle hepatic vein

Right hepatic vein

Hepatic vein confluence/IVC

Left hepatic vein

Left hepatic vein

Normal chaotic pulsatile left hepatic vein Doppler waveform

- 40
- 20
cm/s
- 20
- 40

(Top) Subcostal, transverse, grayscale ultrasound of the left hepatic vein as it enters the hepatic vein confluence. A degree of cranial angulation of the transducer is generally required to evaluate this part of the liver. The left hepatic vein runs between the medial and lateral segments of the left lobe and is frequently duplicated. (Middle) Subcostal, transverse, color Doppler ultrasound of the hepatic vein confluence. (Bottom) Spectral Doppler ultrasound image of the left hepatic vein as it enters the hepatic vein confluence. Note the normal chaotic pulsatile Doppler waveform which results from a combination of phasic variation and transmission of right atrial pulsations into the vein.

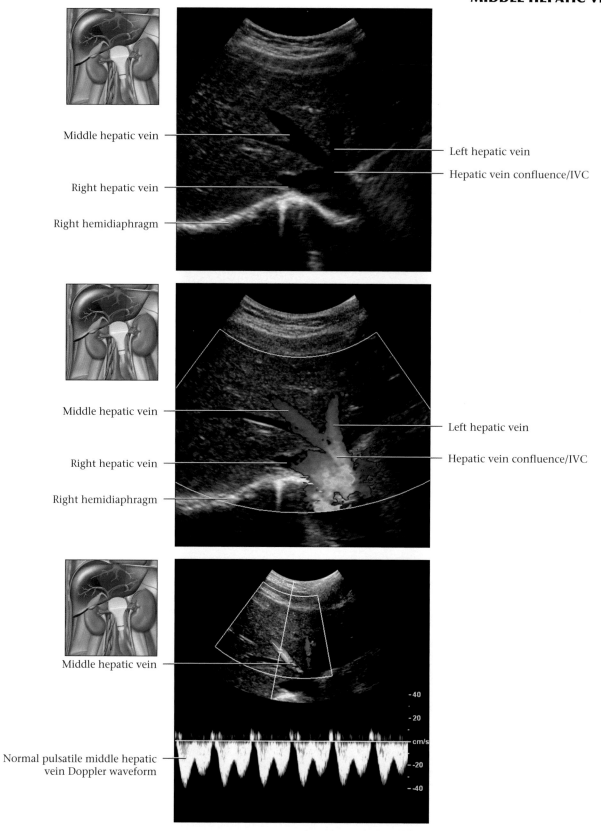

Middle hepatic vein

Right hepatic vein

Right hemidiaphragm

Left hepatic vein

Hepatic vein confluence/IVC

Middle hepatic vein

Right hepatic vein

Right hemidiaphragm

Left hepatic vein

Hepatic vein confluence/IVC

Middle hepatic vein

Normal pulsatile middle hepatic vein Doppler waveform

(Top) Subcostal, transverse, grayscale ultrasound (with cranial angulation) of the middle hepatic vein as it enters the hepatic vein confluence. The middle hepatic vein lies in a sagittal or parasagittal plane between the right and left hepatic lobes. (Middle) Transverse color Doppler ultrasound image of the middle hepatic vein as it enters the hepatic vein confluence. (Bottom) Spectral Doppler ultrasound image of the middle hepatic vein as it enters the hepatic vein confluence. Note the normal chaotic pulsatile Doppler waveform which results from a combination of phasic variation and transmission of right atrial pulsations into the vein.

LIVER

RIGHT HEPATIC VEIN

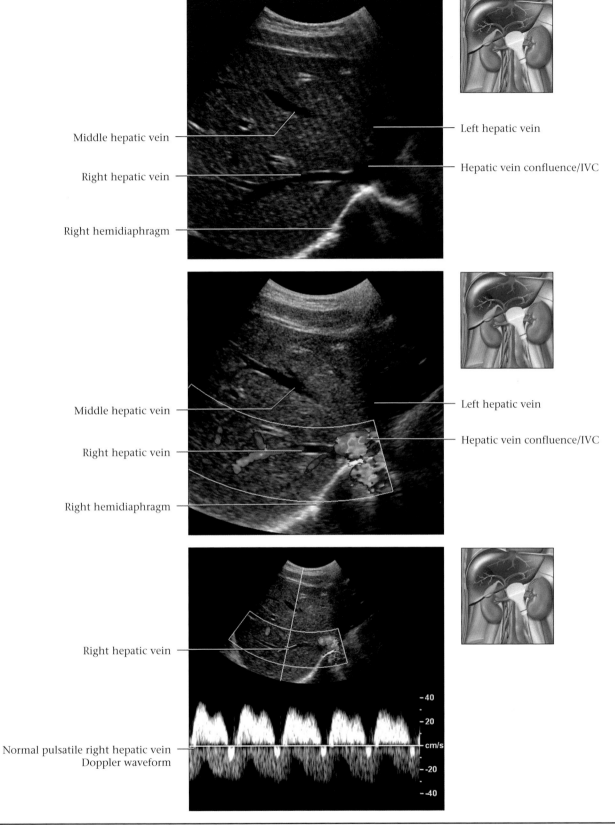

Middle hepatic vein

Right hepatic vein

Right hemidiaphragm

Left hepatic vein

Hepatic vein confluence/IVC

Middle hepatic vein

Right hepatic vein

Right hemidiaphragm

Left hepatic vein

Hepatic vein confluence/IVC

Right hepatic vein

Normal pulsatile right hepatic vein Doppler waveform

(Top) Subcostal, transverse, grayscale ultrasound of the right hepatic vein as it enters the hepatic vein confluence. The right hepatic vein runs in a coronal plane between the anterior and posterior segments of the right hepatic lobe and may be absent in 6%. (Middle) Transverse color Doppler ultrasound of the right hepatic vein as it enters the hepatic vein confluence. (Bottom) Spectral Doppler ultrasound of the right hepatic vein as it enters the hepatic vein confluence. Note the normal chaotic pulsatile Doppler waveform which results from a combination of phasic variation and transmission of right atrial pulsations into the vein.

LIVER

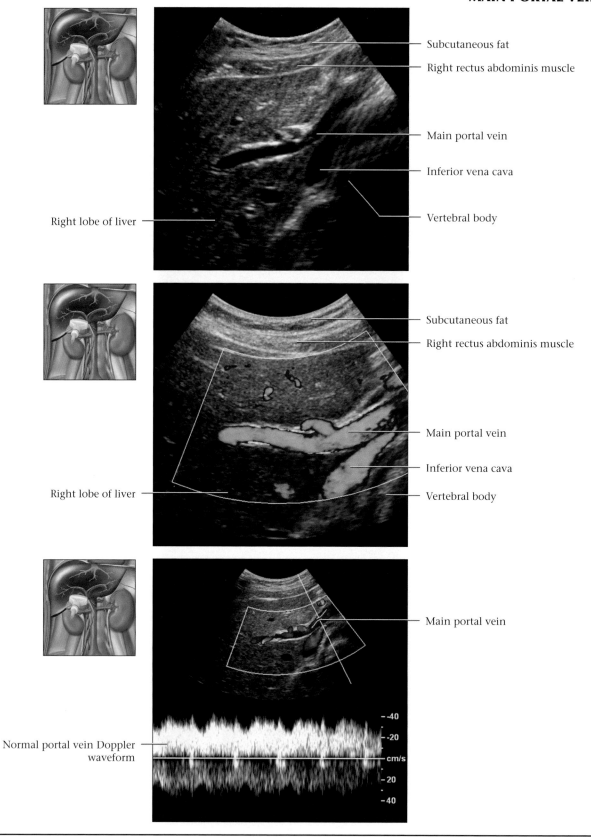

Subcutaneous fat

Right rectus abdominis muscle

Main portal vein

Inferior vena cava

Right lobe of liver

Vertebral body

Subcutaneous fat

Right rectus abdominis muscle

Main portal vein

Inferior vena cava

Right lobe of liver

Vertebral body

Main portal vein

Normal portal vein Doppler waveform

-40
-20
cm/s
-20
-40

(Top) Subcostal, transverse, grayscale ultrasound of the main portal vein and inferior vena cava. (Middle) Subcostal, transverse, power Doppler ultrasound of the main portal vein and inferior vena cava. (Bottom) Spectral Doppler ultrasound of the main portal vein showing normal phasic waveform. Normal portal waveform has an undulating appearance due to variations in respiration and cardiac activity.

LIVER

MAIN PORTAL VEIN

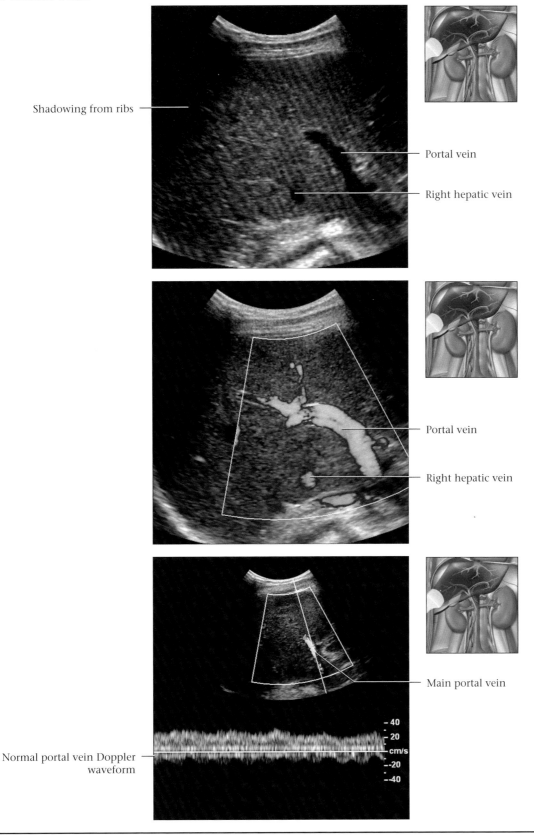

Shadowing from ribs

Portal vein

Right hepatic vein

Portal vein

Right hepatic vein

Main portal vein

Normal portal vein Doppler waveform

(Top) Intercostal grayscale ultrasound of the main portal vein. It is important to maintain the transducer parallel to the intercostal space to minimize shadowing from ribs. (Middle) Intercostal power Doppler ultrasound of the main portal vein. (Bottom) Spectral Doppler ultrasound of the main portal vein showing normal phasic waveform. Normal portal flow is hepatopetal, absent or reverse flow may be seen in portal hypertension. The mean flow velocity is 15-18 cm/sec with a wide normal range.

LIVER

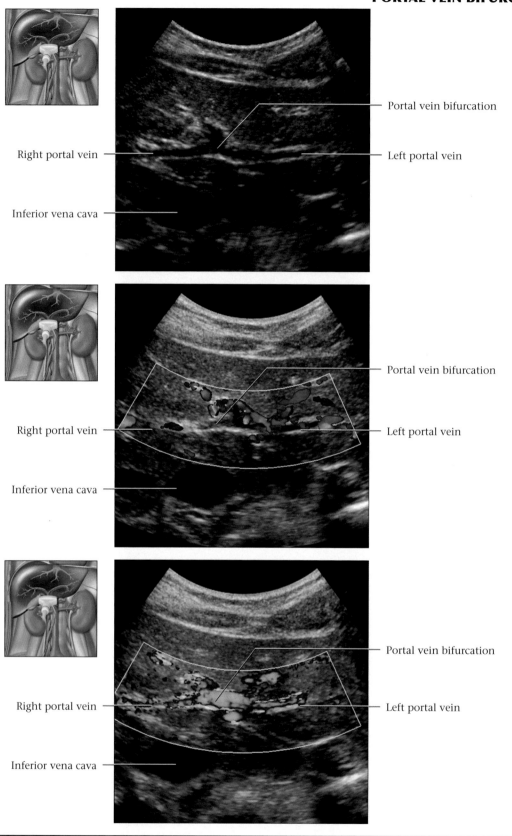

Right portal vein — Portal vein bifurcation

Left portal vein

Inferior vena cava

Right portal vein — Portal vein bifurcation

Left portal vein

Inferior vena cava

Right portal vein — Portal vein bifurcation

Left portal vein

Inferior vena cava

(Top) Subcostal, transverse, grayscale ultrasound of the portal vein bifurcation. **(Middle)** Color Doppler ultrasound of the portal vein bifurcation. Note the relative absence of color signal in the portal vein bifurcation on this view as it is almost at 90 degrees with the transducer. **(Bottom)** Power Doppler ultrasound of the portal vein bifurcation. Note the relative abundance of flow signal in the portal vein bifurcation when compared with the color Doppler image as power Doppler is less dependent on the Doppler angle. However, it is unable to provide information about flow direction.

LIVER

LEFT PORTAL VEIN

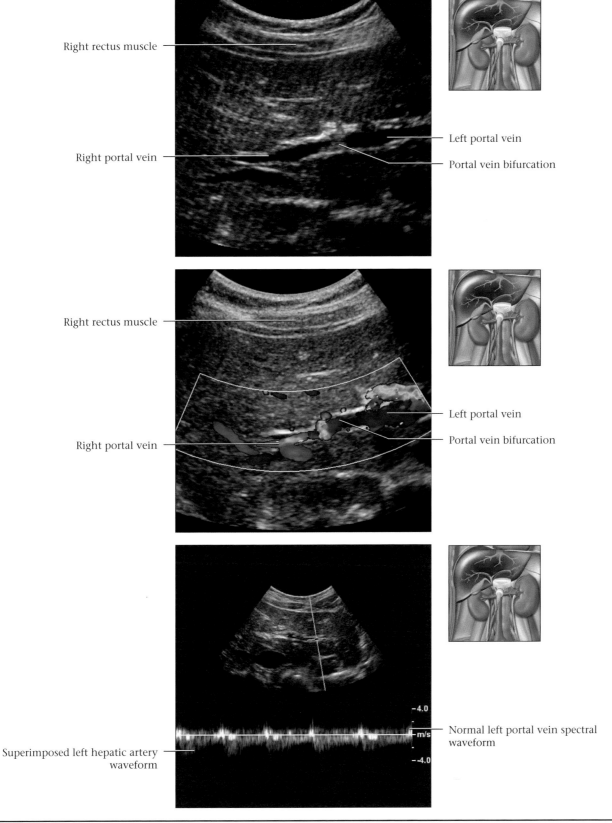

Right rectus muscle

Right portal vein

Left portal vein

Portal vein bifurcation

Right rectus muscle

Left portal vein

Right portal vein

Portal vein bifurcation

Superimposed left hepatic artery waveform

Normal left portal vein spectral waveform

−4.0

m/s

−4.0

(**Top**) Subcostal, transverse, grayscale ultrasound of the left portal vein as it branches out from the portal vein bifurcation. (**Middle**) Color Doppler ultrasound of the left portal vein as it branches out from the portal vein bifurcation. (**Bottom**) Spectral Doppler ultrasound of the left portal vein shows superimposed spectral waveform from the left hepatic artery. Branches of the portal vein can be traced towards the porta hepatis.

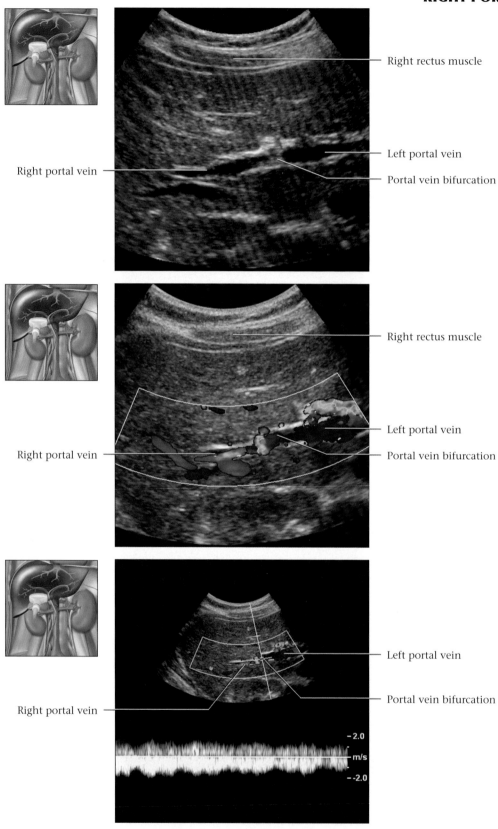

Right rectus muscle

Right portal vein

Left portal vein

Portal vein bifurcation

Right rectus muscle

Right portal vein

Left portal vein

Portal vein bifurcation

Left portal vein

Portal vein bifurcation

Right portal vein

− 2.0

− m/s

− −2.0

(Top) Subcostal, transverse, grayscale ultrasound of the right portal vein as it branches out from the portal vein bifurcation. (Middle) Color Doppler ultrasound of the right portal vein as it branches out from the portal vein bifurcation. (Bottom) Spectral Doppler ultrasound of the right portal vein showing normal phasic pattern. Portal vein branches decrease in size as they branch away from the porta hepatis.

LIVER

COMMON HEPATIC ARTERY

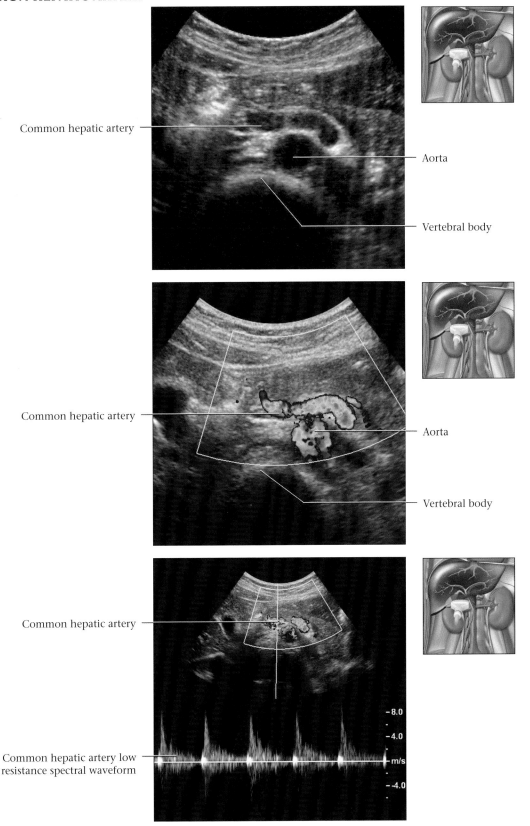

Common hepatic artery

Aorta

Vertebral body

Common hepatic artery

Aorta

Vertebral body

Common hepatic artery

Common hepatic artery low
resistance spectral waveform

−8.0

−4.0

−m/s

−4.0

(Top) Transverse grayscale ultrasound of the common hepatic artery above its origin from the celiac axis (not imaged) and hooking towards the right. There are wide variations of sites of origin of the common hepatic artery. The sonologist must be aware of these variations, but they are best assessed by CT angiogram, digital subtraction angiography and magnetic resonance angiography. **(Middle)** Transverse color Doppler ultrasound of the common hepatic artery. **(Bottom)** Spectral Doppler ultrasound waveform of the common hepatic artery showing low resistance flow characteristics with a moderate amount of continuous forward flow throughout diastole.

LIVER

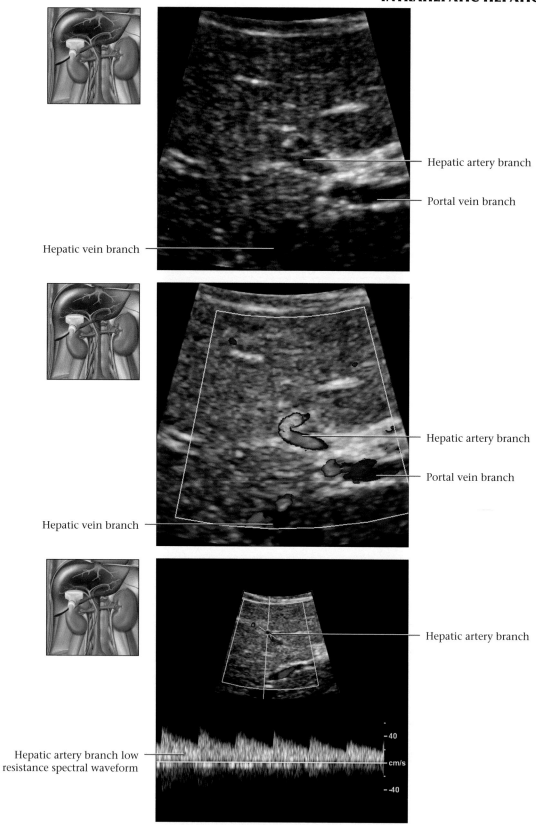

Hepatic artery branch

Portal vein branch

Hepatic vein branch

Hepatic artery branch

Portal vein branch

Hepatic vein branch

Hepatic artery branch

Hepatic artery branch low
resistance spectral waveform

-40

cm/s

-40

(Top) Zoomed grayscale ultrasound of a hepatic artery branch, a portal vein branch and a hepatic vein branch. Note the reflective wall of the portal vein branch and the lack of reflective wall of the hepatic vein branch. **(Middle)** Zoomed color Doppler ultrasound of a hepatic artery branch, a portal vein branch and a hepatic vein branch. Note the color flow within these branches. **(Bottom)** Spectral Doppler ultrasound waveform of the hepatic artery branch showing low resistance flow characteristics with a large amount of continuous forward flow throughout diastole.

LIVER

PORTAL HYPERTENSION

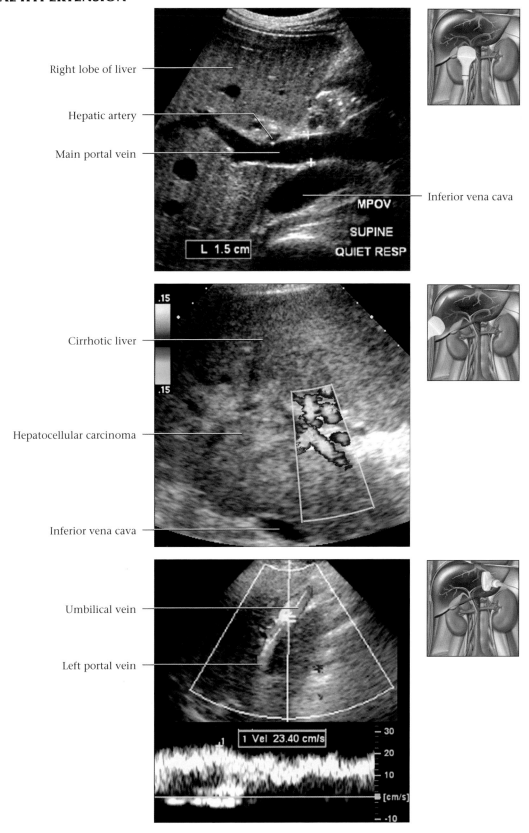

Right lobe of liver

Hepatic artery

Main portal vein

Inferior vena cava

MPOV

SUPINE

QUIET RESP

L 1.5 cm

Cirrhotic liver

Hepatocellular carcinoma

Inferior vena cava

Umbilical vein

Left portal vein

1 Vel 23.40 cm/s

(Top) Subcostal grayscale transverse ultrasound shows a dilated main portal vein 15 mm in caliber, characteristic of portal vein hypertension. The normal portal vein should not be more than 13 mm in diameter. (Middle) Oblique color Doppler ultrasound shows cavernous transformation of the portal vein in a case of portal hypertension. There are numerous collateral veins in the porta hepatis. Note the cirrhotic liver parenchyma with a ill-defined mass representing a hepatocellular carcinoma. (Bottom) Sagittal color Doppler ultrasound shows patency of the umbilical vein coming frpom the left portal vein. The huge collateral courses along the inferior border of the liver and towards the anterior abdominal wall. Note the high peak velocity (23 cm/sec).

LIVER

— Left lobe of liver

— Left portal vein

— Right lobe of liver

Main portal vein (with color flow and intraluminal echoes) —

— Right lobe of liver

— Right portal vein

(**Top**) Transverse color Doppler ultrasound of the left portal vein with absent color flow, indicating thrombosis. (**Middle**) Oblique color Doppler ultrasound of the main portal vein with color flow as well as echoes within the lumen. Features are suggestive of non-occlusive thrombosis. (**Bottom**) Oblique spectral Doppler of the same patient as previous image. There is color flow within the right portal vein and normal flow velocity (15 cm/sec), indicating that the previously imaged main portal vein thrombosis is not substantially occlusive.

LIVER

TRANSPLANT HEPATIC ARTERY STENOSIS

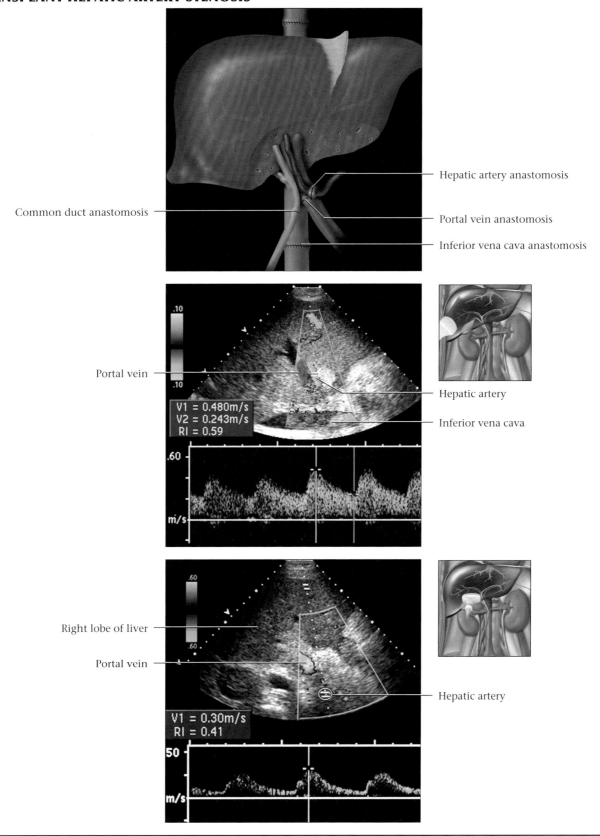

Common duct anastomosis

Hepatic artery anastomosis

Portal vein anastomosis

Inferior vena cava anastomosis

Portal vein

V1 = 0.480m/s
V2 = 0.243m/s
RI = 0.59

Hepatic artery

Inferior vena cava

Right lobe of liver

Portal vein

V1 = 0.30m/s
RI = 0.41

Hepatic artery

(Top) Graphic shows the typical anastomoses in a liver transplant. These are end-to-end anastomoses for the inferior vena cava, portal vein and common duct. The hepatic artery is reconstructed creating a "fish-mouth" anastomosis. **(Middle)** Oblique pulsed Doppler ultrasound on first post transplant day shows normal hepatic artery Doppler waveform at porta hepatis. **(Bottom)** Oblique pulsed Doppler ultrasound two days post transplant shows damped hepatic arterial Doppler waveforms due to stenosis. Peak systolic velocity is 30 cm/s. Resistive index is 0.41.

BILIARY SYSTEM

Terminology

Abbreviations
- Extrahepatic biliary structures
  - Gallbladder (GB)
  - Cystic duct (CD)
  - Right hepatic (RH) and left hepatic (LH) ducts
  - Common hepatic duct (CHD)
  - Common bile duct (CBD)

Definitions
- Proximal/distal biliary tree
  - Proximal represents portion of biliary tree that is in relative proximity to liver and hepatocytes
  - Distal refers to caudal end closer to bowel
- Central/peripheral
  - Central denotes biliary ducts close to porta hepatis
  - Peripheral refers to higher order branches of intrahepatic biliary tree extending to hepatic parenchyma

Imaging Anatomy

Overview
- Biliary ducts convey bile from liver to duodenum
  - Bile is produced continuously by liver, stored & concentrated by gallbladder (GB), released intermittently by GB contraction in response to presence of fat in duodenum
  - Hepatocytes form bile → bile canaliculi → interlobular biliary ducts → collecting bile ducts → right & left hepatic ducts → common hepatic duct → common bile duct
- Bile duct forms in free edge of lesser omentum by union of cystic duct and common hepatic duct
  - Length of duct: 5-15 cm depending on point of junction of cystic & common hepatic ducts
  - Duct descends posterior & medial to duodenum, lying on dorsal surface of pancreatic head
  - Bile duct joins with pancreatic duct to form hepaticopancreatic ampulla (of Vater)
  - Ampulla opens into duodenum through major duodenal (hepaticopancreatic) papilla
  - Distal bile duct is thickened into a sphincter (of Boyden) and hepaticopancreatic segment is thickened into a sphincter (of Oddi)
    - Contraction of these sphincters prevents bile from entering duodenum; forces it to collect in GB
    - Relaxation of sphincters in response to parasympathetic stimulation & cholecystokinin (released by duodenum in response to fatty meal)
- Vessels, nerves and lymphatics
  - Arteries
    - Hepatic arteries to intrahepatic ducts
    - Cystic artery to proximal common duct
    - Right hepatic artery to middle part of common duct
    - Gastroduodenal and pancreaticoduodenal arcade to distal common duct
    - Cystic artery to GB (usually from right hepatic artery; variable)
  - Veins

- From intrahepatic ducts → hepatic veins
- From common duct → portal vein (in tributaries)
- From GB directly into liver sinusoids, bypassing portal vein
  - Nerves
    - Sensory: Right phrenic nerve
    - Parasympathetic & sympathetic from celiac ganglion and plexus; contraction of GB & relaxation of biliary sphincters is caused by parasympathetic stimulation, but more important stimulus is from hormone cholecystokinin
  - Lymphatics
    - Same course and name as arterial branches
    - Collect at celiac lymph nodes and node of omental foramen
    - Nodes draining GB are prominent in the porta hepatis and around pancreatic head
- Gallbladder
  - ~ 7-10 cm long, holds up to 50 mL of bile
  - Lies in a shallow fossa on the visceral surface of liver
  - Vertical plane through GB fossa & middle hepatic vein divides left & right hepatic lobes
  - Touches & indents duodenum
  - Fundus is covered with peritoneum & relatively mobile; body & neck are attached to liver & covered by hepatic capsule
  - Fundus: Wide tip of GB, projects below liver edge (usually)
  - Body: Contacts liver, duodenum & transverse colon
  - Neck: Narrowed, tapered and tortuous; joins cystic duct
  - Cystic duct: 3-4 cm long, connects GB to common hepatic duct; marked by spiral folds (of Heister); helps to regulate bile flow to & from GB
- Normal measurement limits of bile ducts
  - CBD/CHD
    - < 6-7 mm in patients without history of biliary disease in most studies
    - Controversy about dilatation related to previous cholecystectomy and old age
  - Intrahepatic ducts
    - Normal diameter of first and higher order branches < 2 mm or < 40% of the diameter of the adjacent portal vein
    - First (i.e., LH duct and RH duct) and second order branches are normally visualized
    - Visualization of third and higher order branches is often abnormal and indicates dilatation

Anatomy-Based Imaging Issues

Imaging Recommendations
- Patient should be fasted for at least 4 hours prior to US examination to ensure GB is not contracted after a meal
- Complete assessment includes scanning the liver, porta hepatis region and pancreas in sagittal, transverse and oblique views
- Subcostal and right intercostal transverse views to align bile ducts and GB along imaging plane for optimal visualization

BILIARY SYSTEM

- Usually structures are better assessed and imaged with patient in full suspended inspiration and in left lateral oblique position
- Harmonic imaging provides improved contrast between bile ducts and adjacent tissues, leading to improved visualization of bile ducts, luminal content and wall
- For imaging of gallstone disease, special maneuvers are recommended
  - Move patient from supine to left lateral decubitus position
    - Demonstrates mobility of gallstones
    - Gravitates small gallstones together to appreciate posterior acoustic shadowing
  - Set the focal zone at the level of posterior acoustic shadowing
    - Maximizes the effect of posterior acoustic shadowing

Imaging Approaches

- Transabdominal ultrasound is an ideal initial investigation for suspected biliary tree or GB pathology
  - Cystic nature of bile ducts and GB, especially if these are dilated, provides inherently high contrast resolution
  - Acoustic window provided by liver and modern state-of-art ultrasound technology provides good spatial resolution
  - Common indications of US for biliary and GB disease include
    - Right upper quadrant/epigastric pain
    - Deranged liver function test or jaundice
    - Suspected gallstone disease
  - Supplemented by various imaging modalities including MR/MRCP and CT
  - US plays a key role in the multimodality evaluation of complex biliary problems

Imaging Pitfalls

- Common pitfalls in the evaluation of GB
  - Posterior shadowing may arise from GB neck, Heister valves of CD or from adjacent gas-filled bowel loops
    - Mimics cholelithiasis
    - Scan after repositioning patient in prone or left lateral decubitus positions
  - Food material within gastric antrum/duodenum
    - Mimics GB filled with gallstones or GB containing milk of calcium
    - During real time scanning carefully evaluate peristaltic activity of involved bowel + oral administration of water
- Common pitfalls in US evaluation of biliary tree
  - Redundancy, elongation or folding of GB neck on itself
    - Mimics dilatation of CHD or proximal CBD
    - Avoided by scanning patient in full suspended inspiration
    - Careful real-time scanning allows separate visualization of CHD/CBD medial to GB neck
  - Presence of gas-filled bowel loops adjacent to distal extrahepatic bile ducts

- Obscure distal biliary tree and render detection of choledocholithiasis difficult
  - Scan with patient in decubitus positions or after oral intake of water
- Gas/particulate material in adjacent duodenum and pancreatic calcification
  - Mimic choledocholithiasis within CBD
- Presence of gas within biliary tree
  - May mimic choledocholithiasis, differentiated by presence of reverberation artifacts
  - Limits US detection of biliary calculus

Key Concepts

- Direct venous drainage of GB into liver bypasses portal venous system, often results in sparing of adjacent liver from generalized steatosis (fatty liver)
- Nodal metastasis from GB carcinoma to peripancreatic nodes may simulate a primary pancreatic tumor
- Sonography: Optimal means of evaluating GB for stones & inflammation (acute cholecystitis); best done in fasting state (distends GB)
- Intrahepatic bile ducts follow branching pattern of portal veins
  - Usually lie immediately anterior to portal vein branch; confluence of hepatic ducts just anterior to bifurcation of right & main portal veins

Clinical Implications

Clinical Importance

- In patients with obstructive jaundice, US plays a key role
  - Differentiates biliary obstruction from liver parenchymal disease
  - Determines presence, level and cause of biliary obstruction
- Common variations of biliary arterial & ductal anatomy result in challenges to avoid injury at surgery
  - CD may run in common sheath with bile duct
  - Anomalous right hepatic ducts may be severed at cholecystectomy
- Close apposition of GB to duodenum can result in fistulous connection with chronic cholecystitis and erosion of gallstone into duodenum
- Obstruction of common bile duct is common
  - Gallstones in distal bile duct
  - Carcinoma arising in pancreatic head or bile duct
  - Result is jaundice due to back up of bile salts into bloodstream

Embryologic Events

- Abnormal embryological development of fetal ductal plate can lead to spectrum of liver & biliary abnormalities including
  - Polycystic liver disease
  - Congenital hepatic fibrosis
  - Biliary hamartomas
  - Caroli disease
  - Choledochal cysts

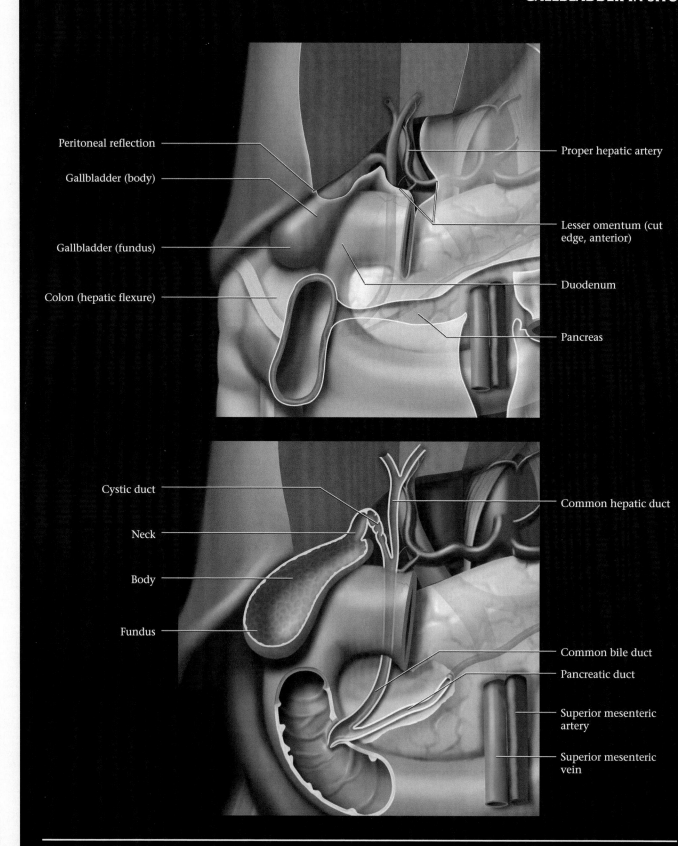

Peritoneal reflection

Gallbladder (body)

Gallbladder (fundus)

Colon (hepatic flexure)

Proper hepatic artery

Lesser omentum (cut edge, anterior)

Duodenum

Pancreas

Cystic duct

Neck

Body

Fundus

Common hepatic duct

Common bile duct

Pancreatic duct

Superior mesenteric artery

Superior mesenteric vein

(Top) The gallbladder is covered with peritoneum, except where it is attached to the liver. The extrahepatic bile duct, hepatic artery & portal vein run in the lesser omentum. The fundus of the gallbladder extends beyond the anterior-inferior edge of the liver and can be in contact with the hepatic flexure of the colon. The body (main portion of the gallbladder) is in contact with the duodenum. **(Bottom)** The neck of the gallbladder narrows before entering the cystic duct, which is distinguished by its tortuous course and irregular lumen. The duct lumen is irregular due to redundant folds of mucosa, called the spiral folds (of Heister), that are believed to regulate the rate of filling and emptying of the gallbladder. The cystic duct joins the hepatic duct to form the common bile duct, which passes behind the duodenum & through the pancreas to enter the duodenum.

BILIARY SYSTEM

ANATOMIC VARIATIONS OF THE BILIARY TREE

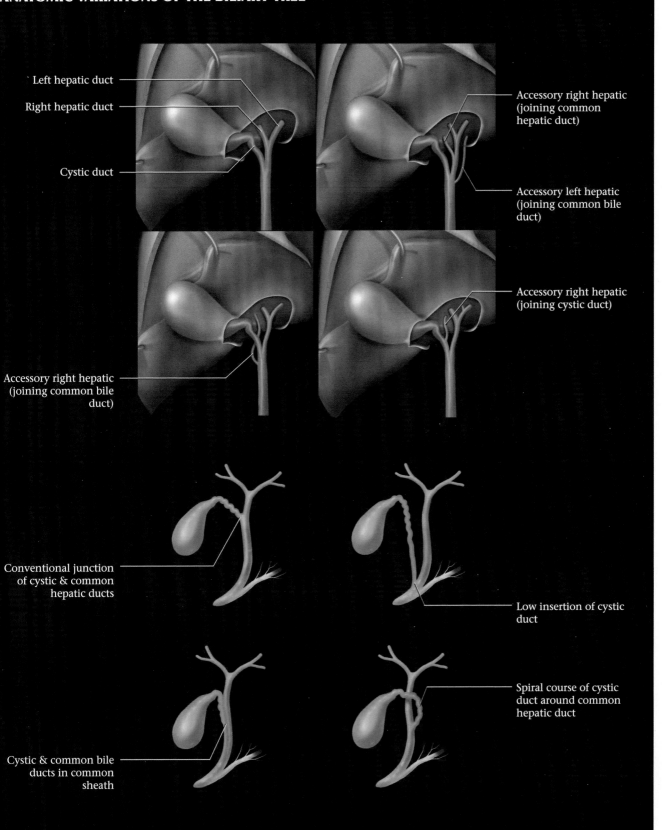

Left hepatic duct

Right hepatic duct

Cystic duct

Accessory right hepatic (joining common hepatic duct)

Accessory left hepatic (joining common bile duct)

Accessory right hepatic (joining cystic duct)

Accessory right hepatic (joining common bile duct)

Conventional junction of cystic & common hepatic ducts

Low insertion of cystic duct

Spiral course of cystic duct around common hepatic duct

Cystic & common bile ducts in common sheath

(Top) Graphic shows the conventional arrangement of the extrahepatic bile ducts, but variations are common (20% of population) and may lead to inadvertent ligation or injury at surgery such as cholecystectomy, where the cystic duct is clamped and transected. Most accessory ducts are on the right side and usually enter the common hepatic duct, but may enter the cystic or common bile duct. Accessory left ducts enter the common bile duct. While referred to as "accessory", these ducts are the sole drainage of bile from at least one hepatic segment. Ligation or laceration can lead to significant hepatic injury or bile peritonitis. (Bottom) The course and insertion of the cystic duct are highly variable, leading to difficulty in isolation and ligation at cholecystectomy. The cystic duct may be mistaken for the common hepatic or common bile duct.

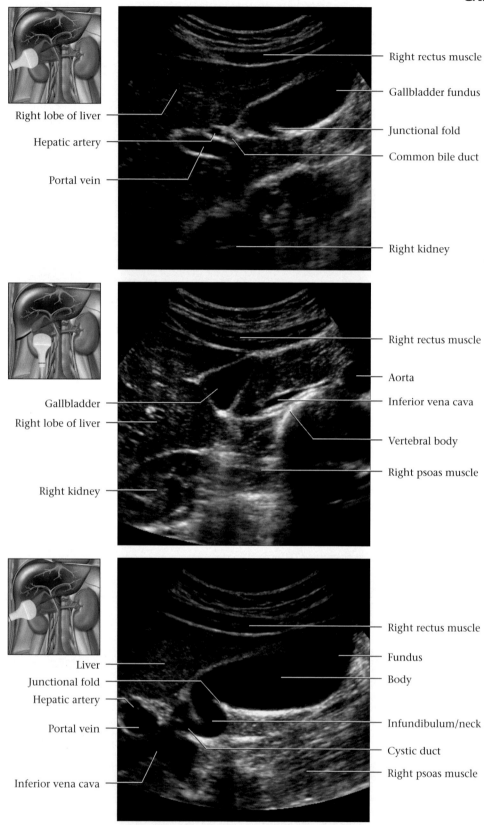

(Top) Subcostal, longitudinal, grayscale ultrasound of the gallbladder with a patient in the left lateral decubitus position. The gallbladder is distended with bile, causing increased transmission of echoes. A patient must be fasted for at least 4 hours to allow for gallbladder distension. **(Middle)** Subcostal transverse ultrasound of the gallbladder, demonstrating its anatomical relationships with the liver and right kidney. **(Bottom)** Zoomed, subcostal, longitudinal, grayscale ultrasound of the gallbladder with better anatomic detail. The normal gallbladder is not more than 5 cm in transverse diameter and ovoid in shape. The wall of a distended gallbladder is less than 3 mm in thickness. Note the echogenic junctional fold between the infundibulum and body of the gallbladder which, when less prominent, may be mistaken for a polyp or gallstone.

LEFT HEPATIC DUCT

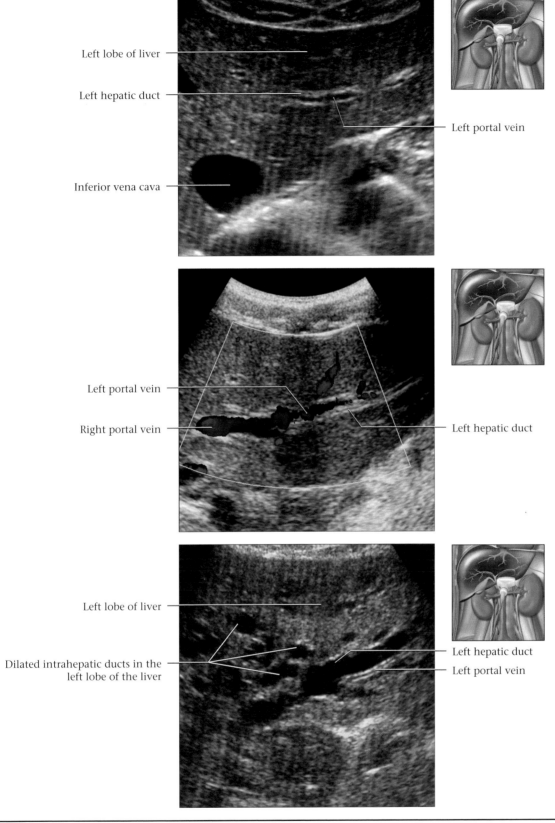

Left lobe of liver

Left hepatic duct

Left portal vein

Inferior vena cava

Left portal vein

Right portal vein

Left hepatic duct

Left lobe of liver

Dilated intrahepatic ducts in the left lobe of the liver

Left hepatic duct

Left portal vein

(**Top**) Subxiphoid, transverse, grayscale ultrasound shows the left portal vein and the anteriorly located diminutive left hepatic duct. Normal intrahepatic ducts are less than 2 mm in caliber. (**Middle**) Subxiphoid, transverse, color Doppler ultrasound shows an anatomic variant: The left hepatic duct is identified posterior to the left portal vein and shows no color flow. (**Bottom**) Subxiphoid, transverse, grayscale ultrasound shows a dilated left hepatic duct, which is identified anterior to the portal vein. Dilated intrahepatic ducts have irregular walls and exhibit posterior acoustic enhancement.

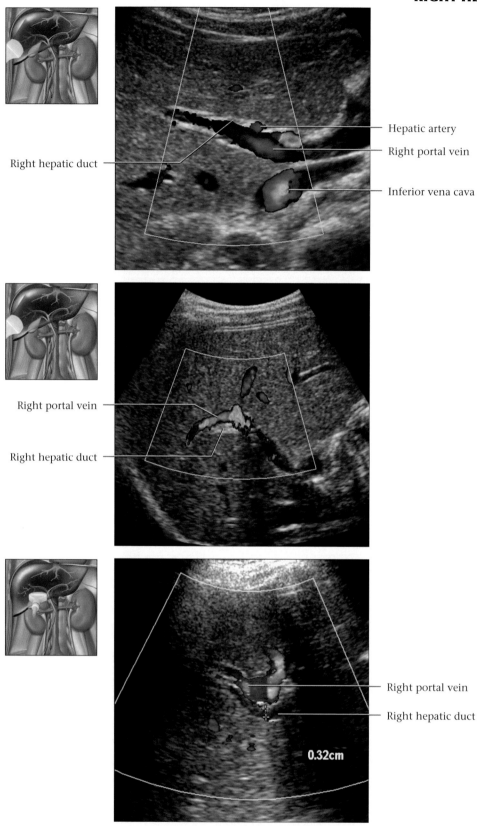

Right hepatic duct

Hepatic artery

Right portal vein

Inferior vena cava

Right portal vein

Right hepatic duct

Right portal vein

Right hepatic duct

0.32cm

(Top) Intercostal, oblique, grayscale ultrasound of the right lobe of the liver. Note the right portal vein and the anteriorly located right hepatic duct. **(Middle)** Intercostal, oblique, color Doppler ultrasound demonstrates an anatomic variant of the relationship of the right portal vein with the right intrahepatic duct. The intrahepatic duct is identified as the tubular structure posterior to the right portal vein. No color flow within. **(Bottom)** Intercostal, transverse, color Doppler ultrasound shows a mildly dilated right intrahepatic duct (3.2 mm) which is posterior to the right portal vein. An intrahepatic duct caliber > 2 mm or > 40% the diameter of the accompanying portal vein is considered to be dilated.

BILIARY SYSTEM

DUCTAL CONFLUENCE

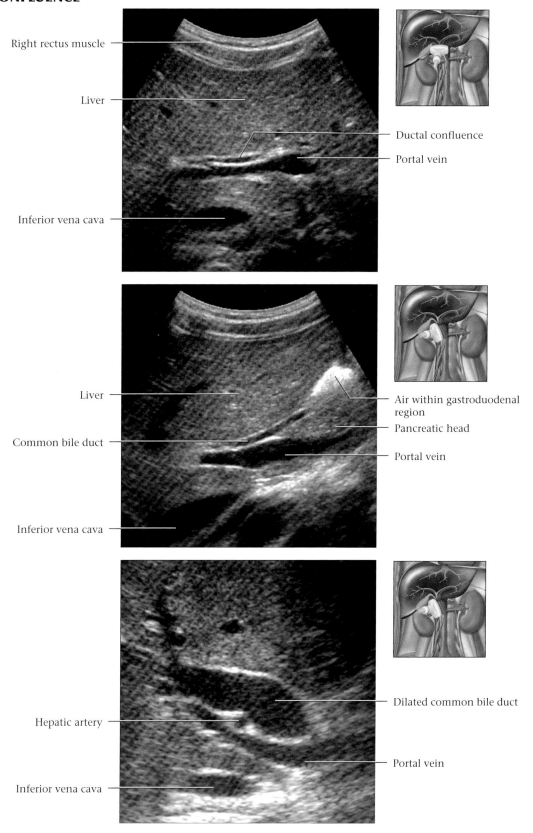

Right rectus muscle

Liver

Inferior vena cava

Ductal confluence

Portal vein

Liver

Common bile duct

Inferior vena cava

Air within gastroduodenal region

Pancreatic head

Portal vein

Dilated common bile duct

Hepatic artery

Portal vein

Inferior vena cava

(Top) Subcostal transverse grayscale ultrasound shows the confluence of the right and left hepatic ducts. **(Middle)** Subcostal, longitudinal, grayscale ultrasound shows the common bile duct and the portal vein in the hepatoduodenal ligament. The portal vein serves as an excellent landmark for the common bile duct, as the CBD is normally identified anterior to the portal vein. Note that the distal CBD pierces the pancreatic head. **(Bottom)** Subcostal, longitudinal, grayscale ultrasound shows a dilated common bile duct, localized anterior to the portal vein. The hepatic artery, which is part of the portal triad, is imaged end on as it crosses between the portal vein and common bile duct.

BILIARY SYSTEM

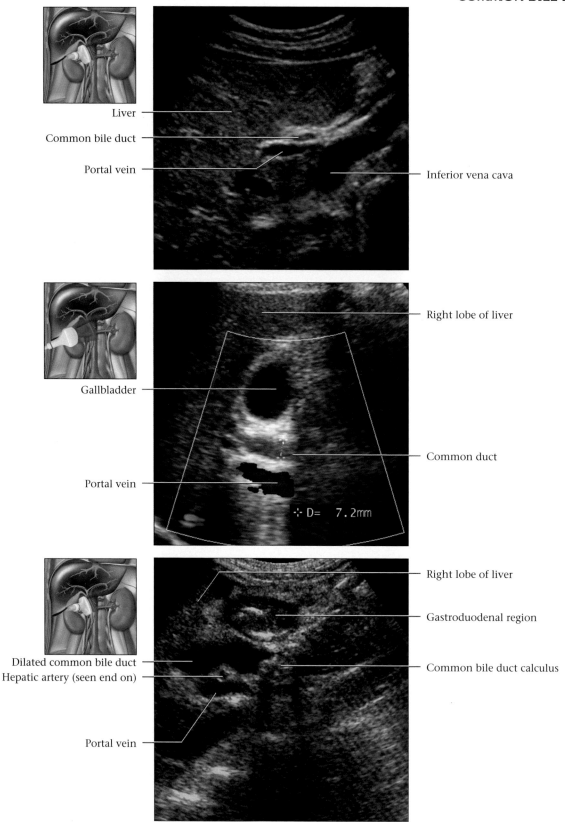

Liver

Common bile duct

Portal vein

Inferior vena cava

Right lobe of liver

Gallbladder

Common duct

Portal vein

∴ D= 7.2mm

Right lobe of liver

Gastroduodenal region

Dilated common bile duct
Hepatic artery (seen end on)

Common bile duct calculus

Portal vein

(**Top**) Subxiphoid, longitudinal, grayscale ultrasound in the right paramedian location shows the common bile duct anterior to the portal vein. The common bile duct has an average diameter of 4 mm. It gradually tapers distally as it pierces the pancreatic head. (**Middle**) Subcostal, longitudinal, color Doppler ultrasound shows the common bile duct anterior to the portal vein. The common bile duct is 7 mm in diameter, still within the normal range of 4-8 mm. The common bile duct becomes more prominent with age and may measure up to 10 mm in the elderly. (**Bottom**) Subcostal, longitudinal, grayscale ultrasound of a dilated common bile duct (1.5 cm) with a hyperechoic calculus exhibiting posterior acoustic shadowing.

BILIARY SYSTEM

INTRALUMINAL ECHOES

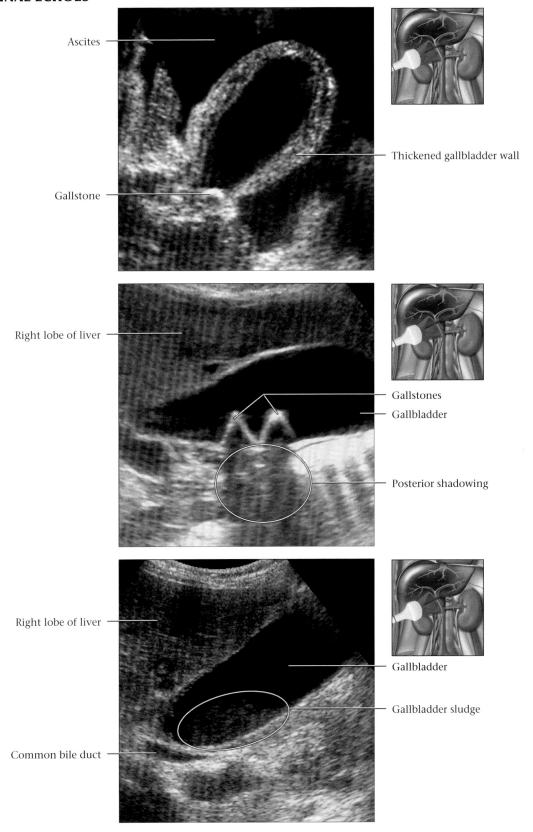

Ascites

Thickened gallbladder wall

Gallstone

Right lobe of liver

Gallstones

Gallbladder

Posterior shadowing

Right lobe of liver

Gallbladder

Gallbladder sludge

Common bile duct

(Top) Subcostal, longitudinal, grayscale ultrasound of a patient with massive ascites shows diffusely thickened gallbladder wall and a small stone in the infundibulum. The causes of wall thickening are many and include cholecystitis, hypoalbuminemia and chronic heart failure. **(Middle)** Subcostal, longitudinal, grayscale ultrasound of the gallbladder shows 2 intraluminal bright foci with posterior acoustic shadowing, the typical appearance of gallstones. There is high absorption as well as reflection of the echoes constituting acoustic shadowing. **(Bottom)** Subcostal, longitudinal, grayscale ultrasound shows echogenic bile/sludge, appearing as medium level echoes within the gallbladder and disrupting its normally anechoic appearance.

SPLEEN

Gross Anatomy

Overview
- Spleen is the the largest lymphatic organ
  - Size is variable
    - Usually not more than 12 cm long, 8 cm wide, or 5 cm thick
    - Usual volume range 100-250 cm³, mean 150 cm³ in adults
    - Volume > 470 cm³ = splenomegaly
  - Functions
    - Manufactures lymphocytes, filters blood (removes damaged red blood cells & platelets)
    - Acts as blood reservoir: Can expand or contract in response to changes in blood volume
- Histology
  - Soft organ with fibroelastic capsule entirely surrounded by peritoneum, except at splenic hilum
  - Trabeculae: Extensions of the capsule into the parenchyma; carry arterial & venous branches
  - Pulp: Substance of the spleen; white pulp = lymphoid nodules; red pulp = sinusoidal spaces containing blood
  - Splenic cords (plates of cells) lie between sinusoids; red pulp veins drain sinusoids
- Relations and vessels
  - Spleen contacts the posterior surface of the stomach and is connected via the gastrosplenic ligament (GSL)
    - GSL is the left anterior margin of the lesser sac
    - GSL carries the short gastric & left gastroepiploic arteries and venous branches to spleen
  - Contacts the pancreatic tail and surface of left kidney and is connected to these by the splenorenal ligament (SRL)
    - SRL carries splenic arterial and venous branches to spleen
    - SRL is the left posterior margin of the lesser sac (omental bursa)
  - Splenic vein runs in groove along dorsal surface of pancreatic body and tail
    - Receives the inferior mesenteric vein (IMV)
    - Combined splenic and IMV join superior mesenteric vein to form portal vein
  - Splenic artery (from celiac), often very tortuous

Imaging Anatomy

Internal Structures-Critical Contents
- Echo pattern
  - Very homogeneous similar to liver
  - Echogenicity
    - Spleen > liver > kidney
- Architecture
  - Characterized by radiating pattern of segmental arteries and veins
  - Splenic vein
    - Normal diameter 5-10 mm; peak systolic velocity 9-18 cm/s
    - Main trunk of splenic vein is a useful landmark for locating the pancreas
    - Pancreas lies anterior to the splenic vein

- Tail of pancreas can be seen anterior to the splenic vein using spleen as acoustic window
- Diameter increases between 50-100% from quiet respiration to deep inspiration - increase < 20% suggests portal hypertension
- Spectral Doppler waveform typically shows band-like flow profile with minimal respiratory fluctuations
  - Splenic artery
    - Because of tortuous course, flow in this vessel is typically turbulent with low pulsatility Doppler signal and ample diastolic flow
    - Normal diameter 4-8 mm; peak systolic velocity 70-110 cm/s

Anatomy-Based Imaging Issues

Imaging Recommendations
- Patient positioned supine or decubitus position (left side up) with left arm raised
- Transducer placed parallel to the ribs in the 10th or 11th intercostal space in left mid axillary line searching for best window
- End expiration may be helpful - lung base may obscure spleen in full inspiration
- Spleen poorly accessed from posterior (obscured by left lung base), anterior or subcostal approach (obscured by stomach and colon)

Key Concepts
- Spleen has highly variable size and shape
  - Imaging accurately detects splenomegaly and may suggest its cause (e.g., with cirrhosis = portal hypertension; with lymphadenopathy = lymphoma, mononucleosis, etc.)
- Spleen is commonly injured in blunt trauma, especially with fracture of the left lower ribs
  - Parenchymal laceration & capsular tear often result in substantial intraperitoneal bleeding
- Spleen texture
  - Easily indented & displaced by masses and even loculated fluid collections

Embryology

Practical Implications
- Accessory spleen/splenunculus/splenule found in 10-30% of population
  - Usually small, near splenic hilum
  - Can enlarge & simulate mass, especially after splenectomy
- Spleen may be on a long mesentery
  - "Wandering spleen" may be found in any abdominal or pelvic location
- Asplenia and polysplenia
  - Rare congenital conditions associated with other cardiovascular anomalies, situs inversus, etc.
  - Polysplenia can be simulated by splenosis (peritoneal implantation of splenic tissue that may follow traumatic splenic injury)

SPLEEN

SPLEEN & RELATIONS

Gastric impression

Stomach

Renal impression

OR

Prominent medial lobulation

Kidney

Stomach

Spleen

Lesser omentum

Gastrosplenic ligament

Splenic artery

Splenic vein

Splenorenal ligament

Inferior mesenteric vein

Root of transverse mesocolon

(Top) Graphic shows the medial surface of the spleen & representative axial sections at three levels through the parenchyma. The spleen is of variable shape & size, even within the same individual, varying with states of nutrition and hydration. It is a soft organ that is easily indented by adjacent organs. The medial surface is often quite lobulated as it is interposed between the stomach & the kidney. **(Bottom)** The liver is retracted upward & the stomach transected to reveal the pancreas and spleen. The splenic artery & vein course along the body of the pancreas, & the tail of the pancreas lies within the splenorenal ligament. The gastrosplenic ligament carries the short gastric & left gastroepiploic vessels to the stomach and spleen. The splenic vein receives the inferior mesenteric vein & joins the superior mesenteric vein behind the neck of the pancreas to form the portal vein.

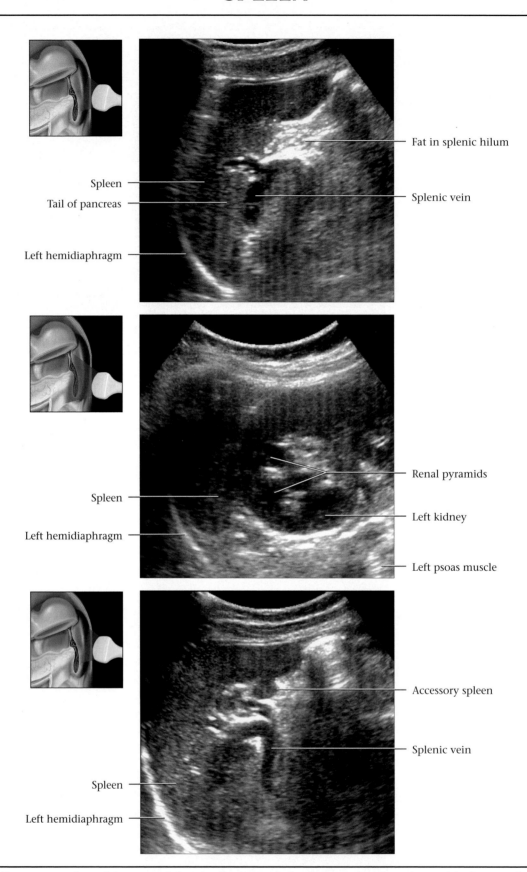

Spleen
Tail of pancreas
Left hemidiaphragm

Fat in splenic hilum
Splenic vein

Spleen
Left hemidiaphragm

Renal pyramids
Left kidney
Left psoas muscle

Accessory spleen

Splenic vein

Spleen
Left hemidiaphragm

(Top) Oblique, posterolateral, intercostal, longitudinal, grayscale ultrasound of the spleen with the transducer placed parallel to the intercostal space. The patient is positioned in the left-side-up decubitus position with examination during full expiration. Note the tail of the pancreas can be imaged using the spleen as an acoustic window. **(Middle)** Oblique, posterolateral, intercostal ultrasound shows the spleen and its relationship to the upper pole of the left kidney with the transducer placed parallel to the intercostal space. **(Bottom)** Oblique, posterolateral, intercostal, grayscale ultrasound of an accessory spleen. Accessory spleens are rounded, well-defined masses commonly found (10-30% of population) in or near the splenic hilum. They are homogeneous and isoechoic to the splenic parenchyma. Other synonyms include splenunculi and splenules.

SPLEEN

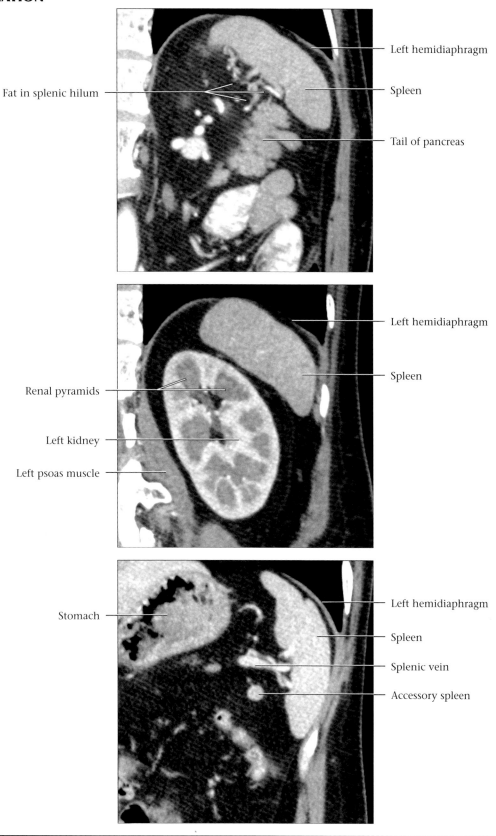

Left hemidiaphragm

Spleen

Tail of pancreas

Fat in splenic hilum

Left hemidiaphragm

Spleen

Renal pyramids

Left kidney

Left psoas muscle

Stomach

Left hemidiaphragm

Spleen

Splenic vein

Accessory spleen

(Top) Oblique, correlative, multiplanar reconstruction CT image of the spleen. Note the fat around the splenic hilum and the extension of the pancreatic tail towards the splenic hilum. This allows the pancreatic tail to be visualized by ultrasound using the spleen as an acoustic window. (Middle) Oblique, correlative, multiplanar reconstruction CT showing the relationship between the spleen and the left kidney. (Bottom) Oblique, correlative, multiplanar reconstruction CT of accessory spleen in the splenic hilum. The accessory spleen simulates the appearance of a normal spleen on imaging. This identical appearance prevents it from being mistaken for pathology.

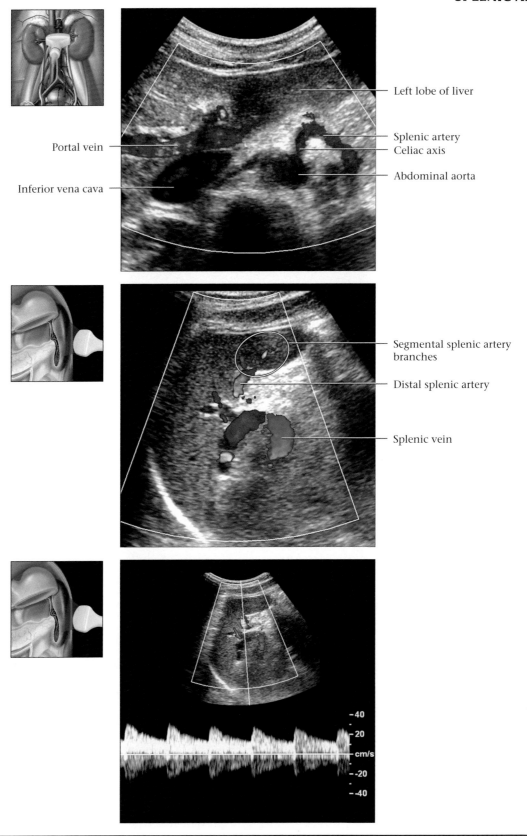

Left lobe of liver

Portal vein

Splenic artery
Celiac axis

Inferior vena cava

Abdominal aorta

Segmental splenic artery branches

Distal splenic artery

Splenic vein

(Top) Transverse power Doppler ultrasound image shows the origin of the splenic artery arising from the celiac axis. Note the tortuous course of the splenic artery as it arises from the celiac axis. **(Middle)** Oblique, intercostal, color Doppler image demonstrating the arteries and veins in the splenic hilum. Note the radiating pattern of segmental arteries. **(Bottom)** Spectral Doppler waveform of the distal splenic artery imaged through the spleen. Because of a tortuous course, flow in this vessel is typically turbulent with low pulsatility Doppler signal and ample diastolic flow.

SPLEEN

SPLENIC VEIN

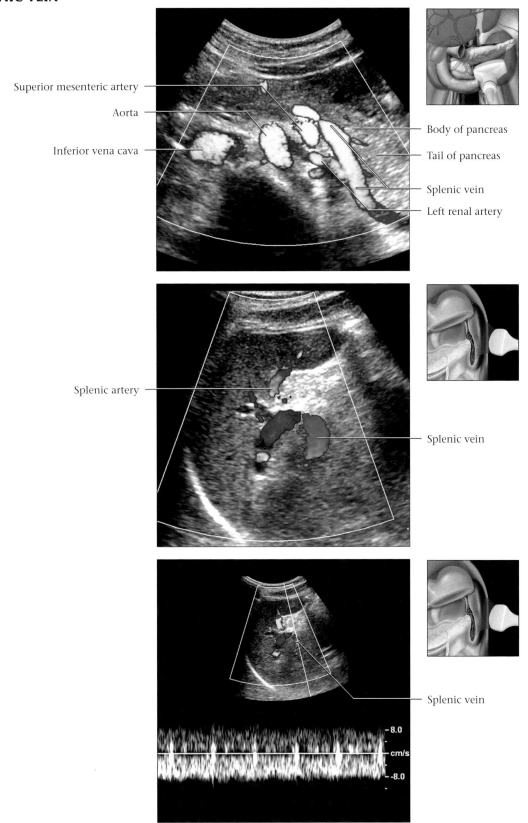

Superior mesenteric artery

Aorta

Inferior vena cava

Body of pancreas

Tail of pancreas

Splenic vein

Left renal artery

Splenic artery

Splenic vein

Splenic vein

(Top) Transverse power Doppler of the main trunk of the splenic vein. The main trunk of splenic vein is a useful landmark for locating the pancreas as the pancreas lies anterior to the splenic vein. **(Middle)** Oblique, intercostal, color Doppler ultrasound demonstrating the arteries and veins in the splenic hilum. Color Doppler is less sensitive than power Doppler in the detection of flow. However, it provides useful information on flow direction which is unavailable using power Doppler. **(Bottom)** Spectral Doppler waveform of the splenic vein in the splenic hilum. Image obtained using the spleen as an acoustic window via the posterolateral intercostal window. Spectral Doppler waveform of the splenic vein shows typical band-like flow profile with minimal respiratory fluctuations. Normal peak systolic velocity of the splenic vein is 9-18 cm/s.

SPLENOMEGALY & FOCAL SPLENIC LESIONS

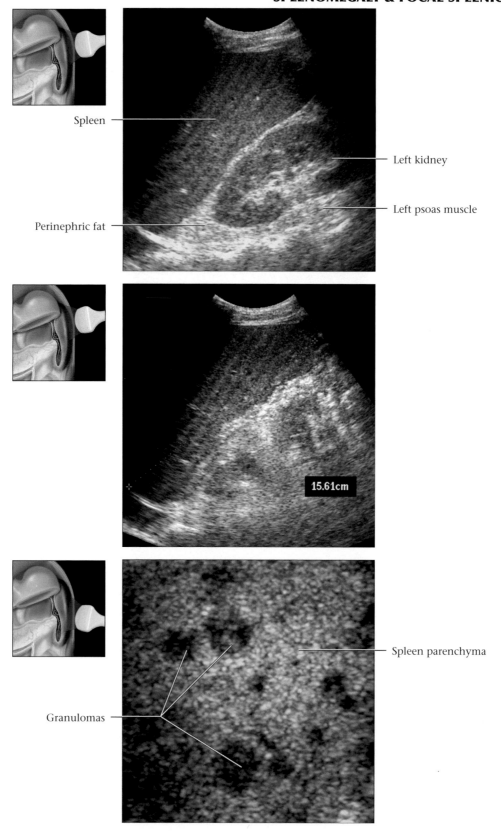

Spleen

Left kidney

Left psoas muscle

Perinephric fat

15.61cm

Spleen parenchyma

Granulomas

(Top) Oblique, posterolateral, grayscale ultrasound shows an enlarged spleen spanning the left kidney. The spleen, when enlarged, provides a better acoustic window for evaluating the left kidney than when it is normal in size. Note that the echogenicity of the spleen is usually higher than the kidney. **(Middle)** Oblique, posterolateral, grayscale ultrasound of the spleen with craniocaudal span obtained at 15.6 cm. Splenomegaly is noted when splenic length is more than 12 cm. Spleen size is variable, though usually not more than 12 cm long, 8 cm wide, or 5 cm thick. Splenomegaly can also be diagnosed if the splenic volume is greater than 470 cubic cm. **(Bottom)** Zoomed, intercostal, grayscale ultrasound of the spleen shows several granulomas (hypoechoic lesions) disrupting the normal homogeneous echo pattern of the spleen.

SPLENIC TRAUMA

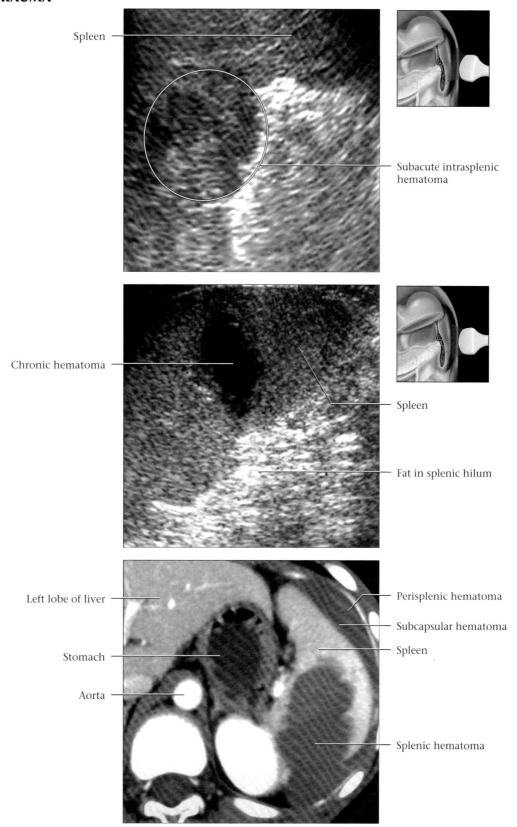

Spleen

Subacute intrasplenic hematoma

Chronic hematoma

Spleen

Fat in splenic hilum

Left lobe of liver

Perisplenic hematoma

Subcapsular hematoma

Stomach

Spleen

Aorta

Splenic hematoma

(Top) Zoomed, oblique, grayscale ultrasound reveals a focal ill-defined hypoechoic area representing a subacute intrasplenic hematoma disrupting the normal homogeneous echo pattern of the spleen. (Middle) Longitudinal grayscale ultrasound shows a well-defined, hypoechoic, liquefied, chronic, splenic hematoma disrupting the normal homogeneous echo pattern of the spleen. Note the lower echogenicity of the chronic splenic hematoma when compared with the subacute intrasplenic hematoma in the previous image. (Bottom) Axial CECT at the level of the stomach and spleen shows a large, hypodense, non-enhancing, intraparenchymal, splenic hematoma along with subcapsular and perisplenic blood.

SPLEEN

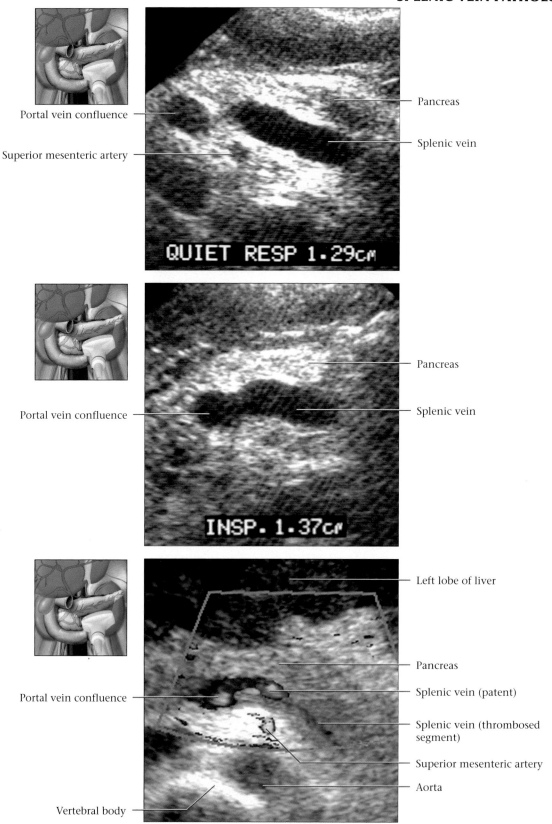

Pancreas

Portal vein confluence

Superior mesenteric artery

Splenic vein

QUIET RESP 1.29cm

Pancreas

Portal vein confluence

Splenic vein

INSP. 1.37cm

Left lobe of liver

Pancreas

Splenic vein (patent)

Portal vein confluence

Splenic vein (thrombosed segment)

Superior mesenteric artery

Aorta

Vertebral body

(Top) Subxiphoid, transverse, grayscale ultrasound of the splenic vein shows splenic vein diameter of 13 mm. Normal diameter of the splenic vein is 5-10 mm. (Middle) Subxiphoid, transverse, grayscale ultrasound of the same patient as previous image, taken during inspiration. The normal splenic vein diameter increases between 50-100% from quiet respiration to deep inspiration - increase < 20% suggests portal hypertension. There is only a 0.8 mm increase in splenic vein caliber. (Bottom) Subxiphoid, transverse, color Doppler ultrasound shows absent flow in the splenic vein at the pancreatic tail level, instead internal echoes are identified, characteristic of thrombosis. There is flow within the proximal splenic vein at the pancreatic head and body level.

SPLEEN

SPLENIC VARICES & INFARCTION

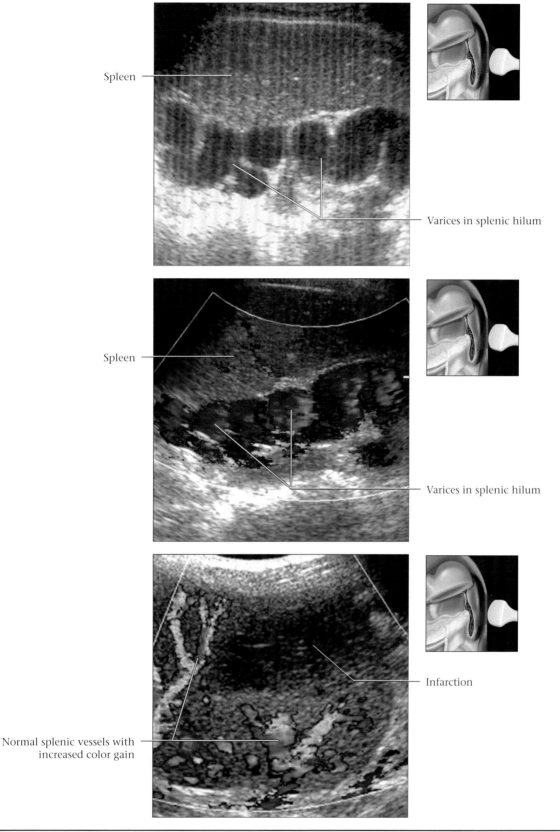

Spleen

Varices in splenic hilum

Spleen

Varices in splenic hilum

Infarction

Normal splenic vessels with
increased color gain

(Top) Longitudinal, oblique, grayscale ultrasound of an enlarged spleen reveals tubular hypoechoic structures along the splenic hilum which are dilated collaterals. **(Middle)** Transverse, transabdominal, color Doppler ultrasound further demonstrates the tortuous course and flow of the dilated splenic hilar collaterals. **(Bottom)** Oblique color Doppler ultrasound shows a hypoechoic zone of infarction in the periphery of the spleen, with absent blood flow in the area. The color gain is increased for more sensitive pick up of vessels/color flow within the splenic parenchyma.

PANCREAS

Gross Anatomy

Overview

- Pancreas: Accessory digestive gland lying in retroperitoneum behind stomach
  - Exocrine function: Pancreatic acinar cells secrete pancreatic juice → pancreatic duct → duodenum
  - Endocrine: Pancreatic islet cells (of Langerhans) secrete insulin, glucagon & other polypeptides → portal venous system

Divisions

- Head: Thickest part; lies to right of superior mesenteric artery and vein (SMA, SMV)
  - Attached to "C" loop of duodenum (2nd & 3rd parts)
  - Uncinate process: Head extension, posterior to SMV
  - Bile duct lies along posterior surface of head, joins with pancreatic duct (of Wirsung) to form hepatopancreatic ampulla (of Vater)
  - Main pancreatic & bile ducts empty into major papilla in 2nd portion of duodenum
- Neck: Thinnest part; lies anterior to SMA, SMV
  - SMV joins splenic vein behind pancreatic neck to form portal vein
- Body: Main part; lies to left of SMA, SMV
  - Splenic vein lies in groove on posterior surface of body
  - Anterior surface is covered with peritoneum forming back surface of omental bursa (lesser sac)
- Tail: Lies between layers of splenorenal ligament in splenic hilum

Internal Structures

- Pancreatic duct (of Wirsung) runs length of pancreas, turning inferiorly through head to join bile duct
- Accessory pancreatic duct (of Santorini) opens into duodenum at minor duodenal papilla
  - Usually communicates with main pancreatic duct
  - Variations are common, including a dominant accessory duct draining most pancreatic juice
- Vessels, nerves and lymphatics
  - Arteries to head mainly from gastroduodenal artery
    - Pancreaticoduodenal arcade of vessels around head also supplied by SMA branches
  - Arteries to body & tail from splenic artery
  - Veins are tributaries of SMV and splenic vein → portal vein
  - Autonomic nerves from celiac and superior mesenteric plexus
    - Parasympathetic stimulation of pancreatic secretion, but pancreatic juice secretion is mostly under hormonal control (secretin, from duodenum)
  - Lymphatics follow blood vessels
    - Collect in splenic, celiac, superior mesenteric and hepatic nodes

Imaging Anatomy

Overview

- Pancreas can be localized on ultrasound by

  - Typical parenchymal architecture - homogeneously isoechoic/hyperechoic echo pattern when compared with overlying liver
  - Surrounding anatomical landmarks - body anterior to splenic vein; neck anterior to SMA/SMV
- Variations in reflectivity related to degree of fatty infiltration; uncinate process and posterior pancreatic head are relatively echo-poor in 25% of subjects (lack of intraparenchymal fat)

Anatomy-Based Imaging Issues

Imaging Recommendations

- Use 2-5 MHz transducers
- Techniques to combat overlying stomach and bowel gas include
  - Displacement of intervening bowel gas by gentle firm graded compression with transducer
  - Overnight fasting
  - Non effervescent fluid can be given orally to fill gastric fundus
    - Scanning delayed for a few minutes to allow fluid to settle
    - Patient can lie on left side to allow imaging of body and tail of pancreas
    - Patient can then be turned to right to allow gastric fluid to flow to stomach antrum and duodenum allowing imaging of head and uncinate process
- CT is preferred imaging modality for imaging of pancreas
- MRCP or ERCP useful for defining pancreatic duct

Imaging Pitfalls

- Ultrasound examination of pancreas is often limited by overlying bowel gas

Key Concepts

- Shape, size & texture of pancreas are quite variable
  - Largest in young adults
  - Atrophy and fatty infiltration with age (> 70), obesity, diabetes, corticosteroids, Cushing disease
  - Pancreatic duct also becomes more prominent with age (< 3 mm diameter)
  - Focal bulge or mass effect is abnormal
- Location behind lesser sac
  - Acute pancreatitis often results in lesser sac fluid (not = pseudocyst)
- Pancreas lies in anterior pararenal space (APS)
  - Inflammation (from pancreatitis) easily spreads to duodenum & descending colon (also lie in APS)
  - Inflammation easily spreads into mesentery & mesocolon (roots of these lie just ventral to pancreas)
- Obstruction of pancreatic duct
  - Relatively common result of chronic pancreatitis (fibrosis &/or stone occluding pancreatic duct), or pancreatic ductal carcinoma
- Acute pancreatitis
  - Relatively common result of gallstone (lodged in hepatopancreatic ampulla causing bile to reflux into pancreas) or damage from alcohol abuse

PANCREAS

Gastroduodenal artery

Posterior superior
pancreaticoduodenal
artery

Anterior superior
pancreaticoduodenal
artery

Base of transverse
mesocolon

Duodenum

Stomach (cut &
removed)

Spleen

Superior (dorsal)
pancreatic artery

Splenic artery

Great pancreatic artery

Transverse colon

Duodeno-jejunal
junction

Superior mesenteric
artery & vein

Base of small bowel
mesentery

Graphic shows the arterial supply to the body & tail of the pancreas through terminal branches of the splenic artery, which are variable in number & size. The two largest are usually the dorsal (superior) and great pancreatic arteries, which arise from the proximal & distal splenic artery, respectively. The arteries to the pancreatic head and duodenum come from the pancreaticoduodenal arcades that receive flow from the celiac and superior mesenteric arteries. The superior mesenteric vessels pass behind the neck of the pancreas and in front of the third portion of the duodenum. The root of the transverse mesocolon and small bowel mesentery arise from the surface of the pancreas and transmit the blood vessels to the small bowel & transverse colon. The splenic vein runs along the dorsal surface of the pancreas. The splenic vessels and pancreatic tail insert into the splenic hilum.

PANCREAS

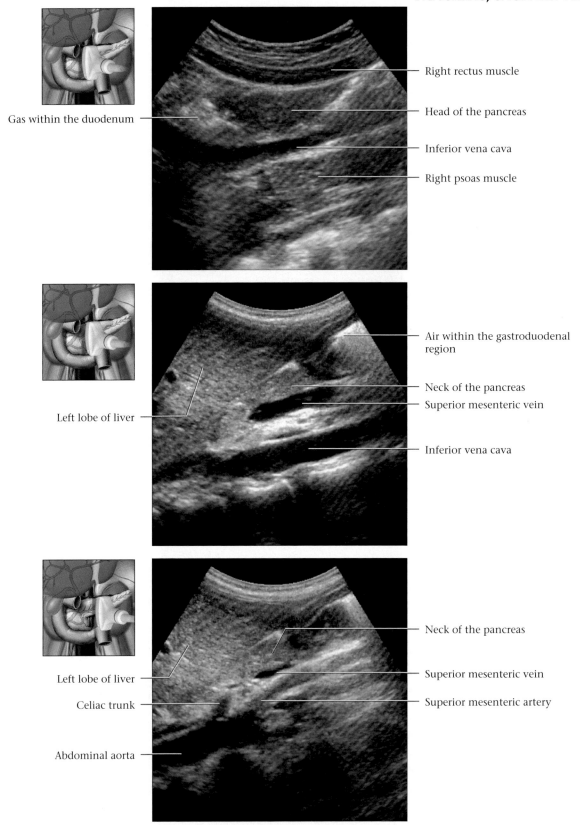

Gas within the duodenum — Right rectus muscle

Head of the pancreas

Inferior vena cava

Right psoas muscle

Left lobe of liver — Air within the gastroduodenal region

Neck of the pancreas
Superior mesenteric vein

Inferior vena cava

Neck of the pancreas

Left lobe of liver

Superior mesenteric vein

Celiac trunk

Superior mesenteric artery

Abdominal aorta

(Top) Longitudinal, transabdominal, grayscale ultrasound at the epigastrium, right paramedian region. Note the relationship of the pancreatic head with the posteriorly located inferior vena cava. (Middle) Longitudinal, transabdominal, grayscale ultrasound at the epigastrium, right paramedian region, continuing medially from the previous image. Note the superior mesenteric vein coming into view - this is a good landmark for locating the neck of the pancreas on the sagittal ultrasound. (Bottom) Longitudinal, transabdominal, grayscale ultrasound at the epigastrium, right paramedian region slightly more medial to the previous image. The origin of the superior mesenteric artery arising from the abdominal aorta is brought into view. The SMA is also a useful marker for identifying the neck of the pancreas on sagittal ultrasound.

PANCREAS

SAGITTAL CT CORRELATION

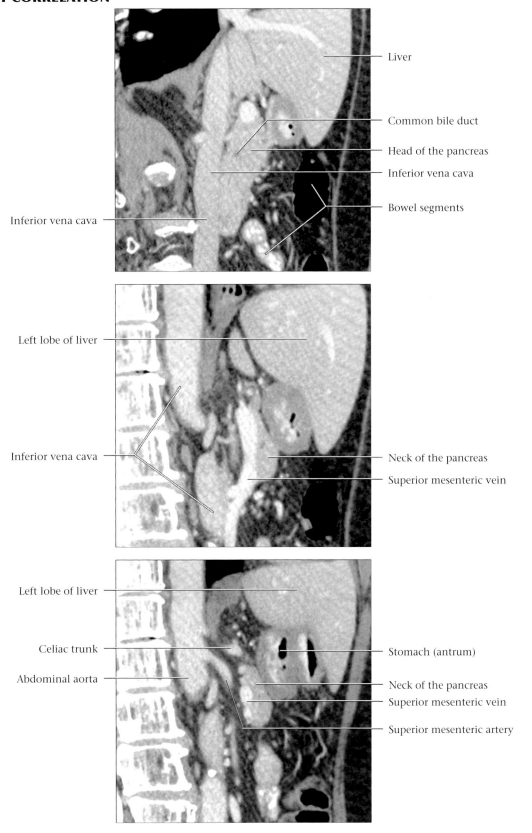

Liver

Common bile duct

Head of the pancreas

Inferior vena cava

Bowel segments

Inferior vena cava

Left lobe of liver

Inferior vena cava

Neck of the pancreas

Superior mesenteric vein

Left lobe of liver

Celiac trunk

Abdominal aorta

Stomach (antrum)

Neck of the pancreas

Superior mesenteric vein

Superior mesenteric artery

(**Top**) Correlative, reconstructed, contrast-enhanced, longitudinal CT image of the pancreatic head. The inferior vena cava serves as a good landmark for identifying the head of the pancreas, which lies anterior to it. Note the overlying air-filled bowel segments which on ultrasound may obscure the pancreas. (**Middle**) Correlative, contrast-enhanced, longitudinal CT at the level of the superior mesenteric vein as it descends. The neck is the thinnest portion of the pancreas and lies anterior to the superior mesenteric vein. (**Bottom**) Correlative, contrast-enhanced, longitudinal CT image at the origin of the superior mesenteric artery which serves as another landmark for identifying the neck of the pancreas. Note the anteriorly located antrum of the stomach, which may be distended with fluid and used as an acoustic window for evaluating the pancreas.

PANCREAS

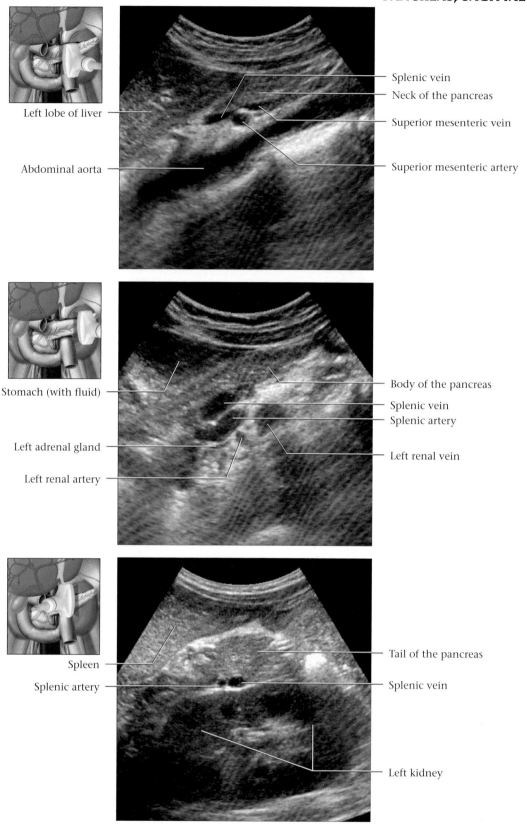

(Top) Left lobe of liver — Abdominal aorta — Splenic vein — Neck of the pancreas — Superior mesenteric vein — Superior mesenteric artery

(Middle) Stomach (with fluid) — Left adrenal gland — Left renal artery — Body of the pancreas — Splenic vein — Splenic artery — Left renal vein

(Bottom) Spleen — Splenic artery — Tail of the pancreas — Splenic vein — Left kidney

(Top) Longitudinal, transabdominal, grayscale ultrasound at the midline epigastrium, revealing the SMA that has taken off from the abdominal aorta, its relationship with the splenic vein, and the anteriorly located pancreatic neck. The inferior mesenteric vein joins the splenic vein here. **(Middle)** Longitudinal, transabdominal, grayscale ultrasound at the epigastrium, left paramedian region, sweeping the transducer laterally from the top image. The body of the pancreas lies to the left of the SMA (not shown). The stomach lies superiorly and may be filled with fluid for use as an acoustic window. The splenic vein maintains its course behind the pancreas. **(Bottom)** Longitudinal, transabdominal, grayscale ultrasound at the epigastrium, continuing the scan laterally from the middle image. The pancreatic tail is identified between the spleen and the left kidney.

PANCREAS

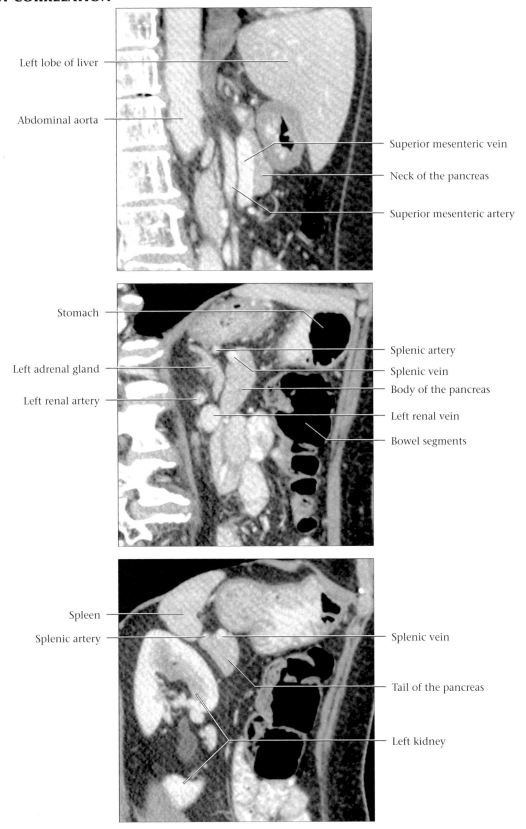

Left lobe of liver

Abdominal aorta

Superior mesenteric vein

Neck of the pancreas

Superior mesenteric artery

Stomach

Splenic artery

Left adrenal gland

Splenic vein

Body of the pancreas

Left renal artery

Left renal vein

Bowel segments

Spleen

Splenic artery

Splenic vein

Tail of the pancreas

Left kidney

(Top) Correlative, reconstructed, contrast-enhanced, longitudinal CT at the plane of the superior mesenteric artery and vein. The two vessels are landmarks for the pancreatic neck on a sagittal image. **(Middle)** Correlative, contrast-enhanced, longitudinal CT at the pancreatic body level, just to the left of the superior mesenteric artery and vein. The splenic artery is superior and posterior to the splenic vein. Overlying bowel segments may limit ultrasound examination of this part of the pancreas. **(Bottom)** Correlative, contrast-enhanced, longitudinal CT at the pancreatic tail level. Note the position of the pancreatic tail relative to the spleen and left kidney. Overlying bowel gas may obscure this portion of the pancreas if ultrasound examination is performed via the anterior approach. Thus a lateral, oblique, intercostal approach using the spleen as an acoustic window may be better for pancreatic tail examination.

PANCREAS

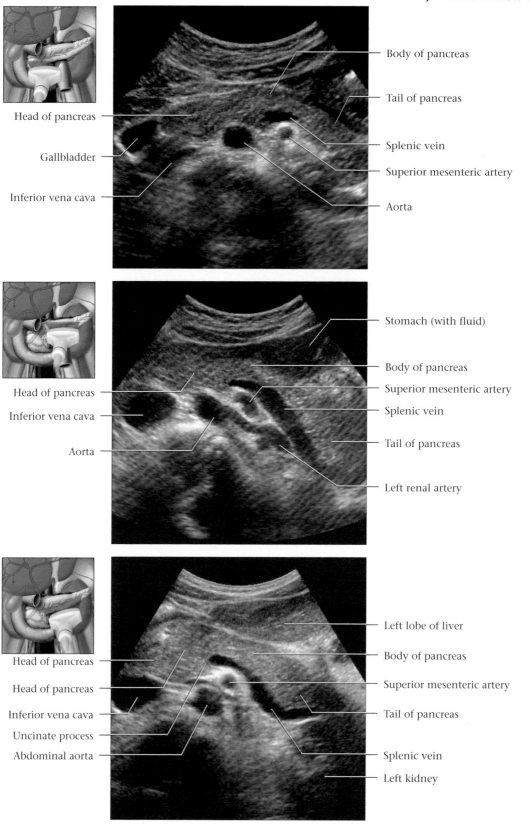

Body of pancreas

Tail of pancreas

Head of pancreas

Splenic vein

Gallbladder

Superior mesenteric artery

Inferior vena cava

Aorta

Stomach (with fluid)

Body of pancreas

Head of pancreas

Superior mesenteric artery

Inferior vena cava

Splenic vein

Aorta

Tail of pancreas

Left renal artery

Left lobe of liver

Head of pancreas

Body of pancreas

Head of pancreas

Superior mesenteric artery

Inferior vena cava

Tail of pancreas

Uncinate process

Abdominal aorta

Splenic vein

Left kidney

(**Top**) Transverse transabdominal grayscale ultrasound at the epigastrium. Anatomically, the pancreatic axis from head to tail is directed superiorly and to the left. This lower transverse section demonstrates the bulk of the pancreatic head. (**Middle**) Transverse, transabdominal, grayscale ultrasound at the epigastrium, slightly higher compared with the previous image. Note the pancreatic body and tail have now come into view. (**Bottom**) Oblique, transabdominal, grayscale ultrasound at the epigastrium. The transducer is tilted slightly cranially and laterally to the left to follow the pancreatic axis, thus imaging the pancreas in its entirety. The splenic vein courses along the posterior pancreas and provides an excellent landmark in locating the pancreas. The superior mesenteric artery is more posteriorly located and has a characteristic dot-shape as it is imaged end on.

PANCREAS

TRANSVERSE CT CORRELATION

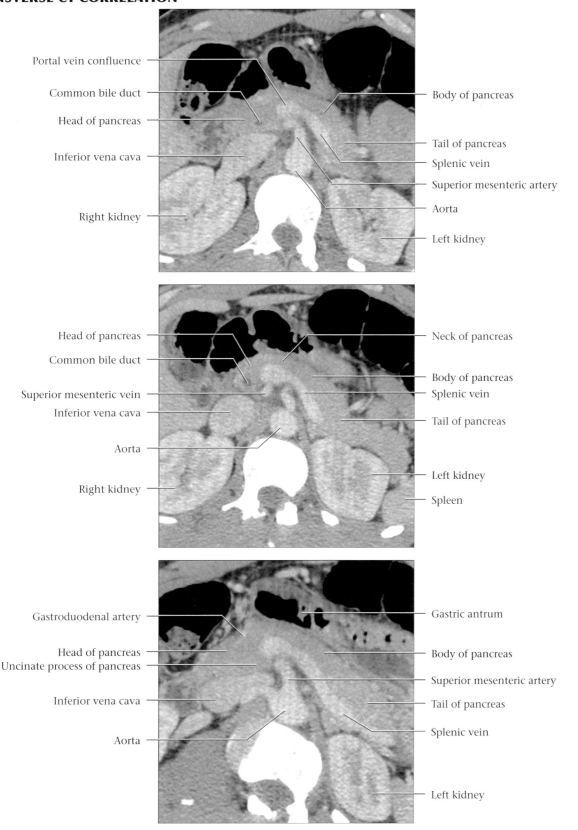

Portal vein confluence

Common bile duct

Head of pancreas

Inferior vena cava

Right kidney

Body of pancreas

Tail of pancreas

Splenic vein

Superior mesenteric artery

Aorta

Left kidney

Head of pancreas

Common bile duct

Superior mesenteric vein

Inferior vena cava

Aorta

Right kidney

Neck of pancreas

Body of pancreas

Splenic vein

Tail of pancreas

Left kidney

Spleen

Gastroduodenal artery

Head of pancreas
Uncinate process of pancreas

Inferior vena cava

Aorta

Gastric antrum

Body of pancreas

Superior mesenteric artery

Tail of pancreas

Splenic vein

Left kidney

(Top) Transverse, correlative, contrast-enhanced CT of the pancreas at the level of the origin of the superior mesenteric artery. Note the common bile duct within the pancreatic head before it exits into the duodenum. **(Middle)** Transverse, correlative, contrast-enhanced CT of the pancreas. Note the course of the pancreatic tail, which goes posteriorly and forms close relations with the left kidney and spleen. **(Bottom)** Oblique, correlative, contrast-enhanced CT following the pancreatic axis and demonstrating its head, body and tail. The splenic vein courses along the posterior pancreas, following its contour. The anteriorly located stomach may be distended with fluid and used as an acoustic window during ultrasound.

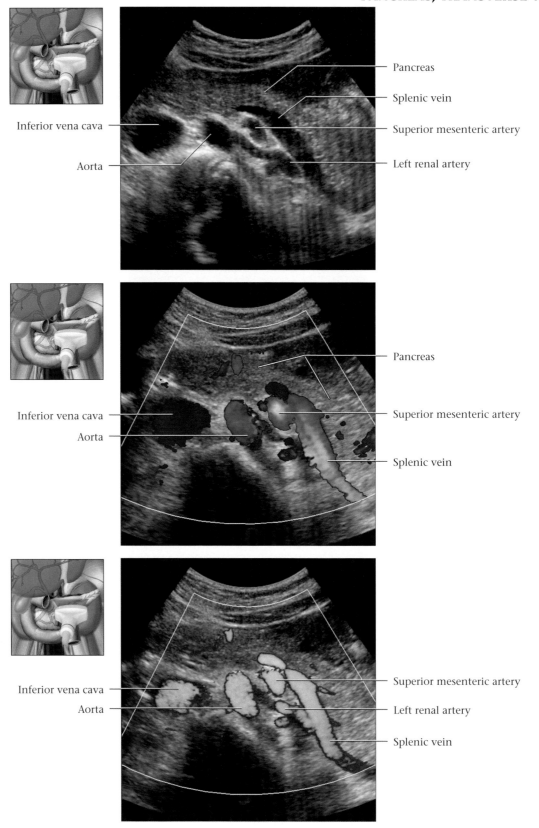

(Top) Transverse, subxiphoid, grayscale ultrasound. The left renal artery courses posterior to the superior mesenteric artery and splenic vein as it descends to enter the left renal hilum. (**Middle**) Transverse, subxiphoid, color Doppler ultrasound. This image was taken with a small amount of cranial tilt so that blue indicates flow towards the transducer and red away from the transducer. Note therefore that aorta flow is blue and IVC flow is red. The splenic vein is red in its proximal portion but exhibits blue color distally, owing to its course. The left renal artery is almost at right angles to the transducer and therefore flow is not well seen. (**Bottom**) Transverse, subxiphoid, power Doppler ultrasound demonstrates the vessels posterior to the pancreas. Power Doppler is more sensitive for detecting vascular flow but fails to provide information on flow direction.

PANCREAS

PANCREATITIS

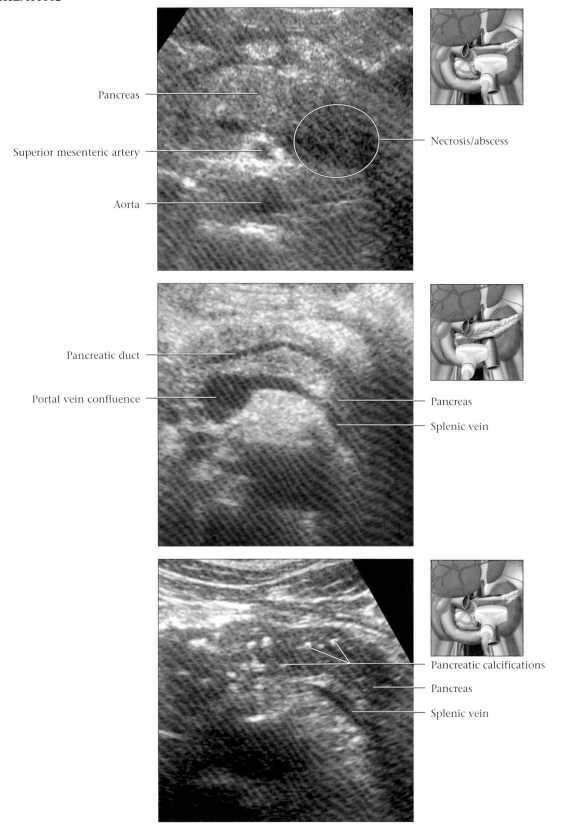

Pancreas

Superior mesenteric artery

Aorta

Necrosis/abscess

Pancreatic duct

Portal vein confluence

Pancreas

Splenic vein

Pancreatic calcifications

Pancreas

Splenic vein

(Top) Transverse grayscale ultrasound shows a bulky hypoechoic pancreas in a patient with acute pancreatitis. There is a focal hypoechoic region in the pancreatic body representing necrosis or phlegmon/abscess formation. Normal pancreatic AP diameters are < 2.5 cm at the pancreatic head level, and < 2.0 cm at the pancreatic body. The pancreas atrophies with age and acute pancreatitis may still be suspected in elderly patients with normal size pancreas. **(Middle)** Transverse grayscale ultrasound of a similar patient shows a slightly edematous pancreas with a mildly dilated pancreatic duct. The normal pancreatic duct is 2.0-2.5 mm in diameter although it may be 3 mm in caliber at the pancreatic head level. **(Bottom)** Transverse grayscale ultrasound shows a normal-sized pancreas with calcifications in the pancreatic head and body suggestive of chronic pancreatitis.

CYSTIC AND SOLID PANCREATIC LESIONS

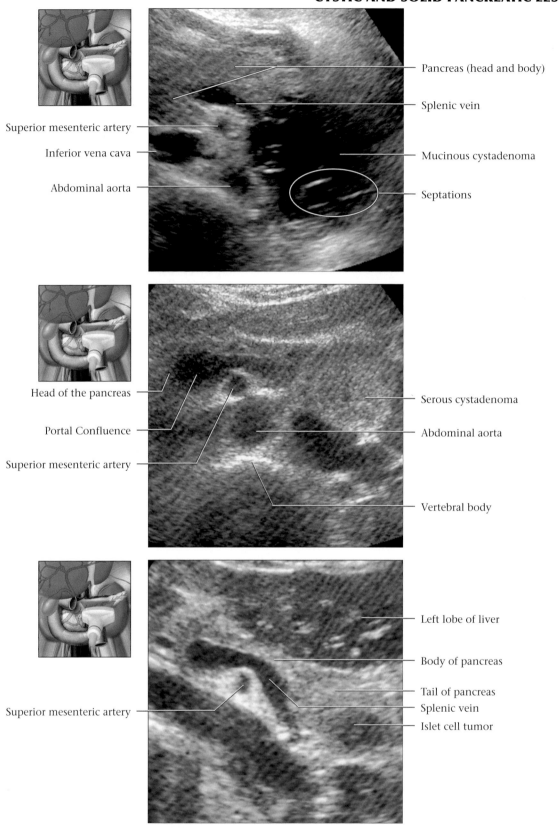

Pancreas (head and body)

Splenic vein

Mucinous cystadenoma

Septations

Superior mesenteric artery

Inferior vena cava

Abdominal aorta

Head of the pancreas

Portal Confluence

Superior mesenteric artery

Serous cystadenoma

Abdominal aorta

Vertebral body

Left lobe of liver

Body of pancreas

Tail of pancreas

Splenic vein

Islet cell tumor

Superior mesenteric artery

(Top) Transverse, transabdominal, grayscale ultrasound shows a well-defined, predominantly cystic mass in the pancreatic tail. Note the presence of internal septations within this lesion. These features are typical of a mucinous cystic neoplasm. (Middle) Transverse, transabdominal, grayscale ultrasound shows a well-circumscribed, solid, slightly hyperechoic mass in the pancreatic tail of a known serous cystadenoma. Note the absence of pancreatic ductal dilatation or calcification within the lesion. (Bottom) Transverse, transabdominal, grayscale ultrasound shows a well-defined, solid, hypoechoic mass in the pancreatic tail. The patient presented with hypoglycemia. Surgery confirmed a pancreatic insulinoma.

PANCREAS

DUCTAL PATHOLOGIES

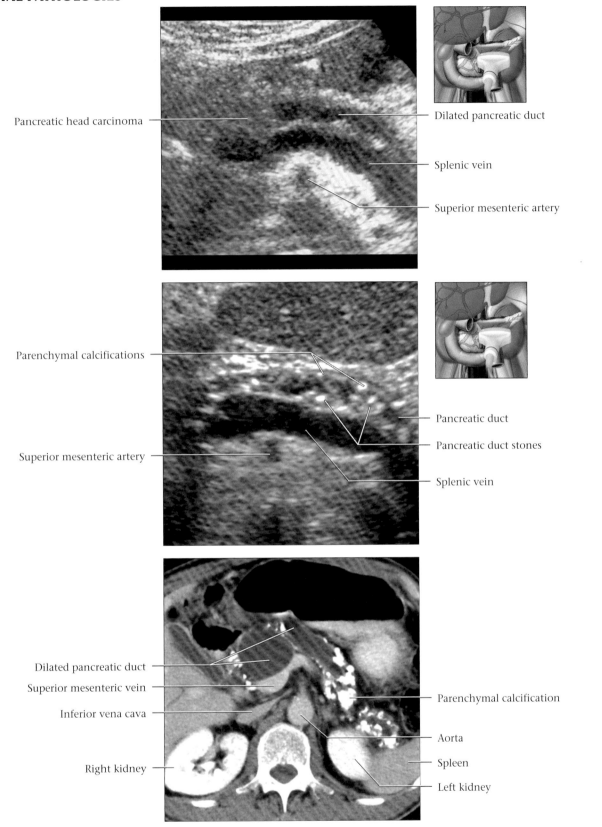

Pancreatic head carcinoma

Dilated pancreatic duct

Splenic vein

Superior mesenteric artery

Parenchymal calcifications

Pancreatic duct

Pancreatic duct stones

Superior mesenteric artery

Splenic vein

Dilated pancreatic duct

Superior mesenteric vein

Inferior vena cava

Parenchymal calcification

Aorta

Spleen

Right kidney

Left kidney

(Top) Transverse, subxiphoid, grayscale ultrasound shows a grossly dilated pancreatic duct (~ 5 mm) secondary to an ill-defined pancreatic head carcinoma. (Middle) Transverse, subxiphoid, grayscale ultrasound shows an atrophic pancreas with parenchymal calcifications. The pancreatic duct is dilated with intraductal stones. (Bottom) Axial contrast-enhanced CT shows an an atrophic pancreas with parenchymal calcification. Note the dilatation of the pancreatic duct in the head and body of the pancreas.

KIDNEYS

Gross Anatomy

Overview
- Kidneys are paired, bean-shaped, retroperitoneal organs
  - Function: Remove excess water, salts and wastes of protein metabolism from blood

Anatomic Relationships
- Lie in retroperitoneum, within perirenal space, surrounded by renal fascia (of Gerota)
- Each kidney is ~ 10-15 cm in length, 5 cm in width
- Both kidneys lie on quadratus lumborum muscles, lateral to psoas muscles

Internal Structures
- Kidneys can be considered hollow with renal sinus occupied by fat, renal pelvis, calices, vessels and nerves
- Renal hilum: Where artery enters, vein and ureter leave renal sinus
- Renal pelvis: Funnel-shaped expansion of upper end of ureter
  - Receives major calices (infundibula) (2 or 3), each of which receives minor calices (2-4)
- Renal papilla: Pointed apex of the renal pyramid of collecting tubules that excrete urine
  - Each papilla indents a minor calyx
- Renal cortex: Outer part, contains renal corpuscles (glomeruli, vessels), proximal portions of collecting tubules & loop of Henle
- Renal medulla: Inner part, contains renal pyramids, distal parts of collecting tubules and loops of Henle
- Vessels, nerves, and lymphatics
  - Artery
    - Usually one for each kidney
    - Arise from aorta at about L1-2 vertebral level
  - Vein
    - Usually one for each kidney
    - Lies in front of renal artery and renal pelvis
  - Nerves
    - Autonomic from renal and aorticorenal ganglia and plexus
  - Lymphatics
    - To lumbar (aortic and caval) nodes

Imaging Anatomy

Overview
- Well-defined retroperitoneal bean-shaped structures which move with respiration

Internal Structures-Critical Contents
- Renal capsule
  - Normal kidneys are well-defined due to presence of renal capsule and are less reflective than surrounding fat
- Renal cortex
  - Renal cortex has reflectivity that is less than adjacent liver or spleen
  - If renal cortex brighter than normal liver (echogenic), then high suspicion of renal parenchymal disease
- Medullary pyramids

- Medullary pyramids are less reflective than renal cortex
- Corticomedullary differentiation
  - Margin between cortex and pyramids is usually well-defined in normal kidneys
  - Margin between cortex and pyramids may be lost in presence of generalized parenchymal inflammation or edema
- Renal sinus
  - Echogenic due to fat that surrounds blood vessels and collecting systems
  - Outline of renal sinus is variable - can vary from smooth to irregular
  - Renal sinus fat may increase in obesity, steroid use and sinus lipomatosis
  - Renal sinus fat may decrease in cachectic patient and neonates
  - If sinus echoes are indistinct in a non-cachectic patient, tumor infiltration or edema should be considered
- Collecting system (renal pelvis and calices)
  - Not usually visible in dehydrated patient
  - May be seen as physiological "splitting" of renal sinus echoes in patients with a full bladder, undergoing diuresis
  - Physiological "splitting" of renal sinus echoes is common in pregnancy
    - Cause of dilatation of pelvicaliceal system may be due to mechanical obstruction by enlarging uterus, hormonal factors, increased blood flow and parenchymal hypertrophy
    - May occur as early as 12 weeks into pregnancy
    - Seen in up to 75% of right kidneys at 20 weeks into pregnancy, less common on the left side
    - Obvious dilatation of pelvicaliceal system can be seen in two thirds of patients at 36 weeks
    - Changes usually resolve within 48 hours after delivery
  - Possible obstruction can be excluded by performing post micturition images of collecting system
    - AP diameter of renal pelvis in adults should be < 10 mm
- Renal arteries
  - Normal caliber 5-8 mm
  - Two thirds of kidneys are supplied by a single renal artery arising from aorta
  - One third of kidneys are supplied by two or more renal arteries arising from aorta
    - Main renal artery may be duplicated
    - Accessory renal arteries may arise from aorta superior or inferior to main renal artery
    - Accessory renal arteries may enter kidney either in hilum or at poles
    - Extrahilar accessory renal arteries may arise from the ipsilateral renal artery, ipsilateral iliac artery, aorta or retroperitoneal arteries
  - Spectral Doppler
    - Open systolic window, rapid systolic upstroke occasionally followed by a secondary slower rise to peak systole with subsequent diastolic delay but persistent forward flow in diastole
    - Continuous diastolic flow is present due to low resistance in renal vascular bed

KIDNEYS

- Low resistance flow pattern is also present in intrarenal branches
- Normal PSV 60-140 cm/s, not more than 180 cm/s
- Resistivity index (RI) is (peak systolic velocity - end diastolic velocity)/peak systolic velocity; normal < 0.7
- Pulsatility index (PI) is (peak systolic velocity - end diastole velocity)/mean velocity, normal < 1.8
- Renal veins
  - Normal caliber 4-9 mm
  - Formed from tributaries that coalesce at renal hilum
  - Right renal vein is relatively short and drains directly into IVC
  - Left renal vein receives left adrenal vein from above and left gonadal vein from below
  - Left renal vein crosses midline between aorta and superior mesenteric artery
  - Spectral Doppler
    - Normal PSV 18-33 cm/s
    - Spectral Doppler in right renal vein mirrors pulsatility in IVC
    - Spectral Doppler in left renal vein may show only slight variability of velocities consequent upon cardiac and respiratory activity

Size

- Bipolar length is found by rotating transducer around its vertical axis such that the longest craniocaudal length can be identified
- Normal size between 10-15 cm
- Volume measurements
  - May be more accurate, but time consuming
  - 3D ellipsoidal formula can be used for volume estimation - length x AP diameter x transverse diameter x 0.5
  - Consistency and changes in volume over time more important

Anatomy-Based Imaging Issues

Imaging Recommendations

- Right kidney
  - Liver used as acoustic window
  - Transducer placed in subcostal or intercostal position
  - Varying degree of respiration is useful
  - Raising patient's right side and scanning laterally/posterolaterally may be useful
- Left kidney
  - More difficult to visualize due to bowel gas from small bowel and splenic flexure
  - Usually easier to search for left kidney using a posterolateral approach with left side raised
  - Full right lateral decubitus with pillow under right flank and left arm extended above head may be useful in difficult cases
    - Spleen can be used as acoustic window for imaging upper pole of left kidney
  - Posterior approach
    - Useful for intervention procedures (renal biopsy, nephrostomy)

- Image quality may be impaired by thick paraspinal muscles and ribs shadowing
- Renal arteries
  - Origins best seen from midline anterior approach
  - Right renal artery can usually be followed to kidney
  - Left renal artery often requires posterolateral coronal transducer scanning position for visualization
- Renal veins
  - Best seen on transverse scan from anterior approach
  - May also be seen on coronal scan from posterolateral coronal

Key Concepts

- Accessory renal vessels
  - Must be accounted for in planning surgery (e.g., resection, transplantation)
  - These are often best seen using multidetector row CT, magnetic resonance angiogram or digital subtraction angiography rather than ultrasound

Clinical Implications

Clinical Importance

- Renal colic
  - Calculi, or "stones" may form within and obstruct the renal calices or ureter
  - Renal carcinoma
    - Tumor invasion of renal veins → lung metastases (common), plus bone and systemic metastases
    - Strong renal fascia usually prevents direct invasion of adjacent organs and body wall
  - Renal cysts
    - Extremely common (> 50% of adults have at least one)

Embryology

Embryologic Events

- Congenital anomalies of renal number, position, structure and form are very common
  - Often accompanied by anomalies of other systems
  - VATER acronym - Vertebral, Anorectal, Tracheoesophageal, Radial ray, Renal
  - Congenital absence of kidney
  - Anomalies of position (ectopia) are common
  - Anomalies of structure
    - Congenitally large septum of Bertin (lobar dysmorphism); asymptomatic
    - Fetal lobulations (lobation), single or multiple indentations of the lateral renal contours
    - Partial duplication: Commonly results in enlarged kidney with 2 separate hila, 2 ureters (may join downstream or join bladder separately); duplex kidney = bifid renal pelvis, single ureter
  - Autosomal dominant polycystic disease: Common hereditary disorder characterized by multiple renal cysts, progressive renal failure & various systemic manifestations (such as cerebral aneurysms)

KIDNEYS

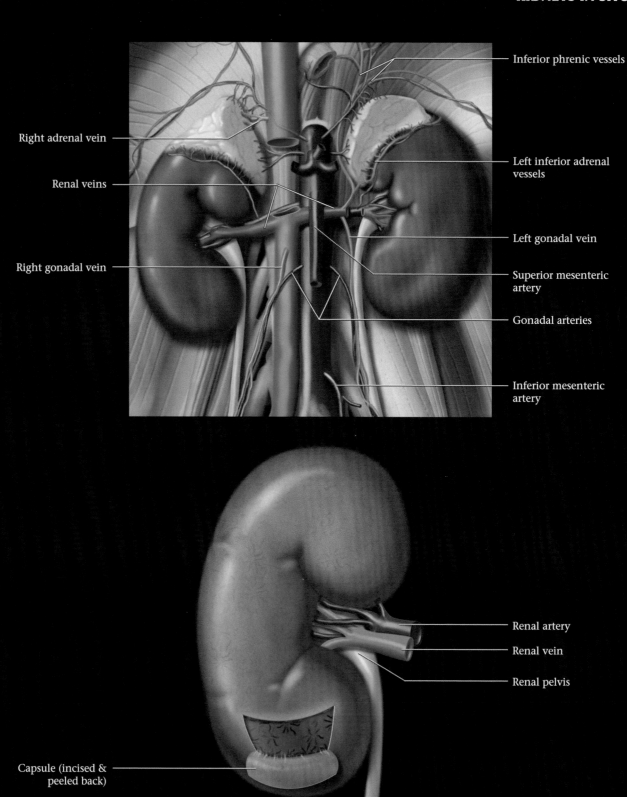

Inferior phrenic vessels

Right adrenal vein

Left inferior adrenal vessels

Renal veins

Left gonadal vein

Right gonadal vein

Superior mesenteric artery

Gonadal arteries

Inferior mesenteric artery

Renal artery

Renal vein

Renal pelvis

Capsule (incised & peeled back)

(Top) The kidneys are retroperitoneal organs that lie lateral to the psoas and "on" the quadratus lumborum muscles. The oblique course of the psoas muscles results in the lower pole of the kidney lying lateral to the upper pole. The right kidney usually lies 1-2 cm lower than the left, due to inferior displacement by the liver. The adrenal glands lie above and medial to the kidneys, separated by a layer of fat and connective tissue. Peritoneum covers much of the anterior surface of the kidneys. The right kidney abuts the liver, hepatic flexure of colon and duodenum, while the left kidney is in close contact with the pancreas (tail), spleen, and splenic flexure. **(Bottom)** The fibrous capsule is stripped off with difficulty. Subcapsular hematomas do not spread far along the surface of the kidney, but compress the renal parenchyma, unlike most perirenal collections.

KIDNEYS

KIDNEY ARTERIES & INTERIOR ANATOMY

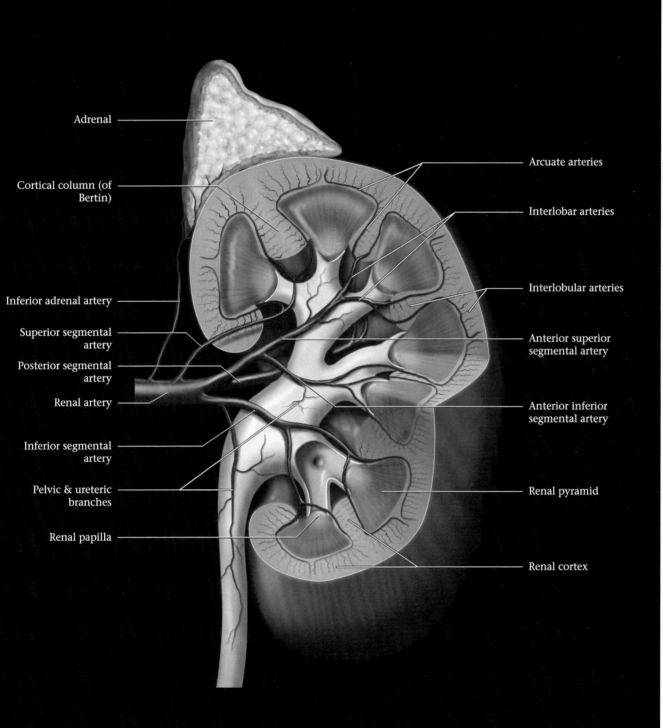

Adrenal

Cortical column (of Bertin)

Inferior adrenal artery

Superior segmental artery

Posterior segmental artery

Renal artery

Inferior segmental artery

Pelvic & ureteric branches

Renal papilla

Arcuate arteries

Interlobar arteries

Interlobular arteries

Anterior superior segmental artery

Anterior inferior segmental artery

Renal pyramid

Renal cortex

The kidney is usually supplied by a single renal artery, the first branch of which is the inferior adrenal artery. It then divides into five segmental arteries only one of which, the posterior segmental artery, passes dorsal to the renal pelvis. The segmental arteries divide into the interlobar arteries that lie in the renal sinus fat. Each interlobar artery branches into 4 to 6 arcuate arteries that follow the convex outer margin of each renal pyramid. The arcuate arteries give rise to the interlobular arteries that lie within the renal cortex, including the cortical columns (of Bertin) that invaginate between the renal pyramids. The interlobular arteries supply the afferent arterioles to the glomeruli. The arterial supply to the kidney is vulnerable as there are no effective anastomoses between the segmental branches, each of which supplies a wedge-shaped segment of parenchyma.

KIDNEYS

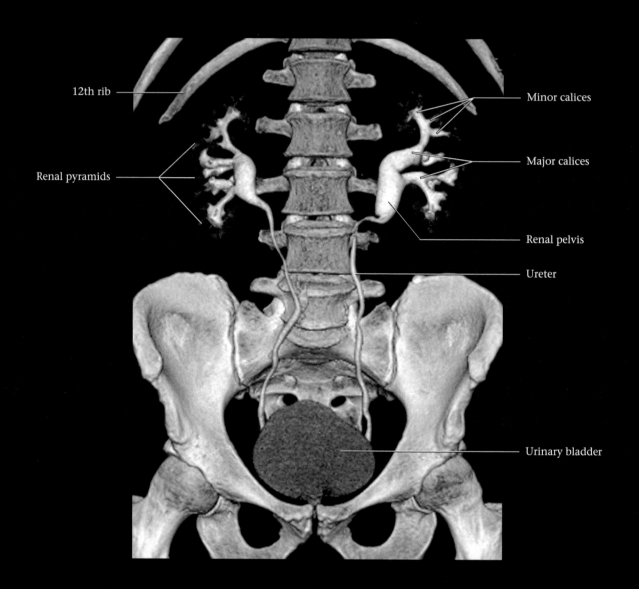

12th rib

Minor calices

Renal pyramids

Major calices

Renal pelvis

Ureter

Urinary bladder

A coronal reconstruction of a series of axial CT sections can be viewed as a surface-rendered 3D image to simulate an excretory urogram. The window levels and workstation controls have been set to display optimally the renal collecting system. The color scale is arbitrary; in this case, opacified urine is displayed as "white". Less dense urine within the renal tubules in the pyramids and the diluted urine within the bladder are displayed as "red". The CT scan was obtained in suspended inspiration, resulting in caudal displacement of the kidneys. In the supine position at quiet breathing, the upper poles of the kidneys usually lie in front of the 12th ribs.

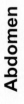

KIDNEYS

Anterior renal fascia

Lateroconal fascia

Psoas (major) muscle

Posterior renal fascia

Latissimus dorsi muscle

Quadratus lumborum muscle

Liver

Adrenal gland

Anterior renal fascia

Posterior renal fascia

Hepatorenal fossa (Morison pouch)

Peritoneum

Iliac crest

Transverse colon

(Top) The anterior and posterior layers of the renal fascia envelope the kidneys and adrenals along with the perirenal fat. Medial to the kidneys, the course of the renal fascia is variable (and controversial). The posterior layer usually fuses with the psoas or quadratus lumborum fascia. The perirenal spaces do not communicate across the abdominal midline. However, the renal & lateroconal fasciae are laminated structures that may be distended with fluid collections to form interfascial planes that do communicate across the midline and also inferiorly to the extraperitoneal pelvis. (Bottom) A sagittal section through the right kidney shows the renal fascia enveloping the kidney and adrenal gland. Inferiorly the anterior and posterior renal fasciae come close together at about the level of the iliac crest. Note the adjacent peritoneal recesses.

Abdomen

IV

KIDNEYS

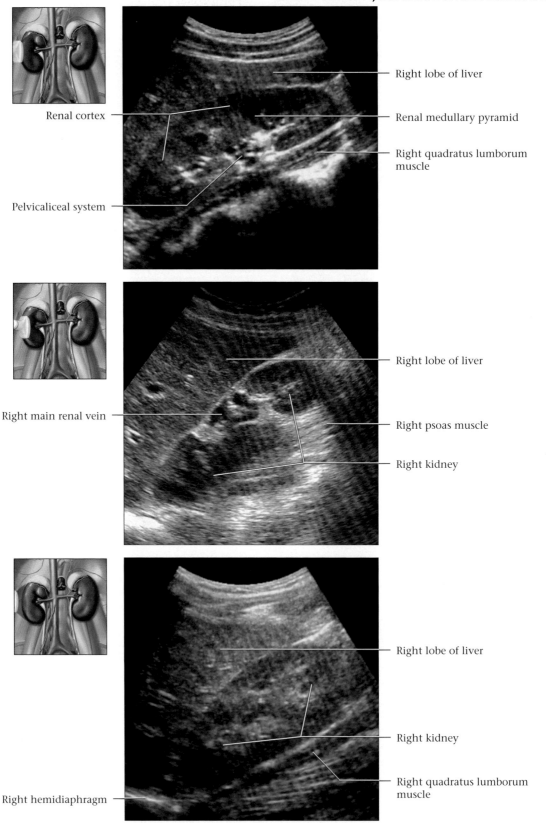

Right lobe of liver

Renal cortex

Renal medullary pyramid

Right quadratus lumborum muscle

Pelvicaliceal system

Right lobe of liver

Right main renal vein

Right psoas muscle

Right kidney

Right lobe of liver

Right kidney

Right quadratus lumborum muscle

Right hemidiaphragm

(Top) Longitudinal grayscale ultrasound of the right kidney using the liver as an acoustic window. This approach usually provides excellent visualization of the right kidney and is useful for measuring bipolar renal length. **(Middle)** Longitudinal, oblique, grayscale ultrasound of the right kidney using the liver as an acoustic window. This view was obtained with a bit more medial angulation (when compared with the previous image). **(Bottom)** Longitudinal, oblique, grayscale ultrasound of the right kidney using the liver as an acoustic window. This view was obtained with a bit more lateral angulation (when compared with the previous two images) and cuts through the renal parenchyma on the lateral aspect of the right kidney. Note the more centrally located pelvicaliceal system is not demonstrated.

KIDNEYS

RIGHT KIDNEY, CT CORRELATION

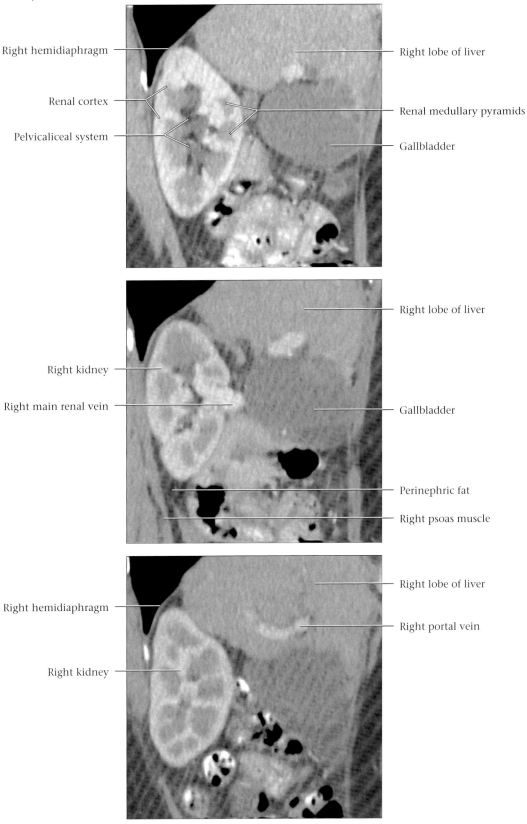

Right hemidiaphragm — Right lobe of liver

Renal cortex — Renal medullary pyramids

Pelvicaliceal system — Gallbladder

Right kidney — Right lobe of liver

Right main renal vein — Gallbladder

Perinephric fat

Right psoas muscle

Right hemidiaphragm — Right lobe of liver

Right portal vein

Right kidney

(Top) Correlative, longitudinal, CT multiplanar reconstruction image of the right kidney through planes that are commonly used when examining the patient with ultrasound. Like ultrasound, multidetector row CT now allows evaluation of kidneys in many planes, however, ionizing radiation and the use of intravenous contrast are its limiting factors, particularly in children. **(Middle)** Correlative, longitudinal, oblique, CT multiplanar reconstruction image of the right kidney cutting through the right renal vein. The plane of this image is angulated more medially when compared with the previous image. **(Bottom)** Correlative, longitudinal, oblique, CT multiplanar reconstruction image of the right kidney cutting through the right portal vein. The plane of this image is angulated more laterally when compared with the previous two images.

KIDNEYS

RIGHT KIDNEY, ANTERIOR ABDOMEN SCAN

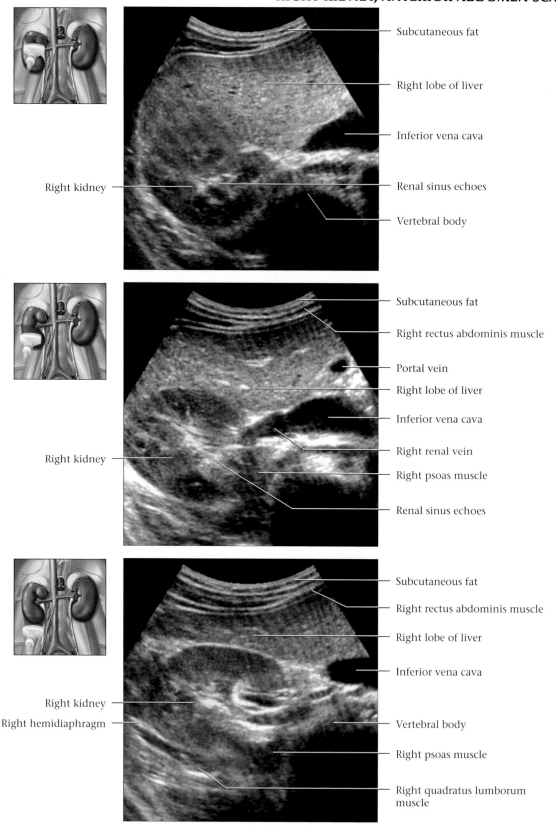

Subcutaneous fat

Right lobe of liver

Inferior vena cava

Renal sinus echoes

Vertebral body

Right kidney

Subcutaneous fat

Right rectus abdominis muscle

Portal vein

Right lobe of liver

Inferior vena cava

Right renal vein

Right psoas muscle

Renal sinus echoes

Right kidney

Subcutaneous fat

Right rectus abdominis muscle

Right lobe of liver

Inferior vena cava

Vertebral body

Right psoas muscle

Right kidney

Right hemidiaphragm

Right quadratus lumborum muscle

(Top) Transverse grayscale ultrasound of the upper pole of the right kidney. (Middle) Transverse grayscale ultrasound of the mid pole of the right kidney shows the renal hilum with the renal vein. Note that the pelvicaliceal system within the renal sinus echoes is not usually visible in the normal individual. (Bottom) Transverse grayscale ultrasound of the lower pole of the right kidney. The renal parenchymal echogenicity is less than the adjacent liver or spleen. If the renal parenchyma is brighter than normal liver, suspect renal parenchymal disease.

Abdomen

KIDNEYS

RIGHT KIDNEY, CT CORRELATION

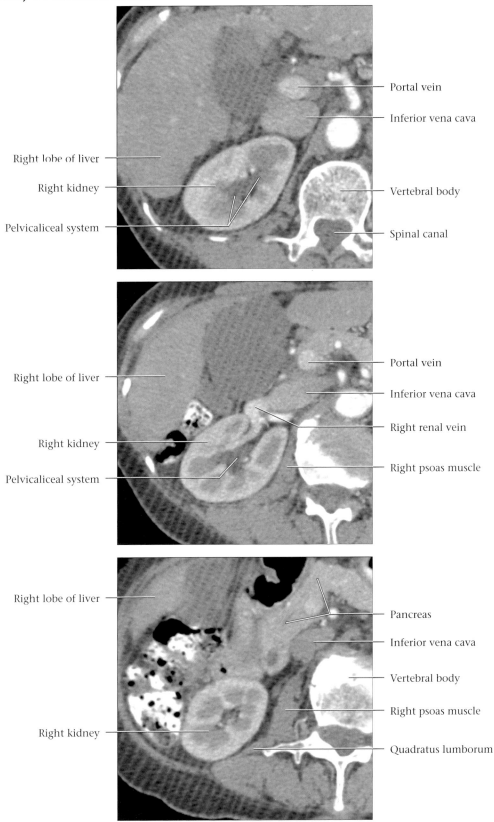

(Top) First in a series of three correlative transverse CT images of the right kidney from the upper pole through the kidney to the lower pole through planes commonly used when examining the patient with ultrasound. This image shows the upper pole of the right kidney. Multidetector row CT with examination in different phases following intravenous contrast injection allows superb differentiation between renal cortex and medulla. (Middle) Correlative transverse CT of the mid pole of the right kidney shows the renal hilum with the renal vein. (Bottom) Correlative transverse CT image of the lower pole of the right kidney.

KIDNEYS

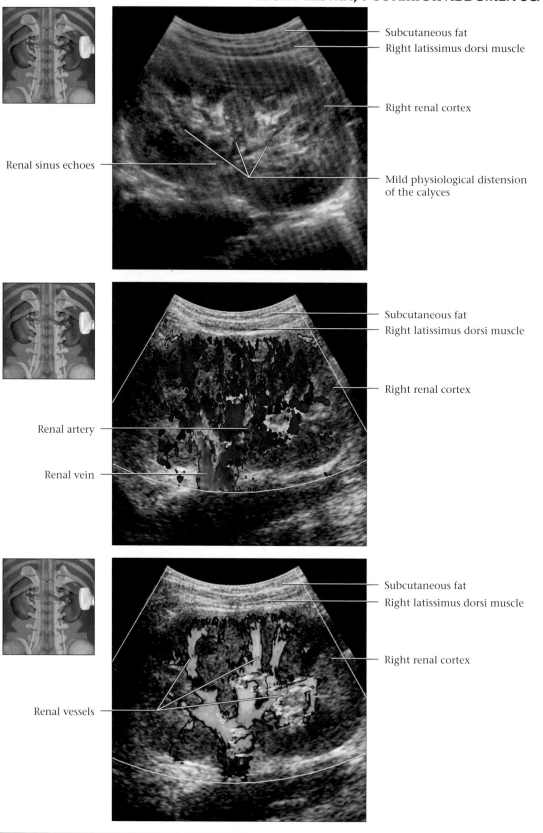

Subcutaneous fat
Right latissimus dorsi muscle

Right renal cortex

Renal sinus echoes

Mild physiological distension of the calyces

Subcutaneous fat
Right latissimus dorsi muscle

Right renal cortex

Renal artery

Renal vein

Subcutaneous fat
Right latissimus dorsi muscle

Right renal cortex

Renal vessels

(Top) Longitudinal grayscale ultrasound of the right kidney scanning from the posterior approach shows mild physiological distension of the calyces. It is a good way for standardizing renal length measurements in children. (Middle) Posterior longitudinal color Doppler ultrasound of the right kidney. This evaluation of the position of major vessels is useful to avoid major vessels during renal interventional procedures such as renal biopsy or nephrostomy. (Bottom) Posterior longitudinal power Doppler ultrasound of the right kidney. Note power Doppler does not provide information about direction of flow within vessels.

KIDNEYS

RIGHT KIDNEY, POSTERIOR ABDOMEN SCAN

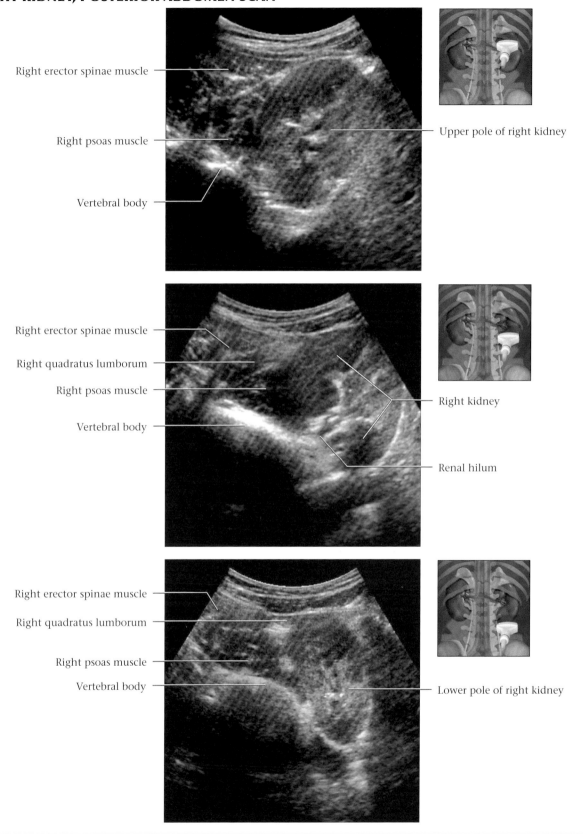

Right erector spinae muscle

Right psoas muscle

Vertebral body

Upper pole of right kidney

Right erector spinae muscle

Right quadratus lumborum

Right psoas muscle

Vertebral body

Right kidney

Renal hilum

Right erector spinae muscle

Right quadratus lumborum

Right psoas muscle

Vertebral body

Lower pole of right kidney

(Top) Transverse grayscale ultrasound of the right kidney scanning from the posterior approach. Scanning through the posterior approach is useful while performing interventional procedures such as nephrostomy or renal biopsy. However, visualization/image quality may be impaired by thick paraspinal muscles and rib shadowing. This image shows the upper pole of the right kidney. **(Middle)** Transverse grayscale ultrasound from the posterior approach shows the mid pole of the right kidney. **(Bottom)** Transverse grayscale ultrasound from the posterior approach shows the lower pole of the right kidney.

KIDNEYS

RIGHT MAIN RENAL ARTERY AND VEIN

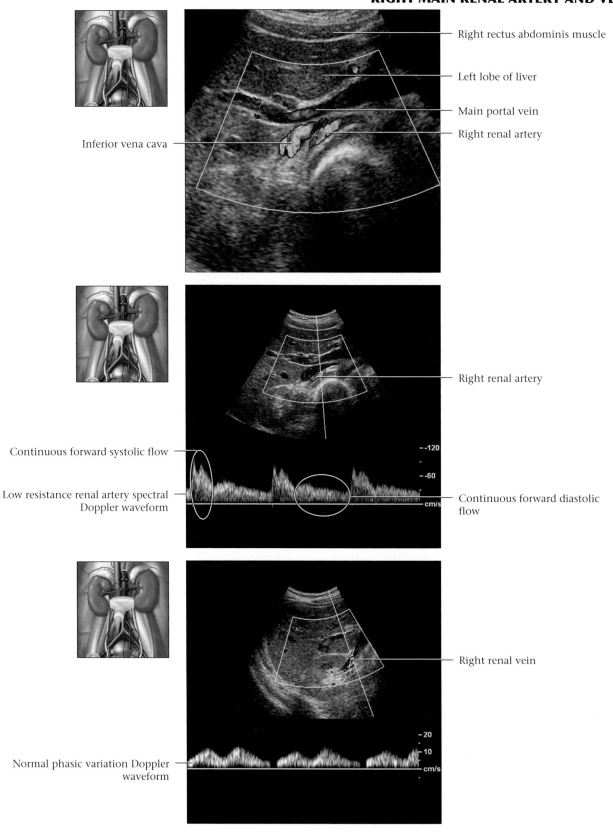

Right rectus abdominis muscle

Left lobe of liver

Main portal vein

Right renal artery

Inferior vena cava

Right renal artery

Continuous forward systolic flow

Low resistance renal artery spectral Doppler waveform

Continuous forward diastolic flow

Right renal vein

Normal phasic variation Doppler waveform

(Top) Transverse color Doppler of the right renal artery. Note the right renal artery lies posterior to the inferior vena cava. The right renal vein, which is not shown on this image, lies anterior to the right renal artery. The renal artery normally measures 5-8 mm in caliber. (Middle) Spectral Doppler waveform of the right renal artery. Note the low resistance renal waveform with continuous forward systolic and diastolic flow. Normal PSV ranges from 60-140 cm/s, not more than 180 cm/s. Normal resistivity index is < 0.7 and normal pulsatility index is < 1.8. In many centers, magnetic resonance imaging is increasingly used for assessment of the main renal arteries. (Bottom) Spectral Doppler waveform of the right renal vein which mirrors the pulsatility in the IVC. The renal vein normally measures 4-9 mm in caliber. Normal PSV ranges from 18-33 cm/s.

KIDNEYS

RIGHT INTRARENAL ARTERY AND VEIN

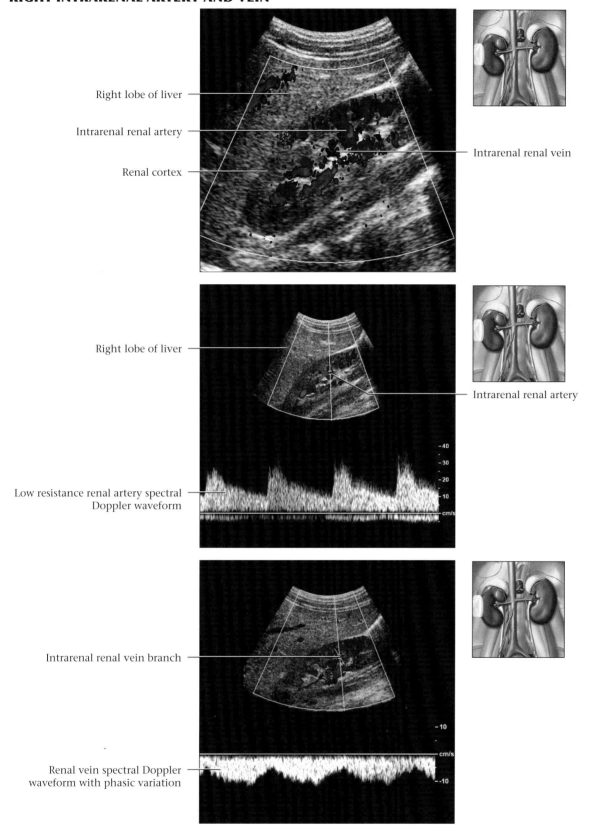

Right lobe of liver

Intrarenal renal artery

Renal cortex

Intrarenal renal vein

Right lobe of liver

Intrarenal renal artery

Low resistance renal artery spectral Doppler waveform

Intrarenal renal vein branch

Renal vein spectral Doppler waveform with phasic variation

(Top) Longitudinal color Doppler ultrasound of the right kidney shows renal artery branches as red and renal vein branches as blue. (Middle) Spectral Doppler waveform of a right intrarenal renal artery branch. Note the low resistance Doppler waveform with continuous diastolic flow similar to that seen in the more proximal renal artery. (Bottom) Spectral Doppler waveform of a right intrarenal renal vein branch. Note the phasic variation similar to that seen in the more central/proximal renal vein.

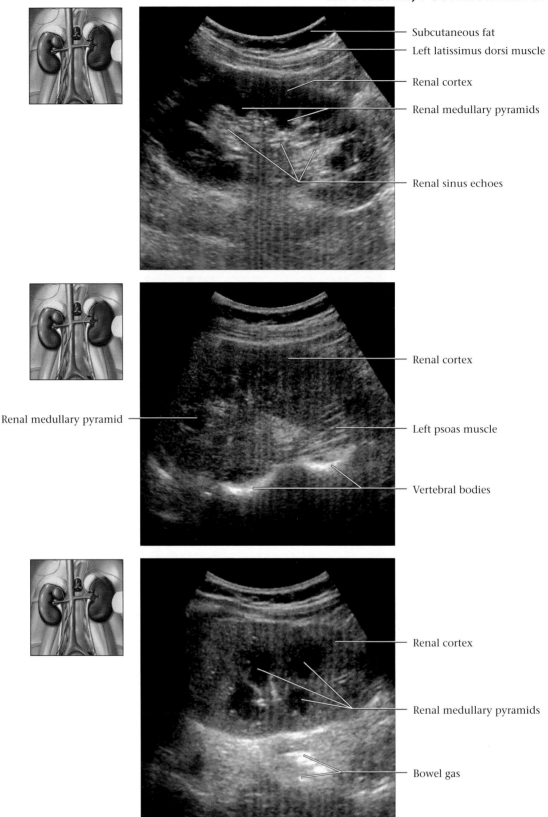

Subcutaneous fat

Left latissimus dorsi muscle

Renal cortex

Renal medullary pyramids

Renal sinus echoes

Renal medullary pyramid

Renal cortex

Left psoas muscle

Vertebral bodies

Renal cortex

Renal medullary pyramids

Bowel gas

(Top) Longitudinal grayscale ultrasound of the left kidney scanning from the posterolateral approach. This approach avoids interference from bowel gas shadowing. (Middle) Longitudinal grayscale ultrasound of the left kidney scanning from the posterolateral approach with the transducer angling more posteriorly when compared with the previous image. Note the left psoas muscle. (Bottom) Longitudinal grayscale ultrasound of the left kidney scanning from the posterolateral approach with the transducer angling more anteriorly when compared with the previous two images.

KIDNEYS

LEFT KIDNEY, CT CORRELATION

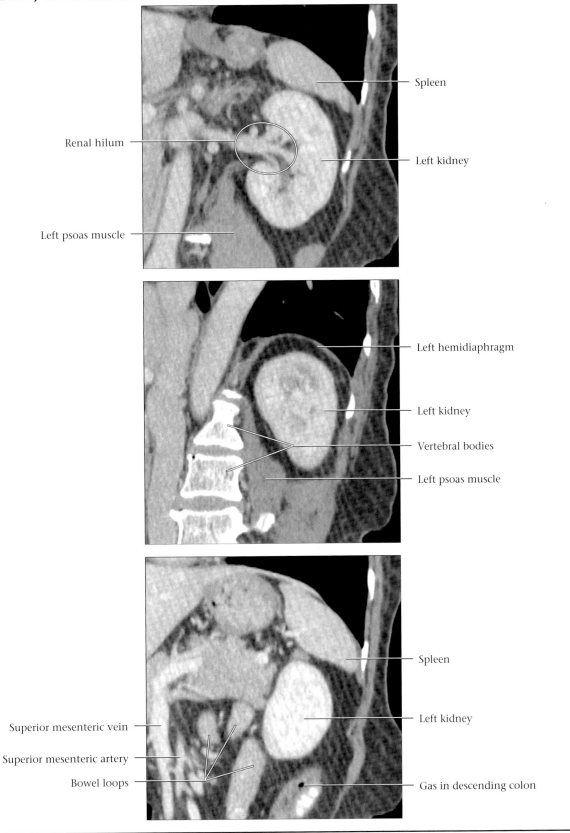

Spleen

Renal hilum

Left kidney

Left psoas muscle

Left hemidiaphragm

Left kidney

Vertebral bodies

Left psoas muscle

Spleen

Left kidney

Superior mesenteric vein

Superior mesenteric artery

Bowel loops

Gas in descending colon

(Top) First in a series of three correlative, oblique, multiplanar reconstruction, longitudinal CT images of the left kidney through planes commonly used when examining the patient with ultrasound. The clear visualization of the kidney, renal pedicle and surrounding structures, make multidetector row CT the imaging modality of choice (over ultrasound) in patients suspected to have renal injury. **(Middle)** Correlative, oblique, multiplanar reconstruction, longitudinal CT image of the left kidney in a plane more posterior to the previous image. **(Bottom)** Correlative, oblique, multiplanar reconstruction, longitudinal CT image of the left kidney in a plane more anterior to the previous two images.

KIDNEYS

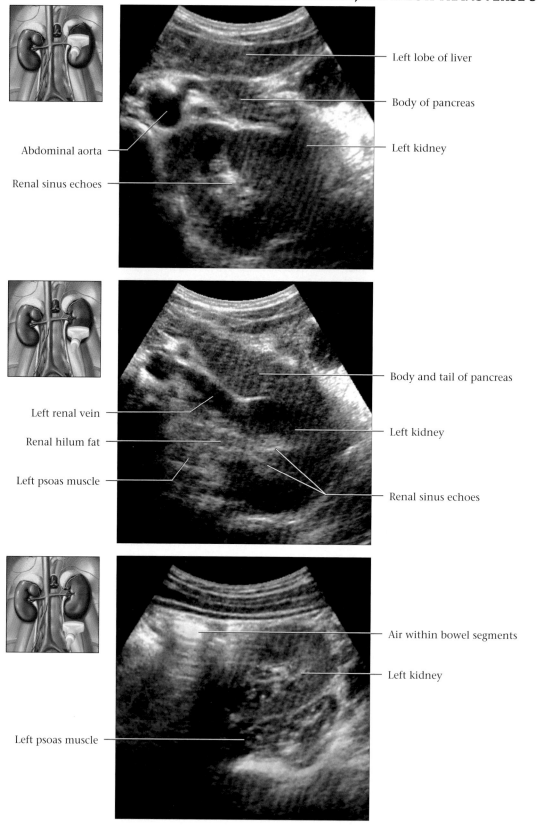

Left lobe of liver

Body of pancreas

Left kidney

Abdominal aorta

Renal sinus echoes

Body and tail of pancreas

Left kidney

Left renal vein

Renal hilum fat

Left psoas muscle

Renal sinus echoes

Air within bowel segments

Left kidney

Left psoas muscle

(Top) Transverse grayscale ultrasound of the upper pole of the left kidney using the anterior approach. Note the image quality is limited by interference from gas in the stomach and bowel. The presence of bowel loops anteriorly also limits the use of this approach for interventional procedures on the left kidney. (Middle) Transverse grayscale ultrasound of the mid pole of the left kidney using the anterior approach. (Bottom) Transverse grayscale ultrasound of the lower pole of the left kidney using the anterior approach.

KIDNEYS

LEFT KIDNEY, CT CORRELATION

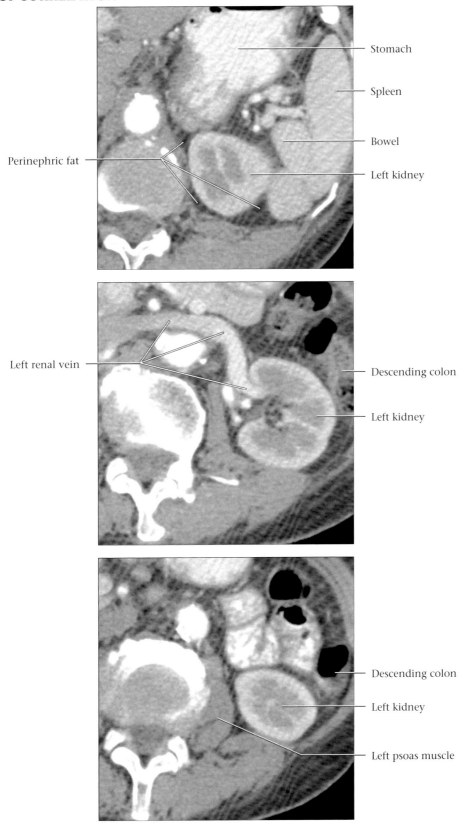

(Top) First in a series of three correlative transverse CT images of the left kidney through planes commonly used when examining the kidney using the anterior approach. Note the relationship of the spleen to the upper pole of the left kidney, allowing it to be used as an acoustic window, particularly in patients with splenomegaly. This transverse CT image shows the upper pole of the left kidney. (Middle) Correlative transverse CT image of the mid pole of the left kidney at the level of the left renal vein. (Bottom) Correlative transverse CT image of the lower pole of the left kidney.

KIDNEYS

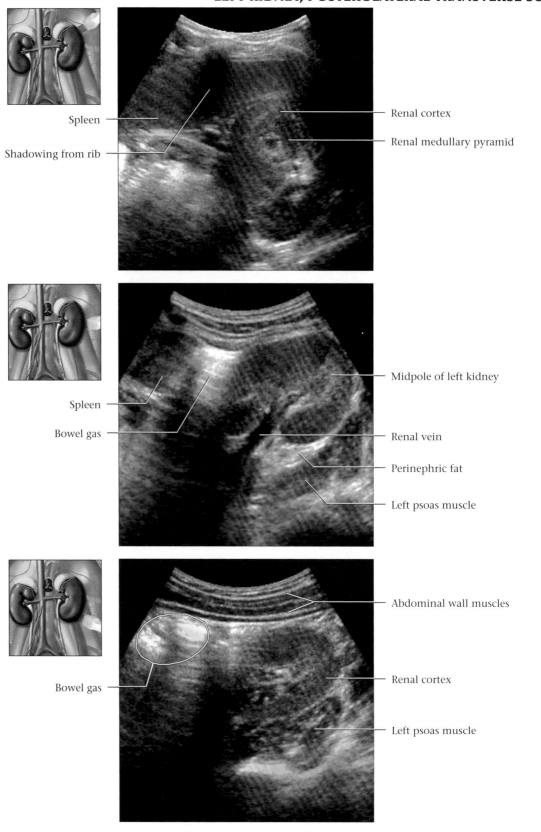

Spleen

Shadowing from rib

Renal cortex

Renal medullary pyramid

Spleen

Bowel gas

Midpole of left kidney

Renal vein

Perinephric fat

Left psoas muscle

Bowel gas

Abdominal wall muscles

Renal cortex

Left psoas muscle

(Top) Transverse grayscale ultrasound of the upper pole of the left kidney using the posterolateral approach. Note the proximity of the kidney to the skin surface and the absence of intervening bowel loops. (Middle) Transverse grayscale ultrasound of the mid pole of the left kidney using the posterolateral approach. (Bottom) Transverse grayscale ultrasound of the lower pole of the left kidney using the posterolateral approach.

KIDNEYS

LEFT KIDNEY, POSTERIOR ABDOMEN SCAN

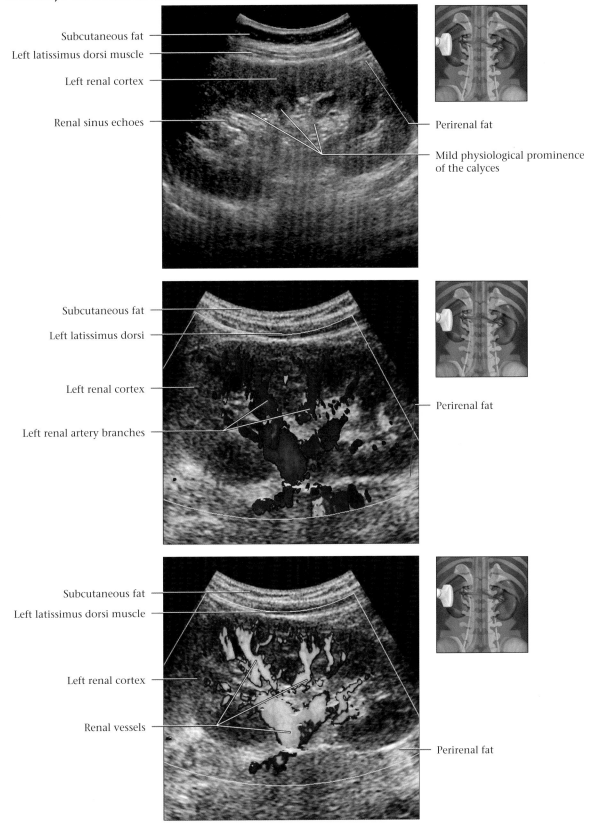

(Top) Image labels:
- Subcutaneous fat
- Left latissimus dorsi muscle
- Left renal cortex
- Renal sinus echoes
- Perirenal fat
- Mild physiological prominence of the calyces

(Middle) Image labels:
- Subcutaneous fat
- Left latissimus dorsi
- Left renal cortex
- Left renal artery branches
- Perirenal fat

(Bottom) Image labels:
- Subcutaneous fat
- Left latissimus dorsi muscle
- Left renal cortex
- Renal vessels
- Perirenal fat

(Top) Longitudinal grayscale ultrasound of the left kidney scanning from the posterior approach shows mild physiological distension of the calyces. This is a useful view for performing renal interventional procedures such as renal biopsy or nephrostomy. It is also a good way for standardizing renal length measurements in children. **(Middle)** Posterior, longitudinal, color Doppler ultrasound of the left kidney. This assessment of the position of major vessels is useful for avoiding major vessels when performing renal interventional procedures such as renal biopsy or nephrostomy. **(Bottom)** Posterior, longitudinal, power Doppler ultrasound of the left kidney. Note the absence of information about flow direction on power Doppler.

KIDNEYS

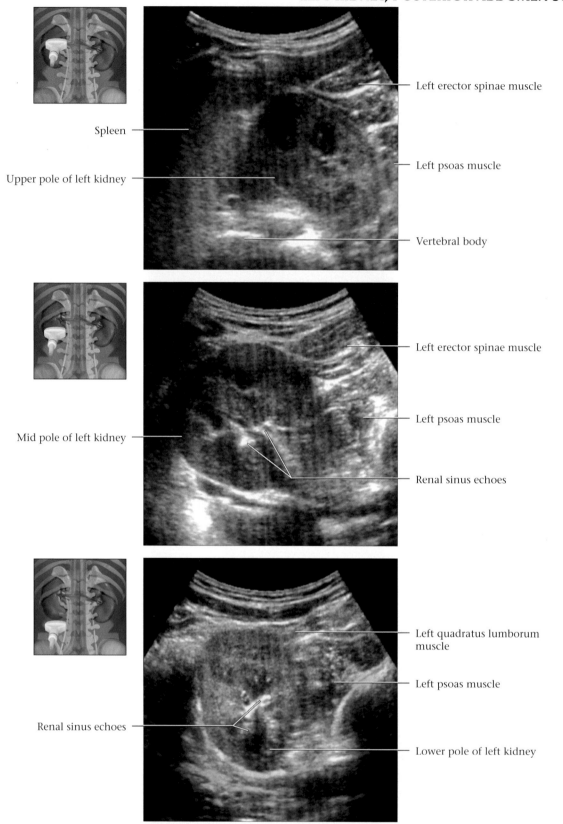

Spleen

Upper pole of left kidney

Left erector spinae muscle

Left psoas muscle

Vertebral body

Mid pole of left kidney

Left erector spinae muscle

Left psoas muscle

Renal sinus echoes

Renal sinus echoes

Left quadratus lumborum muscle

Left psoas muscle

Lower pole of left kidney

(Top) Transverse grayscale ultrasound of the upper pole of the left kidney using the posterior approach. Note the proximity of the kidney to the skin surface, absence of intervening bowel/other major structures, making this a suitable approach for renal interventional procedures. (Middle) Transverse grayscale ultrasound of the mid pole of the left kidney using the posterior approach. (Bottom) Transverse grayscale ultrasound of the lower pole of the left kidney using the posterior approach.

KIDNEYS

LEFT MAIN RENAL ARTERY AND VEIN

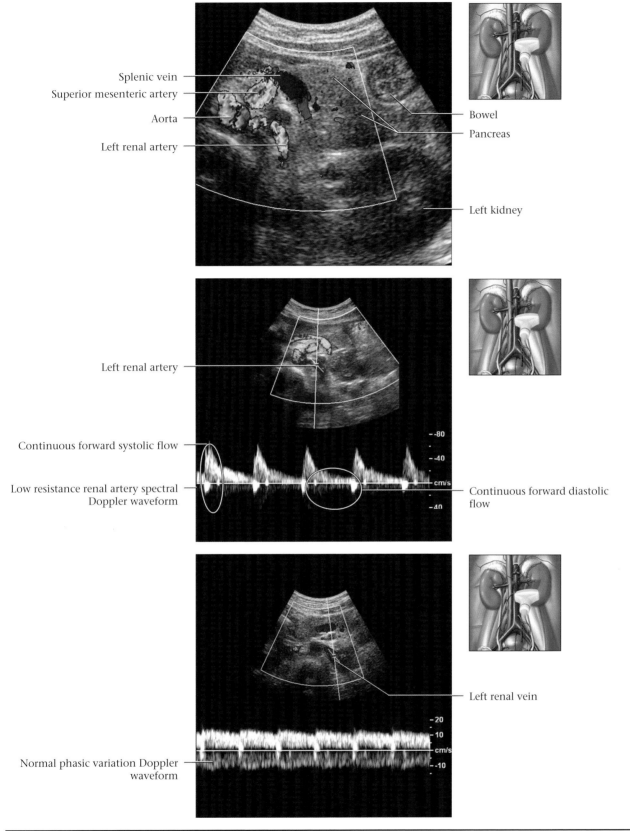

Splenic vein
Superior mesenteric artery
Aorta
Left renal artery

Bowel
Pancreas

Left kidney

Left renal artery

Continuous forward systolic flow

Low resistance renal artery spectral Doppler waveform

Continuous forward diastolic flow

Left renal vein

Normal phasic variation Doppler waveform

(Top) Transverse color Doppler image of the left renal artery. Note the left renal artery arises from just around or below the level of the superior mesenteric artery. The normal caliber of the renal artery ranges from 5-8 mm. (Middle) Spectral Doppler waveform of the left renal artery. Note the low resistance renal waveform with continuous forward systolic and diastolic flow. Normal PSV ranges from 60-140 cm/s, not more than 180 cm/s. Normal resistivity index is < 0.7 and normal pulsatility index is < 1.8. In many centers, magnetic resonance imaging is increasingly used for assessment of the main renal arteries. (Bottom) Spectral Doppler waveform of the left renal vein which shows only slight variability of the velocities consequent upon cardiac and respiratory activity. The renal vein normally measures 4-9 mm in caliber. Normal PSV is 18-33 cm/s.

KIDNEYS

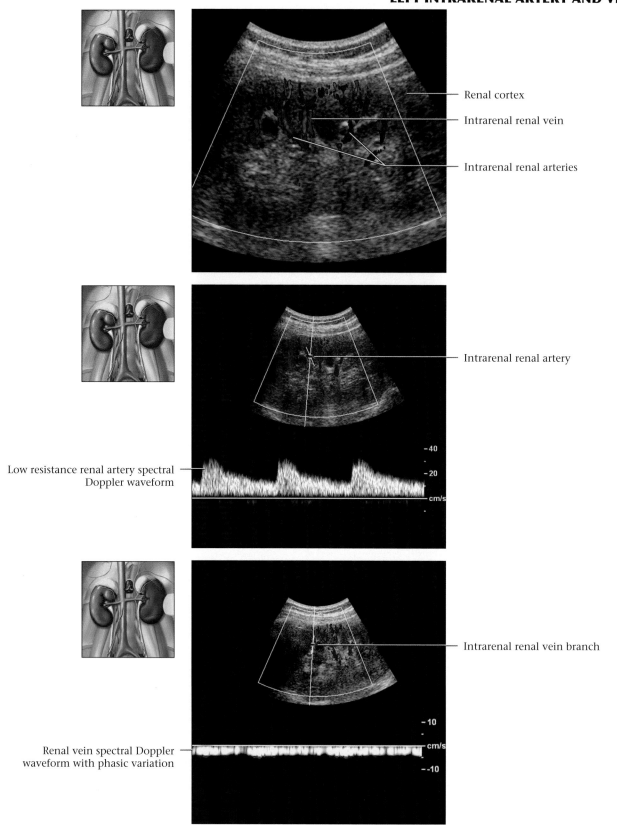

Renal cortex

Intrarenal renal vein

Intrarenal renal arteries

Intrarenal renal artery

Low resistance renal artery spectral Doppler waveform

Intrarenal renal vein branch

Renal vein spectral Doppler waveform with phasic variation

(Top) Longitudinal color Doppler ultrasound image of the left kidney shows renal artery branches as red and renal vein branches as blue. (Middle) Spectral Doppler waveform of a left intrarenal renal artery branch. Note the low resistance Doppler waveform with continuous diastolic flow similar to that seen in the more proximal renal artery. (Bottom) Spectral Doppler waveform of a left intrarenal renal vein branch. Note the phasic variation similar to that seen in the more central/proximal renal vein.

KIDNEYS

HYPERTROPHIED COLUMN OF BERTIN

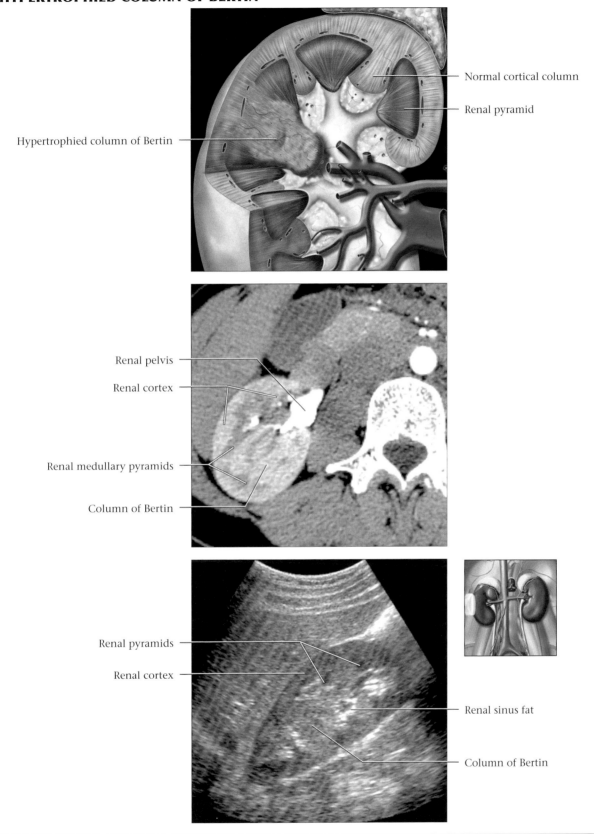

Normal cortical column

Renal pyramid

Hypertrophied column of Bertin

Renal pelvis

Renal cortex

Renal medullary pyramids

Column of Bertin

Renal pyramids

Renal cortex

Renal sinus fat

Column of Bertin

(Top) Graphic shows a hypertrophied column of Bertin which is a rounded enlargement of the septal cortical tissue that separates the renal pyramids. This is normal tissue with the same imaging features as other renal cortex, but it may protrude into the renal sinus fat simulating a renal mass. (Middle) This corticomedullary phase CT image shows a rounded, prominent "mass" of cortical tissue projecting deep into the renal sinus, seemingly compressing and displacing the renal pyramids in the midpole of the right kidney. The opacified urine is the result of a prior "timing bolus" of contrast material. (Bottom) A sagittal sonogram shows a rounded "mass", a hypertrophied column of Bertin, projecting into and displacing renal sinus fat. This has the same echogenicity as other cortical tissue. The location, between the upper and midpole of the kidney, is typical.

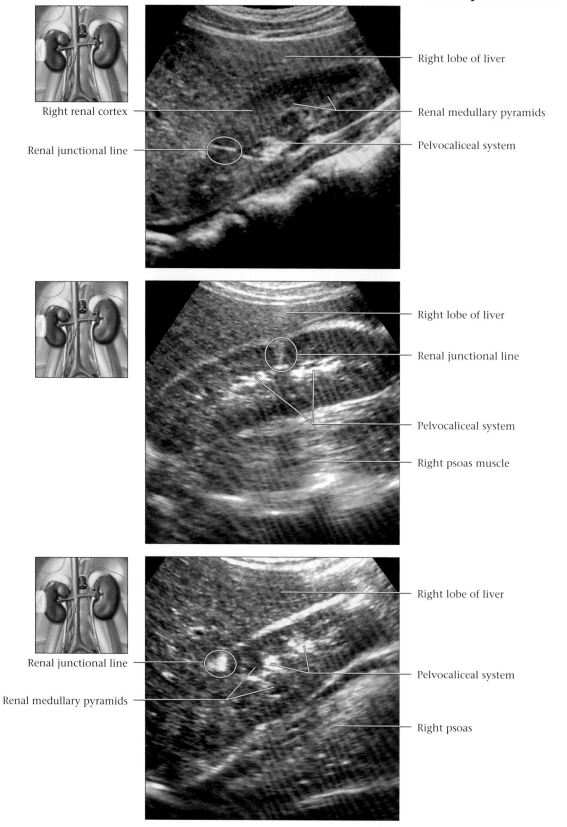

(Top) Longitudinal grayscale ultrasound of the right kidney shows the typical location of a renal junctional line at the anterosuperior aspect of the right kidney. (Middle) Longitudinal, transabdominal, grayscale ultrasound reveals another variation of the renal junctional line, seen at the middle third of the kidney, which is a less common location compared to the previous image. (Bottom) Longitudinal, transabdominal, grayscale ultrasound shows a renal junctional line as a triangular echogenic focus near the junction of the upper and middle third of the right kidney.

FETAL LOBATION

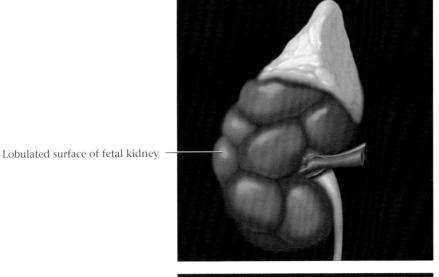

Lobulated surface of fetal kidney

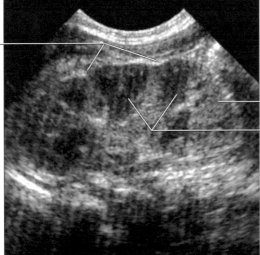

Fetal lobulations

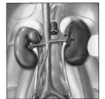

Left renal cortex

Renal medullary pyramids

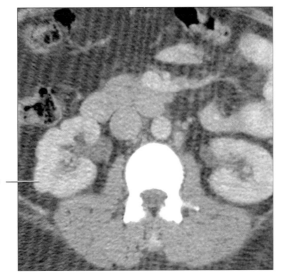

Right kidney

(Top) Graphic shows the typical lobulated appearance of the kidney in fetal life, reflecting the development of the kidney from numerous lobes, each consisting of a renal pyramid and its associated cortex. This may persist into infancy and occasionally into adult life, though to a lesser degree. Note that the adrenal gland is relatively large compared with the kidney in fetal life and childhood. **(Middle)** Intercostal, longitudinal, grayscale ultrasound of the left kidney in a neonate shows fetal lobulations along the contour of the kidney. **(Bottom)** A more caudal section shows the lobulated surface of the right kidney.

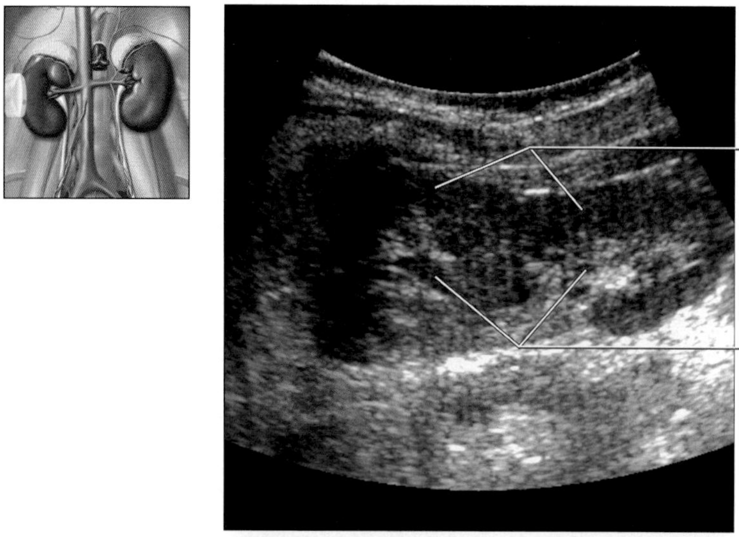

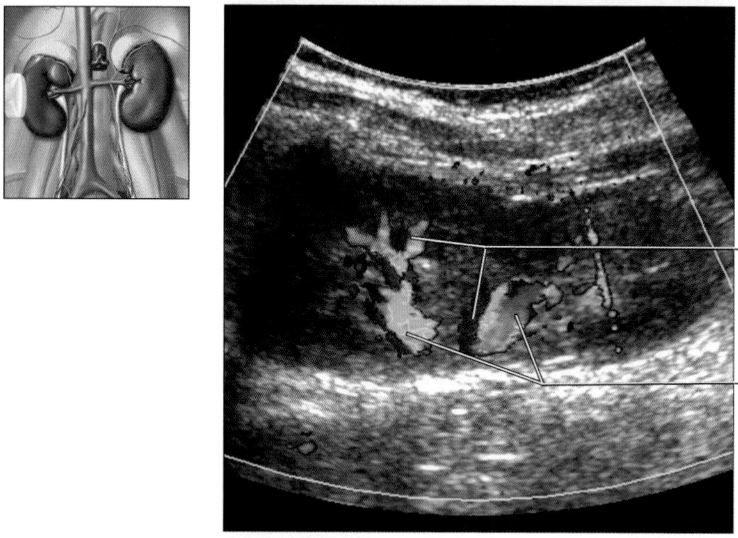

Renal cortex

Pelvocaliceal systems

Intrarenal arteries

Renal veins

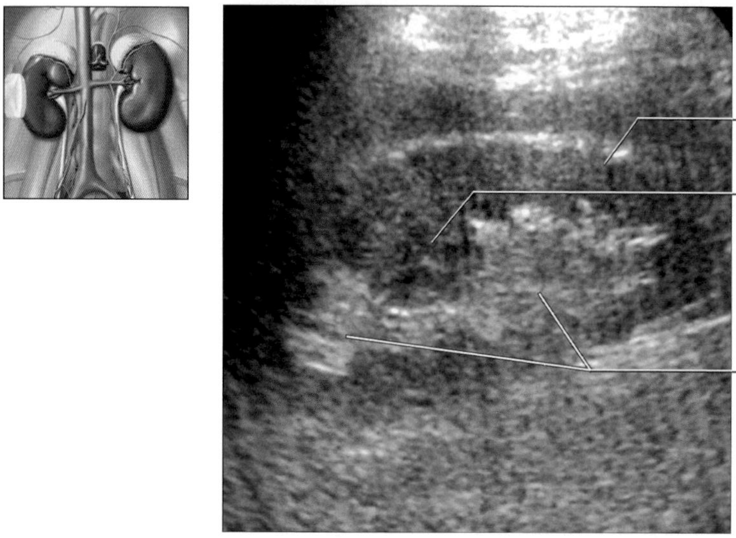

Renal parenchyma

Hypertrophied column of Bertin

Pelvocaliceal system

(Top) Longitudinal, transabdominal, grayscale ultrasound of the right kidney shows 2 central echo complexes representing 2 pelvocaliceal systems and an intervening renal parenchyma in a case of duplex kidney. A duplex kidney may be longer than its counterpart and may be associated with a single or a double ureter. When hydronephrosis is present, it is usually seen in the upper moiety. **(Middle)** Longitudinal, transabdominal, color Doppler ultrasound of the duplex kidney shows vascular distribution in the 2 pelvocaliceal systems. **(Bottom)** Longitudinal grayscale ultrasound of the right kidney shows renal parenchyma indenting on the pelvicaliceal kystem. Compare with the duplex kidney images and note the renal parenchyma does not completely intervene and separate the central echo complex. This is a case of hypertrophied column of Bertin.

KIDNEYS

HORSESHOE KIDNEY

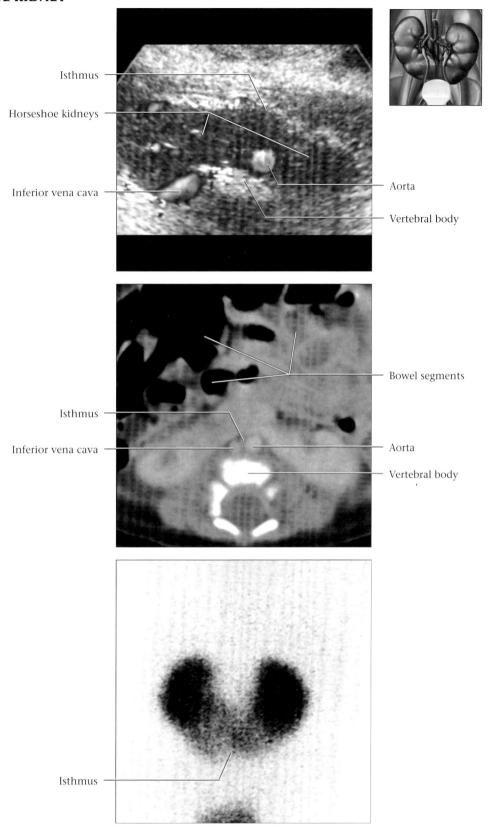

(Top) Transverse, transabdominal ultrasound of horseshoe kidneys shows the isthmus of the kidneys and its relationships with the aorta, inferior vena cava and spine. **(Middle)** Axial CT image of horseshoe kidneys with the isthmus crossing over the aorta and inferior vena cava. **(Bottom)** Tc-99m DMSA scan shows symmetrical midline fusion of a horseshoe kidney with a characteristic U-shape.

RENAL ARTERY STENOSIS

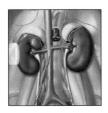

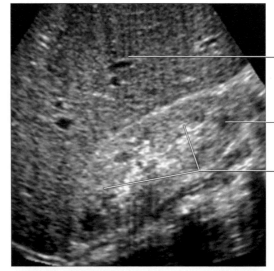

— Right lobe of liver

— Renal medullary pyramid

— Right kidney with echogenic parenchyma

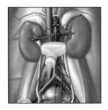

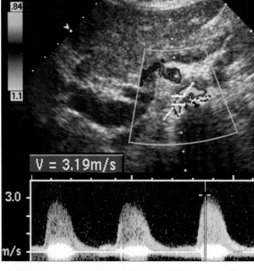

V = 3.19m/s

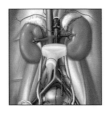

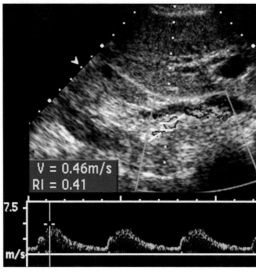

V = 0.46m/s
RI = 0.41

(Top) Longitudinal grayscale ultrasound of the right kidney shows a small kidney with increased renal parenchymal echogenicity. The appearance is suggestive of medical renal disease; the causes are many and may include renal artery stenosis. (Middle) Pulsed Doppler ultrasound of the right renal artery shows color aliasing in the proximal right renal artery which registers a peak systolic velocity of 319 cm/sec, consistent with high grade stenosis. The renal aortic ratio was 4.0. (Bottom) Transverse pulsed Doppler ultrasound at the right renal hilar region of the same patient as previous two images. Note the damped Doppler waveforms (parvus tardus) demonstrated distal to the right renal artery stenosis.

KIDNEYS

RENAL VEIN THROMBOSIS

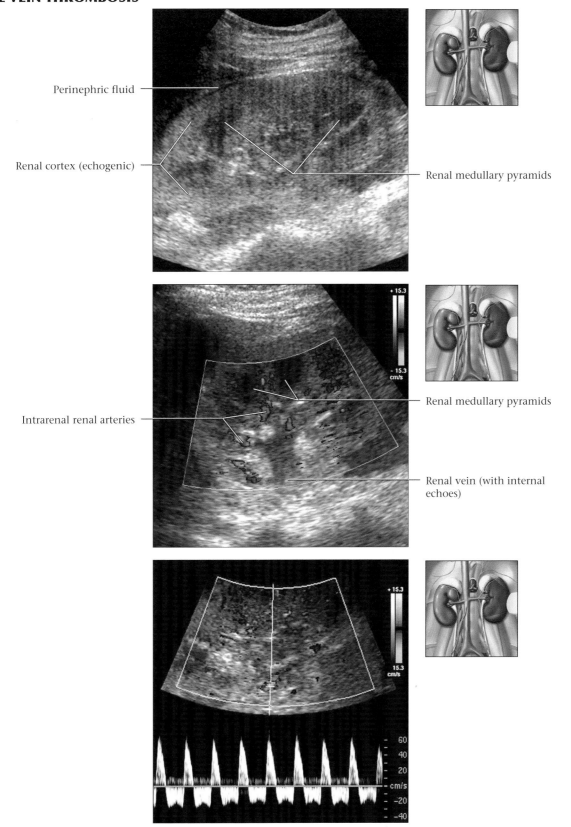

Perinephric fluid

Renal cortex (echogenic)

Renal medullary pyramids

Intrarenal renal arteries

Renal medullary pyramids

Renal vein (with internal echoes)

(Top) Longitudinal, transabdominal, grayscale ultrasound shows a bulky kidney with increased cortical echogenicity, and minimal perinephric fluid. **(Middle)** Longitudinal, transabdominal, color Doppler ultrasound reveals echogenic material distending the renal vein and absent venous blood flow. **(Bottom)** Corresponding, oblique, pulsed Doppler ultrasound shows striking diastolic flow reversal in the renal artery. The findings in this image and the previous two are characteristic of renal vein thrombosis.

EXTRARENAL PELVIS VS. HYDRONEPHROSIS

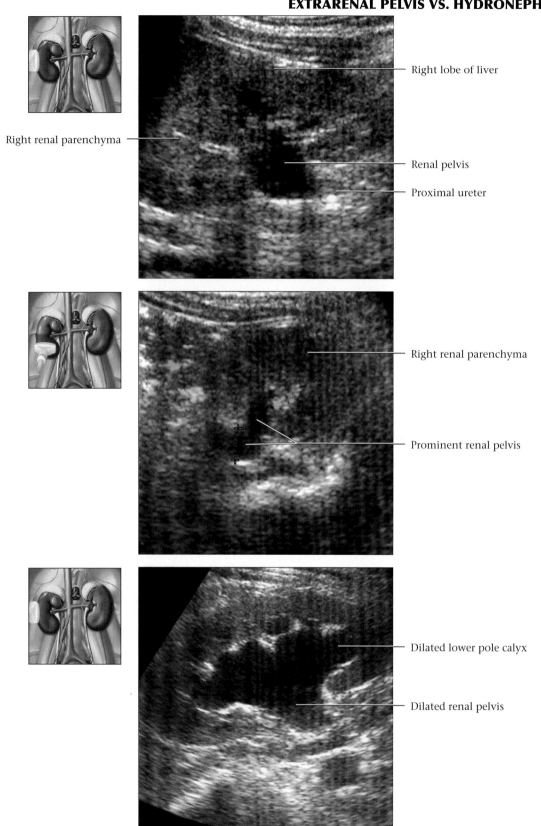

Right renal parenchyma

Right lobe of liver

Renal pelvis

Proximal ureter

Right renal parenchyma

Prominent renal pelvis

Dilated lower pole calyx

Dilated renal pelvis

(Top) Longitudinal, transabdominal, grayscale ultrasound shows a prominent pelvis with no obstructing element. The proximal ureter is not dilated. (Middle) Transverse, transabdominal, grayscale ultrasound of the right kidney in the same patient as previous image. The renal pelvis diameter is 7 mm and still within normal limit. A diameter of > 1.0 cm is considered dilated. (Bottom) Longitudinal, transabdominal, grayscale ultrasound shows a grossly dilated pelvocaliceal system. Renal pelvis diameter is more than 1 cm. A search for an obstructive element must be attempted when this is encountered.

KIExDNEYS

FOCAL BACTERIAL NEPHRITIS

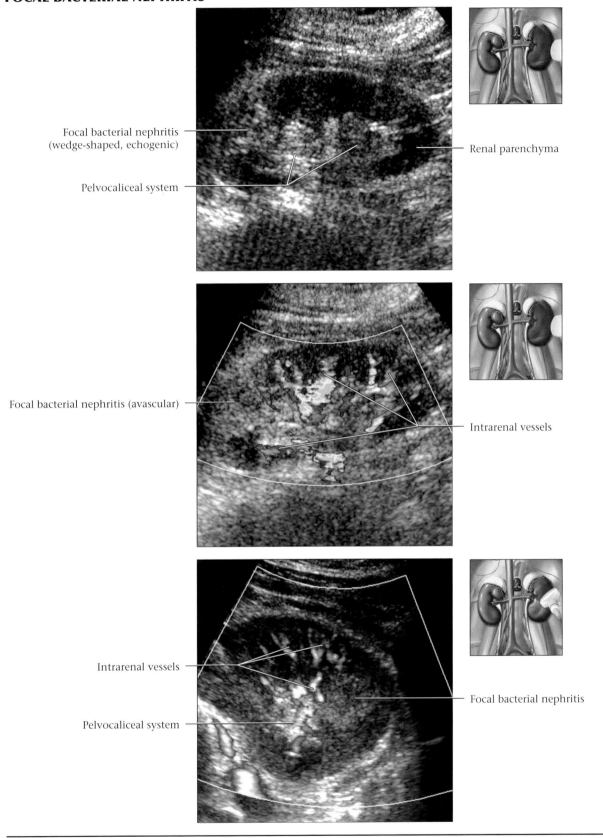

Focal bacterial nephritis (wedge-shaped, echogenic)

Pelvocaliceal system

Renal parenchyma

Focal bacterial nephritis (avascular)

Intrarenal vessels

Intrarenal vessels

Pelvocaliceal system

Focal bacterial nephritis

(Top) Longitudinal, transabdominal, grayscale ultrasound shows a wedge-shaped echogenic area in a febrile patient with flank pain. **(Middle)** Longitudinal, transabdominal, color Doppler ultrasound reveals absent vascular flow in the parenchyma. In the proper clinical setting, sonographic findings are diagnostic of focal bacterial nephritis. **(Bottom)** Transverse, transabdominal, power Doppler of the kidney of another case of focal bacterial nephritis. There is an echogenic focus devoid of vascular flow despite power Doppler sensitivity to vascularity. Sonographic findings overlap with renal metastasis and angiomyolipoma.

Abdomen

IV

97

ADRENALS

Gross Anatomy

Overview
- Adrenal (suprarenal) glands are part of the endocrine and neurological systems
  - Lie within the perirenal space bilaterally, bounded by the renal (perirenal) fascia
  - Lie above and medial to kidneys

Relations
- Right adrenal is more apical in location
  - Lies anterolateral to right crus of diaphragm, medial to liver, posterior to inferior vena cava (IVC)
  - Often pyramidal in shape, inverted "V" shape on transverse section
- Left adrenal is more caudal, lies medial to upper pole of left kidney, lateral to left crus of diaphragm, posterior to splenic vein & pancreas
  - Often crescentic in shape, "lambda" or triangular on transverse section

Divisions
- Adrenal cortex
  - Derived from mesoderm
  - Secretes corticosteroids (cortisol, aldosterone) and androgens
- Adrenal medulla
  - Derived from neural crest
  - Part of the sympathetic nervous system
  - Chromaffin cells secrete catecholamines (mostly epinephrine) into bloodstream
- Vessels, nerves & lymphatics
  - Arteries
    - Superior adrenal arteries: (6-8) from inferior phrenic arteries
    - Middle adrenal artery: (1) from abdominal aorta
    - Inferior adrenal artery: (1) from renal arteries
  - Veins
    - Right adrenal vein drains into IVC
    - Left adrenal vein drains into left renal vein (usually after joining left inferior phrenic vein)
  - Nerves
    - Extensive sympathetic connection to adrenal medulla
    - Presynaptic sympathetic fibers from paravertebral ganglia end directly on the secretory cells of medulla
  - Lymphatics
    - Drain to lumbar (aortic and caval) nodes

Anatomy-Based Imaging Issues

Imaging Recommendations
- Transducer: 2-5 MHz
  - High frequency (7.5-10 MHz) linear transducer may be used in neonates
- Complex shape of the adrenal glands requires multiplanar evaluation
- Ultrasound may be used for initial screening and detection of adrenal lesions, followed by CT/MR for further characterization
- Right adrenal gland
  - Intercostal transverse approach, using the liver as acoustic window
  - Direct anterior abdomen scanning is limited by overlying bowel loops
- Left adrenal gland
  - Intercostal at the mid-axillary line, using the spleen or left kidney as acoustic window
  - In pediatric subjects and thin adults, direct transabdominal ultrasound at the epigastrium
    - Stomach may be distended with fluid to serve as acoustic window

Clinical Implications

Clinical Importance
- Rich blood supply of adrenals reflects important endocrine function
  - Adrenal glands are common site for hematologic metastases (lung, breast, melanoma, etc.)
- Adrenal glands are designed to respond to stress (trauma, sepsis, surgery, etc.) by secreting more cortisol & epinephrine
  - Overwhelming stress may result in adrenal hemorrhage, acute adrenal insufficiency (Addisonian crisis)

Key Concepts
- Adrenal (cortical) adenomas
  - Very common (at least 2% of general population), but usually cause no symptoms
  - Usually contain abundant intra & intercellular lipid (precursor to steroid hormones)
  - Best evaluated by CT and MR sequences that show lipid-rich mass
- Cushing syndrome
  - Due to excess cortisol
  - Signs: Truncal obesity, hirsutism, hypertension, abdominal striae
  - Causes: Pituitary tumors (→ ACTH), exogenous (medications) > adrenal adenoma > carcinoma
- Conn syndrome (excess aldosterone)
  - Signs: Hypertension, hypokalemic alkalosis
  - Causes: Adrenal adenomas > hyperplasia > carcinoma
- Addison syndrome (adrenal insufficiency)
  - Signs: Hypotension, weight loss, altered pigmentation
  - Causes: Autoimmune > adrenal metastases > adrenal hemorrhage > adrenal infection
- Pheochromocytoma (tumor of adrenal medulla)
  - Signs: Headache, palpitations, excessive perspiration
  - 90% arise in adrenal, 90% unilateral, 90% benign
    - Similar tumor arising in other chromaffin cells of sympathetic ganglia is called paraganglioma
  - May occur in syndromes, including
    - Multiple endocrine neoplasia (often with thyroid & parathyroid tumors)
    - Neurofibromatosis
    - Von Hippel Lindau (along with renal & pancreatic cysts and tumors, CNS hemangioblastomas)

ADRENAL GLANDS IN SITU

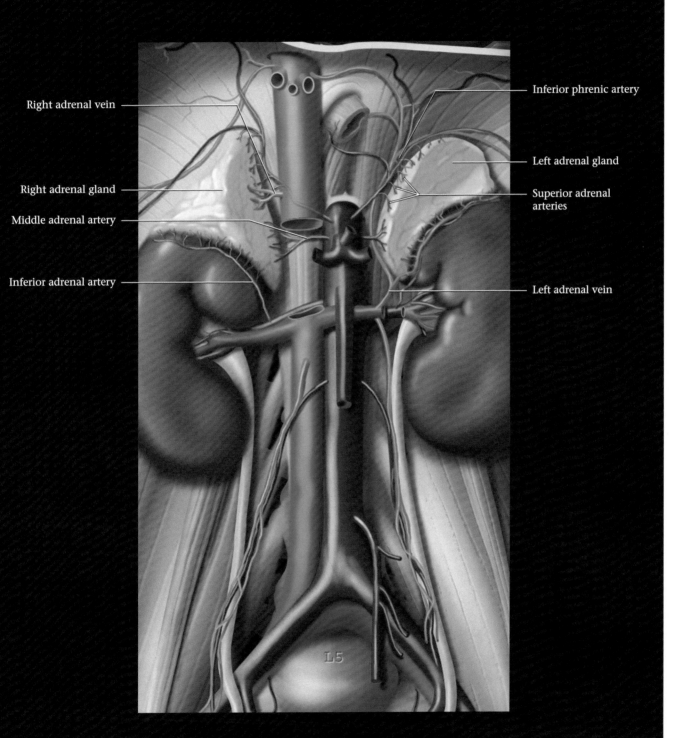

Right adrenal vein

Right adrenal gland

Middle adrenal artery

Inferior adrenal artery

Inferior phrenic artery

Left adrenal gland

Superior adrenal arteries

Left adrenal vein

L5

Graphic shows the adrenal glands rest atop the kidneys, with an interposed layer of fat. Reflecting their critical role in maintaining homeostasis and responding to stress, the adrenal glands have a very rich vascular supply. The superior adrenal arteries are short branches of the inferior phrenic arteries bilaterally. The middle adrenal arteries are short vessels arising from the aorta. The inferior adrenal arteries are branches of the renal arteries. The left adrenal vein drains into the left renal vein, while the right adrenal vein drains directly into the IVC. The size of the adrenal glands is somewhat exaggerated in this illustration, to facilitate demonstration of the vascular anatomy.

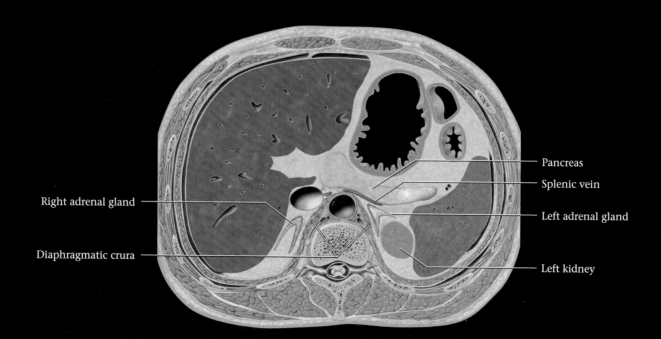

Pancreas

Splenic vein

Right adrenal gland

Left adrenal gland

Diaphragmatic crura

Left kidney

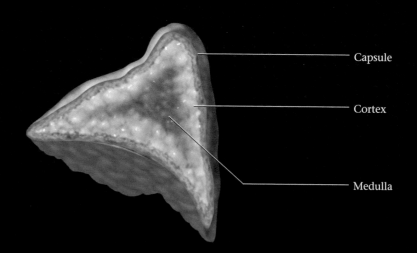

Capsule

Cortex

Medulla

(Top) Graphic shows the right adrenal gland is often more cephalic in location, and lies above the right kidney, while the left adrenal gland lies partly in front of the upper pole of the left kidney. The left adrenal gland lies directly posterior to the splenic vein and body of pancreas, and lateral to the left crus of the diaphragm. The right adrenal gland lies lateral to the crus, medial to the liver, and directly behind the inferior vena cava. **(Bottom)** The adrenal gland is essentially two organs in a single structure. The cortex is an endocrine gland, secreting primarily cortisol, aldosterone, and androgenic steroids. All of these hormones are derived from cholesterol, which imparts the characteristic lipid-rich appearance and imaging characteristics of the gland. The adrenal medulla is part of the autonomic nervous system and secretes epinephrine and norepinephrine.

ADRENALS

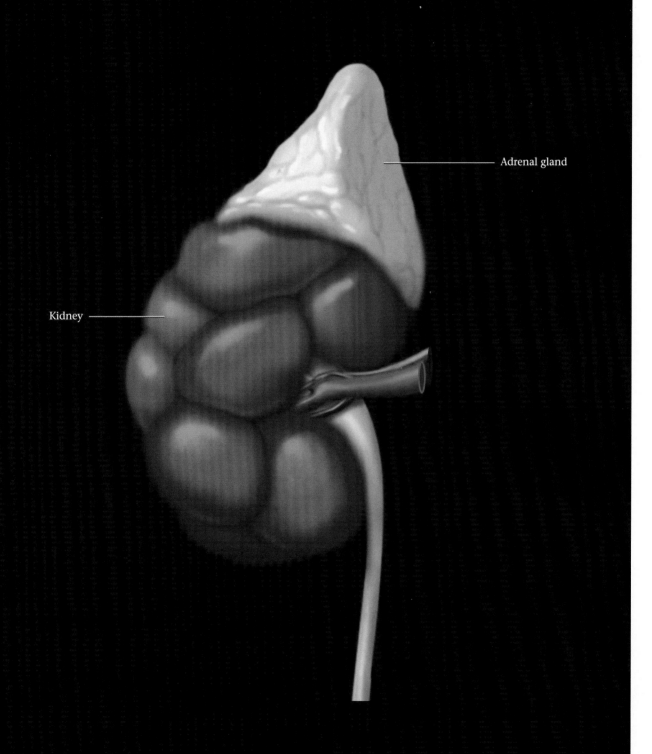

Adrenal gland

Kidney

Graphic shows the appearance of the adrenal gland and kidney in the fetus and neonate. The adrenal gland is much larger relative to the kidney than in the adult, making it easier to scan on ultrasound. The kidney has a lobulated appearance, reflecting the ongoing fusion of the individual renal lobes, each comprised of one renal pyramid and its associated renal cortex.

ADRENALS

Liver

Portal vein

Inferior vena cava

Right adrenal gland

Perinephric fat

Right kidney

Portal vein

Aorta

Liver

Inferior vena cava

Vertebral body

Right adrenal gland

Crus of the right hemidiaphragm

Right kidney

Inferior vena cava

Crus of the hemidiaphragm

Genu of the right adrenal gland

Vertebral body

Lateral limb of the right adrenal gland

Medial limb of the right adrenal gland

Right kidney

(Top) Transabdominal, longitudinal, grayscale US with some lateral angulation of the transducer to include the right kidney in the image. The right adrenal gland is thin (< 1 cm in thickness), hypoechoic and enclosed by perinephric fat. Note its anatomical relationships with the anteriorly located inferior vena cava and posteriorly located superior pole of the right kidney. (Middle) Transabdominal, transverse, grayscale US shows the inverted Y-shaped right adrenal gland. The inferior vena cava is a useful landmark as the right adrenal is seen just posteriorly. The adrenal gland is more easily visualized in pediatric subjects or adults with thin habitus. (Bottom) Zoomed, transverse, grayscale US of the right adrenal gland. Note the medially located crus of the right hemidiaphragm which may be mistaken for the gland. The crus is more hypoechoic and its contour hugs the vertebral body.

ADRENALS

RIGHT ADRENAL GLAND CT CORRELATION

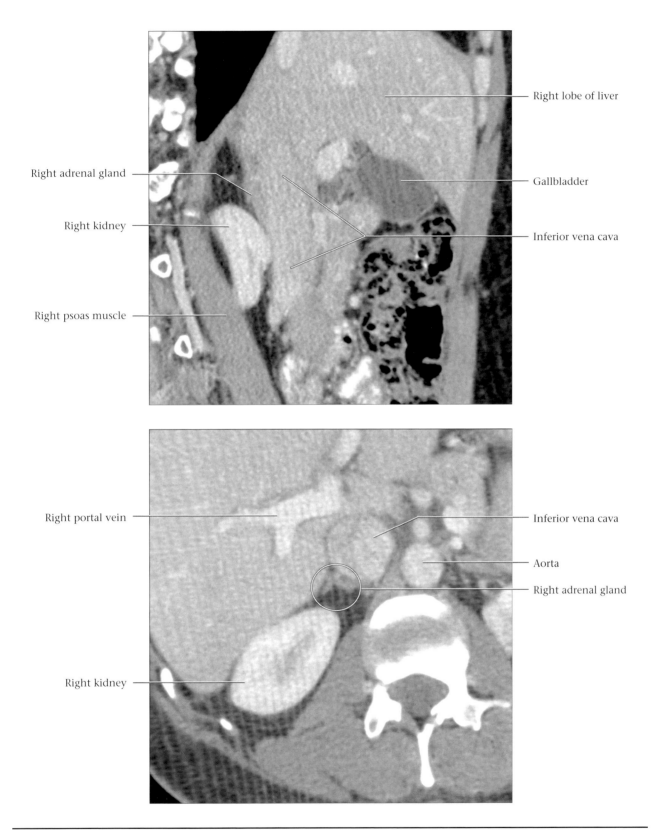

(Top) Sagittal, correlative, contrast-enhanced CT demonstrates the relationship of the right adrenal gland with the anteriorly located inferior vena cava and posteriorly located superior portion of the right kidney. Note the overlying bowel segments, which on transabdominal ultrasound may obscure the adrenal gland making the examination suboptimal. (Bottom) Axial, correlative, contrast-enhanced CT demonstrates the genu of the right adrenal gland and its proximal medial and lateral limbs. CT better depicts the normally thin right adrenal gland. Although the right adrenal gland may be easily identified in thin subjects and the pediatric population, scanning in obese patients is more challenging.

ADRENALS

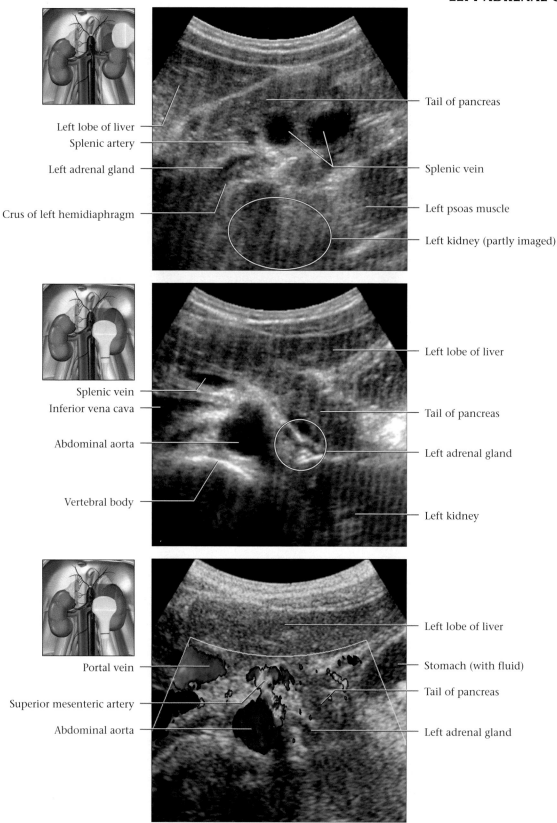

Tail of pancreas

Left lobe of liver

Splenic artery

Left adrenal gland

Splenic vein

Crus of left hemidiaphragm

Left psoas muscle

Left kidney (partly imaged)

Left lobe of liver

Splenic vein

Inferior vena cava

Tail of pancreas

Abdominal aorta

Left adrenal gland

Vertebral body

Left kidney

Left lobe of liver

Portal vein

Stomach (with fluid)

Superior mesenteric artery

Tail of pancreas

Abdominal aorta

Left adrenal gland

(Top) Longitudinal grayscale ultrasound at the epigastrium, left paramedian region. The left lobe of the liver and the pancreatic body/tail combined serve as an acoustic window for imaging the hypoechoic left adrenal gland. (Middle) Subxiphoid, transverse, grayscale ultrasound at the epigastrium, level of the pancreatic body and tail. The left adrenal gland is seen as a lambda structure and surrounded by hyperechoic perirenal fat. It is anterior to the left kidney and to the left of the abdominal aorta. (Bottom) Subxiphoid transverse color Doppler ultrasound at the epigastrium further differentiates the left adrenal gland from the adjacent vessels which exhibit color flow.

ADRENALS

LEFT ADRENAL GLAND CT CORRELATION

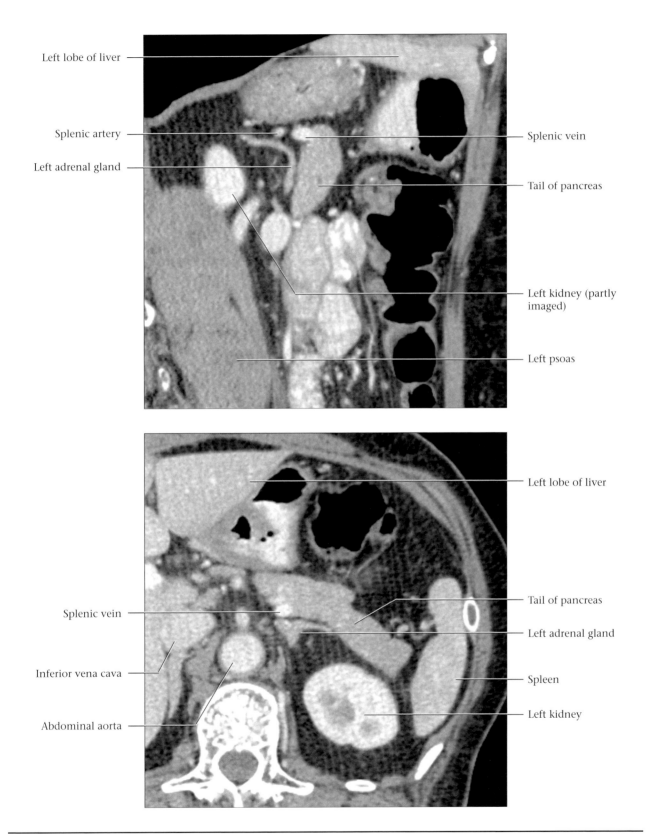

Left lobe of liver

Splenic artery

Left adrenal gland

Splenic vein

Tail of pancreas

Left kidney (partly imaged)

Left psoas

Left lobe of liver

Splenic vein

Inferior vena cava

Abdominal aorta

Tail of pancreas

Left adrenal gland

Spleen

Left kidney

(Top) Sagittal, correlative, contrast-enhanced CT shows the left adrenal gland between the anteriorly located tail of the pancreas and the posteriorly located upper pole of the left kidney. Note the overlying bowel segments which may limit US examination of the left adrenal gland when using an anterior approach. **(Bottom)** Axial correlative contrast-enhanced CT shows the left adrenal gland surrounded by fat. The genu, proximal medial and lateral limbs form an inverted-Y configuration.

ADRENALS

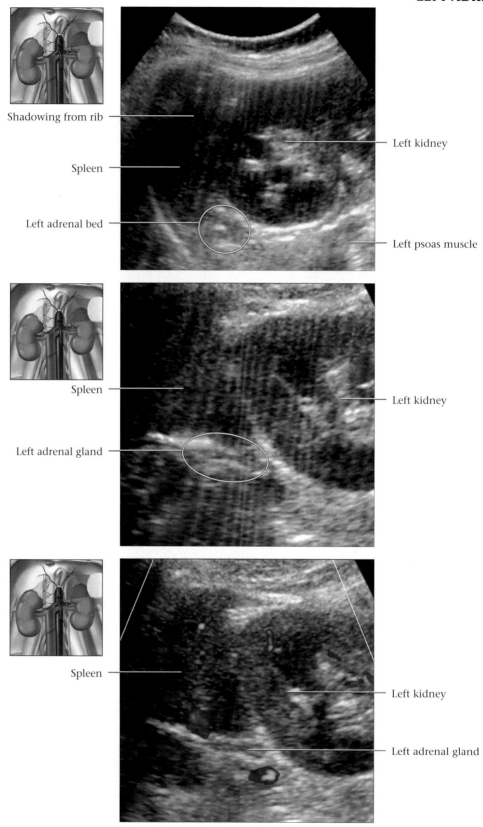

Shadowing from rib

Spleen

Left adrenal bed

Left kidney

Left psoas muscle

Spleen

Left adrenal gland

Left kidney

Spleen

Left kidney

Left adrenal gland

(Top) Posterolateral, oblique, grayscale ultrasound of the left adrenal bed in an adult using the spleen and the superior pole of the left kidney as acoustic windows. The transducer is placed along the intercostal space to avoid shadowing from ribs. Note the suboptimal evaluation of the left adrenal gland owing to its deep location using this approach. (Middle) Zoomed posterolateral oblique grayscale ultrasound of the left adrenal gland. The left adrenal gland is thin and hypoechoic, not more than 1 cm in thickness and is located posterosuperior to the left kidney and posteroinferior to the spleen. (Bottom) Posterolateral oblique power Doppler ultrasound of the left adrenal gland, which better identifies the gland from nearby vessels.

ADRENALS

LEFT ADRENAL GLAND CT CORRELATION

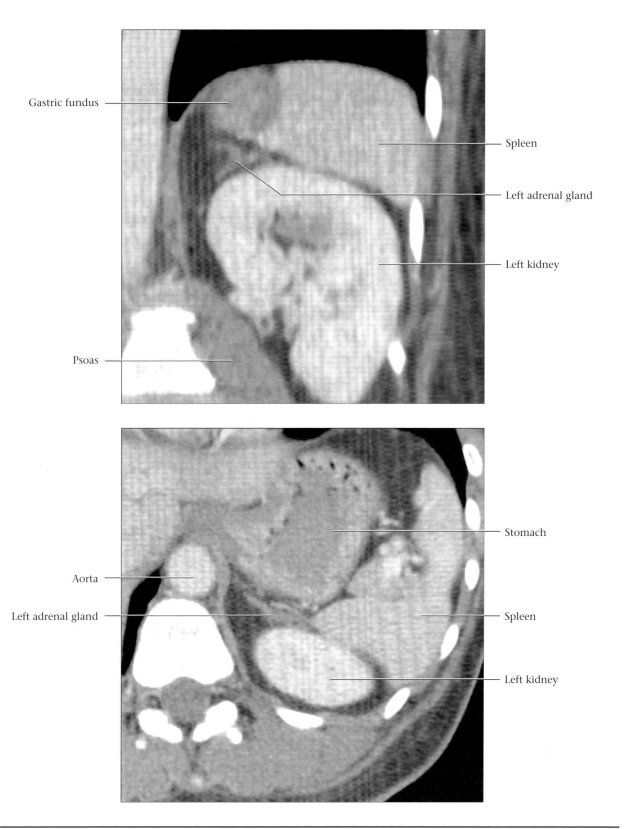

(Top) Correlative contrast-enhanced CT reformation through the intercostal plane used in ultrasound for examining the left adrenal gland. The relationship of the spleen, left kidney and left adrenal gland is better demonstrated. (Bottom) Axial, correlative, contrast-enhanced CT shows the left adrenal gland anteromedial to the superior portion of the left kidney and medial to the spleen. The diagonal course of the ribs creates difficulty in producing a similar image on ultrasound.

ADRENALS

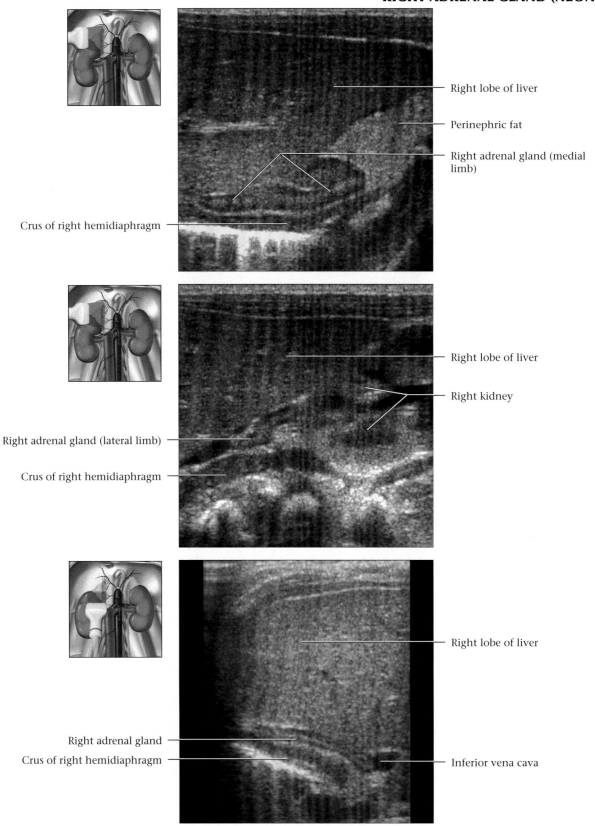

Right lobe of liver

Perinephric fat

Right adrenal gland (medial limb)

Crus of right hemidiaphragm

Right lobe of liver

Right kidney

Right adrenal gland (lateral limb)

Crus of right hemidiaphragm

Right lobe of liver

Right adrenal gland

Crus of right hemidiaphragm

Inferior vena cava

(Top) Transabdominal, longitudinal, grayscale ultrasound of the right adrenal gland using the liver as acoustic window. Using a high frequency linear transducer better demonstrates the right adrenal gland in neonates and infants; it has a trilaminar appearance with a hyperechoic medulla and hypoechoic cortex. (Middle) Transabdominal, longitudinal, grayscale ultrasound of the right adrenal gland using the liver as acoustic window. The transducer is angulated slightly more laterally to reveal the lateral limb of the right adrenal gland. The crus of the right hemidiaphragm is seen posteriorly and is more hypoechoic and lacks the adrenal gland's trilaminar appearance. (Bottom) Intercostal, transverse, grayscale US of the right adrenal gland using the liver as acoustic window. Note the posteriorly located crus of the right hemidiaphragm which may be mistaken for the gland.

ADRENALS

LEFT ADRENAL GLAND (NEONATE)

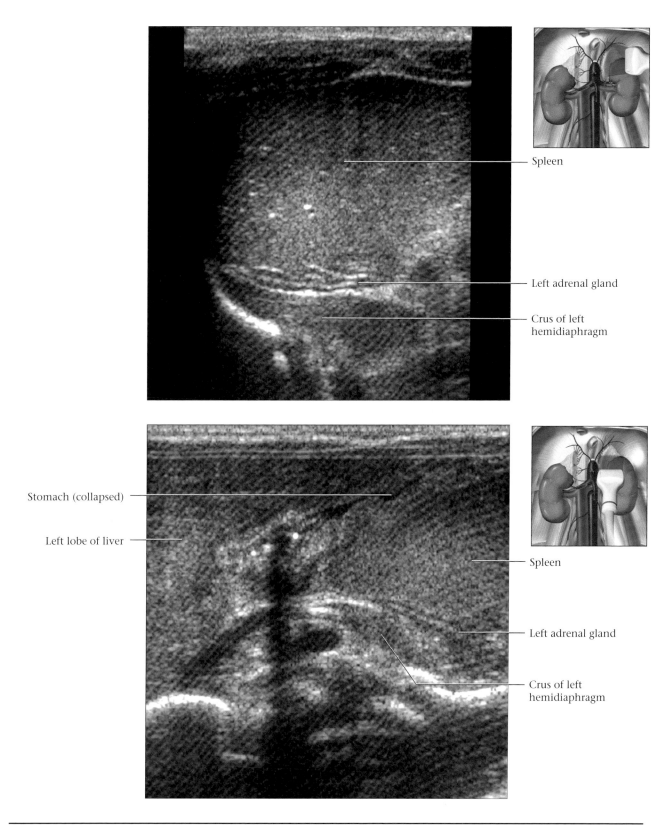

Spleen

Left adrenal gland

Crus of left hemidiaphragm

Stomach (collapsed)

Left lobe of liver

Spleen

Left adrenal gland

Crus of left hemidiaphragm

(Top) Intercostal, oblique, grayscale ultrasound of the left adrenal gland using the spleen as acoustic window. The gland is identified between the spleen and crus of the hemidiaphragm. (Bottom) Transverse, transabdominal, grayscale ultrasound through the spleen shows the left adrenal gland. Its trilaminar appearance is maintained.

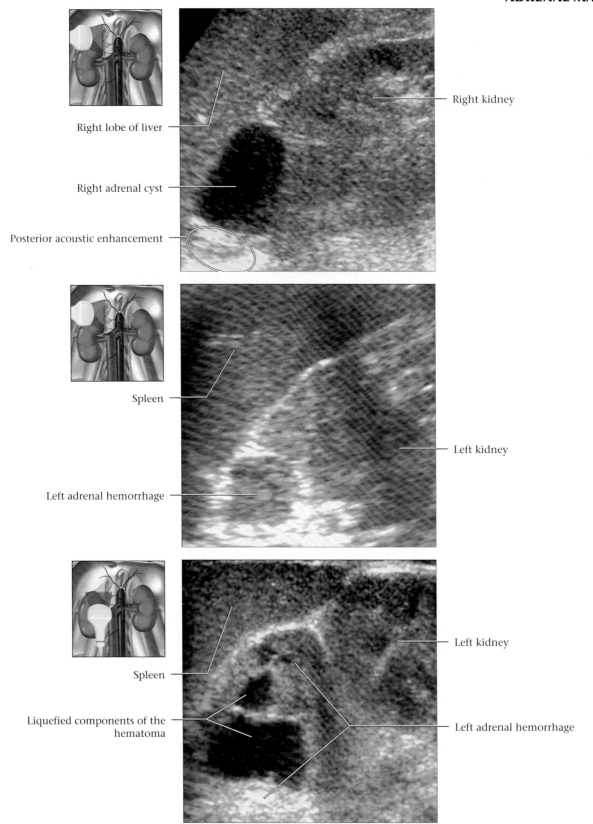

Right kidney

Right lobe of liver

Right adrenal cyst

Posterior acoustic enhancement

Spleen

Left kidney

Left adrenal hemorrhage

Spleen

Left kidney

Liquefied components of the hematoma

Left adrenal hemorrhage

(Top) Transabdominal, longitudinal, grayscale ultrasound of the right adrenal gland shows a hypoechoic focus in the right adrenal bed. Posterior acoustic enhancement suggests through-transmission of echoes, typical of fluid-filled cysts. **(Middle)** Oblique, transabdominal, grayscale ultrasound shows a small acute left adrenal hemorrhage. Echogenicity varies with stage of the bleed, and a hyperechoic mass lesion represents an acute hematoma. The adrenal gland appears nodular with loss of its normal linear appearance. Adrenal gland thickness of > 1 cm is considered abnormal. **(Bottom)** Transabdominal, transverse, grayscale ultrasound shows a large well-defined left adrenal hematoma, likely subacute as evidenced by central anechoic areas of liquefaction.

ADRENALS

ADRENAL MASSES

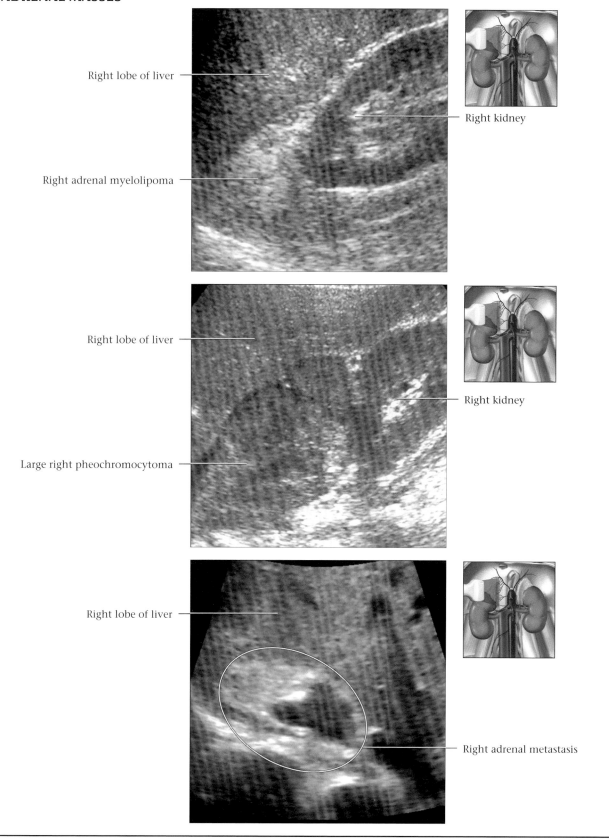

Right lobe of liver

Right kidney

Right adrenal myelolipoma

Right lobe of liver

Right kidney

Large right pheochromocytoma

Right lobe of liver

Right adrenal metastasis

(Top) Longitudinal, transabdominal, grayscale ultrasound shows a bulky right adrenal gland with inhomogeneous hyperechoic appearance similar to fatty deposits and suggestive of myelolipoma. (Middle) Longitudinal, transabdominal, grayscale ultrasound shows a large, lobulated, right adrenal gland/mass isoechoic with the right renal cortex in a case of pheochromocytoma. (Bottom) Longitudinal transabdominal grayscale ultrasound of the right adrenal bed shows an echogenic lesion with cystic/necrotic component in a patient with lung carcinoma.

AORTA AND INFERIOR VENA CAVA

Terminology

Abbreviations
- Inferior vena cava (IVC); superior mesenteric artery (SMA); superior mesenteric vein (SMV); superior vena cava (SVC); inferior mesenteric artery (IMA); peak systolic velocity (PSV)

Definitions
- "Proximal" and "distal" in arterial and venous systems apply to position of arterial and venous segment in relation to heart (rather than direction of flow)
- Aneurysm is a focal increase in caliber of artery with diameter of dilated segment measuring at least 1.5 times greater than adjacent unaffected segments

Gross Anatomy

Overview
- Abdominal aorta
  - Enters abdomen at T12 level, bifurcates at L4
  - Level of origins of major branches: Celiac axis (T12), SMA (L1), renal arteries (L1/2), IMA (L3), common iliac arteries (L4)
- Inferior vena cava
  - Blood from alimentary tract passes through portal venous system before entering IVC through hepatic veins
  - Begins at L5 level with union of common iliac veins
  - Leaves abdomen via IVC hiatus in diaphragm at T8 level
  - IVC tributaries correspond to paired visceral and parietal branches of aorta
  - IVC development has complex embryology
    - Various anomalies are common (up to 10% of population), especially at and below level of renal veins
    - All are variations of persistence/regression of embryologic sub- and supracardinal veins

Imaging Anatomy

Overview
- Not all branches of abdominal aorta and tributaries of IVC can be well seen on ultrasound examination
- Major arterial branches of abdominal aorta seen on ultrasound
  - Celiac artery, common hepatic artery, splenic artery, SMA, IMA, renal arteries, common iliac arteries
- Major venous tributaries draining into IVC
  - Common iliac veins, renal veins, hepatic veins

Internal Structures-Critical Contents
- Abdominal aorta
  - Normal PSV: 60-110 cm/s
  - Spectral Doppler waveform
    - Upper: Narrow, well-defined systolic complex with forward flow during diastole
    - Mid: Reduced diastolic flow
    - Distal: Absent diastolic flow, similar to lower limb arteries
  - Normal caliber 15-25 mm
    - Upper: 22 mm above renal arteries
    - Middle: 18 mm below renal arteries
    - Lower: 15 mm above bifurcation
  - Best ultrasound imaging plane: Both transverse and longitudinal
- Celiac axis
  - Normal PSV: 98-105 cm/s
  - Spectral Doppler demonstrates low resistance flow with high end-diastolic velocities
  - Flow velocity not dependent on food intake
  - Normal caliber 6-10 mm
  - Best ultrasound imaging plane: Transverse plane - to show typical T-shaped bifurcation
- Common hepatic artery
  - Normal PSV: 70-120 cm/s
  - Spectral Doppler shows low resistance flow characteristics with large amount of continuous flow in diastole
  - Normal caliber 4-10 mm
  - Best ultrasound imaging plane
    - Start transverse midline to follow common hepatic artery to right of T-shaped bifurcation from celiac axis
    - Gastroduodenal artery may be seen to arise from common hepatic artery along the anterosuperior aspect of pancreas, thereafter the common hepatic artery becomes the proper hepatic artery
- Splenic artery
  - Normal PSV 70-110 cm/s
  - Spectral Doppler shows typically turbulent flow due to tortuosity of vessel
  - Normal diameter 4-8 mm
  - Best ultrasound imaging plane
    - Transverse midline approach - shows the proximal portion of artery well
    - Intercostal through the spleen using it as an acoustic window - useful for showing the distal splenic artery around hilum
- SMA
  - Normal PSV: 97-142 cm/s
  - Spectral Doppler demonstrates high impedance flow with low diastolic velocities during fasting due to relative vasoconstriction
  - End diastolic velocity increases after meal due to vasodilation of mesenteric branches - typically 30-90 minutes after meals
  - Normal caliber 5-8 mm
  - Best ultrasound imaging plane
    - Longitudinal midline approach - best for evaluation of SMA blood flow
    - Transverse plane - useful for identifying the short anteriorly directed stump, shows dot-like appearance, surrounded by a distinctive triangular mantle of fat
- IMA
  - Normal PSV: 93-189 cm/s
  - Spectral Doppler demonstrates high impedance flow with low diastolic velocities during fasting due to relative vasoconstriction
  - End diastolic velocity increases after meal due to vasodilation of mesenteric branches
  - Normal caliber 1-5 mm

- Best imaging plane: Transverse plane following line of aorta - origin of IMA arises from below origins of renal arteries and may be anterior or slightly to left of midline
- Renal arteries
  - Normal PSV: 60-140 cm/s, not more than 180 cm/s
  - Spectral Doppler demonstrates open systolic window, rapid systolic upstroke occasionally followed by a secondary slower rise to peak systole with subsequent gradual diastolic delay but with persistent forward flow in diastole
  - Normal caliber 5-8 mm
  - Best imaging plane
    - Transverse anterior midline approach - best for identification of origins of renal arteries
    - Posterolateral approach using kidneys as acoustic window - useful for visualization of distal portions of renal arteries
- Common iliac arteries
  - Normal spectral Doppler shows characteristic triphasic waveform
    - Initial high velocity peak forward flow phase resulting from cardiac systole
    - Brief phase of reverse flow in early diastole
    - Low velocity forward flow in diastole
  - Normal caliber 8-12 mm
  - Best imaging plane: Transverse anterior approach and oblique anterior approach along the long axis of iliac arteries
  - Stenosis causing 1-19% diameter reduction
    - Triphasic waveform with minimal spectral waveform broadening
    - PSV increase < 30% relative to adjacent proximal segment; proximal and distal waveform remain normal
  - Stenosis causing 20-49% diameter reduction
    - Triphasic waveform usually maintained, though reverse flow component may be diminished
    - Spectral broadening is prominent with filling in of the area under systolic peak
    - PSV 30-100% increase relative to adjacent proximal segment, proximal and distal segment remain normal
  - Stenosis causing 50-99% diameter reduction
    - Monophasic waveform with loss of reverse flow component, forward flow throughout cardiac cycle
    - Extensive spectral broadening
    - PSV > 100% increase relative to adjacent proximal segment
    - Distal waveform is monophasic with reduced systolic velocity
  - Occlusion
    - No flow, preocclusive thump may be heard proximal to site of obstruction
    - Distal waveforms are monophasic with reduced systolic velocities
- Inferior vena cava
  - Normal PSV: 44-118 cm/s
  - Spectral Doppler shows slow flow that varies with respiration and cardiac pulsation
  - Normal caliber 5-29 mm during quiet inspiration

- Best imaging plane: Both transverse and longitudinal
- Common iliac veins
  - Spectral Doppler shows five normal characteristics
    - Spontaneous flow, phasic flow, flow ceases with Valsalva maneuver, flow augmentation with distal compression, unidirectional flow towards heart
  - Best imaging plane: Transverse anterior approach and oblique anterior approach along the long axis of iliac veins
- Renal veins
  - Normal PSV: 18-33 cm/s
  - Right renal vein is relatively short and drains directly into IVC
  - Left renal vein runs a slightly longer course - receives left gonadal vein, usually courses anterior to aorta before joining IVC
  - Spectral Doppler of right renal vein mirrors pulsatility of IVC
  - Spectral Doppler of left renal vein may show only slight variability of flow velocities consequent upon cardiac and respiratory activity
  - Normal caliber 4-9 mm
  - Best imaging plane: Transverse anterior approach
- Hepatic veins
  - Normal PSV: 16-40 cm/s
  - Spectral Doppler shows triphasic waveform due to transmitted cardiac activity
  - Best imaging plane: Transverse/oblique subcostal approach with cranial angulation

Anatomy-Based Imaging Issues

Imaging Recommendations
- Use 2-5 MHz transducer
- Fasting for 12 hours is recommended to reduce interference by bowel gas - satisfactory Doppler signal for aorta and IVC can be obtained in up to 90% of patients
- Imaging patient in the morning after an overnight fast is most convenient protocol
- Lateral decubitus position and graded compression to displace intervening bowel gas may be useful
- Angle correction is crucial in spectral Doppler assessment
- Detailed delineation of branches of aorta and IVC better assessed on CTA or MRA
- Digital subtractive angiography usually reserved for when intervention may be required (e.g., embolization of mesenteric artery branches in GI bleed, renal artery stenting, etc.)

Imaging Pitfalls
- Bowel gas, patient body habitus and operator dependence are main factors contributing to suboptimal ultrasound examination of aorta and IVC

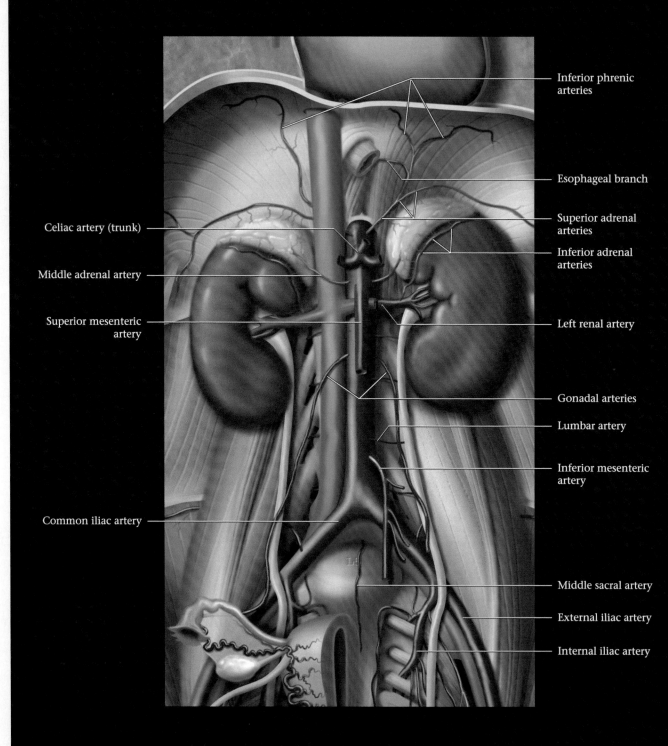

Celiac artery (trunk)

Middle adrenal artery

Superior mesenteric artery

Common iliac artery

Inferior phrenic arteries

Esophageal branch

Superior adrenal arteries

Inferior adrenal arteries

Left renal artery

Gonadal arteries

Lumbar artery

Inferior mesenteric artery

Middle sacral artery

External iliac artery

Internal iliac artery

Graphic shows the major arteries to the gastrointestinal tract arise as unpaired vessels from the aortic midline plane and include the celiac, superior and inferior mesenteric arteries. Branches to the urogenital and endocrine organs arise as paired vessels in the lateral plane and include the renal, adrenal, and gonadal (testicular or ovarian) arteries. The diaphragm and posterior abdominal wall are supplied by paired branches in the posterolateral plane, including the inferior phrenic and lumbar arteries (four pairs, only one of which is labeled in this graphic). The anterior abdominal wall is supplied by the inferior epigastric and deep circumflex iliac arteries, both branches of the external iliac artery. The inferior epigastric artery turns superiorly to run in the rectus sheath, where it anastomoses with the superior epigastric artery, a terminal branch of the internal mammary (thoracic) artery.

Abdomen

IV

114

COMMON VARIATIONS OF THE IVC

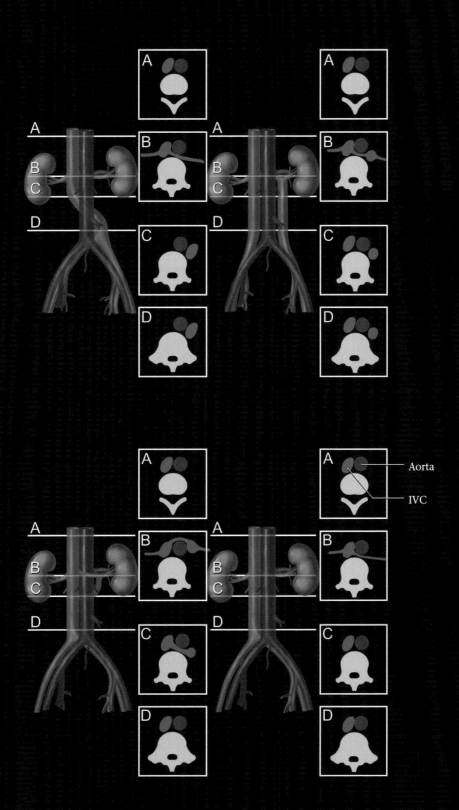

(Top) First two of four graphics illustrating common variations of the IVC. The labeled lines on the frontal graphics correspond to the levels of the axial sections. The left graphic shows transposition of the IVC, in which the infrarenal portion of the IVC lies predominantly to the left side of the aorta. A more common anomaly is shown on the right graphic, a "duplication" of the IVC in which the left common iliac vein continues in a cephalad direction without crossing over to join the right iliac vein. Instead, it joins the left renal vein, and then crosses over to the right. The suprarenal IVC has a conventional course and appearance. **(Bottom)** The left graphic shows a circumaortic left renal vein, with the smaller, more cephalic vein passing in front of the aorta & the larger vein passing behind & caudal. The right graphic shows a completely retroaortic renal vein.

AORTA AND INFERIOR VENA CAVA

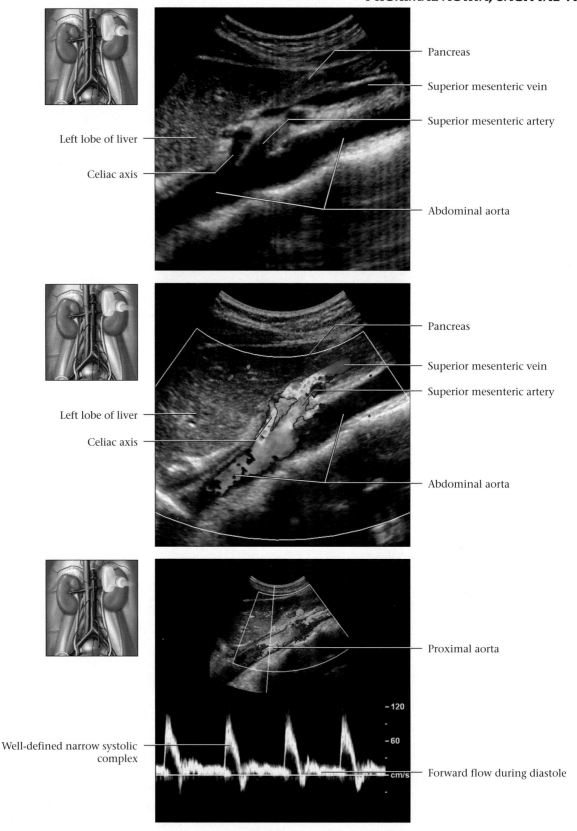

Pancreas

Superior mesenteric vein

Superior mesenteric artery

Left lobe of liver

Celiac axis

Abdominal aorta

Pancreas

Superior mesenteric vein

Superior mesenteric artery

Left lobe of liver

Celiac axis

Abdominal aorta

Proximal aorta

Well-defined narrow systolic complex

Forward flow during diastole

− 120

− 60

cm/s

(Top) Longitudinal grayscale ultrasound of the proximal abdominal aorta shows the origins of the celiac axis and superior mesenteric artery. The origin of the celiac axis is usually seen at T12 while the origin of the SMA is usually seen at L1 immediately below the origin of the celiac axis on this view. The normal diameter of the abdominal aorta is 15-25 mm, and the average diameter of the proximal abdominal aorta above the renal arteries is around 22 mm. (Middle) Longitudinal color Doppler ultrasound of the proximal abdominal aorta shows the origins of the celiac axis and superior mesenteric artery. Apart from assessment of flow through the aorta, this is also a useful view for assessment of the flow in the SMA. (Bottom) Spectral Doppler ultrasound of the proximal aorta shows narrow well-defined systolic complex with forward flow during diastole.

MIDDLE AND DISTAL AORTA, SAGITTAL VIEW

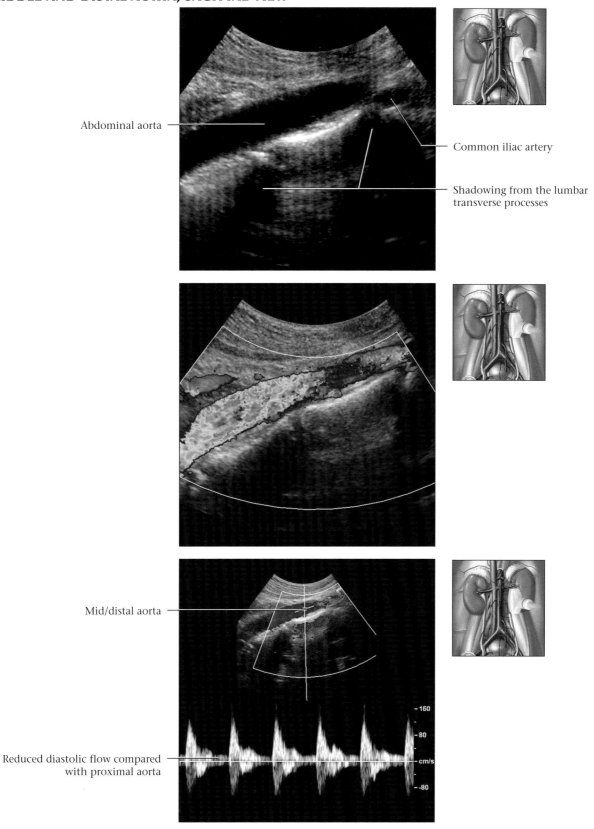

Abdominal aorta

Common iliac artery

Shadowing from the lumbar transverse processes

Mid/distal aorta

Reduced diastolic flow compared with proximal aorta

(Top) Longitudinal grayscale ultrasound of the mid/distal abdominal aorta shows one of the common iliac arteries coming off the aortic bifurcation. The aortic bifurcation is usually seen at the L4 level. The average diameter of the mid portion of the abdoinal aorta is around 18 mm below the renal arteries and 15 mm above the aortic bifurcation. **(Middle)** Color Doppler ultrasound of the mid/distal abdominal aorta shows one of the common iliac arteries coming off the aortic bifurcation. **(Bottom)** Spectral Doppler ultrasound of the mid/distal abdominal aorta shows reduced diastolic flow compared sith the proximal aorta. The spectral Doppler waveform to be expected in the distal abdominal aorta usually shows absent diastolic flow, similar to that seen in the lower limb arteries.

Abdomen

IV

117

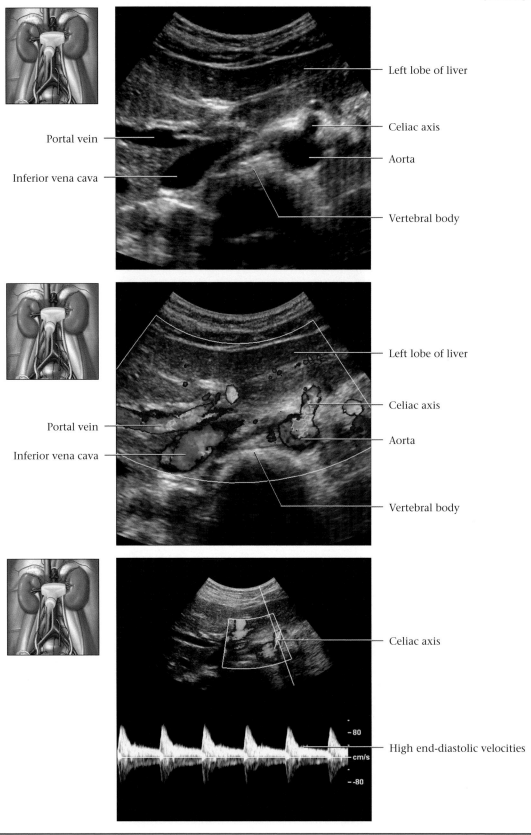

Left lobe of liver

Celiac axis

Aorta

Vertebral body

Portal vein

Inferior vena cava

Left lobe of liver

Celiac axis

Aorta

Vertebral body

Portal vein

Inferior vena cava

Celiac axis

High end-diastolic velocities

(Top) Transverse grayscale ultrasound of the abdominal aorta at the level of the celiac axis via a midline approach. The celiac axis is the first branch of the abdominal aorta seen arising anteriorly, usually at the level of T12. The normal caliber of the celiac axis is between 6-10 mm. Note the normal position of the IVC, to the right of the abdominal aorta. (Middle) Transverse color Doppler ultrasound of the abdominal aorta at the level of the celiac axis via a midline approach. As the celiac axis is perpendicular to the transducer, a small amount of cranial angulation was used to improve the color Doppler signal obtained. (Bottom) Spectral Doppler ultrasound of the celiac axis shows low resistance flow with high end-diastolic velocities. Flow velocity in the celiac axis is not dependent on food intake, and the normal PSV ranges from 98-105 cm/s.

SPLENIC ARTERY

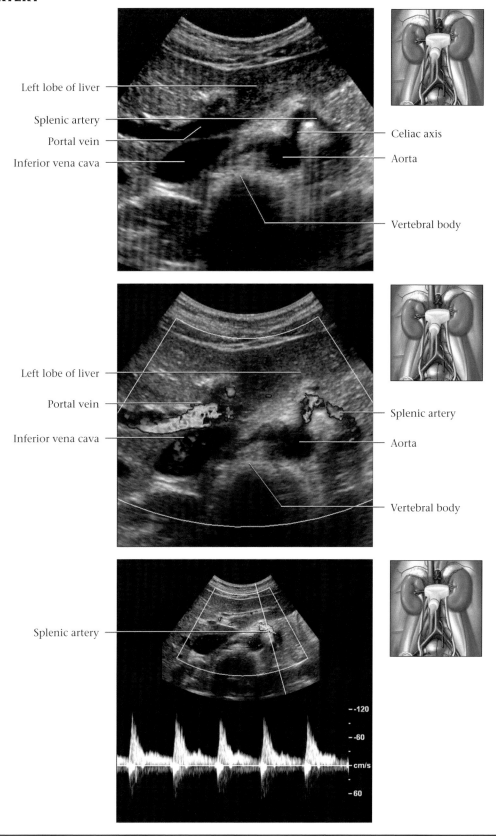

Left lobe of liver

Splenic artery

Portal vein

Inferior vena cava

Celiac axis

Aorta

Vertebral body

Left lobe of liver

Portal vein

Inferior vena cava

Splenic artery

Aorta

Vertebral body

Splenic artery

--120

--60

cm/s

-60

(**Top**) Transverse grayscale ultrasound via a midline approach shows the origin of the splenic artery as it branches from the celiac axis and hooks to the left. This is usually the best view for visualizing the proximal portion of the splenic artery. The more distal splenic artery is tortuous in its course. An intercostal approach using the spleen as an acoustic window may be useful for showing the distal splenic artery around the hilum. The normal caliber of the splenic artery ranges from 4-8 mm. (**Middle**) Transverse color Doppler ultrasound via a midline approach shows flow within the proximal splenic artery. (**Bottom**) Spectral Doppler ultrasound of the proximal splenic artery shows typically turbulent flow due to tortuosity of the vessel. The normal PSV in the splenic artery ranges between 70-110 cm/s.

Abdomen

IV

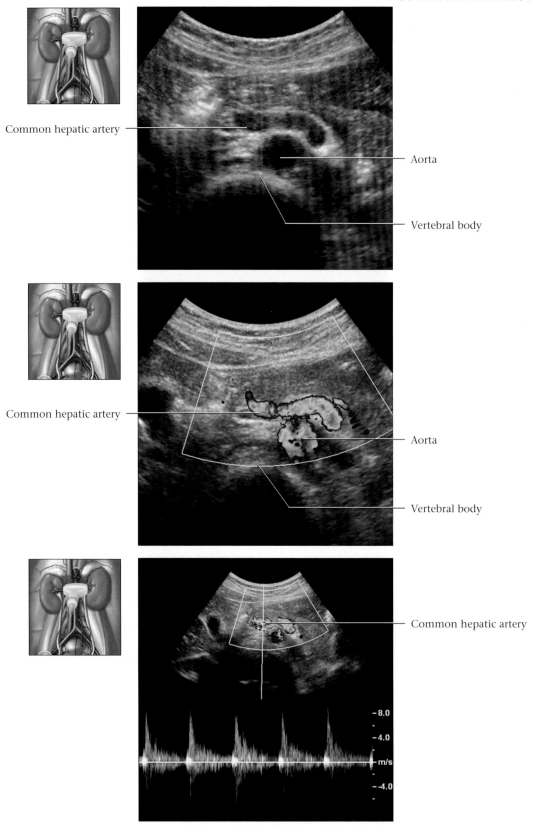

Common hepatic artery

Aorta

Vertebral body

Common hepatic artery

Aorta

Vertebral body

Common hepatic artery

-8.0

-4.0

- m/s

-4.0

(Top) Transverse grayscale ultrasound via a midline approach shows the proximal portion of the common hepatic artery as it branches to the right, off the T-shaped bifurcation of the celiac axis (not imaged). The normal diameter of the common hepatic artery ranges from 4-10 mm. **(Middle)** Color Doppler ultrasound shows flow within the proximal portion of the common hepatic artery. The gastroduodenal artery may be seen to arise from the common hepatic artery along the anterosuperior aspect of the pancreas, thereafter the common hepatic artery becomes the proper hepatic artery. **(Bottom)** Spectral Doppler ultrasound of the common hepatic artery shows low resistance flow characteristics with large amount of continuous flow in diastole. The normal PSV for the common hepatic artery ranges from 70-120 cm/s.

SUPERIOR MESENTERIC ARTERY

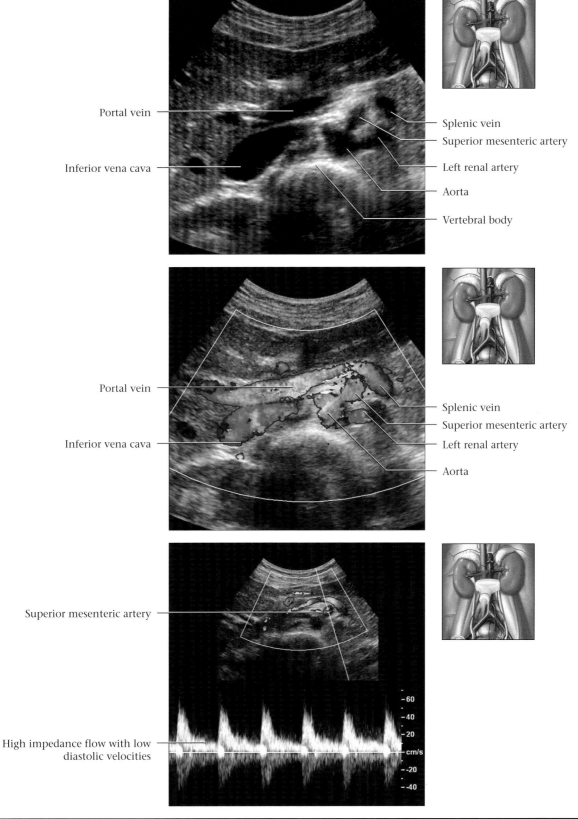

Portal vein
Inferior vena cava
Splenic vein
Superior mesenteric artery
Left renal artery
Aorta
Vertebral body

Portal vein
Inferior vena cava
Splenic vein
Superior mesenteric artery
Left renal artery
Aorta

Superior mesenteric artery
High impedance flow with low diastolic velocities

-60
-40
-20
cm/s
-20
-40

(Top) Transverse grayscale ultrasound of the origin of the superior mesenteric artery seen arising anteriorly from the aorta. The origin of the SMA is usually seen at L1 between the celiac axis (T12) and the renal arteries (L1/2). The normal caliber of the SMA ranges between 5-8 mm. (Middle) Transverse color Doppler ultrasound of the proximal SMA. The transducer has been angled slightly cranially with the arterial blood coming towards the transducer shown in red and the venous blood going away from the transducer shown in blue. (Bottom) Spectral Doppler ultrasound image of the proximal portion of the SMA. High impedance flow with low diastolic velocities is observed during fasting due to relative vasoconstriction. End diastolic velocity increases after meals due to vasodilation of the mesenteric branches, typically 30-90 minutes after meals.

RIGHT RENAL ARTERY

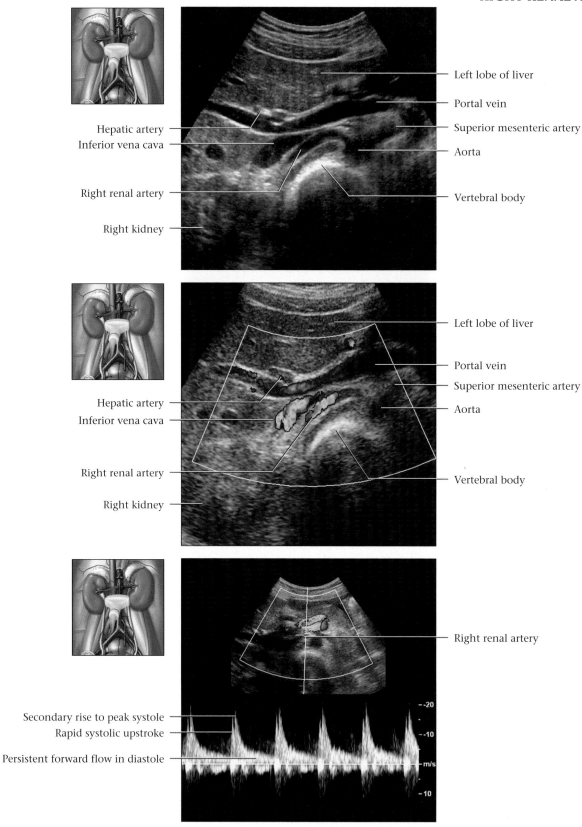

Left lobe of liver

Portal vein

Superior mesenteric artery

Aorta

Vertebral body

Hepatic artery

Inferior vena cava

Right renal artery

Right kidney

Left lobe of liver

Portal vein

Superior mesenteric artery

Aorta

Vertebral body

Hepatic artery

Inferior vena cava

Right renal artery

Right kidney

Right renal artery

Secondary rise to peak systole

Rapid systolic upstroke

Persistent forward flow in diastole

(Top) Transverse grayscale ultrasound shows the proximal right renal artery as it branches from the aorta and courses behind the IVC. This midline anterior approach is usually the best for evaluating the origin of the renal arteries. The normal diameter of the renal arteries ranges from 5-8 mm. The renal arteries arise around the L1/2 level at or below the level of the SMA. **(Middle)** Transverse color Doppler ultrasound of the abdominal aorta shows the proximal right renal artery as it branches from the aorta and courses behind the IVC. **(Bottom)** Spectral Doppler ultrasound of the right renal artery shows open systolic window, rapid systolic upstroke followed by a secondary slower rise to peak systole with subsequent gradual diastolic delay but with persistent forward flow in diastole. The normal PSV ranges from 60-140 cm/s, but not more than 180 cm/s.

LEFT RENAL ARTERY

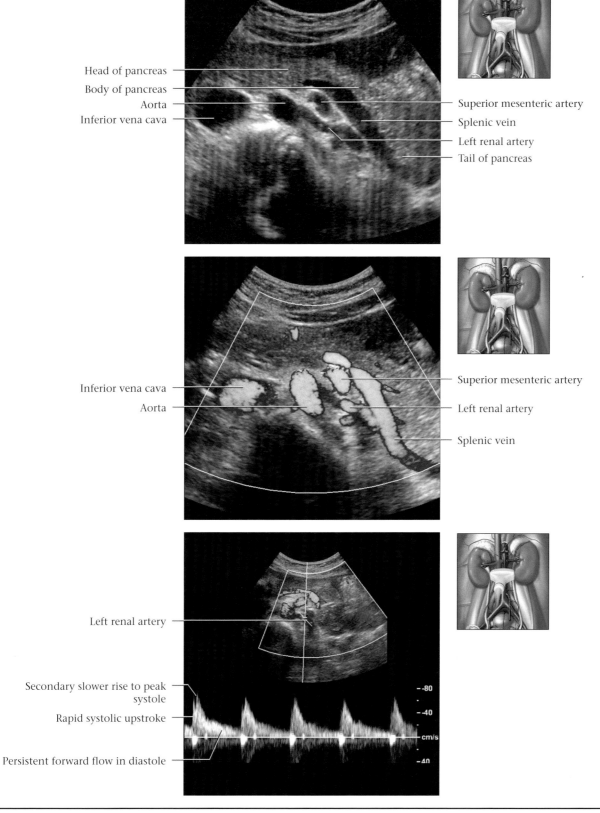

Head of pancreas
Body of pancreas
Aorta
Inferior vena cava

Superior mesenteric artery
Splenic vein
Left renal artery
Tail of pancreas

Inferior vena cava
Aorta

Superior mesenteric artery
Left renal artery
Splenic vein

Left renal artery

Secondary slower rise to peak systole
Rapid systolic upstroke
Persistent forward flow in diastole

-80
-40
cm/s
-40

(Top) Transverse grayscale ultrasound shows the proximal left renal artery as it branches from the aorta and courses posterior to the SMA and splenic vein. This midline anterior approach is usually the best for evaluating the origin of the renal arteries. The normal diameter of the renal arteries ranges from 5-8 mm. The renal arteries arise around the L1/2 level. **(Middle)** Power Doppler ultrasound shows flow in the proximal left renal artery as it branches from the aorta and courses posterior to the SMA and splenic vein. **(Bottom)** Spectral Doppler ultrasound of the left renal artery shows open systolic window, rapid systolic upstroke followed by a secondary slower rise to peak systole with subsequent gradual diastolic delay but with persistent forward flow in diastole. The normal PSV ranges from 60-140 cm/s, but not more than 180 cm/s.

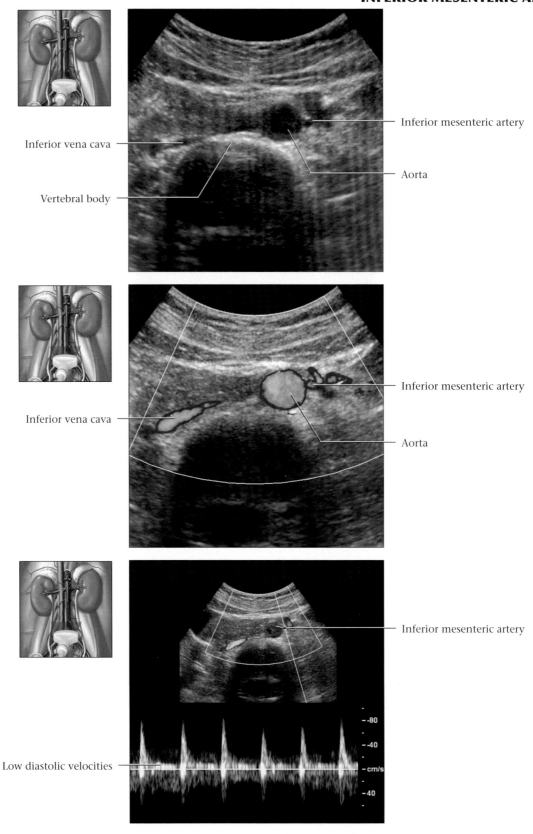

Inferior vena cava

Inferior mesenteric artery

Aorta

Vertebral body

Inferior vena cava

Inferior mesenteric artery

Aorta

Inferior mesenteric artery

Low diastolic velocities

(Top) Transverse grayscale ultrasound of the distal abdominal aorta at the level of the origin of the inferior mesenteric artery. The IMA arises from the anterior or left anterolateral aspect (as in the above case) of the abdominal aorta at the L3 level. The transverse plane following the line of the aorta is the best imaging plane for identification of the origin of the IMA. The normal caliber of the IMA ranges from 1-4 mm. **(Middle)** Transverse power Doppler ultrasound shows flow in the proximal inferior mesenteric artery. **(Bottom)** Spectral Doppler ultrasound of the inferior mesenteric artery shows high impedance flow with low diastolic velocities during fasting due to relative vasoconstriction. End diastolic velocity increases after meal due to vasodilation of the mesenteric branches. Normal PSV ranges from 93-189 cm/s.

Abdomen

IV

AORTA AND INFERIOR VENA CAVA

AORTIC BIFURCATION

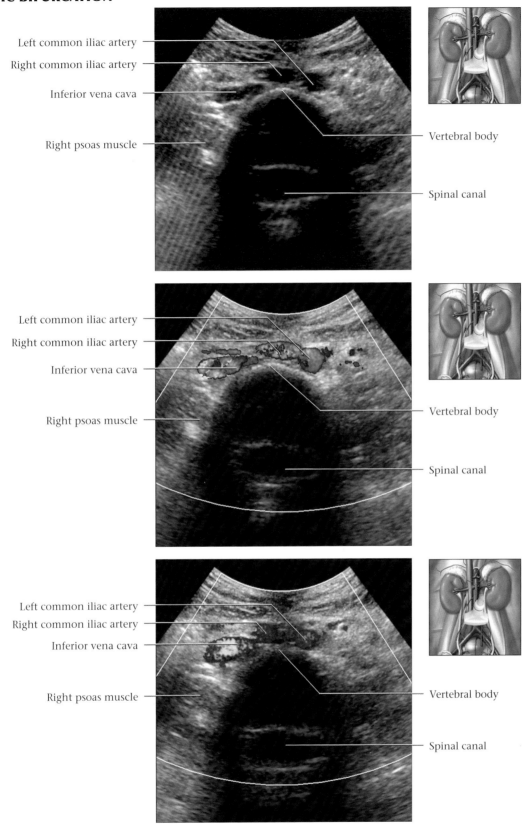

(Top) Transverse grayscale ultrasound of the aortic bifurcation shows the origins of the right and left common iliac arteries. The aortic bifurcation is usually seen at the L4 level. **(Middle)** Transverse color Doppler ultrasound shows flow in the origins of the right and left common iliac arteries. **(Bottom)** Transverse power Doppler ultrasound shows flow in the origins of the right and left common iliac arteries. Power Doppler is less angle dependent and demonstrates flow more readily, particularly in vascular structures that are close to a right angle with the transducer.

RIGHT COMMON ILIAC ARTERY

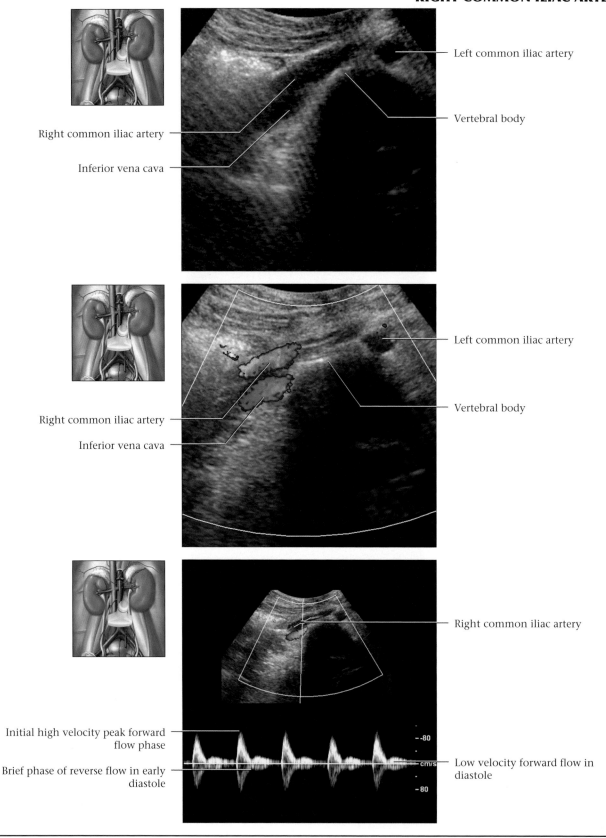

Left common iliac artery

Vertebral body

Right common iliac artery

Inferior vena cava

Left common iliac artery

Vertebral body

Right common iliac artery

Inferior vena cava

Right common iliac artery

Initial high velocity peak forward flow phase

Brief phase of reverse flow in early diastole

Low velocity forward flow in diastole

(Top) Oblique grayscale ultrasound shows the course of the right common iliac artery as it branches off the aortic bifurcation. The proximal common iliac artery is first identified on the transverse plane and the transducer is then angulated along the long axis of the right common iliac artery. The normal diameter of the common iliac arteries ranges from 8-12 mm. (Middle) Oblique color Doppler ultrasound shows flow in the proximal right common iliac artery. (Bottom) Spectral Doppler image of the right common iliac artery shows triphasic waveform. Initial high velocity peak forward flow phase resulting from cardiac systole, brief phase of reverse flow in early diastole, low velocity forward flow in diastole.

LEFT COMMON ILIAC ARTERY

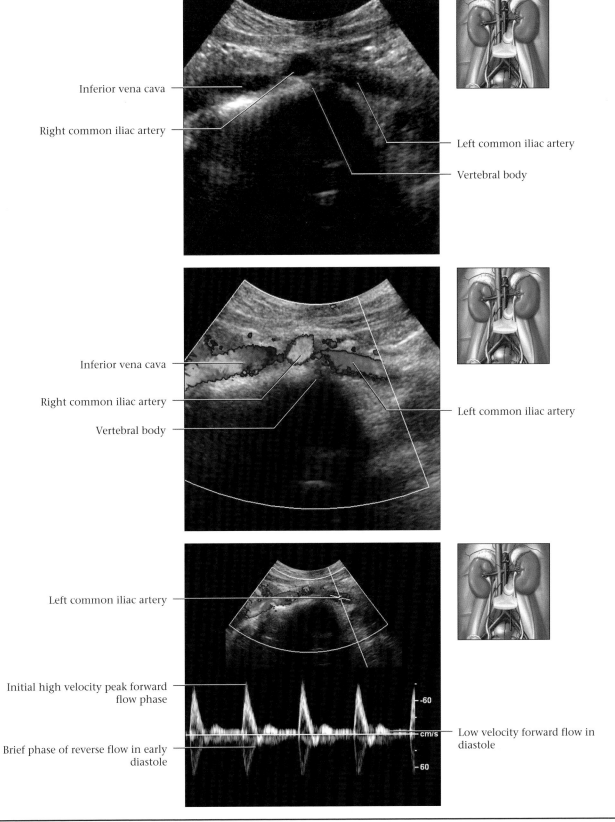

Inferior vena cava

Right common iliac artery

Left common iliac artery

Vertebral body

Inferior vena cava

Right common iliac artery

Vertebral body

Left common iliac artery

Left common iliac artery

Initial high velocity peak forward flow phase

Low velocity forward flow in diastole

Brief phase of reverse flow in early diastole

-60

cm/s

-60

(Top) Oblique grayscale ultrasound shows the course of the left common iliac artery as it branches off the aortic bifurcation. The proximal common iliac artery is first identified on the transverse plane and the transducer is then angulated along the long axis of the left common iliac artery. The normal diameter of the common iliac arteries ranges from 8-12 mm. (Middle) Oblique color Doppler ultrasound shows flow in the proximal left common iliac artery. (Bottom) Spectral Doppler ultrasound of the left common iliac artery shows characteristic triphasic waveform. Initial high velocity peak forward flow phase resulting from cardiac systole, brief phase of reverse flow in early diastole, low velocity forward flow in diastole.

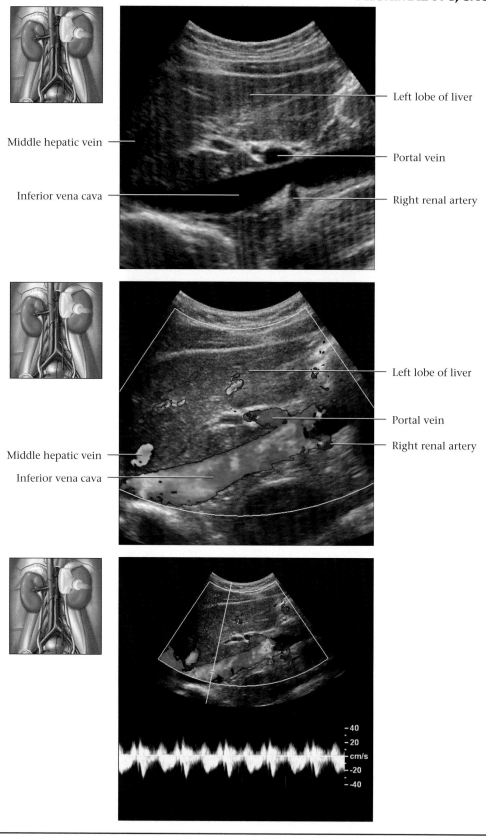

Left lobe of liver

Middle hepatic vein

Portal vein

Inferior vena cava

Right renal artery

Left lobe of liver

Portal vein

Right renal artery

Middle hepatic vein

Inferior vena cava

-40
-20
cm/s
-20
-40

(Top) Longitudinal grayscale ultrasound of the epigastric region shows the proximal IVC. The normal caliber of the IVC ranges from 5-29 mm during quiet respiration with the diameter being larger in the proximal portion. The diameter increases by about 10% during deep inspiration. (Middle) Longitudinal color Doppler ultrasound of the epigastric region shows flow within the proximal IVC (shown in blue). (Bottom) Spectral Doppler ultrasound of the proximal IVC showing slow flow that varies with respiration and cardiac pulsation. The pulsatile Doppler flow pattern contributed by atrial pressure changes is more apparent in the proximal portion of the IVC. The normal PSV ranges from 48-115 cm/s.

AORTA AND INFERIOR VENA CAVA

MID-INFERIOR VENA CAVA, SAGITTAL VIEW

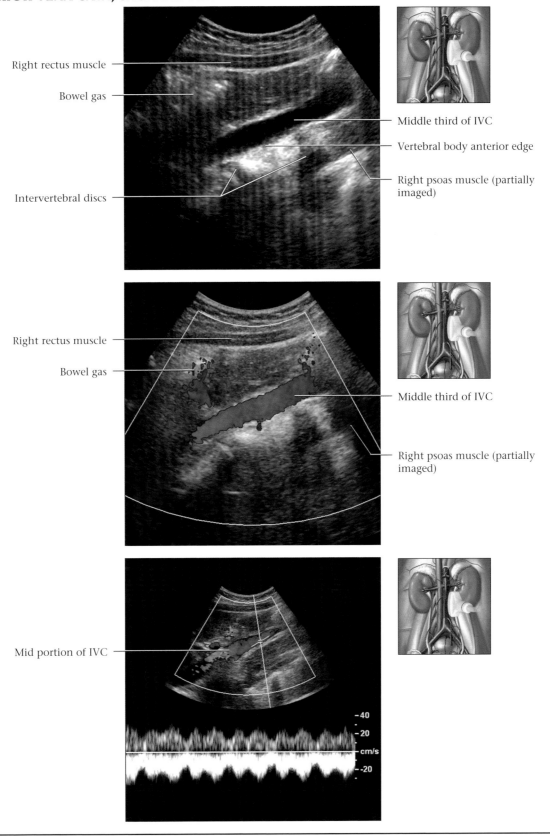

Right rectus muscle

Bowel gas

Intervertebral discs

Middle third of IVC

Vertebral body anterior edge

Right psoas muscle (partially imaged)

Right rectus muscle

Bowel gas

Middle third of IVC

Right psoas muscle (partially imaged)

Mid portion of IVC

−40

−20

cm/s

−20

(Top) Longitudinal grayscale ultrasound of the epigastric region shows the middle portion of the IVC, lying to the right of the lumbar vertebrae. Therefore the right psoas may be included in the image. The normal caliber of the IVC ranges from 5-29 mm during quiet respiration with the diameter being larger in the proximal portion. The diameter increases by about 10% during deep inspiration. (Middle) Longitudinal color Doppler ultrasound shows flow in the mid portion of the IVC. (Bottom) Spectral Doppler ultrasound of the mid portion of the IVC shows less pulsatility than that seen in the proximal IVC. This is due to the reduction in influence of the right atrium.

DISTAL IVC, SAGITTAL VIEW

— Right rectus abdominis muscle

— Bowel

— Distal inferior vena cava

— Anterior edge of vertebral body

— Intervertebral discs

— Right rectus abdominis muscle

— Distal inferior vena cava

— Anterior edge of vertebral body

— Intervertebral discs

— Distal IVC

(Top) Longitudinal grayscale ultrasound of the distal IVC below the level of the renal veins. Left-sided IVC and other congenital anomalies are encountered in the IVC below the renal veins in about 10% of the population. The diameter of the distal IVC is normally smaller than that seen in the proximal IVC. Note that in this subject, the anterior border of the vertebral bodies and the intervertebral discs can be visualized. (Middle) Longitudinal color Doppler ultrasound shows flow in the distal IVC above the common iliac vein confluence. (Bottom) Spectral Doppler ultrasound of the distal IVC shows only variations from respiration with no influence from the right atrium, unlike that seen in the proximal IVC.

AORTA AND INFERIOR VENA CAVA

PROXIMAL IVC, TRANSVERSE VIEWS

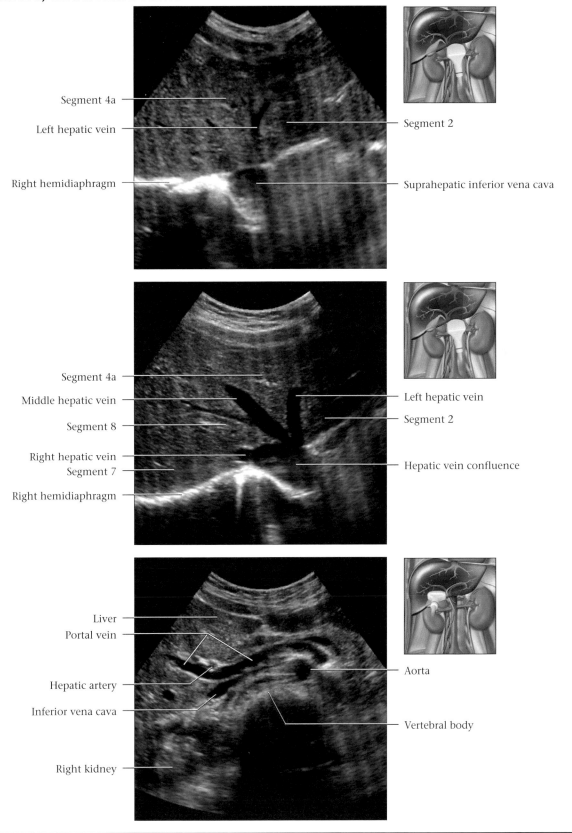

Segment 4a

Left hepatic vein

Right hemidiaphragm

Segment 2

Suprahepatic inferior vena cava

Segment 4a

Middle hepatic vein

Segment 8

Right hepatic vein

Segment 7

Right hemidiaphragm

Left hepatic vein

Segment 2

Hepatic vein confluence

Liver

Portal vein

Hepatic artery

Inferior vena cava

Right kidney

Aorta

Vertebral body

(**Top**) Transverse grayscale ultrasound with cranial angulation shows the suprahepatic IVC proximal to the hepatic confluence. The IVC leaves the abdomen via the IVC hiatus in the diaphragm at the T8 level. (**Middle**) Transverse grayscale ultrasound shows the hepatic vein confluence. Cranial angulation is often required to produce this image, and is a very useful view for designation of the segments of the liver. The middle hepatic vein defines the plane that separates the right and left lobe of the liver. The right hepatic vein defines the plane that separates the anterior and posterior segments of the right lobe. The left hepatic vein defines the plane that separates the medial and lateral segments of the left lobe. (**Bottom**) Transverse grayscale ultrasound shows the distal intrahepatic IVC at the level of the extrahepatic portal vein.

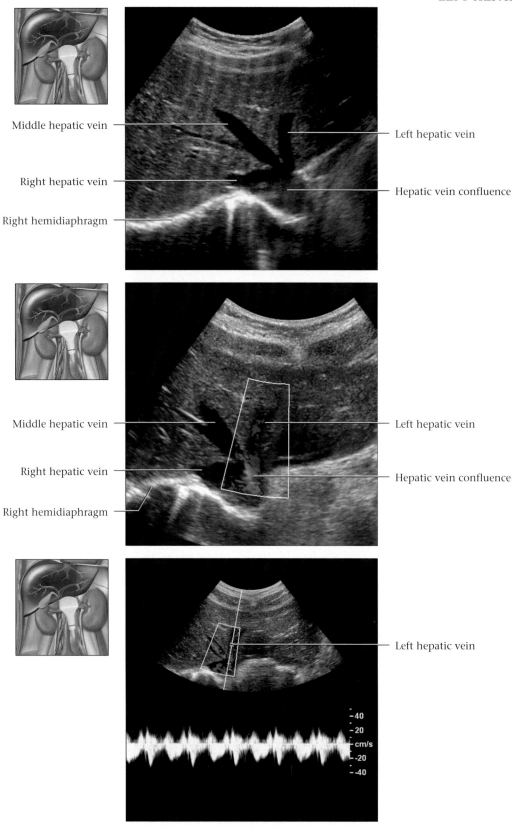

Middle hepatic vein — Left hepatic vein

Right hepatic vein — Hepatic vein confluence

Right hemidiaphragm

Middle hepatic vein — Left hepatic vein

Right hepatic vein — Hepatic vein confluence

Right hemidiaphragm

Left hepatic vein

(Top) Transverse grayscale ultrasound shows the left hepatic vein as it drains into the hepatic vein confluence. It may join the middle hepatic vein before joining the proximal IVC. The left hepatic vein runs between the medial and lateral segments of the left lobe and is frequently duplicated. **(Middle)** Transverse color Doppler ultrasound shows flow within the left hepatic vein. **(Bottom)** Spectral Doppler ultrasound of the left hepatic vein shows the normal chaotic pulsatile waveform which results from a combination of phasic variation and transmission of right atrial pulsations to the vein. The normal PSV in hepatic veins ranges from 16-40 cm/s.

MIDDLE HEPATIC VEIN

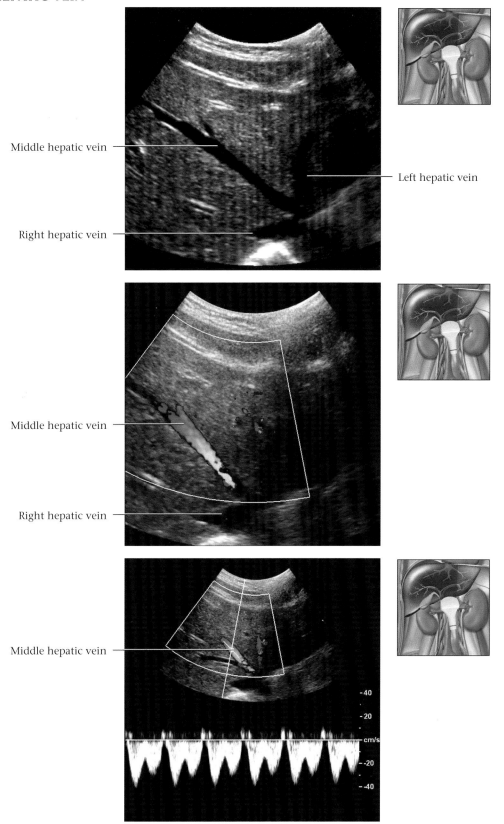

Middle hepatic vein

Left hepatic vein

Right hepatic vein

Middle hepatic vein

Right hepatic vein

Middle hepatic vein

(**Top**) Transverse grayscale ultrasound of the middle hepatic vein as it drains directly into the hepatic vein confluence. The middle hepatic vein lies in a sagittal or parasagittal plane between the right and left lobes of the liver. (**Middle**) Color Doppler ultrasound shows flow within the middle hepatic vein. (**Bottom**) Spectral Doppler ultrasound of the middle hepatic vein shows the normal chaotic pulsatile waveform which results from a combination of phasic variation and transmission of right atrial pulsations to the vein. The normal PSV in hepatic veins ranges from 16-40 cm/s.

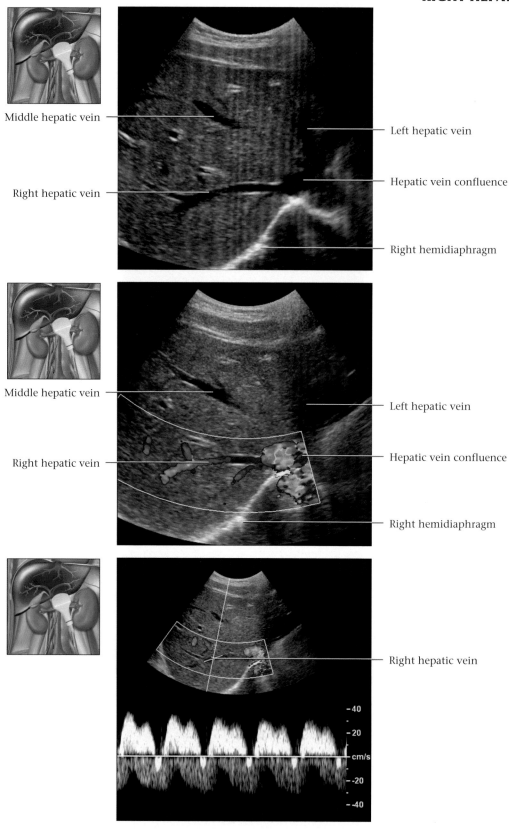

Middle hepatic vein

Right hepatic vein

Left hepatic vein

Hepatic vein confluence

Right hemidiaphragm

Middle hepatic vein

Right hepatic vein

Left hepatic vein

Hepatic vein confluence

Right hemidiaphragm

Right hepatic vein

-40

-20

cm/s

-20

-40

(Top) Transverse grayscale ultrasound of the right hepatic as it enters the hepatic vein confluence. The right hepatic vein runs in a coronal plane between the anterior and posterior segments of the right lobe of liver and may be absent in 6% of the population. **(Middle)** Transverse color Doppler ultrasound shows flow in the right hepatic vein. Note that the mid portion of the vein is perpendicular to the transducer, thereby creating an area of lack of signal in the mid portion of the vein. **(Bottom)** Spectral Doppler ultrasound of the right hepatic vein shows the normal chaotic pulsatile waveform which results from a combination of phasic variation and transmission of right atrial pulsations to the vein. The normal PSV in hepatic veins ranges from 16-40 cm/s.

RIGHT RENAL VEIN

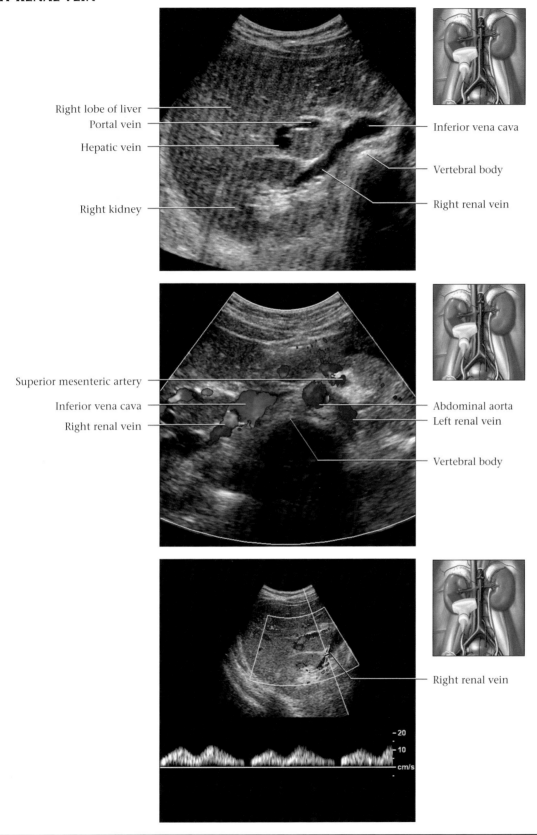

Right lobe of liver
Portal vein
Hepatic vein
Right kidney

Inferior vena cava
Vertebral body
Right renal vein

Superior mesenteric artery
Inferior vena cava
Right renal vein

Abdominal aorta
Left renal vein
Vertebral body

Right renal vein

(Top) Transverse grayscale ultrasound of the right renal vein utilizing the liver as an acoustic window. This is usually the best approach for imaging the proximal right renal vein. The right renal vein is relatively short and drains directly into the IVC. The normal caliber of the right renal vein is between 4-9 mm. **(Middle)** Transverse color Doppler ultrasound shows flow in the right renal vein. The image is obtained with slight cranial angulation so that flow towards the transducer is registered as red (right renal vein, aorta, SMA, left renal vein) and flow away from the transducer in the IVC is registered as blue. **(Bottom)** Spectral Doppler ultrasound of the right renal vein mirroring the pulsatility in the IVC. The normal PSV ranges from 18-33 cm/s.

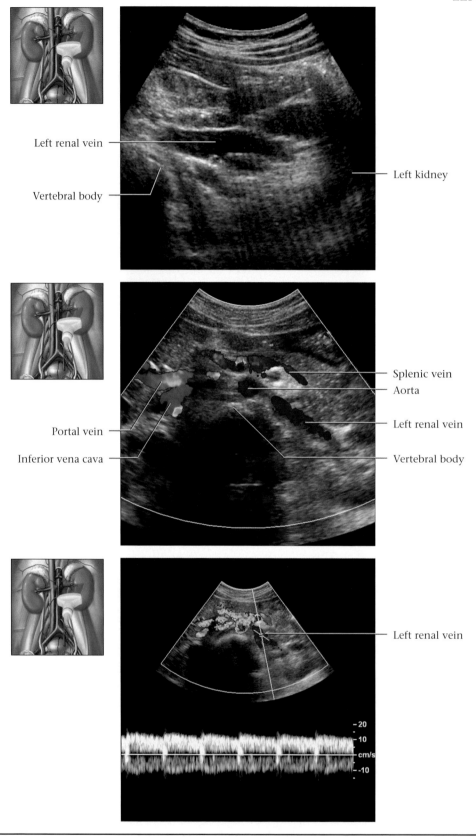

Left renal vein

Vertebral body

Left kidney

Splenic vein

Aorta

Left renal vein

Portal vein

Inferior vena cava

Vertebral body

Left renal vein

(Top) Transverse grayscale ultrasound of the left renal vein via the anterior approach. This approach may be affected by intervening bowel loops. The left renal vein has a longer course to the IVC compared with the right renal vein. The normal caliber of the left renal vein is between 4-9 mm. **(Middle)** Transverse color Doppler ultrasound with slight cranial angulation shows flow in the left renal vein in red. Flow towards the transducer is shown in red (aorta, splenic vein) and flow away from the transducer is shown in blue (IVC, portal vein). Note that the left renal vein usually courses anterior to the aorta before entering the IVC. **(Bottom)** Spectral Doppler of the left renal vein shows slight variability of flow velocities consequent upon cardiac and respiratory activity.

AORTA AND INFERIOR VENA CAVA

COMMON ILIAC VEINS

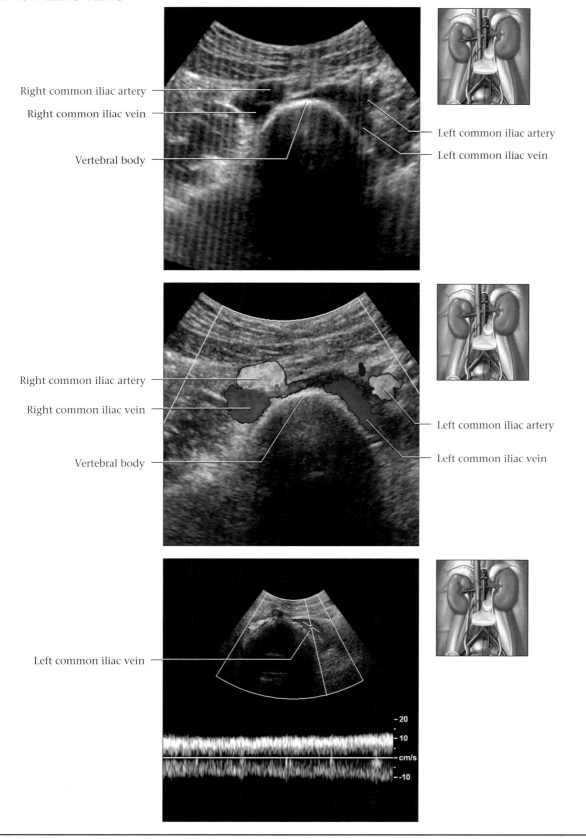

Right common iliac artery

Right common iliac vein

Vertebral body

Left common iliac artery

Left common iliac vein

Right common iliac artery

Right common iliac vein

Vertebral body

Left common iliac artery

Left common iliac vein

Left common iliac vein

(Top) Transverse grayscale ultrasound shows the common iliac veins just below where they converge to form the inferior vena cava. Note at this level the common iliac arteries are located anterior to the common iliac veins. Examination of the common iliac veins with ultrasound is often limited by intervening bowel loops and patient's body habitus. **(Middle)** Transverse color Doppler ultrasound of the proximal common iliac veins below the origin of the IVC shows flow in the common iliac veins in blue and flow in the common iliac arteries in red. **(Bottom)** Spectral Doppler ultrasound of the left common iliac vein. The normal spectral Doppler of the common iliac veins has 5 characteristics: Spontaneous flow, phasic flow, flow ceases with Valsalva maneuver, flow augmentation with distal compression and unidirectional flow towards the heart.

Abdomen

IV

137

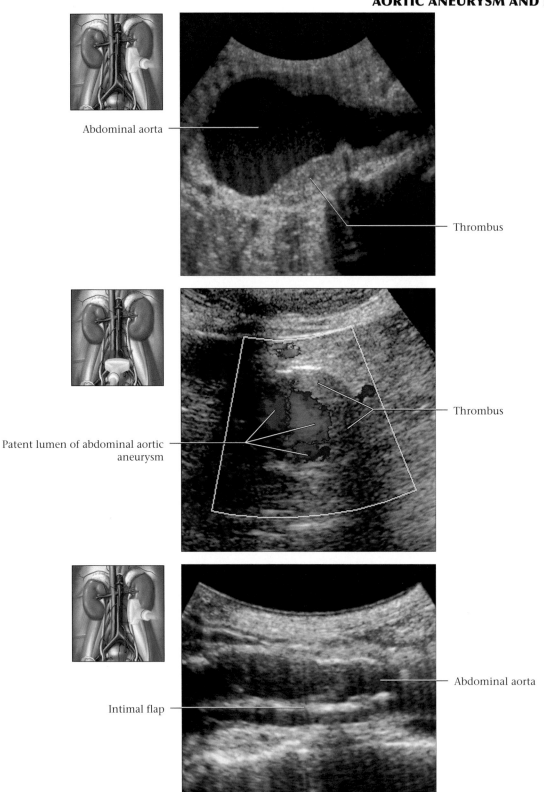

Abdominal aorta

Thrombus

Patent lumen of abdominal aortic aneurysm

Thrombus

Intimal flap

Abdominal aorta

(Top) Oblique, transabdominal, grayscale ultrasound shows a distal abdominal aortic aneurysm with no involvement of the bifurcation. A vessel is considered aneurysmal when it is dilated to 1.5 times or more compared to normal adjacent segments. The abdominal aorta is considered to be dilated when its caliber exceeds 3 cm. **(Middle)** Transverse color Doppler ultrasound shows an abdominal aortic aneurysm with circumferential mural thrombus in the lumen of an aortic aneurysm. **(Bottom)** Longitudinal grayscale ultrasound shows dissection of the abdominal aorta with an echogenic intimal flap. Dissection in the abdominal aorta is more commonly seen as an extension of a dissection of the thoracic aorta rather than a localized event in the abdominal aorta.

AORTA AND INFERIOR VENA CAVA

INFERIOR VENA CAVA OBSTRUCTION

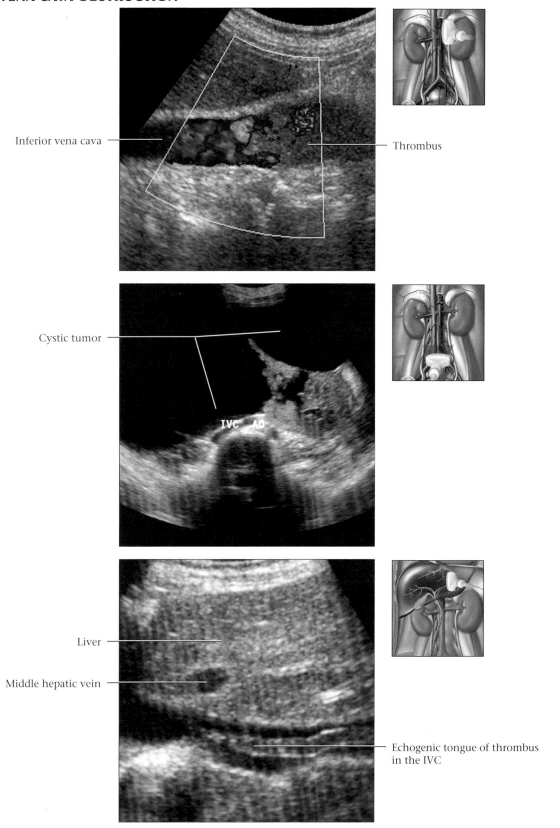

Inferior vena cava — Thrombus

Cystic tumor

IVC AO

Liver

Middle hepatic vein

Echogenic tongue of thrombus in the IVC

(Top) Longitudinal color Doppler ultrasound showing thrombosis within the inferior vena cava. Tumors such as renal cell carcinoma and hepatocellular carcinoma have a propensity to invade venous structures and are both causes of tumor thrombus extension into the IVC. Note the color Doppler flow within the thrombus, suggesting it is a tumor thrombus rather than a bland stasis/occlusive thrombus. (Middle) Transverse transabdominal grayscale ultrasound shows a large complex cystic tumor compressing the inferior vena cava. (Bottom) Longitudinal grayscale ultrasound shows an echogenic "tongue" of thrombus extending from the iliac veins into the partially patent inferior vena cava. This patient is at high risk of pulmonary embolism.

Gross Anatomy

Divisions

- Esophagus - cervical and thoracic segments
- Stomach
  - Hollow muscular organ between esophagus and small intestine
  - Location: Left upper intraperitoneal region, bordered superiorly by left hemidiaphragm, posterolaterally by spleen, posteroinferiorly by pancreas
    - Greater omentum attached from greater curvature and drapes over small and large intestines
    - Lesser omentum attached from lesser curvature to porta hepatis, covers lesser sac
  - Function
    - Gastric acid production for breakdown of large molecules of food into smaller molecules in preparation for small intestinal absorption
    - Storage of food
  - Sections
    - Gastroesophageal junction/cardia, lower esophageal sphincter
    - Fundus and body: Delineated by a horizontal plane passing through cardia
    - Antrum/pylorus: Lower section facilitating entry of gastric contents into duodenum
  - Curvatures
    - Greater curvature: Lateral wall of stomach
    - Lesser curvature: Medial wall of stomach
  - Rugae/internal ridges increase surface area for digestion
  - Arterial supply
    - Right and left gastric arteries supply lesser curvature
    - Right and left gastroepiploic arteries supply greater curvature
    - Short gastric artery supplies fundus
  - Venous drainage
    - Follow arteries and drain into portal vein and its tributaries
- Small bowel
  - Between stomach and large intestine
  - ~ 4-7 meters in length
  - Centrally located in abdomen
  - Intraperitoneal except for 2nd-4th portions of duodenum
  - Function: Further breakdown of food molecules from stomach with eventual absorption
  - Intraluminal extensions called plicae circulares increase surface area for absorption
    - Abundant in proximal small bowel, decrease in number in distal small bowel loops
  - Duodenum
    - C-shaped hollow tube connecting stomach with jejunum
    - Begins with duodenal bulb, ends in ligament of Treitz (duodenojejunal junction)
    - Arterial supply and venous drainage: Superior and inferior pancreaticoduodenal artery, pancreaticoduodenal veins
  - Jejunum
    - Connects duodenum with ileum
    - ~ 2.5 meters in length
    - Begins at ligament of Treitz
    - Along with ileum, suspended by mesentery
    - Arterial supply and venous drainage: Superior mesenteric artery and vein
  - Ileum
    - Connects jejunum with ascending colon
    - ~ 3.5 meters in length
    - Along with jejunum, suspended by mesentery
    - Arterial supply and venous drainage: Superior mesenteric artery and vein
- Large bowel
  - Between small bowel and anus
  - ~ 1.5 meters in length
  - Peripherally located in abdomen
    - Cecum and appendix, transverse colon and rectosigmoid are intraperitoneal
    - Ascending colon, descending colon and middle rectum are retroperitoneal
    - Distal rectum is extraperitoneal
  - Function: Absorption of remaining water, storage and elimination of waste
  - Sections
    - Ascending colon: Located in right side of abdomen, includes cecum where appendix arises
    - Hepatic flexure: Turn of colon at liver
    - Transverse colon: Traverses upper abdomen
    - Splenic flexure: Turn of colon at spleen
    - Descending colon: Left side of abdomen
    - Sigmoid/rectum: At posterior pelvis
  - With taenia coli: Three bands of smooth muscle just under serosa
    - Haustration: Sacculations in colon resulting from contraction of taenia coli
    - Epiploic appendages: Small fat accumulations on viscera
  - Arterial supply
    - Superior mesenteric artery supplies colon from appendix through splenic flexure
    - Ileocolic branch supplies cecum
    - Right colic branch supplies ascending colon
    - Middle colic branch supplies transverse colon
    - Inferior mesenteric artery supplies descending colon through rectum
    - Left colic branch supplies descending colon
    - Sigmoid branches supply sigmoid
    - Superior rectal artery supplies superior rectum
    - Middle and inferior rectum are supplied by arteries of same name originating from internal iliac artery
  - Venous drainage
    - Superior and inferior mesenteric veins
- Anus
  - External opening of rectum
    - Termination of gastrointestinal tract
  - With sphincters for controlling defecation
  - Internal anal sphincter
    - Thin ring of smooth muscle surrounding anal canal, deep to submucosa
    - Under involuntary control
    - Continuous with muscularis propria of rectum
    - Forms an incomplete ring in females
  - External anal sphincter

BOWEL

- Thick ring of skeletal muscle around internal anal sphincter
- Under voluntary control
- Three parts from superior to inferior: Deep, superficial and subcutaneous
  - Longitudinal muscle
    - Thin muscle between internal and external anal sphincters
    - Conjoined muscle from muscularis propria of rectum and levator ani

Histology

- Bowel wall throughout gastrointestinal tract has uniform general histology, comprising of 4 layers
  - Mucosa
    - Functions for absorption and secretion
    - Composed of epithelium and loose connective tissue
    - Lamina propria
    - Muscularis mucosa
  - Submucosa
    - Consists of fibrous connective tissue
    - Contains Meissner plexus
  - Muscularis externa
    - Muscular layer responsible for peristalsis or propulsion of food through gut
    - Contains Auerbach plexus
  - Serosa
    - Epithelial lining continuous with peritoneum

Imaging Anatomy

Overview

- Except for a few cases, bowel segments are not targeted for ultrasound examinations but may provide additional information when in their fluid-distended state
- Normal measurements of bowel caliber
  - Small bowel < 3 cm
  - Large bowel
    - Cecum < 9 cm
    - Transverse colon < 6 cm
- Five layers of bowel wall may be identified on ultrasound as alternating echogenic/sonolucent appearance ("gut signature")
  - Lamina propria: Echogenic
  - Muscularis mucosa: Sonolucent
  - Submucosa: Echogenic
  - Muscularis propria/externa: Sonolucent
  - Serosa: Echogenic
- Normal bowel wall thickness < 3 mm

Anatomy-Based Imaging Issues

Imaging Recommendations

- Transducer: 2-5 MHz for general scanning over abdomen
  - High frequency (7.5 MHz) linear transducer to examine pylorus in neonates, appendix in pediatric patients and thin adults
  - 7.5 MHz rectal transducer which produces a panoramic display of 360 degrees

- Scan over entire abdomen to check for any abnormally distended bowel loop with increased caliber and/or thickened walls
  - Small bowel segments are central
  - Colonic segments are peripheral
  - Appendix and cecum normally located in right lower quadrant

Imaging Pitfalls

- Most of the time, bowel segments have intraluminal air precluding ultrasound evaluation
- In infants suspected of hypertrophic pyloric stenosis, stomach must be emptied
  - Distended stomach displaces the gastroduodenal region inferiorly, and pylorus may be poorly visualized
  - Minimal examination time of 15 minutes, observing for peristalsis
- An inflamed retrocecal appendix is more challenging to demonstrate
  - Cecal gas may obscure underlying inflammatory changes

Clinical Implications

Clinical Importance

- Transabdominal ultrasound is a good screening modality for investigation of cases of hypertrophic pyloric stenosis, intussusception and appendicitis
- Hypertrophic pyloric stenosis
  - Usually infants 3-6 weeks old with non-bilious projectile vomiting
  - Palpation of olive-sized mass not a frequent clinical finding
  - US shows thickened muscle > 4 mm, diameter of > 15 mm and pyloric canal length of > 17 mm with retrograde, hyperperistaltic or absent contractions
- Intussusception
  - Usually children 6 months – 2 years old
  - Telescoping of one bowel loop into an adjacent segment
    - Location in children: Ileocolic > > > ileoileocolic > ileoileal > colocolic
    - Location in adults: Ileoileal > ileocolic
  - Alternating sonolucent and hyperechoic bowel walls of a loop within a loop
- Appendicitis
  - Patients with right lower quadrant pain and tenderness, and fever
  - US shows edematous non-compressible appendix with diameter ≥ 7 mm ± surrounding hypoechoic inflammatory changes
    - Other findings: Appendicolith, thickening of cecal wall, periappendiceal abscess
    - Gut signature is well-demonstrated
- Transanal endosonography may be used in evaluation of obstetric anal sphincter trauma and fistula in ano

GASTROINTESTINAL TRACT IN SITU

Esophagus
Right hemidiaphragm
Aorta
Stomach
Transverse colon
Descending colon
Ascending colon
Small intestine
Cecum
Sigmoid
Appendix
Rectum

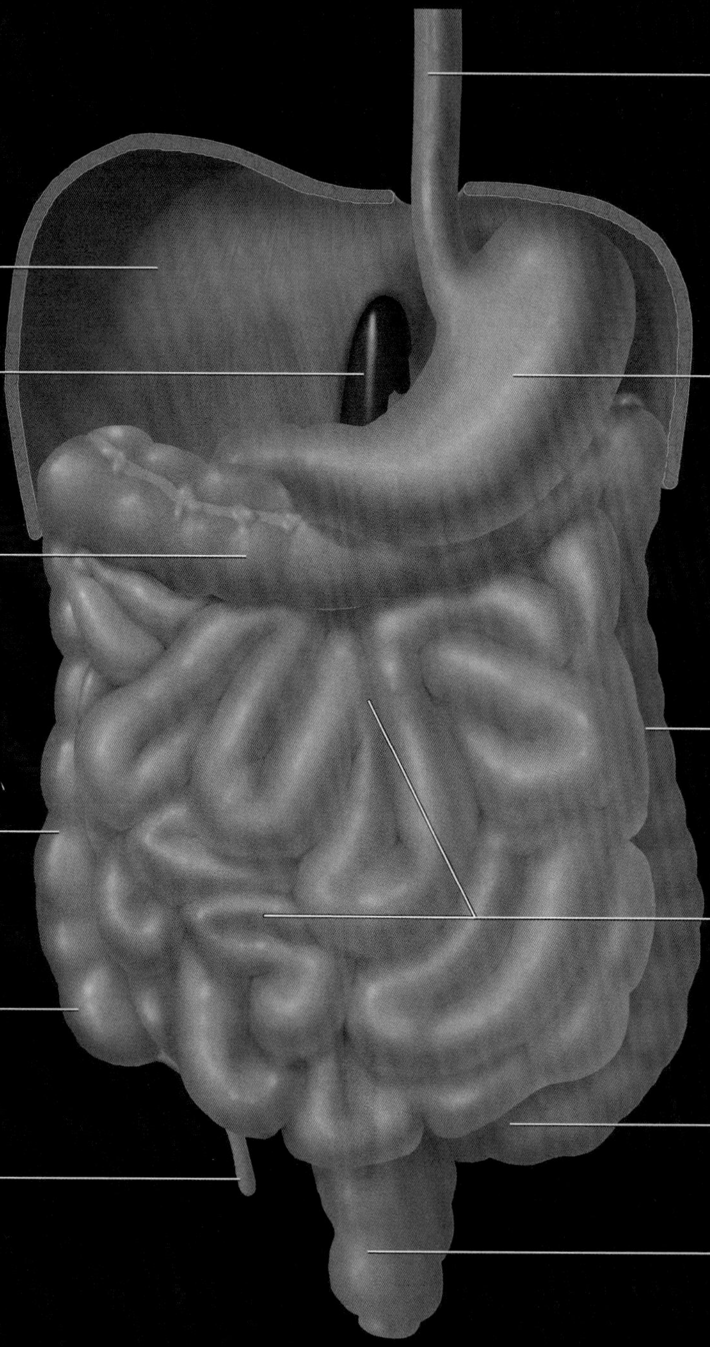

Graphic shows the gastrointestinal tract in situ. The liver and the greater omentum have been removed. Note the relatively central location of the small intestine compared with the peripherally located large intestine. Most of the bowel segments are intraperitoneal apart from the 2nd-4th parts of the duodenum, the ascending and descending colon, and middle third of the rectum which are retroperitoneal. The distal third of the rectum is extraperitoneal.

BOWEL

Liver (left lobe)

Falciform ligament

Fundus

Cardia

Gallbladder

Duodenal bulb

Body

Pylorus

Gastroepiploic artery branches

Antrum

Gastrocolic ligament

Transverse colon

Greater omentum

Hepatogastric ligament

Left gastric artery

Hepatoduodenal ligament

Pyloric sphincter

Celiac artery

Inner (oblique) muscle layer

Middle (circular) muscle layer

Outer (longitudinal) muscle layer

(Top) Graphic shows the stomach and proximal duodenum in situ. The liver and gallbladder have been retracted upward. Note that the lesser curvature and anterior wall of the stomach touch the underside of the liver, and the gallbladder abuts the duodenal bulb. The greater curvature is attached to the transverse colon by the gastrocolic ligament, which continues inferiorly as the greater omentum, covering most of the colon and small bowel. (Bottom) Graphic shows the lesser omentum extending from the stomach to the porta hepatis, and divided into the broader and thinner hepatogastric ligament and the thicker hepatoduodenal ligament. The lesser omentum carries the portal vein, hepatic artery, common bile duct and lymph nodes. The free edge of the lesser omentum forms the ventral margin of the epiploic foramen. Note the layers of gastric muscle; middle circular layer is thickest.

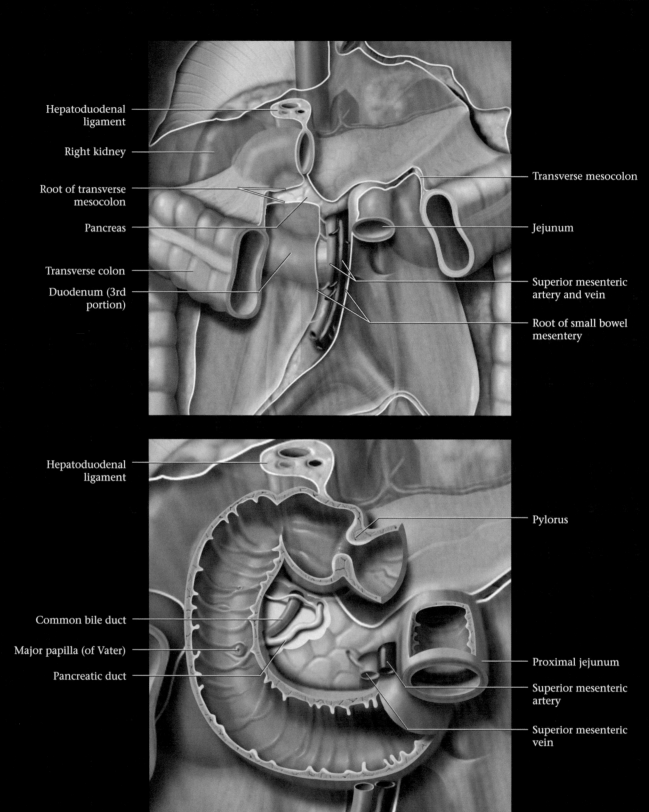

(Top) The duodenum is retroperitoneal, except for the bulb (1st part). The proximal jejunum is intraperitoneal. The hepatoduodenal ligament attaches the duodenum to the porta hepatis and contains the portal triad (bile duct, hepatic artery, portal vein). The root of the transverse mesocolon and mesentery both cross the duodenum. The third portion of the duodenum crosses in front of the aorta and IVC, and behind the superior mesenteric vessels. The second portion of the duodenum is attached to the pancreatic head and lies close to the hilum of the right kidney. **(Bottom)** Graphic shows the duodenal bulb suspended by the hepatoduodenal ligament. The duodenal-jejunal flexure is suspended by the ligament of Treitz, an extension of the right crus. The major pancreaticobiliary papilla enters the medial wall of the second portion of the duodenum.

SMALL INTESTINE

Celiac artery

Superior mesenteric artery

Ileocolic artery

Jejunal straight arteries

Jejunal arterial arcades

Ileal straight arteries

Liver

Stomach

Transverse colon

Greater omentum

Pancreas

Superior mesenteric artery

Duodenum (3rd part)

Aorta

Inferior vena cava

Small bowel loops

(Top) Graphic shows the vascular supply of the entire small intestine from the superior mesenteric artery (SMA). The small bowel segments are displaced inferiorly. The SMA arises from the anterior abdominal aorta, and gives off the inferior pancreaticoduodenal branch that supplies the duodenum & pancreas. Arising from the left side of the SMA are numerous branches to the jejunum & ileum. Jejunal arteries are generally larger and longer than those of the ileum. After a straight course the arteries form multiple intercommunicating curvilinear arcades. **(Bottom)** Graphic shows sagittal section of the central abdomen revealing the jejunum and ileum suspended in a radial pattern by mesentery. Note the overlying greater omentum, attached from the inferior portion of the stomach to drape the small bowel segments and transverse colon.

Abdomen

IV

145

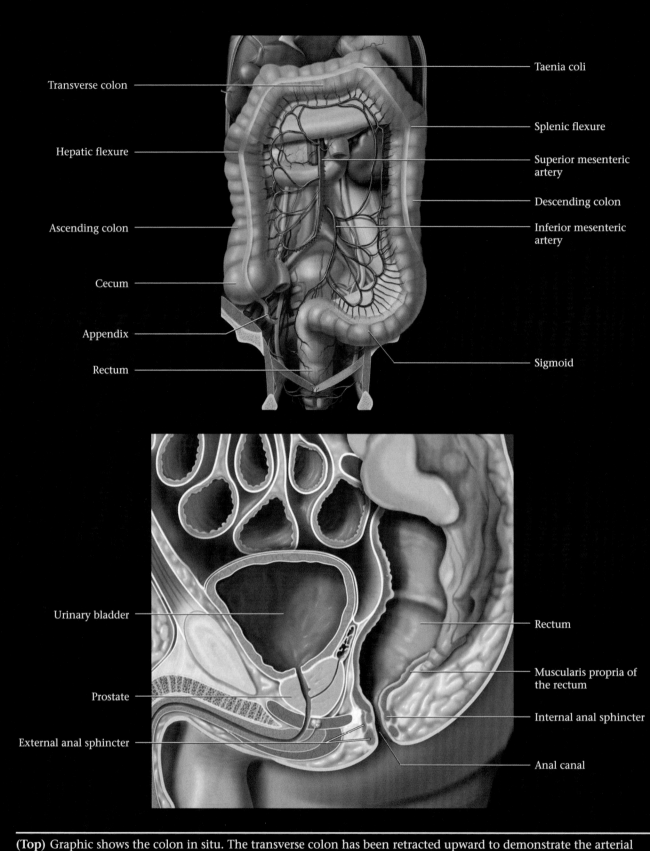

Transverse colon

Hepatic flexure

Ascending colon

Cecum

Appendix

Rectum

Taenia coli

Splenic flexure

Superior mesenteric artery

Descending colon

Inferior mesenteric artery

Sigmoid

Urinary bladder

Prostate

External anal sphincter

Rectum

Muscularis propria of the rectum

Internal anal sphincter

Anal canal

(Top) Graphic shows the colon in situ. The transverse colon has been retracted upward to demonstrate the arterial supply of the colon from the superior and inferior mesenteric arteries. The SMA supplies the colon from the appendix through the splenic flexure, and the IMA supplies the descending colon through the rectum. Note the band of smooth muscle (taenia coli) running along the length of the intestine, which terminates in the vermiform appendix. These result in sacculations/haustrations along the colon, giving it a segmented appearance. **(Bottom)** Graphic shows longitudinal section of a male pelvis. The anus is the external opening of the rectum and terminal end of the gastrointestinal tract. The internal anal sphincter (IAS) is a thin involuntary muscle deep to the submucosa. The external anal sphincter is thicker, encircles the IAS and is under voluntary control.

BOWEL

STOMACH

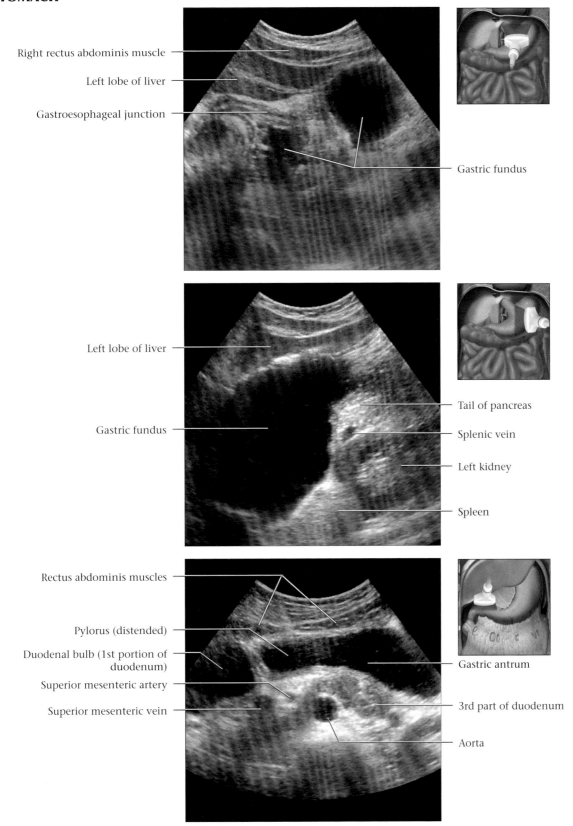

Right rectus abdominis muscle

Left lobe of liver

Gastroesophageal junction

Gastric fundus

Left lobe of liver

Gastric fundus

Tail of pancreas

Splenic vein

Left kidney

Spleen

Rectus abdominis muscles

Pylorus (distended)

Duodenal bulb (1st portion of duodenum)

Superior mesenteric artery

Superior mesenteric vein

Gastric antrum

3rd part of duodenum

Aorta

(**Top**) Transverse, subxiphoid, grayscale ultrasound demonstrates the gastroesophageal region and the medially located fluid-filled gastric fundus. Note the anterior wall of the stomach touches the underside of the left lobe of the liver. (**Middle**) Transabdominal, longitudinal, grayscale ultrasound at the left upper quadrant shows a fluid-distended gastric fundus and its anatomic relationships with the adjacent organs. The tail of the pancreas is immediately inferoposterior, left lobe of the liver is anterosuperior, while the spleen and left kidney are posterior. (**Bottom**) Transverse, transabdominal, grayscale ultrasound of the gastroduodenal region, with an open pylorus. When distended, the gastric antrum and duodenal bulb may be displaced to a more inferior location. Thus instead of visualizing the pancreas posteriorly, the 3rd portion of the duodenum is included in this image.

BOWEL

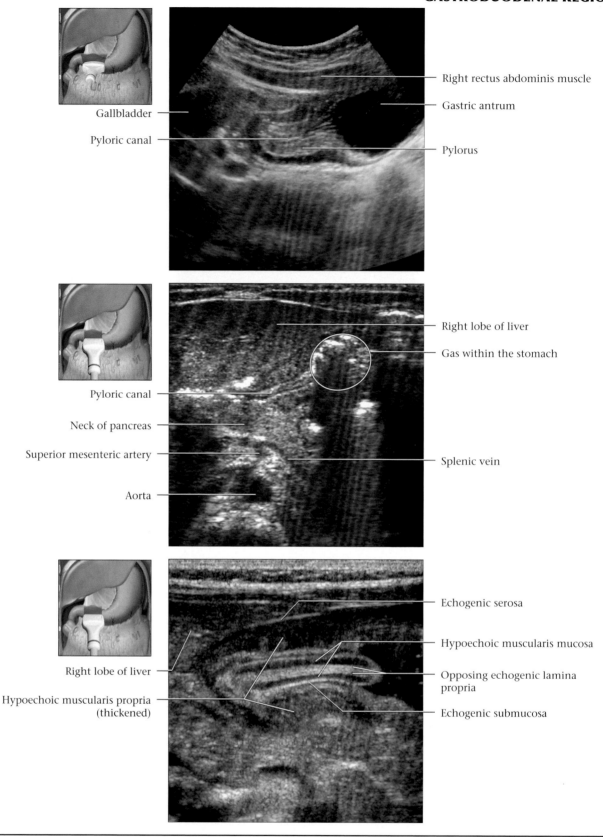

Right rectus abdominis muscle

Gastric antrum

Gallbladder

Pyloric canal

Pylorus

Right lobe of liver

Gas within the stomach

Pyloric canal

Neck of pancreas

Superior mesenteric artery

Splenic vein

Aorta

Echogenic serosa

Hypoechoic muscularis mucosa

Opposing echogenic lamina propria

Right lobe of liver

Hypoechoic muscularis propria (thickened)

Echogenic submucosa

(Top) Transverse, transabdominal, grayscale ultrasound of the gastroduodenal region in an adult shows peristaltic contraction of the pylorus. **(Middle)** Transverse, transabdominal, grayscale ultrasound of the normal pylorus of an infant. The gastric antrum and duodenal bulb are non-distended, and the pancreas is identified posteriorly. The pylorus is collapsed and its canal, lined by thin echogenic mucosa (lamina propria) is normally < 17 mm long. Normal pyloric muscle thickness < 3 mm with overall pyloric caliber (serosa to serosa) of < 15 mm. **(Bottom)** Transverse, transabdominal, grayscale ultrasound in a 6 week old with projectile non-bilious vomiting. The pyloric muscle is thickened to 7 mm and the pyloric canal is 24 mm long. Note the prominent alternating sonolucent and echogenic layers of the bowel wall, constituting the "gut signature."

BOWEL

DUODENUM

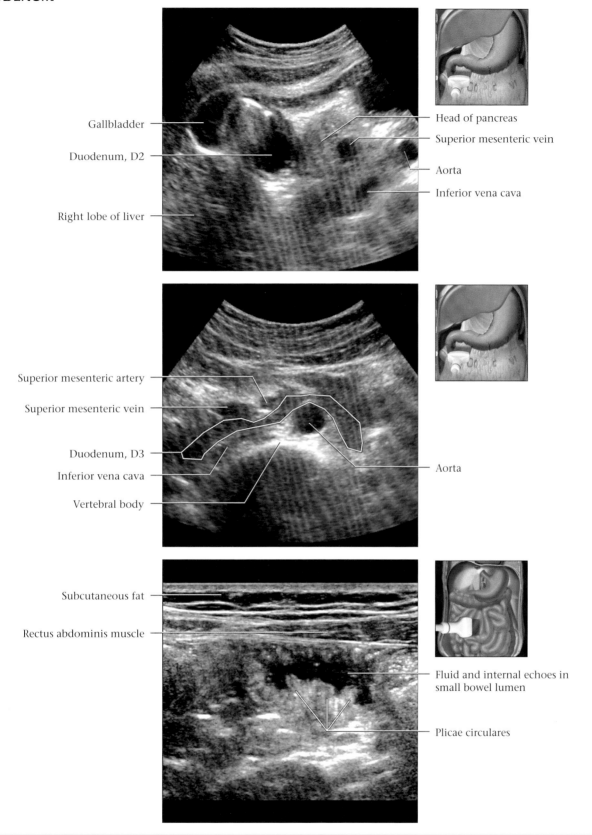

Gallbladder

Duodenum, D2

Right lobe of liver

Head of pancreas

Superior mesenteric vein

Aorta

Inferior vena cava

Superior mesenteric artery

Superior mesenteric vein

Duodenum, D3

Inferior vena cava

Vertebral body

Aorta

Subcutaneous fat

Rectus abdominis muscle

Fluid and internal echoes in small bowel lumen

Plicae circulares

(Top) Transverse, transabdominal, grayscale ultrasound shows fluid-distended second part of the duodenum (D2), identified lateral to the head of the pancreas. The major duodenal papilla in its medial side (not demonstrated) marks the opening of the ampulla of Vater. (Middle) Transverse, transabdominal, grayscale ultrasound at a lower level shows collapsed third portion of the duodenum (D3). D3 crosses in front of the aorta and IVC, and behind the superior mesenteric vessels. Its distal portion hugs and follows the contour of the abdominal aorta. (Bottom) Longitudinal transabdominal grayscale ultrasound at the central abdomen. Occasionally small bowel loops may be seen especially when they are distended with fluid, revealing luminal folds (plicae circulares) which increase the surface area for absorption.

BOWEL

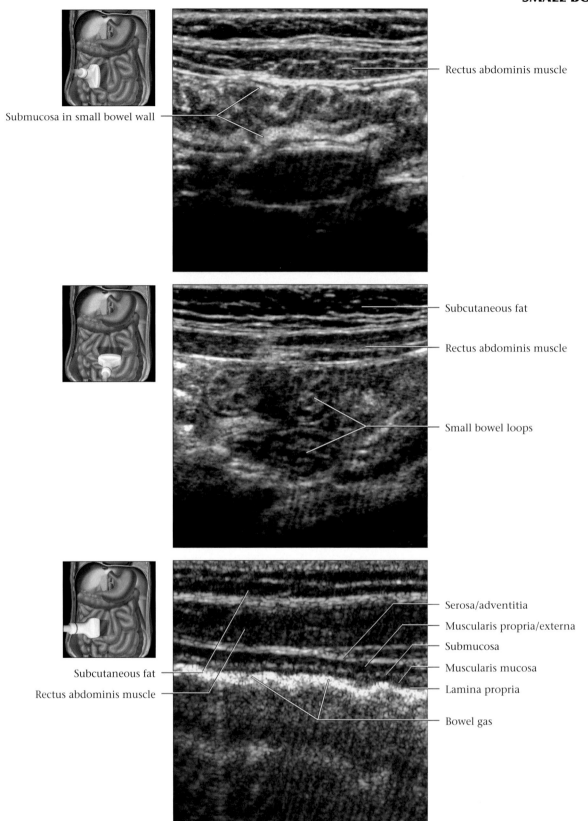

Submucosa in small bowel wall

Rectus abdominis muscle

Subcutaneous fat

Rectus abdominis muscle

Small bowel loops

Subcutaneous fat
Rectus abdominis muscle

Serosa/adventitia
Muscularis propria/externa
Submucosa
Muscularis mucosa
Lamina propria

Bowel gas

(Top) Longitudinal, transabdominal, grayscale ultrasound at the central abdomen shows non-distended small bowel segments close to the anterior abdominal wall. The thick echogenic layer is the submucosa of the bowel wall sandwiched between the hypoechoic muscularis mucosa and muscularis propria. The echogenic lamina propria and serosa are very thin and not visible on this image. **(Middle)** Transverse, transabdominal, grayscale ultrasound shows small bowel loops seen end on. **(Bottom)** Longitudinal, transabdominal, grayscale ultrasound illustrates the gut signature in the anterior wall of a bowel loop with intraluminal gas. The lamina propria is very thin and echogenic and not easily identified due to bowel gas echoes.

BOWEL

APPENDIX

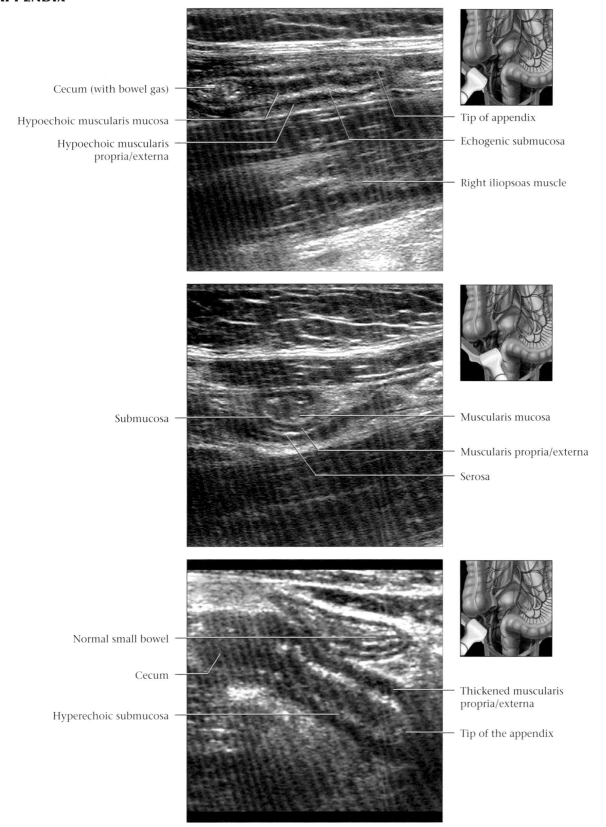

Cecum (with bowel gas)

Hypoechoic muscularis mucosa

Hypoechoic muscularis propria/externa

Tip of appendix

Echogenic submucosa

Right iliopsoas muscle

Submucosa

Muscularis mucosa

Muscularis propria/externa

Serosa

Normal small bowel

Cecum

Hyperechoic submucosa

Thickened muscularis propria/externa

Tip of the appendix

(Top) Oblique, transabdominal, grayscale ultrasound at the right lower quadrant. The normal appendix is infrequently visualized and may be seen in thin adults. The appendix is a blind-ended tubular structure which exhibits peristalsis. (Middle) Transverse, transabdominal, grayscale ultrasound reveals cross-section of the normal appendix. It has a diameter of < 6 mm and may be compressed on application of transducer pressure. The thin lamina propria is not clearly identified, but the rest of the gut signature is noted. (Bottom) Oblique transabdominal ultrasound shows a blind-ending, tubular, dilated and non-compressible acutely inflamed appendix. The adjacent small bowel is compressible.

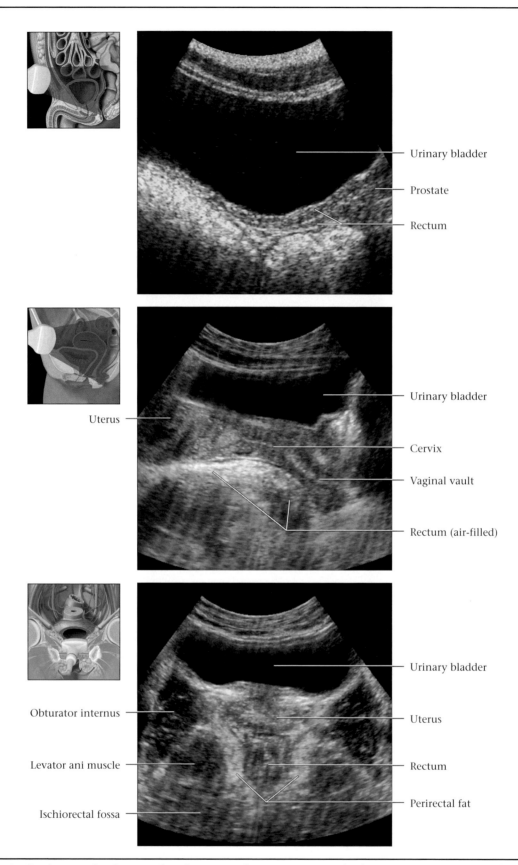

Urinary bladder

Prostate

Rectum

Uterus

Urinary bladder

Cervix

Vaginal vault

Rectum (air-filled)

Obturator internus

Urinary bladder

Uterus

Levator ani muscle

Rectum

Ischiorectal fossa

Perirectal fat

(**Top**) Longitudinal grayscale ultrasound at the suprapubic region in a male shows an empty rectum which is immediately posterior to the urinary bladder. (**Middle**) Longitudinal grayscale ultrasound at the suprapubic region of a female demonstrates the relationship of the pelvic organs, from anterior to posterior: Urinary bladder, uterus, rectum. Air within the rectum causes ring down artifact. (**Bottom**) Transverse grayscale ultrasound obtained by swinging the probe caudally. The relationships of the urinary bladder, uterus and rectum are maintained. The pelvic floor muscles are visible in this image.

BOWEL

ANUS, FEMALE

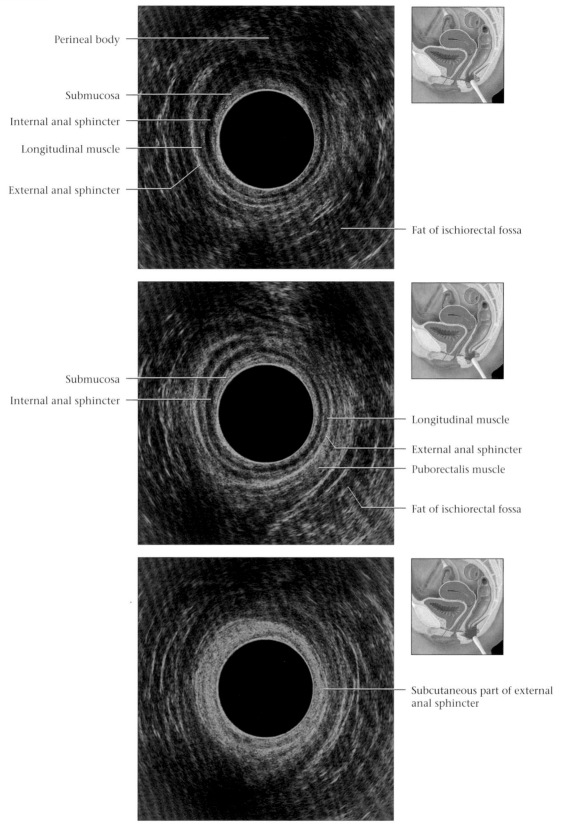

Perineal body

Submucosa

Internal anal sphincter

Longitudinal muscle

External anal sphincter

Fat of ischiorectal fossa

Submucosa

Internal anal sphincter

Longitudinal muscle

External anal sphincter

Puborectalis muscle

Fat of ischiorectal fossa

Subcutaneous part of external anal sphincter

(Top) First of three transanal endosonography images in a female, taken at high, middle and low levels. The internal anal sphincter is a hypoechoic ring identified deep to the submucosa. It is continuous with the muscularis propria of the rectum, which has fibers conjoined with those of the levator ani to form the longitudinal muscle. **(Middle)** The external anal sphincter is less well-defined and more echogenic and does not form a complete ring in the female. It is identified deep to the longitudinal muscle. **(Bottom)** At the lower level, only the subcutaneous part of the external anal sphincter is visible.

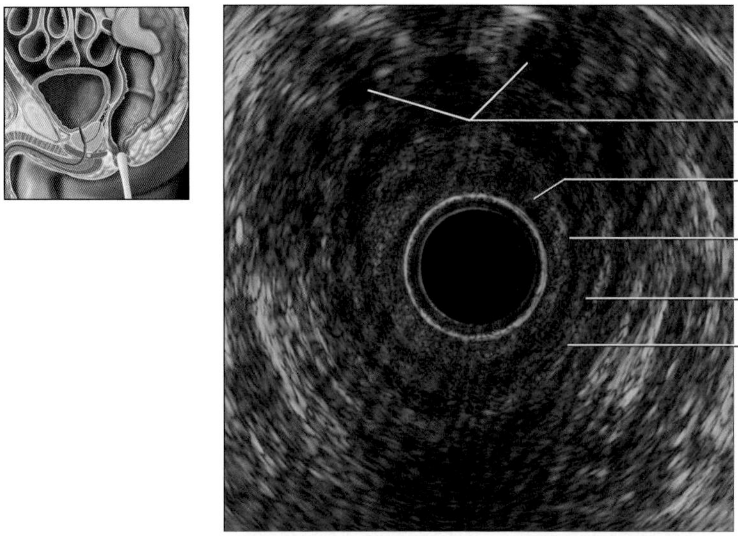

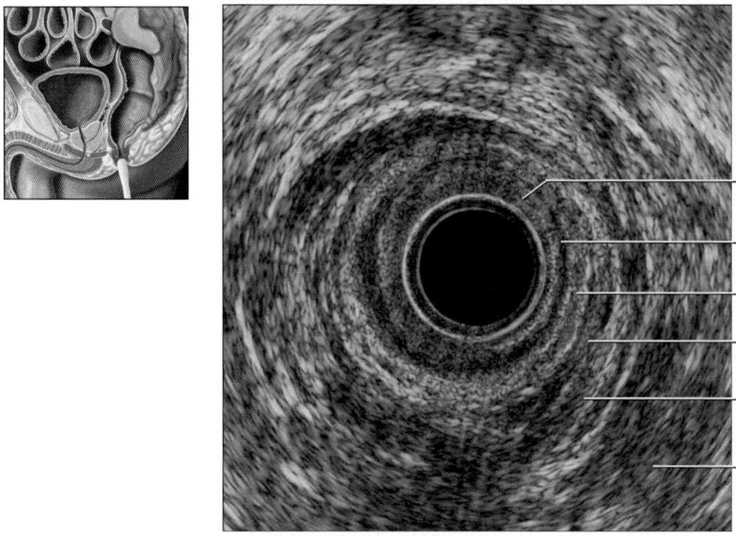

Transverse perineal muscle

Submucosa

Internal anal sphincter

Longitudinal muscle

External anal sphincter

Submucosa

Internal anal sphincter

Longitudinal muscle

External anal sphincter

Puborectalis muscle

Fat of ischiorectal fossa

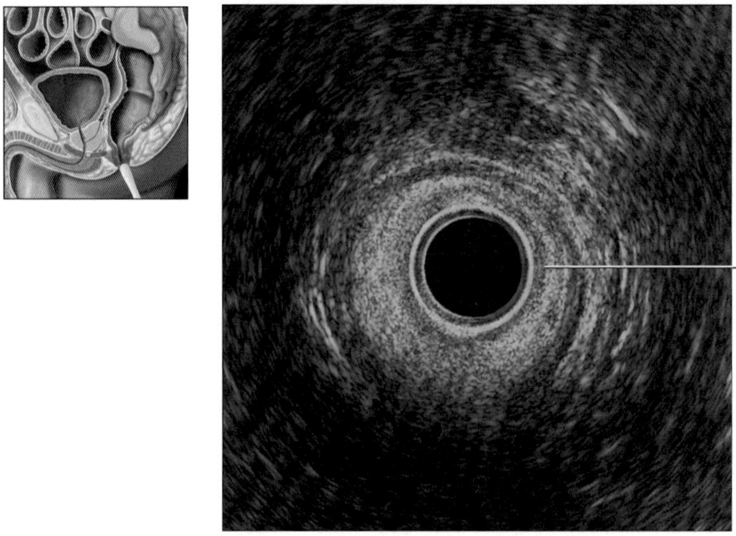

Subcutaneous part of external anal sphincter

(Top) First of three transanal endosonography images in a male taken at high, middle and low levels. The internal anal sphincter appears as a thin black ring encircling the submucosa, and it is continuous with the muscularis propria of the rectum. Likewise the outer longitudinal muscle is an extension of the muscularis propria in the rectum conjoined with fibers from the levator ani. **(Middle)** The external anal sphincter is less well-defined and more echogenic and in males forms a complete ring. **(Bottom)** At the lower level, the subcutaneous part of the external anal sphincter is visible on ultrasound.

BOWEL

SAMPLE CASES

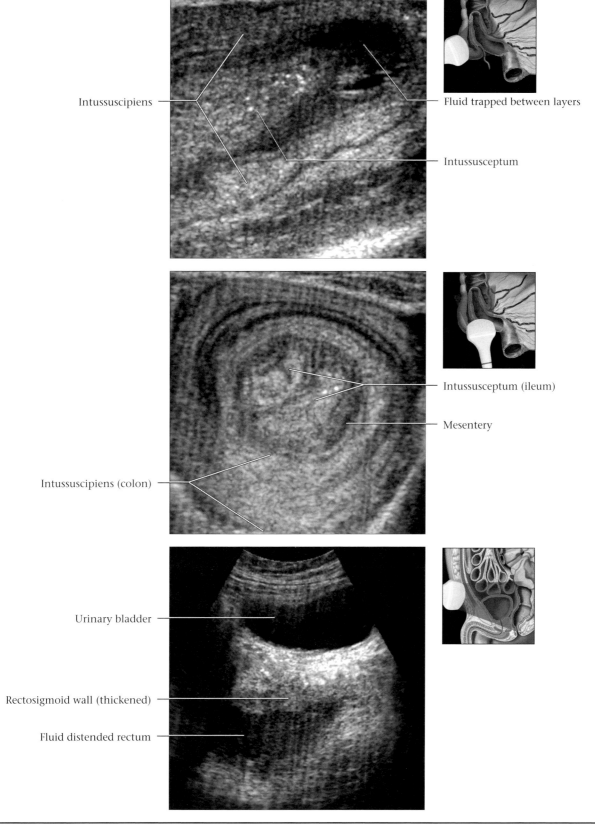

Intussuscipiens

Fluid trapped between layers

Intussusceptum

Intussusceptum (ileum)

Mesentery

Intussuscipiens (colon)

Urinary bladder

Rectosigmoid wall (thickened)

Fluid distended rectum

(Top) Longitudinal, transabdominal, grayscale ultrasound shows multilayered appearance of intussusception, giving the "pseudokidney" sign. Minimal fluid is trapped between the layers. **(Middle)** Transverse, transabdominal, grayscale ultrasound shows classical "coiled spring" appearance of ileo-colic intussusception. The inner intussusceptum is separated from the outer intussuscipiens by mesentery. **(Bottom)** Longitudinal grayscale ultrasound at the suprapubic region of a male patient reveals fluid-distended rectosigmoid, which lies behind the urinary bladder. Note the abnormally thickened wall, > 3 mm. Histopathology revealed rectosigmoid adenocarcinoma.

ABDOMINAL LYMPH NODES

Gross Anatomy

Overview

- Major lymphatic vessels and nodal chains lie along major blood vessels (aorta, IVC, iliac) and have same names (e.g., common iliac nodes)
- Lymph from alimentary tract, liver, spleen and pancreas passes along celiac, superior mesenteric chains to nodes with similar names (e.g., celiac nodes)
  - Efferent vessels from alimentary nodes form intestinal lymphatic trunks
  - Cisterna chyli (chyle cistern)
    - Formed by confluence of intestinal lymphatic trunks and right and left lumbar lymphatic trunks (which receive lymph from non-alimentary viscera, abdominal wall and lower extremities)
    - May be discrete sac or plexiform convergence
- Thoracic duct: Inferior extent is chyle cistern at the L1-2 level
  - Formed by the convergence of main lymphatic ducts of abdomen
  - Ascends through aortic hiatus in diaphragm to enter posterior mediastinum
  - Ends by entering junction of left subclavian and internal jugular veins
- Lymphatic system drains surplus fluid from extracellular spaces and returns it to bloodstream
  - Has important function in defense against infection, inflammation and tumor via lymphoid tissue present in lymph nodes, gut wall, spleen and thymus
  - Absorbs and transports dietary lipids from intestine to thoracic duct and bloodstream
- Lymph nodes
  - Composed of cortex and medulla
  - Invested in fibrous capsule which extends into the nodal parenchyma to form trabeculae
  - Internal honeycomb structure filled with lymphocytes that collect and destroy pathogens
  - Hilum: In concave side, with artery and vein, surrounded by fat

Abdominopelvic Nodes

- Named after the adjacent vessel
- Preaortic nodes
  - Celiac nodes
    - Drainage from gastric nodes, hepatic nodes and pancreaticosplenic nodes
  - Superior mesenteric nodes
    - Drainage from mesenteric nodes
  - Inferior mesenteric nodes
    - Drainage from mesenteric nodes
- Lateral aortic nodes
  - Drainage from kidneys, adrenal glands, ureter, posterior abdominal wall, testes and ovary, uterus and fallopian tubes
- Retroaortic nodes
  - Drainage from the posterior abdominal wall
- External iliac nodes
  - Primary drainage from inguinal nodes
  - Flow into common iliac nodes
- Internal iliac nodes

- Drainage from inferior pelvic viscera, deep perineum and gluteal region
- Flow into common iliac nodes
- Common iliac nodes
  - Drainage from external iliac, internal iliac and sacral nodes
  - Flow into lumbar (lateral aortic) chain of nodes
- Superficial inguinal nodes
  - In superficial fascia parallel to inguinal ligament, along cephalad portion of greater saphenous vein
  - Receive lymphatic drainage from superficial lower extremity, superficial abdominal wall and perineum
  - Flow into deep inguinal and external iliac nodes
- Deep inguinal nodes
  - Along medial side of femoral vein, deep to fascia lata and inguinal ligament
  - Receive lymphatic drainage from superficial inguinal and popliteal nodes
  - Flow into external iliac nodes

Imaging Anatomy

Overview

- Ultrasound is useful for assessing the size and appearance of enlarged lymph nodes especially in children or thin adults
  - CT is the imaging procedure of choice for standard and repeatable examination of the retroperitoneum
- Normal diameter of lymph node varies depending on location
  - Shortest diameter
    - Abdomen < 1 cm
    - Retrocrural < 0.6 cm
    - Pelvic < 1.5 cm

Anatomy-Based Imaging Issues

Imaging Recommendations

- Transducer: 2-5 MHz
- Patient examined in supine position
  - Fasting for at least 4 hours may help decrease overlying bowel gas
- Graded compression technique, to clear overlying bowel loops
- Nodes are named according to the adjacent vessel

Clinical Implications

Clinical Importance

- Lymphoma
  - 10% of lymphoma patients have disease in normal nodes
  - Discrete hypoechoic or anechoic nodes
- Metastatic lymphadenopathy
  - More echogenic and heterogeneous nodes compared to lymphomatous nodes
- Infectious/reactive lymphadenopathy
  - Non-specific sonographic features

RETROPERITONEAL LYMPH NODES

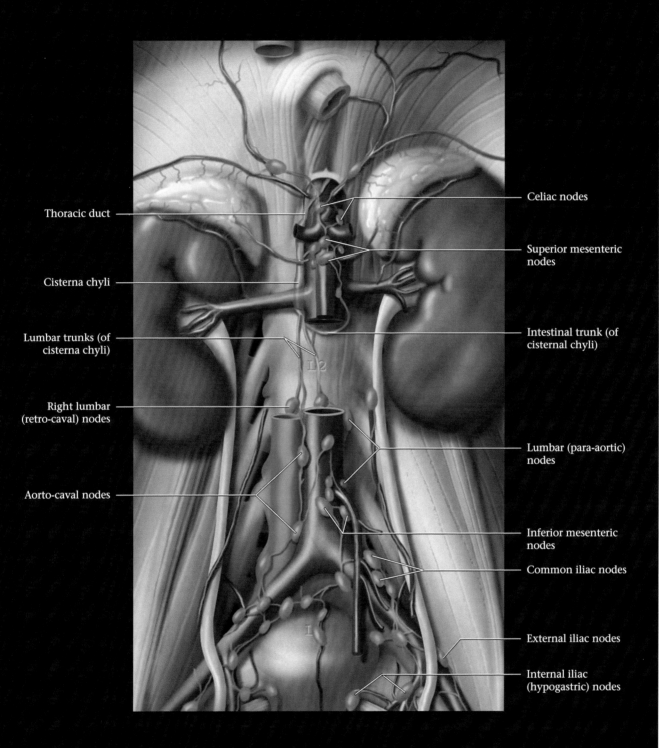

Thoracic duct

Cisterna chyli

Lumbar trunks (of cisterna chyli)

Right lumbar (retro-caval) nodes

Aorto-caval nodes

Celiac nodes

Superior mesenteric nodes

Intestinal trunk (of cisternal chyli)

Lumbar (para-aortic) nodes

Inferior mesenteric nodes

Common iliac nodes

External iliac nodes

Internal iliac (hypogastric) nodes

Graphic shows that the major lymphatics and lymph nodes of the abdomen are located along, and share the same name as the major blood vessels, such as the external iliac nodes, celiac and superior mesenteric nodes. The para-aortic and para-caval nodes are also referred to as the lumbar nodes and receive afferents from the lower abdominal viscera, abdominal wall and lower extremities; they are frequently involved in inflammatory and neoplastic processes. The lumbar trunks join with an intestinal trunk (at about the L1 level) to form the cisterna chyli, which may be a discrete sac or a plexiform convergence. The cisterna chyli and other major lymphatic trunks join to form the thoracic duct which passes through the aortic hiatus to enter the mediastinum. After picking up additional lymphatic trunks within the thorax, the thoracic duct empties into the left subclavian or innominate vein.

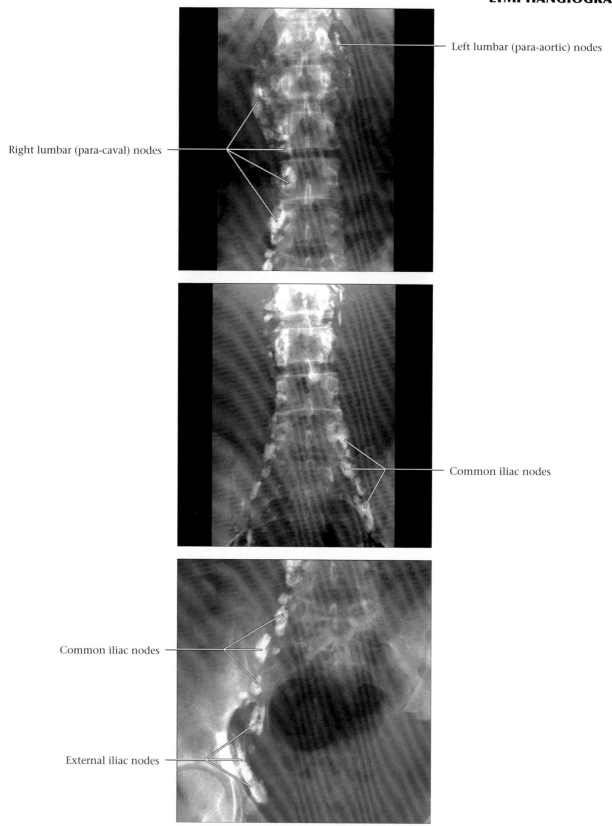

Left lumbar (para-aortic) nodes

Right lumbar (para-caval) nodes

Common iliac nodes

Common iliac nodes

External iliac nodes

(Top) First of three images from a lymphangiogram, in which iodinated oil is slowly infused into the lymphatics of the foot to produce opacification of the lymph channels and nodes. Note the sub-centimeter (short axis) diameter of these normal retroperitoneal lymph nodes. (Middle) Lymphatic channels and lymph nodes parallel the course of major blood vessels and share similar names, such as these common iliac nodes. (Bottom) With the availability of CT, MR and PET (positron emission tomography), lymphangiograms are performed much less frequently than in the past.

ABDOMINAL LYMPH NODES

NON-ENLARGED NODES

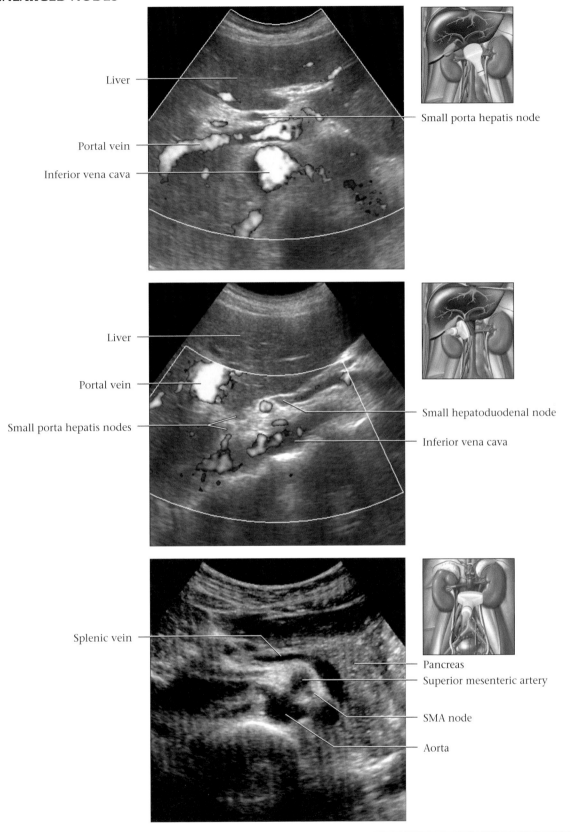

Liver

Small porta hepatis node

Portal vein

Inferior vena cava

Liver

Portal vein

Small hepatoduodenal node

Small porta hepatis nodes

Inferior vena cava

Splenic vein

Pancreas

Superior mesenteric artery

SMA node

Aorta

(Top) Transverse, subcostal, power Doppler ultrasound using the liver as an acoustic window shows a small avascular node in the porta hepatic region. It is < 1 cm and is considered non-enlarged. **(Middle)** Longitudinal, subcostal, power Doppler ultrasound shows small nodes in the porta and hepatoduodenal ligament. The porta hepatis node is identified nearer to the hepatic hilum. **(Bottom)** Transverse transabdominal ultrasound at the level of the pancreas. There is a small node lateral to the superior mesenteric artery. Abdominal nodes < 1 cm in short axis diameter are considered non-enlarged.

ABDOMINAL LYMPH NODES

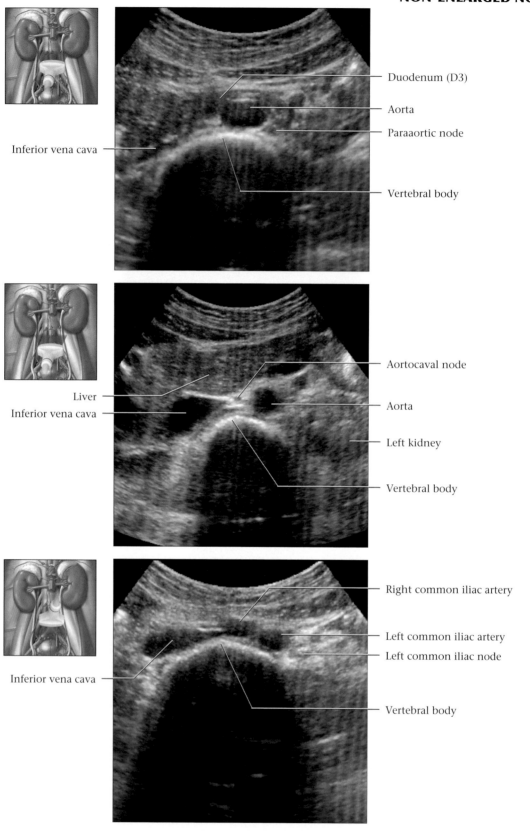

Duodenum (D3)

Aorta

Paraaortic node

Vertebral body

Inferior vena cava

Aortocaval node

Aorta

Left kidney

Vertebral body

Liver

Inferior vena cava

Right common iliac artery

Left common iliac artery

Left common iliac node

Vertebral body

Inferior vena cava

(Top) Transverse, transabdominal, grayscale ultrasound reveals a lymph node to the left of the abdominal aorta, which is < 1 cm in diameter and considered normal. Ten percent of patients with lymphoma will have disease in normal-size lymph nodes. (Middle) Transverse, transabdominal, grayscale ultrasound at the level of the kidneys. There is a tiny hypoechoic node between the aorta and inferior vena cava. (Bottom) Transverse, transabdominal, grayscale ultrasound at the infraumbilical level, shows the aortic bifurcation. A small node is identified adjacent to the left common iliac artery.

ABDOMINAL LYMPH NODES

ENLARGED LYMPH NODES

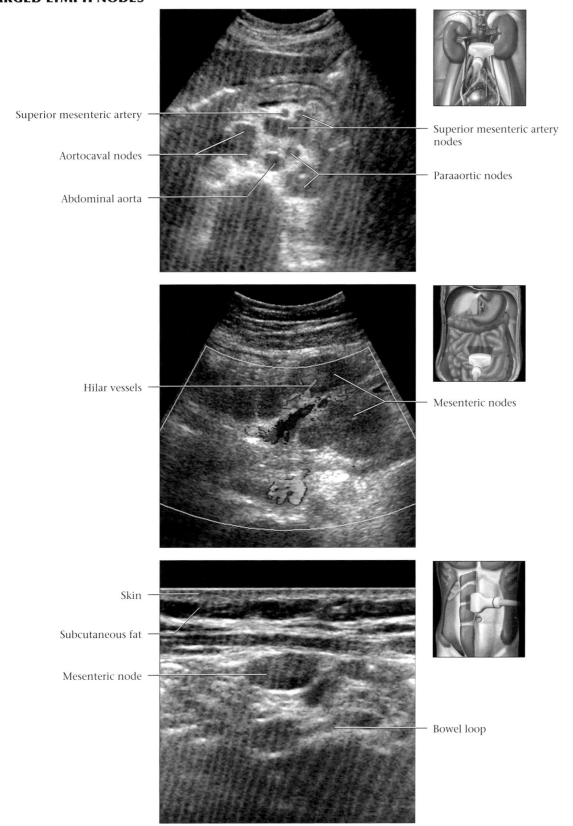

Superior mesenteric artery

Aortocaval nodes

Abdominal aorta

Superior mesenteric artery nodes

Paraaortic nodes

Hilar vessels

Mesenteric nodes

Skin

Subcutaneous fat

Mesenteric node

Bowel loop

(Top) Transverse, transabdominal, grayscale ultrasound shows multiple enlarged pre-aortic and lateral para-aortic lymph nodes. There are enlarged nodes along the superior mesenteric artery and along the anterior and lateral abdominal aorta. (Middle) Transverse, transabdominal, color Doppler ultrasound reveals a conglomeration of hypoechoic nodes with hilar vascularity. Mesenteric nodes are readily identified due to their more superficial location compared to retroperitoneal nodes. (Bottom) Longitudinal, transabdominal, grayscale ultrasound reveals a small node close to the anterior abdominal wall. Small mesenteric nodes are frequently encountered during abdominal ultrasound examinations in children.

PERITONEAL SPACES AND STRUCTURES

Terminology

Definitions
- Peritoneal cavity: Potential space in abdomen between visceral and parietal peritoneum, usually containing only small amount of peritoneal fluid (for lubrication)
- Abdominal cavity: Not synonymous with peritoneal cavity
  - Contains all of abdominal viscera (intra- and retroperitoneal)
  - Limited by abdominal wall muscles, diaphragm and (arbitrarily) by pelvic brim

Gross Anatomy

Divisions
- Greater sac of peritoneal cavity
- Lesser sac (omental bursa)
  - Communicates with greater sac via epiploic foramen (of Winslow)
  - Bounded anteriorly by caudate lobe, stomach and greater omentum; posteriorly by pancreas, left adrenal and kidney; on the left by splenorenal and gastrosplenic ligaments; on the right by epiploic foramen and lesser omentum

Compartments
- Supramesocolic space
  - Divided into right and left supramesocolic spaces which are separated by falciform ligament
    - Right supramesocolic space: Composed of right subphrenic space, right subhepatic space and lesser sac
    - Left supramesocolic space: Divided into left perihepatic spaces (anterior and posterior) and left subphrenic (anterior perigastric and posterior perisplenic)
- Inframesocolic compartment
  - Divided into right inframesocolic space, left inframesocolic space, paracolic gutters and pelvic cavity
  - Pelvic cavity is the most dependent part of peritoneal cavity in erect and supine positions

Peritoneum
- Thin serous membrane consisting of a single layer of squamous epithelium (mesothelium)
  - Parietal peritoneum lines abdominal wall
  - Visceral peritoneum (serosa) lines abdominal organs

Mesentery
- Double layer of peritoneum that encloses an organ and connects it to abdominal wall
- Covered on both sides by mesothelium and has a core of loose connective tissue containing fat, lymph nodes, blood vessels and nerves passing to and from viscera
- Most mobile parts of intestine have mesentery, while ascending and descending colon are considered retroperitoneal (covered only by peritoneum on their anterior surface)
- Root of mesentery is its attachment to posterior abdominal wall

- Root of small bowel mesentery is ~ 15 cm in length and passes from left side of L2 vertebra downward and to the right; contains superior mesenteric vessels, nerves and lymphatics
- Transverse mesocolon crosses almost horizontally in front of pancreas, duodenum and right kidney

Omentum
- Multi-layered fold of peritoneum that extends from stomach to adjacent organs
- Lesser omentum joins lesser curve of stomach and proximal duodenum to liver
  - Hepatogastric and hepatoduodenal ligament components contain common bile duct, hepatic and gastric vessels and portal vein
- Greater omentum
  - 4 layered fold of peritoneum hanging from greater curve of stomach like an apron, covering transverse colon and much of small intestine
    - Contains variable amounts of fat and abundant lymph nodes
    - Mobile and can fill gaps between viscera
    - Acts as barrier to generalized spread of intraperitoneal infection or tumor

Ligaments
- All double layered folds of peritoneum other than mesentery and omentum are peritoneal ligaments
- Connect one viscus to another (e.g., splenorenal ligament) or a viscus to abdominal wall (e.g., falciform ligament)
- Contain blood vessels or remnants of fetal vessels

Folds
- Reflections of peritoneum with defined borders, often lifting peritoneum off abdominal wall (e.g., median umbilical fold covers urachus and extends from dome of urinary bladder to umbilicus)

Peritoneal Recesses
- Dependent pouches formed by peritoneal reflections
- Many have eponyms (e.g., Morrison's pouch for posterior subhepatic [hepatorenal] recess; pouch of Douglas for rectouterine recess)

Anatomy-Based Imaging Issues

Imaging Recommendations
- Transducer: 2-5 MHz
  - High frequency linear transducer may be used to evaluate parietal peritoneum of anterior abdominal wall
- Patient examined supine with additional decubitus positions to determine if fluid collection is free or loculated
- Peritoneal cavity and its various mesenteries and recesses are usually not apparent on imaging studies unless distended or outlined by intraperitoneal fluid or air

PERITONEAL CAVITY

Liver (caudate lobe)

Lesser omentum

Lesser sac

Pancreas

Superior mesenteric artery

Duodenum (3rd portion)

Transverse mesocolon

Small bowel mesentery

Stomach

Gastrocolic ligament

Transverse colon

Greater omentum

Graphic of a sagittal section of the abdomen shows the peritoneal cavity artificially distended, as with air. Note the margins of the lesser sac in this plane, including caudate lobe of the liver, stomach and gastrocolic ligament anteriorly, and pancreas posteriorly. The hepatogastric ligament is part of the lesser omentum, and carries the hepatic artery and portal vein to the liver. The mesenteries are multi-layered folds of peritoneum that enclose a layer of fat, and convey blood vessels, nerves, and lymphatics to the intraperitoneal abdominal viscera. The greater omentum is a 4 layered fold of peritoneum that extends down from the stomach, covering much of the colon and small intestine. The layers are generally fused together caudal to the transverse colon. The gastrocolic ligament is part of the greater omentum.

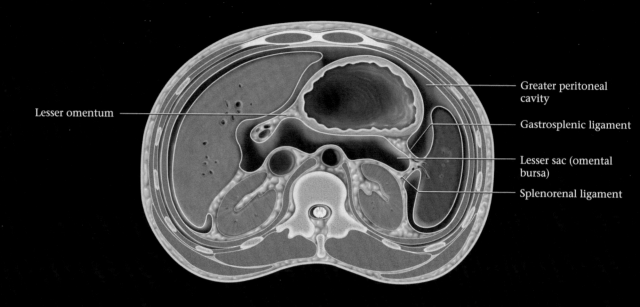

Lesser omentum

Greater peritoneal cavity

Gastrosplenic ligament

Lesser sac (omental bursa)

Splenorenal ligament

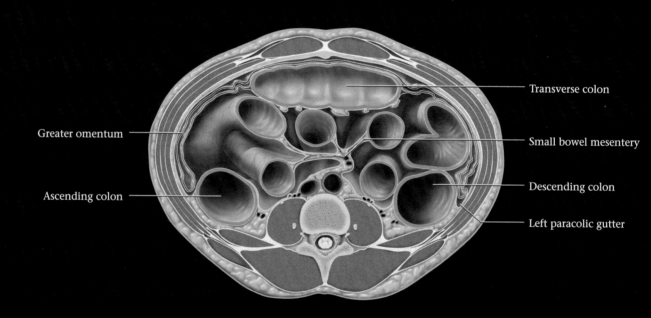

Greater omentum

Ascending colon

Transverse colon

Small bowel mesentery

Descending colon

Left paracolic gutter

(Top) The borders of the lesser sac (omental bursa) include the lesser omentum, which conveys the common bile duct, hepatic and gastric vessels. The left border includes the gastrosplenic ligament (with short gastric vessels) and the splenorenal ligament (with splenic vessels). (Bottom) The paracolic gutters are formed by reflections of peritoneum covering the ascending and descending colon and the lateral abdominal wall. Note the innumerable potential peritoneal recesses lying between the bowel loops and their mesenteric leaves. The greater omentum covers much of the bowel like an apron.

PERITONEAL SPACES AND STRUCTURES

PERITONEAL DIVISIONS AND COMPARTMENTS

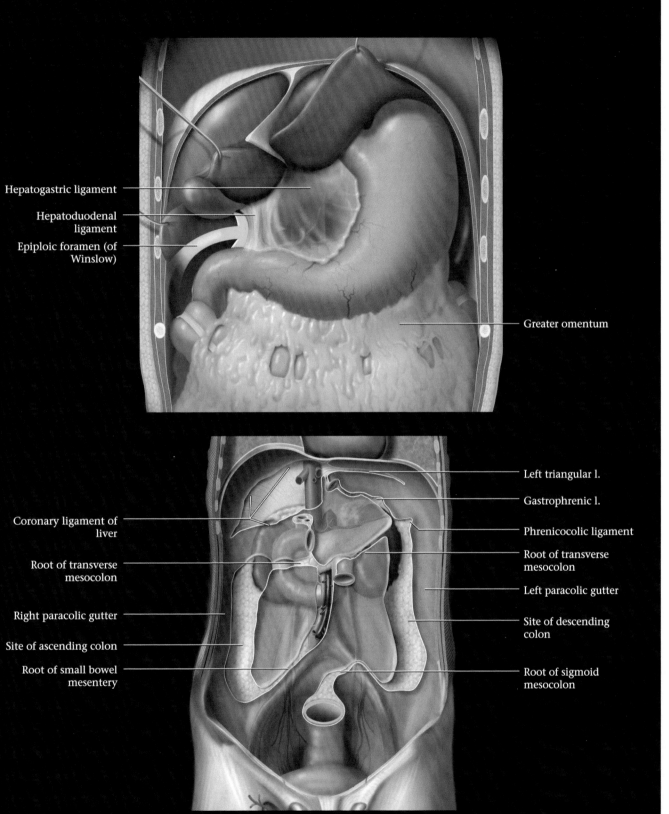

Hepatogastric ligament

Hepatoduodenal ligament

Epiploic foramen (of Winslow)

Greater omentum

Left triangular l.

Gastrophrenic l.

Coronary ligament of liver

Phrenicocolic ligament

Root of transverse mesocolon

Root of transverse mesocolon

Right paracolic gutter

Left paracolic gutter

Site of ascending colon

Site of descending colon

Root of small bowel mesentery

Root of sigmoid mesocolon

(Top) The liver has been retracted upward. The lesser omentum is comprised of the hepatoduodenal and hepatogastric ligaments. It forms part of the anterior wall of the lesser sac, and conveys the common bile duct, hepatic and gastric vessels, and the portal vein. The aorta and celiac artery can be seen through the lesser omentum, as they lie just posterior to the lesser sac. **(Bottom)** Frontal view of the abdomen with all of the intraperitoneal organs removed. The root of the transverse mesocolon divides the peritoneal cavity into supramesocolic and inframesocolic spaces that communicate only along the paracolic gutters. The coronary and triangular ligaments suspend the liver from the diaphragm. The superior mesenteric vessels traverse the small bowel mesentery whose root crosses obliquely from the upper left to the lower right posterior abdominal wall.

PERITONEAL SPACES AND STRUCTURES

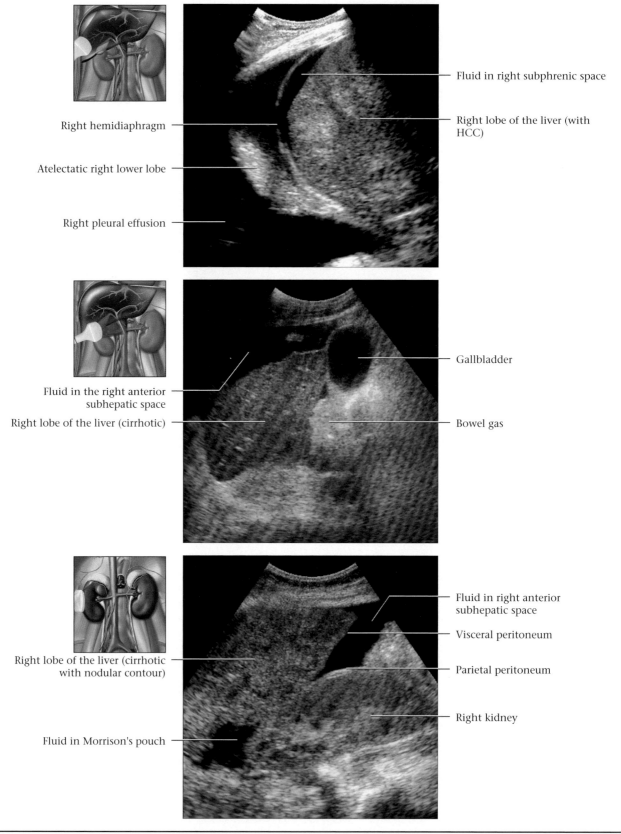

Right hemidiaphragm

Atelectatic right lower lobe

Right pleural effusion

Fluid in right subphrenic space

Right lobe of the liver (with HCC)

Fluid in the right anterior subhepatic space

Right lobe of the liver (cirrhotic)

Gallbladder

Bowel gas

Right lobe of the liver (cirrhotic with nodular contour)

Fluid in Morrison's pouch

Fluid in right anterior subhepatic space

Visceral peritoneum

Parietal peritoneum

Right kidney

(Top) Intercostal, oblique, grayscale ultrasound (in a patient with hepatocellular carcinoma) shows the dome of the right lobe of the liver and minimal fluid in the right subphrenic region, separated from the right-sided pleural effusion by the right diaphragmatic leaf. (Middle) Subcostal oblique longitudinal, grayscale ultrasound of the right hepatic lobe shows fluid in the right anterior subhepatic space. Note the small cirrhotic liver with a nodular contour. Ascites may be a manifestation of portal hypertension. (Bottom) Longitudinal, transabdominal, grayscale ultrasound shows fluid in the right, posterior, subhepatic space. Other names for this space are Morrison's pouch and hepatorenal fossa. This space is continuous with the right anterior subhepatic space and right paracolic gutter.

PERITONEAL SPACES AND STRUCTURES

RIGHT SUPRAMESOCOLIC SPACE: LESSER SAC

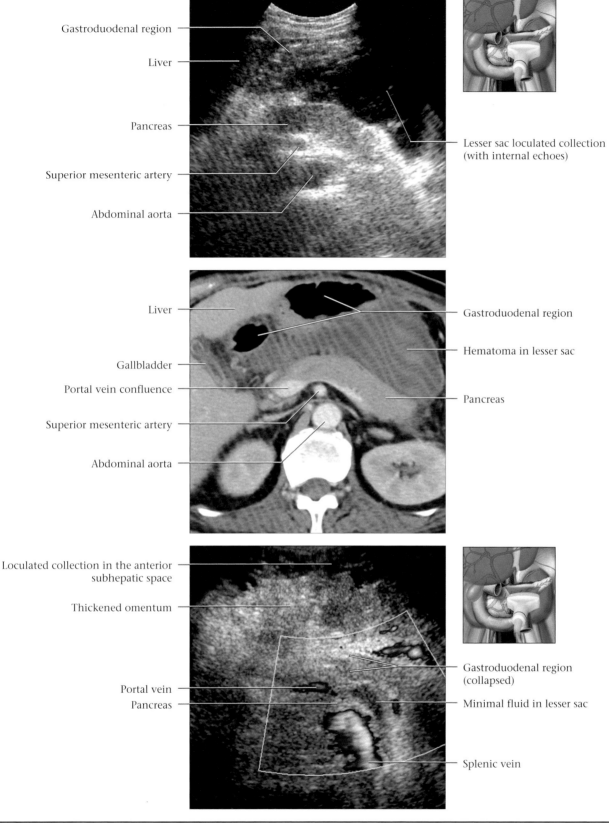

(Top) Subxiphoid, transverse, grayscale ultrasound reveals fluid collection (hematoma) in the lesser sac, which extends to the left, behind the stomach and anterior to the pancreas. The lesser sac is part of the right supramesocolic space and communicates with the rest of the peritoneal cavity through the epiploic foramen (of Winslow). **(Middle)** Axial, contrast-enhanced, correlative CT demonstrates the lesser sac hematoma situated between the stomach and pancreas. **(Bottom)** Subxiphoid, transverse, power Doppler ultrasound in a different patient shows trace fluid in the lesser sac. A larger collection is identified in the right, anterior, subhepatic space. The heterogeneous lesion, between the anterior subhepatic collection and the gastroduodenal region, is the thickened omentum due to peritoneal carcinomatosis.

PERITONEAL SPACES AND STRUCTURES

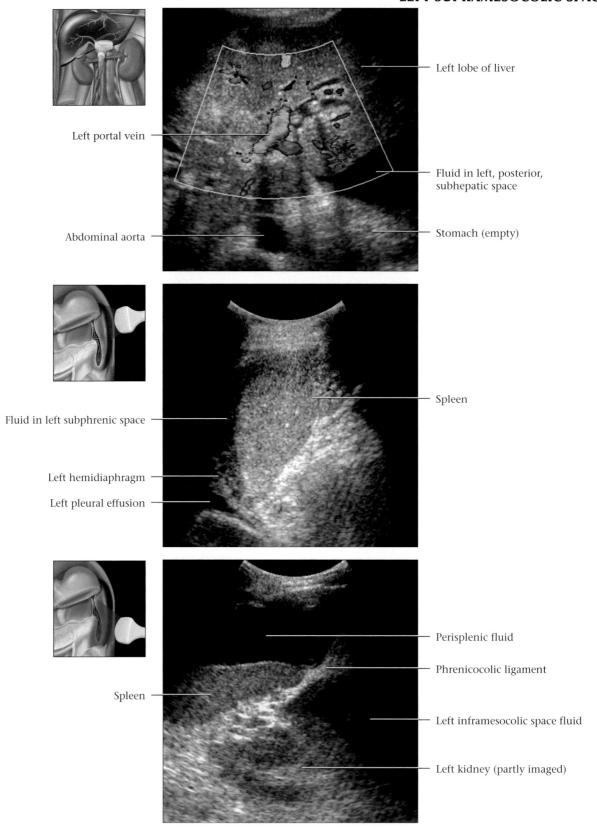

Left lobe of liver

Left portal vein

Fluid in left, posterior, subhepatic space

Abdominal aorta

Stomach (empty)

Spleen

Fluid in left subphrenic space

Left hemidiaphragm

Left pleural effusion

Perisplenic fluid

Phrenicocolic ligament

Spleen

Left inframesocolic space fluid

Left kidney (partly imaged)

(Top) Subxiphoid, transverse, color Doppler ultrasound shows fluid posterior to the left lobe of the liver, localized to the left, posterior, subhepatic space. Incidental calculi are seen within a dilated intrahepatic biliary duct. **(Middle)** Intercostal grayscale ultrasound of the spleen reveals minimal fluid just under the left hemidiaphragm. The left subphrenic space is separated from the right subphrenic space by the falciform ligament. **(Bottom)** Intercostal, oblique, grayscale ultrasound of the left upper quadrant reveals fluid in the perisplenic space. Fluid is also identified in the left inframesocolic space, anterior to the left kidney. The two collections are separated by the phrenicocolic ligament, which suspends the spleen and attaches to the left hemidiaphragm and proximal descending colon.

PERITONEAL SPACES AND STRUCTURES

INFRAMESOCOLIC SPACE

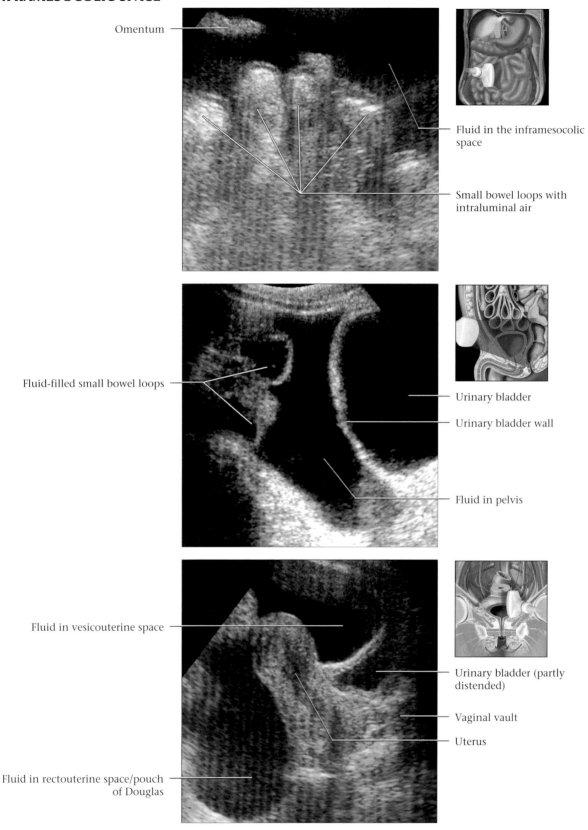

Omentum

Fluid in the inframesocolic space

Small bowel loops with intraluminal air

Fluid-filled small bowel loops

Urinary bladder

Urinary bladder wall

Fluid in pelvis

Fluid in vesicouterine space

Urinary bladder (partly distended)

Vaginal vault

Uterus

Fluid in rectouterine space/pouch of Douglas

(**Top**) Transabdominal, longitudinal, grayscale ultrasound of the central abdomen reveals massive ascites with floating small bowel loops. Note the echogenic and thin omentum. The left inframesocolic space is larger compared to the right and communicates directly with the pelvic cavity. (**Middle**) Longitudinal grayscale ultrasound at the suprapubic region of a male patient demonstrates intraperitoneal fluid between bowel loops and a distended urinary bladder. (**Bottom**) Longitudinal grayscale ultrasound shows fluid in the pelvis of a female patient. Owing to the presence of the uterus, the pelvic cavity is divided into the vesicouterine and rectouterine (pouch of Douglas) spaces.

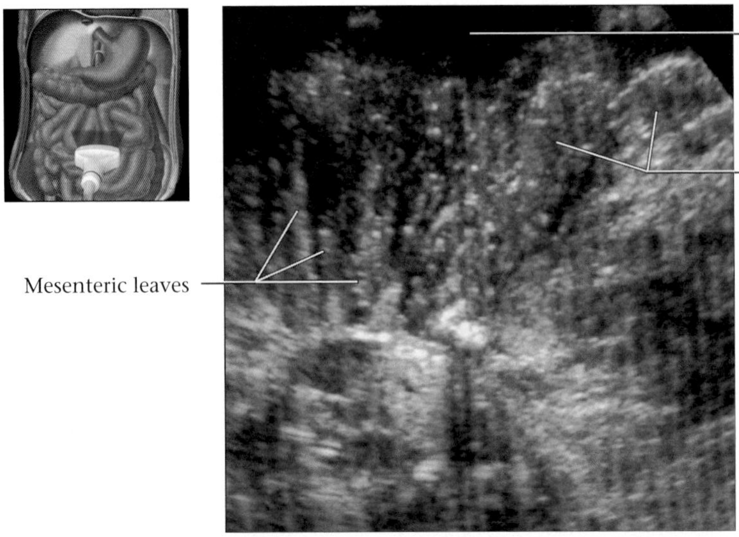

PERITONEAL SPACES AND STRUCTURES

Fluid in inframesocolic space

Small bowel loops

Mesenteric leaves

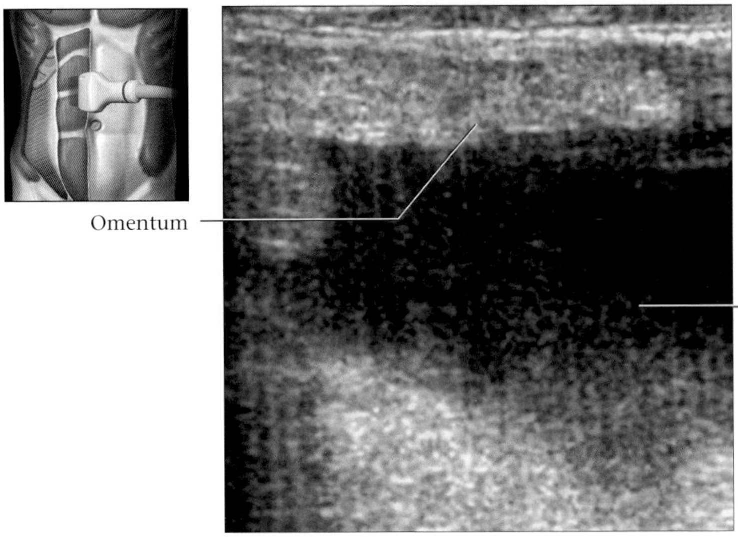

Omentum

Fluid

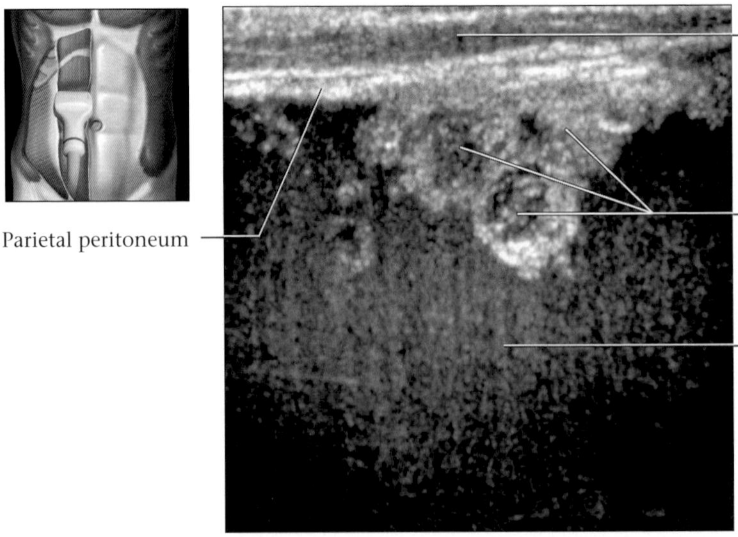

Rectus muscle

Peritoneal deposits

Parietal peritoneum

Fluid

(Top) Transverse, transabdominal, grayscale ultrasound shows echogenic small bowel loops. The mesenteric leaves are echogenic and markedly thickened and exhibit classic sunburst appearance. (Middle) Longitudinal, transabdominal, grayscale ultrasound shows a tongue of thickened omentum and ascites in a patient with peritoneal tuberculosis. (Bottom) Transverse transabdominal ultrasound shows nodular peritoneal deposits along the thickened parietal peritoneum in another patient with peritoneal carcinomatosis. A normal peritoneum may be seen as a pencil-thin echogenic structure apposed to the anterior abdominal wall but is normally not imaged unless thickened.

PERITONEAL SPACES AND STRUCTURES

PERITONEAL PATHOLOGIES

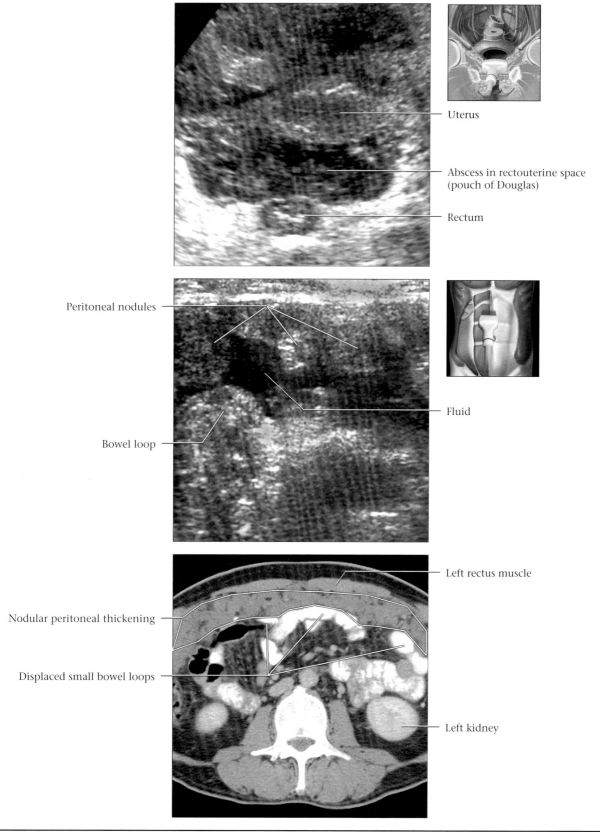

Uterus

Abscess in rectouterine space (pouch of Douglas)

Rectum

Peritoneal nodules

Fluid

Bowel loop

Left rectus muscle

Nodular peritoneal thickening

Displaced small bowel loops

Left kidney

(Top) Transverse, transabdominal, grayscale ultrasound shows a pelvic abscess in a case of ileal perforation. Note echogenic fluid with internal echoes around the uterus and rectum. (Middle) Longitudinal, transabdominal, grayscale ultrasound shows nodular hypoechoic peritoneal deposits, which are well-delineated due to the presence of adjacent anechoic ascites. (Bottom) Transverse contrast-enhanced CT shows enhancing "cake-like", nodular, peritoneal thickening due to metastases. The bowel loops are displaced away from the anterior abdominal wall.

ABDOMINAL WALL & PARASPINAL STRUCTURES

Terminology

Definitions
- Abdomen is the region between diaphragm and pelvis

Gross Anatomy

Anatomic Boundaries
- Anterior abdominal wall bounded superiorly by xiphoid process and costal cartilages of 7th-10th ribs
- Anterior wall bounded inferiorly by iliac crest, iliac spine, inguinal ligament and pubis
- Inguinal ligament is inferior edge of aponeurosis of the external oblique muscle

Muscles of Anterior Abdominal Wall
- Consist of three flat muscles (external, internal oblique and transverse abdominal), and one strap-like muscle (rectus)
- Combination of muscles and aponeuroses (sheet-like tendons) act as a corset to confine and protect abdominal viscera
- Linea alba is a fibrous raphe stretching from xiphoid to pubis
  - Forms central anterior attachment for abdominal wall muscles
  - Formed by interlacing fibers of aponeuroses of the oblique and transverse abdominal muscles
  - Rectus sheath is also formed by these aponeuroses as they surround rectus muscle
- External oblique muscle
  - Largest and most superficial of the 3 flat abdominal muscles
  - Origin: External surfaces of ribs 5-12
  - Insertion: Linea alba, iliac crest, pubis via a broad aponeurosis
- Internal oblique muscle
  - Middle of the 3 flat abdominal muscles
  - Runs at right angles to external oblique
  - Origin: Posterior layer of thoracolumbar fascia, iliac crest and inguinal ligament
  - Insertion: Ribs 10-12 posteriorly, linea alba via a broad aponeurosis, pubis
- Transverse abdominal muscle
  - Innermost of the 3 flat abdominal muscles
  - Origin: Lowest six costal cartilages, thoracolumbar fascia, iliac crest, inguinal ligament
  - Insertion: Linea alba via broad aponeurosis, pubis
- Rectus abdominis muscle
  - Origin: Pubic symphysis and pubic crest
  - Insertion: Xiphoid process and costal cartilages 5-7
  - Rectus sheath: Strong fibrous compartment that envelops each rectus muscle
  - Rectus sheath contains superior and inferior epigastric vessels
- Actions of anterior abdominal wall muscles
  - Support and protect abdominal viscera
  - Help flex and twist trunk, maintain posture
  - Increase intra-abdominal pressure for defecation, micturition and childbirth
  - Stabilize pelvis during walking, sitting up
- Transversalis fascia

- Lies deep to abdominal wall muscles and lines entire abdominal wall
- Is separated from parietal peritoneum by layer of extraperitoneal fat

Muscles of Posterior Abdominal Wall
- Consist of psoas (major and minor), iliacus and quadratus lumborum
- Psoas: Long thick, fusiform muscle lying lateral to vertebral column
  - Origin: Transverse processes and bodies of vertebrae T12-L5
  - Insertion: Lesser trochanter of femur (passing behind inguinal ligament)
  - Action: Flexes thigh at hip joint; bends vertebral column laterally
- Iliacus: Large triangular sheet of muscle lying along lateral side of psoas
  - Origin: Superior part of iliac fossa
  - Insertion: Lesser trochanter of femur (after joining with psoas tendon)
  - Action: "Iliopsoas muscle" flexes thigh
- Quadratus lumborum: Thick sheet of muscle lying adjacent to transverse processes of lumbar vertebrae
  - Invested by lumbodorsal fascia
  - Origin: Iliac crest and transverse processes of lumbar vertebrae
  - Insertion: 12th rib
  - Actions: Stabilizes position of thorax and pelvis during respiration, walking
    - Bends trunk to side

Paraspinal Muscles
- Also called erector spinae muscles
  - Invested by lumbodorsal fascia
- Composed of three columns
  - Iliocostalis: Lateral
  - Longissimus: Intermediate
  - Spinalis: Medial
- Origins: Sacrum, ilium, and spines of lumbar and 11th-12th thoracic vertebrae
- Insertions: Ribs and vertebrae with additional muscle slips joining columns at successively higher levels
- Action: Extends vertebral column

Anatomy-Based Imaging Issues

Imaging Recommendations
- Transducer: High frequency (7-10 MHz) linear transducer for anterior abdominal wall and paraspinal muscles
  - 3-5 MHz for posterior abdominal wall muscles
- Patient position: Supine for examination of anterior and lateral abdominal wall
  - Patient may be asked to perform Valsalva maneuver to increase abdominal pressure and exaggerate abdominal wall hernia for better visualization
  - Patient examined in prone position for ultrasound of paraspinal muscles
- Comparison with contralateral side to check for symmetry

ANTERIOR ABDOMINAL WALL

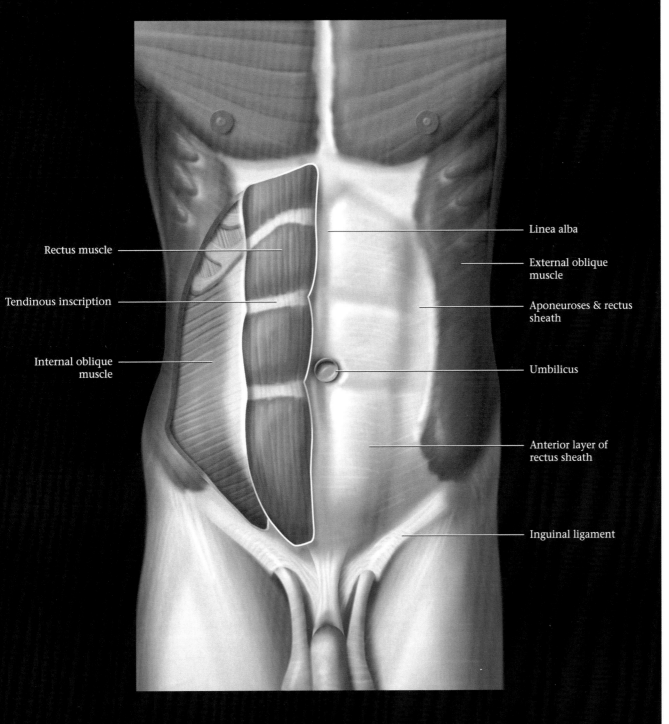

Rectus muscle

Tendinous inscription

Internal oblique muscle

Linea alba

External oblique muscle

Aponeuroses & rectus sheath

Umbilicus

Anterior layer of rectus sheath

Inguinal ligament

Graphic shows the aponeuroses of the internal and external oblique and transverse abdominal muscles are two-layered and interweave with each other, covering the rectus muscle, constituting the rectus sheath and linea alba. About midway between the umbilicus and symphysis, at the arcuate line, the posterior rectus sheath ends (arcuate line), and the transversalis fascia is the only structure between the rectus muscle and parietal peritoneum.

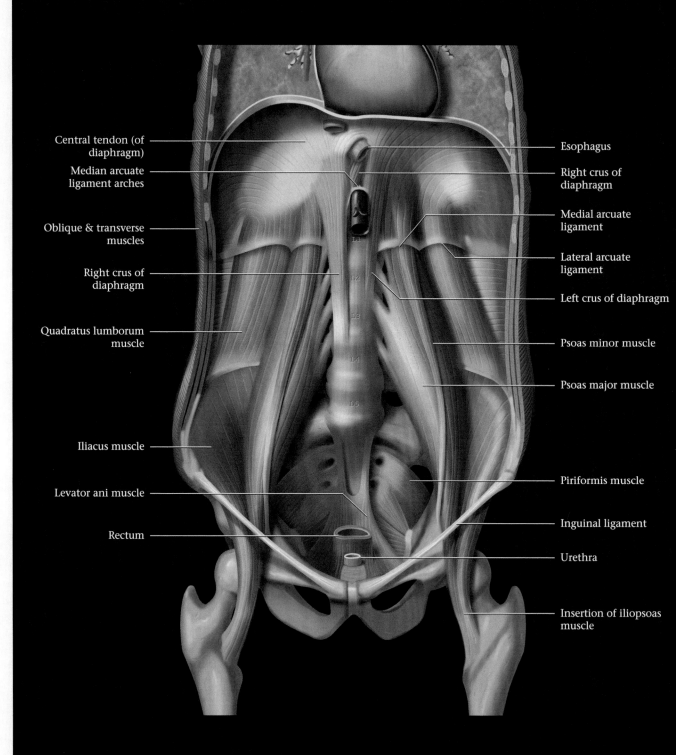

Central tendon (of diaphragm)

Median arcuate ligament arches

Oblique & transverse muscles

Right crus of diaphragm

Quadratus lumborum muscle

Iliacus muscle

Levator ani muscle

Rectum

Esophagus

Right crus of diaphragm

Medial arcuate ligament

Lateral arcuate ligament

Left crus of diaphragm

Psoas minor muscle

Psoas major muscle

Piriformis muscle

Inguinal ligament

Urethra

Insertion of iliopsoas muscle

Graphic shows the lumbar vertebrae are covered and attached by the anterior longitudinal ligament, and the diaphragmatic crura are closely attached to it, as are the origins of the psoas muscles, which also arise from the transverse processes. Iliacus muscle arises from the iliac fossa of pelvis and inserts into the tendon of the psoas major, constituting iliopsoas muscle, which inserts onto the lesser trochanter. Quadratus lumborum arises from the iliac crest and inserts onto the 12th rib and transverse processes of the lumbar vertebrae. Diaphragmatic and transverse abdominal fibers interlace. Psoas and quadratus lumborum pass behind diaphragm under medial and lateral arcuate ligaments.

ABDOMINAL WALL & PARASPINAL STRUCTURES

MUSCLES OF BACK IN SITU

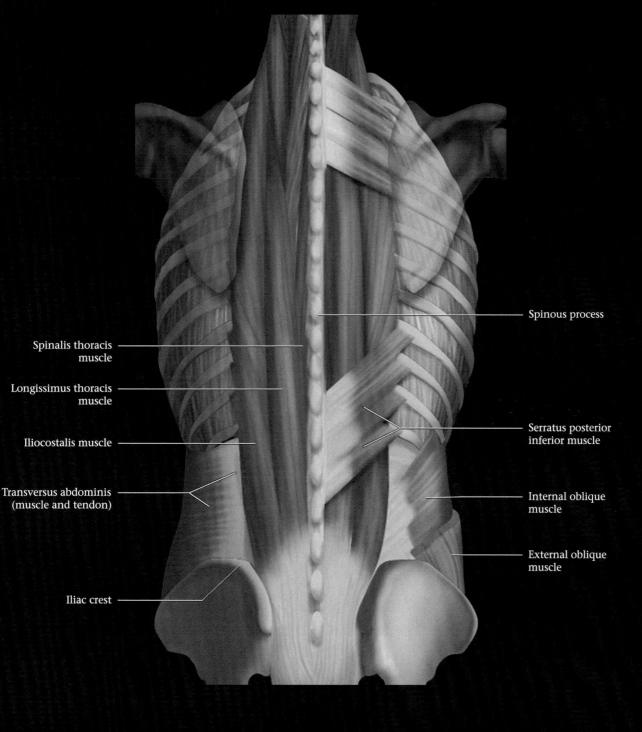

Spinous process

Spinalis thoracis muscle

Longissimus thoracis muscle

Iliocostalis muscle

Serratus posterior inferior muscle

Transversus abdominis (muscle and tendon)

Internal oblique muscle

External oblique muscle

Iliac crest

Graphic shows the paraspinal muscles and muscles of the back. The latissimus dorsi muscles are not included. The erector spinae have thick tendinous origins from the sacral and iliac crests and the lumbar and 11th to 12th thoracic spinous processes. Superiorly the muscle becomes fleshy and in the upper lumbar region subdivides to become the iliocostalis, longissimus and spinalis muscles (from lateral to medial), tapering as they insert into the vertebrae and ribs. The erector muscles flank the spinous processes and span the length of the posterior thorax and abdomen. They are responsible for extension sif of the vertebral column.

ABDOMINAL WALL & PARASPINAL STRUCTURES

Subcutaneous fat

Skin

Linea alba

Right rectus

Liver

Left rectus abdominis muscle

Skin

Subcutaneous fat

Rectus abdominis muscle

Superior epigastric vessels

Liver

Subcutaneous fat

Rectus abdominis muscle

Tendinous insertion of rectus abdominis to the symphysis pubis

Bowel segments with intraluminal gas

(Top) Transverse extended field of view, grayscale ultrasound of the midline anterior abdominal wall shows the paired rectus abdominis muscles separated by the linea alba. The rectus abdominis muscles are comparable in echogenicity and thickness. The surrounding rectus sheath is seen as a fine, thin, echogenic structure around the muscles. (Middle) Transverse color Doppler ultrasound of a rectus abdominis muscle shows arteries within the muscle. At the upper abdomen these are branches of the superior epigastric artery and at the lower abdomen comprise branches of the inferior epigastric arteries. These anastomose at the umbilicus. (Bottom) Longitudinal extended field of view, grayscale ultrasound shows the distal rectus abdominis muscle and its tendinous insertion into the symphysis pubis. Note how the rectus abdominis muscle tapers distally.

ABDOMINAL WALL & PARASPINAL STRUCTURES

ANTEROLATERAL ABDOMINAL WALL

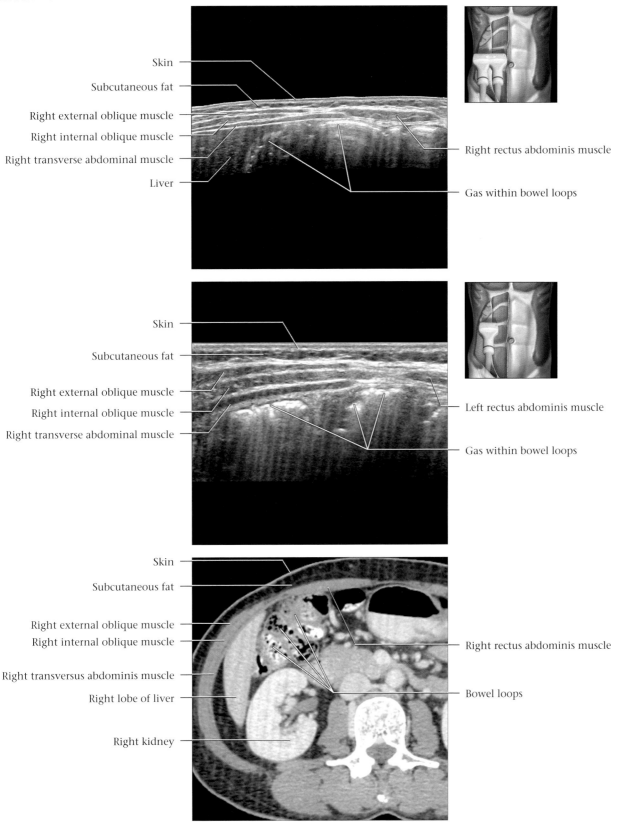

(Top) Transverse extended field of view (EFOV), grayscale ultrasound shows the relationship of the medially located rectus abdominis and the laterally located oblique and transverse abdominal muscles. Medially the external and internal oblique, and the transversus abdominal muscles form aponeuroses that comprise the rectus sheath. **(Middle)** Transverse grayscale ultrasound at the right anterolateral abdominal wall shows the relationship of the lateral abdominal wall muscles in better detail. Note the oblique and transverse abdominal muscles taper medially as they become aponeuroses. **(Bottom)** Correlative, axial, contrast-enhanced CT illustrates the muscles of the abdominal wall. The rectus abdominis muscle in the anterior abdominal wall, and the oblique and transverse abdominal muscles in the anterolateral abdominal wall and their aponeuroses are shown.

ABDOMINAL WALL & PARASPINAL STRUCTURES

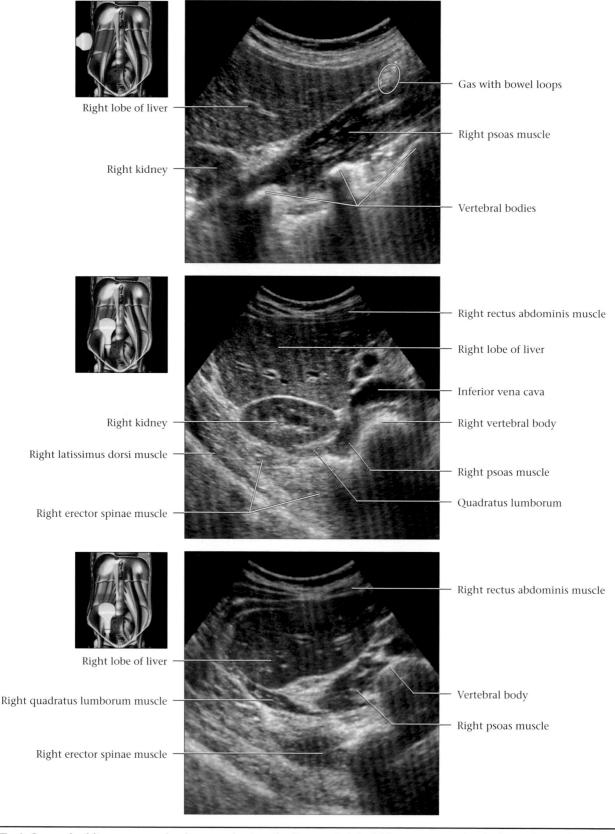

(Top) Coronal, oblique, grayscale ultrasound using the liver and right kidney as acoustic windows shows the right psoas muscle, which originates from the lumbar spine and inserts into the proximal femur. **(Middle)** Transverse grayscale ultrasound at right upper abdomen using liver and kidney as acoustic windows. The kidney is identified lateral to the psoas and anterior to the quadratus lumborum. The psoas is identified along the paravertebral region in its entire abdominal course. The quadratus lumborum originates from the iliolumbar ligament and iliac crest to insert into the last rib and lumbar transverse processes. It is easily identified as the muscle on which the kidney rests. **(Bottom)** Transverse grayscale ultrasound of the right upper abdomen, continuing the scan inferiorly. The relationship of the posterior abdominal wall muscles are maintained.

ABDOMINAL WALL & PARASPINAL STRUCTURES

POSTERIOR ABDOMINAL WALL, CT CORRELATION

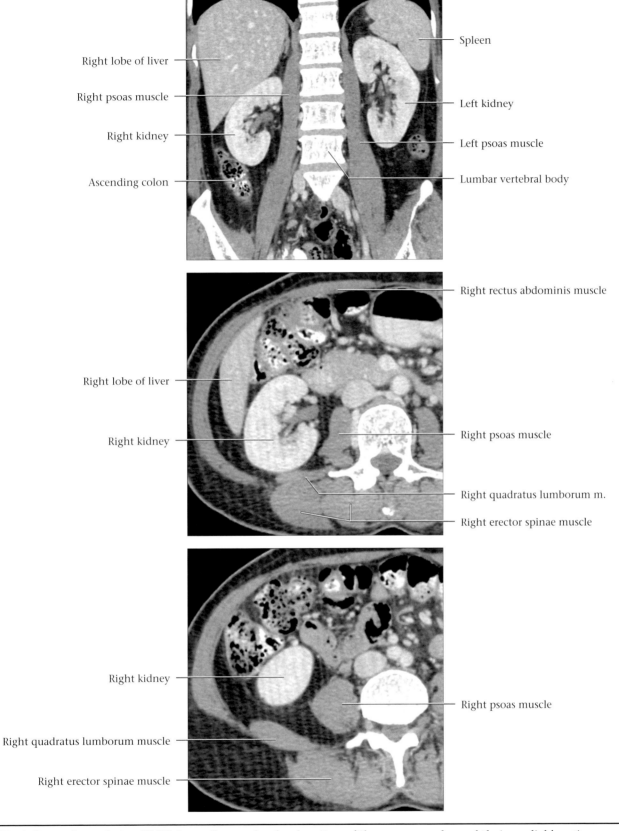

Spleen

Right lobe of liver

Right psoas muscle

Left kidney

Right kidney

Left psoas muscle

Ascending colon

Lumbar vertebral body

Right rectus abdominis muscle

Right lobe of liver

Right kidney

Right psoas muscle

Right quadratus lumborum m.

Right erector spinae muscle

Right kidney

Right psoas muscle

Right quadratus lumborum muscle

Right erector spinae muscle

(Top) Coronal correlative CECT shows the paralumbar location of the psoas muscles and their medial location relative to the kidneys. The psoas muscles originate from the lumbar and 12th thoracic vertebral bodies and their transverse processes and run past the pelvic brim where they course inferolaterally to be joined by the iliacus muscle. **(Middle)** Axial correlative CECT better illustrates the anatomic relationships of the kidney with the posterior abdominal wall muscles. The kidney is lateral to the psoas muscle and rests upon the quadratus lumborum muscle. The posterior erector spinae muscles are immediately posterior to the quadratus lumborum, and the two muscles are invested by lumbodorsal fascia. **(Bottom)** Axial correlative CECT at the level of the inferior pole of the right kidney. The psoas muscle and quadratus lumborum muscles, seen in their mid-sections, are now thicker.

ABDOMINAL WALL & PARASPINAL STRUCTURES

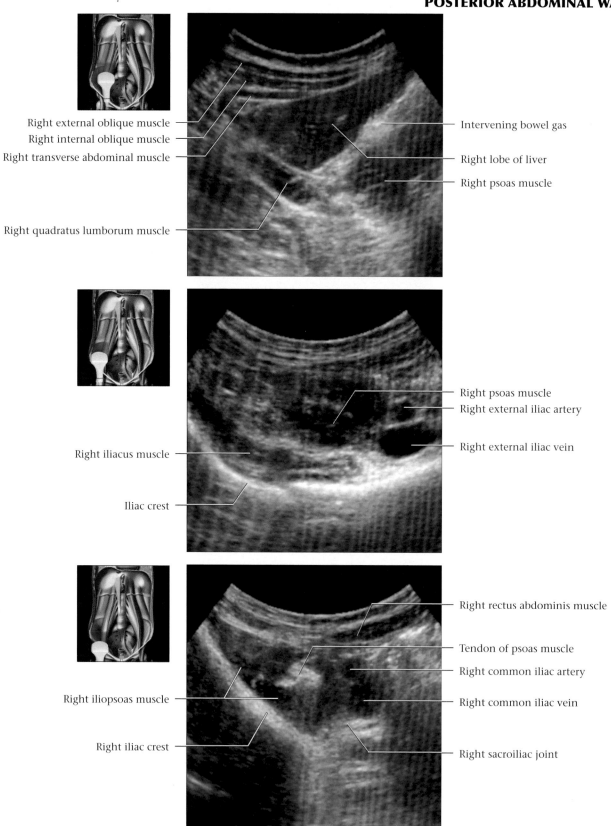

Right external oblique muscle
Right internal oblique muscle
Right transverse abdominal muscle

Right quadratus lumborum muscle

Intervening bowel gas
Right lobe of liver
Right psoas muscle

Right iliacus muscle

Iliac crest

Right psoas muscle
Right external iliac artery
Right external iliac vein

Right iliopsoas muscle

Right iliac crest

Right rectus abdominis muscle
Tendon of psoas muscle
Right common iliac artery
Right common iliac vein
Right sacroiliac joint

(Top) Transverse grayscale ultrasound in the lower abdominal region shows the right psoas muscle, composed of the psoas minor which rests upon the psoas major. The two muscles cannot be separated clearly on ultrasound. Owing to their depth, the paraspinal muscles cannot be demonstrated in detail. **(Middle)** Transverse grayscale ultrasound of the right lower abdomen, continued from previous image. The distal psoas muscle has diminished in size. It rests on the medial portion of the iliacus muscle; the latter is a flat muscle that fills the iliac fossa. Both continue inferiorly together. **(Bottom)** Distally, the fibers from the iliacus muscle converge and insert into the lateral side of the psoas muscle to form the iliopsoas muscle.

ABDOMINAL WALL & PARASPINAL STRUCTURES

POSTERIOR ABDOMINAL WALL, CT CORRELATION

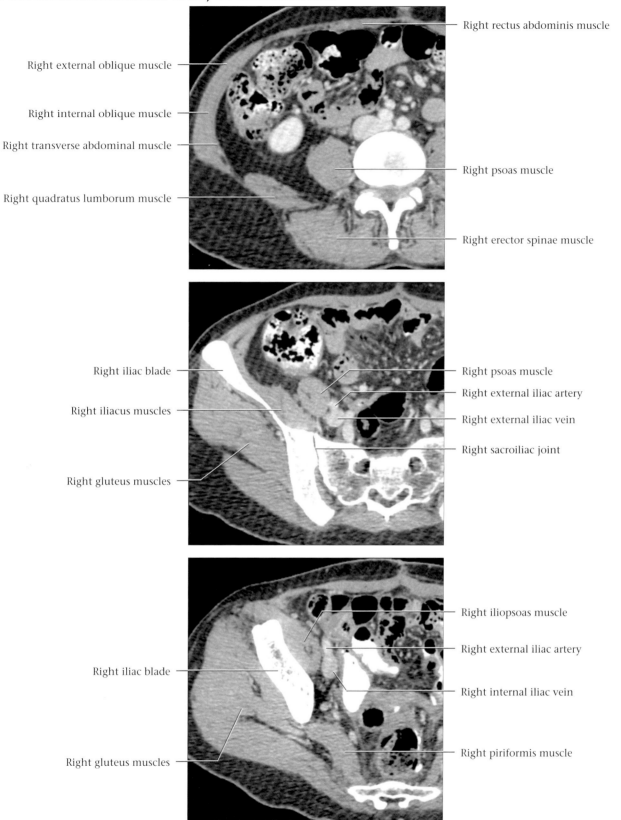

Right rectus abdominis muscle

Right external oblique muscle

Right internal oblique muscle

Right transverse abdominal muscle

Right psoas muscle

Right quadratus lumborum muscle

Right erector spinae muscle

Right iliac blade

Right psoas muscle

Right external iliac artery

Right iliacus muscles

Right external iliac vein

Right sacroiliac joint

Right gluteus muscles

Right iliopsoas muscle

Right external iliac artery

Right iliac blade

Right internal iliac vein

Right piriformis muscle

Right gluteus muscles

(Top) Axial correlative CECT at the level of the inferior pole of the kidney. The quadratus lumborum muscle is more laterally located and the psoas muscle is directly anterior to the erector spinae muscle. (Middle) Axial correlative CECT shows the psoas muscle has begun its dorsolateral course and is now anterior to the iliacus muscle. The iliacus muscle is easily identified as a flat muscle filling the iliac fossa, arising from the upper two-thirds of the iliac fossa, inner lip of the iliac crest, anterior sacroiliac and the iliolumbar ligaments, and base of the sacrum. (Bottom) Axial correlative CECT shows the psoas and iliacus muscles have converged and are now indistinguishable from one another. The resultant iliopsoas muscle passes beneath the inguinal ligament and becomes tendinous as it inserts into the lesser trochanter of the femur.

ABDOMINAL WALL & PARASPINAL STRUCTURES

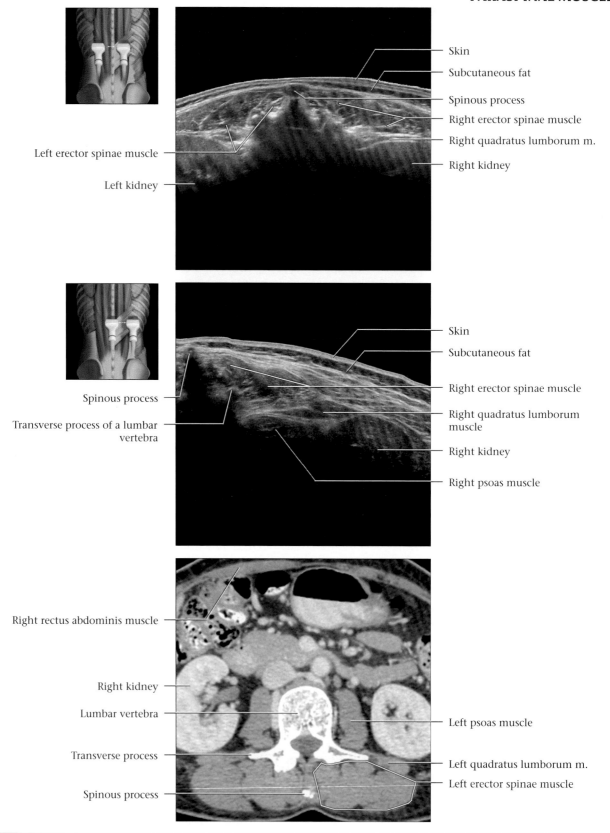

(Top) Transverse EFOV grayscale US of the back (with patient prone) shows the erector spinae muscles flanking the spinous process. They are invested by lumbodorsal fascia, which also invests the anteriorly located quadratus lumborum muscle. The kidneys are partially demonstrated. (Middle) Transverse EFOV grayscale US of the right erector spinae muscle (with patient prone). The three columns (iliocostalis, longissimus and spinalis muscles, from lateral to medial) comprising the erector spinae are not clearly separated from one another on ultrasound. They are identified collectively as a thick fleshy muscle lateral to the spinous process. (Bottom) Axial correlative CECT of the paraspinal muscles at the level of the kidneys. The erector spinae muscles originate from a broad and thick tendon which originates from the sacrum and iliac crest, lumbar and 11th and 12th thoracic spinous processes.

ABDOMINAL WALL & PARASPINAL STRUCTURES

PATHOLOGY

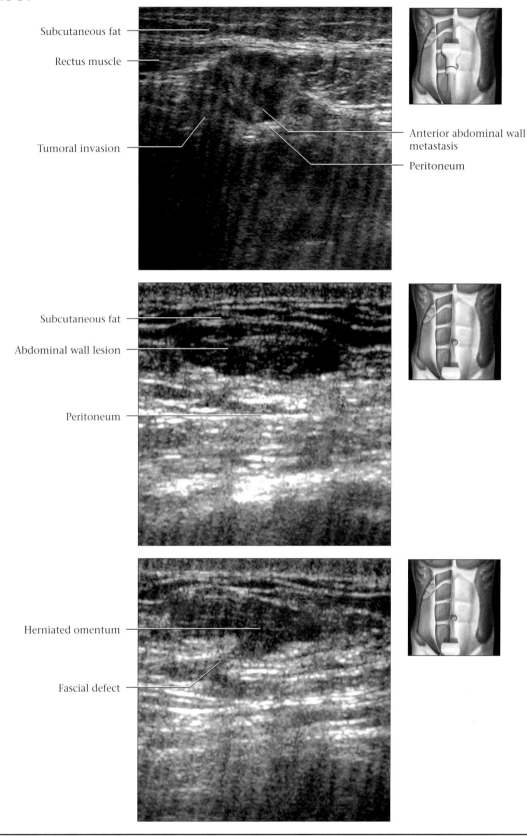

Subcutaneous fat

Rectus muscle

Tumoral invasion

Anterior abdominal wall metastasis

Peritoneum

Subcutaneous fat

Abdominal wall lesion

Peritoneum

Herniated omentum

Fascial defect

(**Top**) Transverse, transabdominal, grayscale ultrasound shows a small heterogeneous nodule in the anterior abdominal wall in a patient with abdominal wall metastasis. Note ill-defined border near the peritoneum suspicious of tumoral invasion. (**Middle**) Transverse, transabdominal, grayscale ultrasound shows a well-defined, ovoid, hypoechoic, anterior abdominal wall nodule. (**Bottom**) Transverse transabdominal ultrasound in the same patient as previous image with Valsalva maneuver. There is a fascial defect in the abdominal wall, with omental herniation. Dynamic maneuvers such as Valsalva can accentuate a hernia, improving detection and diagnosis.

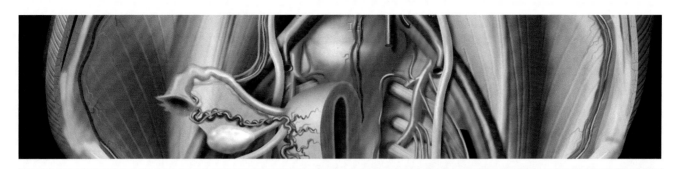

SECTION V: Pelvis

URETERS AND BLADDER

Gross Anatomy

Ureter
- Muscular tubes (25-30 cm long) that carry urine from kidneys to bladder
  - Course along posterior abdominal wall in retroperitoneum, just behind parietal peritoneum
    - Proximal ureters lie in perirenal space
    - In lower abdomen, lie on psoas muscles
  - In pelvis, lie along lateral walls near internal iliac vessels
    - At the level of ischial spines, ureters curve anteromedially to enter bladder at level of seminal vesicles (men) or cervix (women)
    - Ureterovesical junction: Ureters pass obliquely through muscular wall of bladder, creating a valve effect with bladder distension, preventing reflux of urine
  - Three points of physiological narrowing: Ureteropelvic junction, pelvic brim and ureterovesical junction
- Vessels, nerves and lymphatics
  - Arterial branches are numerous and variable, arising from aorta, and renal, gonadal, internal iliac, vesical, rectal arteries
    - Arterial branches anastomose along length of ureter
  - Venous branches & lymphatics follow the arteries with similar names
  - Innervation
    - Autonomic from adjacent plexuses
    - Cause ureteral peristalsis
    - Also carry pain (stretch) receptors; "stone" in abdominal ureter perceived as back & flank pain; stone in pelvic ureter causes lower abdominal & groin pain
  - Lymphatics to external & internal iliac nodes (pelvic ureter), aorto-caval nodes (abdomen)

Bladder
- Hollow, distensible viscus with a strong muscular wall
- Lies in extraperitoneal (retroperitoneal) pelvis
- Peritoneum covers dome of bladder
  - Reflections of peritoneum form deep recesses in the pelvic peritoneal cavity
  - Rectovesical pouch is the most dependent recess in men (and in women following hysterectomy)
  - Vesicouterine pouch and rectouterine pouch (of Douglas) are most dependent in women
- Bladder is surrounded by loose connective tissue and fat
  - Perivesical space (contains bladder and urachus)
  - Prevesical space (of Retzius) between bladder and symphysis pubis
    - Communicates superiorly with infrarenal retroperitoneal compartment
    - Communicates posteriorly with presacral space
  - Spaces can expand to contain large amounts of fluid (as in extraperitoneal rupture of the bladder, and hemorrhage from pelvic fractures)
- Wall of bladder composed mostly of detrusor muscle

- Trigone of bladder: Triangular structure at base of bladder with apices marked by 2 ureteral orifices and internal urethral orifice
- Vessels, nerves and lymphatics
  - Arteries from internal iliac
    - Superior vesical arteries and other branches of internal iliac arteries in both sexes
  - Venous drainage
    - Men: Vesical & prostatic venous plexuses → internal iliac and internal vertebral veins
    - Women: Vesical and uterovaginal plexuses → internal iliac vein
  - Autonomic innervation
    - Parasympathetic from pelvic splanchnic & inferior hypogastric nerves (causes contraction of detrusor muscle and relaxation of internal urethral sphincter to permit emptying of the bladder)
    - Sensory fibers follow parasympathetic nerves

Imaging Anatomy

Overview
- Normal ureters are small in caliber (2-8 mm) and are nearly impossible to appreciate on ultrasound largely due to obscuration by overlying bowel gas
- Fluid-distended urinary bladder permits through-transmission of echoes and appears anechoic with posterior acoustic enhancement
- Urinary bladder changes in shape and position depending on volume of urine within
  - In its non-distended state, urinary bladder is retropubic in location, lying anterior to uterus (females) or rectum (males)
  - In markedly distended state urinary bladder may occupy abdominopelvic area
  - Urinary bladder wall also changes in thickness depending on state of distension of urinary bladder, and is normally 3-5 mm in thickness

Anatomy-Based Imaging Issues

Imaging Recommendations
- Transducer: 2-5 MHz
- Ureters
  - Ureters are normally not seen on ultrasound unless they are dilated; when dilated, overlying bowel gas may still limit ureteral evaluation in transabdominal approach; use other windows
    - Kidneys serve as windows for imaging the proximal ureters in the coronal oblique plane
    - Continue scan inferiorly on anterior abdomen to follow course of ureter
    - Middle portion of ureter may be identified in pediatric patients or thin adults using transabdominal approach
    - Visualize distal ureters using urinary bladder as window
    - Terminations/ureterovesical junctions of distal ureters are in the posterolateral regions of urinary bladder and do not exhibit color signal on color Doppler

URETERS AND BLADDER

○ Ureteral caliber may slightly increase as result of overfilled urinary bladder
- When mild proximal ureteral dilatation is encountered (usually in conjunction with prominent pelvocaliceal system) and no cause for obstruction is identified, ask patient to void and then rescan ureters to evaluate any decrease in caliber
- Bladder
  ○ Recommend fluid intake prior to examination to ensure moderate distension of urinary bladder, or perform scan when patient reports full bladder sensation
    - Overdistended urinary bladder may give patient significant discomfort during examination
    - In a fully distended state, urinary bladder is easily visualized using transabdominal approach
    - With smaller volumes, caudal angulation of transducer is needed to visualize urinary bladder in its retropubic location
  ○ Examine patient in supine position with transducer on suprapubic region
    - Perform scanning in sagittal and transverse planes
    - Patient may be placed in decubitus position, especially to determine mobility of intravesical lesions, if present
  ○ Nature of cystic structure in pelvis may be ascertained by asking patient to void or by inserting Foley catheter
  ○ Additional transvaginal ultrasound may be employed in women for detailed examination of urinary bladder wall
  ○ Advantages of ultrasound
    - High spatial resolution of bladder wall
    - Real-time imaging for assessment of urine jets with color Doppler imaging (i.e., dynamic functional assessment); important after ureteric surgery for treating reflux
    - Real-time imaging guidance for placement of percutaneous suprapubic catheters, percutaneous nephrostomy tubes, biopsies, etc.
    - Provides radiation-free, real-time assessment of bladder during micturition
    - Color Doppler interrogation allows assessment of vascularity of bladder wall and/or lesion

Imaging Pitfalls
- Bladder
  ○ Reverberation artifacts are commonly encountered behind anterior wall of urinary bladder
    - Appear as regularly spaced lines at increasing depth
    - Give false impression of solid structure in a fluid-filled urinary bladder
    - Result from repeated reflection of ultrasound signals between highly reflective interfaces close to transducer
    - May be reduced or avoided by changing the scanning angle or by moving the transducer or using spacer
  ○ Due to volume-dependent changes in appearance of urinary bladder and its wall, perform examination when

- Urinary bladder is in distended state
- Patient claims full bladder sensation

Clinical Implications

Clinical Importance
- Ureters are often injured inadvertently during abdominal or gynecological surgery due to retraction
  ○ Causing interruption of their fragile, short arterial supply
- Ectopic ureter
  ○ Usually (80%) associated with complete ureteral duplication
  ○ Much more common in females (10x)
  ○ Ureter from upper renal pole often becomes obstructed & inserts ectopically (not at trigone)
  ○ Causes constant urine dribbling in females (ectopic insertion below urethral sphincter)
  ○ Weigert-Meyer rule: Ureter from upper pole inserts inferior & medial to lower pole ureter
- Ureterocele: Cystic dilation of distal ureter due to poor outflow
  ○ Simple (orthotopic) at trigone, with single ureter
  ○ Ectopic; inserts below trigone
- Ureteral duplication
  ○ Bifid ureter drains a duplex kidney; ureters unite before entering bladder
- Extraperitoneal bladder rupture
  ○ Urine and blood distend prevesical space; looks like a "molar tooth" on transverse CT section
  ○ Urine often tracks posteriorly into presacral space, superiorly into retroperitoneal abdomen
  ○ Usually caused by pelvic fractures
- Intraperitoneal bladder rupture
  ○ Urine flows up paracolic gutters into peritoneal recesses and surrounds intestine
  ○ Usually caused by blunt trauma to an overdistended bladder
- Fetal urachus forms conduit between umbilicus and bladder
  ○ Usually becomes obliterated → median umbilical ligament
  ○ May persist as channel "cyst" or diverticulum
  ○ May become infected or lead to carcinoma
- Bladder diverticula are common
  ○ Congenital: Hutch diverticulum
    - Near ureterovesical junction
  ○ Acquired (usually due to bladder outlet obstruction)
    - Clue: Bladder wall hypertrophy
  ○ Can lead to infection, stones, tumor

URETERS AND BLADDER

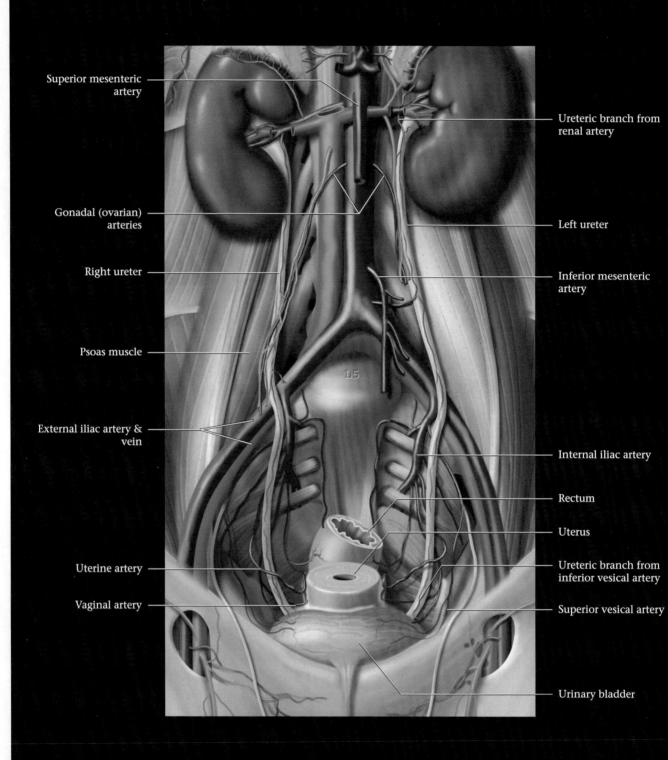

Superior mesenteric artery

Ureteric branch from renal artery

Gonadal (ovarian) arteries

Left ureter

Right ureter

Inferior mesenteric artery

Psoas muscle

L5

External iliac artery & vein

Internal iliac artery

Rectum

Uterus

Uterine artery

Ureteric branch from inferior vesical artery

Vaginal artery

Superior vesical artery

Urinary bladder

The ureters receive numerous and highly variable arterial branches from the aorta, and the renal, gonadal, and internal iliac arteries. These vessels are short and can be easily ruptured by retraction of the ureter during surgical procedures. The arterial supply to the bladder is also quite variable. Both genders receive supply from the superior vesical arteries and from various branches of the internal iliac arteries. Branches to the prostate & seminal vesicles (men) also send branches to the inferior bladder wall. In women, branches to the vagina send arteries to the base of the bladder. Note how the ureters deviate anteriorly as they cross the external (or common) iliac vessels & pelvic brim. This may constitute a point of relative narrowing where the passage of ureteral calculi (stones) may be impeded. In the abdomen the ureters course along the psoas muscles.

URINARY BLADDER

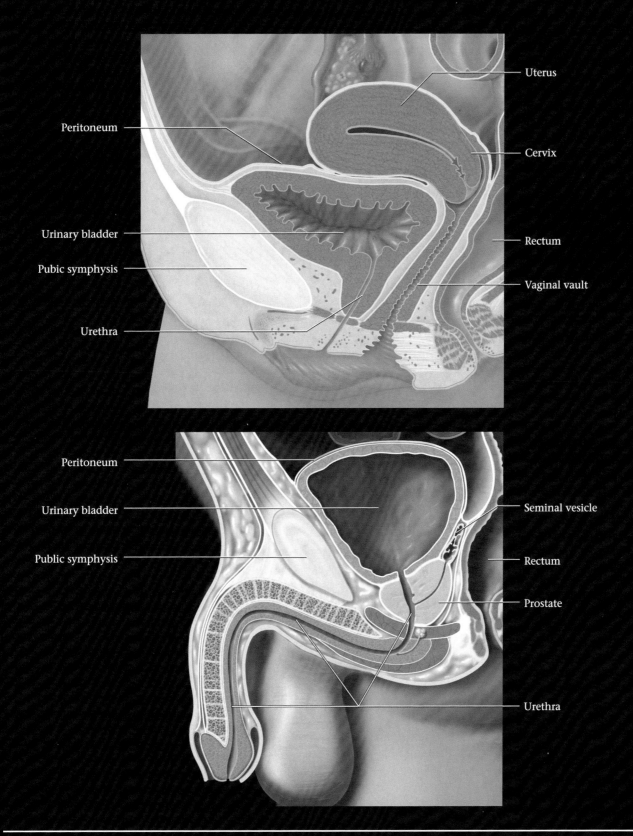

Peritoneum

Urinary bladder

Pubic symphysis

Urethra

Uterus

Cervix

Rectum

Vaginal vault

Peritoneum

Urinary bladder

Public symphysis

Seminal vesicle

Rectum

Prostate

Urethra

(Top) Graphic of a sagittal section of the female bladder shows that it rests almost directly on the muscular floor of the pelvis. The dome of the bladder is covered with peritoneum.The bladder is surrounded by a layer of loose fat and connective tissue (the prevesical & perivesical spaces) that communicate superiorly with the retroperitoneum. Note the vaginal vault/uterus in the female pelvis which intervenes between the urinary bladder and rectum. **(Bottom)** Graphic of a sagittal section of the male bladder shows that it rests on the prostate, which separates it from the muscular pelvic floor. The bladder wall is muscular, strong, and very distensible. In males the urinary bladder is directly anterior to the rectum.

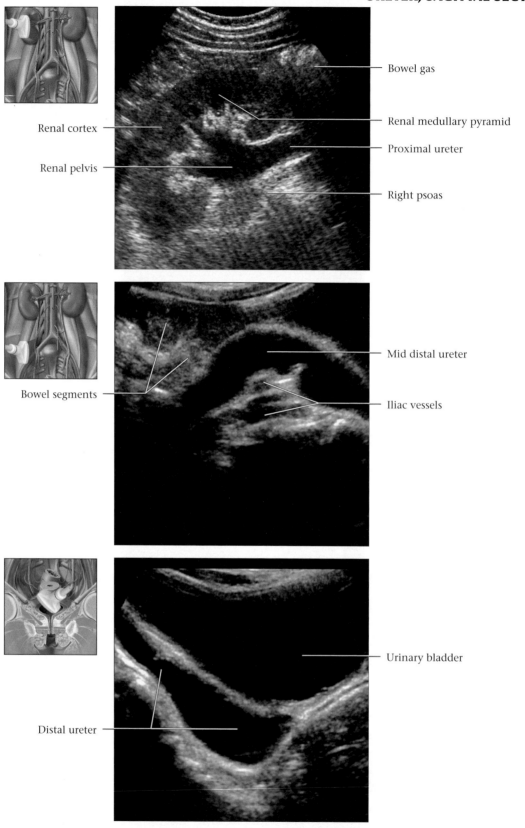

(Top) Longitudinal, transabdominal, grayscale ultrasound of the right kidney shows dilated pelvicaliceal system and proximal ureter. The ureter is normally not visible on ultrasound unless it is dilated. (Middle) Longitudinal, transabdominal, grayscale ultrasound at the right mid-abdomen shows continuation of the hydroureter with a dilated mid and distal segment. Note the anterior location of the ureter relative to the iliac vessels. Distally the ureter dips posteriorly as it passes the pelvic brim. Note the overlying bowel segments which often limit the evaluation of the ureter using this approach. (Bottom) Oblique, transabdominal, grayscale ultrasound at the suprapubic region, right paramedian side. The dilated distal ureter continues its posterior course to follow the contour of the pelvis, then runs anteromedially to terminate in the ureterovesical junction.

URETERS AND BLADDER

CT CORRELATION, URETERS

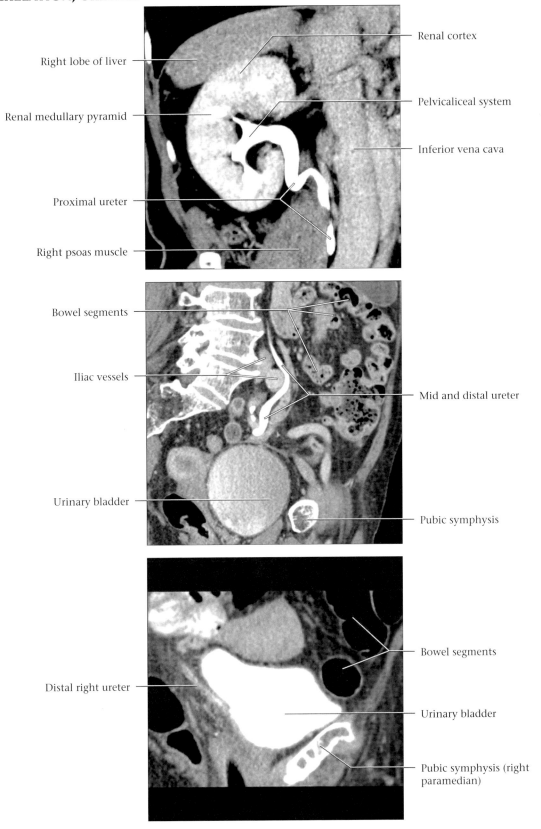

Right lobe of liver

Renal medullary pyramid

Proximal ureter

Right psoas muscle

Renal cortex

Pelvicaliceal system

Inferior vena cava

Bowel segments

Iliac vessels

Urinary bladder

Mid and distal ureter

Pubic symphysis

Distal right ureter

Bowel segments

Urinary bladder

Pubic symphysis (right paramedian)

(Top) Longitudinal, contrast-enhanced, correlative CT shows a normal caliber proximal ureter and normal kinking at a level inferior to the kidney. The ureter is better demonstrated in delayed CT scans when it contains contrast. CT is superior to ultrasound in delineating the course of the ureter. **(Middle)** Oblique, correlative, contrast-enhanced CT reformation shows the course of the right ureter along the retroperitoneum. The ureter crosses over the iliac vessels, its distal segment dipping posteriorly as it passes the pelvic brim. Note the anteriorly located bowel loops which usually obscure the ureter during transabdominal ultrasound. **(Bottom)** Longitudinal, correlative, contrast-enhanced CT demonstrating the distal right ureter as it enters the urinary bladder at its posterolateral region. Contrast partially opacifies the distal ureteric lumen.

URETER, TRANSVERSE SECTIONS

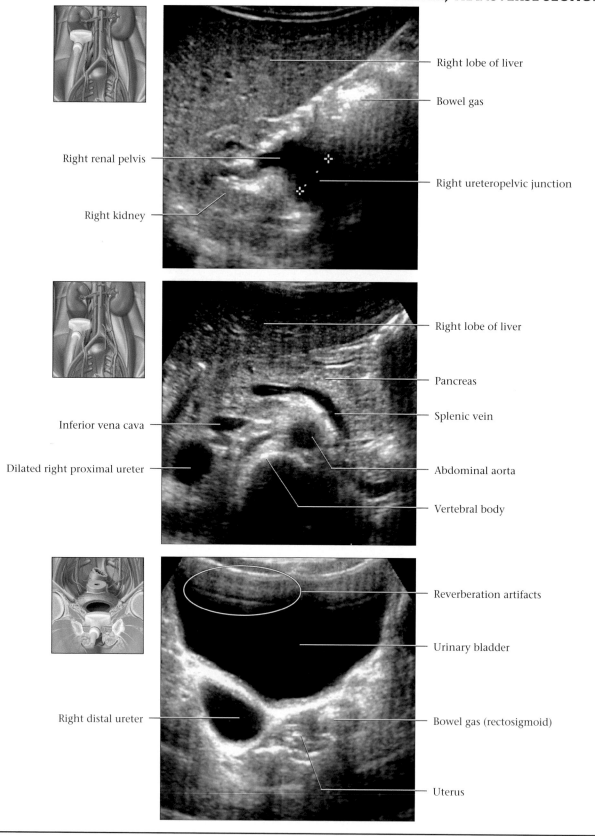

Right lobe of liver

Bowel gas

Right renal pelvis

Right ureteropelvic junction

Right kidney

Right lobe of liver

Pancreas

Splenic vein

Inferior vena cava

Abdominal aorta

Dilated right proximal ureter

Vertebral body

Reverberation artifacts

Urinary bladder

Right distal ureter

Bowel gas (rectosigmoid)

Uterus

(Top) Transverse, transabdominal, grayscale ultrasound at the level of the right renal hilum demonstrating a dilated right ureteropelvic junction (1 cm). (Middle) Transverse, transabdominal, grayscale ultrasound at the level of the pancreas. Note the anatomic relationships of the dilated right proximal ureter, which is identified in the right paravertebral region and posterolateral to the head of the pancreas and inferior vena cava. (Bottom) Transverse, transabdominal, grayscale ultrasound at the suprapubic region of a female shows the dilated distal ureter on the right side. Note the posterolateral location of the distal ureter relative to the urinary bladder. Note also reverberation artifacts in the anterior portion of the urinary bladder (not to be mistaken for a lesion).

URETERS AND BLADDER

CT CORRELATION, URETERS

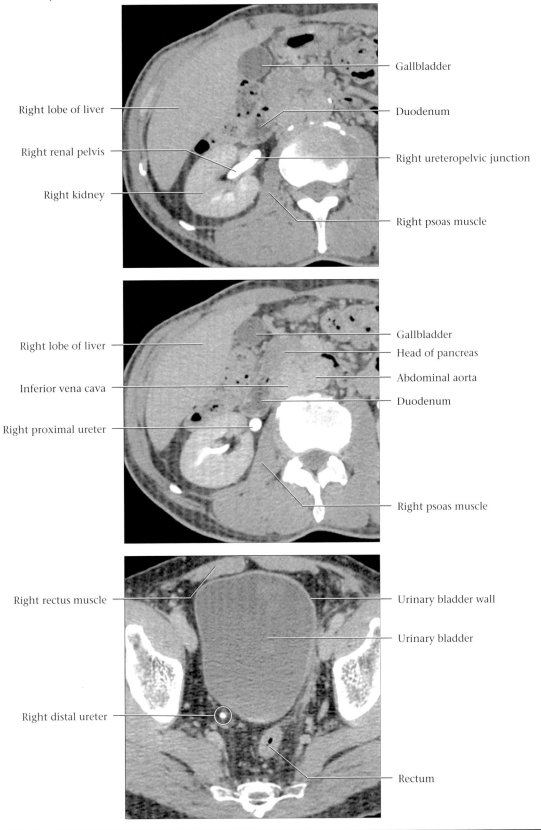

Gallbladder

Right lobe of liver

Duodenum

Right renal pelvis

Right ureteropelvic junction

Right kidney

Right psoas muscle

Right lobe of liver

Gallbladder

Head of pancreas

Inferior vena cava

Abdominal aorta

Duodenum

Right proximal ureter

Right psoas muscle

Right rectus muscle

Urinary bladder wall

Urinary bladder

Right distal ureter

Rectum

(Top) Axial, contrast-enhanced, correlative CT shows the origin of the proximal ureter from the renal pelvis. (Middle) Axial, contrast-enhanced, correlative CT shows the the proximal ureter at the level of the right inferior kidney and its relationship with the duodenum (fluid-filled) and inferior vena cava. The ureter is demonstrated adjacent to the right psoas muscle. (Bottom) Axial, contrast-enhanced, correlative CT shows the posterolateral location of the right distal ureter relative to the urinary bladder. Note the rectum is posteriorly located to the urinary bladder in this male patient. CT readily demonstrates the course of the normal ureter (particularly when filled with contrast) whereas bowel gas obscures good visualization of normal ureters on ultrasound.

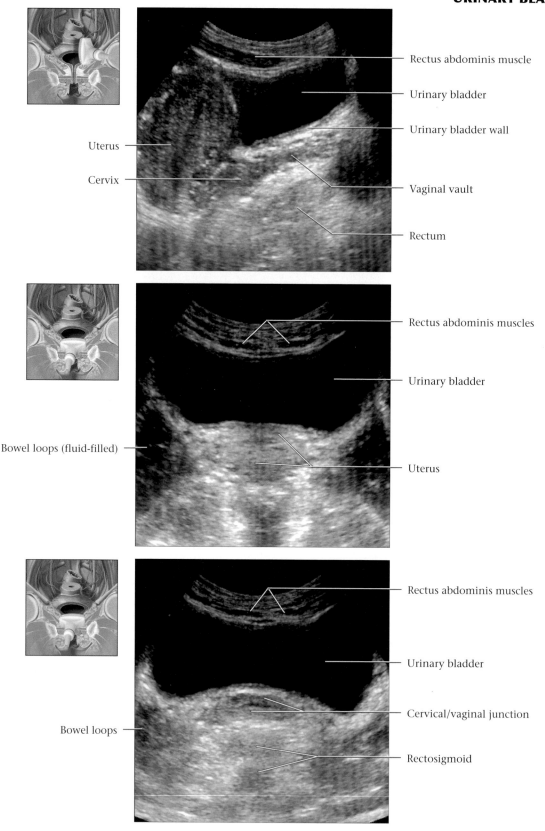

(Top) Longitudinal transabdominal grayscale ultrasound at the suprapubic region shows the anteriorly located urinary bladder relative to the the uterus. Note the anechoic appearance of the urinary bladder due to its fluid-filled state, permitting through transmission of echoes. The urinary bladder wall is 3 mm thick in the distended state and not more than 5 mm in the partly distended state. **(Middle)** Transverse, transabdominal, grayscale ultrasound at the suprapubic region at the uterine body level. The transducer must be angled caudally to image the urinary bladder, especially when it is not well-distended and assumes a retropubic location. **(Bottom)** Transverse, transabdominal, grayscale ultrasound at the suprapubic region shows the urinary bladder at the cervix level. The transducer is angled more caudally compared with the middle image.

URETERS AND BLADDER

URINARY TRACT CALCULI AND DEBRIS

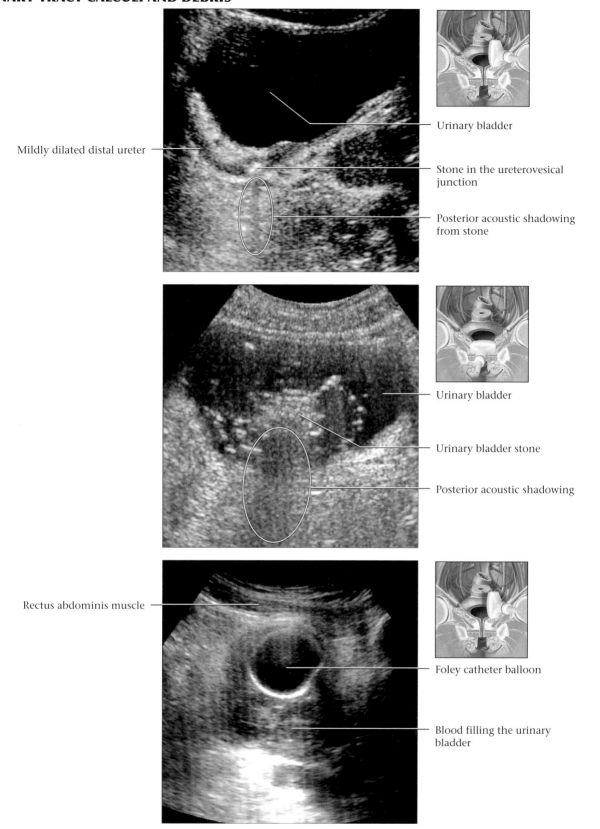

Mildly dilated distal ureter

Urinary bladder

Stone in the ureterovesical junction

Posterior acoustic shadowing from stone

Urinary bladder

Urinary bladder stone

Posterior acoustic shadowing

Rectus abdominis muscle

Foley catheter balloon

Blood filling the urinary bladder

(Top) Longitudinal, transabdominal, grayscale ultrasound shows a mildly distended distal ureter secondary to a small calculus at the ureterovesical junction. (Middle) Transverse, transabdominal, grayscale ultrasound shows a large lobulated echogenic calculus within the urinary bladder exhibiting posterior acoustic shadowing. (Bottom) Longitudinal, transabdominal, grayscale ultrasound shows medium to high level echoes (blood) filling the urinary bladder in a patient with gross hematuria. Examination in both supine and decubitus positions helps to evaluate mobility of bladder lesions.

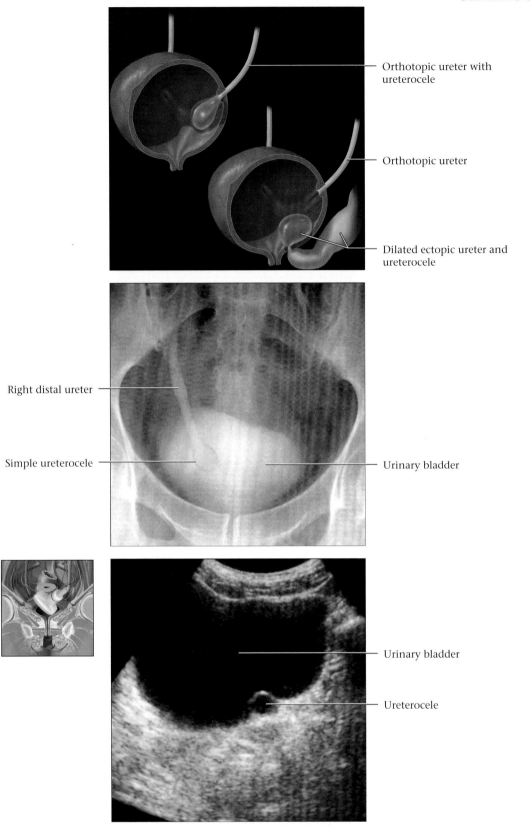

(Top) Graphic illustrates orthotopic ureterocele in a single ureter system (left, upper) and ectopic ureterocele in a duplicated ureter system (right, lower). Note the hydroureter accompanying the ectopic ureterocele. **(Middle)** A frontal radiograph from an excretory urogram shows a dilated right ureter that terminates in a cystic dilation, outlined by thin dark rim of ureterocele wall, within the bladder. This appearance of a simple ureterocele has been likened to the head of a spring onion or a cobra. **(Bottom)** Oblique, transabdominal, grayscale ultrasound shows typical ureterocele as a thin-walled sac within the urinary bladder.

URINARY BLADDER WALL THICKENING

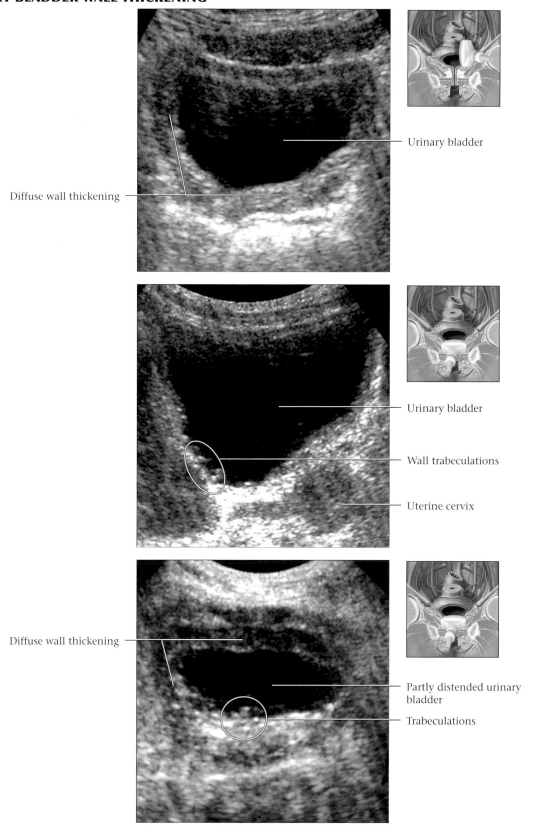

Urinary bladder

Diffuse wall thickening

Urinary bladder

Wall trabeculations

Uterine cervix

Diffuse wall thickening

Partly distended urinary bladder

Trabeculations

(Top) Longitudinal, transabdominal, grayscale ultrasound at the suprapubic region shows diffuse smooth urinary bladder wall thickening (7 mm) in a patient reporting full bladder sensation, post-fluid intake of 500 mL. The contour of the urinary bladder is maintained. **(Middle)** Transverse, transabdominal, grayscale ultrasound shows an irregular inner bladder outline compatible with trabeculations in a patient with chronic outflow obstruction. A normal urinary bladder may assume similar wall trabeculations in a non-distended state. **(Bottom)** Transverse, transabdominal, grayscale ultrasound at the suprapubic region shows the appearance of an under-filled urinary bladder which exhibits diffuse urinary bladder wall thickening and trabeculations. The urinary bladder must be examined in a fully distended state or when the patient reports full bladder sensation.

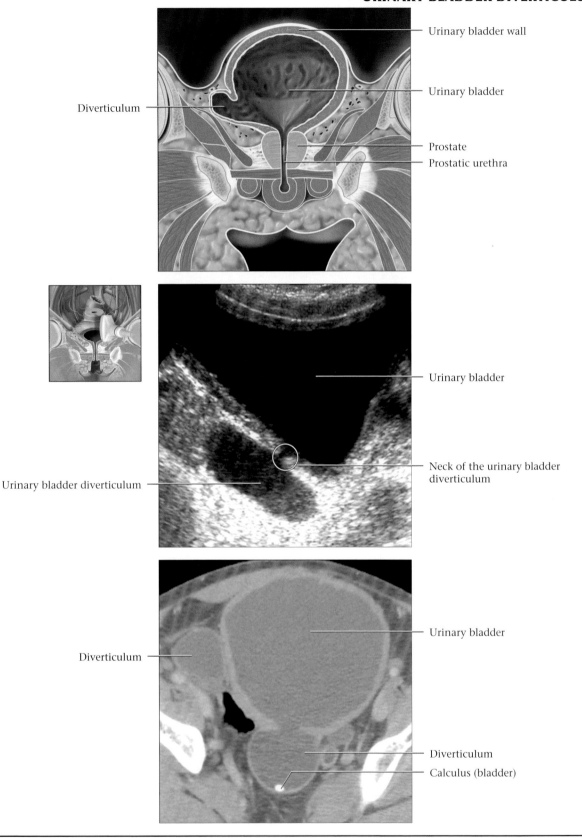

Urinary bladder wall

Urinary bladder

Prostate

Prostatic urethra

Diverticulum

Urinary bladder

Neck of the urinary bladder diverticulum

Urinary bladder diverticulum

Urinary bladder

Diverticulum

Diverticulum

Calculus (bladder)

(**Top**) Graphic shows a diverticulum arising from the lateral urinary bladder wall, due to herniation of the mucosa and submucosa through the muscular wall. (**Middle**) Longitudinal, transabdominal, grayscale ultrasound shows Hutch congenital diverticulum arising from the posterolateral wall of the urinary bladder with a narrow neck. (**Bottom**) Axial non-enhanced CT of an elderly man with hematuria and dysuria shows multiple urinary bladder diverticula with a calculus in the dependent position within one of the diverticula.

URINARY BLADDER CARCINOMA

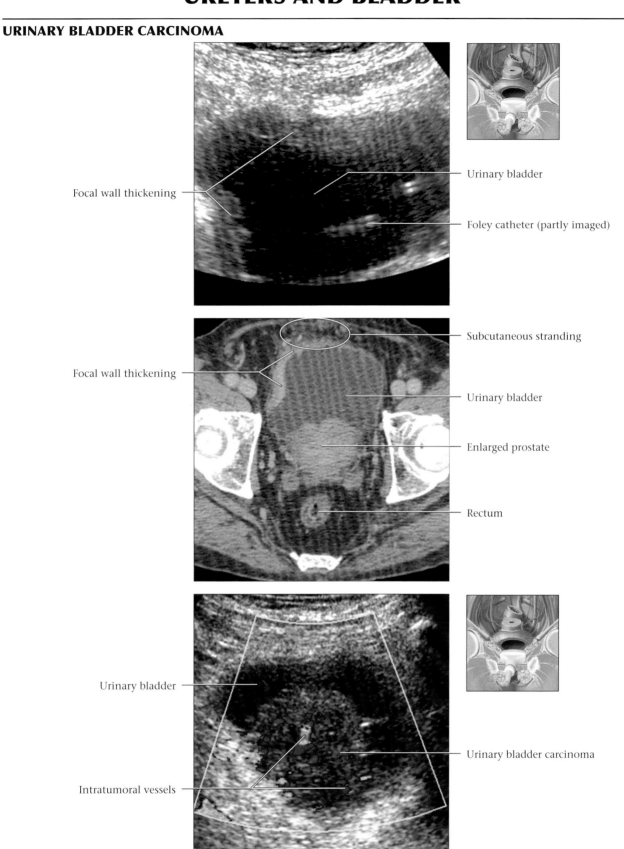

Focal wall thickening

Urinary bladder

Foley catheter (partly imaged)

Subcutaneous stranding

Focal wall thickening

Urinary bladder

Enlarged prostate

Rectum

Urinary bladder

Urinary bladder carcinoma

Intratumoral vessels

(Top) Transverse, transabdominal, grayscale ultrasound shows irregular eccentric wall thickening in the anterior and right lateral wall of the urinary bladder in a proven case of transitional cell carcinoma. (Middle) Axial, correlative, CECT of the same patient more clearly demonstrates the thickened anterior and right lateral walls of the urinary bladder. Note the overlying subcutaneous stranding, not visible on ultrasound, suggestive of tumoral invasion. The prostate is nodular and enlarged. (Bottom) Transverse color Doppler ultrasound in a different patient with proven urinary bladder carcinoma shows a large immobile soft tissue tumor at the base of the urinary bladder with characteristic intralesional vascularity.

PROSTATE

Gross Anatomy

Prostate
- Walnut-sized gland located beneath bladder and in front of rectum
  - Normal prostate ~ 3 cm craniocaudal x 4 cm wide x 2 cm anteroposteriorly
  - Surrounded by fibrous prostatic capsule
- Conical in shape with base, apex; anterior, posterior and two inferolateral surfaces
  - Posterior surface separated from rectum by rectovesical septum (Denonvilliers fascia)
  - Anterior surface separated from symphysis pubis by extraperitoneal fat and plexus of veins
    - Connected to pubic bone on either side by puboprostatic ligaments
  - Inferolateral surface separated from levator ani by periprostatic plexus of veins
- Prostatic urethra
  - Prostatic utricle, prostatic ducts and ejaculatory ducts enter prostatic urethra
  - Urethral crest
    - Narrow longitudinal ridge on posterior wall
  - Verumontanum (colliculus seminalis)
    - Median elevation of urethral crest below its summit
    - Openings of prostatic utricle and ejaculatory ducts
  - Prostatic sinus
    - Slightly depressed fossae on each side of verumontanum
    - Multiple openings of prostatic ducts
  - Prostatic utricle
    - Small vestigial blind pouch of prostate gland, about 6 mm long
    - Developed from united lower ends of atrophied Müllerian ducts
    - Homologous with uterus and vagina in female
  - Prostatic urethra is divided into proximal and distal parts by verumontanum
- Neurovascular bundles (NVB)
  - Lie posterolaterally to prostate
  - Separated from prostate by Denonvilliers fascia
  - Carries nerve and vascular supply to corpora cavernosa
- Arterial supply derived from internal pudendal, inferior vesical, and middle rectal arteries
- Prostatic venous plexus
  - Receives blood from dorsal vein of penis
  - Drains into internal iliac veins
- Nerve supply
  - Parasympathetic fibers from pelvic splanchnic nerves (S2-4)
  - Sympathetic fibers from inferior hypogastric plexuses
- Lymphatic drainage chiefly to internal iliac and sacral lymph nodes
  - Some drainage from posterior surface joins with bladder lymphatics, and drains to external iliac lymph nodes

Lobar Anatomy (Lowsley)
- Anatomic descriptions of the prostate
- Lobes: Anterior, median, lateral and posterior

- Median lobe surrounds the prostatic urethra
- Currently used only in the context of benign prostatic hyperplasia, which shows enlargement of the median lobe
- Largely replaced by zonal anatomy

Zonal Anatomy (McNeal)
- Prostate is histologically composed of glandular (acinar) and non-glandular elements
- Two non-glandular elements: Prostatic urethra and anterior fibromuscular stroma
- Glandular prostate consists of outer and inner components
- Inner prostate
  - Periurethral glands
    - < 1% of normal glandular prostate
  - Transitional zone (TZ)
    - ~ 5% of normal glandular prostate
    - Surrounds anterior and lateral aspects of proximal urethra
- Outer prostate
  - Named after anatomic locations relative to the prostatic urethra
  - Central zone (CZ)
    - ~ 25% of normal glandular prostate
    - Funnel-shaped with its widest portion making majority of prostatic base
    - Encloses both periurethral glands and transitional zone
    - Spans the proximal prostatic urethra
    - Ducts drain to region of verumontanum, clustered around entry of ejaculatory ducts
  - Peripheral zone (PZ)
    - ~ 70% of the normal glandular prostate
    - Surrounds both CZ and distal prostatic urethra
    - Spans both proximal and distal prostatic urethra
    - Ducts drain exclusively to distal prostatic urethra
  - Prostate pseudocapsule ("surgical capsule")
    - Visible boundary between CZ and PZ

Seminal Vesicles and Ejaculatory Ducts
- Seminal vesicles
  - Saclike structures located superolaterally to prostate
    - Between fundus of urinary bladder and rectum
  - Secrete fructose-rich, alkaline fluid, which is major component of semen
    - Secretions are energy source for sperm
  - Arterial supply
    - Inferior vesicle and middle hemorrhoidal arteries
  - Venous drainage accompanies arteries
  - Lymphatic drainage
    - Superior portion → external iliac nodes
    - Inferior portion → internal iliac nodes
- Ejaculatory ducts
  - Located on either side of midline
  - Formed by union of seminal vesicle duct and ductus deferens
  - ~ 2.5 cm long
  - Start at base of prostate and run forward and downward through gland
    - Terminate as separate slit-like openings close to utricle

PROSTATE

Imaging Anatomy

Prostate
- Transrectal ultrasound (TRUS)
  - Zones of normal prostate are not sonographically evident
  - TZ becomes distinguishable in BPH as well-demarcated area of heterogeneity
  - TRUS guided biopsy for suspected prostate cancer
- Prostate volume measurement
  - Prolate ellipse volume for 3 unequal axes
    - Width x height x length x 0.523
  - 1 cc of prostate tissue ~ 1 g
  - Prostate weighs ~ 20 g in young men
  - Prostatic enlargement when gland is > 40 g

Seminal Vesicles and Vasa Deferentia
- Cystic appearance on TRUS

Ultrasound Orientation in Transrectal Approach
- Rectum is at the bottom of the screen
  - Beam emanates from the rectum
- Axial ultrasound
  - Top of the screen: Anterior abdominal wall
  - Right of the screen: Left side of the patient
  - Left of the screen: Right side of the patient
- Sagittal ultrasound
  - Top of the screen: Anterior abdominal wall
  - Right of the screen: Head of the patient
  - Left of the screen: Feet of the patient
- Semi-coronal ultrasound
  - Top of the screen: Anterior abdominal wall
  - Right of the screen: Left side of the patient
  - Left of the screen: Right side of the patient
  - True coronal plane is not achieved during transrectal ultrasound

Anatomy-Based Imaging Issues

Imaging Recommendations
- Transducer
  - 5-8 MHz rectal transducer (end-firing or transverse panoramic)
  - 2.5-5 MHz curvilinear transducer for transabdominal ultrasound
  - High frequency (7.5 MHz) linear transducer for transperineal ultrasound
  - Examination performed in at least 2 orthogonal planes (axial/semi-coronal and sagittal)
- Patient position
  - Transrectal ultrasound: Left lateral decubitus, with hips and knees flexed (fetal position)
    - Biopsies of the prostate may be performed using this approach
  - Transabdominal ultrasound: Supine, using the urinary bladder as acoustic window (transvesical)
    - Fluid intake to ensure bladder distension
    - Angle the transducer posteroinferiorly, following the location of the prostate relative to the urinary bladder
  - Transperineal ultrasound: Supine, in lithotomy

- Provides alternative approach to prostate biopsy when transrectal approach is not possible
- Correlate ultrasound findings with clinical history, digital rectal examination results and prostate specific antigen (PSA) levels
  - Variable elevated PSA levels in literature and range from > 2.5-10 ng/mL

Imaging Pitfalls
- Transrectal ultrasound is the preferred approach to imaging the prostate
  - Most common site of prostatic carcinoma (posterior gland) is better evaluated
  - Abnormal vascularity on power Doppler ultrasound may be seen in hypertrophy, inflammation and cancer
    - Useful for directing biopsy
- Transabdominal ultrasound of the prostate is limited to the evaluation of prostate size

Transrectal Biopsy of the Prostate
- Most transrectal transducers have needle guidance system
- Local anesthesia injected in neurovascular bundles or into gland itself
- Common minor complications
  - Hematuria, hematochezia and hematospermia (may last for months)

Clinical Implications

Zonal Distribution of Prostatic Disease
- Prostate carcinoma
  - 70% of adenocarcinomas arise in PZ
  - 20% in TZ
  - 10% in CZ
- Benign prostatic hypertrophy (BPH)
  - Originates in TZ
  - Compresses CZ and PZ
  - Causes bladder outlet obstruction because of urethral compression

Spread of Prostate Carcinoma
- Predictors of extracapsular extension of prostatic carcinoma
  - Asymmetry of NVB
  - Obliteration of rectoprostatic angle
  - Irregular bulge in prostatic contour
- Up to 80% of prostatic cancers in the peripheral zone are hypoechoic
  - Hyperechoic cancers are uncommon
  - Isoechoic cancers usually occur in the transitional zone
    - Identified by mass effect (gland asymmetry, bulging)
- Rarely spreads posterior to seminal vesicles across Denonvilliers fascia to involve rectum
- 90% of prostatic metastases involve spine

PROSTATE

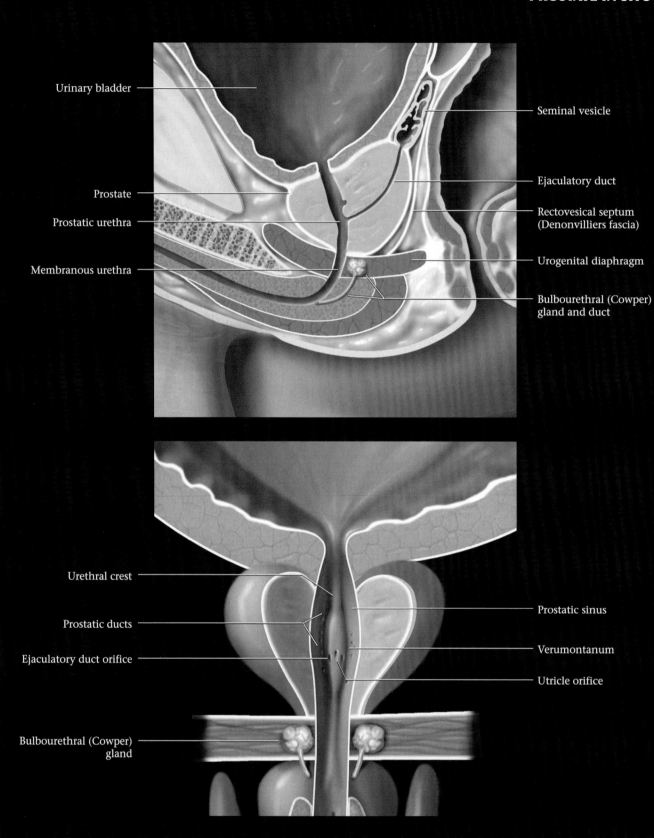

Urinary bladder

Prostate

Prostatic urethra

Membranous urethra

Seminal vesicle

Ejaculatory duct

Rectovesical septum (Denonvilliers fascia)

Urogenital diaphragm

Bulbourethral (Cowper) gland and duct

Urethral crest

Prostatic ducts

Ejaculatory duct orifice

Bulbourethral (Cowper) gland

Prostatic sinus

Verumontanum

Utricle orifice

(Top) Graphic illustrates the relationship between the prostate and the male pelvic organs. The prostate surrounds the upper part of the urethra (prostatic urethra). The base of the prostate is in direct contact with the neck of the urinary bladder and its apex is in contact with the superior fascia of urogenital diaphragm. The posterior surface is separated from the rectum by the rectovesical septum (Denonvilliers fascia). (Bottom) Graphic shows the topography of the posterior wall of the prostatic urethra. The urethral crest is a mucosal elevation along the posterior wall, with the verumontanum being a mound-like elevation in the mid-portion of the crest. The utricle opens midline onto the verumontanum, with the ejaculatory ducts opening on either side. The prostatic ducts are clustered around the verumontanum and open into the prostatic sinuses, which are depressions along the sides of the urethral crest.

PROSTATE

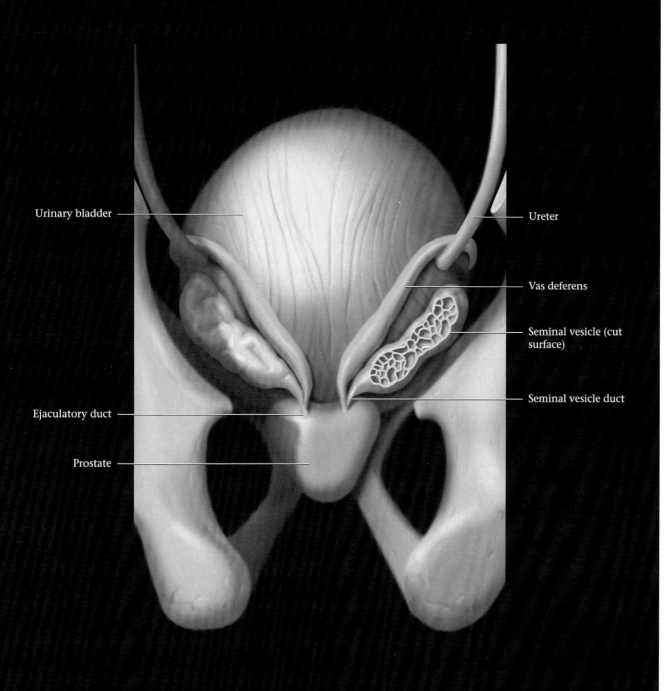

Urinary bladder

Ureter

Vas deferens

Seminal vesicle (cut surface)

Ejaculatory duct

Seminal vesicle duct

Prostate

Graphic shows the posterior view of the prostate gland and seminal vesicles. The cut surface of the seminal vesicle shows its highly convoluted fold pattern. The vas deferens (also called ductus deferens) crosses superior to the ureterovesical junction, continues along the posterior surface of the urinary bladder, medial to the seminal vesicle. At the base of the prostate, it is directed forward and is joined at an acute angle by the duct of the seminal vesicle to form the ejaculatory duct. The ejaculatory ducts course anteriorly and downward through the prostate to slit-like openings on either side of the orifice of the prostatic utricle.

Graphic depiction of the prostate with axial drawings of the zonal anatomy at three different levels. The TZ (in blue) is anterolateral to the verumontanum. The CZ (in orange) surrounds the ejaculatory ducts, and encloses the periurethral glands and the TZ. It is conical in shape and extends downward to about the level of the verumontanum. The PZ (in green) surrounds the posterior aspect of the CZ in the upper half of the gland and the urethra in the lower half, below the verumontanum. The prostatic pseudocapsule is a visible boundary between the CZ & PZ. The anterior fibromuscular stroma (in yellow) covers the anterior part of the gland and is thicker superiorly and thins inferiorly in the prostatic apex.

PROSTATE

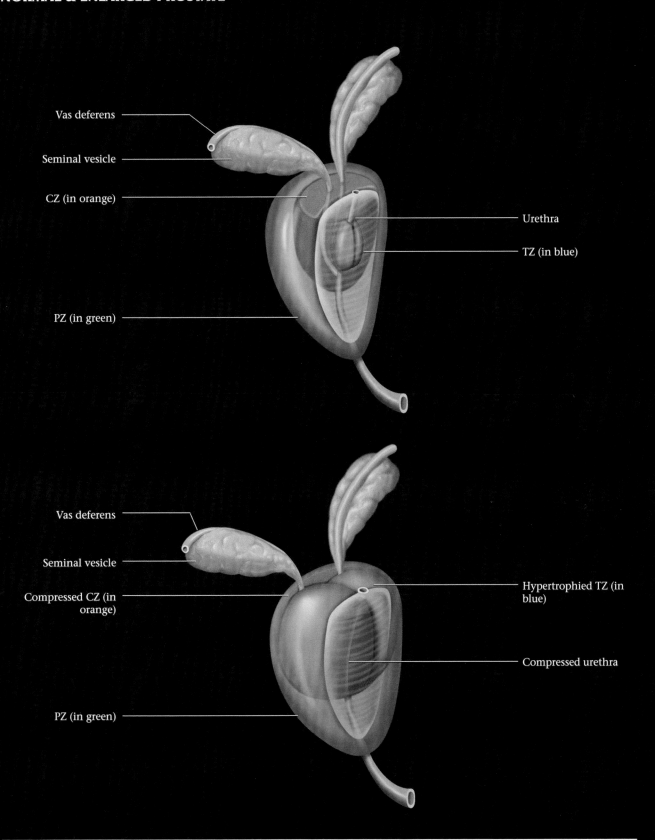

Vas deferens

Seminal vesicle

CZ (in orange)

Urethra

TZ (in blue)

PZ (in green)

Vas deferens

Seminal vesicle

Compressed CZ (in orange)

Hypertrophied TZ (in blue)

Compressed urethra

PZ (in green)

(Top) First of two graphics comparing zonal anatomy in a young man to an older man with benign prostatic hyperplasia (BPH). The transitional zone in young men is small in size, comprising about 5% of the volume of the glandular tissue of the prostate. It surrounds the anterolateral aspect of the urethra at the level of verumontanum in a horseshoe fashion. **(Bottom)** With the development of BPH, there is enlargement of the transitional zone. This causes enlargement of the prostate and compression of the central and peripheral zones. BPH mainly involves the transitional zone, though other zones may also be involved. The enlarged transitional zone causes compression of the prostatic urethra, the primary reason for development of urinary obstructive symptoms in patients with BPH.

PROSTATE

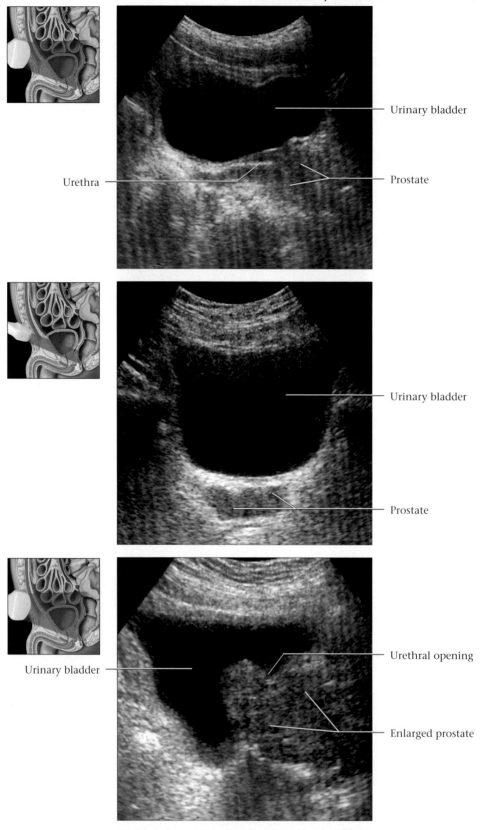

Urinary bladder

Urethra — — Prostate

Urinary bladder

Prostate

Urinary bladder — — Urethral opening

— Enlarged prostate

(Top) Transvesical, longitudinal, grayscale ultrasound of the prostate, angulating the transducer inferoposteriorly. The proximal urethra is echogenic and lined by calcifications. This approach is limited to examining the anterior portion of the prostate. The posterior portion or peripheral zone, which is the most common site for prostate carcinoma, is not clearly visualized, making this an unsuitable approach for prostate cancer investigation. (Middle) Transabdominal, transverse, grayscale ultrasound of the prostate through the urinary bladder. Normal size prostate has volume (CC x TS x AP x 0.52) < 40 g. (Bottom) Transabdominal, longitudinal, grayscale ultrasound shows an enlarged prostate indenting the urinary bladder. The notch-like opening of the urethra is well-demonstrated.

PROSTATE

SEMINAL VESICLES AND VAS DEFERENS

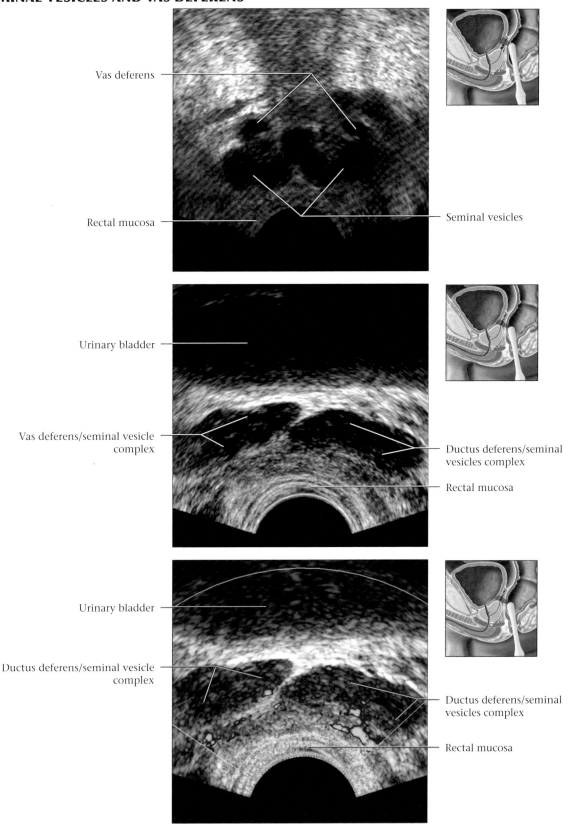

Vas deferens

Rectal mucosa

Seminal vesicles

Urinary bladder

Vas deferens/seminal vesicle complex

Ductus deferens/seminal vesicles complex

Rectal mucosa

Urinary bladder

Ductus deferens/seminal vesicle complex

Ductus deferens/seminal vesicles complex

Rectal mucosa

(Top) Transrectal, axial, grayscale ultrasound above the base of the prostate reveals the vas deferens (seen end on as dot-like structures) which is medial to the seminal vesicles. The seminal vesicles are usually 1 cm in AP diameter, but may sometimes be longer. (Middle) Transrectal, axial, grayscale ultrasound just above the base of the prostate (slightly inferior level compared with the top image). The vas deferens and seminal vesicles, which are both cystic in appearance, are seen more closely to and indistinguishable from each other. (Bottom) Transrectal, axial, power Doppler ultrasound shows the flow of vessels in the ductus deferens and seminal vesicle region. Power Doppler is less dependent on insonation angle but more sensitive to flow without providing information on its direction.

Urethra

Prostate

Rectal wall

Urinary bladder

Anterior fibromuscular stroma (hyperechoic)

Urethral sphincter (hypoechoic)

Central/transitional zone

Urethra

Peripheral zone

Surgical capsule

Rectal wall

Central zone

Urethral artery

Capsular arteries

(Top) Transverse, transrectal, grayscale ultrasound of the base of a normal prostate gland. The zonal anatomy of a normal prostate is not sonographically evident. The urethra is seen end on as a hypoechoic dot due to the surrounding smooth muscle of the sphincter. (Middle) Transverse, transrectal, grayscale ultrasound at the mid-gland level of the prostate. At this level the urethra is surrounded by transitional zone, which in turn is surrounded by peripheral zone. The hypoechoic surgical capsule is subtly demonstrated, separating the two zones. (Bottom) Transrectal, axial, power Doppler ultrasound reveals flow in the centrally located urethral artery and the peripherally located capsular arteries. Both arise from the prostatic artery which in turn arises from the inferior vesical branch of the internal iliac artery.

PROSTATE

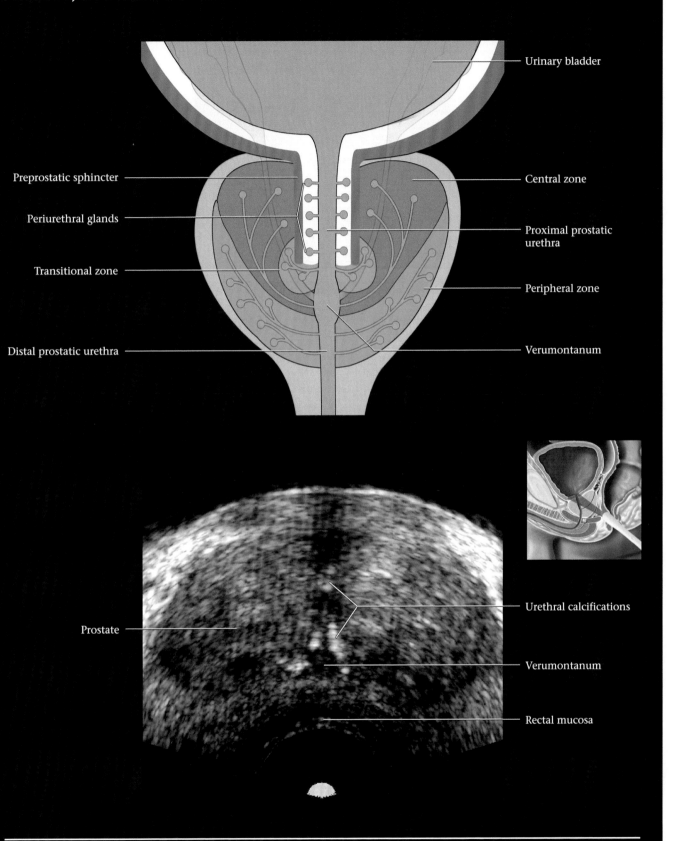

Preprostatic sphincter

Periurethral glands

Transitional zone

Distal prostatic urethra

Urinary bladder

Central zone

Proximal prostatic urethra

Peripheral zone

Verumontanum

Prostate

Urethral calcifications

Verumontanum

Rectal mucosa

(Top) Graphic illustrates the zonal anatomy of the prostate in the coronal plane. The proximal half of the prostatic urethra is surrounded by preprostatic sphincter, which extends inferiorly to the level of the verumontanum. The periurethral glands are in the urethral submucosa. The TZ is a downward extension of the periurethral glands around the verumontanum. **(Bottom)** Semi-coronal, transrectal, grayscale ultrasound shows the midline hypoechoic urethra which is continuous with the verumontanum, forming the "Eiffel tower" sign. The anterior shadowing is due to thick periprostatic sphincter. Echogenic foci/calcification line the urethra. A true coronal ultrasound is not possible in transrectal ultrasound but may be achieved with transperineal approach.

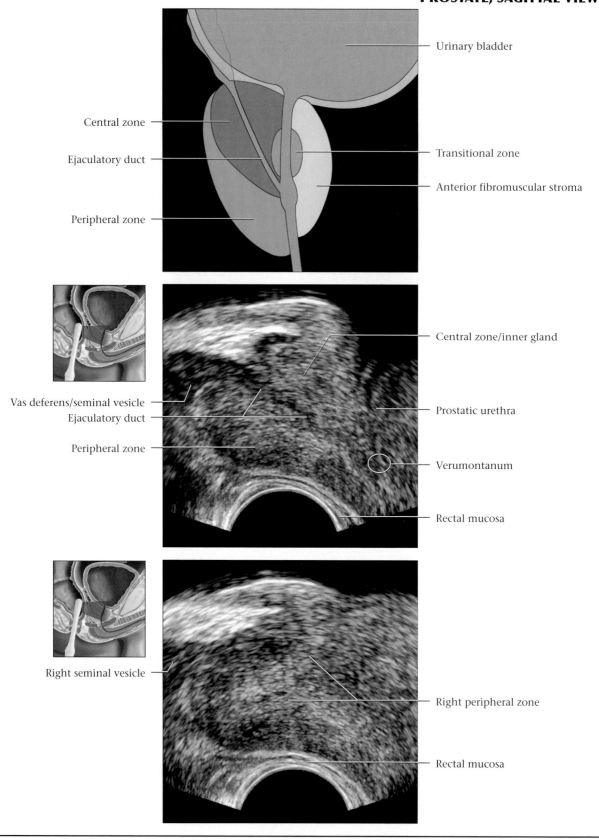

Urinary bladder

Central zone

Ejaculatory duct

Peripheral zone

Transitional zone

Anterior fibromuscular stroma

Vas deferens/seminal vesicle

Ejaculatory duct

Peripheral zone

Central zone/inner gland

Prostatic urethra

Verumontanum

Rectal mucosa

Right seminal vesicle

Right peripheral zone

Rectal mucosa

(Top) Graphic illustrates the zonal anatomy of the prostate in the sagittal plane. The outer prostate is composed of CZ and PZ. The CZ surrounds the proximal urethra posterosuperiorly, enclosing both the periurethral glands and the TZ. It forms most of the prostatic base. The PZ surrounds both the CZ and the distal prostatic urethra. **(Middle)** True sagittal grayscale ultrasound reveals the course of the prostatic urethra (proximal) anterior to the central zone. The ejaculatory duct starts at the base of the prostate and runs forward and downward through the gland. It terminates into the urethra at the verumontanum, which anatomically defines the proximal and distal segments of the prostatic urethra. **(Bottom)** Transrectal, parasagittal, grayscale ultrasound reveals mostly peripheral zone tissue, which constitutes 70% of the glandular elements of the prostate.

PROSTATIC CALCIFICATIONS

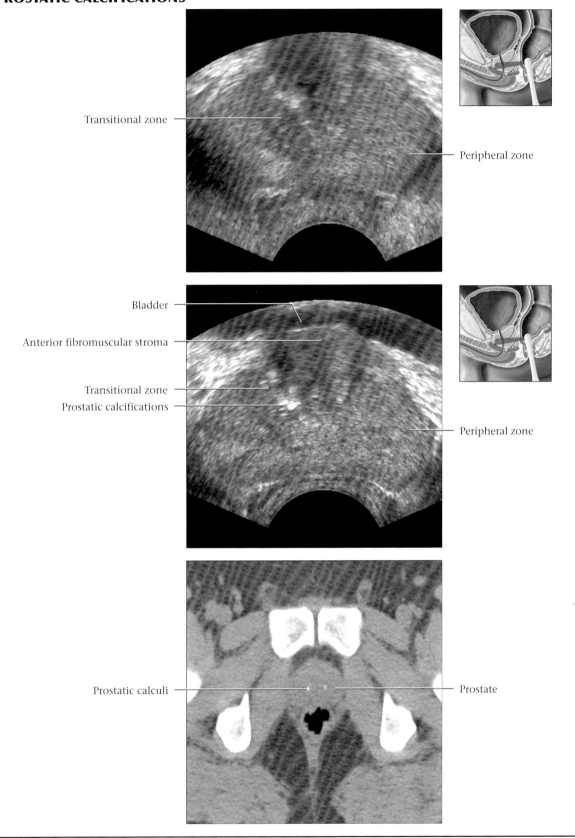

Transitional zone

Peripheral zone

Bladder

Anterior fibromuscular stroma

Transitional zone

Prostatic calcifications

Peripheral zone

Prostatic calculi

Prostate

(**Top**) First of two transverse transrectal ultrasounds of the prostate shows a heterogeneous, slightly enlarged, transitional zone. As BPH begins to develop, the transitional zone becomes distinguishable by ultrasound. It has a heterogeneous echogenicity with visible cysts, nodules and calcifications. (**Middle**) Focal areas of calcifications with shadowing are seen in the transitional zone of this patient. (**Bottom**) Axial non-enhanced CT of a normal-sized prostate shows prostatic calculi. Prostatic calculi are most often asymptomatic, but may be associated with some other disease process (BPH, prostatic carcinoma, metabolic abnormalities). They may be solitary but usually occur in clusters. CT images cannot show the zonal anatomy of the prostate but can show prostatic enlargement, and mass effect on adjacent structures.

TESTES

Gross Anatomy

Testis

- Densely packed seminiferous tubules separated by thin fibrous septae
  - 200-300 lobules in adult testis
  - Each has 400-600 seminiferous tubules
  - Total length of seminiferous tubules 300-980 meters
- Seminiferous tubules converge posteriorly to form larger ducts (tubuli recti)
  - Drain into rete testis at testicular hilum
- Rete testis converges posteriorly to form 15-20 efferent ductules
  - Penetrate posterior tunica albuginea at mediastinum to form head of epididymis
- Tunica albuginea forms thick fibrous capsule around testis
- Mediastinum testis is a thickened area of tunica albuginea where ducts, nerves, and vessels enter and exit testis
- Testicular appendage (appendix testis)
  - Small, nodular protuberance from surface of testis
  - Remnant of the Müllerian system

Epididymis

- Crescent-shaped structure running along posterior border of testis
- Efferent ductules form head (globus major)
  - Unite to form single, long, highly convoluted tubule in body of epididymis
- Tubule continues inferiorly to form epididymal tail (globus minor)
  - Attached to lower pole of testis by loose areolar tissue
- Tubule emerges at acute angle from tail as vas deferens (also known as ductus deferens)
  - Continues cephalad within spermatic cord
  - Eventually merges with duct of seminal vesicle to form ejaculatory duct
- Epididymal appendage (appendix epididymis)
  - Small nodular protuberance from surface of epididymis
  - Remnant of Wolffian system

Spermatic Cord

- Contains vas deferens, nerves, lymphatics, and connective tissue
- Begins at internal (deep) inguinal ring and exits through external (superficial) inguinal ring into scrotum
- Arteries
  - Testicular artery
    - Branch of aorta
    - Primary blood supply to testis
  - Deferential artery
    - Branch of inferior or superior vesicle artery
    - Arterial supply to vas deferens
  - Cremasteric artery
    - Branch of inferior epigastric artery
    - Supplies muscular components of cord and skin
- Venous drainage
  - Pampiniform plexus
    - Interconnected network of small veins
    - Merges to form testicular vein
    - Left testicular vein drains to left renal vein
    - Right testicular vein drains to inferior vena cava
- Lymphatic drainage
  - Testis follows venous drainage
    - Right side drains to interaortocaval chain
    - Left side drains to left para-aortic nodes near renal hilum
  - Epididymis may also drain to external iliac nodes
  - Scrotal skin drains to inguinal nodes

Embryology

- Testis develop from genital ridges, which extend from T6-S2 in embryo
- Composed of 3 cell lines (germ cells, sertoli cells, Leydig cells)
- Germ cells
  - Form in wall of yolk sac and migrate along hindgut to genital ridges
  - Form spermatogenic cells in mature testes
- Sertoli cells
  - Supporting network for developing spermatozoa
  - Form tight junctions (blood-testis barrier)
  - Secrete Müllerian inhibiting factor
    - Causes paramesonephric (Müllerian) ducts to regress
    - Embryologic remnant may remain as appendix testis
- Leydig cells
  - Principal source of testosterone production
  - Lies within interstitium
  - Causes differentiation of mesonephric duct (Wolffian) ducts
    - Each duct forms epididymis, vas deferens, seminal vesicle, ejaculatory duct
    - An embryologic remnant may remain as appendix epididymis
- Scrotum derived from labioscrotal folds
  - Folds swell under influence of testosterone to form twin scrotal sacs
    - Point of fusion is median raphe, which extends from anus, along perineum to ventral surface of penis
  - Processus vaginalis, a sock-like evagination of peritoneum, elongates through the abdominal wall into twin sacs
    - Aids in descent of testes, along with gubernaculum (ligamentous cord extending from testis to labioscrotal fold)
    - Results in component layers of adult scrotum
- Testicular descent
  - Between 7-12th week of gestation, testes descend into pelvis
    - Remain near internal inguinal ring until 7th month, when they begin descent through inguinal canal into twin scrotal sacs
    - Testes remain retroperitoneal throughout descent
    - Testes intimately associated with posterior wall of processus vaginalis
  - Component layers of spermatic cord and scrotum form during descent through abdominal wall

TESTES

○ Transversalis fascia ⇒ internal spermatic fascia
- Transversus abdominis muscle is discontinuous inferiorly and does not contribute to formation of scrotum
○ Internal oblique muscle ⇒ cremasteric muscle and fascia
○ External oblique muscle ⇒ external spermatic fascia
○ Dartos muscle and fascia embedded in loose areolar tissue below skin
○ Processus vaginalis closes and forms tunica vaginalis
- Mesothelial-lined sac around anterior and lateral sides of testis
- Visceral layer of tunica vaginalis blends imperceptibly with tunica albuginea

Anatomy-Based Imaging Issues

Imaging Recommendations
- Palpation of scrotal contents and taking history prior to US examination
- Transducer: High frequency (7.5-10 MHz) linear transducer
- Patient in supine position
  ○ Penis lies on anterior abdominal wall
  ○ Towel draped over thighs to elevate scrotum
  ○ Additional positions with patient upright or with patient performing Valsalva maneuver

Imaging Anatomy

- Testes
  ○ Ovoid, homogeneous, medium-level, granular echotexture
  ○ Mediastinum testis may appear as prominent echogenic line emanating from posterior testis
  ○ Blood flow
    - Testicular artery pierces tunica albuginea and arborizes over periphery of testis
    - Multiple, radially-arranged vessels travel along septae
    - May have prominent transmediastinal artery
    - Low-velocity, low-resistance wave form on Doppler imaging, with continuous forward flow in diastole
- Epididymis
  ○ Isoechoic to slightly hyperechoic compared with testis
  ○ Best seen in longitudinal plane
  ○ Head has rounded or triangular configuration
  ○ Head 10-12 mm, body and tail often difficult to visualize
- Spermatic cord
  ○ May be difficult to differentiate from surrounding soft tissues
  ○ Evaluate for varicocele with color Doppler

Clinical Implications

Hydrocele
- Fluid between visceral and parietal layers of tunica vaginalis

- Small amount of fluid is normal
- Larger hydroceles may be either congenital (patent processus vaginalis) or acquired

Cryptorchidism
- Failure of testes to descend completely into scrotum
- Most lie near external inguinal ring
- Associated with decreased fertility and testicular carcinoma
  ○ Risk of carcinoma is increased for both testes, even if other side is normally descended

Varicocele
- Idiopathic or secondary to abdominal mass
  ○ Idiopathic more common on left
- Vessel diameter > 3 mm abnormal
- Always evaluate with provocative maneuvers, such as Valsalva

Dilated Rete Testes
- Clusters of dilated tubules in the mediastinum testis
- Empty into the epididymis
- Often associated with epididymal cysts

Torsion
- Occurs most commonly when tunica vaginalis completely surrounds testis and epididymis
  ○ Testis is suspended from spermatic cord like "bell-clapper", rather than being anchored posteriorly
- Normal grayscale appearance with early torsion
  ○ Becomes heterogeneous and enlarged with infarction
- Doppler required for diagnosis
  ○ Some flow may be seen even if torsed but will be decreased compared to normal side
  ○ Venous flow compromised first, then diastolic flow, finally systolic flow

Testicular Microlithiasis
- Calcifications in testicular parenchyma
- Association with testicular carcinoma
  ○ Controversial whether risk factor

Testicular Carcinoma
- Most common malignancy in young men
  ○ 95% are germ cell tumors
    - Seminoma (most common pure tumor), embryonal, yolk sac tumor, choriocarcinoma, teratoma
    - Mixed germ cell tumor (components of 2 or more cell lines) most common overall
  ○ Remainder of primary tumors are sex cord (Sertoli cells) or stromal (Leydig cells)
  ○ Lymphoma, leukemia and metastases are more common in older men
- Most metastasize via lymphatics in predictable fashion
  ○ Right-sided first echelon nodes: Interaortocaval chain at second vertebral body
  ○ Left-sided first echelon nodes: Left paraaortic nodes in area bounded by renal vein, aorta, ureter and inferior mesenteric artery

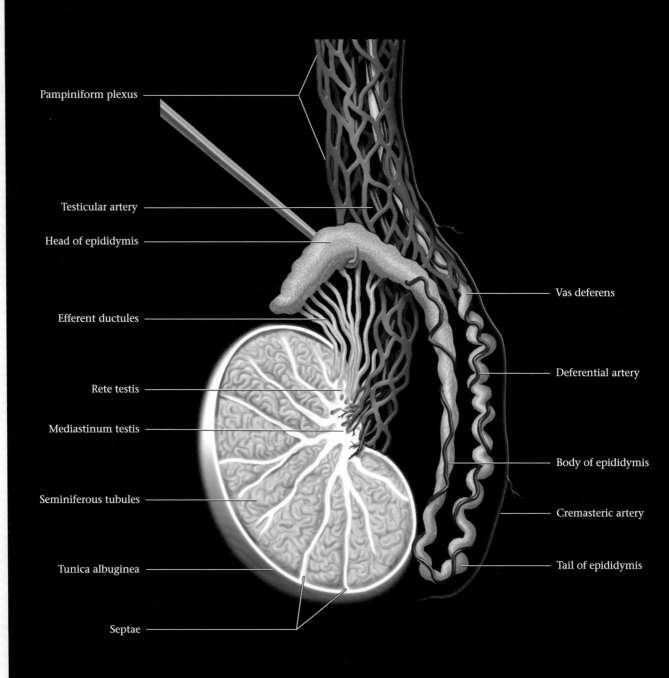

Pampiniform plexus

Testicular artery

Head of epididymis

Efferent ductules

Rete testis

Mediastinum testis

Seminiferous tubules

Tunica albuginea

Septae

Vas deferens

Deferential artery

Body of epididymis

Cremasteric artery

Tail of epididymis

Graphic shows the testis is composed of densely packed seminiferous tubules, which are separated by thin fibrous septae. These tubules converge posteriorly, eventually draining into the rete testis. The rete testis continues to converge to form the efferent ductules, which pierce through the tunica albuginea at the mediastinum testis and form the head of the epididymis. Within the epididymis these tubules unite to form a single, highly-convoluted tubule in the body, which finally emerges from the tail as the vas deferens. In addition to the vas deferens, other components of the spermatic cord include the testicular artery, deferential artery, cremasteric artery, pampiniform plexus, lymphatics and nerves.

TESTES

EPIDIDYMIS & SCROTAL WALL LAYERS IN SITU

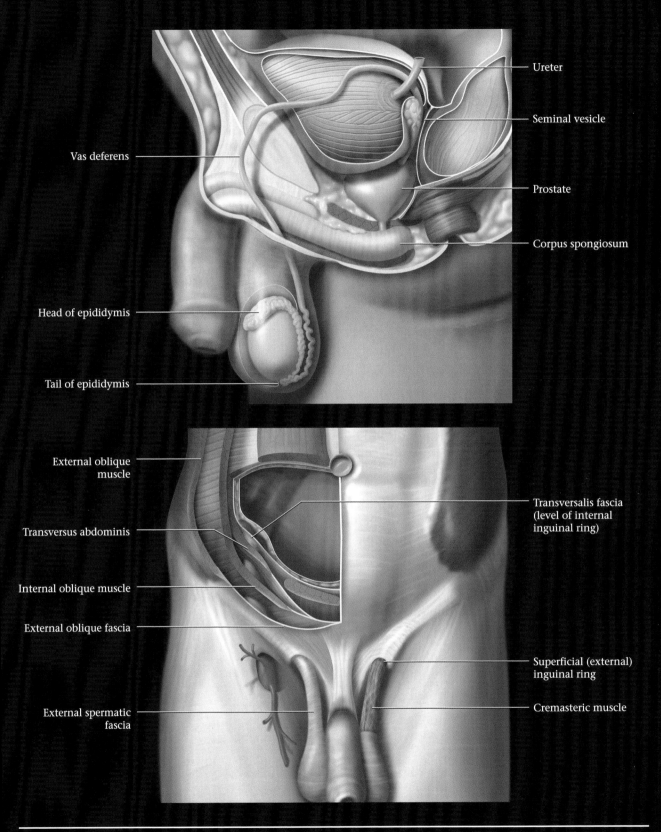

Ureter

Seminal vesicle

Vas deferens

Prostate

Corpus spongiosum

Head of epididymis

Tail of epididymis

External oblique muscle

Transversalis fascia (level of internal inguinal ring)

Transversus abdominis

Internal oblique muscle

External oblique fascia

Superficial (external) inguinal ring

External spermatic fascia

Cremasteric muscle

(Top) Graphic shows the tail of the epididymis is loosely attached to the lower pole of the testis by areolar tissue. The vas deferens (also referred to as ductus deferens) emerges from the tail at an acute angle and continues cephalad as part of the spermatic cord. After passing through the inguinal canal, the vas deferens courses posteriorly to unite with the duct of the seminal vesicle to form the ejaculatory duct. These narrow ducts have thick, muscular walls composed of smooth muscle, which reflexly contract during ejaculation and propel sperm forward. **(Bottom)** The muscle layers of the pelvic wall have been separated to show the spermatic cord as it passes through the inguinal canal. The cremasteric muscle is derived from the internal oblique muscle, while the external spermatic fascia is formed by the fascia of the external oblique muscle.

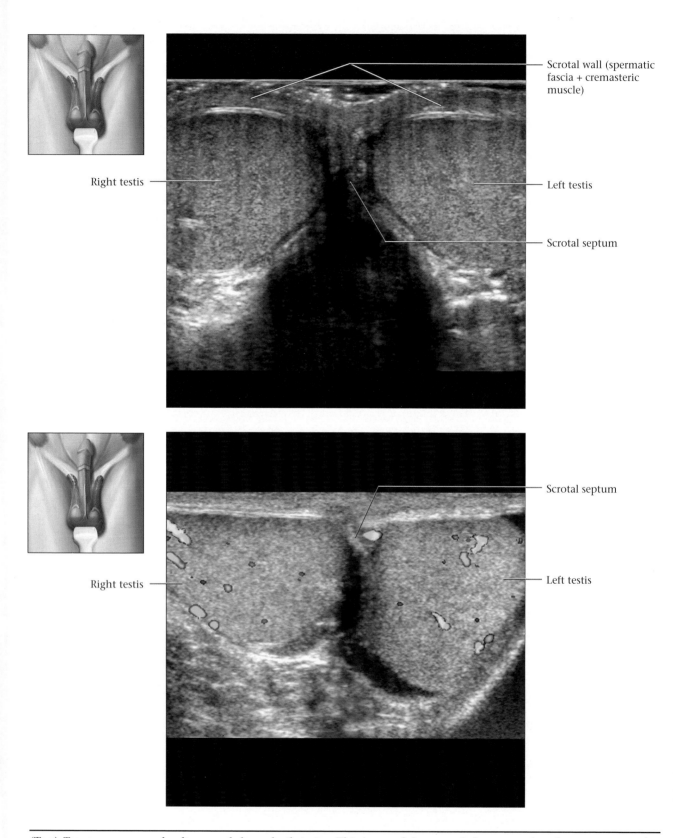

Right testis

Left testis

Scrotal wall (spermatic fascia + cremasteric muscle)

Scrotal septum

Right testis

Left testis

Scrotal septum

(Top) Transverse grayscale ultrasound shows both testes. This is a useful approach for comparing the appearance of the testes, which should have similar, homogeneous, medium-level, granular echotexture. (Bottom) Transverse color Doppler ultrasound of the testes. It is important to compare flow between testes to determine if the symptomatic side has increased or decreased flow, when compared to the asymptomatic side. This approach also helps to globally evaluate edema, hematoma or abnormality in the scrotal wall.

TESTES

TESTIS, SAGITTAL VIEW

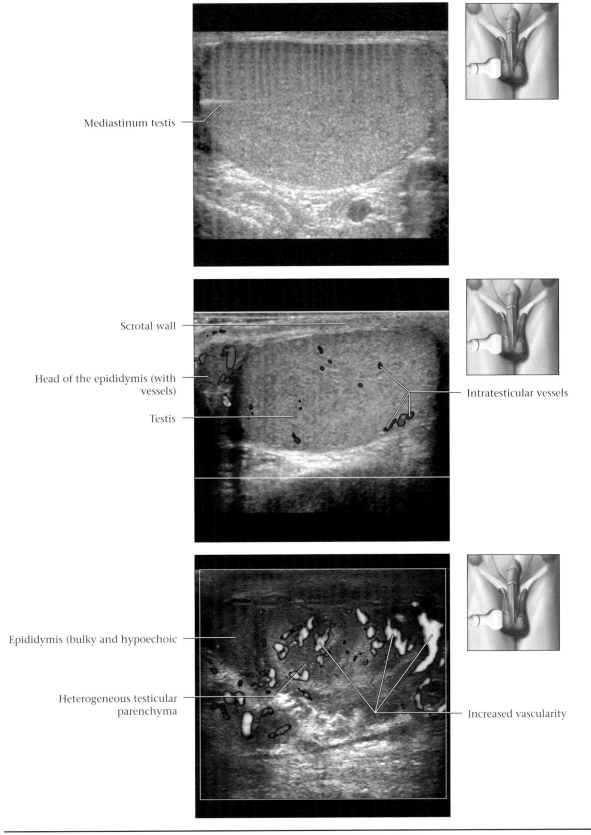

Mediastinum testis

Scrotal wall

Head of the epididymis (with vessels)

Testis

Intratesticular vessels

Epididymis (bulky and hypoechoic

Heterogeneous testicular parenchyma

Increased vascularity

(Top) Longitudinal grayscale ultrasound shows the ovoid shape of the testis. The tunica albuginea may form an echogenic linear band where it invaginates at the mediastinum testis. The mediastinum testis has a craniocaudal linear course and is where the efferent ductules, vessels and lymphatics pierce through the capsule. **(Middle)** Longitudinal color Doppler ultrasound shows normal modest vascularity of the testis. **(Bottom)** Longitudinal power Doppler ultrasound shows heterogeneous echotexture of testicular parenchyma and abnormally increased testicular vascularity. Note also the bulky and hypoechoic epididymis. This is a case of epididymo-orchitis.

TESTES

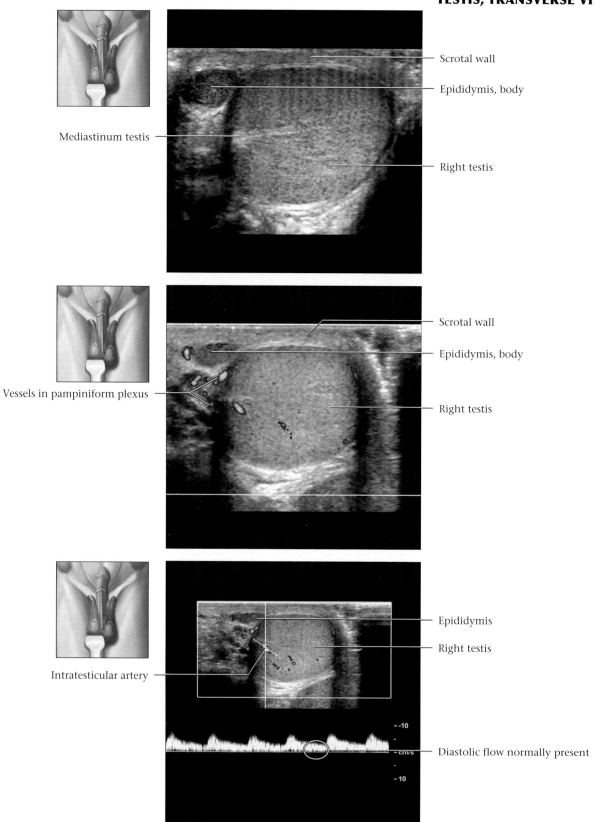

Top image labels:
- Scrotal wall
- Epididymis, body
- Mediastinum testis
- Right testis

Middle image labels:
- Scrotal wall
- Epididymis, body
- Vessels in pampiniform plexus
- Right testis

Bottom image labels:
- Epididymis
- Right testis
- Intratesticular artery
- Diastolic flow normally present

(Top) Transverse grayscale ultrasound of the right scrotum demonstrates the anatomic relationship of the testis and epididymis. Image obtained at the superior pole of the testis, thus the epididymis is seen anterolaterally. Note the mediastinum testis, arising from the central and lateral portion of the testis. (Middle) Transverse color Doppler ultrasound again shows normal paucity of testicular vascularity. Some vessels are also identified in the epididymis. More vessels can be identified along the mediastinum testis. (Bottom) Pulsed Doppler ultrasound of an intratesticular artery shows low resistance with low systolic and end-diastolic flow velocities. Normal peak systolic velocity of 12 cm/sec and end diastolic velocity of 4 cm/sec.

TESTES

EPIDIDYMIS, HEAD

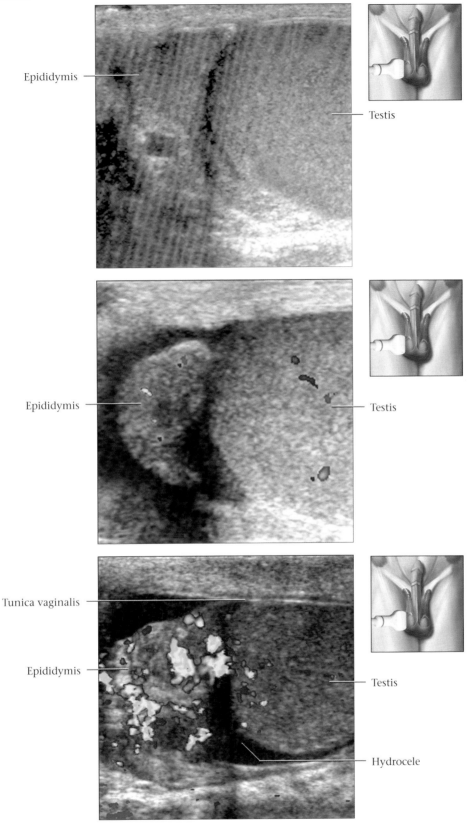

Epididymis — Testis

Epididymis — Testis

Tunica vaginalis — Epididymis — Testis — Hydrocele

(Top) Longitudinal grayscale ultrasound shows the epididymal head, which is demonstrated superior to the testis and typically has a triangular or slightly rounded configuration. **(Middle)** Color Doppler ultrasound of the epididymal head which shows minimal vascularity compared with the testis. **(Bottom)** Color Doppler ultrasound of a patient with acute epididymitis. The epididymal head is enlarged and hyperemic, with a marked increase in color flow. The testis is normal and flow was symmetric with the other testis. Most infections occur from direct extension of pathogens retrograde, via the vas deferens, from a lower urinary tract source. Thus, the epididymis becomes infected before the testis.

Epididymal head (partly imaged) —

— Epididymal body

— Epididymal tail

— Pampiniform venous plexus & ductus deferens

Vessels in pampiniform plexus —

— Epididymal tail

— Epididymis (body and tail)

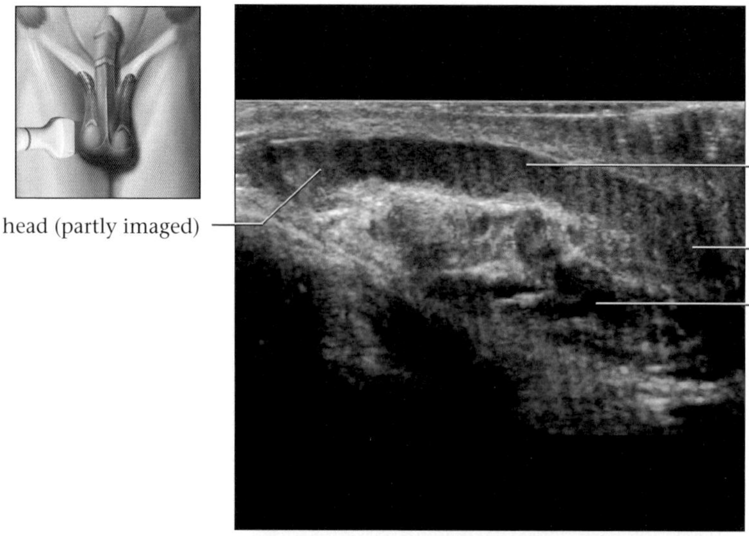

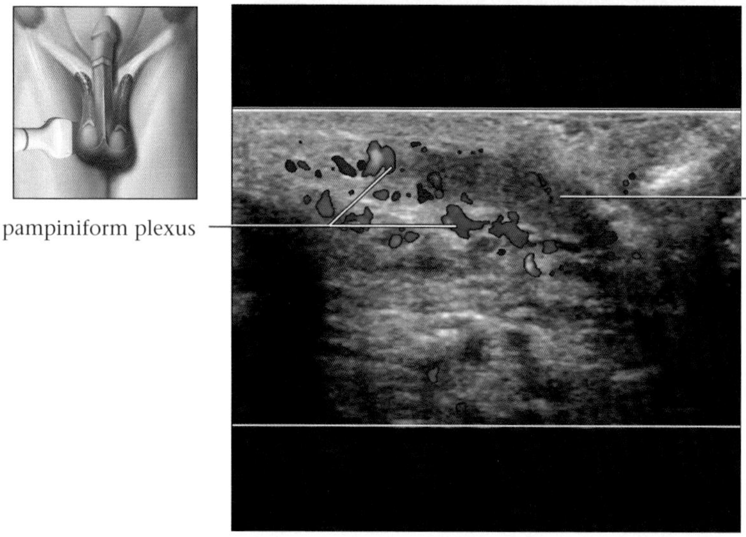

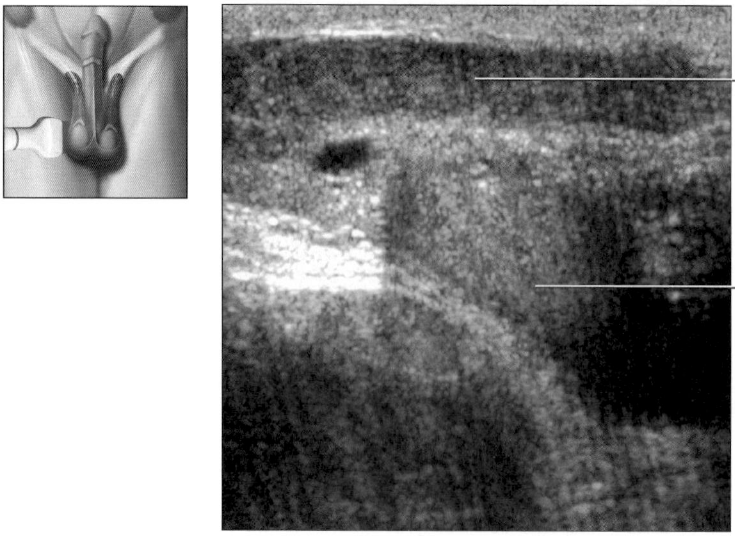

— Testis

(**Top**) Longitudinal grayscale ultrasound of the epididymis. Image obtained by directing the ultrasound beam at the posterolateral portion of the scrotum, following the axis of the epididymal body. (**Middle**) Longitudinal color Doppler ultrasound better demonstrates the relationship of the epididymal tail with the pampiniform plexus, which is located more medially. (**Bottom**) Longitudinal grayscale ultrasound of the scrotum shows an enlarged and hypoechoic body and tail of the epididymis, suggestive of epididymitis. The use of high resolution transducer is essential to evaluate the superficially located structures. In patients with acute scrotum, transducer must be placed gently as excessive transducer pressure is painful.

TESTES

TESTICULAR AND EPIDIDYMAL APPENDAGE

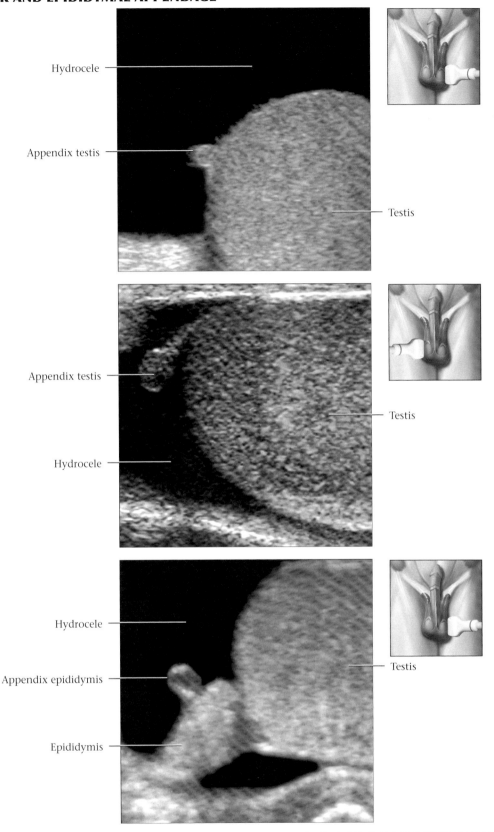

Hydrocele

Appendix testis

Testis

Appendix testis

Testis

Hydrocele

Hydrocele

Appendix epididymis

Testis

Epididymis

(Top) Longitudinal grayscale ultrasound of the testis in a patient with a hydrocele shows a small, nodular protuberance from the surface of the testis. It is isoechoic to normal testicular parenchyma. This is the appendix testis, which is a remnant of the Müllerian system. **(Middle)** Longitudinal grayscale ultrasound of a slightly larger and pedunculated appendix testis. The normal testicular appendage is not more than 6 mm wide. **(Bottom)** Longitudinal grayscale ultrasound of the upper testis and epididymis shows a small, cystic "tag" of tissue projecting from the epididymis. This is an appendix epididymis, which is a remnant of the Wolffian system. Both the appendix testis and appendix epididymis are usually not visible sonographically, unless there is a hydrocele. They are usually of no clinical significance; however, they can rarely torse and be a cause of scrotal pain.

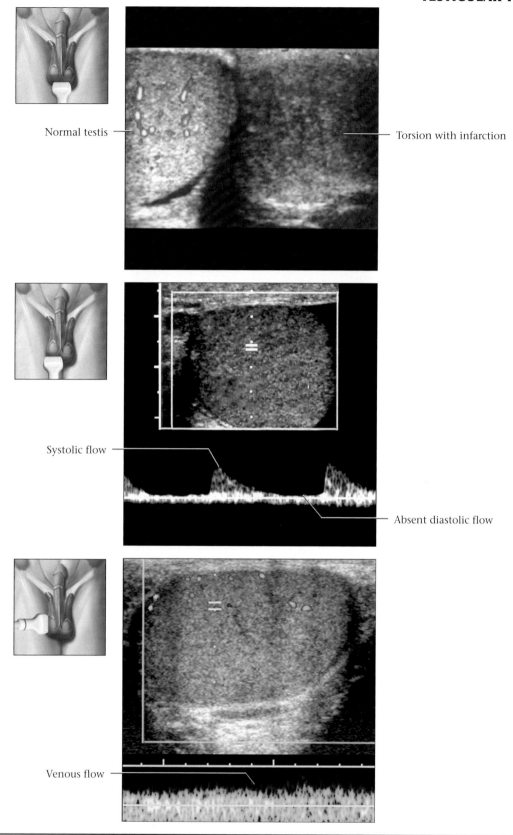

Normal testis — Torsion with infarction

Systolic flow — Absent diastolic flow

Venous flow

(Top) Transverse power Doppler ultrasound in a patient with left testicular torsion and infarction. The left testis is enlarged and hypoechoic compared to the normal right side. Flow is seen in the surrounding scrotal skin but none is present within the testis itself. (Middle) Pulsed-wave Doppler shows systolic flow but absent diastolic flow. Venous flow was absent as well. Because veins are more compressible, their flow is compromised first. This is followed by loss of diastolic flow and finally systolic flow. Complete loss of blood flow may not be seen unless the cord has twisted at least 540 degrees. (Bottom) Pulsed-wave venous Doppler shows normal venous flow. In evaluating an acutely painful testis, both arterial and venous flow should be documented, as incomplete torsion may compromise venous flow but not arterial flow.

TESTES

VARICOCELE

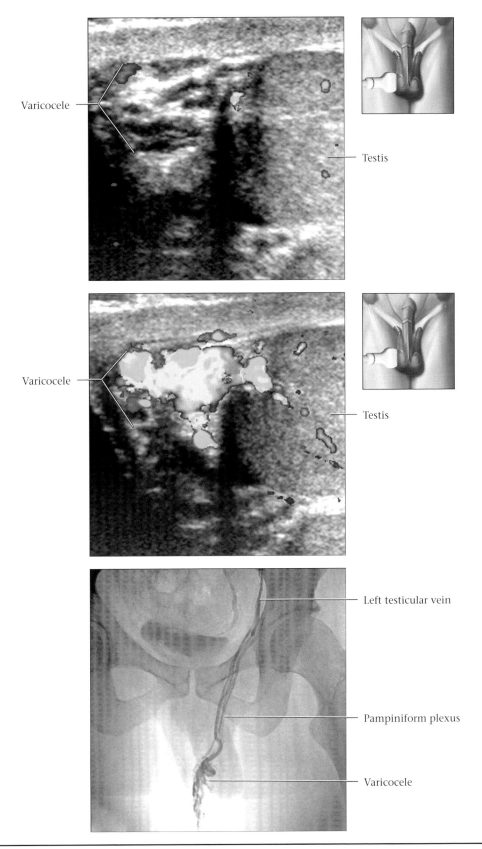

Varicocele

Testis

Varicocele

Testis

Left testicular vein

Pampiniform plexus

Varicocele

(Top) First of three images in a patient with infertility and a left-sided varicocele. Normal vessel diameter should not exceed 3 mm. Color Doppler ultrasound at rest shows parallel channels with little to no flow. Often flow is so slow it is not discernible by Doppler. **(Middle)** Color Doppler ultrasound shows filling of the varicocele with the Valsalva maneuver. Other provocative maneuvers, such as scanning in the upright position, can also be used to help make the diagnosis. **(Bottom)** Angiogram confirms the varicocele, which was subsequently embolized.

TESTES

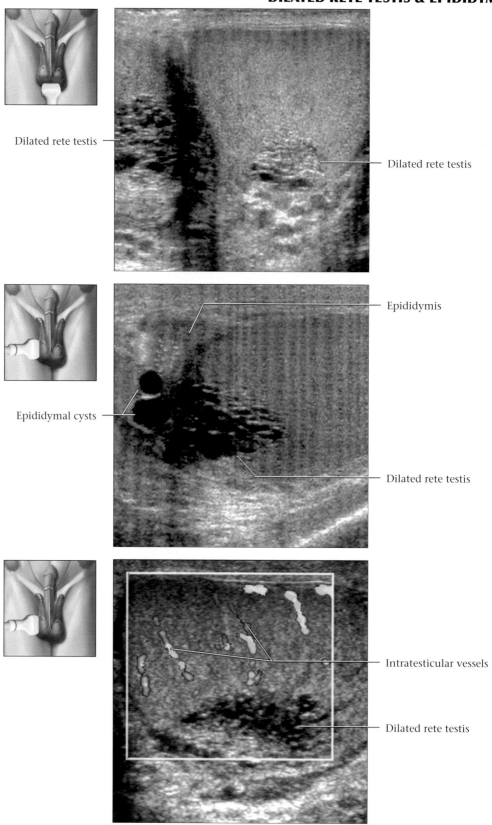

Dilated rete testis

Dilated rete testis

Epididymis

Epididymal cysts

Dilated rete testis

Intratesticular vessels

Dilated rete testis

(Top) First of three ultrasound images in a patient with tubular ectasia of the rete testis. The rete testis is normally not seen unless dilated. Dilatation is thought to occur secondary to obstruction in the epididymis or efferent ductules. Tubular ectasia is located posteriorly by the mediastinum and is frequently bilateral. It may give an impression of a mass, but careful scanning shows the "mass" is actually a series of dilated tubules. **(Middle)** Longitudinal grayscale ultrasound of the right side shows two epididymal cysts. These are frequently associated with dilatation of the rete testis. **(Bottom)** Longitudinal color Doppler ultrasound of the left testis shows no flow within these cystic spaces. Note the radiating pattern of the intratesticular vessels.

TESTES

TESTICULAR MASSES

Testis

Microlithiases

Tunica vaginalis

Testicular mass

Tumoral and peritumoral vessels

Testis

Lacerated testicular parenchyma

Ruptured tunica albuginea

Tunica albuginea

(Top) Longitudinal grayscale ultrasound of the scrotum reveals testicular microlithiases, with multiple, small, echogenic, non-shadowing foci diffusely scattered throughout the testicular parenchyma. These are found to have significant association with testicular carcinoma. (Middle) Longitudinal power Doppler ultrasound shows a small, well-defined hypoechoic vascular testicular mass suggestive of a small testicular carcinoma. (Bottom) Longitudinal ultrasound shows a heterogeneous testis with irregular, poorly defined hypoechoic foci. Note interruption of tunica albuginea indicating testicular rupture. In patients with testicular trauma, apply gentle transducer pressure as the scrotum is quite tender.

PENIS AND MALE URETHRA

Imaging Anatomy

Penis

- Composed of three cylindrical shafts
  - Two corpora cavernosa: Main erectile bodies
    - On dorsal surface of penis
    - Diverge at root of penis (crura) and are invested by ischiocavernosus muscles
    - Chambers traversed by numerous trabeculae, creating sinusoidal spaces
    - Multiple fenestrations between the two corpora, creating multiple anastomotic channels
  - One corpus spongiosum: Contains urethra
    - On ventral surface, in the groove created by corpora cavernosa
    - Becomes penile bulb (urethral bulb) at root and is invested by bulbospongiosus muscle
    - Forms glans penis distally
    - Also erectile tissue but of far less importance
- Tunica albuginea forms capsule around each corpora
  - Thinner around spongiosum than cavernosa
- All three corpora surrounded by a deep fascia (Buck fascia) and a superficial fascia (Colles fascia)
- Suspensory ligament of penis (part of fundiform ligament) is an inferior extension of abdominal rectus sheath
- Main arterial supply from internal pudendal artery
  - Cavernosal artery runs within center of each corpus cavernosum
    - Gives off helicine arteries, which fill trabecular spaces
    - Primary source of blood for erectile tissue
  - Paired dorsal penile arteries run between tunica albuginea of corpora cavernosa and Buck fascia
    - Supplies glans penis and skin
  - Multiple anastomoses between cavernosal and dorsal penile arteries
- Venous drainage of corpora cavernosa
  - Emissary veins in corpora pierce through tunica albuginea ⇒ circumflex veins ⇒ deep dorsal vein of penis ⇒ retropubic venous plexus
  - Superficial dorsal vein drains skin and glans penis
- Primary innervation from terminal branches of internal pudendal nerve

Normal Erectile Function

- Neurologically mediated response eliciting smooth muscle relaxation of cavernosal arteries, helicine arteries and cavernosal sinusoids
- Blood flows from helicine arteries into sinusoidal spaces
- Sinusoids distend, eventually compressing emissary veins against rigid tunica albuginea
  - Venous compression prevents egress of blood from corpora, which maintains erection
- Ultrasound can be used to evaluate erectile function
  - Doppler evaluation of cavernosal arteries performed after injection of vasodilating agent
  - In flaccid state there is little diastolic flow
  - At onset of erection, there is dilatation of cavernosal arteries
    - Increase in both systolic and diastolic flow
  - At maximum erection, venous drainage is blocked

- Doppler waveform changes to high resistance with reversal of diastolic flow
  - Normal measurements
    - Peak systolic velocity > 30 cm/sec
    - Cavernosal artery diameter increase > 75%

Urethra

- Divided into four sections: Prostatic, membranous, bulbous and penile
  - Posterior urethra: Prostatic and membranous
  - Anterior urethra: Bulbous and penile
- Prostatic urethra
  - Verumontanum is 1 cm ovoid mound along ureteral crest (smooth muscle ridge on posterior wall)
  - Prostatic utricle, prostatic ducts and ejaculatory ducts enter in this segment
  - Lined by transitional cells
    - Remainder of urethra lined by columnar cells, except glans which has squamous epithelium
- Membranous urethra
  - Short course through urogenital diaphragm
    - Level of external urethral sphincter
  - Contains bulbourethral glands (Cowper glands)
    - Ducts travel distally ~ 2 cm to enter bulbous urethra
- Bulbous urethra
  - Below urogenital diaphragm to suspensory ligament of penis at penoscrotal junction
- Penile urethra
  - Pendulous portion, distal to suspensory ligament
  - Fossa navicularis: Widening at glans penis
  - Both penile and bulbous urethra lined by mucosal urethral glands (glands of Littré)
- Two points of fixations: Urogenital diaphragm (membranous urethra) and penoscrotal junction

Anatomy-Based Imaging Issues

Imaging Recommendations

- Transducer: High frequency (7.5-10 MHz) linear transducer provides best detail
- Patient is supine with penis in anatomic position, lying on the anterior abdominal wall
- Transducer placed on the ventral side of the penis
  - Corpus spongiosum easily compressed therefore copious amount of gel should be used with gentle compression during scanning
- For erectile dysfunction studies, a vasodilating agent (papaverine, phentolamine or prostaglandin E1) is injected into the dorsal 2/3 of shaft
  - Velocity measurements taken beginning 5 minutes from injection
  - Effect of drug may wear off in 20-30 minutes
- Imaging of the anterior urethra is optimal with distension
  - For longer examination, a viscous lidocaine gel may be injected in retrograde fashion
  - Patient may be asked to void during scanning
- Posterior urethra is best imaged by transrectal ultrasound of the prostate

PENIS

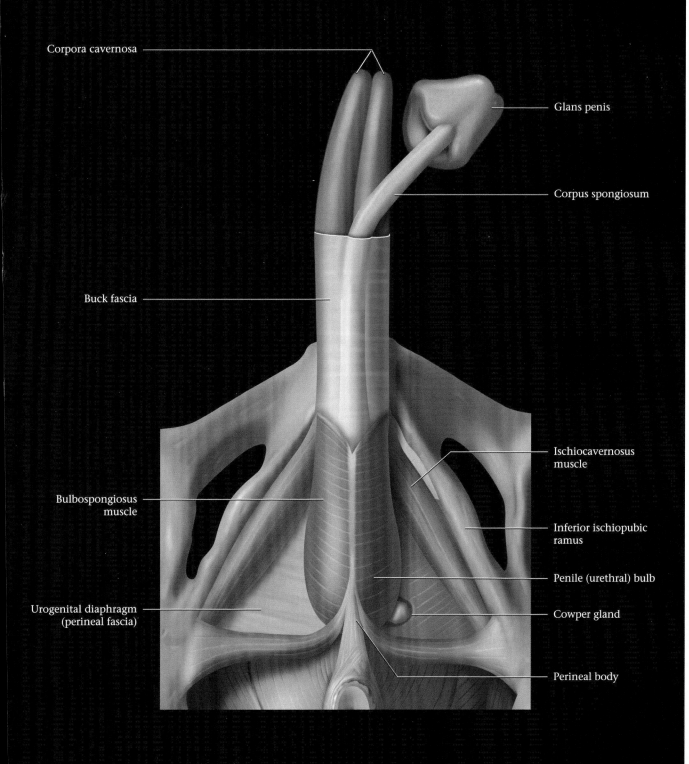

Corpora cavernosa

Glans penis

Corpus spongiosum

Buck fascia

Ischiocavernosus muscle

Bulbospongiosus muscle

Inferior ischiopubic ramus

Penile (urethral) bulb

Urogenital diaphragm (perineal fascia)

Cowper gland

Perineal body

Graphic shows that at the root of the penis, the corpora split into a triradiate form. The crura of the corpora cavernosa diverge and each crus is invested by an ischiocavernosus muscle. The corpus spongiosum remains midline and is invested by the bulbospongiosus muscle. It widens at its attachment to the urogenital diaphragm and is called the penile or urethral bulb. The root of the penis is firmly anchored between the urogenital diaphragm above and Colles fascia below (cut away to show perineal muscles). Additional supports include fascial attachments to the medial surface of the pubic rami and and pubic symphysis.

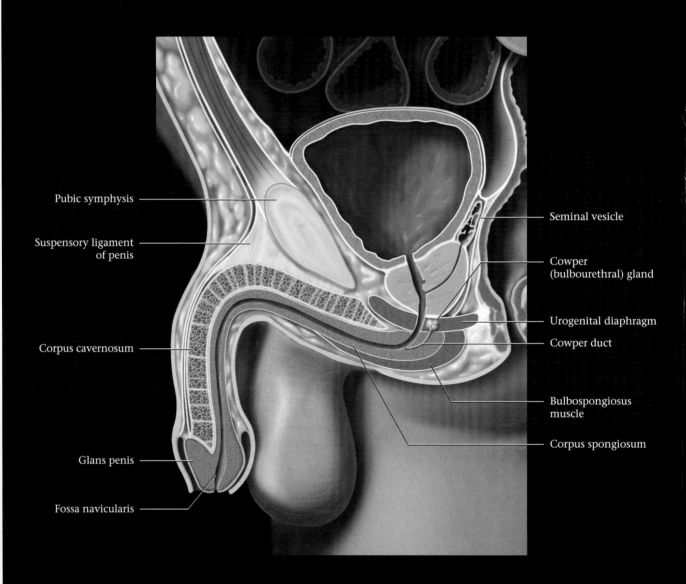

Pubic symphysis

Suspensory ligament
of penis

Corpus cavernosum

Glans penis

Fossa navicularis

Seminal vesicle

Cowper
(bulbourethral) gland

Urogenital diaphragm

Cowper duct

Bulbospongiosus
muscle

Corpus spongiosum

Sagittal midline graphic shows the course of the urethra. The anterior urethra runs within the corpus spongiosum. The external (pendulous) portion of the penis begins below the pubic symphysis, at the penoscrotal junction. It is fixed at this position by the suspensory ligament of the penis, which is part of the fundiform ligament, an inferior extension of the rectus sheath. The proximal (internal) urethral sphincter extends from the bladder neck to above the verumontanum. The distal, or external sphincter, has both intrinsic and extrinsic components. The intrinsic component is composed of concentric smooth muscle extending from the distal prostatic urethra through the membranous urethra. The surrounding extrinsic component is composed of striated muscle and is under voluntary control.

PENIS AND MALE URETHRA

MALE URETHRA

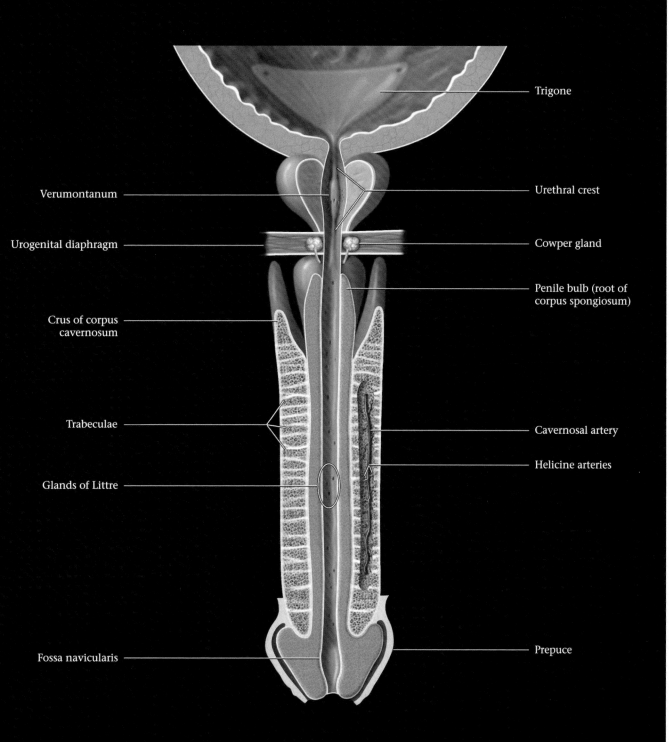

Trigone

Verumontanum

Urethral crest

Urogenital diaphragm

Cowper gland

Penile bulb (root of corpus spongiosum)

Crus of corpus cavernosum

Trabeculae

Cavernosal artery

Helicine arteries

Glands of Littre

Fossa navicularis

Prepuce

Graphic shows the posterior wall of the urethra from the bladder base to the fossa navicularis. The verumontanum is the most prominent portion of the urethral crest. The prostatic utricle (an embryologic remnant of the Müllerian system) enters in the center of the verumontanum, along with the ejaculatory ducts, which are just distal on either side. Cowper glands are within the urogenital diaphragm but their ducts course distally approximately 2 cm to enter the bulbous urethra. Multiple, small, mucosal glands (glands of Littré) line the mucosa of the anterior urethra. The corpora cavernosa are the primary erectile bodies. They are traversed by numerous trabeculae, creating sinusoidal spaces. The cavernosal artery runs within the center of each corpus cavernosum and gives rise to the helicine arteries, which flow into the sinusoids.

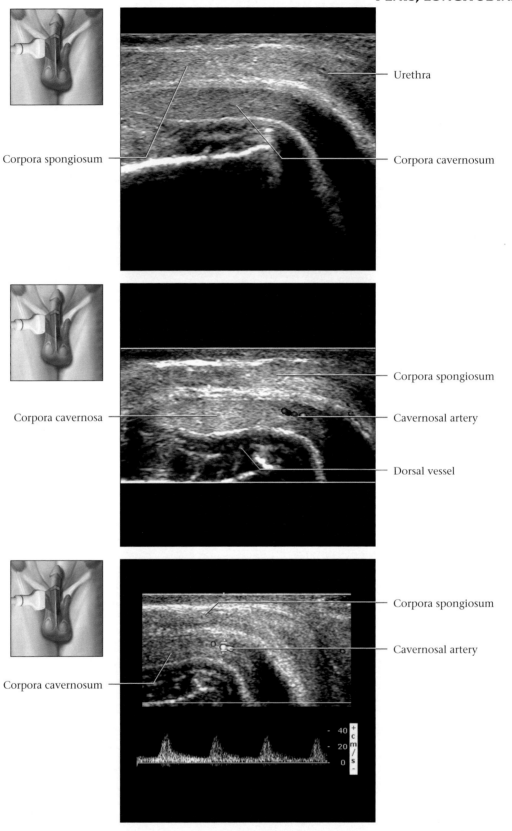

Urethra

Corpora spongiosum

Corpora cavernosum

Corpora cavernosa

Corpora spongiosum

Cavernosal artery

Dorsal vessel

Corpora spongiosum

Cavernosal artery

Corpora cavernosum

(Top) Longitudinal grayscale (GS) ultrasound of the penis. The penis lies on the anterior abdominal wall and is scanned on the ventral side. The urethra is identified within the substance of the corpora spongiosum. One of the paired corpora cavernosa, which is more hypoechoic relative to the spongiosum, is shown. (Middle) Longitudinal power Doppler ultrasound reveals the cavernosal artery within the corpora cavernosa. One of the vessels in the dorsal penis is imaged. (Bottom) Normal pulsed Doppler waveform of the cavernosal artery shows a peak systolic velocity of 34 cm/sec (normal value > 30 cm/s). Normal end diastolic velocity < 3 cm/sec.

URETHRA, LONGITUDINAL VIEW

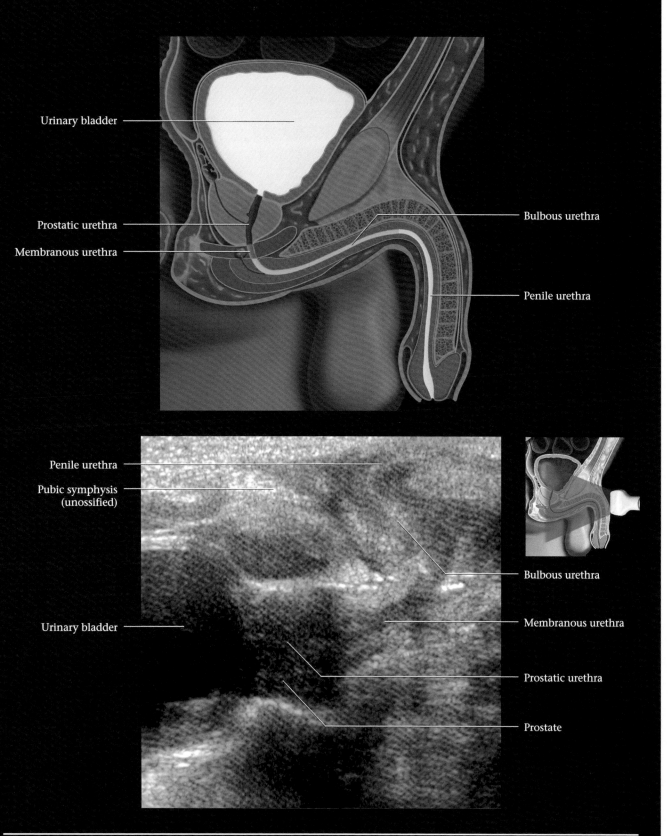

Urinary bladder

Prostatic urethra

Membranous urethra

Bulbous urethra

Penile urethra

Penile urethra

Pubic symphysis (unossified)

Urinary bladder

Bulbous urethra

Membranous urethra

Prostatic urethra

Prostate

(Top) Graphic shows the urethra's two major divisions: Anterior and posterior urethra, each with two parts. The posterior urethra is composed of the prostatic and membranous portions, and the anterior urethra is composed of the bulbous and penile portions. The prostatic urethra begins at the bladder base and extends to the apex of the prostatic gland. The membranous urethra traverses the urogenital diaphragm. It is the shortest portion of the urethra but the area most vulnerable to injury. The bulbous urethra extends from the bottom of the urogenital diaphragm to the suspensory ligament of the penis. The penile urethra is distal to the suspensory ligament and travels through the pendulous portion of the penis. It widens into the fossa navicularis at the distal glans. (Bottom) Longitudinal transpelvic/perineal ultrasound of a male neonate shows the urethral segments.

CORPORA CAVERNOSA, LONGITUDINAL VIEW

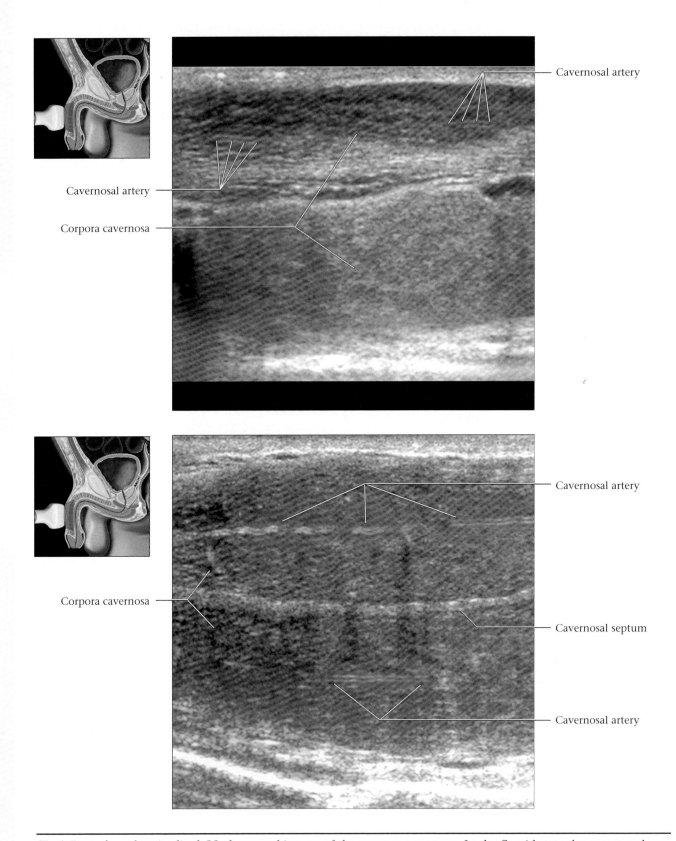

Cavernosal artery

Cavernosal artery

Corpora cavernosa

Cavernosal artery

Corpora cavernosa

Cavernosal septum

Cavernosal artery

(Top) First of two longitudinal GS ultrasound images of the corpora cavernosa. In the flaccid state the cavernosal arteries are tortuous, and can only be intermittently visualized in the longitudinal plane. Magnified views of the cavernosal artery should be used for vessel diameter measurements. Most measure < 1 mm in the flaccid state.
(Bottom) In the erect state, the cavernosal arteries assume a straighter course and can be easily imaged. The diameter should increase by 75% with erection. Failure to increase in size and an abnormal Doppler waveform is strong evidence of arteriogenic impotence. Despite the fact that each corpora is sheathed within its own tunica albuginea, there is significant communication across the septum between the two corpora cavernosa. Therefore when performing a study, only one corpus cavernosum needs to be injected with the vasodilating agent.

PENIS AND MALE URETHRA

PENIS, TRANSVERSE VIEW

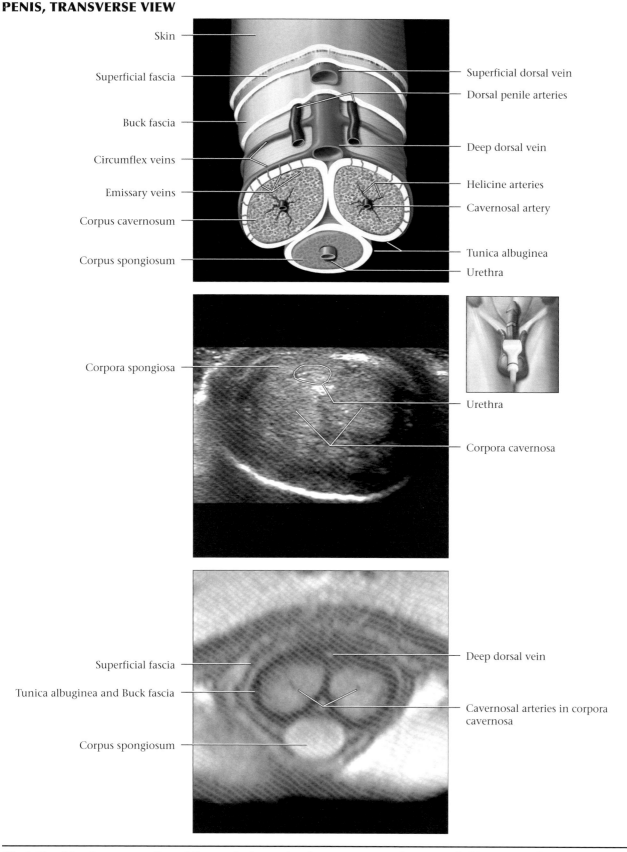

(**Top**) Graphic of a cross-section of the penis shows the three corpora, each surrounded by tunica albuginea. The cavernosal arteries run within the corpora cavernosa to become helicine arteries, which fill the sinusoids; drainage via the emissary veins ⇒ circumflex veins ⇒ deep dorsal vein of penis. With erection, emissary veins are compressed against tunica albuginea, occluding venous drainage. (**Middle**) Transverse grayscale ultrasound of the penis, scanning from the ventral side. The urethra assumes a slit-like configuration in its collapsed state and may be distended with fluid or gel during examination. (**Bottom**) T2 MR cross-section of the penis shows the low signal tunica albuginea surrounding each of the corpora (more prominent around the cavernosa). Buck fascia can not be separated from the tunica albuginea.

PENIS AND MALE URETHRA

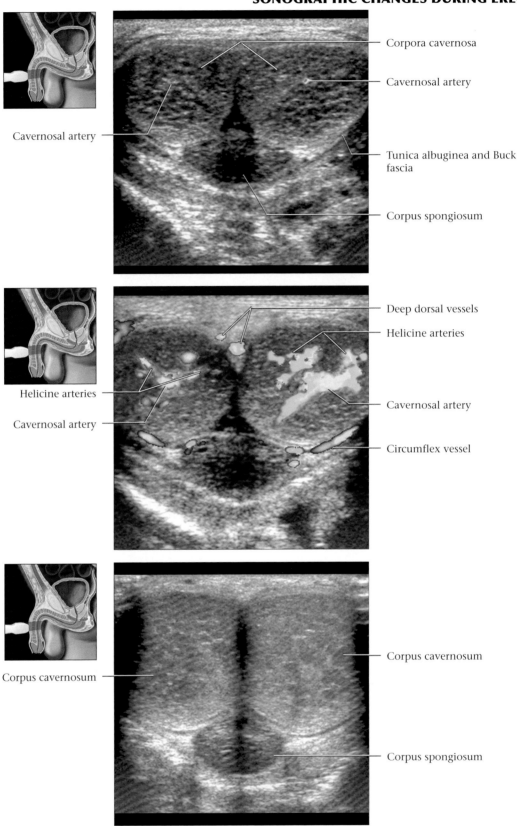

Corpora cavernosa

Cavernosal artery

Cavernosal artery

Tunica albuginea and Buck fascia

Corpus spongiosum

Deep dorsal vessels

Helicine arteries

Helicine arteries

Cavernosal artery

Cavernosal artery

Circumflex vessel

Corpus cavernosum

Corpus cavernosum

Corpus spongiosum

(Top) First of three cross-sectional ultrasound images of the penis shows the changing appearance during a normal erection. The paired corpora cavernosa are the primary erectile bodies. They are composed of a complex network of trabeculae, which create the sinusoids and give a "sponge-like" appearance on ultrasound. Each corpus is surrounded by a tough tunica albuginea, which appears as a thin echogenic line. Buck fascia, which surrounds all three corpora, is intimately associated with the tunica and cannot be distinguished as a separate structure. (Middle) Color Doppler ultrasound at the onset of an erection shows arterial inflow. There is dilation of the cavernosal and helicine arteries, as they begin to fill the sinusoidal spaces. (Bottom) With continued arterial inflow and compressed venous outflow, the corpora become maximally distended and rigid.

PENIS AND MALE URETHRA

ERECTION, CORRELATIVE SPECTRAL WAVEFORM

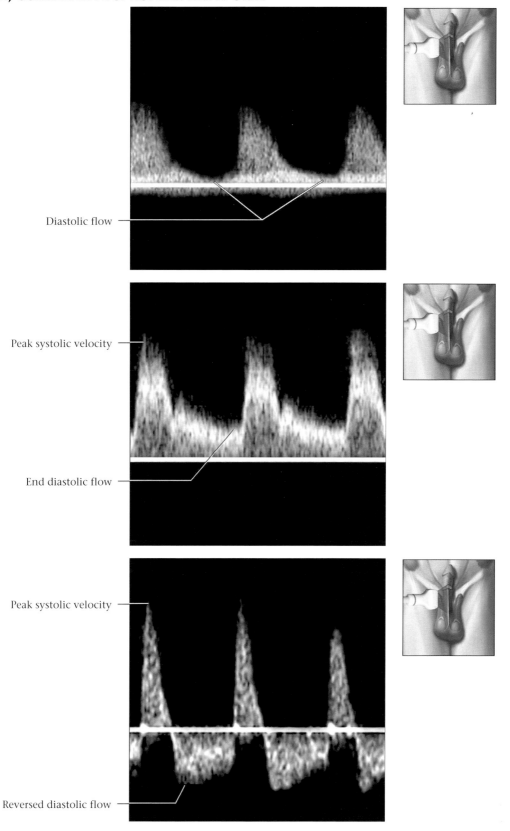

Diastolic flow

Peak systolic velocity

End diastolic flow

Peak systolic velocity

Reversed diastolic flow

(Top) First of 3 Doppler tracings shows changing arterial flow pattern during a normal erection. In the flaccid state, there is little to no diastolic flow. **(Middle)** At onset of erection, there is vasodilation of the cavernosal and helicine arteries (increased inflow), and smooth muscle relaxation within the sinusoids (decreased resistance). This causes a marked increase in both the peak systolic velocity (PSV) & end diastolic flow. **(Bottom)** In the fully erect state, the emissary veins are compressed against the rigid tunica albuginea, preventing outflow of blood. This dramatically increases the arterial resistance resulting in absent or reversed diastolic flow. A PSV > 30 cm/sec is considered normal, while < 25 cm/sec is strong evidence of arteriogenic impotence (25-30 borderline). Venogenic impotence is due to failure of draining vein occlusion. The Doppler trace would show continuous forward flow in diastole.

UTERUS

Terminology

Definitions
- Also referred to as "the womb"
- Major female reproductive organ

Imaging Anatomy

Overview
- Location: Midline in the true pelvis
- Anatomical division
  - Fundus: Uterine roof
  - Body (corpus): Upper 2/3 uterus
  - Cervix: Lower 1/3 uterus
  - Isthmus: Junction of body and cervix
- Position
  - Anteversion: Uterine body bends forward (commonest)
  - Anteflexion: Marked forward bending of the body
  - Retroversion: Uterine body bends backward
  - Retroflexion: Marked backward bending of the body
- Size: Body (corpus uteri) at reproductive age
  - 7.5-9.0 cm (length)
  - 4.5-6.0 cm (breadth)
  - 2.5-4.0 cm (thickness)
- Layers
  - Parametrium
    - Outer/serous layer; part of visceral peritoneum
    - Forms broad ligaments and rectouterine pouch (pouch of Douglas/cul-de-sac)
    - Appears as highly reflective uterine outline
  - Myometrium
    - Middle/muscular layer; forms main bulk of uterus
    - Homogeneous and of low echogenicity
    - Three zones: Inner (hypoechoic); middle (thicker; more echogenic); outer (outlined by arcuate arteries)
  - Endometrium
    - Internal/mucous layer
    - Thickness and echogenicity variable
    - Stratum functionale (inner) - much thicker and with cyclical changes
    - Stratum basale (outer) - thin and hypoechoic
- Peritoneum and ligaments
  - Vesicouterine pouch: Anterior recess between uterus and bladder
  - Rectouterine pouch of Douglas: Posterior recess between vaginal fornix and rectum
  - Broad ligaments
    - Paired; a double fold of peritoneum
    - Contain the fallopian tube superiorly and round ligament, ovaries, ovarian ligament and blood vessels inferiorly
- Vessels
  - Uterine artery (UA) arises from internal iliac artery (IIA) with variable flow resistance
    - High flow resistance: Periovulation, aging, infertility, endometriosis
    - Low flow resistance: Late secretory phase, hormonal therapy, fibroids, malignancy
  - Arcuate artery: Formed by anastomosis of both UAs; seen in the outer third of the myometrium
  - Radial artery: Arises from arcuate arteries penetrating vertically into the myometrium
  - Spiral artery: Arises from radial arteries in stratum functionale which sheds during menstruation
    - Assessment of spiral blood flow is important prior to embryo transfer
    - Absent subendometrial blood flow is always related to failure of implantation
  - Basal artery: Arises from radial arteries nourishing the outer basal layer of the endometrium which do not change during menstruation

Anatomy Relationships
- Anterior: Bladder
- On either side: Ovaries, broad ligaments
- Posterior: Rectouterine pouch of Douglas, rectum

Variations with Age
- Neonatal: Prominent size under effect of residual maternal hormone
- Infantile: Cervix > corpus (2:1)
- Prepubertal: Cervix = corpus (1:1)
- Reproductive: Cervix < corpus (1:2)
- Postmenopausal: Overall reduction in size

Variations with Menstrual Cycle
- Menstrual phase
  - Early: Cystic areas within echogenic endometrium indicating endometrial breakdown
  - Mid: Mixed appearance of cystic areas (blood) and hyperechoic areas (clot or sloughed endometrium)
  - Late: Thin, single-line endometrium
- Proliferative phase
  - Hyperechoic endometrium with thickness < 5 mm
- Periovulatory phase
  - Characteristic "triple-line" endometrium
- Secretory phase
  - Thick and bright endometrial lining < 16 mm

Developmental Anomalies
- Didelphys: Lack of fusion of fundus gives rise to deep fundal notch, double endometria, cervices and vaginas
- Bicornuate: Lack of fusion of fundus; usually double endometria, single cervix and single vagina
- Septate: Mild form of lack of fundal fusion; shallow fundal notch; two endometria separated by thin fibrous septum, single cervix and single vagina
- Unicornis with rudimentary horn: Difficult to recognize sonographically

Anatomy-Based Imaging Issues

Imaging Recommendations
- Transabdominal (TA) scan is good for providing overview of pelvic organs
- Transvaginal (TV) scan is excellent in assessing uterine morphological details

Imaging Pitfalls
- Uterine retroflexion may mimic intramural fibroid on transabdominal scan
  - Transvaginal scan is helpful to rule out the abnormality

UTERUS

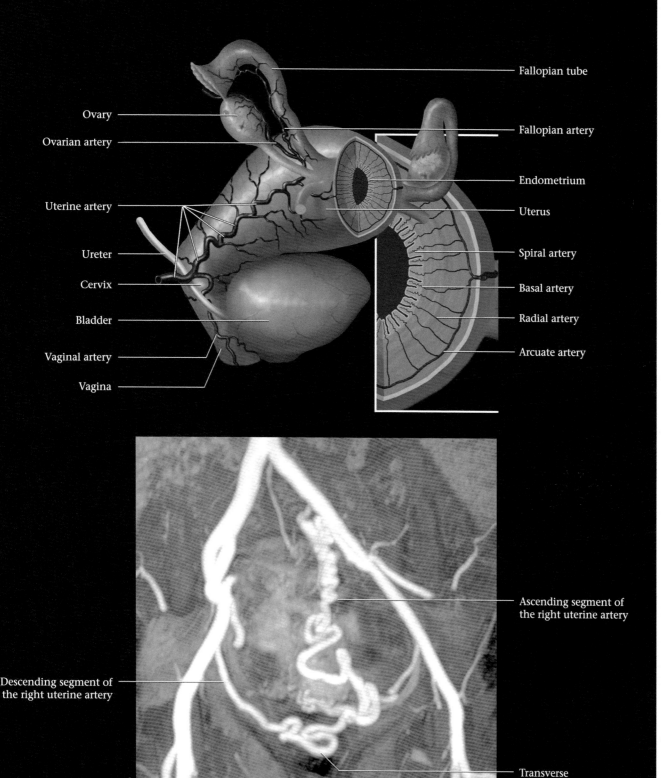

Fallopian tube

Ovary

Ovarian artery

Uterine artery

Ureter

Cervix

Bladder

Vaginal artery

Vagina

Fallopian artery

Endometrium

Uterus

Spiral artery

Basal artery

Radial artery

Arcuate artery

Ascending segment of the right uterine artery

Descending segment of the right uterine artery

Transverse (ligamentous) segment of right uterine artery

(Top) Diagram showing uterine vasculature. The descending segment of uterine artery after branching off from the internal iliac artery runs medially towards the cervix. The ascending segment ascends laterally along the uterine wall to meet the ovarian and fallopian arteries. The transverse segments cross the cardinal ligament and anastomose extensively with each other to form the arcuate arteries which give rise to the radial arteries penetrating the myometrium vertically. The arteries then branch into spiral and basal arteries in the functional and basal layers of the endometrium respectively. (Bottom) MR angiography shows the course of uterine artery branching off from the internal iliac artery.

UTERUS

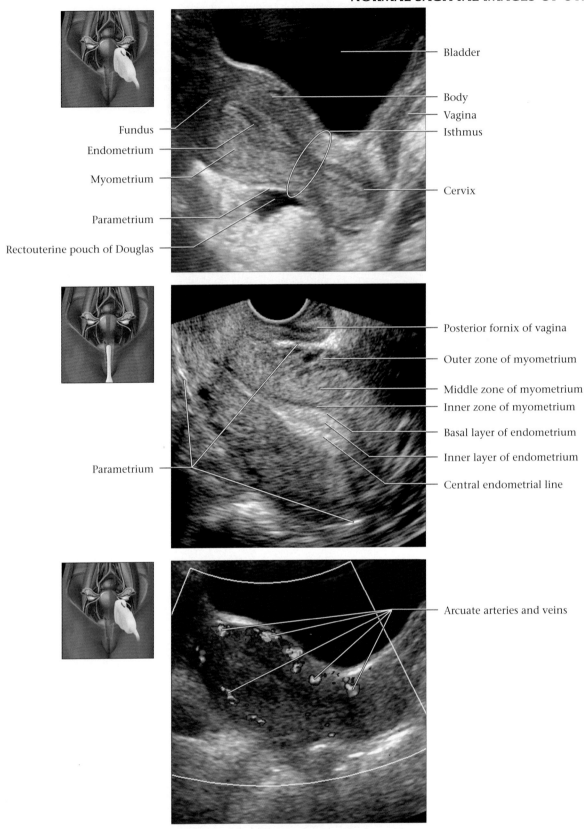

- Bladder
- Body
- Vagina
- Isthmus
- Cervix

Fundus
Endometrium
Myometrium
Parametrium
Rectouterine pouch of Douglas

- Posterior fornix of vagina
- Outer zone of myometrium
- Middle zone of myometrium
- Inner zone of myometrium
- Basal layer of endometrium
- Inner layer of endometrium
- Central endometrial line

Parametrium

- Arcuate arteries and veins

(Top) Longitudinal TA scan showing a normal anteverted uterus. Version refers to the angle the cervix makes with the vagina. In this case, the cervix is angled anteriorly and the uterus continues in a straight line with the cervix. This is the commonest position found in the female pelvis. **(Middle)** Longitudinal TV ultrasound demonstrates different zones in a retroflexed uterus. The smooth muscle within the inner zone of myometrium is more compact making it more hypoechoic (subendometrial halo). Majority of myometrium is homogeneously echogenic, with the outer zone being less echogenic. **(Bottom)** Color Doppler ultrasound, longitudinal TA scan, shows arcuate arteries and veins which run in the outer third of the myometrium.

UTERUS

NORMAL VARIATIONS, UTERINE POSITION

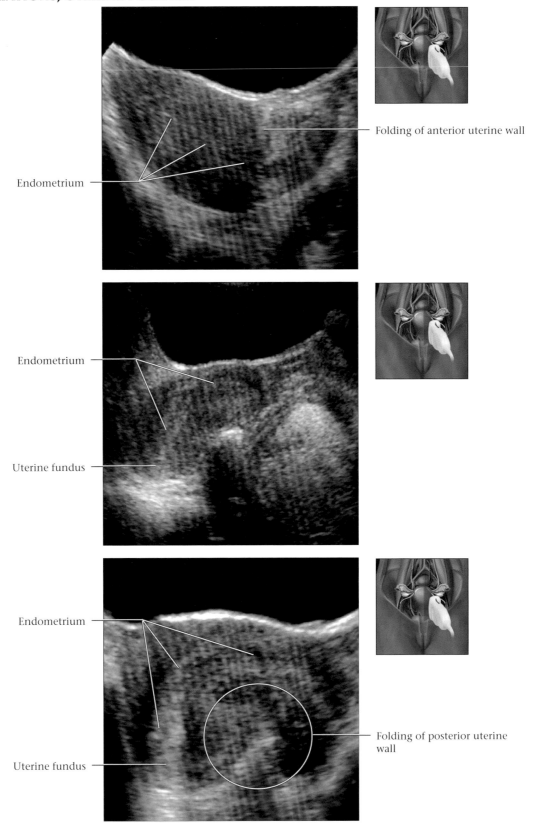

Endometrium ——— Folding of anterior uterine wall

Endometrium ———

Uterine fundus ———

Endometrium ———

Uterine fundus ——— Folding of posterior uterine wall

(Top) Longitudinal TA ultrasound of anteflexed uterus shows the uterine body is angled forward with respect to the cervix. Flexion refers to the angle the uterine body makes with the cervix, i.e. the uterus and the cervix are not in a straight line. (Middle) Uterine retroversion. Note the body of the uterus is bending backward with the uterine fundus pointing posteriorly. (Bottom) Uterine retroflexion. This is an exaggerated uterine retroversion in which the uterus resembles a "boxing glove". Folding of the posterior uterine wall may be confused with an intramural fibroid

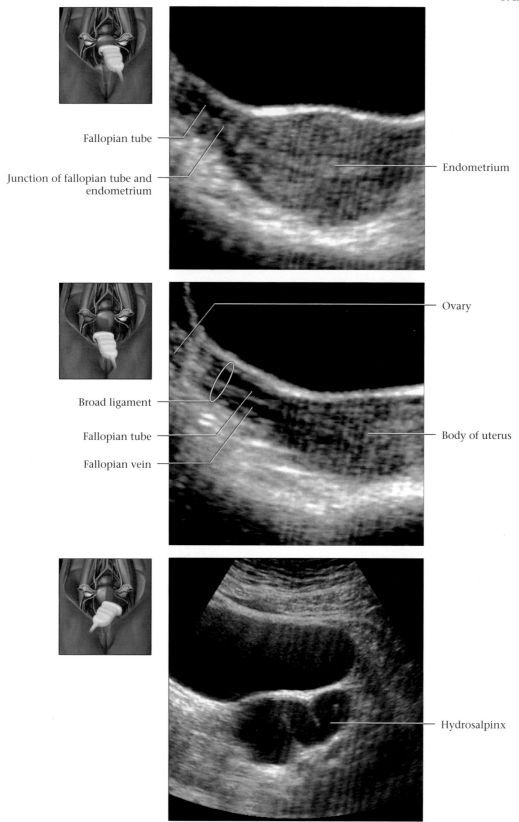

Fallopian tube

Junction of fallopian tube and endometrium

Endometrium

Ovary

Broad ligament

Fallopian tube

Fallopian vein

Body of uterus

Hydrosalpinx

(Top) Transverse TA ultrasound of the uterus at the level where the fallopian tube opens into the endometrial cavity. The fallopian tube has four segments including interstitial, isthmus, ampulla and infundibulum. This image shows the interstitial portion of the tube traversing the myometrial wall at the cornu. (Middle) Normal appearance of broad ligament shows fallopian tube with peristaltic movement and a fallopian vessel running parallel to the tube connecting uterus and ovary. (Bottom) Transverse TA ultrasound shows hydrosalpinx which is a dilated fluid-filled fallopian tube. It is important to elongate the tube during real-time scanning to differentiate it from a cystic ovarian mass.

FALLOPIAN TUBE

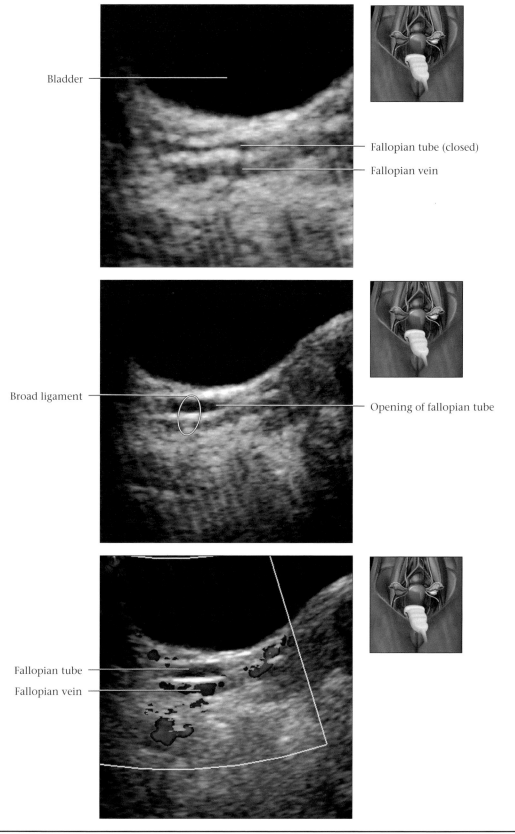

Bladder

Fallopian tube (closed)

Fallopian vein

Broad ligament

Opening of fallopian tube

Fallopian tube

Fallopian vein

(Top) Transverse transabdominal ultrasound of normal fallopian tube. This image and the middle image demonstrate the normal peristalsis of fallopian tube. **(Middle)** The fallopian tube demonstrates peristaltic movement with intermittent opening of the lumen. **(Bottom)** Color Doppler ultrasonography shows a fallopian vessel running parallel to the fallopian tube.

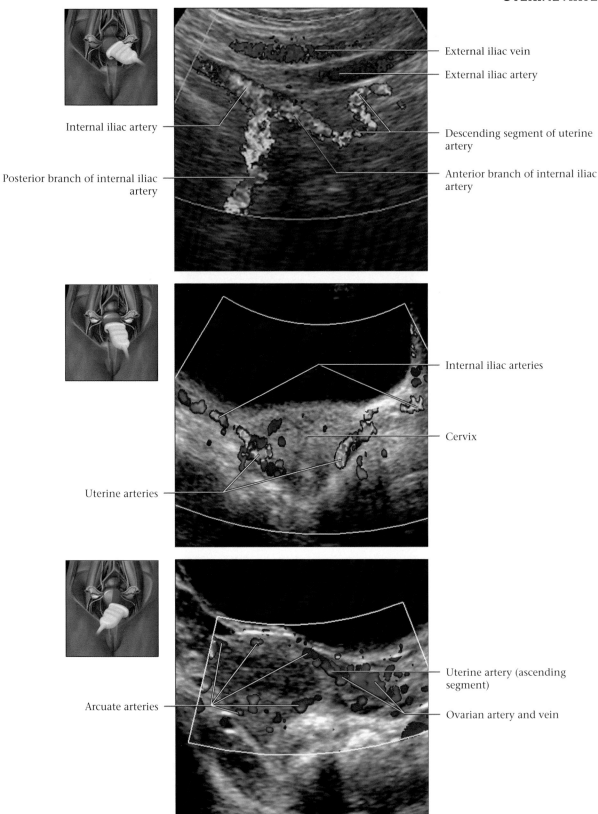

Internal iliac artery

Posterior branch of internal iliac artery

External iliac vein

External iliac artery

Descending segment of uterine artery

Anterior branch of internal iliac artery

Internal iliac arteries

Cervix

Uterine arteries

Arcuate arteries

Uterine artery (ascending segment)

Ovarian artery and vein

(Top) Longitudinal TA color Doppler ultrasound shows the uterine artery arising from the anterior branch of the internal iliac artery at the level of the uterine cervix. Uterine artery can also be assessed with transvaginal ultrasound by locating it lateral to the cervix. **(Middle)** Transverse TA color Doppler ultrasound shows descending branches of both uterine arteries running medially at the level of the cervix. Care must be taken not to confuse these with the iliac arteries which lie more laterally. **(Bottom)** Transverse color Doppler ultrasound at the level of uterine fundus. The UA is seen at the lateral wall of the uterus anastomosing with the ovarian artery. It then courses medially to give rise to the arcuate arteries in the uterus.

UTERINE ARTERY

Anterior segment of internal iliac artery

PS	83.10 cm/s
ED	12.59 cm/s
Accel	783.47 cm/s2
AT	0.090 s

INVERT AC 52

Uterine artery

Uterine artery (ascending segment)

Diastolic notch

(Top) Spectral Doppler imaging of the anterior segment of internal iliac artery which shows relatively high-resistance waveform with narrow systolic envelope, sharp systolic upstroke, high peak systolic velocity and reduced mid- and late-diastolic flow velocity. (Middle) Spectral Doppler imaging of UA. As compared to the top image, the waveform of UA has relatively lower resistance waveform than internal iliac artery with wider systolic envelope and lower peak systolic velocity. (Bottom) Spectral Doppler imaging of UA (ascending segment). The UA typically has a high resistance pattern with low end-diastolic flow and a notch. The UA flow resistance is highest at postovulatory phase and lowest at mid to late secretory phase.

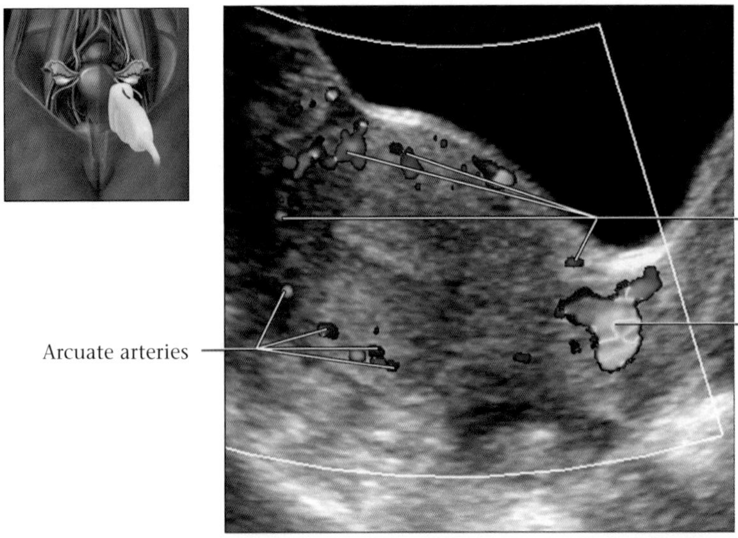

Arcuate veins

Descending trunk of uterine artery

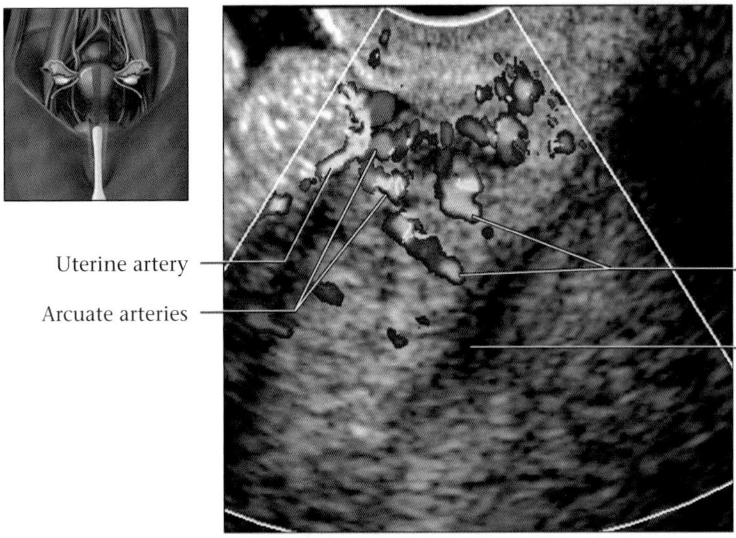

Arcuate arteries

Uterine artery

Arcuate arteries

Radial arteries

Endometrial canal

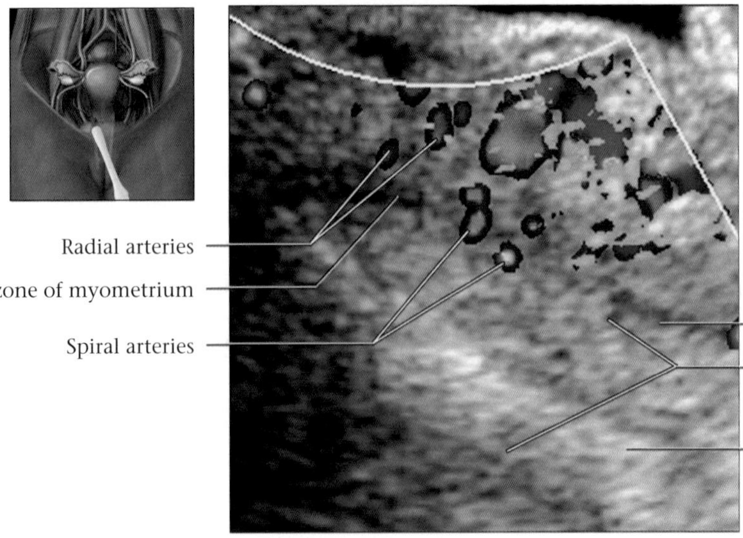

Radial arteries

Inner zone of myometrium

Spiral arteries

Stratum basale

Stratum functionale

Central endometrial line

(Top) Longitudinal TA color Doppler scan shows the arcuate arteries and veins located at the periphery of the uterus. The arcuate arteries commonly calcify with advancing age. **(Middle)** Longitudinal TV color Doppler imaging shows arcuate arteries branching off from the UA. It then gives rise to radial arteries which run vertically in the myometrium. **(Bottom)** Magnified view focusing on the intrauterine vasculature near the junction of myometrium and endometrium. Transvaginal color Doppler image demonstrates the spiral arteries arising from radial arteries and penetrating deep into the stratum functionale of the endometrium which sheds during menstruation.

INTRAUTERINE ARTERIES

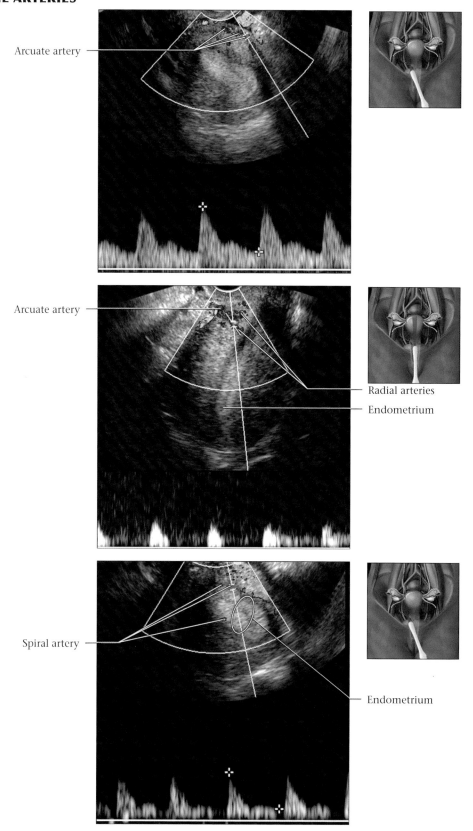

Arcuate artery

Arcuate artery

Radial arteries

Endometrium

Spiral artery

Endometrium

(Top) Transvaginal spectral Doppler image of the arcuate artery demonstrates the typical low-resistance waveform at late secretory phase. It is consistent with the presence of a thick and echogenic endometrium. (Middle) Transvaginal spectral Doppler image of the radial artery. The radial and spiral arteries are usually inconsistently seen during proliferative phase or in postmenopausal women. (Bottom) Transvaginal spectral Doppler waveform of the spiral artery demonstrates low resistance waveform which is normal in late secretory phase. The usual pattern is of a gradual decrease in resistance in the more peripheral arteries.

UTERUS

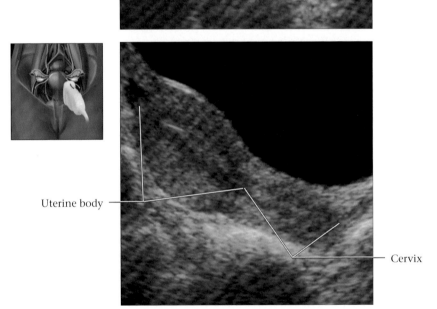

Uterine body

Endometrium

Cervix

Uterine body

Cervix

Uterine body

Cervix

(Top) Longitudinal TA scan of an immediate neonatal uterus (day 4). The uterus is prominent with a bulbous cervix and a rudimentary body. The endometrium is seen as a thin echogenic line which may be due to stimulation by the residual maternal hormones. **(Middle)** Longitudinal TA scan of a prepubertal uterus (5 years old). The uterus demonstrates a tubular appearance with the length of the cervix nearly double that of the uterine body. **(Bottom)** Longitudinal TA scan of an early pubertal uterus (15 years old). The body length of the uterus approximates the cervical length with the endometrium changing in appearance and thickness during the menstrual cycle. At this time, the uterine body grows dramatically until it reaches the adult size.

UTERUS

UTERINE VARIATIONS WITH AGE

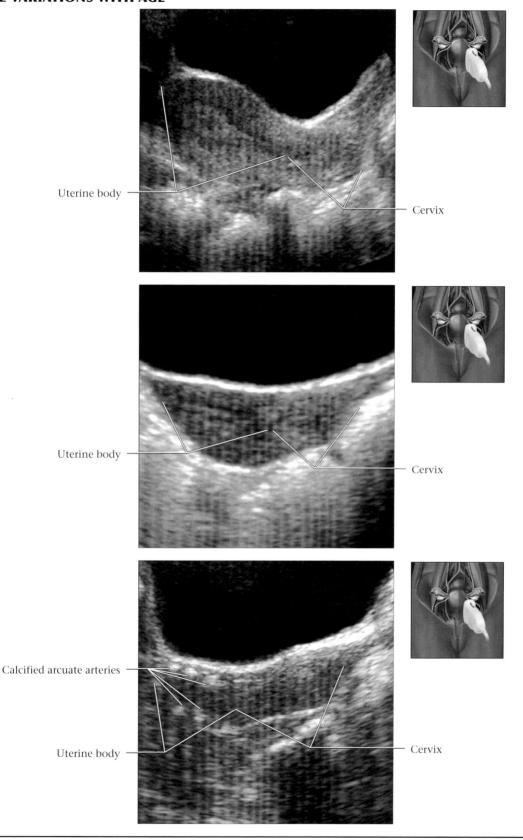

Uterine body — Cervix

Uterine body — Cervix

Calcified arcuate arteries

Uterine body — Cervix

(Top) Longitudinal TA scan of a nulliparous uterus. The normal adult uterus should attain a "pear-shaped" or "hour-glass" appearance with the length of the uterine body doubles that of the cervix. The size of a nulliparous uterus is usually smaller than that of a parous uterus. **(Middle)** Longitudinal TA scan of an early postmenopausal uterus. The uterus is atrophic with prominent reduction in body size relative to the cervix. **(Bottom)** Longitudinal TA scan of a later postmenopausal uterus. Note its cervix to body ratio is similar to that of a prepubertal uterus. The arcuate arteries are commonly calcified and are seen as echogenic foci in the periphery of the uterine body.

CYCLIC CHANGES OF THE ENDOMETRIUM

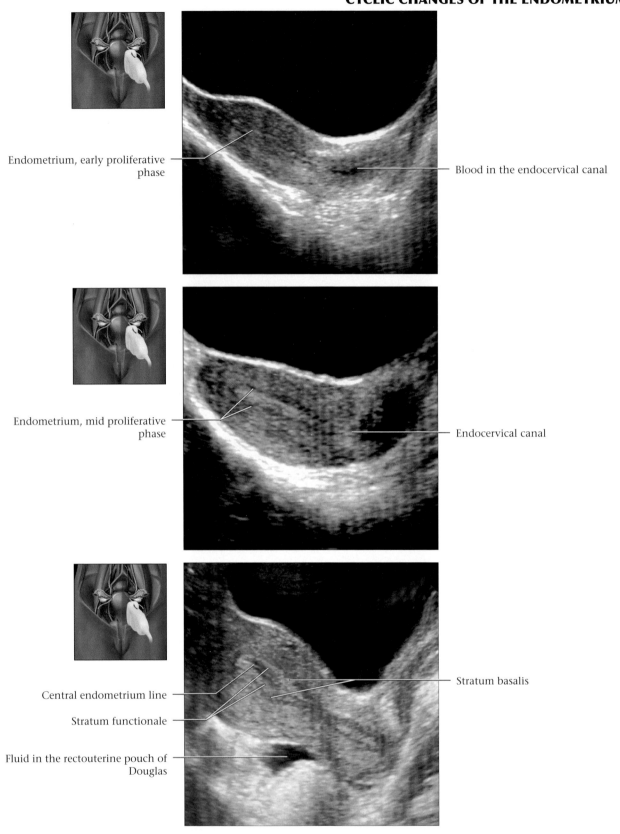

Endometrium, early proliferative phase

Blood in the endocervical canal

Endometrium, mid proliferative phase

Endocervical canal

Central endometrium line

Stratum basalis

Stratum functionale

Fluid in the rectouterine pouch of Douglas

(Top) Longitudinal TA scan of endometrium in the postmenstrual or early proliferative phase. Note the endometrium is thin and echogenic with small amount of blood present in the endocervical canal. (Middle) Longitudinal TA scan of endometrium during mid proliferative phase shows the endometrium progressively thickened and more echogenic. (Bottom) Longitudinal TA scan of uterus in periovulatory phase shows thickening of the stratum functionale with an echogenic central line and layered, "sandwich" appearance of the endometrium. Small amount of free fluid is usually present in the rectouterine pouch of Douglas.

CYCLIC CHANGES OF THE ENDOMETRIUM

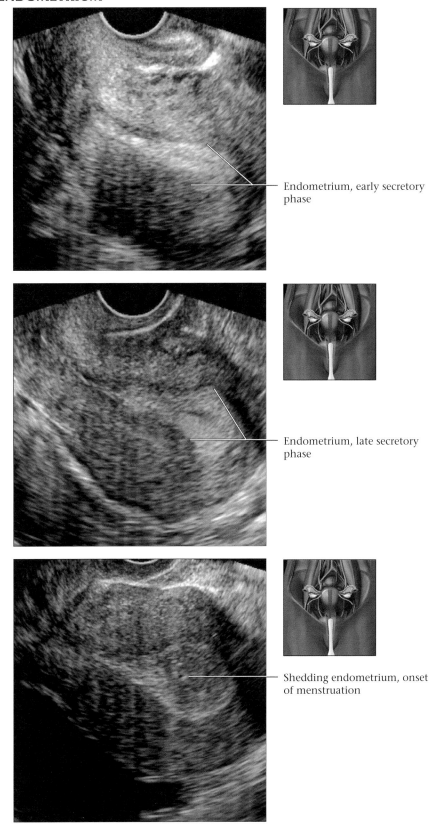

Endometrium, early secretory phase

Endometrium, late secretory phase

Shedding endometrium, onset of menstruation

(**Top**) Cyclic endometrial changes in a retroflexed uterus. Longitudinal TV scan of the endometrium during the early secretory phase. The endometrium becomes progressively thickened and more echogenic. (**Middle**) Longitudinal TV scan in the late secretory phase shows the endometrium is uniformly thickened and echogenic. The normal maximal endometrial thickness should not exceed 1.6 cm. (**Bottom**) Longitudinal TV scan shows an area of hypoechogenicity in a thickened endometrium on day 1 of menstruation, which likely represents the shedding endometrium. Small amount of fluid may be seen within the endometrial cavity.

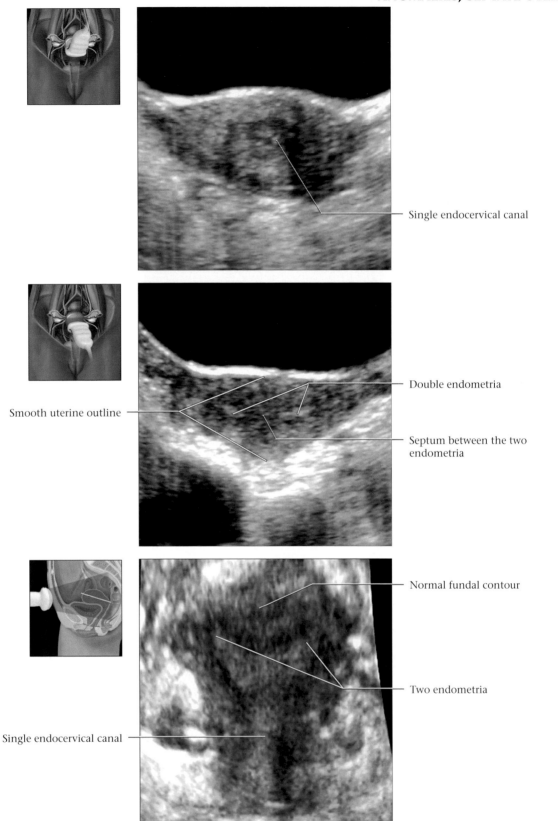

Single endocervical canal

Double endometria

Smooth uterine outline

Septum between the two endometria

Normal fundal contour

Two endometria

Single endocervical canal

(Top) Transverse TA scan of the cervix of a septate uterus. Single endocervical canal is demonstrated with ultrasound appearance indistinct from that of a normal uterus. (Middle) More cephalad transverse scan of the corresponding septate uterus at the level of the fundus shows two distinct endometria. Note the fundal contour is smooth and normal without indentation. The finding is more suggestive of a septate uterus rather than a bicornuate uterus. However, the anomaly is better delineated by 3D ultrasound or MR. (Bottom) 3D ultrasound of previous septate uterus shows the en-face view of the two endometrial echoes and single endocervical canal resembling a letter "Y". A septate uterus can be confidently differentiated from a didelphic or bicornuate uterus by the demonstration of a single endocervical canal and normal smooth fundal contour.

UTERUS

ANOMALIES, DIDELPHIC UTERUS

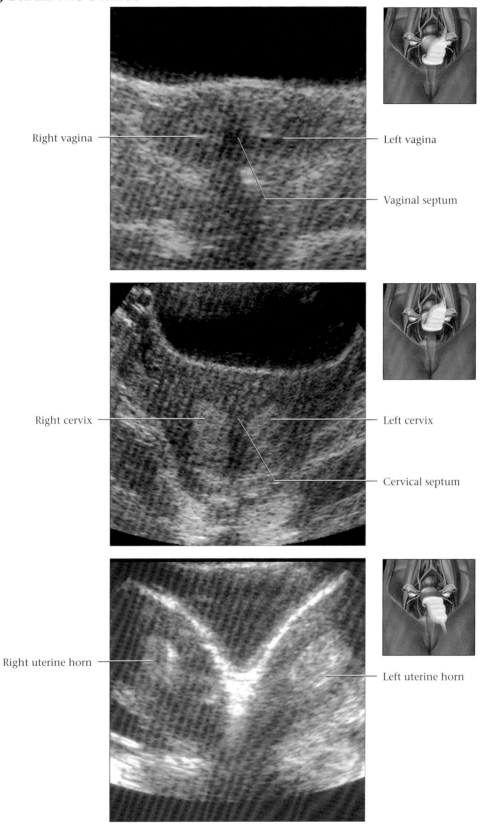

Right vagina — Left vagina

Vaginal septum

Right cervix — Left cervix

Cervical septum

Right uterine horn — Left uterine horn

(Top) Transverse TA scan of didelphic uterus. This malformation has the appearance of two unicornuate uteri lying side-by-side. Two vaginas are identified. A vaginal septum is seen in approximately 75% of cases. **(Middle)** Two distinct cervices are separated by a thick cervical septum. **(Bottom)** There are two separate uterine horns, each with a thick echogenic endometrial echo complex.

CERVIX

Gross Anatomy

Overview

- Begins at inferior narrowing of uterus (isthmus)
  - Supravaginal portion: Endocervix
  - Vaginal portion: Ectocervix
- Endocervical canal: Spindle-shaped cavity communicates with uterine body and vagina
- Internal os: Opening into uterine cavity
- External os: Opening into vagina
- Largely fibrous stroma with high proportion of elastic fibers interwoven with smooth muscle
- Endocervical canal lined by mucous secreting columnar epithelium
  - Epithelium in a series of small V-shaped folds (plicae palmatae)
- Ectocervix lined by stratified squamous epithelium
- Squamocolumnar junction near external os but exact position variable
- Nabothian cysts are commonly seen
  - Represent obstructed mucous-secreting glands
- Entire cervix is extraperitoneal
  - Anterior: Peritoneum reflects over dome of bladder above level of internal os
  - Posterior: Peritoneum extends along posterior vaginal fornix, creating rectouterine pouch (of Douglas)
- Arteries, veins, nerves and lymphatics
  - Arterial supply
    - Descending branch of uterine artery from internal iliac artery
  - Venous drainage
    - To uterine vein and drains into internal iliac vein
  - Lymphatics
    - Drain into internal and external iliac lymph nodes
  - Innervation
    - Sympathetic and parasympathetic nerves from branches of inferior hypogastric plexuses
- Variations with pregnancy
  - Nulliparous: Circular external os, arterial waveform shows high resistivity index (RI)
  - During pregnancy: Changes become apparent by ~ 6 weeks of gestation
    - Softened and enlarged cervix due to engorgement with blood with decreased RI of uterine artery
    - Hypertrophy of mucosa of cervical canal: Increased echogenicity of mucosal layer
    - Increased secretion of mucous glands: Increased volume of mucus ± mucus plug in cervical canal
  - Parous: Larger vaginal part of cervix, external os opens out transversely with an anterior and posterior lips
- Variations with age: Cervix grows less with age than uterus
  - Neonatal: Adult configuration due to residual maternal hormonal stimulation
  - Infantile: Cervix predominant with cervix to corpus length ratio ~ 2:1
  - Prepubertal: Cervix to corpus length ratio ~ 1:1
  - Reproductive: Uterus predominant, cervix to corpus length ratio ≥ 1:2
  - Postmenopausal: Overall reduction in size

Anatomy Relationships

- Anterior
  - Supravaginal cervix: Superior surface of bladder
  - Vaginal cervix: Anterior fornix of vagina
- Posterior
  - Supravaginal cervix: Rectouterine pouch (of Douglas)
  - Vaginal cervix: Posterior fornix of vagina
- Lateral
  - Supravaginal cervix: Bilateral ureters
  - Vaginal cervix: Lateral fornices of vagina
- Ligamentous support: Condensations of pelvic fascia attached to cervix and vaginal vault
  - Transverse cervical (cardinal) ligaments
    - Fibromuscular condensations of pelvic fascia
    - Pass to cervix and upper vagina from lateral walls of pelvis
  - Pubocervical ligaments
    - Two firm bands of connective tissue
    - Extend from posterior surface of pubis, position on either side of neck of bladder and then attach to anterior aspect of cervix
  - Sacrocervical ligaments
    - Fibromuscular condensations
    - Attach posterior aspect of cervix and upper vagina from lower end of sacrum
    - Form two ridges, one on either side of rectouterine pouch of Douglas

Imaging Anatomy

Ultrasound

- Transabdominal scan
  - Mucus within endocervical canal usually creates echogenic interface
  - In periovulatory phase cervical mucus becomes hypoechoic due to high fluid content
  - Mucosal layer: Echogenic
    - Thickness and echogenicity shows cyclical changes similar to endometrium
  - Submucosal layer: Hypoechoic
  - Cervical stroma: Intermediate to echogenic
- Transvaginal scan
  - Not as readily depicted due to proximity of transducer to the cervix
  - Obtain images with withdrawal of probe to mid-vagina

MR

- Important in local staging of cervical cancer
- Uniform intermediate signal on T1WI
- Zonal anatomy on T2WI
  - Endocervical canal: High signal
  - Cervical stroma: Predominately low signal, contiguous with junctional zone
  - Outer layer of smooth muscle (variably present): Intermediate signal
  - Parametrium: Variable signal intensity
    - Cardinal ligament and associated venous plexuses high signal
    - Sacrocervical ligament low signal

CERVIX

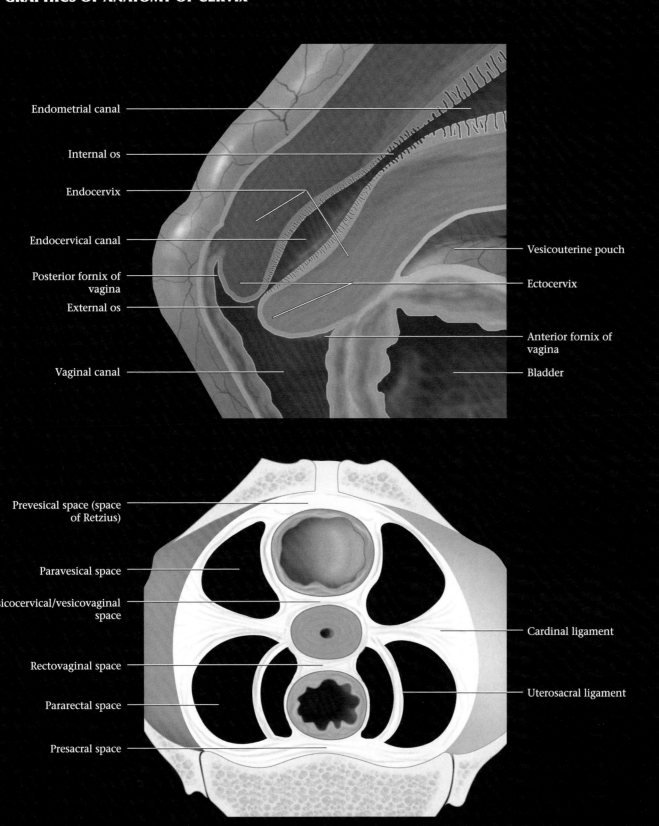

Top image labels:
- Endometrial canal
- Internal os
- Endocervix
- Endocervical canal
- Posterior fornix of vagina
- External os
- Vaginal canal
- Vesicouterine pouch
- Ectocervix
- Anterior fornix of vagina
- Bladder

Bottom image labels:
- Prevesical space (space of Retzius)
- Paravesical space
- Vesicocervical/vesicovaginal space
- Rectovaginal space
- Pararectal space
- Presacral space
- Cardinal ligament
- Uterosacral ligament

(Top) Median sagittal graphic shows the cervix which begins at the isthmus, the inferior narrowing portion, of the uterus. It has a supravaginal portion (endocervix) and a vaginal portion (ectocervix) which divides the vagina into shallow anterior fornix, deep posterior and lateral fornices. **(Bottom)** Schematic representation of the female pelvic ligaments and spaces at the cervical/vaginal junction. The ligaments are visceral ligaments, which are composed of specialized endopelvic fascia and contain vessels, nerves and lymphatics. Some of the main supporting ligaments for the uterus are attached to the cervix which are cardinal and uterosacral ligaments. The spaces are largely filled with loose connective tissue and are used as dissection planes during surgery.

CERVIX

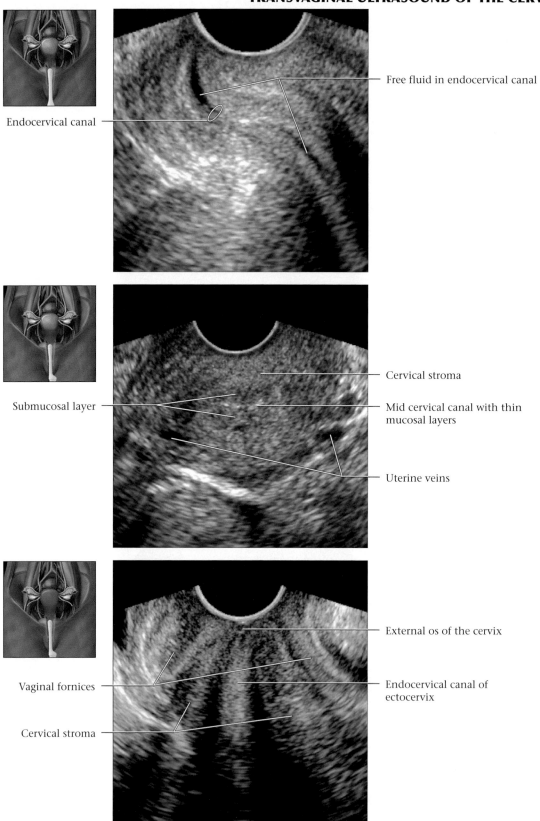

Endocervical canal — Free fluid in endocervical canal

Submucosal layer — Cervical stroma

Mid cervical canal with thin mucosal layers

Uterine veins

Vaginal fornices — External os of the cervix

Cervical stroma — Endocervical canal of ectocervix

(Top) Sagittal transvaginal scan of the cervix shows hypoechoic fluid present in the endocervical canal. The endocervical canal is rich in mucous secreting glands, the mucous secreted is usually slightly echogenic but becomes hypoechoic during periovulatory phase. (Middle) Transverse transvaginal scan of the cervix at the mid endocervical canal shows typical appearance with echogenic mucosal layers, hypoechoic band of submucosal layer and intermediate echogenic stroma. The submucosal layer is filled with mucous secreting gland leading to its hypoechoic appearance. (Bottom) Coronal transvaginal scan shows the transducer in touch with external os. The two lateral vaginal fornices are seen lying on its sides.

CERVIX

TRANSABDOMINAL ULTRASOUND OF THE CERVIX

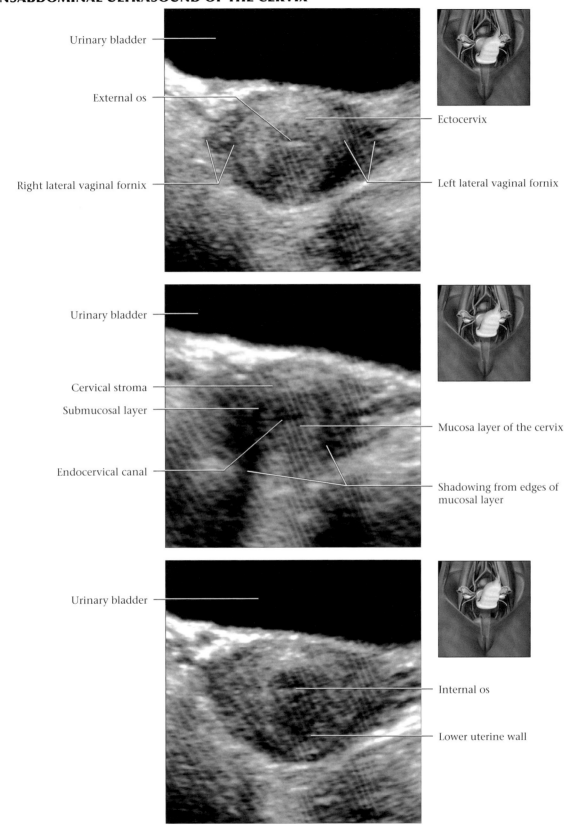

Urinary bladder

External os

Right lateral vaginal fornix

Ectocervix

Left lateral vaginal fornix

Urinary bladder

Cervical stroma

Submucosal layer

Endocervical canal

Mucosa layer of the cervix

Shadowing from edges of mucosal layer

Urinary bladder

Internal os

Lower uterine wall

(Top) Transverse transabdominal scan of the ectocervix at the level of external os. The lateral vaginal fornices are seen as relatively hypoechoic areas on each side of the ectocervix. (Middle) Transverse transabdominal scan of the mid-endocervix shows the mildly thickened and echogenic mucosal layer. Note that, during the menstrual cycle, the thickness and echogenicity of the mucosal layer undergoes changes as the endometrium does. When thickened, it typically casts shadowing from its edges. (Bottom) Transverse transabdominal scan of the upper cervix at the level of the internal os, which opens into the uterine cavity. Identification of the internal os is clinically significant in pregnancy for placental site localization.

CERVIX

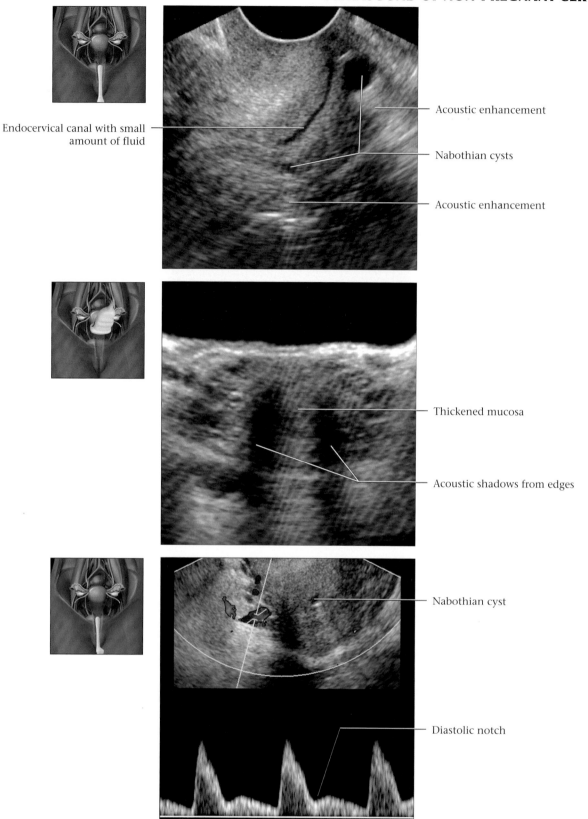

Endocervical canal with small amount of fluid

Acoustic enhancement

Nabothian cysts

Acoustic enhancement

Thickened mucosa

Acoustic shadows from edges

Nabothian cyst

Diastolic notch

(Top) Longitudinal transvaginal ultrasound of cervix and lower uterus shows two Nabothian cysts with marked posterior enhancement. Nabothian cyst is a common sonographic finding in the cervix and is usually anechoic but sometimes can contain internal debris. It is generally of no clinical significance. (Middle) Transverse transabdominal scan at the level of the cervix of a non-pregnant uterus commonly shows thickened mucosal layers casting shadows from its edges. (Bottom) Transverse transvaginal scan shows spectral waveform of the uterine artery at the lateral margin of a non-pregnant cervix shows typical high-resistance flow with a diastolic notch. In normal women, the Doppler waveform usually demonstrates a high resistance pattern except in late secretory phase.

CERVIX

ULTRASOUND OF CERVIX DURING PREGNANCY

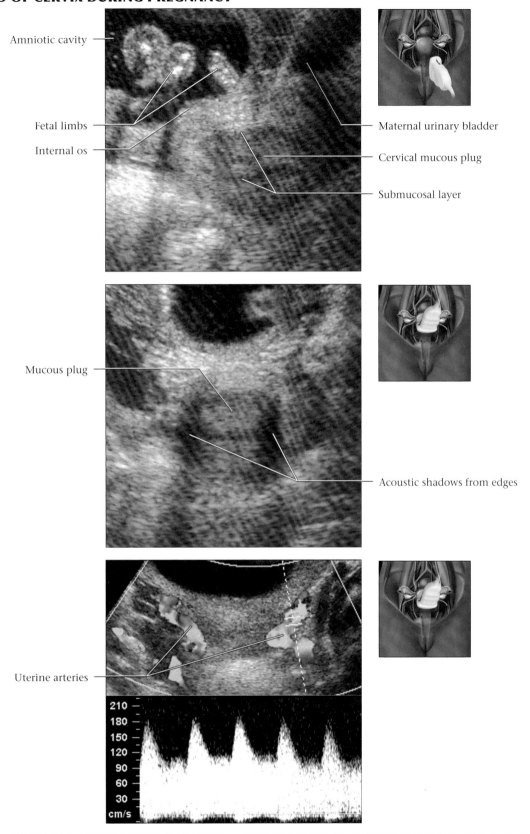

Amniotic cavity

Fetal limbs

Internal os

Maternal urinary bladder

Cervical mucous plug

Submucosal layer

Mucous plug

Acoustic shadows from edges

Uterine arteries

210
180
150
120
90
60
30
cm/s

(Top) Longitudinal transabdominal scan of the cervix during pregnancy. Cervical mucous increases in volume and echogenicity during pregnancy. The mucous is so thick that it forms a plug at the endocervical canal that provides extra support for the competence of cervix during pregnancy. (Middle) Transverse transabdominal scan shows the typical thick and echogenic mucous plug in a pregnant cervix casting dense shadows from its edges. (Bottom) As softening of the cervix due to engorgement with blood becomes apparent by 6 weeks after conception, the changes can be reflected in the uterine artery with high-velocity, low-resistance flow seen on this transabdominal spectral Doppler examination.

VAGINA

Terminology

Abbreviations
- Ultrasound (US), vaginal artery (VA), uterine artery (UA)

Gross Anatomy

Overview
- Muscular tube formed by smooth muscle and elastic connective fibers
- Serves as excretory duct for uterus, female organ for copulation and part of birth canal
- Extends up and back from vestibule of external genitalia to surround the cervix of uterus
- Has anterior and posterior walls, normally in apposition, with longer posterior wall
- Superiorly, cervix projects downward and backward into vagina and divides vagina into a shallow anterior, deep posterior and lateral fornices
- Upper half of vagina lies above pelvic floor, lower half lies within perineum
- Lined with stratified squamous epithelium
- Inner mucosal surface of the wall form rugae when collapsed
- Thin mucosal fold called hymen surrounds the entrance to vaginal orifice
- Outer surface, adventitial coat, is a thin fibrous layer continuous with surrounding endopelvic fascia
- Vasculature
  - Arterial supply
    - VA: Can branch off directly from the internal iliac artery (anterior trunk) or sometimes from the inferior vesical artery or UA
    - Vaginal branches of UA
    - Branches of VA and UA anastomose to form two median longitudinal vessels: Azygos arteries, one in front and one behind the vagina
  - Venous drainage
    - Form venous plexus around vagina
    - Eventually drains to internal iliac veins
- Variations with age
  - Menarche: 7-10 cm long
  - Postmenopausal: Shrinks in length and diameter, fornices virtually disappear

Anatomy Relationships
- Anterior
  - Superior: Bladder base
  - Inferior: Urethra
- Posterior
  - Upper 1/3: Rectouterine pouch of Douglas
  - Middle 1/3: Ampulla of rectum
  - Lower 1/3: Perineal body
- Lateral
  - Upper 1/3: Ureters
  - Middle 1/3: Levator ani and pelvic fascia
  - Lower 1/3: Bulb of vestibule, urogenital diaphragm and bulbospongiosus muscles
- Ligamentous supports
  - Upper 1/3: Levator ani muscles, transverse cervical (cardinal), pubocervical and sacrocervical ligaments
  - Middle 1/3: Urogenital diaphragm
  - Lower 1/3: Perineal body

Imaging Anatomy

Ultrasound
- Transabdominal US with distended bladder is standard imaging technique
  - Caudal angulation on both longitudinal and transverse scans
  - Commonly found at/near sagittal midline of pelvis
  - Length and wall thickness vary in response to bladder and rectal filling
  - Combined thickness of anterior and posterior vaginal walls should not exceed 1 cm for transabdominal scan with distended bladder
  - Characteristic appearance of three parallel lines
    - Highly echogenic mucosa center, may be difficult to visualize if stretched by distended bladder
    - Moderately hypoechoic muscular walls
- Transperineal US with nondistended bladder for assessment of uterine prolapse or for difficult cases
  - Vagina especially the vaginal canal is less well-defined

Embryology
- Uterus and upper vagina are formed from paired Müllerian (paramesonephric) ducts
- Paired ducts meet in midline and fuse, forming uterovaginal canal
- Lower vagina is formed from urogenital sinus

Clinical Implications

Uterine Prolapse
- Ligamentous support of pelvic organs may be damaged or become lax leading to uterine prolapse or prolapse of vaginal walls
- Cystocele: Sagging of bladder with bulging of anterior vaginal wall
- Rectocele: Sagging of ampulla of rectum with bulging of posterior vaginal wall
- Best to be investigated by transperineal US

Müllerian Duct Anomalies
- Failure of Müllerian duct development ± fusion
- Uterus didelphys (class III anomaly) most commonly affects vagina; a vaginal septum seen in ~ 75% of cases

Pelvic Abscess
- Common site: Rectouterine pouch of Douglas
- Feasible for transvaginal US guided drainage of pelvic abscess without doing major operation

Persistent Sexual Arousal Syndrome
- Persistent sexual arousal during sleep in postmenopausal women
- VA blood flow as one of the diagnostic aids
- VA normally shows high resistance flow
- During sexual arousal, increase blood flow to VA with low-resistance spectral waveform

VAGINA

GRAPHICS OF NORMAL VAGINAL ANATOMY

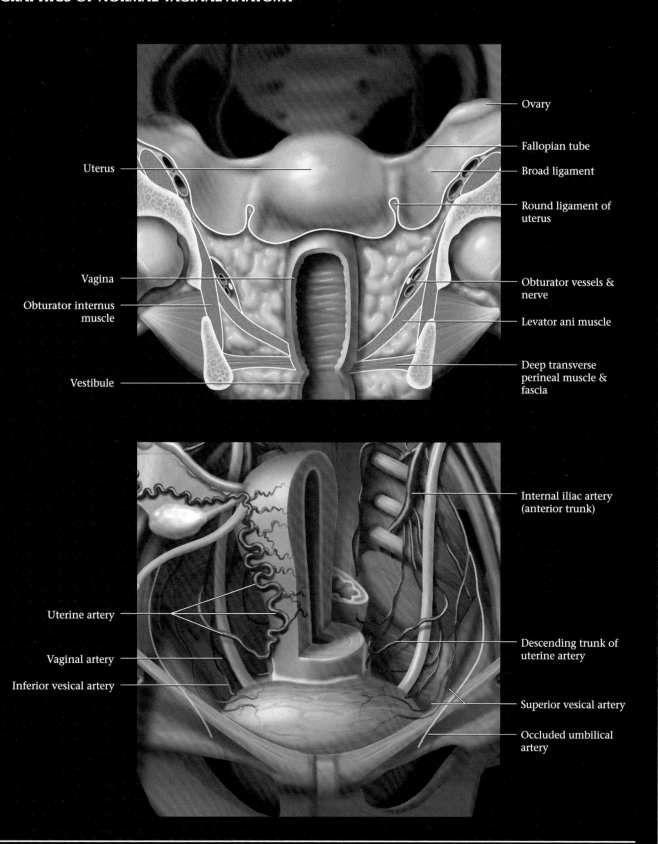

(Top) Coronal view of the pelvic floor in a female at the level of the vagina. The levator ani muscles form the pelvic floor through which the urethra, vagina and rectum pass, and is the main support for the pelvic organs. The deep transverse perineal muscle and fascia, along with the urethral sphincter, form the urogenital diaphragm which is the main support of the lower vagina. **(Bottom)** Frontal graphic of iliac vessels in a female. The internal iliac artery divides into an anterior trunk and posterior trunk. The VA can branch off directly from the anterior trunk of the internal iliac artery or sometimes from the inferior vesical artery or UA. The arterial supply of vagina includes VA and vaginal branch of descending trunk of UA.

VAGINA

Urinary bladder

Urethra

Muscular walls of vagina

Mucosal layer of the vagina

Cervix

Rectum

Acoustic jelly

Vaginal canal
Urinary bladder

Muscular walls of vagina
Cervix, external os

Cervix

Anal canal

Rectovaginal fascia

Urethra

Vesicovaginal fascia

Vaginal wall

Urinary bladder

(Top) Transabdominal midline sagittal scan of vagina shows characteristic triple-line echoes, i.e., hypoechoic muscular walls interfaced by echogenic mucosa. When looking for the vagina using transabdominal scan it is best to view with a distended bladder, to start at midline near the cervical level and tilt the transducer further caudally. (Middle) Longitudinal transvaginal scan of the vagina again shows characteristic triple-line echoes pattern. Using transvaginal sonography, the technique is to use a high frequency vaginal transducer with gradual withdrawal of the transducer so as to outline the vaginal canal with acoustic jelly. (Bottom) Transperineal sagittal scan shows the vagina sandwiched between the urethra anteriorly and the rectum posteriorly. Note the vaginal canal is barely visible in the absence of intraluminal acoustic jelly or fluid.

VAGINA

TRANSVERSE SCAN OF THE VAGINA

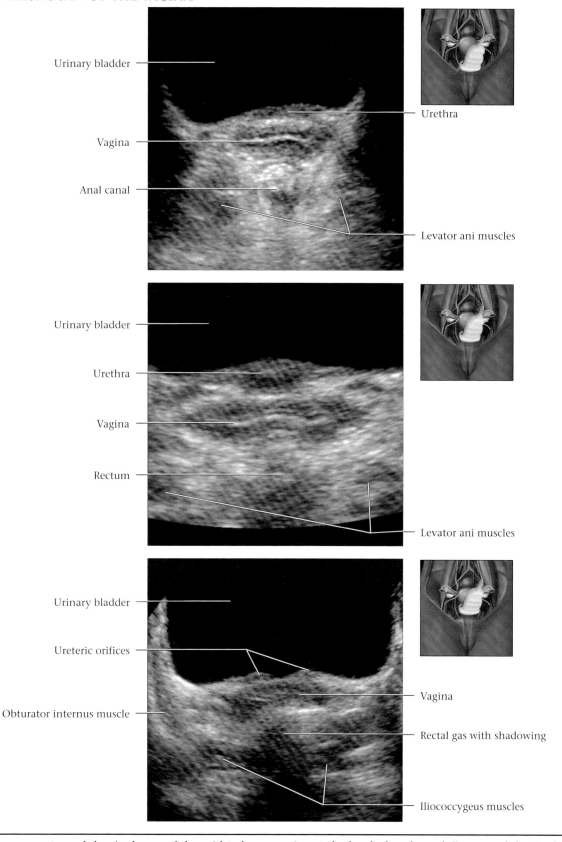

Urinary bladder

Urethra

Vagina

Anal canal

Levator ani muscles

Urinary bladder

Urethra

Vagina

Rectum

Levator ani muscles

Urinary bladder

Ureteric orifices

Vagina

Obturator internus muscle

Rectal gas with shadowing

Iliococcygeus muscles

(**Top**) Transverse transabdominal scan of the mid to lower vagina at the level of anal canal. For transabdominal scan of vagina, caudal angulation of US probe is needed on both longitudinal and transverse scans. Note the vaginal canal is better demonstrated on transabdominal scan because the angle of insonation is more favorable, approaching a right angle. (**Middle**) Transverse transabdominal scan of the mid vagina shows the levator ani muscles adjacent to the posterolateral aspect of vagina. (**Bottom**) Upper vagina at the level of ureteric orifices. The ureters run lateral to the lateral fornices of the vagina, cross anteriorly and then enter into the posterior wall of the bladder. This is a useful plane for the investigation of ureteric jet.

COLOR DOPPLER USG OF VAGINAL ARTERY

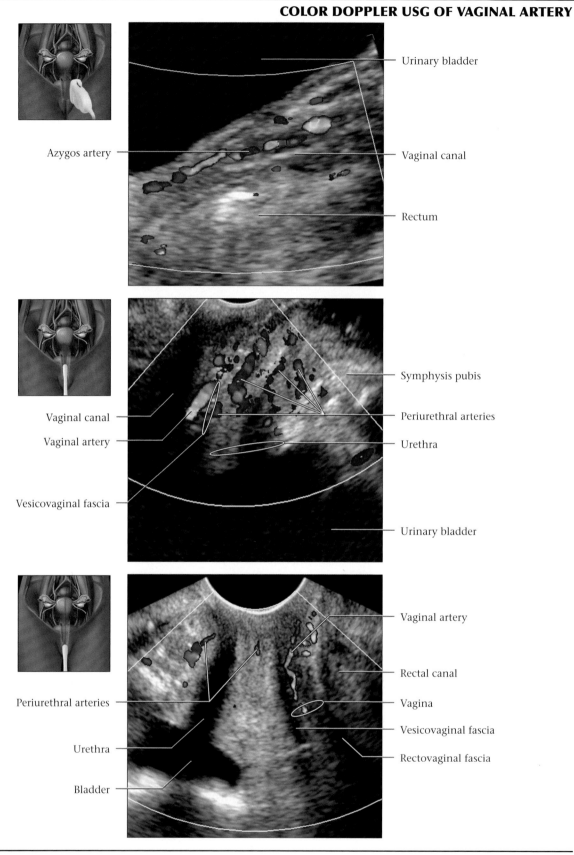

Azygos artery

Urinary bladder

Vaginal canal

Rectum

Vaginal canal

Vaginal artery

Vesicovaginal fascia

Symphysis pubis

Periurethral arteries

Urethra

Urinary bladder

Periurethral arteries

Urethra

Bladder

Vaginal artery

Rectal canal

Vagina

Vesicovaginal fascia

Rectovaginal fascia

(Top) Longitudinal transabdominal color Doppler US of the vagina shows the longitudinally running azygos artery which arises from anastomosis of the vaginal branches of UA and branches of VA. (Middle) Longitudinal transvaginal color Doppler US shows the highly vascularized vagina with multiple small branches of VA running along the vesicovaginal fascia. (Bottom) Transperineal sagittal color Doppler US shows a tortuous branch of the vaginal artery running along the vesicovaginal fascia in the vagina.

VAGINA

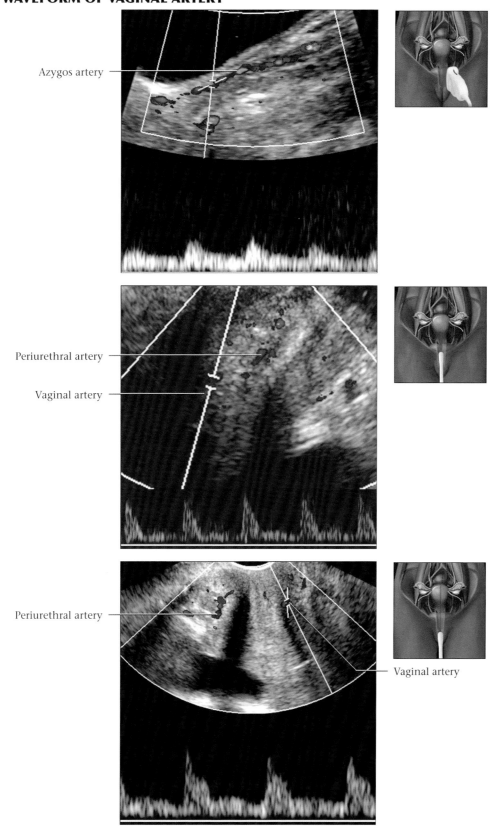

(**Top**) Transabdominal spectral Doppler US of the azygos artery shows low-resistance flow during mid cycle. The findings are most probably due to the influence of cyclical/hormonal change. (**Middle**) Spectral waveform of VA by transvaginal scan shows high-resistance flow which is the most common pattern in normal females. (**Bottom**) Spectral Doppler imaging of VA by transperineal scan. The typical high flow resistance in VA may decrease during sexual arousal, cyclical or hormonal changes. This phenomenon is useful for investigation and management of sexual dysfunction in post-menopausal women.

OVARIES

Terminology

Abbreviations
- Transvaginal (TV) ultrasound
- Transabdominal (TA) ultrasound

Gross Anatomy

Overview
- Ovaries located in true pelvis, although exact position variable
  - Only pelvic organ entirely inside peritoneal sac
  - Laxity in ligaments allows some mobility
  - Location affected by parity, bladder filling, ovarian size and uterine size/position
  - Located within ovarian fossa in nulliparous women
    - Lateral pelvic sidewall below bifurcation of common iliac vessels
    - Anterior to ureter
    - Posterior to broad ligament
  - Position more variable in parous women
    - Ovaries pushed out of pelvis with pregnancy
    - Seldom return to same spot
- Fallopian tube drapes over much of surface
  - Partially covered by fimbriated end
- Composed of medulla and cortex
  - Vessels enter and exit ovary through medulla
  - Cortex contains follicles in varying stages of development
  - Surface covered by specialized peritoneum called germinal epithelium
- Ligamentous supports
  - Suspensory ligament of ovary (infundibulopelvic ligament)
    - Attaches ovary to lateral pelvic wall
    - Contains ovarian vessels and lymphatics
    - Positions ovary in craniocaudal orientation
  - Mesovarium
    - Attaches ovary to broad ligament (posterior)
    - Transmits nerves and vessels to ovary
  - Proper ovarian ligament (utero-ovarian ligament)
    - Continuation of round ligament
    - Fibromuscular band extending from ovary to uterine cornu
  - Mesosalpinx
    - Extends between fallopian tube and proper ovarian ligament
  - Broad ligament
    - Below proper ovarian ligament
- Arterial supply: Dual blood supply
  - Ovarian artery is branch of aorta, arises at L1/2 level
    - Descends to pelvis and enters suspensory ligament
    - Continues through mesovarium to ovarian hilum
    - Anastomoses with uterine artery
  - Both arteries and veins markedly enlarge in pregnancy
- Drainage via pampiniform plexus into ovarian veins
  - Right ovarian vein drains to inferior vena cava
  - Left ovarian vein drains to left renal vein
- Lymphatic drainage follows venous drainage to preaortic lymph nodes at L1 & 2 levels

Physiology
- ~ 400,000 follicles present at birth but only 0.1% (400) mature to ovulation
- Variations in menstrual cycle
  - Follicular phase (days 0-14)
    - Several follicles begin to develop
    - By days 8-12 a dominant follicle develops, while remainder start to regress
  - Ovulation (day 14)
    - Dominant follicle typically 2.0-2.5 cm
  - Luteal phase (days 14-28)
    - Luteinizing hormone induces formation of corpus luteum
    - If fertilization occurs, corpus luteum maintains and enlarges to corpus luteum cyst of pregnancy

Variations with Age
- At birth: Large ovaries ± follicles due to influence of maternal hormones
- Childhood: Volume < 1 cc, follicles < 2 mm diameter
- Above 8 year-old: ≥ 6 follicles of > 4 mm diameter
- Adult, reproductive age: Mean ~ 10 ± 6 cc, max 22 cc
- Postmenopausal: Mean ~ 2-6 cc, max 8 cc

Imaging Anatomy

Ultrasound
- Scan between uterus and pelvic sidewall
  - Ovaries often seen adjacent to internal iliac vessels
- Relatively hypoechoic, scattered coarse pattern compared to uterine myometrium
- Medulla mildly hyperechoic compared to hypoechoic cortex
- Developing follicles anechoic
- Corpus luteum may have thick, echogenic ring
  - Hemorrhage common
    - Variable appearance: Lace-like septations; fluid-fluid level; retracting clot; internal debris
    - No flow on Doppler ultrasound
- Echogenic foci common
  - Non-shadowing, 1-3 mm
  - Represent specular reflectors from walls of tiny unresolved cysts or small vessels in medulla
  - More common in periphery
- Focal calcification may also be seen
- Doppler: Low-velocity, low-resistance arterial waveform
- Volume (0.523 x length x width x height) more accurate than individual measurements

Anatomy-Based Imaging Issues

Imaging Recommendations
- TAS with a full bladder is good for an overview of pelvic organs
- TVS is excellent in assessing detail of the ovaries or for patients who are unable to maintain a full bladder
- Knowledge of last menstrual period is useful for rendering correct diagnosis
- Follow-up scan is recommended to differentiate a physiological cyst from a pathological cyst

OVARIES

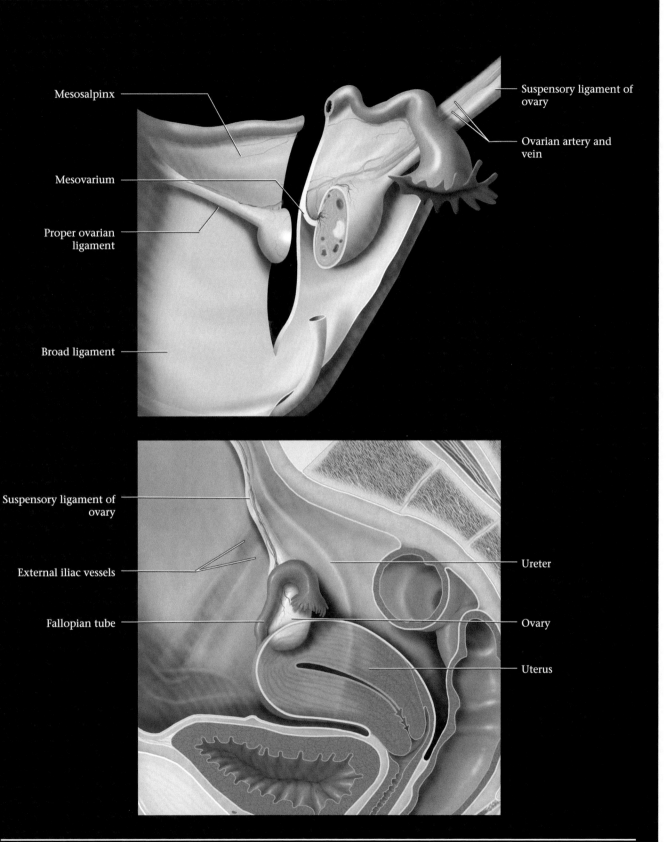

Mesosalpinx

Mesovarium

Proper ovarian ligament

Broad ligament

Suspensory ligament of ovary

Ovarian artery and vein

Suspensory ligament of ovary

External iliac vessels

Fallopian tube

Ureter

Ovary

Uterus

(Top) Posterior view of the ligamentous attachment of the ovary. The ovary is attached to the pelvic sidewall by the suspensory ligament (infundibulopelvic ligament) of the ovary, which transmits the ovarian artery and vein. These vessels enter the ovary through the mesovarium, a specialized ligamentous attachment between the ovary and broad ligament. The ovary is attached to the uterus by the proper ovarian ligament, which divides the mesosalpinx above from the broad ligament below. **(Bottom)** Sagittal graphic of the female pelvis shows the location of the ovary which lies in the ovarian fossa, the area below the iliac bifurcation, posterior to the external iliac vessels and anterior to the ureter.

OVARIES

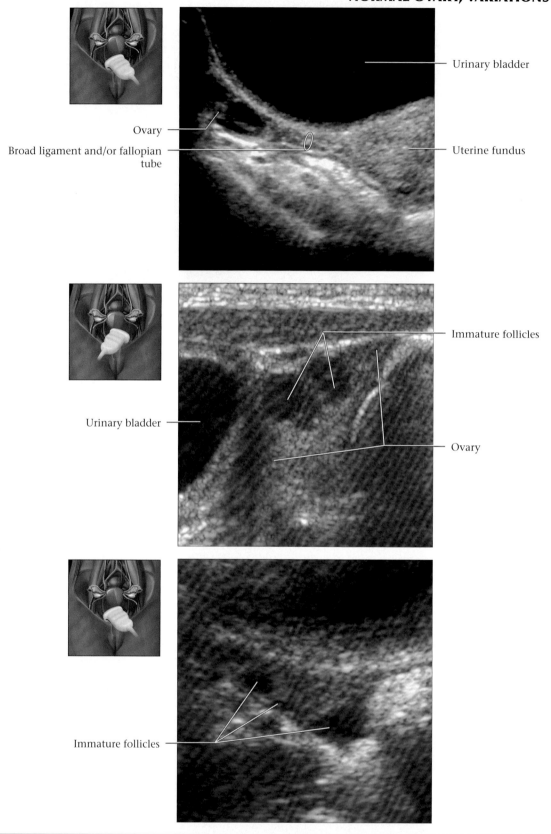

Urinary bladder

Ovary

Broad ligament and/or fallopian tube

Uterine fundus

Immature follicles

Urinary bladder

Ovary

Immature follicles

(Top) Transverse TA ultrasound at the level of the uterine horn shows the ovary is in the vicinity of the uterus and connected to it by the broad ligament. Ovarian ligaments can be lax making ovarian position quite variable, from above the fundus to the posterior rectouterine pouch of Douglas. (Middle) Transverse TA ultrasound of the ovary in a neonate. The size of the ovary is enlarged with prominent immature follicles which are thought to be under the stimulation of residual maternal gonadotrophins. The follicles may persist until 9 months of age or longer. (Bottom) Transverse TA ultrasound of the normal ovary of a 5 year old girl. The ovary is small and slender with immature follicles of variable size (usually less than 0.9 cm). The size of the ovaries change very little in the first 6 years of life.

OVARIES

NORMAL OVARY, VARIATIONS WITH AGE

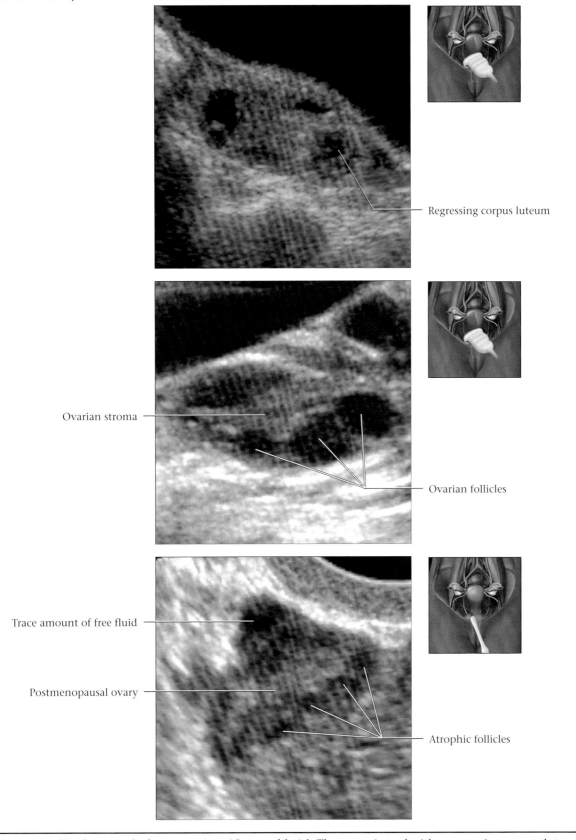

Regressing corpus luteum

Ovarian stroma

Ovarian follicles

Trace amount of free fluid

Postmenopausal ovary

Atrophic follicles

(Top) Transverse TA ultrasound of an ovary in a 15 year old girl. The ovary is oval with a regressing corpus luteum. Note the ovary after puberty will enlarge and the primordial follicles will undergo cyclical development. (Middle) Transverse TA ultrasound of an adult ovary. There are multiple developing follicles of variable size around the echogenic ovarian stroma (medulla) where the ovarian vessels and lymphatics enter and exit. Follicular rupture usually occurs when it reaches the size between 2.0 and 2.5 cm. (Bottom) Longitudinal TV ultrasound of a postmenopausal ovary. The ovary is atrophic with tiny cysts discernible at the periphery. Visualization of postmenopausal ovary is difficult with TAS unless it is surrounded by ascitic fluid. TVS is the method of choice but the detection rate is variable.

OVARIES

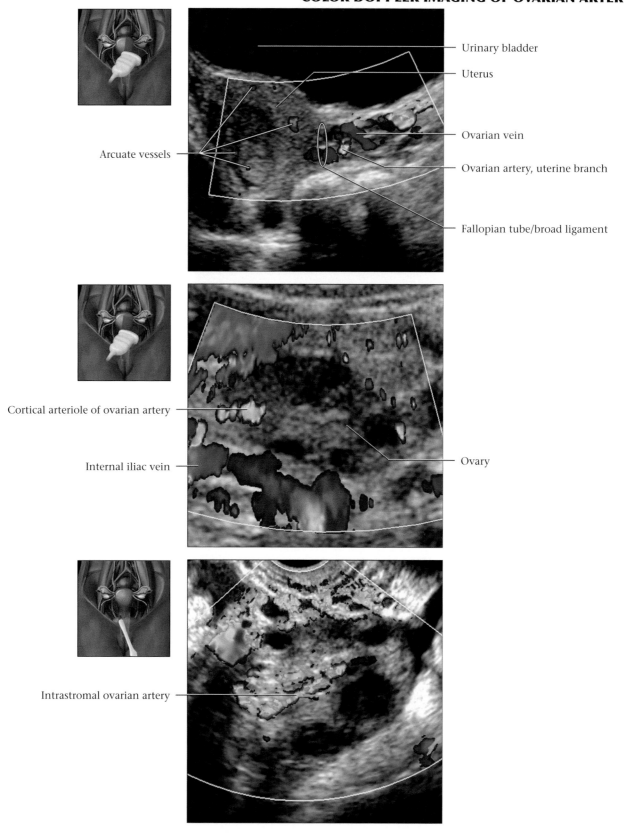

Top image labels:
- Urinary bladder
- Uterus
- Ovarian vein
- Ovarian artery, uterine branch
- Fallopian tube/broad ligament
- Arcuate vessels

Middle image labels:
- Cortical arteriole of ovarian artery
- Internal iliac vein
- Ovary

Bottom image labels:
- Intrastromal ovarian artery

(Top) Transverse TA ultrasound shows the ovarian branch of the uterine artery running in the broad ligament. It begins at the uterine horn and goes to the lower pole of the ovary through the proper ovarian ligament. **(Middle)** Transverse TA ultrasound shows the ovary adjacent to the internal iliac vein. The straight cortical arteriole of the ovarian artery enters into the medulla of the ovary via the hilum. **(Bottom)** Longitudinal color Doppler TV ultrasound shows an intrastromal ovarian artery running in the ovarian medulla. Note ovarian vascularity will progressively increase after menstruation and approach a maximum in the luteal phase.

OVARIES

SPECTRAL WAVEFORM OF OVARIAN ARTERY

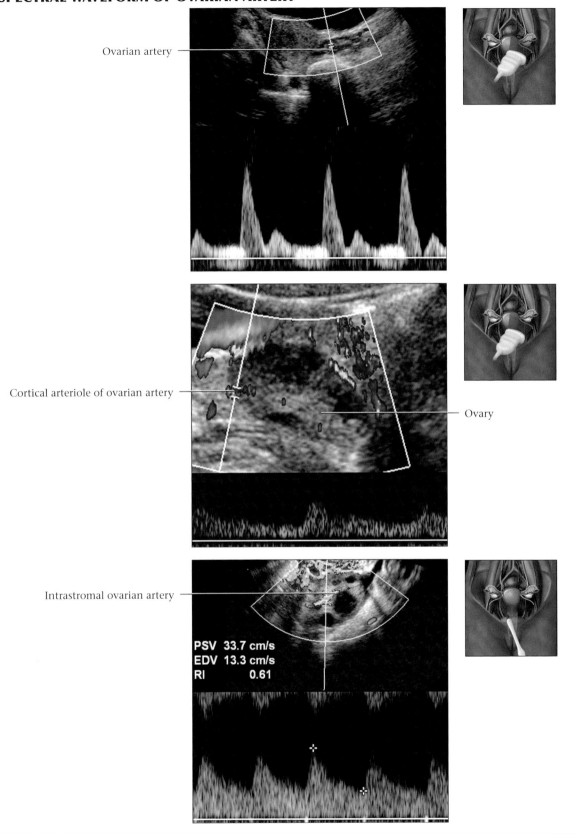

Ovarian artery

Cortical arteriole of ovarian artery

Ovary

Intrastromal ovarian artery

PSV 33.7 cm/s
EDV 13.3 cm/s
RI 0.61

(**Top**) Transverse spectral Doppler TA ultrasound shows a normal ovarian artery with a high-resistance flow pattern suggestive of an inactive state of the ovary. (**Middle**) Transverse spectral Doppler TA ultrasound shows the waveform of the cortical arteriole of the ovarian artery. (**Bottom**) Transverse spectral Doppler TV ultrasound of the intrastromal ovarian artery as a continuation of the straight cortical arteriole shows a typical low-resistance, low-velocity waveform during the luteal phase.

OVARIES

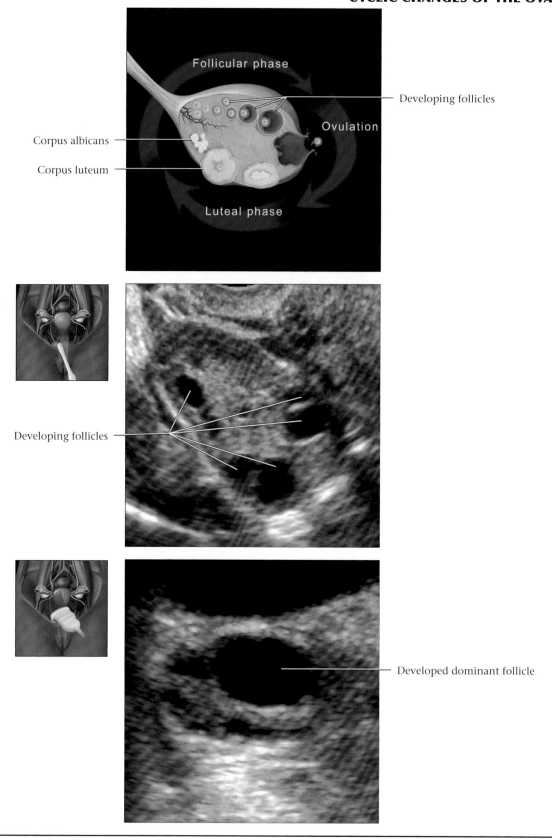

Follicular phase

Developing follicles

Corpus albicans

Ovulation

Corpus luteum

Luteal phase

Developing follicles

Developed dominant follicle

(Top) During the follicular phase of the menstrual cycle, several follicles begin to develop but by days 8-12 a dominant follicle has formed, and the remainder begin to regress. On day 14 the follicle ruptures and the egg is extruded. After ovulation, a corpus luteum forms, and if fertilization does not occur, the corpus luteum degenerates into a corpus albicans. (Middle) Longitudinal TV ultrasound of the ovary at the early follicular phase. Note the developing follicles of variable size are seen at the periphery of the ovary. (Bottom) TA ultrasound shows a dominant follicle developed in the late follicular phase days before ovulation.

OVARIES

CYCLIC CHANGES OF THE OVARY

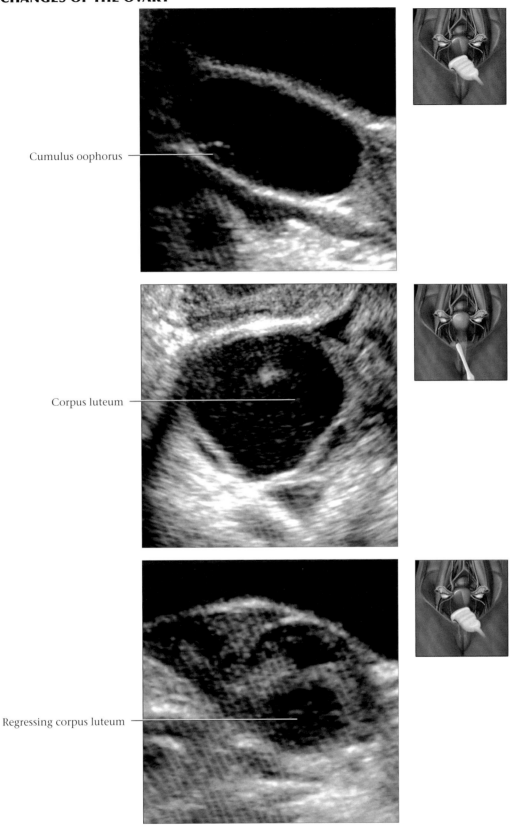

Cumulus oophorus

Corpus luteum

Regressing corpus luteum

(Top) Transverse TA ultrasound of the ovary demonstrates a large mature follicle with a small cyst on its wall representing a cumulus oophorus. The size of a mature follicle can reach up to 25 mm before ovulation. (Middle) Longitudinal TV ultrasound of the ovary shows a dominant follicle immediately after its rupture at ovulation. Note the partially collapsed wall resulting from loss of part of the liquor folliculi and the hypoechoic internal contents representing blood. (Bottom) Transverse TA ultrasound of the ovary shows a regressing corpus luteum with echogenic internal contents and strains of fibrin within its liquefied center.

CYCLIC CHANGES OF INTRAOVARIAN ARTERY

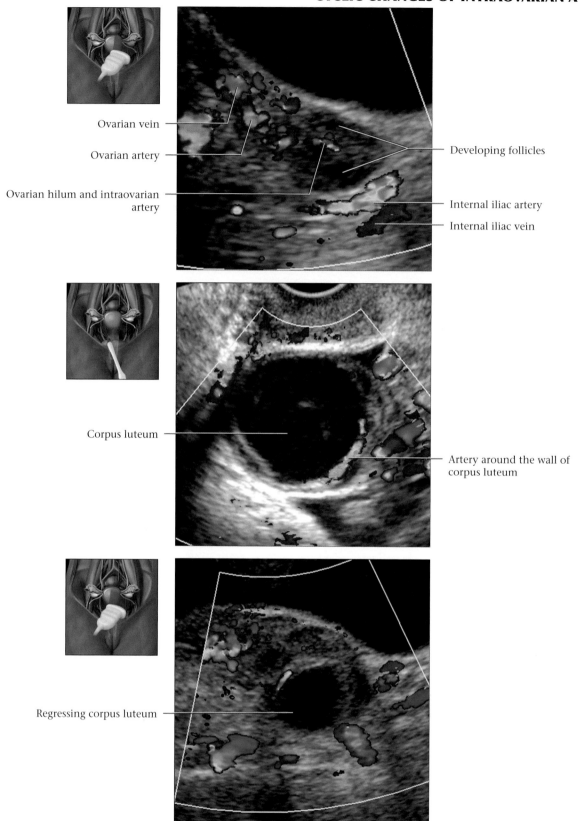

Ovarian vein

Ovarian artery

Ovarian hilum and intraovarian artery

Developing follicles

Internal iliac artery

Internal iliac vein

Corpus luteum

Artery around the wall of corpus luteum

Regressing corpus luteum

(Top) Color Doppler TA ultrasound shows an inactive ovary. The ovary demonstrates a hilar artery surrounded by small developing follicles in the early follicular phase. Note the non-dominant ovary may show similar appearance as an inactive ovary. **(Middle)** Longitudinal TV ultrasound of the ovary in the early luteal phase. A corpus luteum with low-level internal echoes is seen following ovulation. The wall of the corpus luteum usually displays the most intense color pattern. **(Bottom)** Transverse TA ultrasound in mid-luteal phase. The ovary shows a regressing corpus luteum with peripheral vascularity.

OVARIES

CYCLIC CHANGES OF INTRAOVARIAN ARTERY

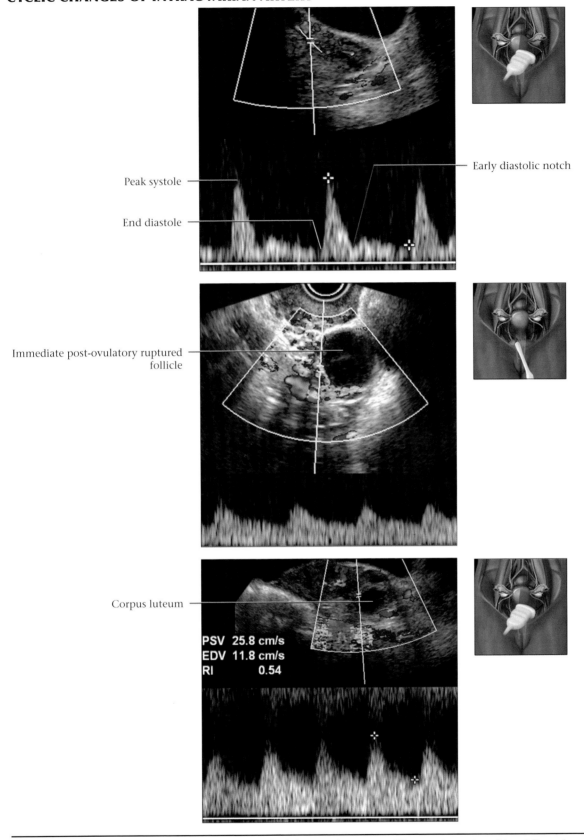

Peak systole

End diastole

Early diastolic notch

Immediate post-ovulatory ruptured follicle

Corpus luteum

PSV 25.8 cm/s
EDV 11.8 cm/s
RI 0.54

(Top) Transverse spectral Doppler TA ultrasound of the ovarian artery. The ovarian artery blood flow shows high-resistance flow pattern with low end-diastolic velocity and an early diastolic notch. This notch indicates initial resistance to forward flow through the ovarian parenchyma. The flow resistance is maximum during the first 8 days of the cycle. **(Middle)** Spectral Doppler TV ultrasound of the intraovarian artery in early luteal phase. The ovarian artery has low-resistance flow which reaches the lowest level in early luteal phase. At this time, the intraovarian vascularity is easily detectable. **(Bottom)** Spectral Doppler of TA ultrasound of the intraovarian artery in mid-luteal phase (opposite image). The ovarian arterial flow is of medium resistance and the flow resistance will gradually increase through to the regenerative phase.

ILIAC ARTERIES AND VEINS

Gross Anatomy

Arteries

- Abdominal aorta
  - Testicular and ovarian arteries originate below renal arteries
  - Median (middle) sacral artery is small, unpaired branch from posterior aspect of distal aorta
  - Divides into common iliac arteries at L4-5
- Common iliac arteries
  - Run anterior to iliac veins and inferior vena cava
  - Usually no major branches
    - Rarely, gives off aberrant iliolumbar or accessory renal arteries
  - Approximately 4 cm long
- External iliac artery
  - No major branches
  - Exits pelvis beneath inguinal ligament
  - Larger than internal iliac artery
  - Inferior epigastric (medial) and deep iliac circumflex (lateral) arteries demarcate junction between external iliac and common femoral arteries
- Internal iliac (hypogastric) artery
  - Principal vascular supply of pelvic organs
  - Divides into anterior and posterior trunk
    - Anterior trunk to pelvic viscera
    - Posterior trunk to pelvic musculature
- Anterior trunk of internal iliac artery
  - Branching pattern quite variable
  - Umbilical artery
    - Only pelvic segment remains patent after birth
    - Remainder becomes fibrous medial umbilical ligament
  - Obturator artery
    - Exits pelvis through obturator canal to supply medial thigh muscles
  - Superior vesicle artery
    - Supplies bladder and distal ureter
    - Gives off branch to ductus deferens in males
  - Inferior vesicle artery (male)
    - May arise from middle rectal artery
    - Supplies prostate, seminal vesicles and lower ureters
  - Uterine artery (female)
    - Passes over ureter at level of cervix ("water under the bridge")
    - Anastomoses with vaginal and ovarian arteries
  - Vaginal artery (female)
  - Middle rectal artery runs above pelvic floor and anastomoses with superior and inferior rectal arteries to supply rectum
    - Also anastomoses with inferior vesicle artery
  - Internal pudendal artery
    - Supplies external genitalia (penis, clitoris) and rectum
  - Inferior gluteal (sciatic) artery
    - Largest and terminal branch of anterior division of hypogastric artery
    - Supplies muscles of pelvic floor, thigh, buttocks and sciatic nerve
- Posterior division of internal iliac artery
  - Iliolumbar artery
    - Ascends laterally to supply iliacus, psoas and quadratus lumborum muscles
  - Lateral sacral artery
    - Runs medially toward sacral foramina to anastomose with middle sacral artery
  - Superior gluteal artery
    - Largest and terminal branch of posterior division
    - Supplies piriformis and gluteal muscles

Veins

- External iliac vein
  - Upward continuation of femoral vein at level of inguinal ligament
  - Receives inferior epigastric, deep iliac circumflex, and pubic veins
- Internal iliac vein begins near upper part of greater sciatic foramen
  - Gluteal, internal pudendal and obturator veins have origins outside pelvis
  - Pelvic viscera drain into multiple, deep pelvic venous plexuses
    - These drain into veins, which roughly parallel pelvic arteries
- Right gonadal vein drains into IVC, left gonadal vein drains into left renal vein
- Common iliac vein is formed by union of external and internal iliac veins
  - Unites with contralateral side to form IVC

Imaging Anatomy

Overview

- CT angiography (CTA) and MR angiography (MRA) are imaging modalities of choice to evaluate pelvic vessels
  - Ultrasound is limited to demonstrating the common iliac, external iliac and proximal internal iliac vessels

Anatomy-Based Imaging Issues

Imaging Recommendations

- Transducer: 2-5 MHz
- Patient examined in supine position
  - Place transducer lateral to the rectus muscles, angulating medially
- Fasting for 4 hours may help decrease overlying bowel gas

Imaging Pitfalls

- Pelvic vessels are usually obscured by overlying bowel gas

Clinical Implications

Clinical Importance

- Abdominal aortic aneurysms may extend to involve the iliac arteries
- Rich, complex collateral circulation helps ensure delivery of blood to pelvic organs and lower limbs in event of proximal obstruction
- Patients with deep venous thrombosis of the lower limbs may have involvement of the iliac veins

ILIAC ARTERIES AND VEINS IN SITU

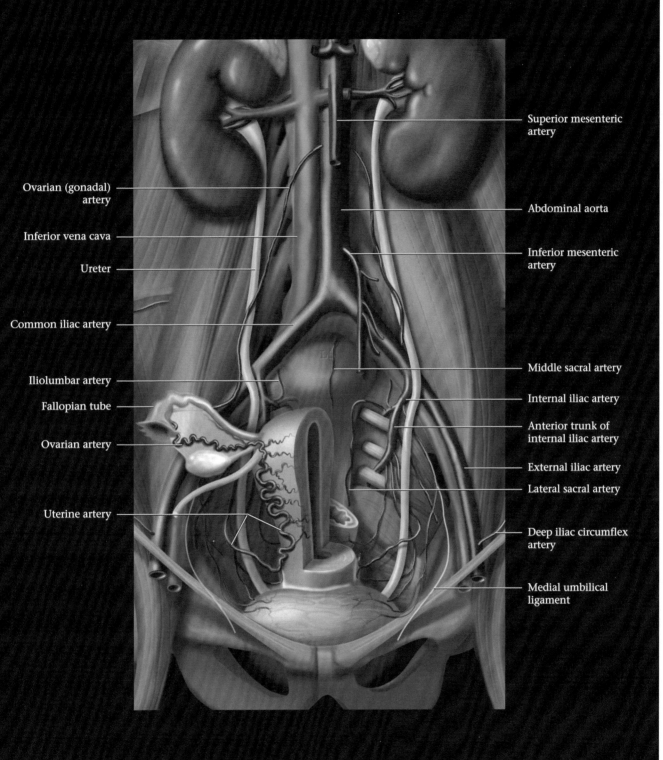

Ovarian (gonadal) artery

Inferior vena cava

Ureter

Common iliac artery

Iliolumbar artery

Fallopian tube

Ovarian artery

Uterine artery

Superior mesenteric artery

Abdominal aorta

Inferior mesenteric artery

Middle sacral artery

Internal iliac artery

Anterior trunk of internal iliac artery

External iliac artery

Lateral sacral artery

Deep iliac circumflex artery

Medial umbilical ligament

Frontal graphic of the abdominal aorta, inferior vena cava, and the iliac vessels in a female. The inferior mesenteric artery is the smallest of the anterior mesenteric branches of the aorta and continues in the pelvis as the superior rectal artery. The paired ovarian arteries arise from the aorta below the renal arteries and pass inferiorly on the posterior abdominal wall to enter the pelvis. The ureters cross anterior to the bifurcation of the common iliac arteries on their way to the urinary bladder. The common iliac artery divides into the external iliac artery, which supplies the lower extremity and the internal iliac (hypogastric) artery, which supplies the pelvis. The internal iliac artery divides into an anterior trunk for the pelvic viscera and a posterior trunk for the muscles of the pelvis.

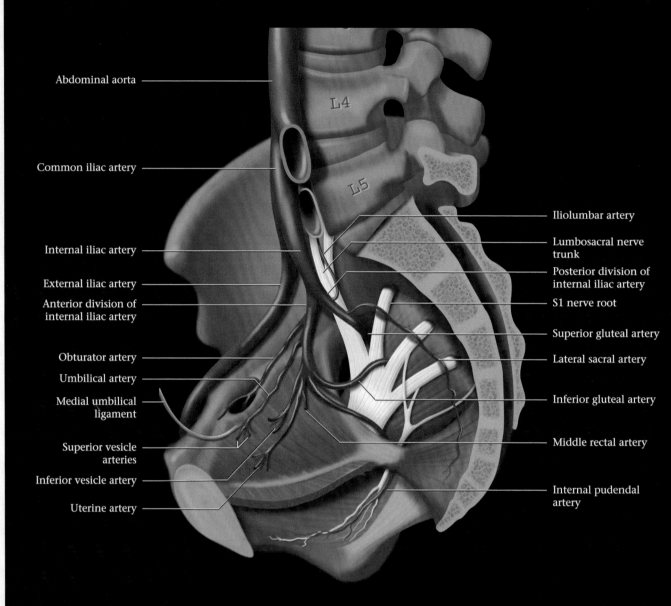

Abdominal aorta

Common iliac artery

Internal iliac artery

External iliac artery

Anterior division of internal iliac artery

Obturator artery

Umbilical artery

Medial umbilical ligament

Superior vesicle arteries

Inferior vesicle artery

Uterine artery

L4

L5

Iliolumbar artery

Lumbosacral nerve trunk

Posterior division of internal iliac artery

S1 nerve root

Superior gluteal artery

Lateral sacral artery

Inferior gluteal artery

Middle rectal artery

Internal pudendal artery

Graphic of the pelvic arteries and their relation to the sacral nerves. The superior gluteal artery passes posteriorly and runs between the lumbosacral trunk and the anterior ramus of the S1 nerve, whereas the inferior gluteal artery usually runs between the S1-2 or S2-3 nerve roots to leave the pelvis through the inferior part of the greater sciatic foramen. Only the proximal portion of the umbilical arteries remains patent after birth, while the distal portion obliterates forming the medial umbilical ligaments. Arteries to the deep pelvic viscera include the superior and inferior vesicle, uterine, middle rectal and internal pudendal. The individual branching pattern is quite variable.

ILIAC ARTERIES AND VEINS

ILIAC VEINS IN SITU

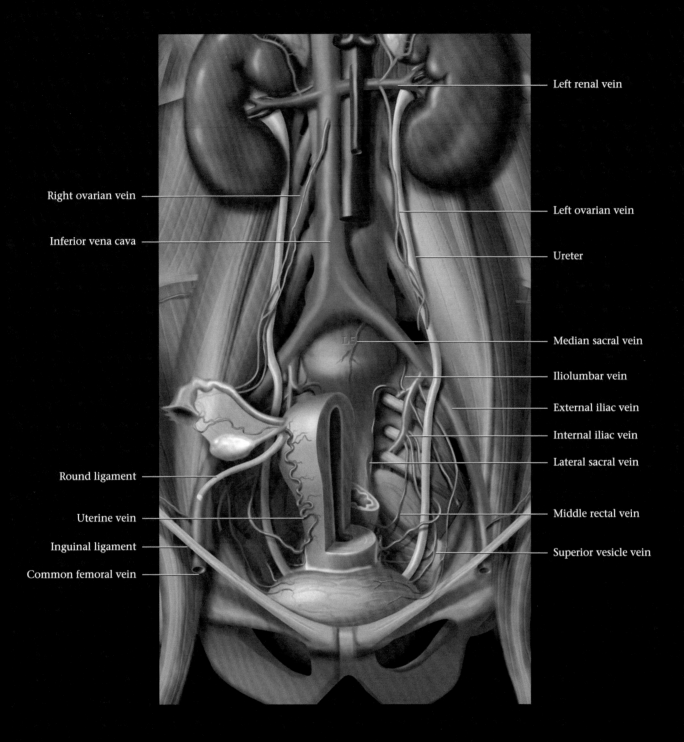

Right ovarian vein

Inferior vena cava

Round ligament

Uterine vein

Inguinal ligament

Common femoral vein

Left renal vein

Left ovarian vein

Ureter

Median sacral vein

Iliolumbar vein

External iliac vein

Internal iliac vein

Lateral sacral vein

Middle rectal vein

Superior vesicle vein

Graphic of the veins of the pelvis. The left ovarian vein drains into the left renal vein, whereas the right ovarian vein drains directly into the inferior vena cava. Multiple intercommunicating pelvic venous plexuses (rectal, vesicle, prostatic, uterine and vaginal) drain mainly to the internal iliac veins. There is a communication between the pelvic veins and the intraspinal epidural plexus of veins through the sacral venous plexus.

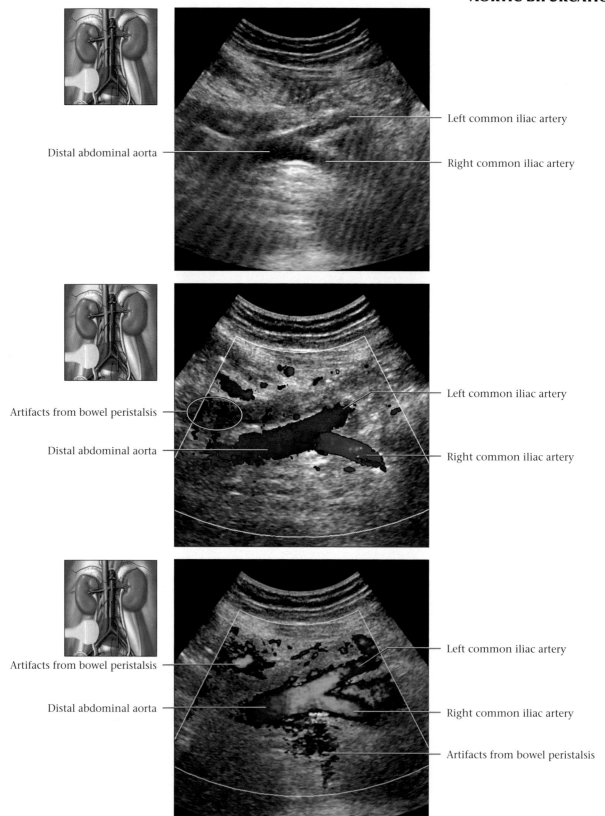

Left common iliac artery

Distal abdominal aorta

Right common iliac artery

Left common iliac artery

Artifacts from bowel peristalsis

Distal abdominal aorta

Right common iliac artery

Left common iliac artery

Artifacts from bowel peristalsis

Distal abdominal aorta

Right common iliac artery

Artifacts from bowel peristalsis

(Top) Coronal grayscale ultrasound shows the bifurcation of the distal aorta into the common iliac arteries. This occurs at the level of L4 vertebra and corresponds to the umbilicus, serving as a useful landmark for transducer placement for common iliac artery insonation. **(Middle)** Coronal color Doppler ultrasound demonstrates color flow in the distal aorta and bifurcation. The right common iliac artery assumes a blue color (as opposed to the red color of the distal aorta and right common iliac artery) owing to its flow direction. Peristalsis of adjacent bowel segments also demonstrates color on color Doppler ultrasound, rendering artifacts. **(Bottom)** Coronal power Doppler is more sensitive than color Doppler in demonstrating blood flow without providing information on flow direction. There is also significant increase in image artifacts from peristalsis.

ILIAC ARTERIES AND VEINS

COMMON ILIAC ARTERY

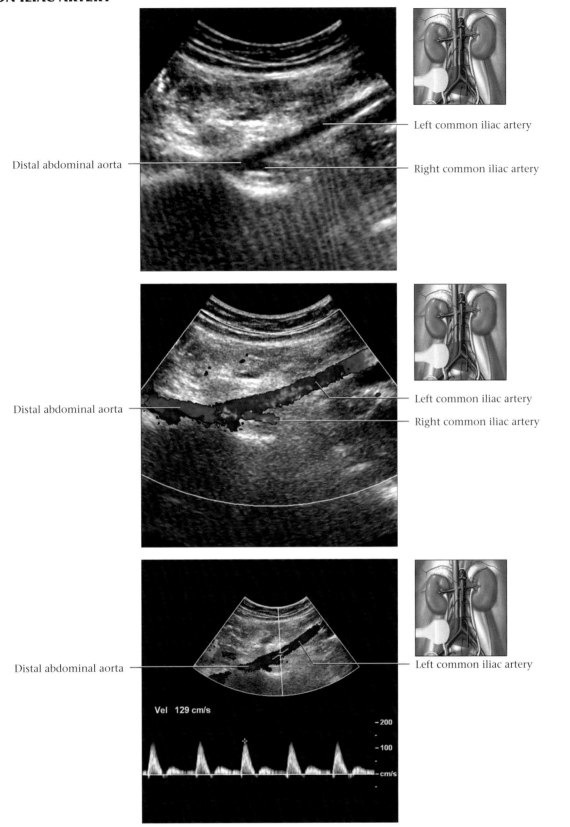

Left common iliac artery

Distal abdominal aorta

Right common iliac artery

Distal abdominal aorta

Left common iliac artery

Right common iliac artery

Distal abdominal aorta

Left common iliac artery

Vel 129 cm/s

−200

−100

−cm/s

(**Top**) Coronal, transabdominal, grayscale ultrasound, angulating the transducer to demonstrate the course of the left common iliac artery. The common iliac artery is about 5 cm long with diameters of 1.3 cm (females) and 1.5 cm (males). (**Middle**) Coronal transabdominal color Doppler of the left common iliac artery (shown in red) with consistent intense color indicating uniform mean flow velocity. This is a useful plane for examining abdominal aortic aneurysms when there is extension into the common iliac arteries. (**Bottom**) Transabdominal, color, pulsed Doppler ultrasound of the left common iliac artery shows peak systolic velocity of 129 cm/sec, within the normal range of 80-187 cm/sec. Note normal triphasic spectral waveform.

ILIAC ARTERIES AND VEINS

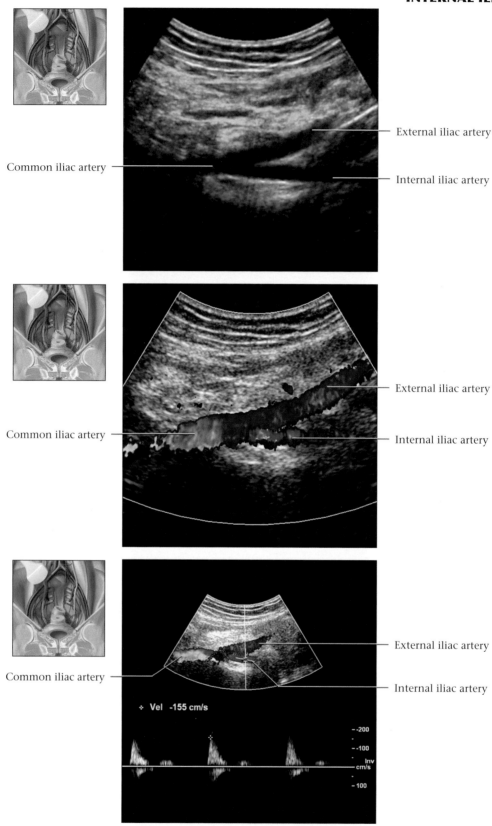

Common iliac artery

External iliac artery

Internal iliac artery

Vel -155 cm/s

(Top) Oblique, transabdominal, grayscale ultrasound of the distal common iliac artery demonstrating its bifurcation into the external iliac and internal iliac arteries. The internal iliac artery has a smaller caliber compared to the external iliac artery and courses more posteriorly. The internal iliac artery divides into 2 trunks, which are usually too deep to be demonstrated on ultrasound. (Middle) Longitudinal, transabdominal color Doppler shows intense color in the distal common iliac (shown in red) and external iliac (shown in red) arteries, suggesting uniform mean velocity in the arterial segments. The branches of the internal iliac artery (shown in blue) supply the wall and viscera of the pelvis, including the reproductive organs. (Bottom) Pulsed Doppler of the internal iliac artery, which is usually investigated in graft kidneys and some cases of erectile dysfunction.

ILIAC ARTERIES AND VEINS

EXTERNAL ILIAC ARTERY

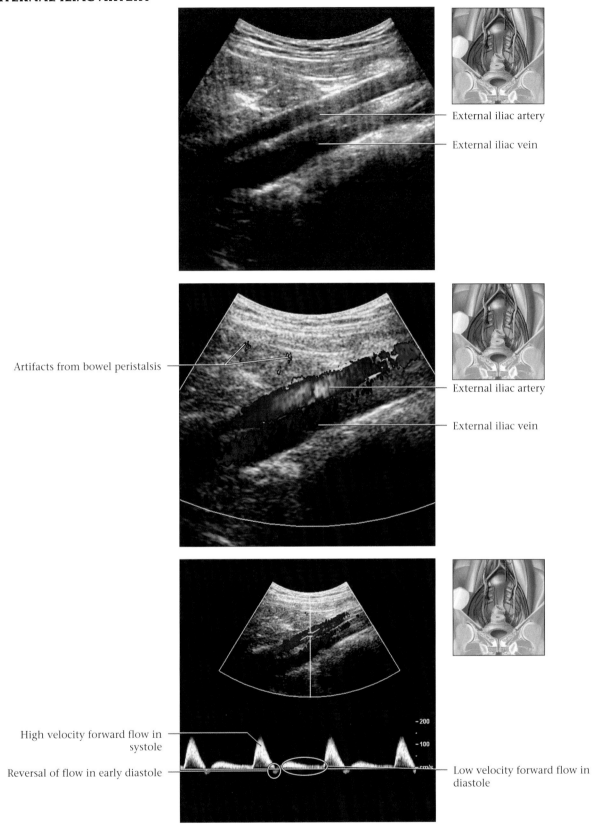

External iliac artery

External iliac vein

Artifacts from bowel peristalsis

External iliac artery

External iliac vein

High velocity forward flow in systole

Reversal of flow in early diastole

Low velocity forward flow in diastole

(Top) Longitudinal, transabdominal, grayscale ultrasound of the external iliac artery, usually easily demonstrated owing to its superficial location and absence of overlying bowel gas. Normal diameters are up to 11 mm in females and 12 mm in males. (Middle) Longitudinal, transabdominal, color Doppler ultrasound shows the relationship of the external iliac artery (shown in red) with the external iliac vein (shown in blue), which is located posteriorly. The two vessels run along the same course as they enter the thigh. (Bottom) Pulsed Doppler ultrasound of the external iliac artery; the waveform resembles those from lower extremity arteries. Note high velocity forward flow during systole and low velocity forward flow during diastole. There is an intervening short reversal of flow in early diastole, due to peripheral resistance. Peak systolic velocity of 129 cm/sec, within the normal range (< 140 cm/sec).

ILIAC VESSELS, TRANSVERSE

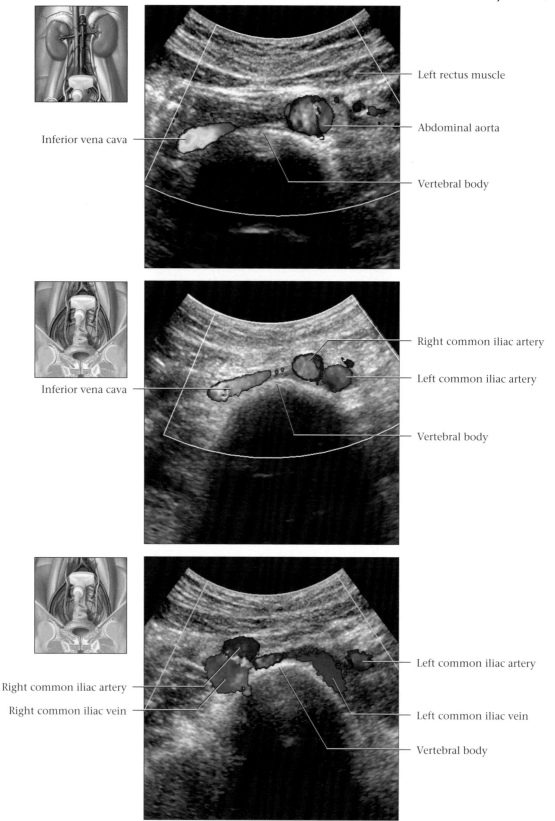

Left rectus muscle

Inferior vena cava

Abdominal aorta

Vertebral body

Inferior vena cava

Right common iliac artery

Left common iliac artery

Vertebral body

Left common iliac artery

Right common iliac artery

Right common iliac vein

Left common iliac vein

Vertebral body

(Top) Transverse, transabdominal, color Doppler ultrasound at the supraumbilical level shows the distal aorta (shown in red) and inferior vena cava (shown in blue), both of which have not yet bifurcated. The inferior vena cava is to the right of the abdominal aorta; a left-sided inferior vena cava is rarely encountered (0.2-0.5%) and may be associated with other vascular anomalies such as circumaortic or retroaortic renal vein. **(Middle)** Transverse, transabdominal, color Doppler ultrasound at the infraumbilical level. The distal aorta has bifurcated into the paired common iliac arteries at the level of L4, occurring more proximally than the formation of the inferior vena cava. **(Bottom)** Transverse, transabdominal, color Doppler ultrasound, continued from the above image. The paired common iliac veins (in blue) are now identified, which run posterior to their arterial counterparts (in red).

ILIAC ARTERIES AND VEINS

ILIAC VESSELS, CT

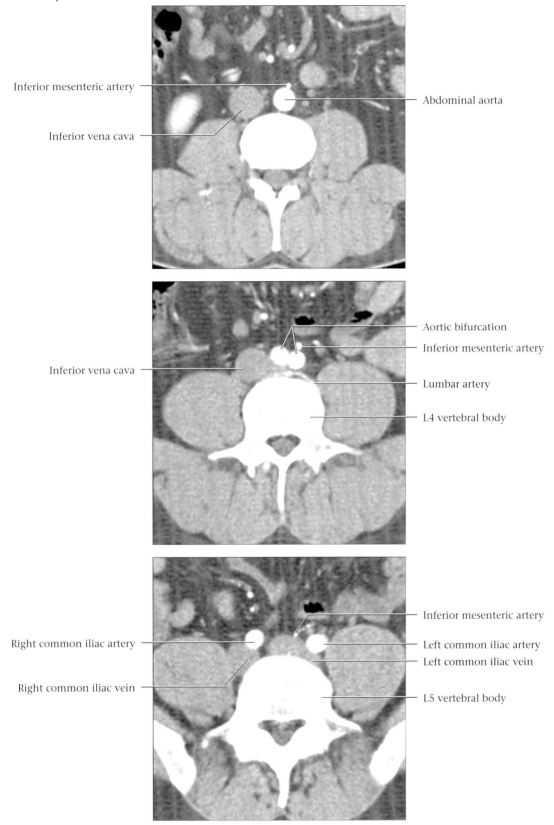

Inferior mesenteric artery — Abdominal aorta

Inferior vena cava

Aortic bifurcation

Inferior mesenteric artery

Inferior vena cava — Lumbar artery

L4 vertebral body

Right common iliac artery — Inferior mesenteric artery

Left common iliac artery

Left common iliac vein

Right common iliac vein — L5 vertebral body

(Top) First of three axial CECT images of the pelvic vessels. The abdominal aorta rests on the vertebral body; its distal portion gives off the inferior mesenteric artery, the smallest of the mesenteric arteries. The inferior vena cava is identified to the right of the abdominal aorta and spine. **(Middle)** The aorta bifurcates at the level of L4 into the two common iliac arteries. Despite its diminutive caliber, the lumbar artery is identified on CT. **(Bottom)** The common iliac arteries usually give off no visceral branches. They may, however, give origin to accessory renal arteries. At this lower level the termination of the common iliac veins are identified just before forming into the inferior vena cava. The left common iliac vein is longer than the right as it traverses the spine to form the IVC, which is located in the right paraspinal region.

ILIAC ARTERIES AND VEINS

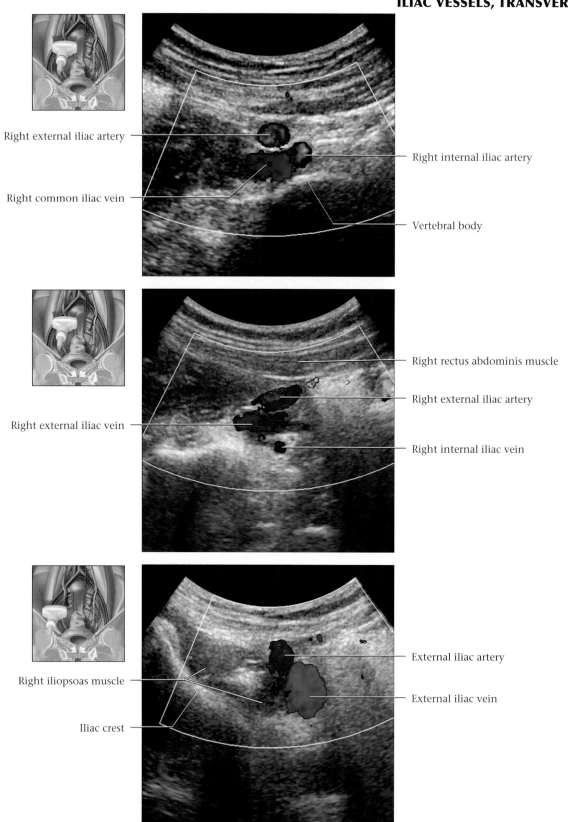

Right external iliac artery

Right common iliac vein

Right internal iliac artery

Vertebral body

Right external iliac vein

Right rectus abdominis muscle

Right external iliac artery

Right internal iliac vein

Right iliopsoas muscle

Iliac crest

External iliac artery

External iliac vein

(Top) Transverse, transabdominal color Doppler showing dichotomous branching of the right common iliac artery into the larger caliber external iliac artery (red) and smaller caliber internal iliac artery (red). The common iliac vein (blue) maintains its posterior location in relation to the two arteries. (Middle) Transverse, transabdominal, color Doppler ultrasound, continued more inferiorly from previous image, demonstrating the right external iliac vein (blue) and smaller internal iliac vein (blue). The right external iliac artery (red) is identified anterior to its venous counterpart. (Bottom) Transverse color Doppler ultrasound at the right iliac fossa. The right vesternal iliac artery (red) and vein (blue) course medial to the psoas major/iliopsoas muscle and maintain their relationship until they exit the pelvis beneath the inguinal ligament. Note the larger diameter of the vein compared to the artery.

ILIAC ARTERIES AND VEINS

ILIAC VESSELS, CT

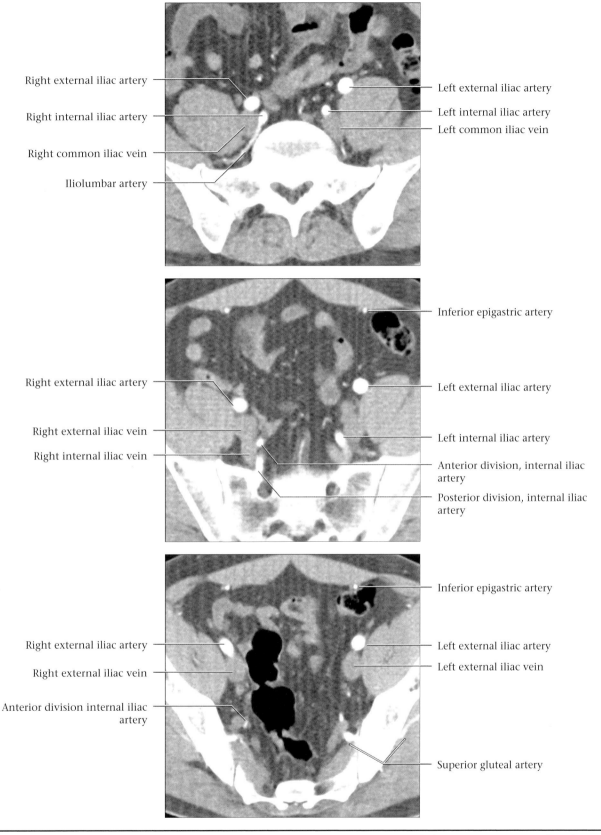

Right external iliac artery

Right internal iliac artery

Right common iliac vein

Iliolumbar artery

Left external iliac artery

Left internal iliac artery

Left common iliac vein

Inferior epigastric artery

Right external iliac artery

Right external iliac vein

Right internal iliac vein

Left external iliac artery

Left internal iliac artery

Anterior division, internal iliac artery

Posterior division, internal iliac artery

Inferior epigastric artery

Right external iliac artery

Right external iliac vein

Anterior division internal iliac artery

Left external iliac artery

Left external iliac vein

Superior gluteal artery

(**Top**) First of three axial CECT images of pelvic vessels. The common iliac arteries bifurcate more proximal to the formation of the common iliac veins. The iliolumbar artery, usually a branch of the posterior trunk of the internal iliac artery, arises in this subject from the main arternal iliac artery. CT is the imaging modality of choice in the examination of smaller pelvic vessels. (**Middle**) The internal iliac artery divides into an anterior and posterior trunk. The anterior trunk mainly supplies the pelvic viscera, whereas the posterior trunk supplies the pelvic musculature. Note their deep location relative to the external iliac vessels, which limits ultrasound examination of internal iliac vessel branches and tributaries. (**Bottom**) The external iliac artery and vein continue in an anterolateral direction as they course out of the pelvis and into the thigh.

ILIAC ARTERIES AND VEINS

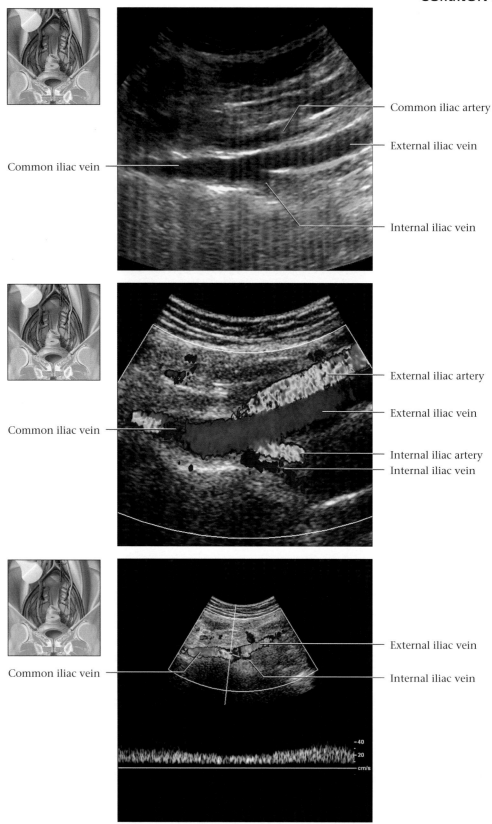

Common iliac vein

Common iliac artery

External iliac vein

Internal iliac vein

Common iliac vein

External iliac artery

External iliac vein

Internal iliac artery

Internal iliac vein

Common iliac vein

External iliac vein

Internal iliac vein

(Top) Longitudinal, transabdominal, grayscale ultrasound shows the external and internal iliac veins converging to form the common iliac vein. (Middle) Longitudinal, transabdominal, color Doppler ultrasound provides information on the direction of blood flow in the pelvic vessels, facilitating identification and differentiation of the veins from arteries. The external iliac vein (shown in blue) is a large caliber vessel seen posterior to its arterial counterpart (shown in multicolor). Note its uniform intensity in color flow. The internal iliac vein (shown in red) is smaller in diameter and directed inferomedially. (Bottom) Pulsed Doppler ultrasound of the common iliac vein shows uniform velocity with mild phasic changes associated with respiration.

ILIAC ARTERIES AND VEINS

INTERNAL ILIAC VEIN

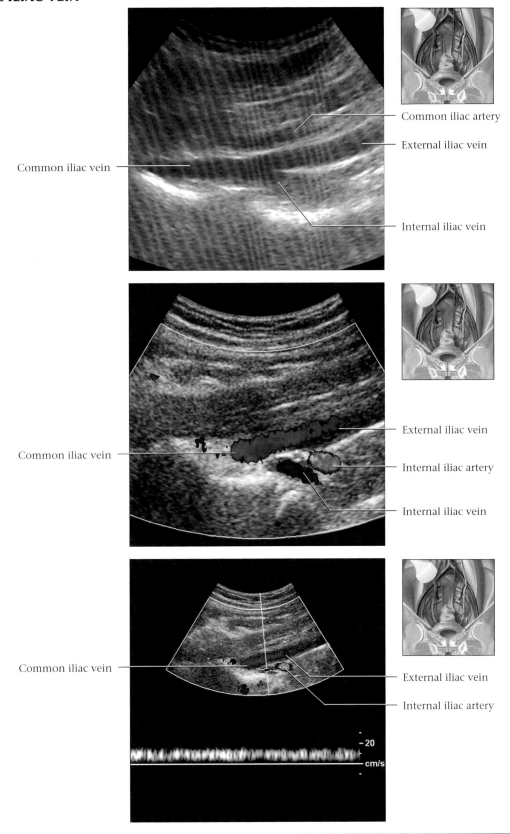

Common iliac artery

External iliac vein

Common iliac vein

Internal iliac vein

External iliac vein

Common iliac vein

Internal iliac artery

Internal iliac vein

External iliac vein

Common iliac vein

Internal iliac artery

− 20

cm/s

(Top) Longitudinal, transabdominal, grayscale ultrasound shows the external and internal iliac veins converging to become the common iliac vein. The internal iliac vein drains various veins from outside the pelvis, the sacrum and from the venous plexuses connected to pelvic viscera. **(Middle)** Longitudinal, transabdominal, color Doppler ultrasound shows a short segment of the internal iliac vein (shown in red) draining into the common iliac vein (shown in blue). Owing to its depth, the internal iliac vein cannot be identified on ultrasound in its entirety. **(Bottom)** Pulsed Doppler ultrasound of the internal iliac vein shows continuous venous flow and uniform velocity devoid of phasic changes and unaffected by respiration.

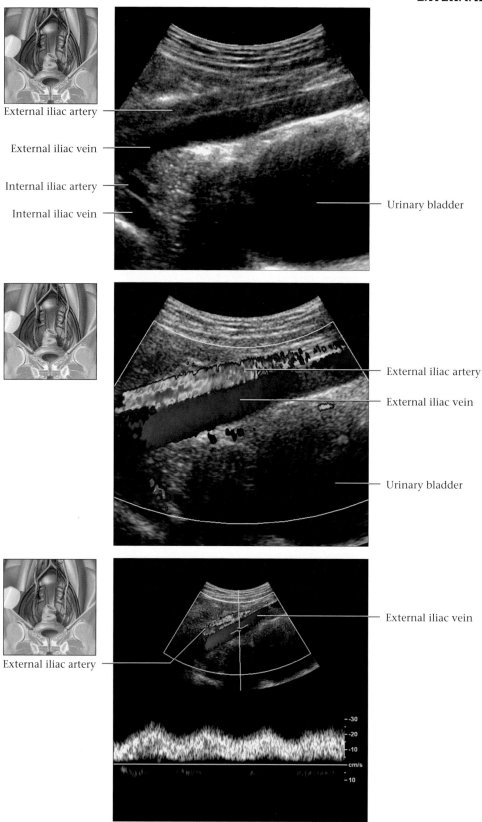

External iliac artery

External iliac vein

Internal iliac artery

Internal iliac vein

Urinary bladder

External iliac artery

External iliac vein

Urinary bladder

External iliac vein

External iliac artery

(Top) Longitudinal, transabdominal, grayscale ultrasound at the lower abdomen. The external iliac vein runs parallel and posterior to the external iliac artery. The two vessels are readily identified owing to their superficial location. The transducer is angulated medially and the urinary bladder is included in the image. **(Middle)** Longitudinal transabdominal color Doppler shows different flow directions in external iliac artery (shown in red) and vein (shown in blue). The artery is anterior to the vein and the two vessels run beneath the inguinal ligament to enter the thigh. Owing to its superficial location, the external iliac vein is easily examined during ultrasound investigation for deep venous thrombosis in the lower limbs. **(Bottom)** Pulsed Doppler ultrasound of the external iliac vein. Normal spectral waveform shows continuous flow and exaggerated phasic changes from deep inspiration/expiration.

ILIAC ARTERIES AND VEINS

ATHEROSCLEROTIC DISEASE

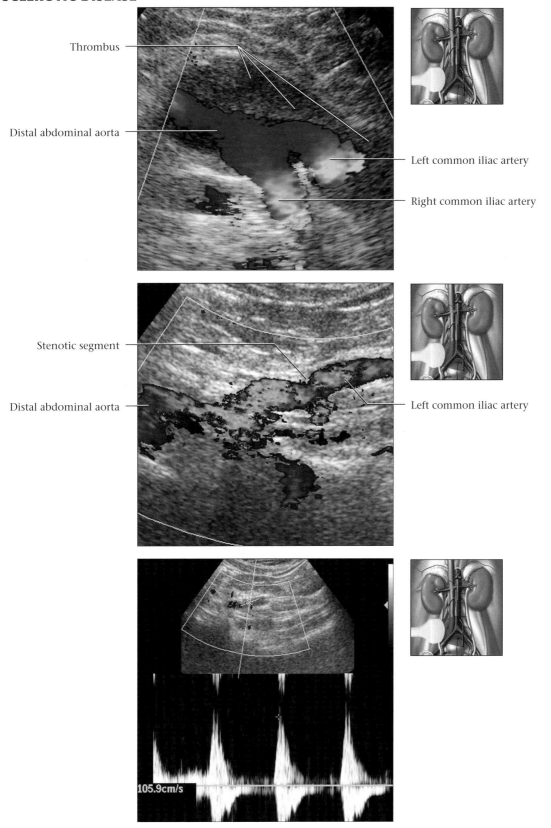

Thrombus

Distal abdominal aorta

Left common iliac artery

Right common iliac artery

Stenotic segment

Distal abdominal aorta

Left common iliac artery

105.9cm/s

(Top) Longitudinal color Doppler ultrasound shows moderate amount of mural thrombus in the infrarenal aorta (shown in blue) just above the bifurcation, causing narrowing of the lumen. The thrombus extends into the left common iliac artery. (Middle) Oblique color Doppler ultrasound shows the common iliac artery with a > 50% diameter reduction. High velocity turbulent flow is seen as "aliasing" artifact on color Doppler imaging at the stenotic segment. (Bottom) Corresponding, oblique, pulsed color Doppler ultrasound shows spectral Doppler trace at the common iliac artery stenosis, with characteristic high velocity bidirectional waveform.

TRANS-PERINEAL ANATOMY

Terminology

Abbreviations
- Longitudinal scan (LS); transverse scan (TS); axial scan (AS); symphysis pubis (SP); ultrasonography (US)

Definitions
- Perineum is divided into anterior and posterior parts by a line drawn across the ischial tuberosities
  - Anterior: Urogenital triangle
  - Posterior: Anal triangle

Imaging Anatomy

Overview
- Symphysis pubis
  - Appears as an echogenic structure with highly reflective surface anterior to the urethra
  - On Valsalva maneuver, inferior margin of SP serves as line of reference for maximal bladder descent, uterovaginal prolapse and rectocele
- Lower urinary tract
  - Urethra and bladder neck: Inverted "funnel"
  - Urethra: Multilayer; cylindrical; posterior to SP
    - Central: Mucosa/submucosa; hypoechoic
    - Concentric: Muscular lissosphincter; echogenic
    - Outer: Striated rhabdosphincter
  - Periurethral artery
    - Identified in urethral mucosa parallel to lumen
    - Resistivity index (RI): Postmenopausal > premenopausal
- Anterior vaginal septum
  - Hypoechoic vesicovaginal fascia between urethra and vagina
- Vagina
  - Posterior to the urethra
  - LS: Hypoechoic structure; poorly defined lumen unless outlined by air, fluid or jelly
  - TS: Visualized as an H-shaped hypoechoic structure
  - Vaginal artery: High RI; ↓ during sexual arousal
- Posterior vaginal septum: Perineal body and rectovesical fascia
  - Perineal body: Fibrous and muscular tissue between anus and lower vagina
  - Rectovesical fascia: Hypoechoic fascia between rectum and mid vagina
- Anus
  - Mucosa: Thin hypoechoic innermost layer
  - Submucosa: Echogenic layer
  - Internal anal sphincter: Concentric hypoechoic ring surrounding the central mucosa
  - External anal sphincter: Hyperechoic ring encircles the internal anal sphincter
- Levator ani muscle
  - Arises from pelvic side wall and is subdivided into
    - Iliococcygeus: Arises from ischial spine to insert into coccyx; lies posterolaterally; usually small
    - Pubococcygeus: Arises from pubic bone; runs posteriorly towards coccyx; surrounds rectum, vagina and bladder opening
    - Puborectalis: Arises from the pubis forming a "sling" around anorectal junction; hyperechoic

Anatomy-Based Imaging Issues

Imaging Recommendations
- Bladder neck position and motility can reliably be assessed by trans-perineal US
- Parting of the labia necessary to improve image quality
- Defecation required for better diagnostic accuracy
- Bladder filling required depending on applications

Imaging Approaches
- Performed with patient in dorsal lithotomy with hips flexed or slightly abducted or in standing position
- 3.5-7 MHz curvilinear transducer is commonly used
- Near-field imaging: Higher frequency transducer used
- 3D US advantages: Produces three orthogonal planes and allows sequential assessment
- Urethra
  - Mid-sagittal scan: Most useful projection
  - Different pelvic floor maneuver: Resting, straining by Valsalva maneuver, contracting by withholding maneuver to demonstrate bladder neck mobility
  - Retrovesical angle between proximal urethra and trigone is useful to assess bladder neck descent
- Anorectal canal
  - Axial scan: Most useful projection
  - Anal sphincter complex is best evaluated with 3D trans-perineal US

Clinical Applications

Stress Urinary Incontinence
- Funneling of the internal urethral meatus on Valsalva or at rest is suggestive of incontinence
- Retrovesical angle > 160° on Valsalva is often associated with funneling
- Bladder neck descent > 2.5 cm on Valsalva is strongly associated with urodynamic stress incontinence
- Color Doppler US may demonstrate urine leakage through the urethra on Valsalva maneuver

Uterovaginal Prolapse
- Anterior compartments (cystocele) better demonstrated than posterior compartment (rectocele)
- True rectocele ⇒ rectovaginal fascial defect
- False rectocele ⇒ intact rectovaginal fascia

Paravaginal Defect
- Lateral defects of the endopelvic fascia
- Well-demonstrated by 3D trans-perineal US

Post-operative Assessment of Uterovaginal Prolapse and Incontinence Surgery
- Status of bladder neck after colposuspension
- Demonstration of fascial and synthetic slings; bulking agents such as Macroplastique

Fecal Incontinence
- Largely due to anal sphincter musculature damage during vaginal delivery
- Anal sphincter defects are best diagnosed with 3D trans-perineal US

TRANS-PERINEAL ANATOMY

PERINEAL ANATOMY AND PELVIC DIAPHRAGM

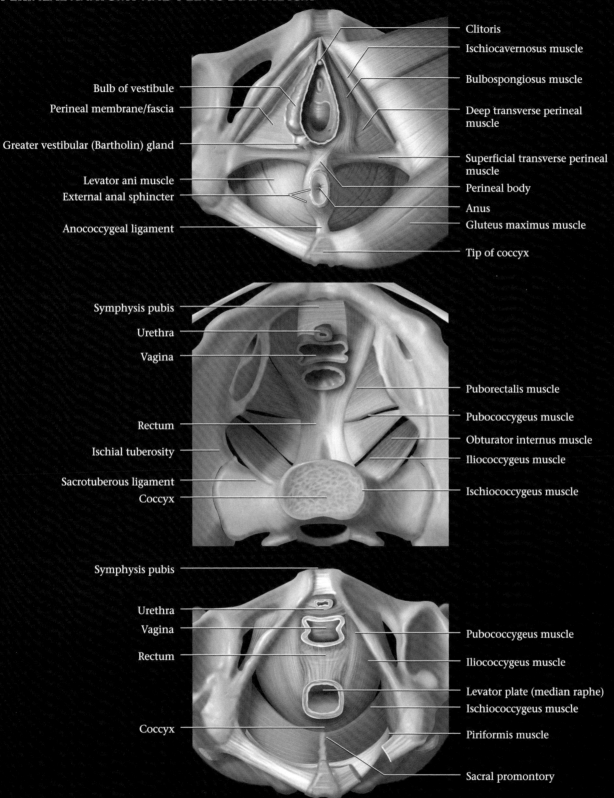

Clitoris

Ischiocavernosus muscle

Bulbospongiosus muscle

Deep transverse perineal muscle

Bulb of vestibule

Perineal membrane/fascia

Greater vestibular (Bartholin) gland

Superficial transverse perineal muscle

Levator ani muscle

Perineal body

External anal sphincter

Anus

Anococcygeal ligament

Gluteus maximus muscle

Tip of coccyx

Symphysis pubis

Urethra

Vagina

Puborectalis muscle

Pubococcygeus muscle

Rectum

Obturator internus muscle

Ischial tuberosity

Iliococcygeus muscle

Sacrotuberous ligament

Coccyx

Ischiococcygeus muscle

Symphysis pubis

Urethra

Vagina

Pubococcygeus muscle

Rectum

Iliococcygeus muscle

Levator plate (median raphe)

Ischiococcygeus muscle

Coccyx

Piriformis muscle

Sacral promontory

(**Top**) Deep dissection of female perineum, inferior view shows the urogenital and anal triangles. The perineum is a diamond-shaped region, bordered by the two ischiopubic rami and the two sacrotuberous ligaments. A horizontal line connecting the two ischial tuberosities divides the perineum into the anterior urogenital triangle and the posterior anal triangle. The perineal body lies at the midpoint of this line, just anterior to the anal canal and provides attachment for muscles and ligaments that support the perineum. (**Middle**) A deeper dissection shows the muscles of the levator ani (puborectalis, pubococcygeus, iliococcygeus) and the more posterior ischiococcygeus muscle. (**Bottom**) Female pelvic diaphragm, superior view shows the passage of urethra, vagina and rectum through the pubococcygeus muscle.

TRANS-PERINEAL ANATOMY

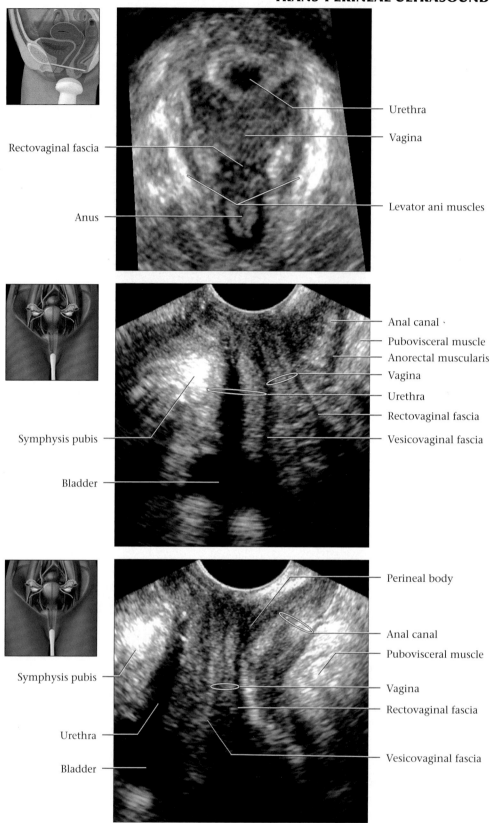

Urethra

Vagina

Rectovaginal fascia

Levator ani muscles

Anus

Anal canal ·

Pubovisceral muscle

Anorectal muscularis

Vagina

Urethra

Rectovaginal fascia

Vesicovaginal fascia

Symphysis pubis

Bladder

Perineal body

Anal canal

Pubovisceral muscle

Vagina

Rectovaginal fascia

Vesicovaginal fascia

Symphysis pubis

Urethra

Bladder

(Top) 3D volume US (axial plane) shows the relationship of the urethra, vagina and anus. The urethra is seen imbedding in the anterior wall of the vagina while the anus is separated from the vagina by the rectovaginal fascia. (Middle) Mid-sagittal scan of the anterior triangle shows the urethra and the vagina. The urethra is seen as a hypoechoic tubular structure immediately posterior to the symphysis pubis and is separated from the vagina by the vesicovaginal fascia. (Bottom) Mid-sagittal scan in the same woman as previous image but tilted more posteriorly to show the vaginal septum. The perineal body is seen as the distal attachment between the ulgina and the anus whereas the rectovaginal fascia is depicted as a hypoechoic lining separating the mid vagina from the rectum. Note the hyperechogenicity of the pubovisceral muscle is similar to that of the symphysis pubis.

TRANS-PERINEAL ANATOMY

TRANS-PERINEAL 3D US OF THE PELVIC FLOOR

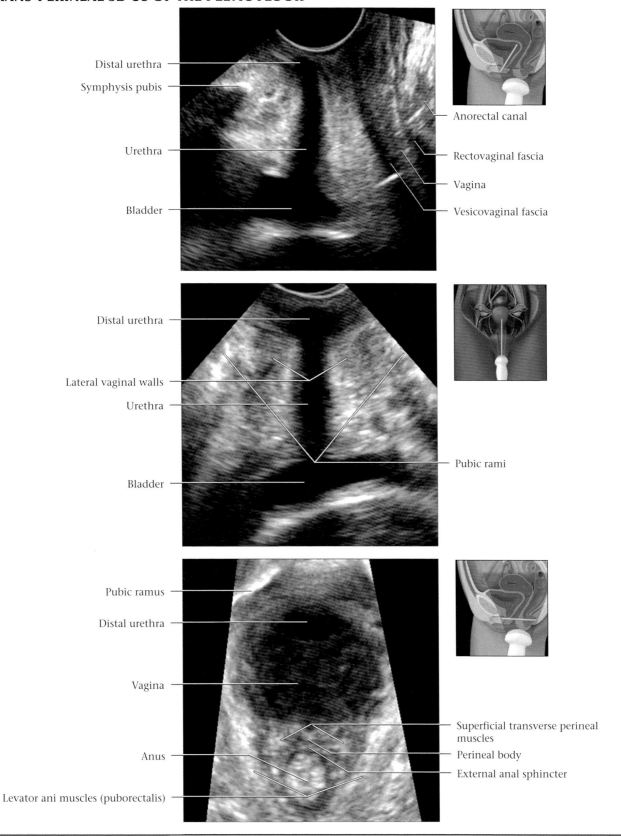

Distal urethra

Symphysis pubis

Urethra

Bladder

Anorectal canal

Rectovaginal fascia

Vagina

Vesicovaginal fascia

Distal urethra

Lateral vaginal walls

Urethra

Bladder

Pubic rami

Pubic ramus

Distal urethra

Vagina

Superficial transverse perineal muscles

Perineal body

Anus

External anal sphincter

Levator ani muscles (puborectalis)

(Top) Mid-sagittal plane of 3D trans-perineal US shows the relationship between the urethra, vagina and anorectal canal. Note the vaginal canal is barely visible unless it is outlined by fluid or acoustic jelly. **(Middle)** Corresponding coronal plane shows the urethra and bladder. Note the lateral walls of the vagina appear as slightly hypoechoic areas on either side of the urethra. **(Bottom)** Corresponding axial plane at the level just caudal to the symphysis pubis shows the distal urethra "resting" on the vagina. The anus is supported by a muscle complex formed by the superficial transverse perineal muscles which insert into the perineal body and external anal sphincter. Note the hyperechoic puborectalis forms a "sling" around the anus.

TRANS-PERINEAL ANATOMY

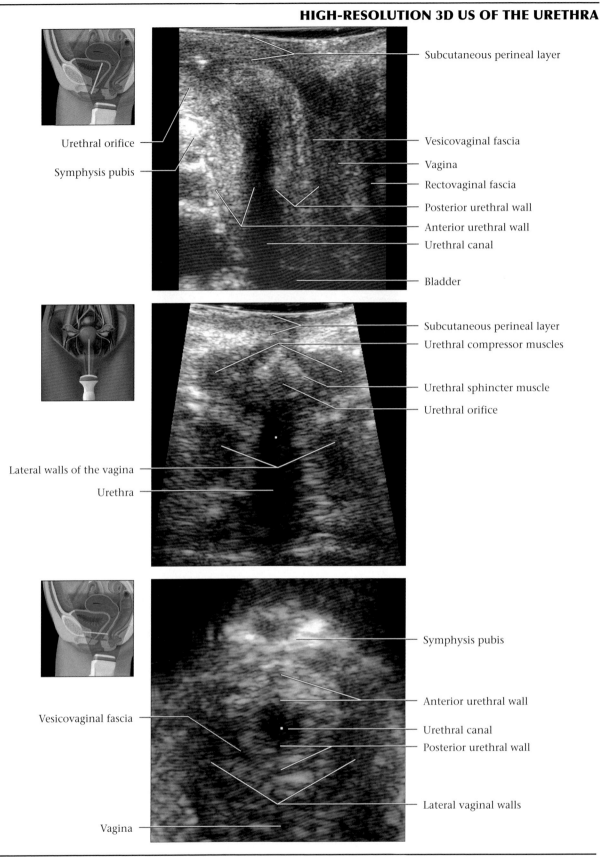

Top image labels:
- Subcutaneous perineal layer
- Urethral orifice
- Symphysis pubis
- Vesicovaginal fascia
- Vagina
- Rectovaginal fascia
- Posterior urethral wall
- Anterior urethral wall
- Urethral canal
- Bladder

Middle image labels:
- Subcutaneous perineal layer
- Urethral compressor muscles
- Urethral sphincter muscle
- Urethral orifice
- Lateral walls of the vagina
- Urethra

Bottom image labels:
- Symphysis pubis
- Anterior urethral wall
- Vesicovaginal fascia
- Urethral canal
- Posterior urethral wall
- Lateral vaginal walls
- Vagina

(Top) Mid-sagittal scan of the urethra using a high-resolution 12 MHz linear 3D transducer. With this technology, the muscular wall of the urethra can be clearly depicted and measurement of the urethral wall thickness is feasible. **(Middle)** Corresponding coronal plane shows the urethral orifice in cross section. The urethral orifice is encircled by the echogenic urethral sphincter muscle and arched over by the urethral compressor muscles. **(Bottom)** Corresponding axial plane shows the urethra in cross section. Although the wall thickness of urethral wall is discernible, differentiation of different layers of the urethra is not feasible with the existing trans-perineal technique.

TRANS-PERINEAL ANATOMY

MEASUREMENT OF BLADDER NECK DESCENT

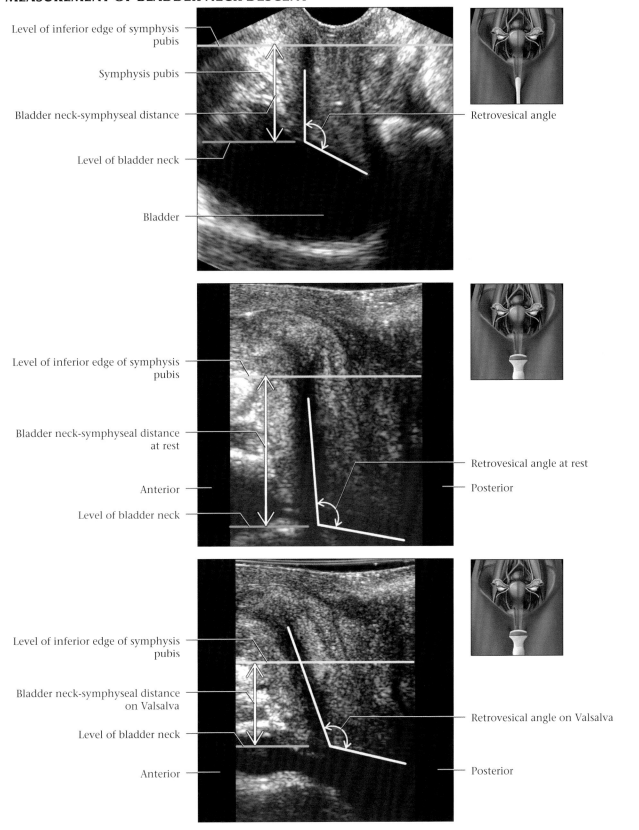

Level of inferior edge of symphysis pubis

Symphysis pubis

Bladder neck-symphyseal distance

Level of bladder neck

Bladder

Retrovesical angle

Level of inferior edge of symphysis pubis

Bladder neck-symphyseal distance at rest

Anterior

Level of bladder neck

Retrovesical angle at rest

Posterior

Level of inferior edge of symphysis pubis

Bladder neck-symphyseal distance on Valsalva

Level of bladder neck

Anterior

Retrovesical angle on Valsalva

Posterior

(**Top**) Mid-sagittal plane of the lower urinary tract demonstrates measurements of bladder neck-symphyseal distance (BSD) and retrovesical angle (RVA) used in the evaluation of bladder neck descent as a cause of urinary stress incontinence. BSD is the distance between the inferior edge of the SP and bladder neck. RVA is the angle between proximal urethra and trigone. A significant change of BSD and RVA between resting and Valsalva maneuver reflects severe bladder neck descent. (**Middle**) Bladder neck position at rest. The RVA measured at rest normally ranges between 90-120 degrees. (**Bottom**) Change of bladder neck position on Valsalva maneuver. The proximal urethra demonstrates a posteroinferior rotational descent which shortens the BSD and widens the RVA. A shortening of BSD > 2.5 cm or a widening of RVA > 160 degrees is indicative of significant bladder descent.

COLOR DOPPLER US, URETHRA AND VAGINA

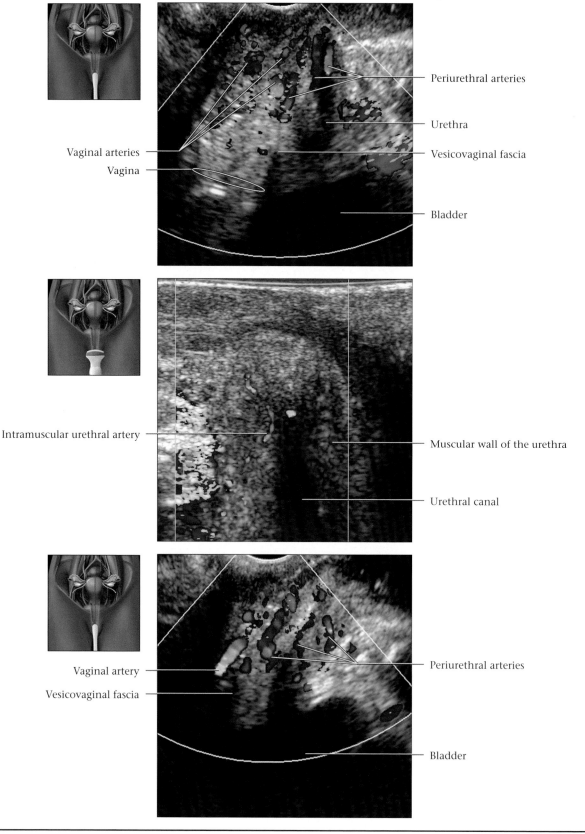

Vaginal arteries — Periurethral arteries

Urethra

Vesicovaginal fascia

Vagina —

Bladder

Intramuscular urethral artery — Muscular wall of the urethra

Urethral canal

Vaginal artery — Periurethral arteries

Vesicovaginal fascia —

Bladder

(Top) Mid-sagittal color Doppler US of the urethra shows two periurethral arteries near the mucosa of the urethra and numerous vessels in the vagina. Care must be taken not to confuse vaginal arteries with periurethral arteries. **(Middle)** High-resolution color Doppler US (mid-sagittal scan) of the urethra shows a small artery running in the muscular layer of the urethra. Note urethral vascularity is influenced by hormonal changes during the menstrual cycle, during pregnancy and postmenopause. It is higher in premenopausal women than those in menopause. **(Bottom)** Mid-sagittal color Doppler US of the vaginal artery which is in the vicinity of the periurethral arteries and is easily confused with them. Special attention should be paid to differentiate vaginal and periurethral arteries. These are separated by the vesicovaginal fascia.

SPECTRAL DOPPLER US, URETHRA AND VAGINA

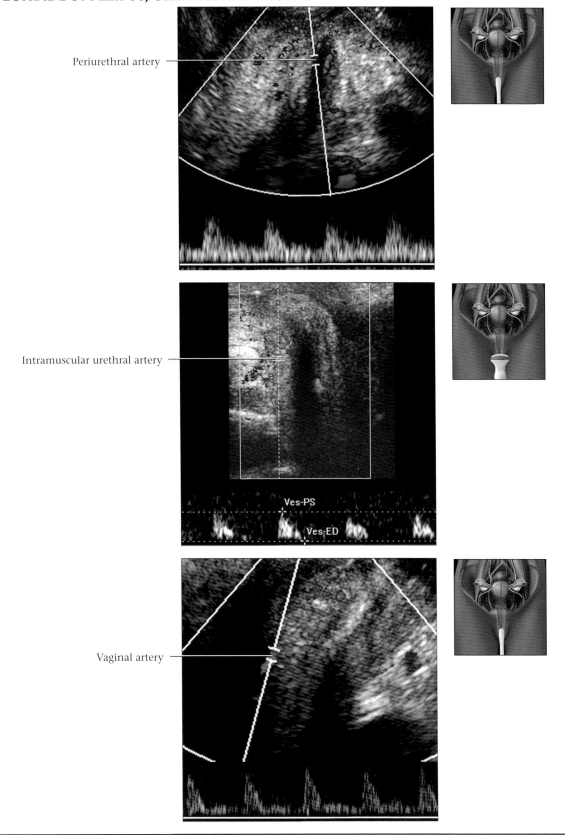

Periurethral artery

Intramuscular urethral artery

Ves-PS

Ves-ED

Vaginal artery

(**Top**) Mid-sagittal spectral Doppler scan of the periurethral artery shows normal, low-resistance blood flow. It has been suggested that decrease in periurethral vascularity is related to stress incontinence in postmenopausal women. (**Middle**) Doppler waveform of intramuscular urethral artery demonstrates high flow resistance with absent diastolic velocity in this artery. (**Bottom**) Doppler waveform of the vaginal artery demonstrates high-resistance blood flow with a low diastolic velocity component. Flow resistance may be lowered during the state of sexual arousal.

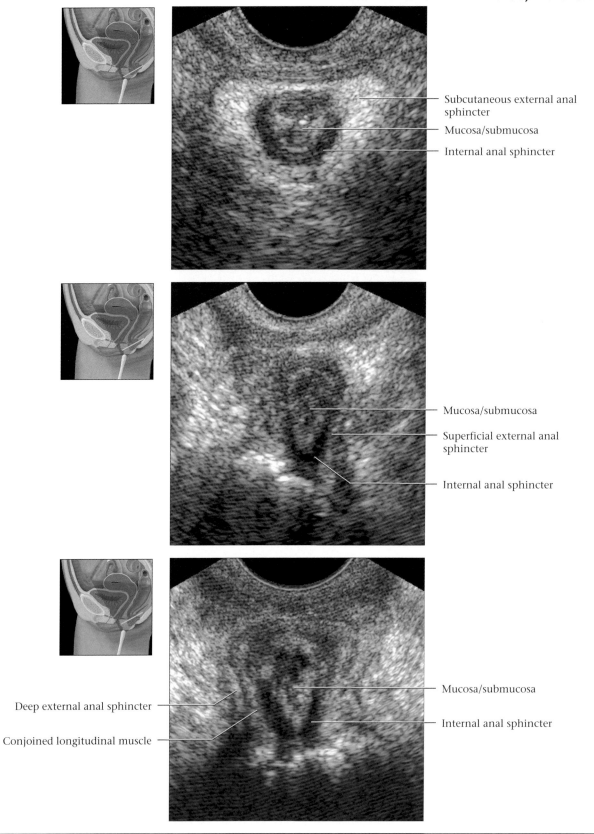

Subcutaneous external anal sphincter

Mucosa/submucosa

Internal anal sphincter

Mucosa/submucosa

Superficial external anal sphincter

Internal anal sphincter

Deep external anal sphincter

Conjoined longitudinal muscle

Mucosa/submucosa

Internal anal sphincter

(Top) 3D ultrasound evaluation of anal orifice. The echogenic mucosa/submucosa of the anus is surrounded by two concentric rings. The inner hypoechoic ring represents the internal anal sphincter (IAS) and the outer hyperechoic ring denotes the subcutaneous external anal sphincter (EAS). **(Middle)** Mid anal canal. The IAS appears as a hypoechoic ring which is asymmetrical in thickness. With advancing age, IAS may lose its uniform thickness and echogenicity. **(Bottom)** High anal canal. The conjoined longitudinal muscle (CLM) is identified as a moderately echogenic band between the IAS and EAS. However, it is not always distinguishable from the EAS along the entire anal canal.

TRANS-PERINEAL ANATOMY

3D VOLUME RENDERED US, VAGINA

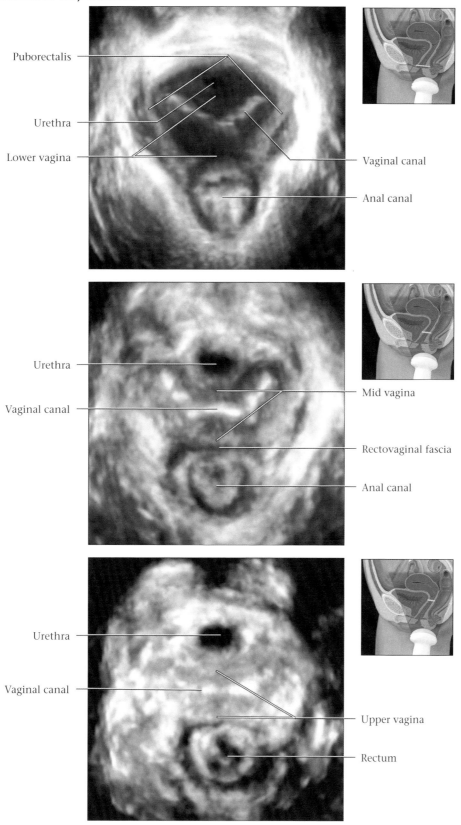

Puborectalis

Urethra

Lower vagina

Vaginal canal

Anal canal

Urethra

Vaginal canal

Mid vagina

Rectovaginal fascia

Anal canal

Urethra

Vaginal canal

Upper vagina

Rectum

(Top) 3D volume rendered Axial scan of the lower vagina at the level of the symphysis pubis. The vagina is "sandwiched" between the urethra and the anus. The vaginal canal is enhanced by acoustic jelly and air bubbles trapped within it following transvaginal scan. It resembles a widened letter "V". (Middle) Axial scan of the mid vagina. The vagina at this level appears as a "cradle" partially invaginating the urethra in its anterior wall. The vaginal canal changes its shape from "V" to "U". (Bottom) Axial scan of the upper vagina. The vagina at this level appears flattened and loses its anterolateral extensions. The vaginal canal becomes an echogenic straight line.

TRANS-PERINEAL ANATOMY

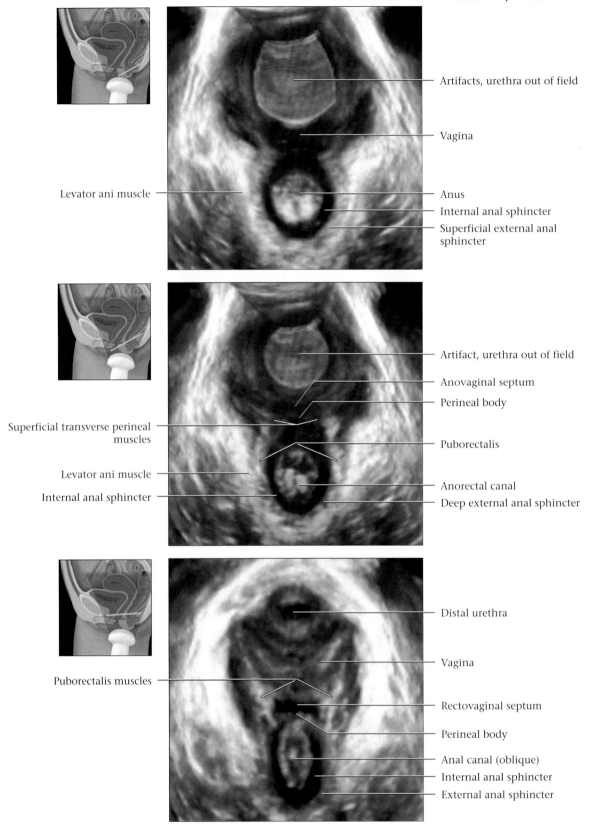

Top image labels:
- Artifacts, urethra out of field
- Vagina
- Anus
- Internal anal sphincter
- Superficial external anal sphincter
- Levator ani muscle

Middle image labels:
- Artifact, urethra out of field
- Anovaginal septum
- Perineal body
- Puborectalis
- Anorectal canal
- Deep external anal sphincter
- Superficial transverse perineal muscles
- Levator ani muscle
- Internal anal sphincter

Bottom image labels:
- Distal urethra
- Vagina
- Rectovaginal septum
- Perineal body
- Anal canal (oblique)
- Internal anal sphincter
- External anal sphincter
- Puborectalis muscles

(Top) Axial scan of mid anal canal. The superficial EAS is seen as an incomplete ring with absent anterior portion. It is a frequent finding either due to a natural gap in normal females or sphincter rupture in multiparous women. **(Middle)** Axial scan of anorectal junction and the perineal body. The deep EAS is seen to be integral with the puborectalis which forms a "sling" around the anorectal junction. The EAS and transverse perineal muscles meet in the perineal body which provides fundamental support to all musculoligamentous components of the pelvis. **(Bottom)** Axial scan of puborectalis muscle in the anterior triangle. The muscles are seen as two echogenic linear structures running alongside the lower vagina and urethra which are projected on an end-on view.

TRANS-PERINEAL ANATOMY

3D VOLUME RENDERED US, PELVIC FLOOR

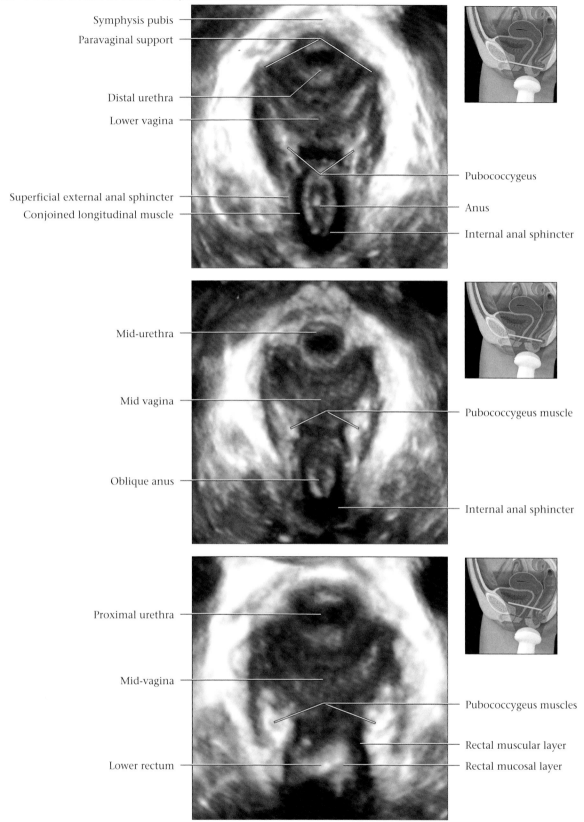

Symphysis pubis

Paravaginal support

Distal urethra

Lower vagina

Superficial external anal sphincter

Conjoined longitudinal muscle

Pubococcygeus

Anus

Internal anal sphincter

Mid-urethra

Mid vagina

Oblique anus

Pubococcygeus muscle

Internal anal sphincter

Proximal urethra

Mid-vagina

Lower rectum

Pubococcygeus muscles

Rectal muscular layer

Rectal mucosal layer

(Top) Axial plane of the paravaginal support. It is seen as the pubovaginal attachment lateral to the urethra. Identification of the paravaginal support is important because disruption of this structure during vaginal delivery may be related to anterior vaginal prolapse and stress urinary incontinence. **(Middle)** Axial scan of the pubococcygeus in the anterior triangle. The echogenic muscle arises from the pubic bone and runs posteriorly towards the ischial spine. It also crosses the midline to form rectal and vaginal hiatus. **(Bottom)** Axial scan of the distal rectum. The rectal wall shows two distinct layers: Innermost echogenic mucosa and outermost hypoechoic muscular layer which is a continuation of IAS and CLM.

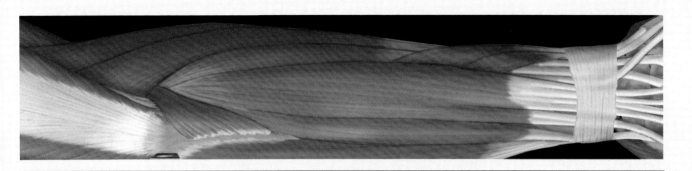

SECTION VI: Upper Limb

STERNOCLAVICULAR & ACROMIOCLAVICULAR JOINTS

Terminology

Abbreviations
- Sternoclavicular (SC) joint
- Acromioclavicular (AC) joint

Gross Anatomy

Sternoclavicular Joint
- Between medial end of clavicle & manubrium
  - Synovial sellar-type (saddle) joint
  - Medial end of clavicle = large & bulbous
  - Much larger than manubrial concavity
  - < Half of medial clavicle articulates with manubrium
    - Stability through capsuloligamentous structures
- Intra-articular disc
  - Attached to joint capsule anteriorly & posteriorly
  - Complete or incomplete ± perforations
  - Thickest posterosuperiorly (3 mm)
- Ligaments of sternoclavicular joint
  - Capsular ligaments
    - Cover anterosuperior & posterior aspects of sternoclavicular joint
    - Prevent upward displacement of medial clavicle, which may be caused by downward force on shoulder
    - Anterior stronger than posterior portion
  - Interclavicular ligament
    - Connects superomedial aspect of clavicle → capsular ligaments & upper manubrium
    - Covers anterosuperior & posterior aspects of joint
    - Prevents excessive upward motion of clavicle
  - Costoclavicular ligaments
    - Unite inferior surface medial end clavicle → upper surface of first rib
    - Anterior fibers arise from anteromedial surface of first rib & resist upward motion
    - Posterior fibers arise lateral to anterior fibers & resist downward motion
- Muscle attachments to medial clavicle & sternum
  - Pectoralis major from anterior aspect medial two-thirds clavicle (clavicular head)
  - Sternocleidomastoid from posterior surface medial third of clavicle (clavicular head)
  - Sternohyoid & sternothyroid muscles separate great vessels from sternoclavicular joint

Acromioclavicular Joint
- Synovial joint between lateral end of clavicle & medial end of acromion
  - Articular surface of clavicle oriented posterolaterally while articular surface of acromion oriented anteromedially
    - Angle of inclination between opposing articular surfaces varies with clavicle over-riding acromion (50%), vertical orientation between acromion & clavicle (25%), clavicle under-riding acromion (5%), & mixed pattern (20%)
    - Maximum width of normal joint on ultrasound = 5 mm if < 35 years & < 4.4 mm if > 35 years
    - Maximum thickness of capsule from bony surface = 2.7 mm if < 35 years & < 3.6 mm if > 35 years
- Intra-articular disc
  - Undergoes rapid degeneration beginning in 2nd decade → marked degeneration of disc by 4th decade
- Ligaments of acromioclavicular joint
  - Superior AC ligament
    - Stronger & thicker (2.0-5.5 mm) than thin or absent inferior AC ligament
    - Inserts along lateral clavicle (8 mm) & medial acromion (10 mm)
  - Coracoclavicular ligaments
    - Conoid & trapezoid ligaments
    - Vary significantly in length & width
    - Conoid ligament located posteromedially
    - Inserts to conoid tubercle, located at point where middle third of clavicle curves into lateral third
    - Mainly prevents upward movement of clavicle
    - Trapezoid ligament located anterolaterally
    - Inserts to trapezoid ridge which runs along inferior surface, of lateral third of clavicle
    - Mainly prevents lateral compression of clavicle against acromion
  - Muscle attachments to lateral clavicle
    - Deltoid → anterior surface lateral third of clavicle
    - Trapezius → posterior surface lateral third of clavicle

Anatomy-Based Imaging Issues

Imaging Recommendations
- High resolution linear transducer
- Align transducer transversely along SC or AC joints
- AC joint laxity can be assessed by pulling down on arm while observing joint width on ultrasound
  - Compare with contralateral side
- Main clinical presentation of SC joint is painless lump
  - Mild degrees of capsular thickening readily apparent clinically since joint just beneath skin surface
    - Mainly due to relative forward positioning of symptomatic SC joint due to axial rotation of upper trunk
    - Occasionally due to mild capsular swelling ± mild subluxation secondary to SC osteoarthropathy
  - Main clinical presentation of AC joint is pain due to osteoarthropathy, AC joint impingement, inflammatory arthropathy & subluxation/dislocation

Imaging Pitfalls
- Sternoclavicular or acromioclavicular joints
  - Normally a step-off between medial clavicle & manubrium &, to lesser degree, between lateral clavicle & acromion
  - Should not be interpreted as subluxation
  - Acromion normally elevates from rest position during arm adduction
  - AC joint index = AC joint width of uninjured side/AC joint width of injured side = 1.0 normally
  - For AC joint injury, AC index = 1.0 for Tossy 1; 0.49 for Tossy II & 0.21 for Tossy III

STERNOCLAVICULAR & ACROMIOCLAVICULAR JOINTS

TRANSVERSE US, STERNOCLAVICULAR JOINT

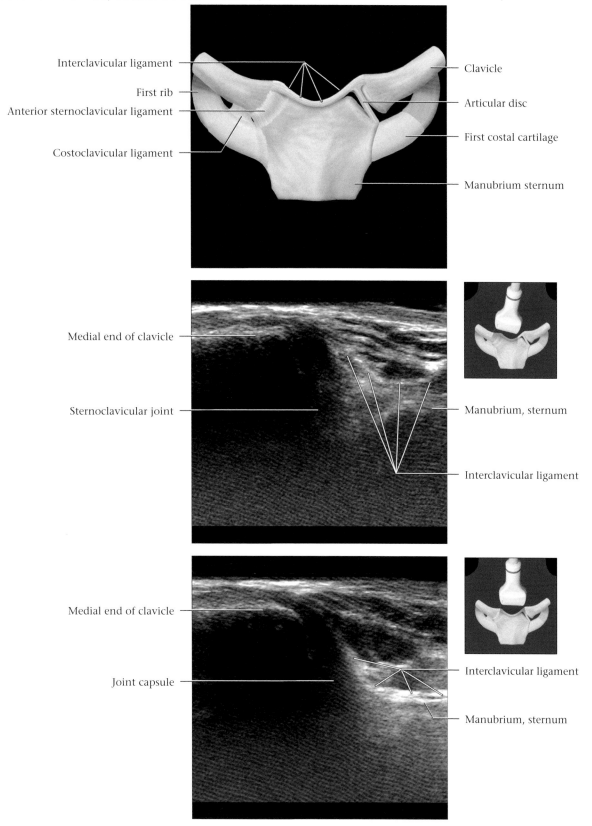

Interclavicular ligament

First rib

Anterior sternoclavicular ligament

Costoclavicular ligament

Clavicle

Articular disc

First costal cartilage

Manubrium sternum

Medial end of clavicle

Sternoclavicular joint

Manubrium, sternum

Interclavicular ligament

Medial end of clavicle

Joint capsule

Interclavicular ligament

Manubrium, sternum

(Top) Graphic showing the anterior aspect of the sternoclavicular joint. Note the joint capsule, articular disc and interclavicular ligament. **(Middle)** Transverse grayscale ultrasound at the anterosuperior aspect of the sternoclavicular joint. The medial clavicle is much larger than the articulating surface of the manubrium. The thin interclavicular ligament is closely applied to the superior aspect of manubrium and its connection with the medial ends of both clavicles is depicted. **(Bottom)** Transverse grayscale ultrasound at the superior aspect of the sternoclavicular joint. The costoclavicular ligament prevents upward movement of the medial clavicle when the lateral clavicle or shoulder is depressed.

LONGITUDINAL US, STERNOCLAVICULAR JOINT

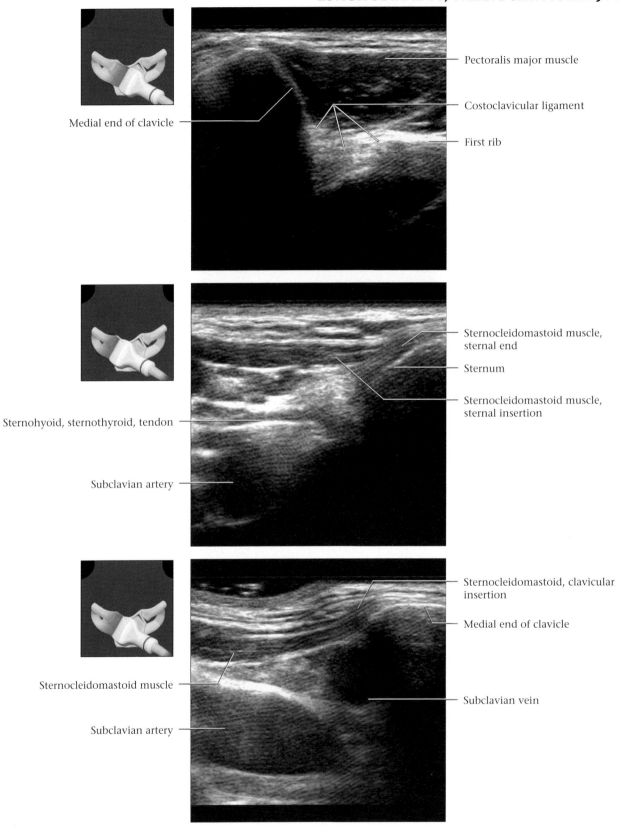

Medial end of clavicle

Pectoralis major muscle

Costoclavicular ligament

First rib

Sternohyoid, sternothyroid, tendon

Subclavian artery

Sternocleidomastoid muscle, sternal end

Sternum

Sternocleidomastoid muscle, sternal insertion

Sternocleidomastoid muscle

Subclavian artery

Sternocleidomastoid, clavicular insertion

Medial end of clavicle

Subclavian vein

(Top) Longitudinal grayscale US at SC joint. Costoclavicular ligament prevents upwards movement of the medial clavicle when shoulder is depressed. Pectoralis major muscle arises from the medial half of the anterior surface of the clavicle as well as from the sternum, upper costal cartilages & upper part of external oblique aponeurosis. **(Middle)** Longitudinal grayscale US at SC joint region. Sternocleidomastoid is attached to the upper surface of the medial end of the clavicle as well as the upper anterior surface of manubrium. Sternohyoid & sternothyroid are attached to the posterior aspect of the sternum as well as the clavicle & 1st costal cartilage. **(Bottom)** Longitudinal grayscale US at SC joint. Great vessels lie posterior to sternoclavicular joint, may get injured in posterior dislocation. All tendinous attachments should be assessed if dislocation is present as they may also be injured.

STERNOCLAVICULAR & ACROMIOCLAVICULAR JOINTS

US, ACROMIOCLAVICULAR JOINT

Superior acromioclavicular l.
Inferior acromioclavicular ligament
Coracoacromial ligament
Coracoclavicular ligament, trapezoid component
Coracohumeral ligament
Transverse humeral ligament
Biceps tendon, long head
Biceps tendon, short head
Latissimus dorsi muscle

Clavicle, distal
Coracoclavicular ligament, conoid band
Coracoid process
Subscapularis muscle
Teres major muscle

Lateral end of clavicle

Coracoclavicular ligament, trapezoid component
Coracoid process

Deltoid muscle
Coracoacromial ligament
Acromion
Supraspinatus muscle
Humeral head

Coracoid process

(Top) Anterior lordotic graphic of the shoulder, superficial dissection. (Middle) Longitudinal grayscale ultrasound of the acromioclavicular joint region. The coracoclavicular ligament is demonstrated but is not clearly depicted on US as on MR exam. These ligaments prevent upward and lateral movement of the clavicle. (Bottom) Transverse grayscale ultrasound at the acromioclavicular joint region showing the coracoacromial ligament. The supraspinatus tendon and intervening bursa can impinge against the coracoacromial ligament during arm abduction.

STERNOCLAVICULAR & ACROMIOCLAVICULAR JOINTS

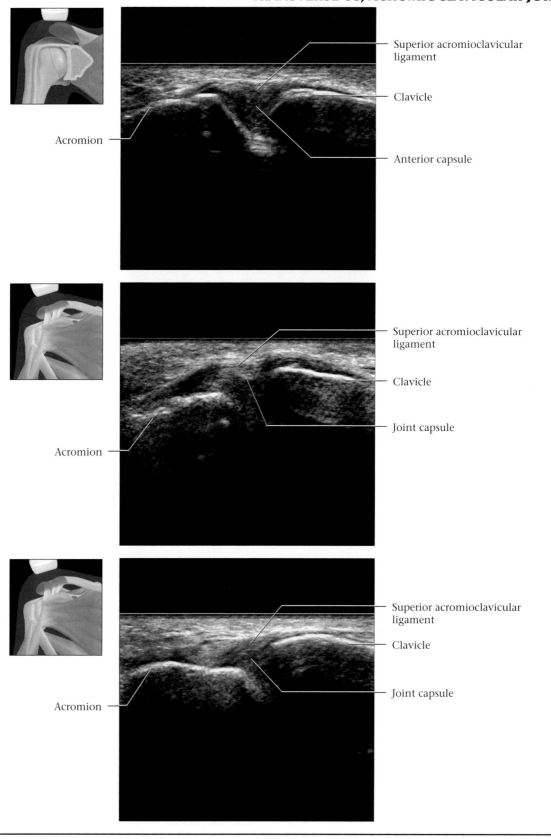

(Top) Transverse grayscale ultrasound at the anterior aspect of the acromioclavicular joint. The joint capsule of the acromioclavicular joint is thin with a strong supporting superior acromioclavicular ligament. **(Middle)** Transverse grayscale ultrasound at the anterosuperior acromioclavicular joint. Separation of the clavicle and acromion can be readily appreciated. Note how opposing bone margins are not vertically aligned. **(Bottom)** Transverse grayscale ultrasound at the superior aspect of the acromioclavicular joint. In this image, the clavicle slightly overrides the acromion. This is a normal configuration.

STERNOCLAVICULAR & ACROMIOCLAVICULAR JOINTS

TRANSVERSE US, ACROMIOCLAVICULAR JOINT

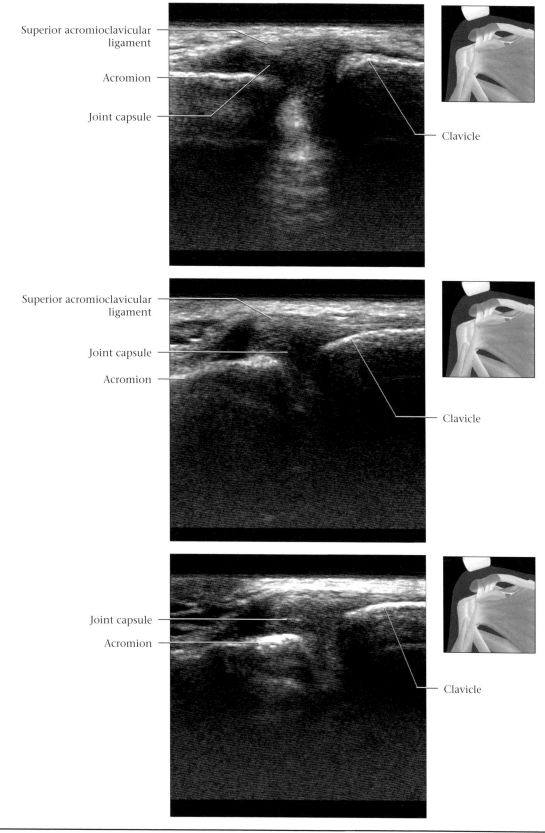

(Top) Transverse grayscale ultrasound at the anterosuperior aspect of the acromioclavicular joint, with arm by the side. Note that the clavicle slightly overrides the acromion. (Middle) Transverse grayscale ultrasound at the acromioclavicular joint, with arm abducted. The acromion is now level with the lateral aspect of the clavicle. Note how the joint capsule bulges superiorly and the opposing bones are approximated with arm abducted. (Bottom) Transverse grayscale ultrasound at the acromioclavicular joint, with arm adducted. The acromion is now depressed relative to this lateral end of the clavicle.

SHOULDER

Terminology

Abbreviations
- Rotator cuff (RC)
- Supraspinatus tendon (SST)
- Infraspinatus tendon (IST)
- Long head biceps tendon (LHBT)
- Subacromial-subdeltoid (SA-SD) bursa
- Acromioclavicular (AC)
- Coracoacromial ligament (CAL)

Imaging Anatomy

Overview
- **Rotator cuff**
  - Consists of supraspinatus, infraspinatus, teres minor & subscapularis muscles & tendons
  - Cuff tendons blend with shoulder joint capsule
  - Supraspinatus & infraspinatus tendons inseparable at insertion
  - Anterior 1.5 cm of tendon comprises supraspinatus tendon insertional area
- **Supraspinatus muscle**
  - Origin: Supraspinatus fossa of scapula
  - Insertion: Superior facet (horizontal orientation) & portion of middle facet of greater tuberosity
    - Broad insertional area
  - Nerve supply: Suprascapular nerve
  - Blood supply: Suprascapular artery & circumflex scapular branches of subscapular artery
  - Action: Abduction of humerus
  - Muscle consists of two distinct portions
    - Anterior portion is larger, fusiform in shape, has dominant tendon & is more likely to tear
    - Posterior portion is flat & has terminal tendon
  - Most commonly injured rotator cuff tendon
- **Infraspinatus muscle**
  - Origin: Infraspinatus fossa of scapula
  - Insertion: Middle facet greater tuberosity
    - Centrally positioned within tendon
  - Nerve supply: Suprascapular nerve, distal fibers
  - Blood supply: Suprascapular artery & circumflex scapular branches of subscapular artery
  - Action: External rotation of humerus & resists posterior subluxation
- **Teres minor muscle**
  - Origin: Lateral scapular border, middle half
  - Insertion: Inferior facet (vertical orientation) of humerus greater tuberosity
  - Nerve supply: Axillary nerve
  - Blood supply: Posterior circumflex humeral artery & circumflex scapular branches of subscapular artery
  - Action: External rotation of humerus
  - Least commonly injured rotator cuff tendon
- **Subscapularis muscle**
  - Origin: Subscapular fossa of scapula
  - Insertion: Lesser tuberosity & up to 40% may insert at surgical neck
  - Nerve supply: Subscapular nerve, upper & lower
  - Blood supply: Subscapularis artery
  - Action: Internal rotation of humerus, also adduction, extension, depression & flexion

- 4-6 tendon slips converge into main tendon; multipennate morphology increases strength
- **Rotator cuff tendon blood supply**
  - Derived from adjacent muscle, bone & bursae
  - Normal hypovascular regions in tendons
    - Termed "critical zone"; about 1 cm proximal to insertion
    - Vulnerable to degeneration & calcific deposition
    - However, the insertional area is more prone to tearing than critical zone
- **Biceps tendon, long head**
  - Origin: Superior glenoid labrum
    - Portions may attach to supraglenoid tubercle, anterosuperior labrum, posterosuperior labrum & coracoid base
  - Courses through superior shoulder joint to bicipital groove
  - Action: Stabilizes & depresses humeral head
  - Anatomic variants
    - Anomalous intra-articular & extra-articular origins from rotator cuff & joint capsule
  - Tendon sheath communicates with glenohumeral joint & normally contains a small amount of fluid
- **Subacromial-subdeltoid fat plane**
  - Subacromial & subdeltoid portions ± subcoracoid extension in some subjects
  - Fat plane is superficial to bursa
  - Can be interrupted or absent in normal patients
  - Attached along free border of coracoacromial ligament & adjacent deep surface of deltoid muscle; also to humerus distal to supraspinatus tendon
- **Rotator cuff interval**
  - Space between supraspinatus & subscapularis tendon through which passes biceps tendons
  - **Borders of rotator interval**
    - Triangular-shaped space
    - Coracohumeral ligament & superior glenohumeral ligament stabilize long head of biceps tendon as it enters bicipital groove
    - Varies in size
    - May not be seen as distinct interspace in some subjects
    - Superior border: Leading edge of supraspinatus
    - Inferior border: Superior aspect subscapularis tendon
    - Lateral border: LHBT & bicipital groove
    - Medial border: Base of coracoid process
  - **Contents of rotator interval**
    - Long head biceps tendon
    - Superior glenohumeral ligament
    - Coracohumeral ligament
- **Coracoacromial ligament**
  - Forms coracoacromial arch along with acromion & coracoid process
    - Reinforces inferior aspect of acromioclavicular joint
  - Extends from distal two-thirds of coracoid to acromion tip
    - Two distinct bands, anterolateral & posteromedial
  - Broad insertion to undersurface acromion
    - Anterolateral band thicker at acromion ± associated with spurs

SHOULDER

Anatomy-Based Imaging Issues

Imaging Approaches

- Tendons best seen when on stretch
  - High resolution linear transducer
  - Long axis (longitudinal) & transverse view of each tendon
  - Each part of tendon needs to be examined; anisotropy will prevent all parts of tendon being seen with one angulation
- Supraspinatus tendon
  - Arm extended & internally rotated
    - Or, if too painful, hand resting on iliac crest
- Infraspinatus & teres minor tendons
  - Arm extended & internally rotated
  - Teres minor tendon located posteroinferior to infraspinatus tendon
- Subscapularis tendon
  - Arm neutral & externally rotated
- Long head biceps tendon
  - Arm neutral & externally rotated
  - Vary degree of external rotation to optimally view biceps
- Subacromial-subdeltoid bursa
  - Stretching tendons may squeeze fluid from area of bursa under inspection
  - Examine in all positions & also in neutral position
  - Fluid collects preferentially just lateral to acromion, lateral to proximal humerus & near coracoacromial ligament
- Coracoid process
  - Neutral position
- Coracoacromial ligament
  - Neutral position
- Supraspinatus & infraspinatus muscles
  - Neutral position with hands resting on thigh
  - Examine thickest part of muscles from behind (in coronal & sagittal planes)
  - Increasing muscle echogenicity (± compared to deltoid), ↓ visibility of central tendon ⇒ > degree of fatty replacement
- Spinoglenoid notch
  - Neutral position

Imaging "Sweet Spots"

- Look particularly at anterior leading edge of supraspinatus tendon for tears
  - Unexplained bursal fluid is a good secondary sign of rotator cuff tear
- Bursa fluid is often best seen with arm in neutral position or decreased internal rotation (hand in back pocket)

Imaging Pitfalls

- **Anisotropy**
  - Echoes are optimally reflected when transducer is parallel to tendon fibers
  - Rotator cuff tendons prone to anisotropy due to curved course
  - If transducer not at right angles to tendon → will appear either isoechoic or hypoechoic to muscle
    - May simulate tendinosis or partial tear
- **Tendon edges**
  - Interfaces of tendons with adjacent structures may simulate tears
  - All tears & other tendon pathology should be confirmed in two planes
- **Acoustic shadowing from tendinous intersections of deltoid**
  - Hypoechoic acoustic shadowing may simulate tendon tear
  - Not seen when same area viewed from a slightly different angle
- **Tendinous interspace at rotator cuff interval**
  - Interspace between leading edge (anterior edge) of supraspinatus & long head biceps tendon may simulate tear
  - Overcome by recognizing ovoid or rounded shape of biceps tendon
  - Rotator cuff best seen with arm in external rotation
- **Focal thinning at supraspinatus - infraspinatus junction**
  - Mild to moderate diffuse thinning of supraspinatus & infraspinatus tendons at their junction is a normal finding
  - Should not be mistaken for tendon attenuation or partial thickness tear
- **Musculotendinous junction**
  - Supraspinatus
    - Hypoechoic muscle extending along superficial aspect of tendon may simulate SA-SD bursal distension
    - Interdigitating tendons of anterior & posterior portions may simulate tendinosis or tear
  - Infraspinatus tendon
    - Muscle fibers surrounding centrally positioned tendon may be confused with tear
  - Subscapularis
    - 4-6 tendon tendon slips converging into main tendon may simulate tendinosis
- **Fibrocartilaginous insertion**
  - Thin layer of fibrocartilage exists between tendon & bone at insertional area
  - > Steepness of insertion, > thickness of fibrocartilaginous layer
  - Thin hypoechoic layer of fibrocartilage may simulate avulsive tear
- **Subacromial-subdeltoid fat plane**
  - Fat plane lies superficial to bursa & deep to deltoid muscle
  - Normal bursa is very thin
  - Thickness of echogenic fat plane variable between patients though usually similar side-to-side
  - May be wrongly interpreted as bursal fluid
    - Look for intrabursal fluid ± hyperemia (latter = feature of inflammatory arthropathy)
  - **Fluid in biceps tendon sheath**
    - Communicates with glenohumeral joint
    - Small to moderate amount of fluid is normal
    - Do not misinterpret as long head biceps tenosynovitis

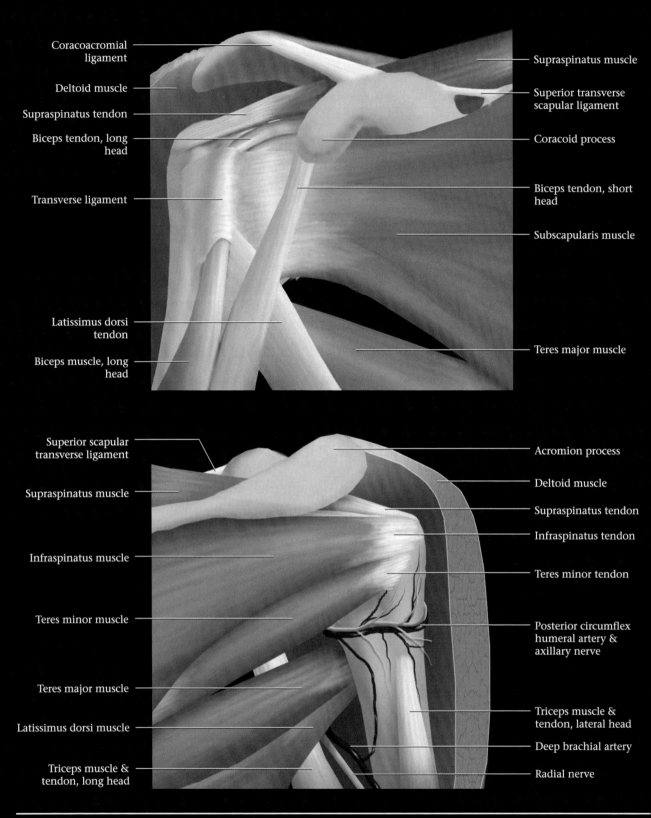

Coracoacromial ligament

Deltoid muscle

Supraspinatus tendon

Biceps tendon, long head

Transverse ligament

Latissimus dorsi tendon

Biceps muscle, long head

Supraspinatus muscle

Superior transverse scapular ligament

Coracoid process

Biceps tendon, short head

Subscapularis muscle

Teres major muscle

Superior scapular transverse ligament

Supraspinatus muscle

Infraspinatus muscle

Teres minor muscle

Teres major muscle

Latissimus dorsi muscle

Triceps muscle & tendon, long head

Acromion process

Deltoid muscle

Supraspinatus tendon

Infraspinatus tendon

Teres minor tendon

Posterior circumflex humeral artery & axillary nerve

Triceps muscle & tendon, lateral head

Deep brachial artery

Radial nerve

(Top) Anterior graphic of the right shoulder demonstrating the rotator cuff & adjacent structures. **(Bottom)** Posterior graphic of the right shoulder demonstrating the rotator cuff & adjacent structures.

SHOULDER

GRAPHICS, DEEP STRUCTURES

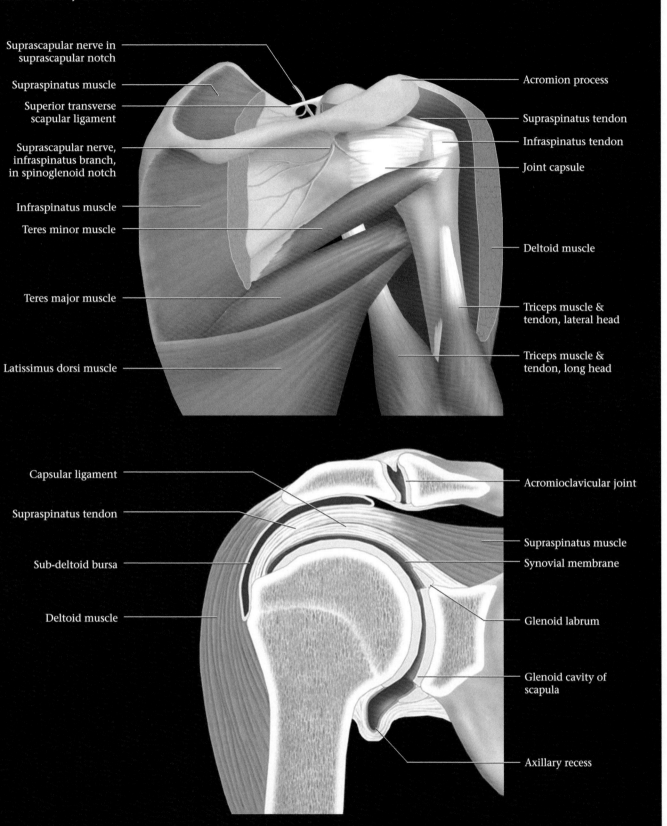

Suprascapular nerve in suprascapular notch

Suprascapular muscle

Superior transverse scapular ligament

Suprascapular nerve, infraspinatus branch, in spinoglenoid notch

Infraspinatus muscle

Teres minor muscle

Teres major muscle

Latissimus dorsi muscle

Acromion process

Supraspinatus tendon

Infraspinatus tendon

Joint capsule

Deltoid muscle

Triceps muscle & tendon, lateral head

Triceps muscle & tendon, long head

Capsular ligament

Supraspinatus tendon

Sub-deltoid bursa

Deltoid muscle

Acromioclavicular joint

Supraspinatus muscle

Synovial membrane

Glenoid labrum

Glenoid cavity of scapula

Axillary recess

(Top) Deep scapulohumeral dissection shows the course of the suprascapular nerve. (Bottom) Graphic shows the coronal section through the shoulder joint.

Deltoid muscle

Labrum, 12:00 position

Infraspinatus tendon

Labrum, 9:00 position

Glenoid fossa

Teres minor muscle and tendon

Inferior glenohumeral ligament complex, posterior band

Inferior glenohumeral ligament complex, axillary pouch

Supraspinatus tendon

Coracohumeral ligament

Biceps tendon

Superior glenohumeral ligament

Subscapularis tendon

Middle glenohumeral ligament

Labrum, 3:00 position

Inferior glenohumeral ligament complex, anterior band

Labrum, 6:00 position

Subscapularis muscle

Sagittal graphic of the glenoid fossa. The labrum lines the edge of the glenoid, increasing the circumference and depth of the shoulder joint.

SHOULDER

LONGITUDINAL US, SUPRASPINATUS INSERTIONAL AREA

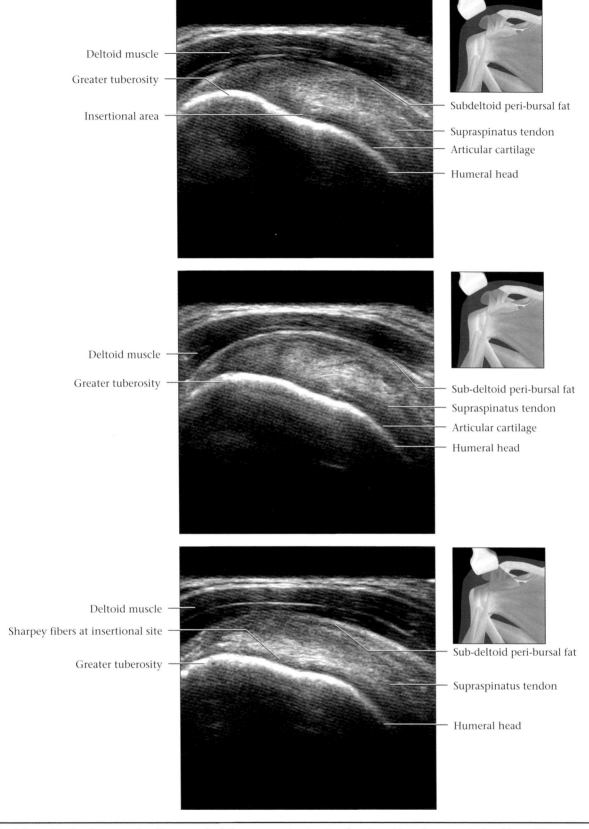

Deltoid muscle

Greater tuberosity

Insertional area

Subdeltoid peri-bursal fat

Supraspinatus tendon

Articular cartilage

Humeral head

Deltoid muscle

Greater tuberosity

Sub-deltoid peri-bursal fat

Supraspinatus tendon

Articular cartilage

Humeral head

Deltoid muscle

Sharpey fibers at insertional site

Greater tuberosity

Sub-deltoid peri-bursal fat

Supraspinatus tendon

Humeral head

(Top) Longitudinal grayscale ultrasound of the supraspinatus tendon insertional area anterior fibers. The supraspinatus inserts over a wide area ("foot print") on the anterior aspect of the greater tuberosity. Many tears of the supraspinatus tendon involve avulsion of the tendon from its insertional site. (Middle) Longitudinal grayscale ultrasound of supraspinatus tendon mid-fibers. There is often a thin hypoechoic line at the insertional area. This is thought to represent Sharpey fibers. (Bottom) Longitudinal grayscale ultrasound of supraspinatus tendon posterior fibers. The anterior, middle, and posterior fibers should be evaluated in turn.

SHOULDER

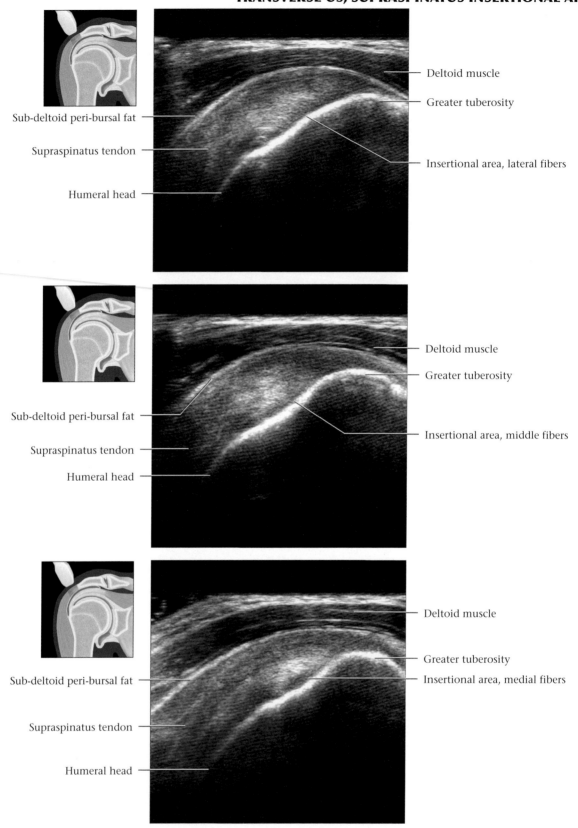

Sub-deltoid peri-bursal fat

Supraspinatus tendon

Humeral head

Deltoid muscle

Greater tuberosity

Insertional area, lateral fibers

Sub-deltoid peri-bursal fat

Supraspinatus tendon

Humeral head

Deltoid muscle

Greater tuberosity

Insertional area, middle fibers

Sub-deltoid peri-bursal fat

Supraspinatus tendon

Humeral head

Deltoid muscle

Greater tuberosity

Insertional area, medial fibers

(Top) Transverse grayscale ultrasound at supraspinatus tendon insertional area. Angulation and slight movement of the transducer will allow visualization of the lateral, middle and medial fibers respectively. The leading anterior edge of the supraspinatus is a common site of tear ("rim rent tear"). (Middle) Transverse grayscale ultrasound of the supraspinatus tendon at the insertional area of mid-fibers. The fibrillar echotexture of the supraspinatus tendon can be seen but is prone to anisotropy. (Bottom) Transverse grayscale ultrasound of supraspinatus medial fibers insertional area. Sub-deltoid peri-bursal fat is variable in depth. The normal bursa cannot be depicted. It is only seen when distended with fluid or thickened due to synovitis.

SHOULDER

TRANSVERSE AND LONGITUDINAL US, SUPRASPINATUS

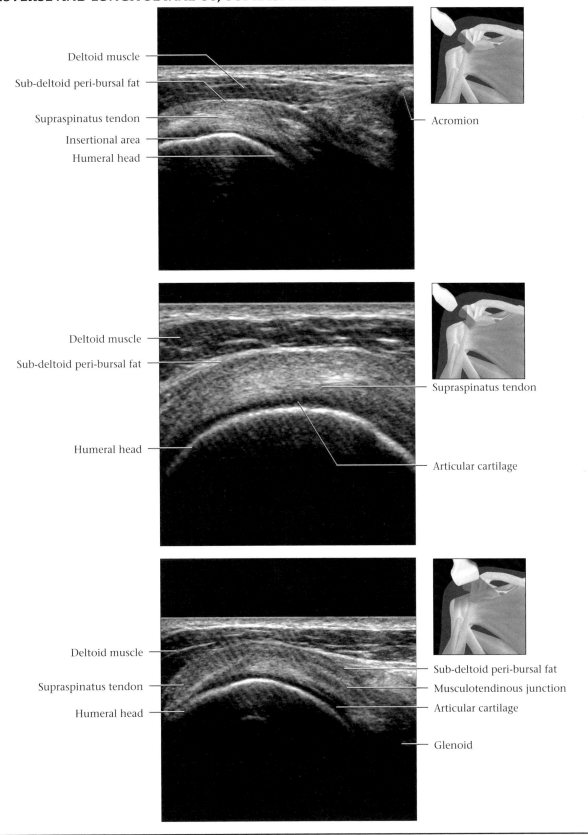

Deltoid muscle
Sub-deltoid peri-bursal fat
Supraspinatus tendon
Insertional area
Humeral head
Acromion

Deltoid muscle
Sub-deltoid peri-bursal fat
Humeral head
Supraspinatus tendon
Articular cartilage

Deltoid muscle
Supraspinatus tendon
Humeral head
Sub-deltoid peri-bursal fat
Musculotendinous junction
Articular cartilage
Glenoid

(Top) Transverse grayscale ultrasound of the supraspinatus tendon just medial to the insertional area. The critical zone is located just medial to the insertional area. This is a relatively hypovascular area. It is prone to calcific tendinosis. It is also prone to tears, though most tears tend to occur at the insertional site. (Middle) Transverse grayscale ultrasound of the supraspinatus medial to the insertional area. The fibrillar pattern of the supraspinatus tendon is prone to anisotropy. With tendinosis, the fibrillar pattern is disrupted. The tendon becomes more hypoechoic and thickened. (Bottom) Longitudinal grayscale ultrasound of the supraspinatus tendon at a slightly more medial aspect. Tears of the musculotendinous junctions are relatively uncommon.

Acromion

Coracohumeral ligament

Supraspinatus tendon

Biceps tendon, long head

Capsule

Synovium

Subscapularis tendon

Infraspinatus tendon

Deltoid muscle

Sub-deltoid peri-bursal fat

Biceps tendon

Subscapularis tendon

Supraspinatus tendon

Humeral head

(Top) Relationship of the coracohumeral ligament with rotator cuff tendons. Portions of the coracohumeral ligament pass superficial & deep to the supraspinatus tendon. The coracohumeral ligament attaches to the superior border of the subscapularis tendon. **(Bottom)** Transverse grayscale ultrasound of the shoulder at the rotator cuff interval. The rotator cuff interval represents the space between the leading anterior edge of the supraspinatus tendon and the adjacent superior edge of the subscapularis. It contains the biceps tendon. This should not be mistaken for a tear of the anterior aspect of the supraspinatus tendon. Patients with adhesive capsulitis may show increased hypoechogenicity and hyperemia of the rotator cuff interval as a result of inflammatory fibrovascular soft tissue.

SHOULDER

TRANSVERSE US, BICEPS TENDON

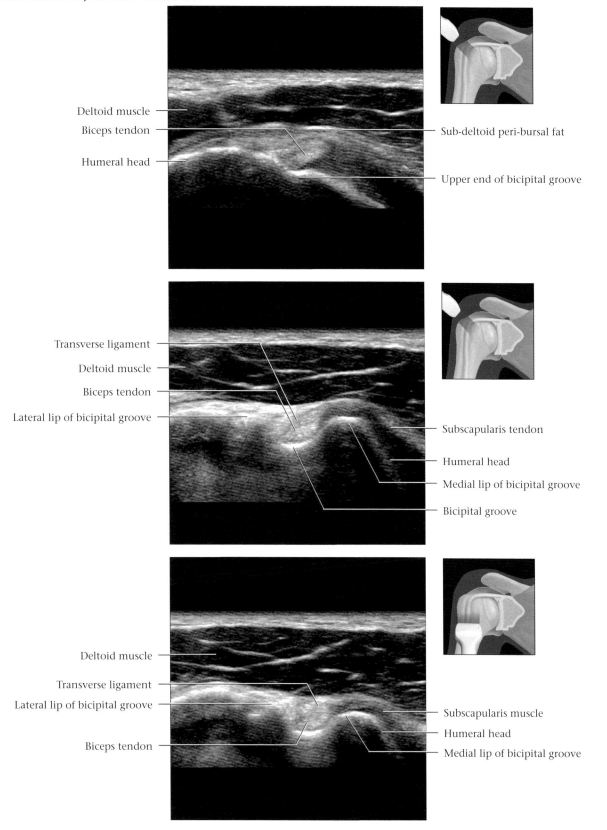

(Top) Labels: Deltoid muscle, Biceps tendon, Humeral head, Sub-deltoid peri-bursal fat, Upper end of bicipital groove

(Middle) Labels: Transverse ligament, Deltoid muscle, Biceps tendon, Lateral lip of bicipital groove, Subscapularis tendon, Humeral head, Medial lip of bicipital groove, Bicipital groove

(Bottom) Labels: Deltoid muscle, Transverse ligament, Lateral lip of bicipital groove, Biceps tendon, Subscapularis muscle, Humeral head, Medial lip of bicipital groove

(Top) Transverse grayscale ultrasound at the superior aspect shows biceps tendon. The bicipital groove forms a fibro-osseus tunnel for the biceps tendon. Normal biceps tendon has an ovoid configuration. With tendinosis, the tendon becomes larger & more rounded in appearance. (Middle) Transverse grayscale US of the biceps tendon. The biceps tendon is held in position by the transverse ligament. The subscapularis tendon inserts into the lesser tuberosity which forms the medial lip of the bicipital groove. The biceps tendon may sublux medially from the groove, & this may be associated with subscapularis tendon injury. (Bottom) Transverse grayscale US shows relations of the biceps tendon. The transverse ligament is not a distinct entity but consists of a fibrous expansion of both the pectoralis major tendon & subscapularis tendon inserting into the lateral lip of the bicipital groove.

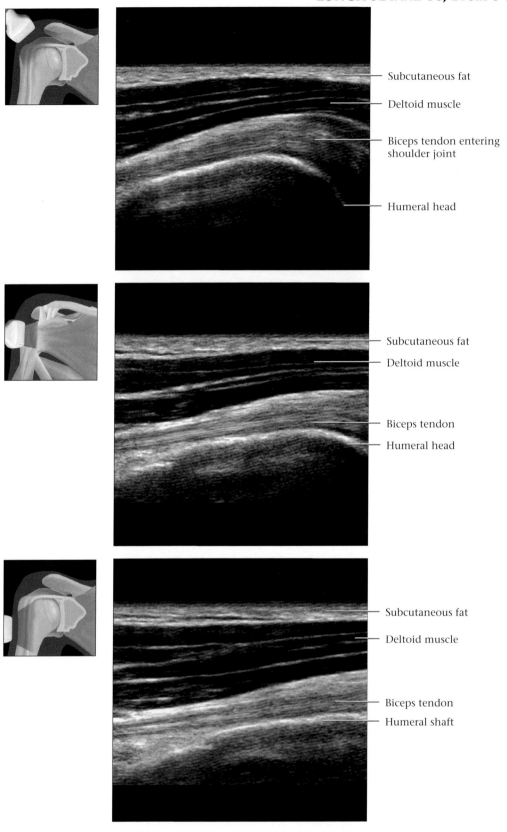

Subcutaneous fat

Deltoid muscle

Biceps tendon entering
shoulder joint

Humeral head

Subcutaneous fat

Deltoid muscle

Biceps tendon

Humeral head

Subcutaneous fat

Deltoid muscle

Biceps tendon

Humeral shaft

(**Top**) Longitudinal grayscale ultrasound of the uppermost section of the biceps tendon. The intra-articular portion of long head of biceps cannot be fully depicted on longitudinal imaging. On longitudinal section, the biceps tendon seems to expand at its upper end as it becomes more ovoid in contour. This location however is also the most common site of biceps tendinosis which also manifests as enlargement of biceps tendon. (**Middle**) Longitudinal grayscale ultrasound of upper section of biceps tendon. A small amount of fluid in the biceps tendon sheath which is continuous with the glenohumeral joint is normal and should not be mistaken for tenosynovitis. No fluid depicted in this image. (**Bottom**) Longitudinal grayscale ultrasound at lower aspect of biceps tendon. Most incomplete tears of biceps tendons are longitudinal in orientation and are best depicted on transverse imaging.

LONGITUDINAL, SUBSCAPULARIS

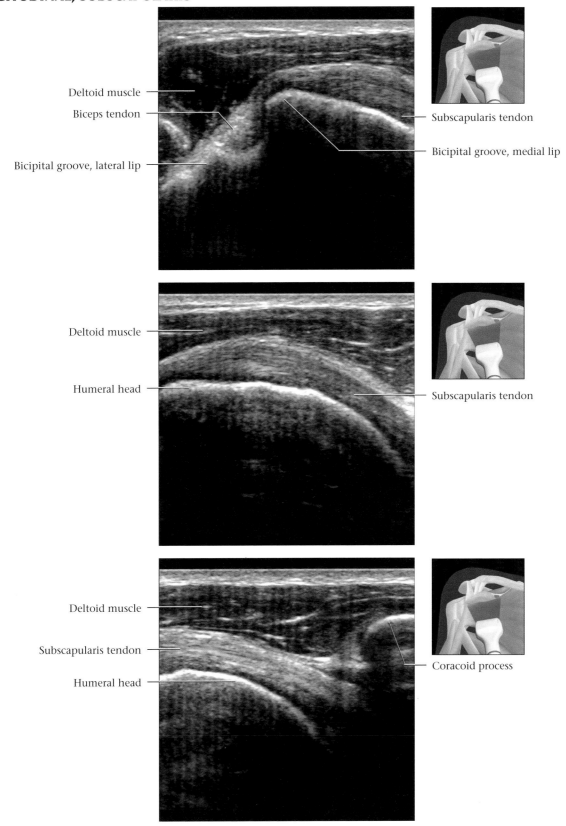

Deltoid muscle

Biceps tendon

Bicipital groove, lateral lip

Subscapularis tendon

Bicipital groove, medial lip

Deltoid muscle

Humeral head

Subscapularis tendon

Deltoid muscle

Subscapularis tendon

Humeral head

Coracoid process

(Top) Longitudinal grayscale ultrasound at the subscapularis insertion. The subscapularis inserts into the medial lip of the bicipital groove but has a fibrous expansion traversing the biceps tendon by which it gains attachment to the lateral lip of the bicipital groove. **(Middle)** Longitudinal grayscale ultrasound at the subscapularis insertional area. Complete tears of the subscapularis are uncommon and usually follow a severe traumatic event. Partial tears are more common and usually involve the superior edge of the tendon. **(Bottom)** Longitudinal grayscale ultrasound of the subscapularis tendon. The subscapularis moves beneath the coracoid process during internal-external rotation. Impingement may occur at this location (subcoracoid impingement).

SHOULDER

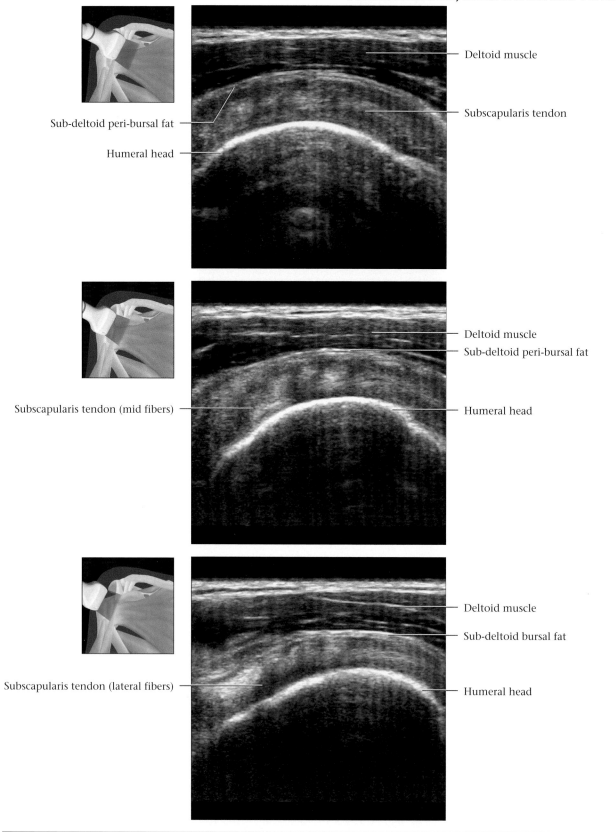

(Top) Transverse grayscale ultrasound of the subscapularis tendon medial fibers. Fiber bundles of the multipennate subscapularis tendon as they converge towards the insertion, give the tendon a mixed echogenic appearance. This is normal and should not be mistaken for tendinosis. (Middle) Transverse grayscale ultrasound of the subscapularis at the level of mid-fibers. (Bottom) Transverse grayscale ultrasound of the subscapularis tendon. Tears of the subscapularis tendon usually occur just proximal to the insertional area. These tears may involve the fascial covering of the biceps tendon, facilitating biceps tendon dislocation.

SHOULDER

LONGITUDINAL AND TRANSVERSE US, INFRASPINATUS

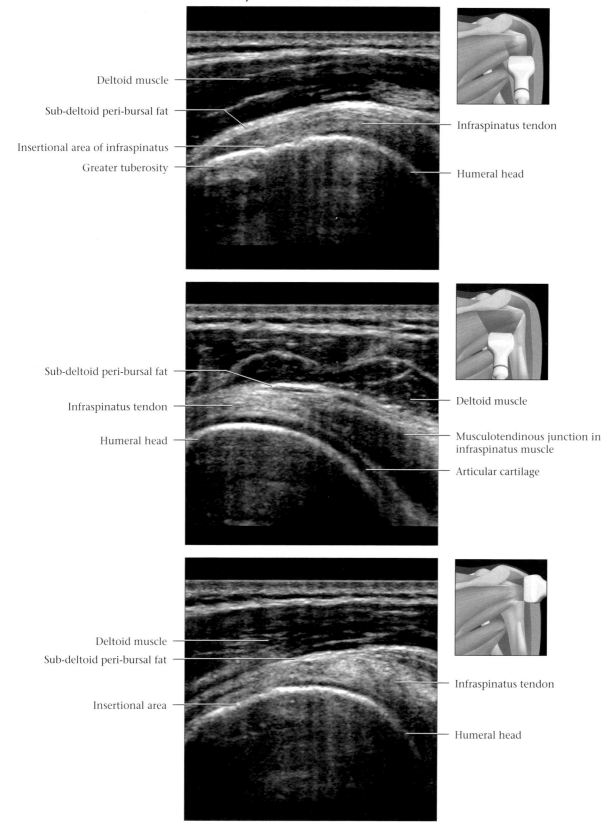

(Top) Longitudinal grayscale ultrasound of the infraspinatus insertional area. The infraspinatus tendon is much less commonly torn then the supraspinatus tendon. Most tears are avulsive-type tears involving the insertional area. (Middle) Longitudinal grayscale ultrasound of the infraspinatus musculotendinous junction. The muscle fibers interdigitate with the tendon at the musculotendinous junction and should not be mistaken for tears/tendinosis. (Bottom) Transverse grayscale ultrasound of the infraspinatus insertional area. All tears of the rotator cuff tendons should be confirmed in both planes (transverse and longitudinal planes).

Deltoid muscle

Teres minor tendon

Articular cartilage

Insertional area of teres minor

Deltoid muscle

Insertional area of teres minor

Humeral head

Teres minor musculotendinous junction

Latissimus dorsi muscle

Teres minor muscle

Infraspinatus muscle

Scapula

(Top) Longitudinal grayscale ultrasound of the teres minor insertional area. The teres minor muscle is usually not torn in isolation, but may be torn in massive rotator cuff tears. It is a small muscle and tendon seen at the postero-inferior edge of the infraspinatus tendon. **(Middle)** Longitudinal grayscale ultrasound of the teres minor insertional area. **(Bottom)** Transverse grayscale ultrasound of the teres minor. The teres minor muscle is best depicted on longitudinal imaging at the inferior aspect of the infraspinatus tendon. Isolated atrophy of the teres minor muscle can occur in quadrilateral space syndrome due to compression of the axillary nerve (some of the deltoid muscle may also be affected).

SHOULDER

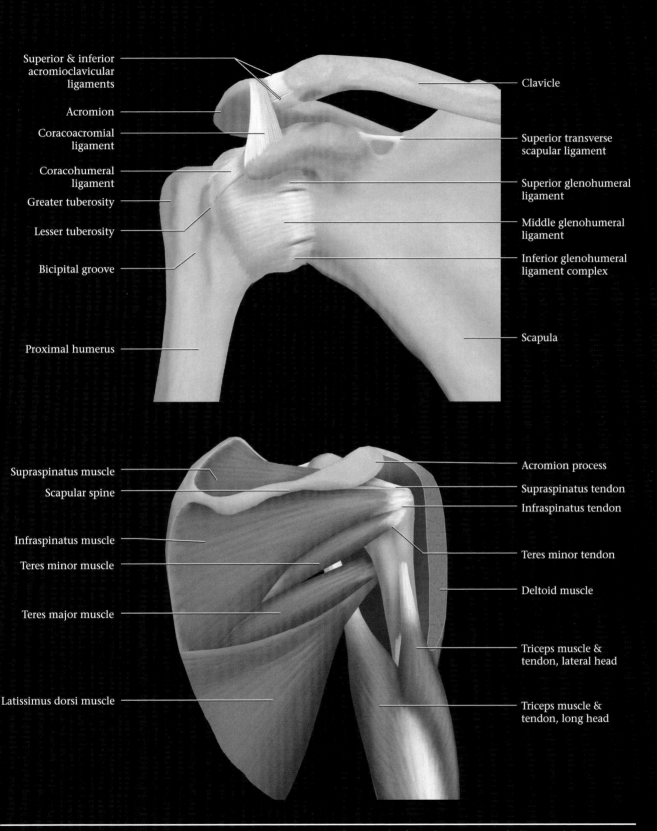

Superior & inferior acromioclavicular ligaments

Acromion

Coracoacromial ligament

Coracohumeral ligament

Greater tuberosity

Lesser tuberosity

Bicipital groove

Proximal humerus

Clavicle

Superior transverse scapular ligament

Superior glenohumeral ligament

Middle glenohumeral ligament

Inferior glenohumeral ligament complex

Scapula

Supraspinatus muscle

Scapular spine

Infraspinatus muscle

Teres minor muscle

Teres major muscle

Latissimus dorsi muscle

Acromion process

Supraspinatus tendon

Infraspinatus tendon

Teres minor tendon

Deltoid muscle

Triceps muscle & tendon, lateral head

Triceps muscle & tendon, long head

(Top) Anterior graphic of the right shoulder, deep dissection. The muscles have been removed. **(Bottom)** Posterior graphic of the shoulder. Superficial scapulohumeral dissection demonstrating the musculature.

SHOULDER

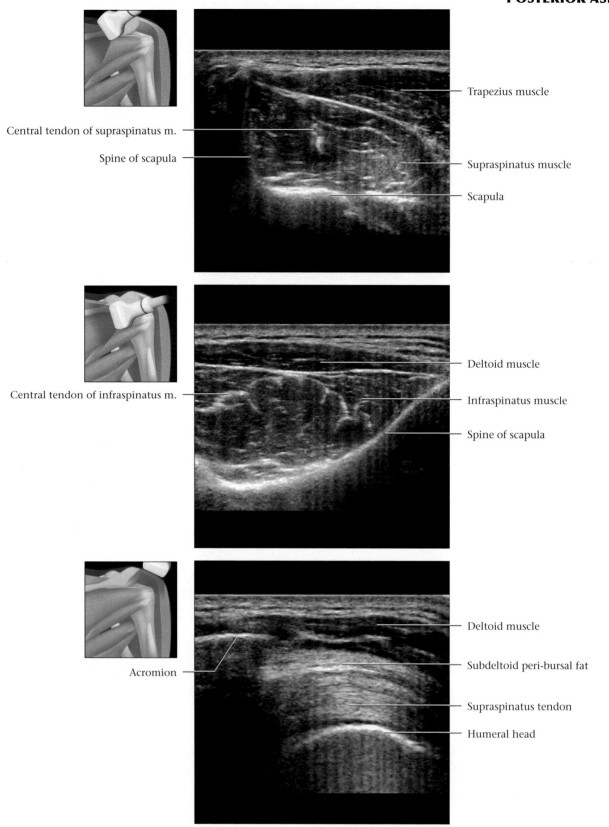

Central tendon of supraspinatus m.

Spine of scapula

Trapezius muscle

Supraspinatus muscle

Scapula

Central tendon of infraspinatus m.

Deltoid muscle

Infraspinatus muscle

Spine of scapula

Acromion

Deltoid muscle

Subdeltoid peri-bursal fat

Supraspinatus tendon

Humeral head

(Top) Longitudinal grayscale US of posterior shoulder at supraspinatus muscle. Muscle atrophy is common in rotator cuff pathology. US is almost as sensitive as MR in depiction of muscle atrophy. Atrophy is seen as reduction in muscle bulk with increase in muscle echogenicity. As a result, central tendon is less readily seen. **(Middle)** Longitudinal grayscale US of shoulder posterior view. Infraspinatus muscle atrophy usually accompanies supraspinatus muscle atrophy to a lesser or greater degree. Muscle bulk is reduced & becomes more echogenic as a result, central tendons are not as clearly seen. **(Bottom)** Longitudinal grayscale US of shoulder. Supraspinatus tendon slides below acromion during abduction. This relationship may be seen either from anterior or posterior aspect of shoulder. Dynamic imaging may reveal impingement of supraspinatus against acromion during abduction.

SHOULDER

POSTERIOR GLENOID LABRUM AND GLENOHUMERAL JOINT

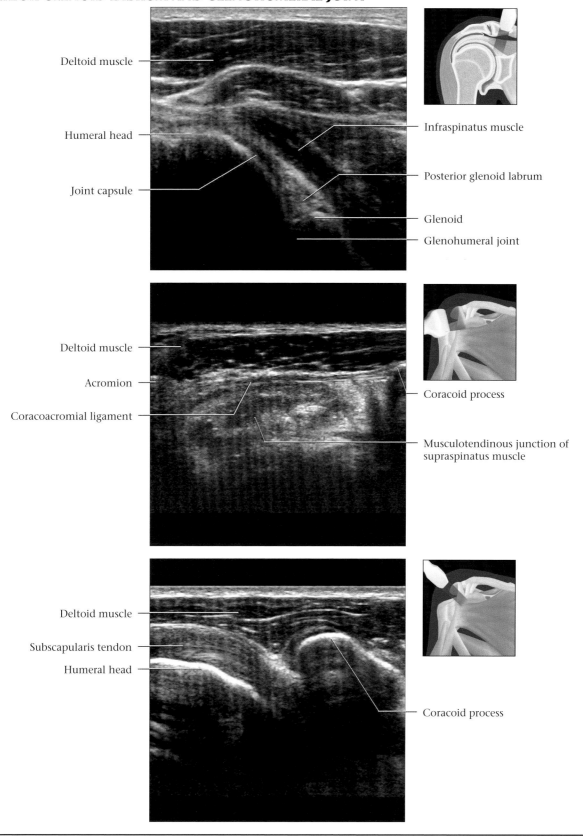

Deltoid muscle

Humeral head

Joint capsule

Infraspinatus muscle

Posterior glenoid labrum

Glenoid

Glenohumeral joint

Deltoid muscle

Acromion

Coracoacromial ligament

Coracoid process

Musculotendinous junction of supraspinatus muscle

Deltoid muscle

Subscapularis tendon

Humeral head

Coracoid process

(Top) Longitudinal grayscale ultrasound of the posterior shoulder. The glenohumeral joint is most easily seen from the posterior aspect. This is a good site for US-guided joint injection. Joint effusions are best seen in this area. (Middle) Longitudinal grayscale ultrasound of the coracoacromial ligament. The coracoacromial ligament extends from the coracoid process to the antero-inferior margin of acromion. Impingement of the supraspinatus tendon and the overlying subacromial-subdeltoid bursa may occur during shoulder abduction. (Bottom) Transverse grayscale ultrasound of the coracoid process. The coracoid process is close to the humeral head and intervening subscapularis. Occasionally, the coraco-humeral distance is reduced and subcoracoid impingement may occur.

AXILLA

Terminology

Definitions
- Fat-filled space between upper limb & thoracic wall

Imaging Anatomy

Extent
- Axilla is shaped like a pyramid with top layers shaved off
- Consists of an apex, a base & four walls
  - Apex
    - Bounded by scapula, 1st rib & mid-third of clavicle
    - Arm communicates with posterior triangle of neck via apex of axilla
  - Anterior wall
    - Composed of pectoralis major & minor muscles
  - Posterior wall
    - Composed of teres major, latissimus dorsi & subscapularis muscles
  - Medial wall
    - Composed of serratus anterior, upper ribs & intercostal spaces
  - Lateral wall
    - Medial and lateral lips of bicipital groove into which anterior & posterior walls are inserted
  - Base
    - Composed of axillary fascia, subcutaneous fat & skin
- Contents of axilla
  - Axillary artery & vein
  - Cords & branches of brachial plexus
  - Coracobrachialis & biceps muscles
  - Lymph nodes & vessels
  - Fat
- Axillary artery
  - Continuation of subclavian artery
  - Lies on posterior wall of axilla
  - Surrounded by cords & branches of brachial plexus
  - Vein lies medial to artery
  - Arterial branches
    - Superior thoracic artery
    - Acromiothoracic artery
    - Lateral thoracic artery
    - Subscapular artery
    - Anterior & posterior circumflex humeral arteries
- Axillary vein
  - Continuation of brachial vein
    - Tributaries correspond to branches of axillary artery & also cephalic vein
- Brachial plexus
  - Cord and terminal branches of brachial plexus pass through axilla
  - Three cords: Lateral, medial & posterior
  - Lateral cord gives rise to
    - Lateral pectoral nerve
    - Musculocutaneous nerve: Pierces coracobrachialis to descend down arm between biceps & brachialis muscles
    - Contributes to median nerve
  - Medial cord gives rise to

- Medial pectoral nerve
- Ulnar nerve
- Contributes to median nerve
- Medial cutaneous nerves of arm & forearm
  - Posterior cord gives rise to
    - Subscapular nerve
    - Thoracodorsal nerve
    - Axillary nerve, passes through quadrilateral space posteriorly around surgical neck of humerus accompanied by posterior circumflex humeral artery
    - Radial nerve

Anatomy Relationships
- **Quadrilateral space**
  - Superior border: Teres minor muscle
  - Inferior border: Teres major muscle
  - Lateral border: Surgical neck of humerus
  - Medial border: Long head of triceps muscle
  - Contents: Axillary nerve & posterior circumflex humeral artery
    - Axillary nerve supplies teres minor muscle, deltoid muscle, posterolateral cutaneous region of shoulder and upper arm
- **Triangular space**
  - Located medial to quadrilateral space
  - Superior border: Teres minor muscle
  - Inferior border: Teres major muscle
  - Lateral border: Long head of triceps muscle
  - Contents: Circumflex scapular artery
    - Branch of subscapular artery supplying infraspinatus fossa

Anatomy-Based Imaging Issues

Key Concepts or Questions
- Quadrilateral space syndrome = neurovascular compression syndrome due to compression of axillary nerve or posterior humeral circumflex artery in quadrilateral space
  - Can have complications that are purely neurologic, purely vascular or both
  - Effects
    - Point tenderness of quadrilateral space
    - Poorly localized shoulder pain ± paresthesia radiating top lateral arm
    - Symptoms aggravated by abduction & external rotation of arm
    - Teres minor ± deltoid atrophy
    - Intermittent ischemic-type pain
  - Due to
    - Humeral fracture
    - Fibrous bands secondary to trauma
    - Muscle hypertrophy ± fibrotic bands seen in throwing athletes, tennis players, or volleyball players
    - Paralabral cysts: Most common cause of mass in this region, high associations with labral tears
    - Glenohumeral joint dislocation
    - Extreme or prolonged abduction of arm during sleep

GRAPHICS, MUSCLES

Supraspinatus muscle

Scapular spine

Infraspinatus muscle

Teres minor muscle

Quadrilateral space

Triangular space

Teres major muscle

Latissimus dorsi muscle

Acromion process

Supraspinatus tendon

Infraspinatus tendon

Teres minor tendon

Deltoid muscle

Triceps muscle & tendon, lateral head

Triceps muscle & tendon, long head

Supraspinatus muscle

Superior transverse scapular ligament

Suprascapular notch

Suprascapular artery & nerve

Spinoglenoid notch

Suprascapular artery, infraspinatus branch

Infraspinatus muscle

Teres minor muscle

Teres major muscle

Latissimus dorsi muscle

Acromion process

Deltoid muscle

Supraspinatus tendon

Infraspinatus tendon

Joint capsule

Posterior circumflex humeral artery & axillary nerve

Deep brachial artery

Radial nerve

Triceps muscle & tendon, lateral head

Triceps muscle & tendon, long head

(Top) Posterior graphic of the shoulder. Superficial scapulohumeral dissection shows the location of the quadrilateral space and triangular space (each outlined in green). **(Bottom)** Graphic of the deep scapulohumeral dissection shows the major neurovascular structures, including those in the quadrilateral space.

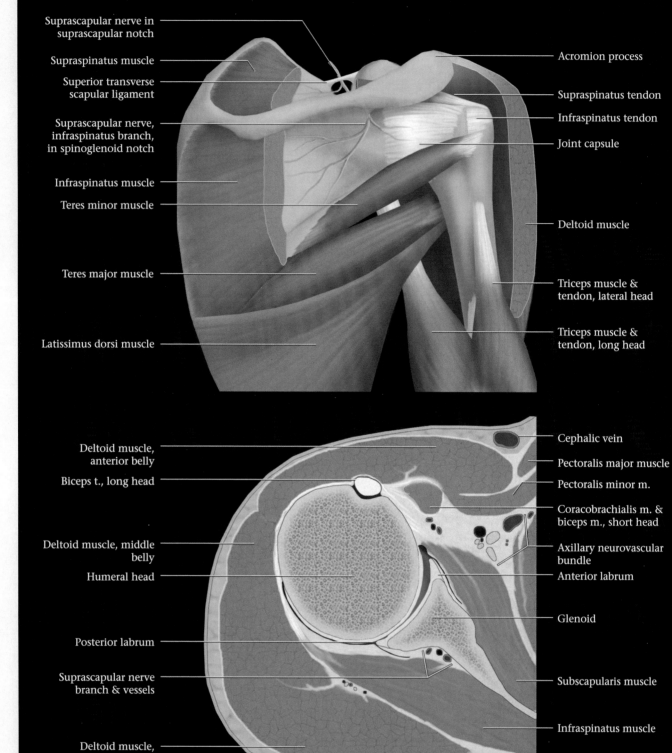

Suprascapular nerve in suprascapular notch

Supraspinatus muscle

Superior transverse scapular ligament

Suprascapular nerve, infraspinatus branch, in spinoglenoid notch

Infraspinatus muscle

Teres minor muscle

Teres major muscle

Latissimus dorsi muscle

Acromion process

Supraspinatus tendon

Infraspinatus tendon

Joint capsule

Deltoid muscle

Triceps muscle & tendon, lateral head

Triceps muscle & tendon, long head

Deltoid muscle, anterior belly

Biceps t., long head

Deltoid muscle, middle belly

Humeral head

Posterior labrum

Suprascapular nerve branch & vessels

Deltoid muscle, posterior belly

Cephalic vein

Pectoralis major muscle

Pectoralis minor m.

Coracobrachialis m. & biceps m., short head

Axillary neurovascular bundle

Anterior labrum

Glenoid

Subscapularis muscle

Infraspinatus muscle

(Top) Graphic of deep scapulohumeral dissection shows the course of the suprascapular nerve. **(Bottom)** Axial graphic shows the location of the suprascapular artery, nerve and vein branches, just below the level of the spinoglenoid notch.

GRAPHICS, RELATIONS OF NEUROVASCULAR STRUCTURES

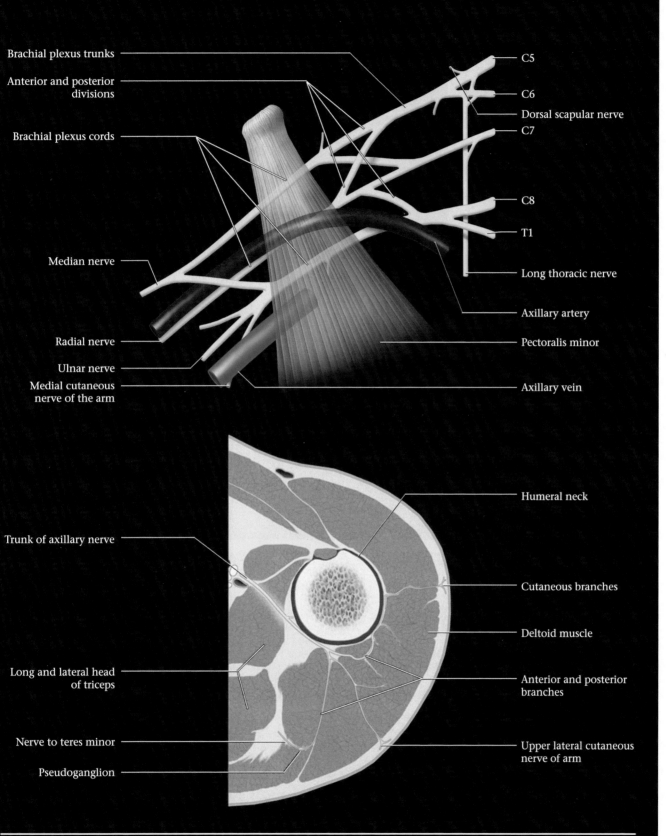

Brachial plexus trunks

Anterior and posterior divisions

Brachial plexus cords

Median nerve

Radial nerve

Ulnar nerve

Medial cutaneous nerve of the arm

C5

C6

Dorsal scapular nerve

C7

C8

T1

Long thoracic nerve

Axillary artery

Pectoralis minor

Axillary vein

Trunk of axillary nerve

Long and lateral head of triceps

Nerve to teres minor

Pseudoganglion

Humeral neck

Cutaneous branches

Deltoid muscle

Anterior and posterior branches

Upper lateral cutaneous nerve of arm

(Top) Graphic shows relations of the brachial plexus in the axilla. The brachial plexus arises from the anterior rami of the C5, C6, C7, C8 and T1 nerves. They first unite to form the superior, middle and inferior trunks. The trunks then divide and reunite to form the lateral, posterior and middle cords. Beyond the lateral margin of the pectoralis minor muscle, they continue as the terminal branches of the plexus (axillary, musculocutaneous, radial, medial and ulnar nerves). **(Bottom)** Graphic shows a section through the upper arm with the axillary nerve and its branches.

AXILLA

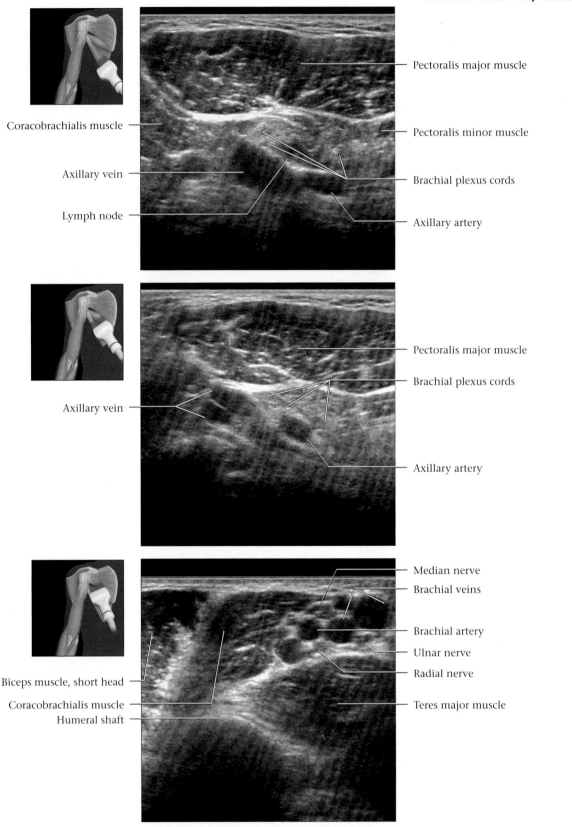

Pectoralis major muscle

Coracobrachialis muscle

Pectoralis minor muscle

Axillary vein

Brachial plexus cords

Lymph node

Axillary artery

Pectoralis major muscle

Brachial plexus cords

Axillary vein

Axillary artery

Median nerve

Brachial veins

Brachial artery

Ulnar nerve

Radial nerve

Biceps muscle, short head

Coracobrachialis muscle

Teres major muscle

Humeral shaft

(Top) Transverse grayscale ultrasound of the proximal axilla with the arm abducted. The contents of the axilla are inspected with the arm fully abducted. (Middle) Transverse grayscale ultrasound of the mid-portion of the axilla. The axillary artery and vein pass the axilla surrounded by the cords of the brachial plexus. The cords (medial, lateral and posterior) are names relative to their location to the axillary artery. Lymph nodes with variably fatty hila are commonly seen in the axilla around the neurovascular bundle. (Bottom) Transverse grayscale ultrasound of the axilla, distal aspect.

AXILLA

TRANSVERSE US, ANTERIOR AXILLARY WALL

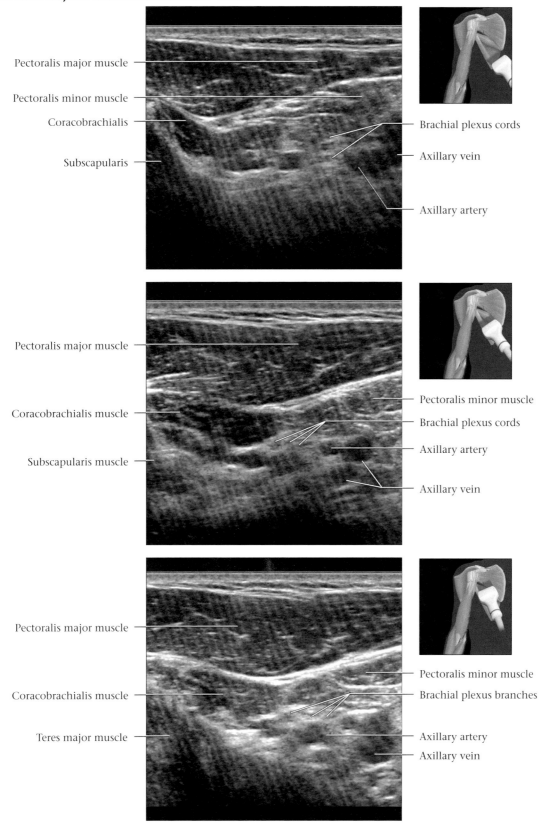

Pectoralis major muscle

Pectoralis minor muscle

Coracobrachialis

Subscapularis

Brachial plexus cords

Axillary vein

Axillary artery

Pectoralis major muscle

Coracobrachialis muscle

Subscapularis muscle

Pectoralis minor muscle

Brachial plexus cords

Axillary artery

Axillary vein

Pectoralis major muscle

Coracobrachialis muscle

Teres major muscle

Pectoralis minor muscle

Brachial plexus branches

Axillary artery

Axillary vein

(Top) Transverse grayscale ultrasound of the upper anterior wall of the axilla. The anterior wall of the axilla can be examined with the arm by the side. **(Middle)** Transverse grayscale ultrasound of mid-section of the anterior wall of the axilla. The anterior wall of the axilla is formed by the pectoralis major and pectoralis minor muscles. **(Bottom)** Transverse grayscale ultrasound of distal anterior axilla.

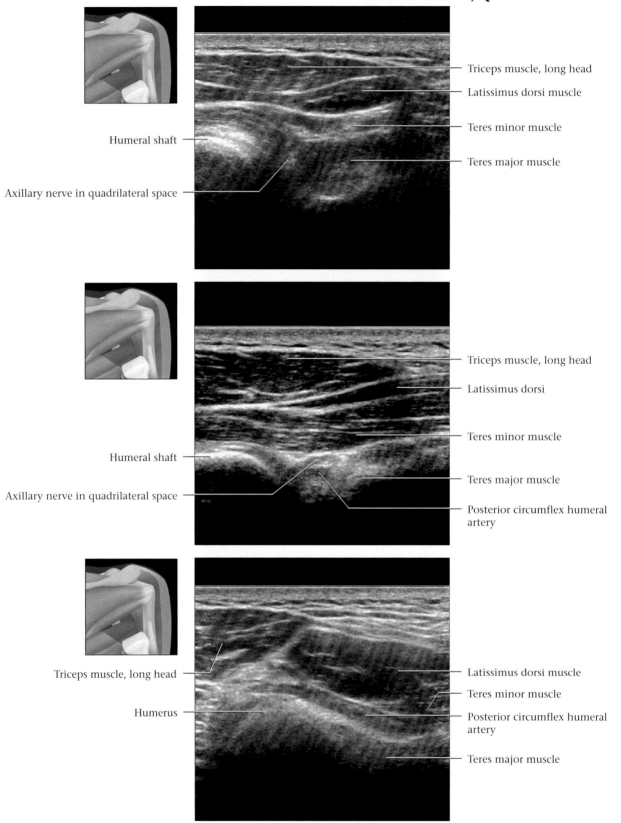

(Top) Transverse grayscale ultrasound of the quadrilateral space. The quadrilateral space (quadrangular space) contains the axillary nerve and posterior circumflex humeral vessels. (Middle) Transverse grayscale ultrasound of the quadrilateral space with the arm adducted. The contents of the space are more easily seen with the arm adducted. (Bottom) Transverse grayscale ultrasound of the posterior circumflex humeral artery posterior to the quadrilateral space.

AXILLA

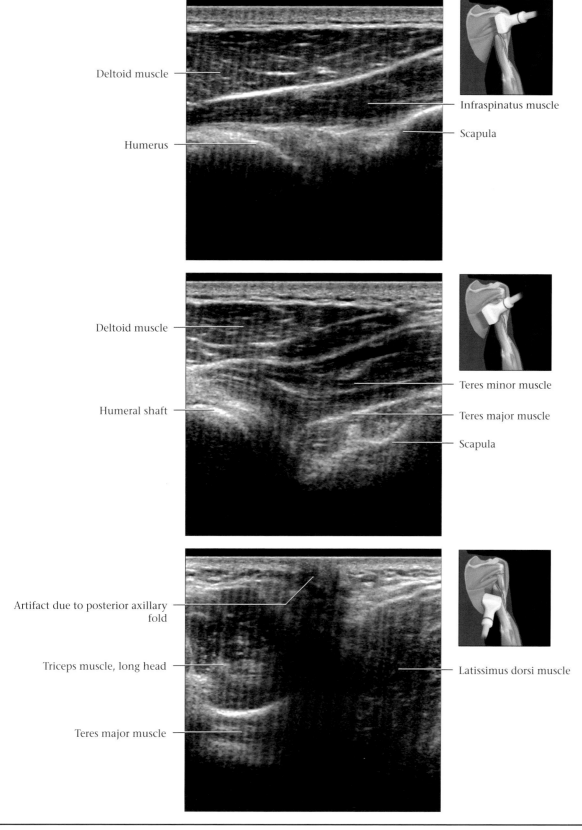

Deltoid muscle

Infraspinatus muscle

Humerus

Scapula

Deltoid muscle

Teres minor muscle

Humeral shaft

Teres major muscle

Scapula

Artifact due to posterior axillary fold

Triceps muscle, long head

Latissimus dorsi muscle

Teres major muscle

(Top) Transverse grayscale ultrasound of the posterior axillary wall, upper aspect. **(Middle)** Transverse grayscale ultrasound of the posterior wall of axilla, middle aspect. The posterior wall of the axilla is composed of teres major, latissimus dorsi and subscapularis muscles. **(Bottom)** Transverse grayscale ultrasound of the axilla, lower most aspect.

ARM

Imaging Anatomy

Overview
- Muscles of the upper arm are divided into anterior & posterior compartments

Anatomy Relationships
- **Anterior compartment of arm**
  - Coracobrachialis muscle
    - Origin: Coracoid process tip, in common with & medial to short head biceps tendon
    - Insertion: Medial surface of humeral mid shaft, between brachialis & triceps muscle origins
    - Nerve supply: Musculocutaneous nerve, perforates muscle
    - Blood supply: Brachial artery, muscular branches
    - Action: Flexes & adducts shoulder, supports humeral head in glenoid
    - Variants: Bony head extending to medial epicondyle, short head extending to lesser tuberosity
  - Biceps muscle, short head
    - Origin: Coracoid process tip, in common with & lateral to coracobrachialis tendon
    - Insertion: Radial tuberosity after joining long head
    - Nerve supply: Musculocutaneous nerve
    - Blood supply: Brachial artery, muscular branches
    - Action: Flexes elbow & shoulder, supinates forearm
  - Biceps muscle, long head
    - Origin: Predominantly supraglenoid tubercle; also superior glenoid labrum & coracoid base
    - Insertion: Radial tuberosity after joining with short head
    - Nerve supply: Musculocutaneous nerve
    - Blood supply: Brachial artery, muscular branches
    - Action: Flexes elbow, supinates forearm
    - Variants, biceps muscle: Third head in 10% arising at upper medial aspect of brachialis muscle, fourth head can arise from lateral humerus, bicipital groove or greater tuberosity
  - Brachialis muscle
    - Origin: Distal half of anterior humeral shaft & two intermuscular septae
    - Insertion: Tuberosity of ulna & anterior surface of coronoid process
    - Nerve supply: Musculocutaneous nerve plus branch of radial nerve
    - Blood supply: Brachial artery, muscular branches & recurrent radial artery
    - Action: Flexes forearm
    - Covers anterior aspect of elbow joint
    - Variants: Doubled; slips to supinator, pronator teres, biceps, lacertus fibrosus or radius
- **Posterior compartment of arm**
  - Triceps muscle, long head
    - Origin: Infraglenoid tubercle of scapula
    - Insertion: Proximal olecranon & deep fascia of arm after joining with lateral & medial heads
    - Nerve supply: Radial nerve
    - Blood supply: Deep brachial artery branches
    - Action: Elbow extension, adducts humerus when arm is extended
  - Triceps muscle, lateral head
    - Origin: Posterior & lateral humeral shaft, lateral intermuscular septum
    - Insertion: Proximal olecranon & deep fascia of arm after joining with long & medial heads
    - Nerve supply: Radial nerve
    - Blood supply: Deep brachial artery branches
    - Action: Elbow extension
  - Triceps muscle, medial head
    - Origin: Posterior humeral shaft from teres major insertion to near trochlea, medial intermuscular septum
    - Insertion: Proximal olecranon & deep fascia of arm after joining with lateral & long heads
    - Nerve supply: Radial & branches of ulnar nerve
    - Blood supply: Deep brachial artery branches
    - Action: Elbow extension
    - Variants, triceps muscle: Fourth head from medial humerus, slip termed the dorso-epitrochlearis extending between triceps & latissimus dorsi
  - Anconeus muscle
    - Origin: Lateral epicondyle of humerus
    - Insertion: Lateral olecranon & posterior ¼ of ulna
    - Nerve supply: Radial nerve
    - Blood supply: Branch of deep brachial artery
    - Action: Assists elbow extension, abducts ulna
- **Fascia**
  - Brachial fascia
    - Continuous with fascia covering deltoid & pectoralis major
    - Varies in thickness being thin over biceps & thick over triceps muscles
    - Lateral intermuscular septum from lower aspect of greater tuberosity to lateral epicondyle
    - Medial intermuscular septum from lower aspect of lesser tuberosity to medial epicondyle
    - Perforated by ulnar nerve, superior ulnar collateral artery & posterior branch of inferior ulnar collateral artery
    - Provides traction on deep fascia of forearm
  - Bicipital fascia
    - Also known as lacertus fibrosus
    - Arises from medial side of distal biceps tendon at level of elbow joint
    - Passes superficial to brachial artery
    - Continuous with deep fascia of forearm

Anatomy-Based Imaging Issues

Imaging Recommendations
- Examine with arm extended, in supine & prone positions
- Transverse plane most helpful to delineate borders of anterior & posterior compartments & relationship to neurovascular structures

Imaging Pitfalls
- Muscle may appear echogenic simulating fatty replacement or edema when beam not aligned parallel to muscle fibers

GRAPHICS, ARM

Acromion

Coracoid process

Transverse ligament

Musculocutaneous nerve

Anterior circumflex humeral artery

Circumflex scapular artery

Coracobrachialis

Subscapularis muscle

Teres major muscle

Biceps muscle, short head

Biceps muscle, long head

Latissimus dorsi

Brachial artery

Lateral antebrachial cutaneous nerve

Median nerve

Biceps tendon

Pronator teres

Brachioradialis

Flexor carpi radialis muscle

Pectoralis major muscle

Biceps m., short head

Cephalic vein

Musculocutaneous n.

Pectoralis major t.

Medial antebrachial n.

Biceps m., long head

Coracobrachialis m.

Basilic vein

Median nerve

Humerus

Brachial vein

Deltoid muscle

Ulnar nerve

Latissimus dorsi t.

Deep brachial artery

Triceps m., lateral head

Medial brachial cutaneous nerve

Teres major muscle

Brachial artery

Radial nerve

Triceps muscle, long head

Brachial vein

(Top) Anterior graphic of arm. **(Bottom)** Upper humeral level.

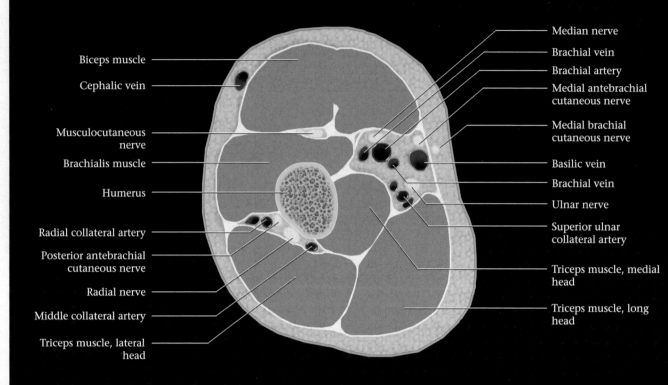

Biceps muscle

Cephalic vein

Musculocutaneous nerve

Brachialis muscle

Humerus

Radial collateral artery

Posterior antebrachial cutaneous nerve

Radial nerve

Middle collateral artery

Triceps muscle, lateral head

Median nerve

Brachial vein

Brachial artery

Medial antebrachial cutaneous nerve

Medial brachial cutaneous nerve

Basilic vein

Brachial vein

Ulnar nerve

Superior ulnar collateral artery

Triceps muscle, medial head

Triceps muscle, long head

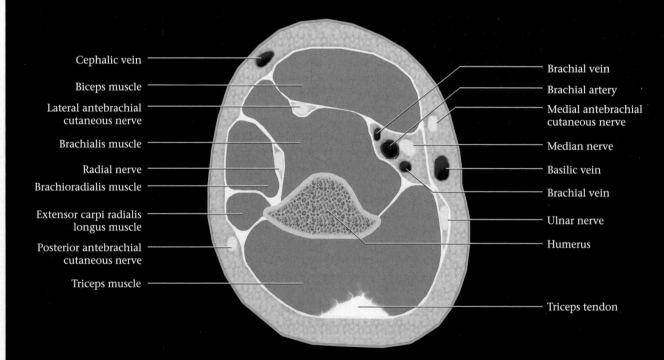

Cephalic vein

Biceps muscle

Lateral antebrachial cutaneous nerve

Brachialis muscle

Radial nerve

Brachioradialis muscle

Extensor carpi radialis longus muscle

Posterior antebrachial cutaneous nerve

Triceps muscle

Brachial vein

Brachial artery

Medial antebrachial cutaneous nerve

Median nerve

Basilic vein

Brachial vein

Ulnar nerve

Humerus

Triceps tendon

(Top) Axial graphic of the right arm at the mid humeral level. **(Bottom)** Axial section at the distal humeral level.

ARM

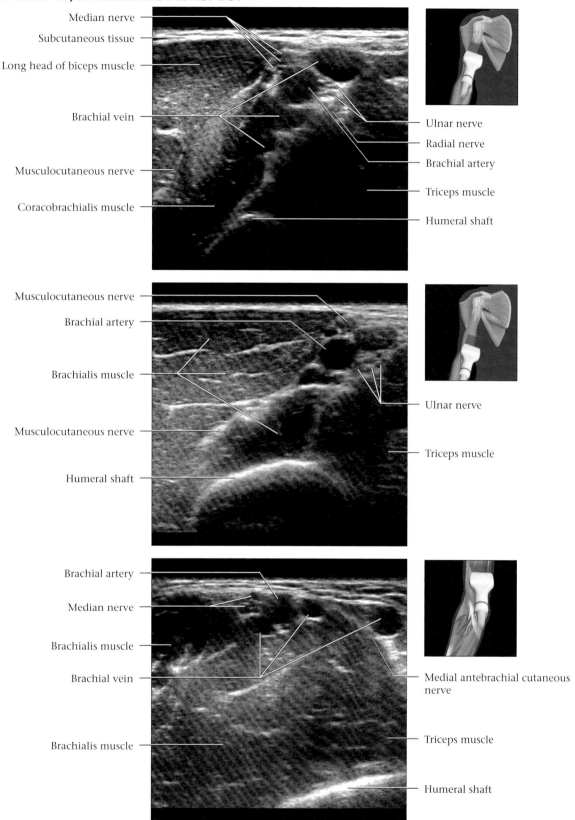

Median nerve

Subcutaneous tissue

Long head of biceps muscle

Brachial vein

Musculocutaneous nerve

Coracobrachialis muscle

Ulnar nerve

Radial nerve

Brachial artery

Triceps muscle

Humeral shaft

Musculocutaneous nerve

Brachial artery

Brachialis muscle

Musculocutaneous nerve

Humeral shaft

Ulnar nerve

Triceps muscle

Brachial artery

Median nerve

Brachialis muscle

Brachial vein

Medial antebrachial cutaneous nerve

Brachialis muscle

Triceps muscle

Humeral shaft

(Top) Transverse grayscale ultrasound of the anteromedial aspect of the upper arm. The terminal branches of the brachial plexus namely, the median nerve, the ulnar nerve and the radial nerve, all lie around the brachial vein and artery. They can be recognized by their position relative to the brachial artery, the radial nerve lying deep, the median nerve laterally and the ulnar nerve medially. (Middle) Transverse grayscale ultrasound of the anteromedial aspect of the mid-arm. Compression of the median or ulnar nerve is uncommon in the mid-arm. The neurovascular bundle helps define the separation of the anterior and posterior compartments of the arm medially. (Bottom) Transverse grayscale ultrasound of the anteromedial aspect of the distal arm. In the distal arm, the median nerve alone is associated with the brachial neurovascular bundle.

TRANSVERSE US, ANTERIOR ASPECT

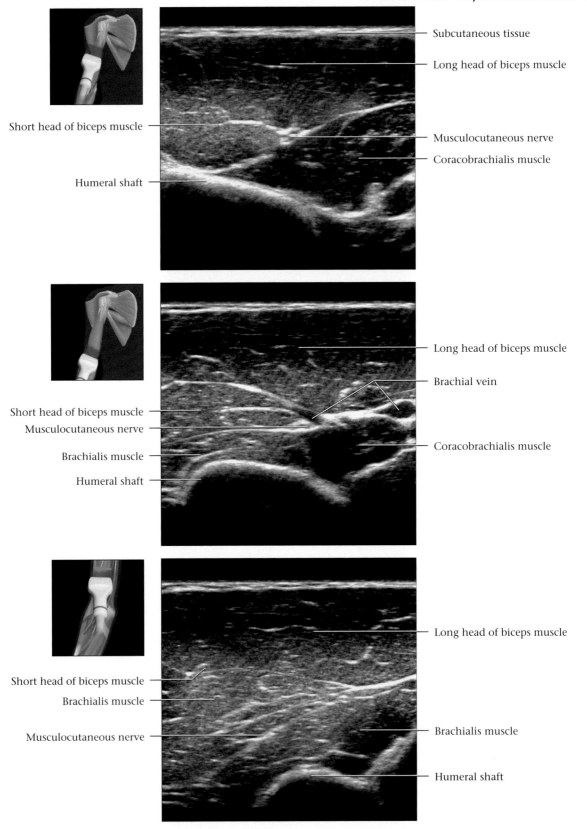

Subcutaneous tissue

Long head of biceps muscle

Short head of biceps muscle

Musculocutaneous nerve

Coracobrachialis muscle

Humeral shaft

Long head of biceps muscle

Brachial vein

Short head of biceps muscle

Musculocutaneous nerve

Brachialis muscle

Coracobrachialis muscle

Humeral shaft

Long head of biceps muscle

Short head of biceps muscle

Brachialis muscle

Musculocutaneous nerve

Brachialis muscle

Humeral shaft

(Top) Transverse grayscale ultrasound of proximal one-third of the arm. The anatomy of the upper arm is quite straight forward. The arm muscles are divided in to two compartments. The anterior compartment is composed of biceps, brachialis and coracobrachialis. The biceps is midline, brachialis is midline and lateral while the coracobrachialis is midline and medial. **(Middle)** Transverse grayscale ultrasound of the mid-third of the anterior arm. Most of the neurovascular bundles in the arm lie anteromedially. **(Bottom)** Transverse grayscale ultrasound of the distal one-third of the anterior arm. The musculocutaneous nerve is the main critical neurovascular structure of the anterior arm lying between the biceps, coracobrachialis and brachialis muscles.

ARM

TRANSVERSE US, ANTEROLATERAL ASPECT

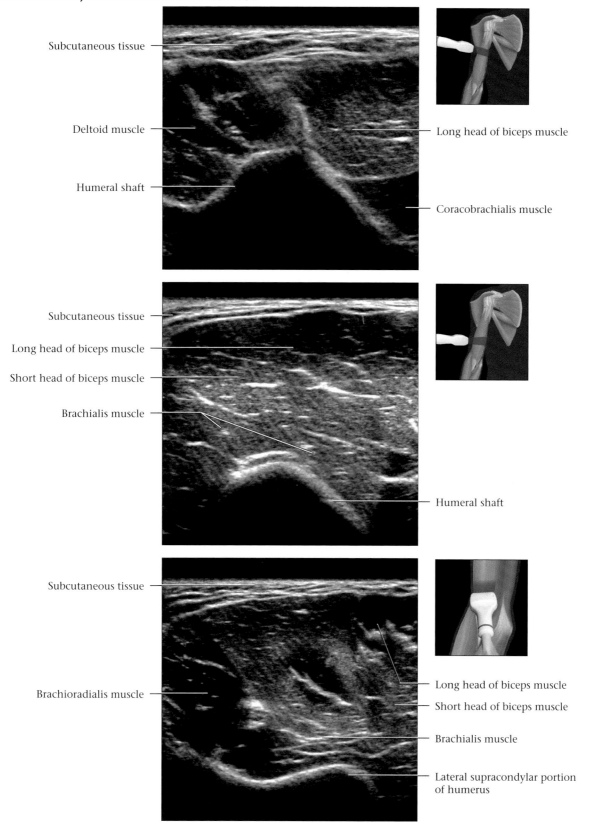

Subcutaneous tissue

Deltoid muscle

Humeral shaft

Long head of biceps muscle

Coracobrachialis muscle

Subcutaneous tissue

Long head of biceps muscle

Short head of biceps muscle

Brachialis muscle

Humeral shaft

Subcutaneous tissue

Brachioradialis muscle

Long head of biceps muscle

Short head of biceps muscle

Brachialis muscle

Lateral supracondylar portion of humerus

(Top) Transverse grayscale ultrasound of the anterolateral aspect of the proximal arm. This is an area prone to injury during contact sports but fortunately there is no neurovascular bundle in the area which would be exposed to injury. (Middle) Transverse grayscale ultrasound of the anterolateral section of the mid-arm. Both the biceps muscle and brachialis muscle may be prone to overuse muscle injury if too vigorous exercise is undertaken. The biceps muscle may appear echogenic if the transducer is aligned at an angle to the transverse plane. (Bottom) Transverse grayscale ultrasound at the anterolateral aspect of the distal arm. Both heads of biceps converge to form the biceps tendon just proximal to the antecubital fossa.

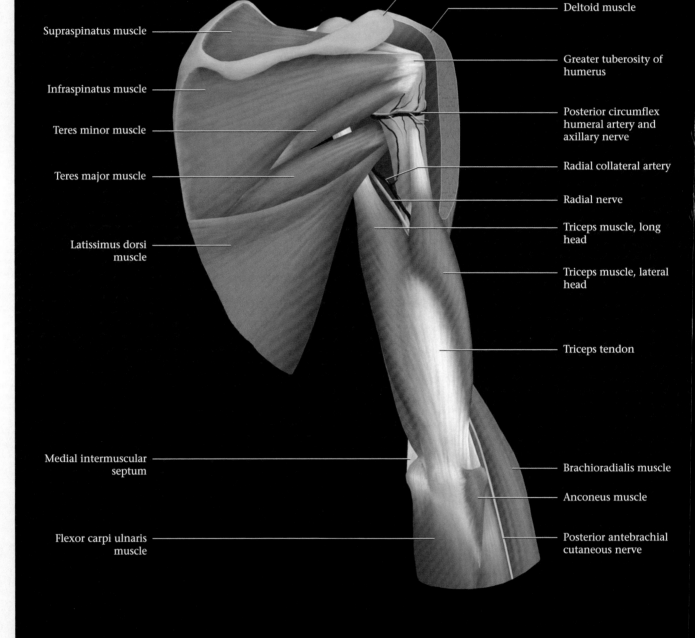

Supraspinatus muscle

Infraspinatus muscle

Teres minor muscle

Teres major muscle

Latissimus dorsi muscle

Medial intermuscular septum

Flexor carpi ulnaris muscle

Acromion

Deltoid muscle

Greater tuberosity of humerus

Posterior circumflex humeral artery and axillary nerve

Radial collateral artery

Radial nerve

Triceps muscle, long head

Triceps muscle, lateral head

Triceps tendon

Brachioradialis muscle

Anconeus muscle

Posterior antebrachial cutaneous nerve

Graphic shows the superficial dissection of the posterior arm.

ARM

TRANSVERSE US, POSTERIOR ASPECT

Triceps muscle, lateral head

Triceps muscle, medial head

Humeral shaft

Radial nerve

Triceps muscle

Radial nerve in spiral groove

Profunda brachii artery

Triceps muscle

Humeral shaft

Brachialis muscle

Triceps muscle

Radial nerve

Profunda brachii artery

Humeral shaft

Brachialis muscle

(Top) Transverse grayscale ultrasound of the posterior upper arm. The triceps muscle occupies nearly the whole of the posterior upper arm. The medial nerve supplies the triceps and supinator muscles. (Middle) Transverse grayscale ultrasound of the posterior mid-arm. The radial nerve runs in the spiral groove on the posterior aspect of the mid-arm. At this level it is prone to injury from humeral shaft fractures, fibrosis or fibrotic bands following trauma or extrinsic compression. (Bottom) Transverse grayscale ultrasound at the posterior aspect of the distal arm. The radial nerve pierces the lateral intermuscular septum just proximal to the lateral epicondyle. It then runs between the brachialis and brachioradialis muscles and passes anterior to the lateral epicondyle. The nerve may be compressed by the lateral intermuscular septum.

ARM VESSELS

Gross Anatomy

Arteries

- Brachial artery
- Continuation of axillary artery
- Extends from lower border of teres major to neck of the radius
- Accompanies median nerve
- Branches of brachial artery in arm
  - Superior ulnar collateral arises medially & descends with ulnar nerve posterior to medial epicondyle → forms anastomosis with branches of ulnar artery
  - Inferior ulnar collateral arises distal to superior ulnar collateral artery, descends anterior to medial epicondyle → forms anastomosis with branches of ulnar artery
  - Profunda brachii: Main branch of brachial artery
    - Arises just distal to teres major, accompanies radial nerve & passes backwards in spiral groove on posterior surface of humerus
    - Gives off further branch, which passes upwards & anastomoses with arteries around shoulder joint
    - Gives two lower medial branches which descend to elbow joint on its medial side & take part in anterior & posterior anastomosis around elbow joint
- Brachial artery lies superficial in its course in arm
- Covered by bicipital aponeurosis at elbow where it may be compressed against medial surface of humerus
- Brachial artery divides at neck of radius → radial artery & ulnar artery
  - High take off of radial artery from brachial artery is a common anatomical variant
  - Radial artery passes inferiorly & laterally, lying on the tendon of the biceps brachii
  - Ulnar artery passes down & medially, deep to pronator teres
  - Within antecubital fossa, radial & ulnar arteries give off recurrent branches to elbow joint

Veins

- Categorized as superficial and deep venous system
  - Veins of upper limb are variable in number & position
- Brachial vein
  - Forms the deep venous system
  - Singular or paired, continue into axillary vein
  - Accompanied by the brachial artery and nerves of upper limb
- Cephalic vein
  - Cephalic vein lies anterolaterally in superficial fascia of antecubital fossa & gives off medial cubital vein which joins the basilic vein
  - Runs in deltopectoral groove → pierces clavipectoral fascia to drain to axillary vein
- Basilic vein
  - Passes upwards on medial side of forearm receiving anterior & posterior tributaries → passes to anteromedial aspect of elbow where it receives medial cubital vein
  - Continues on medial aspect of biceps brachii until it pierces deep fascia to run cranially, medial to brachial artery

- Joins brachial vein & becomes axillary vein at lower border of teres major

Anatomy-Based Imaging Issues

Imaging Recommendations

- Venous examination
  - Examination of upper limb veins is normally performed with patient supine & arm abducted to about 90°
  - Use of high frequency linear transducer (5-10 MHz) is recommended
    - Determination of compressibility & flow pattern is normally performed, normal venous waveform
  - Augmentation of flow is obtained by manual compression of forearm or upper arm
  - Alternatively asking patient to clench their fist to increase venous flow
  - Flow can also be augmented or dampened by deep inspiration
- Arterial examination
  - In patients with possible arterial compression syndromes, arteries are examined in various positions of shoulder abduction so that any compression may be accentuated

Imaging Pitfalls

- Brachial vein duplication is common
- Clavicle can produce mirror artifact of subclavian vessels
- Due to proximity, arm venous flow is affected by respiration
  - Deep inspiration will augment flow
  - Flow can also be augmented by fist clenching (contracting muscles of forearm)
- Angle of insonation should not be > 60° as this will reduce sensitivity of Doppler & color flow signals
- Color signal scale should match flow velocity
- Doppler gate should be located at center of artery or vein as this is the site of peak flow velocity
- Gold standard for assessment of accuracy of arterial Doppler ultrasound with respect to stenoses or occlusion is arteriography
  - Other methods of visualizing the arterial tree are computed tomography angiography & magnetic resonance angiography

Clinical Implications

Clinical Importance

- Brachial artery may be used for access in angiography, either by a high brachial approach or in antecubital fossa where it lies medial to biceps tendon & lateral to median nerve
- Spontaneous thrombosis of axillary vein occasionally occurs following excessive movements of arm at shoulder joint
- Diagnosis of exclusion of deep vein thrombosis in upper or lower limb; spontaneous or related to indwelling catheters
- Vein mapping prior to bypass grafts
- Localization of veins for venous access & cannulation

GRAPHICS, ARTERIES

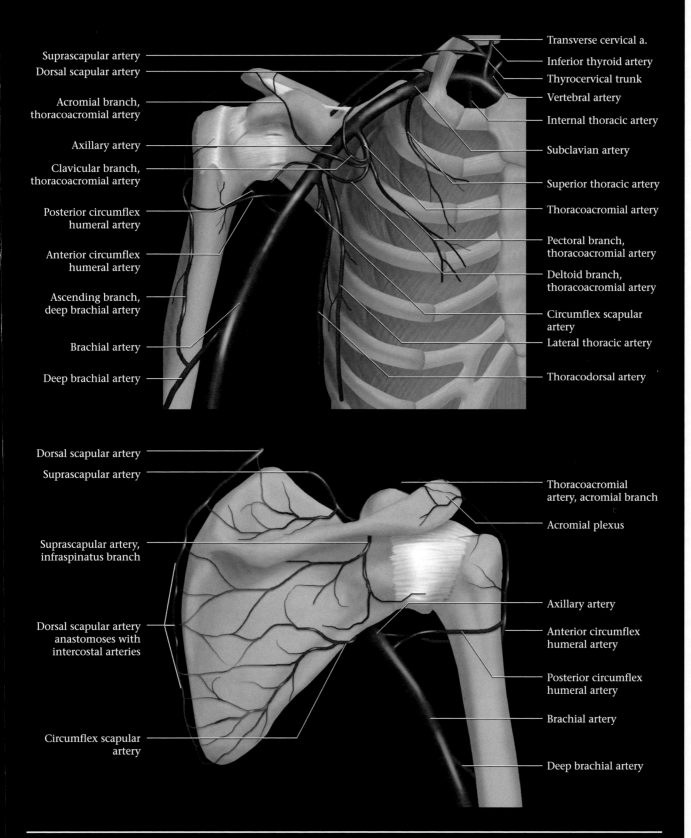

Suprascapular artery
Dorsal scapular artery
Acromial branch, thoracoacromial artery
Axillary artery
Clavicular branch, thoracoacromial artery
Posterior circumflex humeral artery
Anterior circumflex humeral artery
Ascending branch, deep brachial artery
Brachial artery
Deep brachial artery

Transverse cervical a.
Inferior thyroid artery
Thyrocervical trunk
Vertebral artery
Internal thoracic artery
Subclavian artery
Superior thoracic artery
Thoracoacromial artery
Pectoral branch, thoracoacromial artery
Deltoid branch, thoracoacromial artery
Circumflex scapular artery
Lateral thoracic artery
Thoracodorsal artery

Dorsal scapular artery
Suprascapular artery
Suprascapular artery, infraspinatus branch
Dorsal scapular artery anastomoses with intercostal arteries
Circumflex scapular artery

Thoracoacromial artery, acromial branch
Acromial plexus
Axillary artery
Anterior circumflex humeral artery
Posterior circumflex humeral artery
Brachial artery
Deep brachial artery

(Top) Anterior graphic of arterial supply to the shoulder. The shoulder is predominantly supplied by anterior & posterior circumflex humeral, suprascapular & circumflex scapular arteries. **(Bottom)** Posterior graphic of arterial supply to the shoulder. Extensive collateral blood vessels include anastomoses with intercostal arteries.

ARM VESSELS

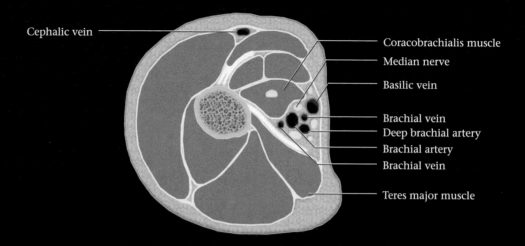

Cephalic vein

Coracobrachialis muscle
Median nerve
Basilic vein

Brachial vein
Deep brachial artery
Brachial artery
Brachial vein

Teres major muscle

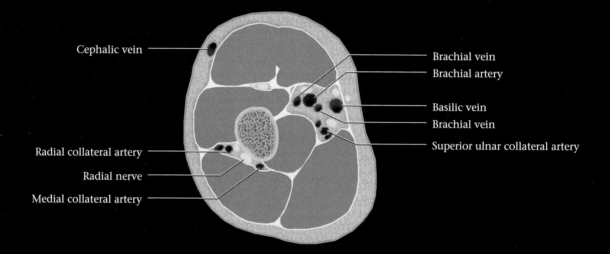

Cephalic vein

Brachial vein
Brachial artery

Basilic vein
Brachial vein

Superior ulnar collateral artery

Radial collateral artery

Radial nerve

Medial collateral artery

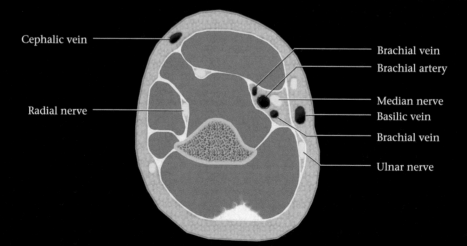

Cephalic vein

Brachial vein
Brachial artery

Median nerve
Basilic vein

Brachial vein

Radial nerve

Ulnar nerve

(Top) Axial graphic of the right arm at the upper arm. **(Middle)** Axial graphic of the right arm at mid-humeral level. **(Bottom)** Axial graphic of the right arm at the distal humeral level.

ARM VESSELS

TRANSVERSE US, PROXIMAL ARM

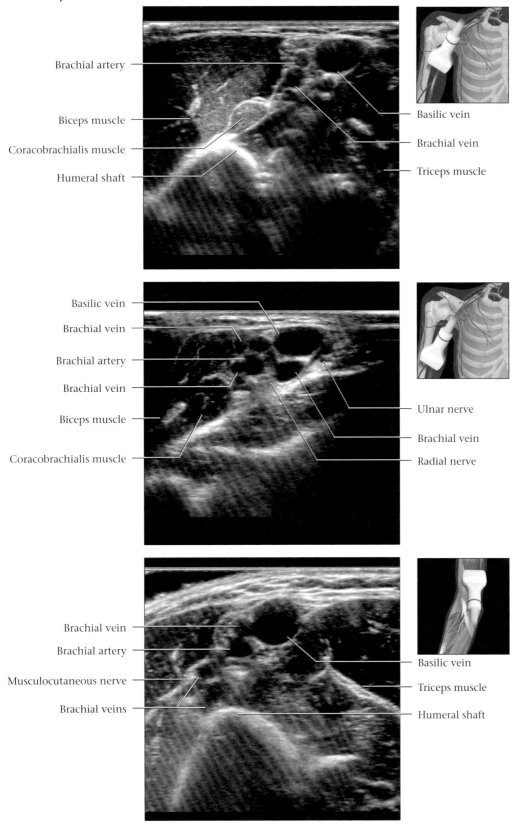

Brachial artery

Biceps muscle

Coracobrachialis muscle

Humeral shaft

Basilic vein

Brachial vein

Triceps muscle

Basilic vein

Brachial vein

Brachial artery

Brachial vein

Biceps muscle

Coracobrachialis muscle

Ulnar nerve

Brachial vein

Radial nerve

Brachial vein

Brachial artery

Musculocutaneous nerve

Brachial veins

Basilic vein

Triceps muscle

Humeral shaft

(Top) Transverse grayscale ultrasound of the vessels of the proximal arm. The basilic vein lies deep to the investing fascia in the arm. The veins are very variable in location and are surrounded by nerves. Hence, ultrasound guidance is helpful when cannulating the veins of the arm. **(Middle)** Transverse grayscale ultrasound of the vessels of the mid-arm. The basilic vein is formed on the ulnar side of the wrist and is joined by the median cubital vein (from cephalic vein at the elbow). In some cases, the brachial artery may bifurcate in the mid-arm or higher. **(Bottom)** Transverse grayscale ultrasound of the vessels of the distal arm. The brachial artery can be seen clinically as a pulsatile vessel in "locomotor brachialis" i.e. in arteriosclerosis.

ARM VESSELS

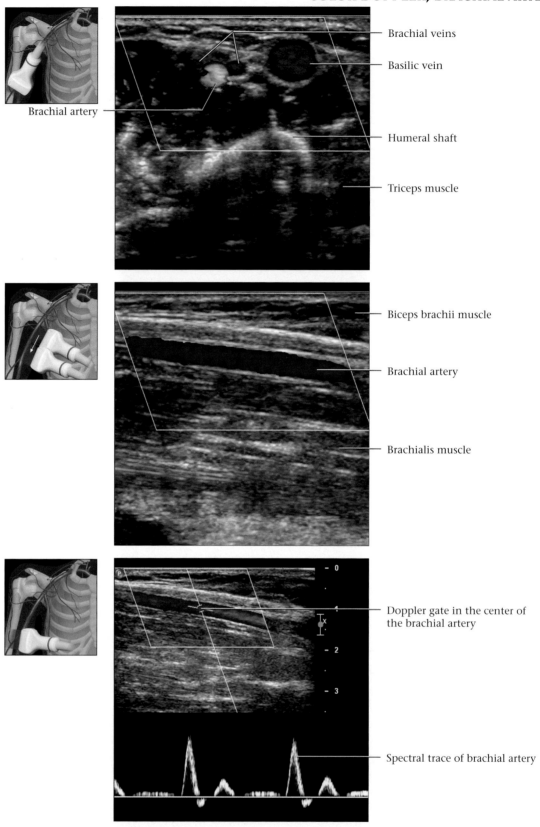

Brachial artery

Brachial veins

Basilic vein

Humeral shaft

Triceps muscle

Biceps brachii muscle

Brachial artery

Brachialis muscle

Doppler gate in the center of the brachial artery

Spectral trace of brachial artery

(Top) Transverse color Doppler ultrasound of the brachial artery. Note the accompanying paired brachial veins. **(Middle)** Longitudinal color Doppler ultrasound of the brachial artery. The normal diameter of the brachial artery at the antecubital fossa ranges between 5.5-6 mm. **(Bottom)** Longitudinal color Doppler spectral analysis ultrasound of the brachial artery. Normal triphasic flow pattern of large arteries is seen, compared to the biphasic flow of more distal arteries, but changes in temperature or even maneuvers such as clenching of the fist, may dramatically change the characteristics of upper extremity waveforms, especially in and near the hands. Peak systolic velocity of the brachial artery ranges from 50-100 cm/sec (average 57 cm/s), end diastolic velocity (EDV) 7-12 cm/s and a pulsatility index (PI) around 5 is considered normal.

ARM VESSELS

LONGITUDINAL COLOR DOPPLER, BRACHIAL VEIN

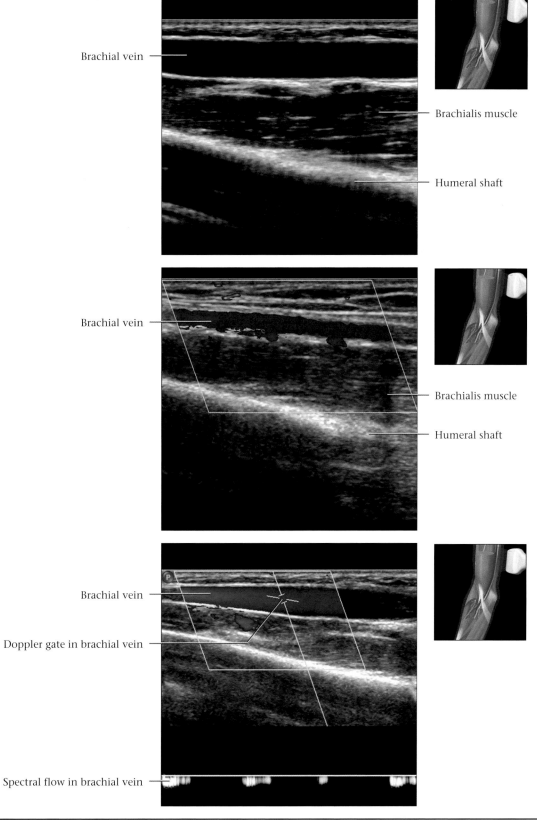

Brachial vein

Brachialis muscle

Humeral shaft

Brachial vein

Brachialis muscle

Humeral shaft

Brachial vein

Doppler gate in brachial vein

Spectral flow in brachial vein

(Top) Longitudinal grayscale ultrasound of the brachial vein. Normal brachial vein in upper arm measures around 2.5-2.7 mm. The venous system of the upper limb is categorized as a superficial and deep system. Brachial vein constitutes the deep venous system. Brachial veins can be paired or singular. (Middle) Longitudinal color Doppler ultrasound of the brachial vein. The ulnar and radial veins collect blood from the deep palmar arch and course in pairs alongside the corresponding arteries. They unite slightly above the elbow joint and flow into the brachial veins which may be either paired or singular. (Bottom) Spectral Doppler ultrasound shows the flow pattern in the brachial vein. The flow is intermittent, because of respiration. Examinations using proximal compression are not clinically relevant. Distal compression, which produces augmentation sounds, to help locate the veins.

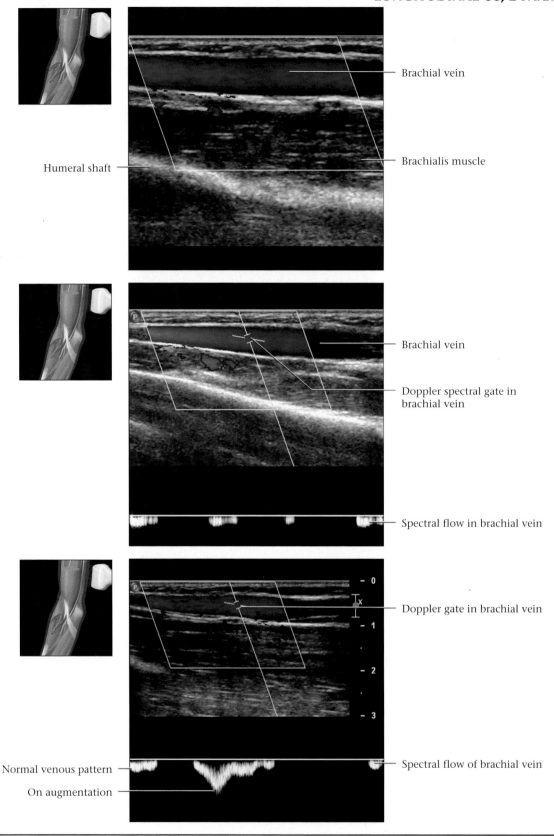

Brachial vein

Brachialis muscle

Humeral shaft

Brachial vein

Doppler spectral gate in brachial vein

Spectral flow in brachial vein

Doppler gate in brachial vein

Normal venous pattern

On augmentation

Spectral flow of brachial vein

(Top) Longitudinal color Doppler ultrasound of the brachial vein. Using Doppler mode, phasic flow during normal respiration is observed. **(Middle)** Spectral Doppler ultrasound shows the flow pattern in the brachial vein. In the upper extremities, including the subclavian vein, the behavior of venous flow during respiration is the opposite of what it is in the lower body region. During inspiration, pressure in the thorax decreases, & the venous blood flows towards the heart. During expiration, the thoracic pressure increases & the flow decreases, or even ceases during deep respiration. **(Bottom)** Spectral Doppler ultrasound shows the phenomenon of augmentation. It demonstrates the patency of the veins. It involves squeezing of the distal arm muscles (which cause motion artifacts from movement of the muscles) which will increase venous flow. Deep inspiration will have the same effect.

ARM VESSELS

CEPHALIC VEIN

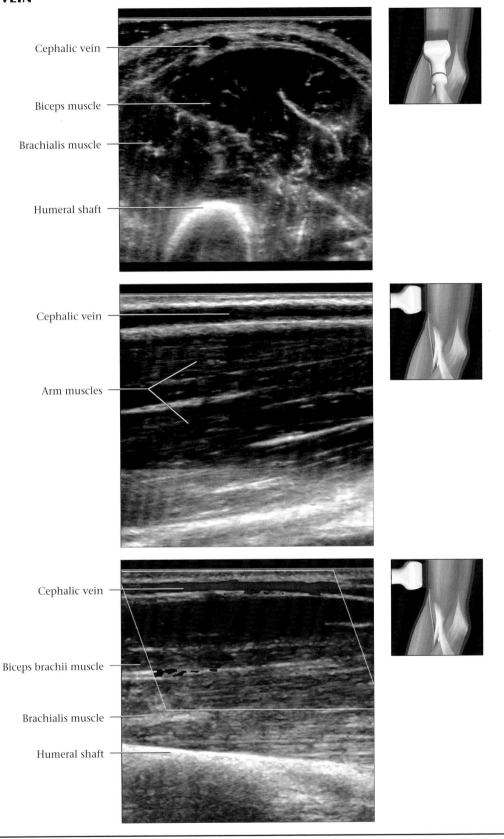

Cephalic vein

Biceps muscle

Brachialis muscle

Humeral shaft

Cephalic vein

Arm muscles

Cephalic vein

Biceps brachii muscle

Brachialis muscle

Humeral shaft

(Top) Transverse grayscale ultrasound at the proximal arm shows the cephalic vein. The normal diameter of the cephalic vein just above the elbow measures 2.5-2.9 mm. **(Middle)** Longitudinal grayscale ultrasound at the proximal arm shows the cephalic vein. The most important collecting veins of the superficial veins of the arm are the cephalic vein and the basilic veins. The cephalic vein from the superficial system unites the brachial and axillary vein confluence. Assessment of valvular insufficiency has no clinical role in the upper limb vessels. **(Bottom)** Longitudinal color Doppler ultrasound in the distal arm shows the cephalic vein. Color flow duplex sonography allows faster documentation of the six important upper arm veins (the paired brachial veins, cephalic veins and basilic veins). Continuous color intensity makes it possible to exclude thromboses.

ELBOW

Terminology

Abbreviations
- Common extensor tendon origin (CETO)
- Common flexor tendon origin (CFTO)
- Ulnar collateral ligament (UCL)
- Radial collateral ligament (RCL)
- Extensor digitorum (ED)
- Extensor carpi radialis brevis (ECRB)

Definitions
- Elbow ligaments = intrinsic ligaments = thickenings of capsule

Gross Anatomy

Joint Capsule Attachments
- Posterior: Humerus proximal to olecranon fossa & capitellum; olecranon process deep to triceps insertion
- Anterior: Humerus proximal to coronoid & radial fossae; coronoid process, annular ligament
  - Anterior & posterior fat pads are intracapsular but extra-synovial
- Synovial recesses
  - Olecranon recesses: Largest; superior, medial, & lateral around olecranon process
  - Anterior humeral recess: Proximal to coronoid fossa
  - Annular recess: Surrounds radial neck
  - Ulnar collateral ligament recess: Deep to ligament
  - Radial collateral ligament recess: Deep to ligament

Ligaments
- **Ulnar collateral ligament**
  - Extends from distal aspect of medial epicondyle → coronoid & olecranon portions of ulna
  - Separated from overlying common flexor tendon by thin layer of fat
  - Three bands; anterior, posterior & transverse
    - Anterior band, most important, cord-like, 4-6 mm thick, taut in extension, anteroinferior aspect medial epicondyle → coronoid process (sublime tubercle)
    - Anterior band divided into superficial & deep layers
    - Posterior band less important, fan-like & thinner, taut in flexion, posteroinferior medial epicondyle → olecranon
    - Transverse band functionally unimportant; forms base of triangle between anterior & posterior bands
- **Radial collateral ligament**
  - Triangular-shaped
  - Apex on lateral epicondyle → blends distally with annular ligament
  - Lies deep to overlying common extensor tendon
  - Provides origin for the superficial head of supinator muscle
- **Anular ligament**
  - Attached to anterior & posterior aspects radial notch of ulna, forming a collar around radial head
    - Anterior attachment becomes taut in supination
    - Posterior attachment becomes taut in extreme pronation
    - Provides origin for superficial head of supinator muscle

Tendons
- **Triceps tendon**
  - Three heads combine to insert onto olecranon process
  - Medial fibers insert exactly on medial margin of olecranon
  - Lateral fibers may fan out as lateral cubital retinaculum to connect with ulna & antebrachial fascia
- **Biceps tendon**
  - Flat tendon forms ≈ 7 cm proximal to elbow joint
  - Twists 90° as it passes deep so that anterior surface faces laterally
    - Expands close to attachment into radial tuberosity; attachment area ≈ 3 cm²
  - Short & long heads have separate adjoined attachments
  - Also attaches to bicipital aponeurosis
    - Bicipital aponeurosis completely encircles ulnar forearm flexor muscles
    - Merges with investing fascia of forearm
    - May be important in stabilizing distal aspect of biceps tendon
- **Common extensor tendon**
  - Arises from lateral epicondyle
  - Superficial to radial collateral ligament
  - Composed of extensor-supinator group: Extensor carpi radialis brevis, extensor carpi radialis longus, extensor digiti minimi, extensor digitorum communis
- **Common flexor tendon**
  - Arises from medial epicondyle
  - Superficial to ulnar collateral ligament
  - Composed of flexor-pronator group: Flexor carpi radialis, flexor carpi ulnaris, flexor digitorum superficialis, pronator teres, palmaris longus

Bursae
- **Subtendinous olecranon bursa**: Between triceps tendon & olecranon
- **Subcutaneous olecranon bursa**: Between skin & olecranon process
- **Bicipitoradial bursa**: Between biceps tendon & radial tuberosity
- **Radioulnar bursa**: Between extensor digitorum & radiohumeral joint

Anatomy-Based Imaging Issues

Imaging Recommendations
- High frequency linear transducer
- Large amount of gel for superficial structures
- Examination usually tailored to site of symptoms
- Lateral elbow best seen with elbow flexed slightly or fully flexed
- Medial elbow best seen with elbow extended
- Biceps tendon best seen in full supination
- Effusion will displace fat pads away from bone

GRAPHIC, CORONAL ELBOW

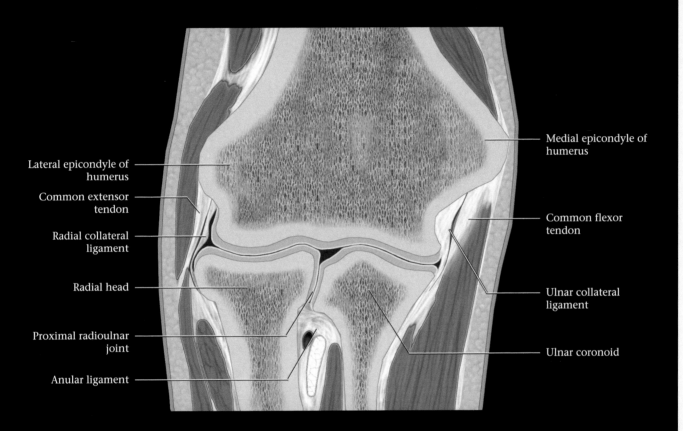

Lateral epicondyle of humerus

Common extensor tendon

Radial collateral ligament

Radial head

Proximal radioulnar joint

Anular ligament

Medial epicondyle of humerus

Common flexor tendon

Ulnar collateral ligament

Ulnar coronoid

Coronal section through the level of the epicondyles shows the collateral ligaments deep to the common tendon groups. Although the radial collateral ligament is shown, the section is too anterior to show the ulnar lateral collateral ligament, which originates just posterior to the radial collateral.

ELBOW

GRAPHICS, PROXIMAL ELBOW CROSS-SECTION

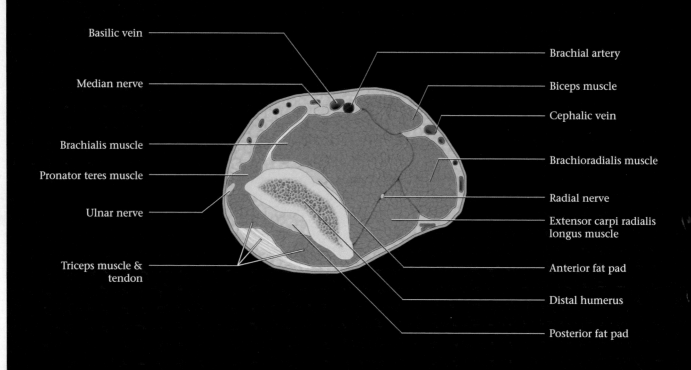

Basilic vein — Brachial artery

Median nerve — Biceps muscle

— Cephalic vein

Brachialis muscle — Brachioradialis muscle

Pronator teres muscle —

Radial nerve

Ulnar nerve — Extensor carpi radialis longus muscle

Anterior fat pad

Triceps muscle & tendon — Distal humerus

Posterior fat pad

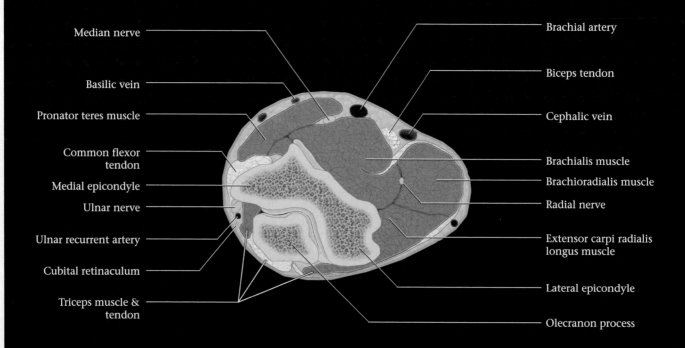

Median nerve — Brachial artery

Basilic vein — Biceps tendon

Pronator teres muscle — Cephalic vein

Common flexor tendon — Brachialis muscle

Medial epicondyle — Brachioradialis muscle

Ulnar nerve — Radial nerve

Ulnar recurrent artery — Extensor carpi radialis longus muscle

Cubital retinaculum — Lateral epicondyle

Triceps muscle & tendon — Olecranon process

(Top) Axial graphic of the supracondylar region of the humerus. The anterior & posterior fat pads are seen in the coronoid & olecranon fossae, respectively. The brachialis muscle accounts for the bulk of the anterior compartment of the distal arm. **(Bottom)** Axial graphic of the epicondylar region of the distal humerus. The triceps muscle thins as its tendon attaches to the olecranon. The ulnar nerve & posterior ulnar recurrent artery are held in the cubital tunnel by the cubital retinaculum (the ligament of Osborn).

ELBOW

GRAPHICS, MID ELBOW CROSS-SECTION

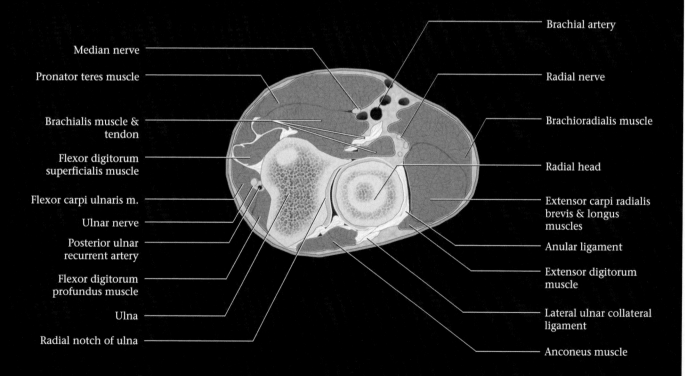

Brachial artery

Median nerve

Pronator teres muscle

Common flexor tendon

Ulnar nerve

Flexor carpi ulnaris m.

Ulnar collateral l.

Triceps muscle & tendon

Cephalic vein

Biceps aponeurosis

Biceps tendon

Radial nerve

Brachioradialis muscle

Brachialis muscle

Extensor carpi radialis longus muscle

Common extensor tendon

Radial collateral l.

Olecranon process

Median nerve

Pronator teres muscle

Brachialis muscle & tendon

Flexor digitorum superficialis muscle

Flexor carpi ulnaris m.

Ulnar nerve

Posterior ulnar recurrent artery

Flexor digitorum profundus muscle

Ulna

Radial notch of ulna

Brachial artery

Radial nerve

Brachioradialis muscle

Radial head

Extensor carpi radialis brevis & longus muscles

Anular ligament

Extensor digitorum muscle

Lateral ulnar collateral ligament

Anconeus muscle

(Top) Axial graphic immediately proximal to the elbow joint. The common extensor tendon overlies the radial collateral ligament & may be difficult to distinguish at this level. The ulnar nerve has exited the cubital tunnel & is entering the flexor carpi ulnaris. **(Bottom)** Axial graphic at the level of the proximal radioulnar joint. The articulating surfaces of the proximal radioulnar joint are well seen as the radial head is held in the radial notch of the ulna by the anular ligament. The lateral ulnar collateral ligament blends with the posterior aspect of the anular ligament.

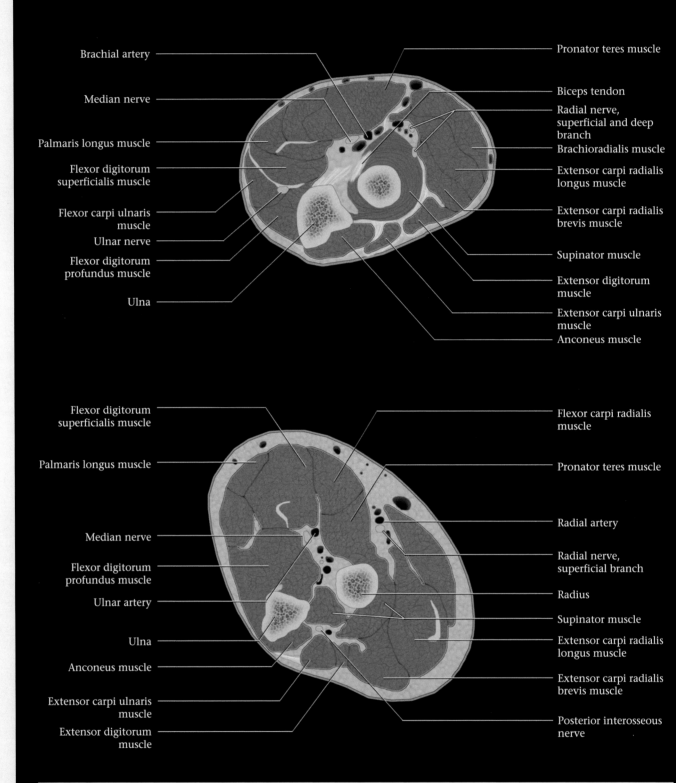

Brachial artery

Median nerve

Palmaris longus muscle

Flexor digitorum superficialis muscle

Flexor carpi ulnaris muscle

Ulnar nerve

Flexor digitorum profundus muscle

Ulna

Pronator teres muscle

Biceps tendon

Radial nerve, superficial and deep branch

Brachioradialis muscle

Extensor carpi radialis longus muscle

Extensor carpi radialis brevis muscle

Supinator muscle

Extensor digitorum muscle

Extensor carpi ulnaris muscle

Anconeus muscle

Flexor digitorum superficialis muscle

Palmaris longus muscle

Median nerve

Flexor digitorum profundus muscle

Ulnar artery

Ulna

Anconeus muscle

Extensor carpi ulnaris muscle

Extensor digitorum muscle

Flexor carpi radialis muscle

Pronator teres muscle

Radial artery

Radial nerve, superficial branch

Radius

Supinator muscle

Extensor carpi radialis longus muscle

Extensor carpi radialis brevis muscle

Posterior interosseous nerve

(Top) Graphic shows the axial elbow at a level immediately above the radial tuberosity. The brachialis tendon inserts on the ulnar tuberosity & the biceps tendon approaches its insertion on the radial tuberosity, which is more distal than the brachialis insertion. **(Bottom)** At the level of the proximal forearm, the muscles are starting to align themselves into the anterior (flexor) compartment, & the posterior (extensor) compartment.

ELBOW

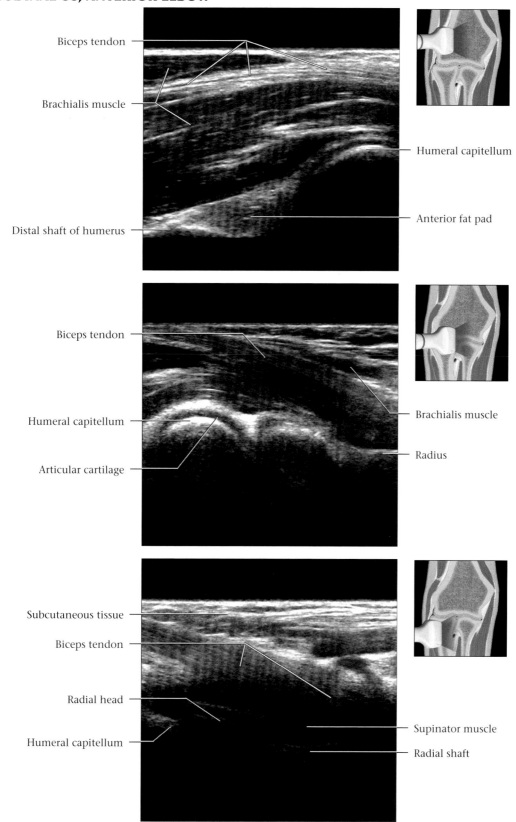

Top image labels: Biceps tendon, Brachialis muscle, Distal shaft of humerus, Humeral capitellum, Anterior fat pad

Middle image labels: Biceps tendon, Humeral capitellum, Articular cartilage, Brachialis muscle, Radius

Bottom image labels: Subcutaneous tissue, Biceps tendon, Radial head, Humeral capitellum, Supinator muscle, Radial shaft

(Top) Longitudinal grayscale ultrasound of the biceps tendon proximal to the elbow. Most biceps tendon tears occur near the shoulder. Tears of the distal end of the biceps tendon are uncommon and mostly occur when unexpected force is applied to the bent arm e.g., fall. (Middle) Longitudinal grayscale ultrasound of the biceps tendon at the elbow. With a torn biceps tendon, a bulge in the arm (Popeye's muscle) may appear. (Bottom) Longitudinal grayscale ultrasound of the biceps tendon just distal to the elbow. The biceps tendon flattens and rotates 90 degrees as it approaches the insertion in the posterior aspect of the radial tuberosity. It is best visualized on longitudinal section with the elbow fully supinated.

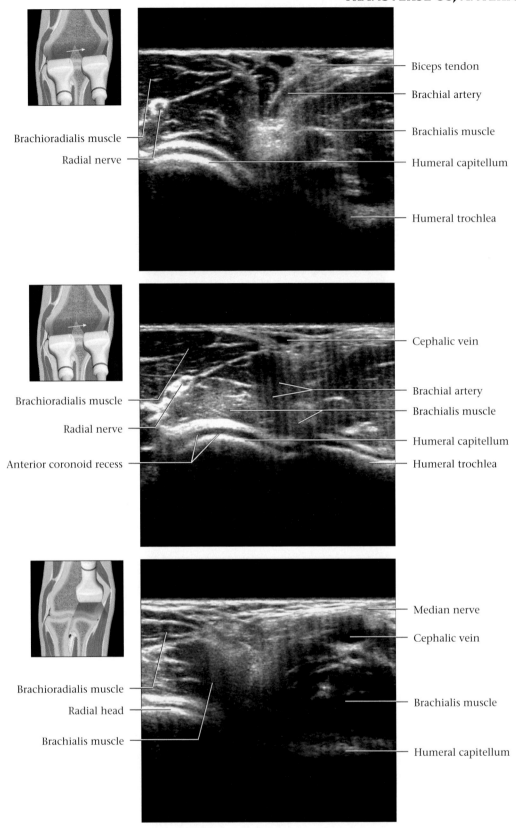

Biceps tendon

Brachial artery

Brachialis muscle

Humeral capitellum

Humeral trochlea

Brachioradialis muscle

Radial nerve

Cephalic vein

Brachial artery

Brachialis muscle

Humeral capitellum

Humeral trochlea

Brachioradialis muscle

Radial nerve

Anterior coronoid recess

Median nerve

Cephalic vein

Brachialis muscle

Humeral capitellum

Brachioradialis muscle

Radial head

Brachialis muscle

(Top) Transverse grayscale ultrasound at the proximal end of the antecubital fossa. Flexion and extension occur at the humero-ulnar articulation while pronation and supination involves pronation of the radius around the ulna. **(Middle)** Transverse grayscale ultrasound at the mid-portion of the antecubital fossa. The median cubital vein unites the cephalic vein with the basilic vein. It is often used for venipuncture and venous access. It lies superficial to the bicipital aponeurosis. **(Bottom)** Transverse grayscale ultrasound at the distal aspect of the antecubital fossa. The elbow joint is supplied by arteries from the profunda brachii, the brachial arteries and recurrent branches of the radial and ulnar arteries.

ELBOW

TRANSVERSE US, ANTECUBITAL FOSSA

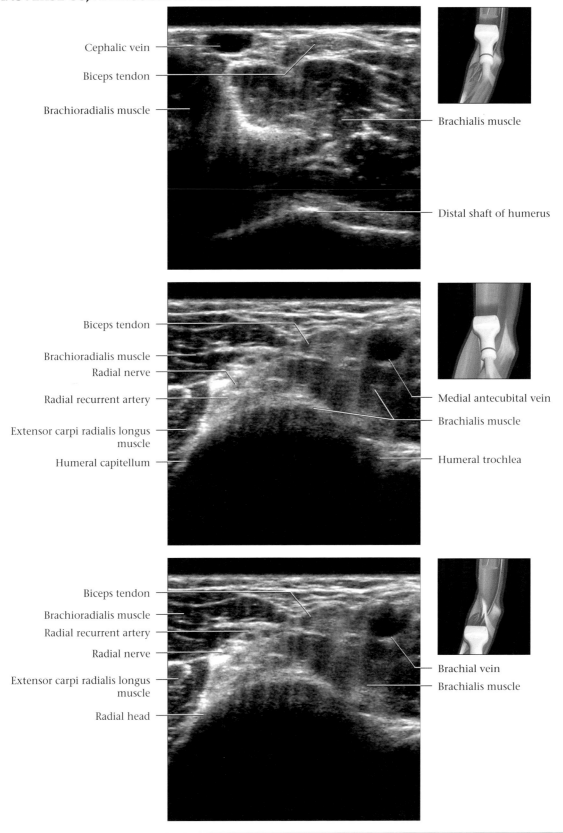

Top image labels:
- Cephalic vein
- Biceps tendon
- Brachioradialis muscle
- Brachialis muscle
- Distal shaft of humerus

Middle image labels:
- Biceps tendon
- Brachioradialis muscle
- Radial nerve
- Radial recurrent artery
- Extensor carpi radialis longus muscle
- Humeral capitellum
- Medial antecubital vein
- Brachialis muscle
- Humeral trochlea

Bottom image labels:
- Biceps tendon
- Brachioradialis muscle
- Radial recurrent artery
- Radial nerve
- Extensor carpi radialis longus muscle
- Radial head
- Brachial vein
- Brachialis muscle

(Top) Transverse grayscale ultrasound of the anterior elbow, proximal antecubital fossa. The antecubital fossa or cubital fossa is the area anterior to the elbow joint. (Middle) Transverse grayscale ultrasound of the antecubital fossa at the mid portion. The antecubital fossa contains the radial nerve, the biceps brachii tendon, the brachial artery and the median nerve from lateral to medial orientation. (Bottom) Transverse grayscale ultrasound at distal antecubital fossa. The bicipital aponeurosis forms the roof of the antecubital fossa. The superficial veins of the elbow lie above the bicipital aponeurosis.

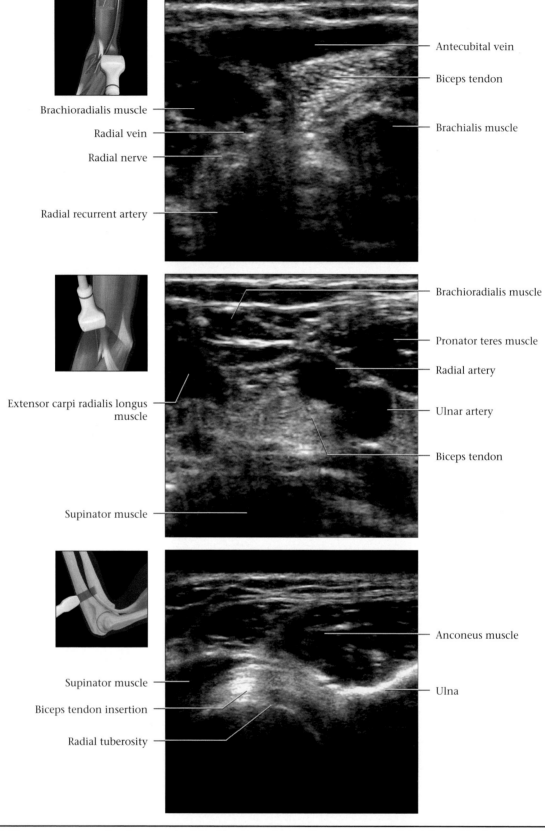

Brachioradialis muscle

Radial vein

Radial nerve

Radial recurrent artery

Antecubital vein

Biceps tendon

Brachialis muscle

Extensor carpi radialis longus muscle

Supinator muscle

Brachioradialis muscle

Pronator teres muscle

Radial artery

Ulnar artery

Biceps tendon

Supinator muscle

Biceps tendon insertion

Radial tuberosity

Anconeus muscle

Ulna

(Top) Transverse grayscale ultrasound of the biceps tendon at the upper antecubital fossa. The biceps tendon forms a few centimeters above the elbow joint. (Middle) Transverse grayscale ultrasound of the biceps tendon at the mid-cubital fossa. The biceps tendon dips deeply and rotates as it passes to its insertion. The distal aspect of the biceps tendon and the insertion is difficult to see on ultrasound of the anterior surface of the elbow. Maximum supination will increase its visibility. (Bottom) Transverse grayscale ultrasound of the biceps tendon insertional area. The insertional area of the biceps tendon is best seen with the elbow flexed and the wrist fully pronated. This positions the radial tuberosity posteriorly allowing the insertional area to be viewed from the posterior aspect as shown here.

ELBOW

ANTEROLATERAL ELBOW

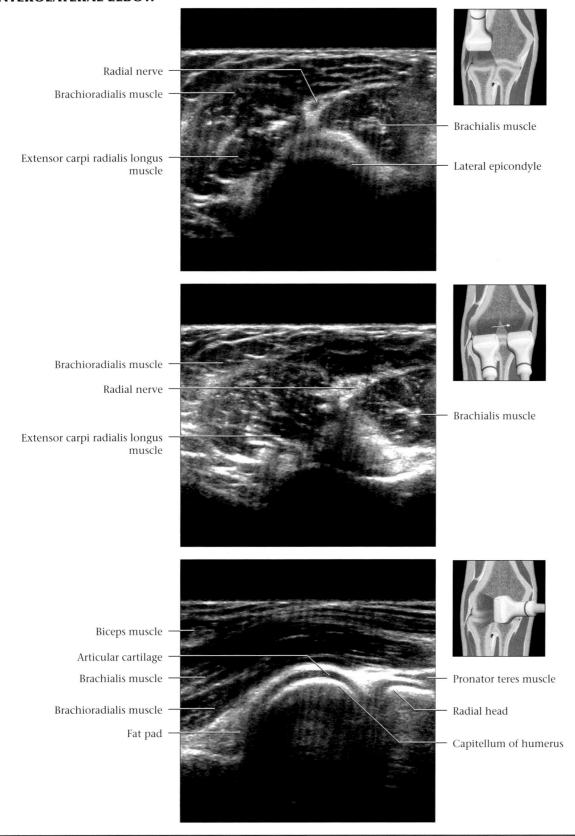

Radial nerve

Brachioradialis muscle

Extensor carpi radialis longus muscle

Brachialis muscle

Lateral epicondyle

Brachioradialis muscle

Radial nerve

Extensor carpi radialis longus muscle

Brachialis muscle

Biceps muscle

Articular cartilage

Brachialis muscle

Brachioradialis muscle

Fat pad

Pronator teres muscle

Radial head

Capitellum of humerus

(Top) Transverse grayscale ultrasound at the proximal anterolateral aspect of the elbow. The radial nerve is located on the anterolateral aspect of the elbow. It can be readily identified deep to the brachioradialis muscle. **(Middle)** Transverse grayscale ultrasound at the mid-section of the anterolateral elbow. The radial nerve passes anterior to the epicondyle deep to the brachioradialis muscle. **(Bottom)** Longitudinal grayscale ultrasound at the anterolateral aspect of the elbow. The fat pads are intracapsular but extrasynovial. The synovial space lies deep to the fat pad on the bone surface. Distension of the fat pads allows these to become visible radiographically in elbow joint effusions.

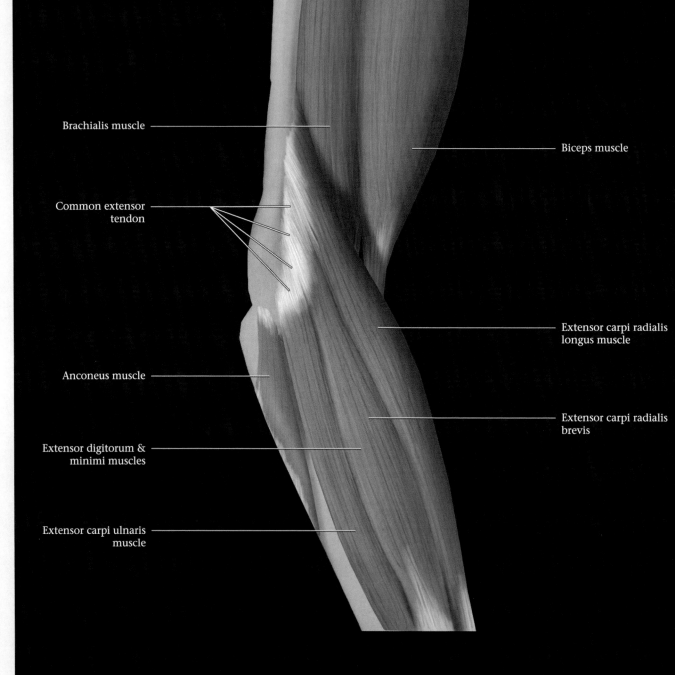

Brachialis muscle

Biceps muscle

Common extensor tendon

Extensor carpi radialis longus muscle

Anconeus muscle

Extensor carpi radialis brevis

Extensor digitorum & minimi muscles

Extensor carpi ulnaris muscle

A side view of the lateral aspect of the elbow shows the extensor-supinator group & its common extensor tendon, attaching to the lateral epicondyle & supracondylar aspect of the humerus. The common extensor tendon is comprised of the extensor carpi radialis brevis, extensor digitorum, extensor digiti minimi, & extensor carpi ulnaris. The extensor digitorum and extensor carpi radialis brevis are very closely aligned in this section.

ELBOW

LONGITUDINAL US, COMMON EXTENSOR ORIGIN

Common extensor tendon origin
Common extensor tendons
Radial head
Radio-humeral joint
Radial collateral ligament

Lateral epicondyle
Humeral capitellum

Common extensor tendons
Anular ligament
Supinator muscle
Radial head

Radial collateral ligament
Common extensor tendon origin

Common extensor tendons
Supinator muscle
Radial head

Humeral capitellum
Radial collateral ligament

(Top) Longitudinal grayscale US at common extensor tendon origin (CETO). CETO has a broad attachment on the posteroinferior aspect of lateral epicondyle. Tendon fibers cannot be separated into individual components at or near the insertion. Fibers from ED make up most of superficial portion while fibers from ECRB make up most of the deep fibers. Contribution from extensor carpi ulnaris and extensor digiti minimi is only small. (Middle) Longitudinal grayscale US at CETO with wrist in neutral position. Radial collateral ligament is less distinct than ulnar collateral ligament. It runs from the inferior aspect of the lateral epicondyle to gain attachment to the anular ligament. (Bottom) Longitudinal grayscale US at CETO with wrist in extension. Wrist extension slightly straightens extensor tendons and dynamic movement during US can help separate movable tendons from fixed radial collateral ligament.

TRANSVERSE US, COMMON EXTENSOR TENDONS

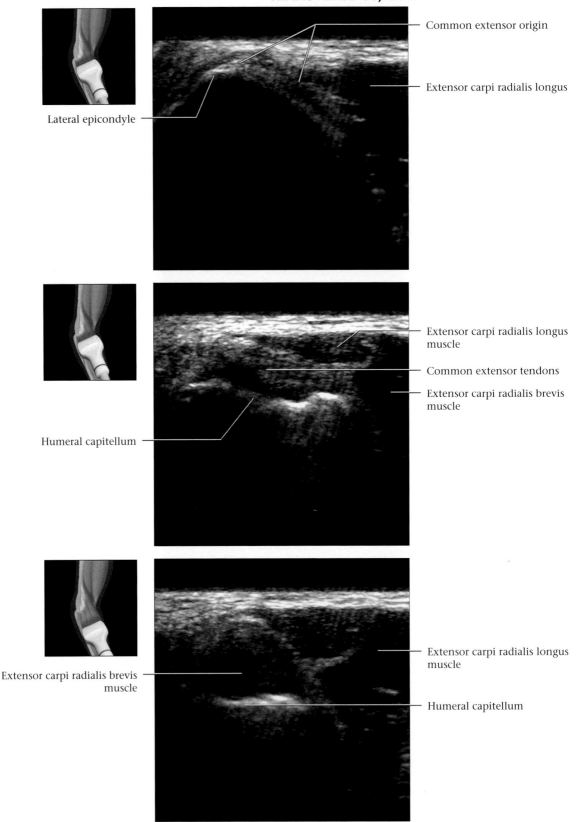

Common extensor origin

Extensor carpi radialis longus

Lateral epicondyle

Extensor carpi radialis longus muscle

Common extensor tendons

Extensor carpi radialis brevis muscle

Humeral capitellum

Extensor carpi radialis brevis muscle

Extensor carpi radialis longus muscle

Humeral capitellum

(Top) Transverse grayscale ultrasound of the common extensor origin. The common extensor tendon gains broad insertion onto the posterior aspect of the lateral epicondyle. (Middle) Transverse grayscale ultrasound of the common extensor origin just distal to their attachment. The tendons begin to diverge just distal to the attachment though they are not yet separate. (Bottom) Transverse grayscale ultrasound of the common extensor tendons even more distal to the above section. Near the elbow joint, the individual components of the tendon begin to be seen.

ELBOW

TRANSVERSE AND LONGITUDINAL US, LATERAL ELBOW

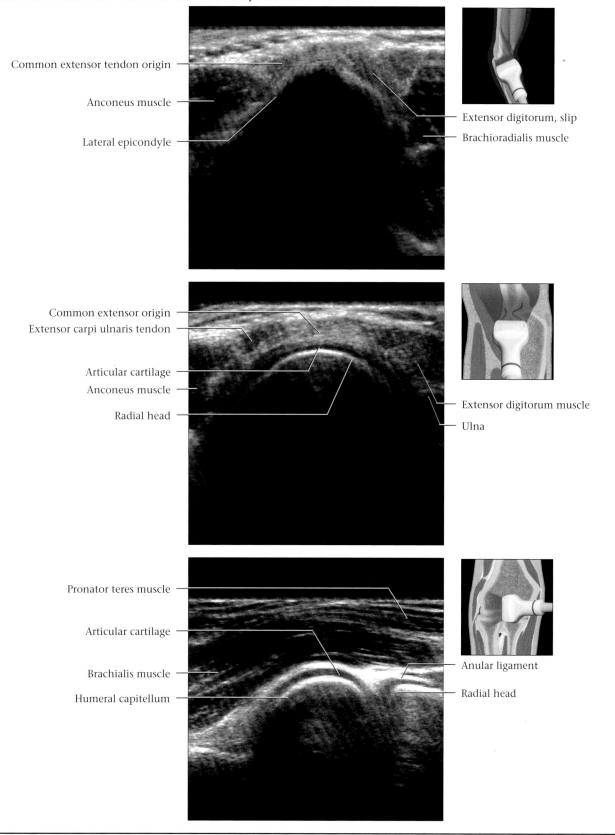

Common extensor tendon origin

Anconeus muscle

Lateral epicondyle

Extensor digitorum, slip

Brachioradialis muscle

Common extensor origin
Extensor carpi ulnaris tendon

Articular cartilage
Anconeus muscle

Radial head

Extensor digitorum muscle

Ulna

Pronator teres muscle

Articular cartilage

Brachialis muscle

Humeral capitellum

Anular ligament

Radial head

(Top) Transverse grayscale ultrasound at the common extensor tendon origin. The tendon caliber is often better appreciated on transverse rather than longitudinal imaging. **(Middle)** Transverse grayscale ultrasound of the common extensor tendons at the level of the radial head. The extensor tendons that originate from the common tendon origin can be traced distally allowing observation of their divisions into separate tendons (extensor digitorum, extensor digiti minimi, extensor carpi ulnaris and extensor carpi radialis brevis). **(Bottom)** Longitudinal grayscale ultrasound of the common extensor tendon origin. The caliber of the common extensor tendons at origin can often be appreciated on transverse imaging.

ELBOW

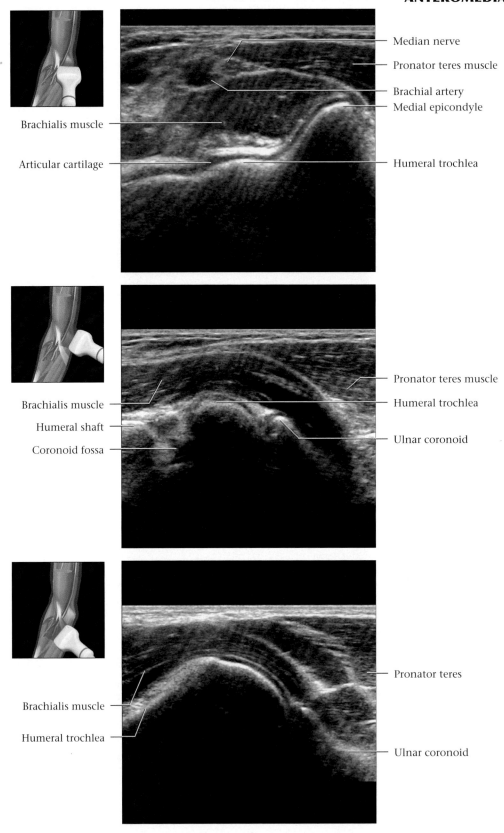

(Top) Transverse grayscale ultrasound of the anteromedial aspect of elbow. The pronator teres has two heads, one from the common flexor origin (medial epicondyle) and supracondylar region and the second head from the medial side of the coronoid process. The median nerve lies deep to the pronator teres and may be trapped between these two heads as it enters the forearm. **(Middle)** Longitudinal grayscale ultrasound of the anteromedial aspect of the elbow. Centrally at the junction of the distal humerus between the coronoid fossa anteriorly and the olecranon fossa posteriorly the humerus is so thin, that it appears as if the bone is absent. **(Bottom)** Longitudinal grayscale ultrasound of the anteromedial aspect of the elbow. The brachialis muscle is clearly applied to the anterior aspect of the elbow joint as it descends to its insertion on the ulnar tuberosity and the coronoid process of ulna.

GRAPHIC, FLEXOR ASPECT

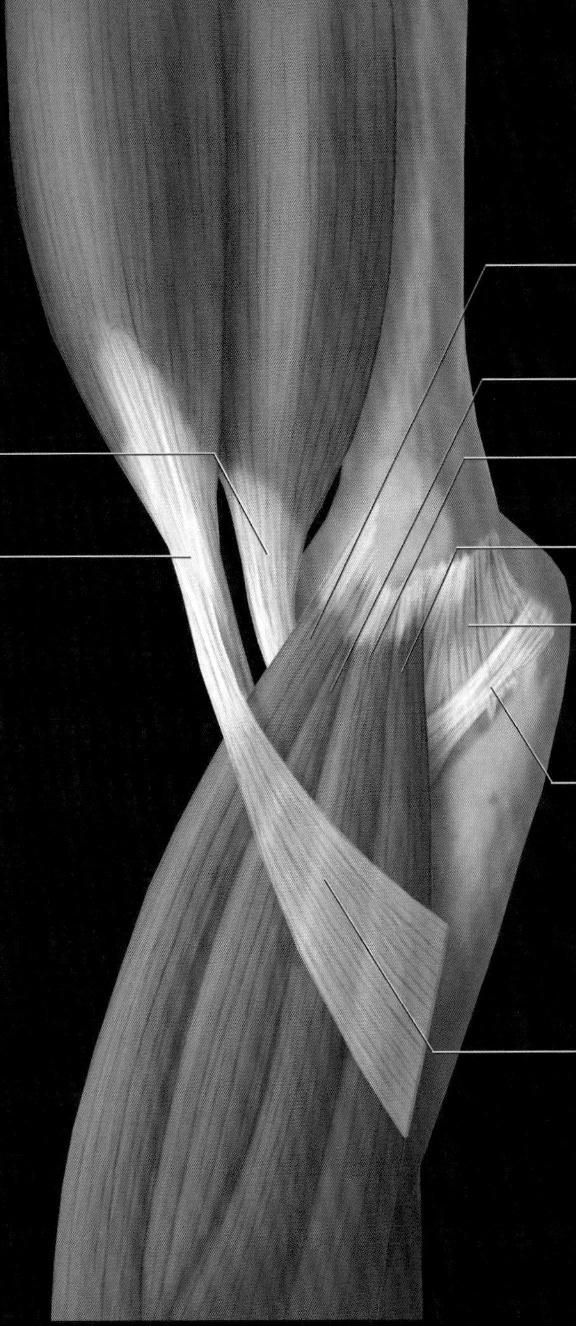

Pronator teres (anterior) & flexor carpi radialis muscle

Palmaris longus muscle

Flexor digitorum superficialis muscle

Flexor carpi ulnaris muscle

Posterior band of ulnar collateral ligament

Transverse band of ulnar collateral ligament

Biceps aponeurosis

Brachialis tendon

Biceps tendon

Side view of the medial aspect of the elbow shows the flexor-pronator group and its common flexor tendon, attaching to the medial epicondyle. The anterior band of the ulnar collateral ligament is deep to the common tendon. The biceps aponeurosis blends with the anterior aspect of the common flexor mass. The flexor digitorum profundus (not shown) arises from the proximal humerus, posterior and deep to the flexor carpi ulnaris, and does not act on the elbow and is not part of the flexor-pronator group.

Posterior band

Anterior band

Transverse band

Radial collateral ligament

Anular ligament

Lateral ulnar collateral ligament

Ulnar collateral ligament

Accessory lateral collateral ligament

Oblique cord

Common flexor tendon

Olecranon

Ulnar nerve

Cubital retinaculum

Posterior ulnar recurrent artery

Triceps muscle & tendon

(Top) Side view of the medial aspect of the elbow shows the three components of the ulnar collateral ligament: Anterior, posterior & transverse band. **(Middle)** Anterior view of the elbow shows the radial collateral ligament complex, which is comprised of radial collateral ligament (provides varus stability), lateral ulnar collateral ligament (provides posterolateral stability), anular ligament (holds radial head against radial notch of the ulna), & accessory lateral collateral ligament (reinforces anular ligament). The oblique cord is part of the proximal radioulnar joint. **(Bottom)** Axial graphic of the cubital tunnel. The ulnar nerve may be compressed within the cubital tunnel ("cubital tunnel syndrome") by a mass, post-traumatic osseous deformity, or aneurysm of the recurrent ulnar artery. The ulnar nerve may also be subluxed out of the cubital tunnel by the adjacent medial head of the triceps.

ELBOW

LONGITUDINAL US, COMMON FLEXOR ORIGIN

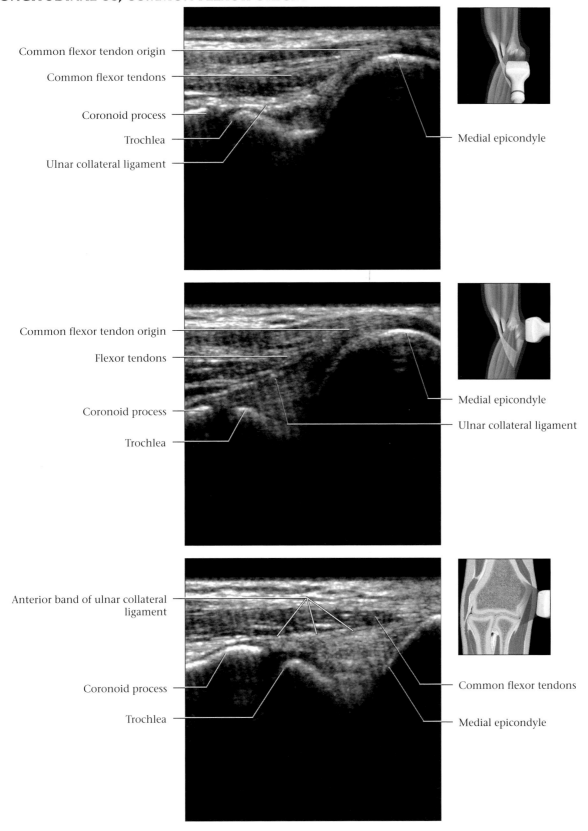

Common flexor tendon origin

Common flexor tendons

Coronoid process

Trochlea

Ulnar collateral ligament

Medial epicondyle

Common flexor tendon origin

Flexor tendons

Coronoid process

Trochlea

Medial epicondyle

Ulnar collateral ligament

Anterior band of ulnar collateral ligament

Coronoid process

Trochlea

Common flexor tendons

Medial epicondyle

(Top) Longitudinal grayscale ultrasound of the origin of the common flexor tendon. The tendon originates from the common flexor tendon origin. These tendons (pronator teres, flexor carpi radialis, palmaris longus, flexor digitorum superficialis, flexor carpi ulnaris) are inseparable at or close to the origin. **(Middle)** Longitudinal grayscale ultrasound of the elbow ulnar collateral ligament. The ulnar collateral ligaments run from the medial epicondyle to the coronoid process. The ulnar collateral ligament lies just deep to the flexor tendons and may be injured along with these tendons. **(Bottom)** Longitudinal grayscale ultrasound of the ulnar collateral ligament anterior band. The anterior band (medial epicondyle-sublime tubercle) is the strongest component of the ulnar collateral ligament.

ELBOW

TRANSVERSE US, COMMON FLEXOR ORIGIN

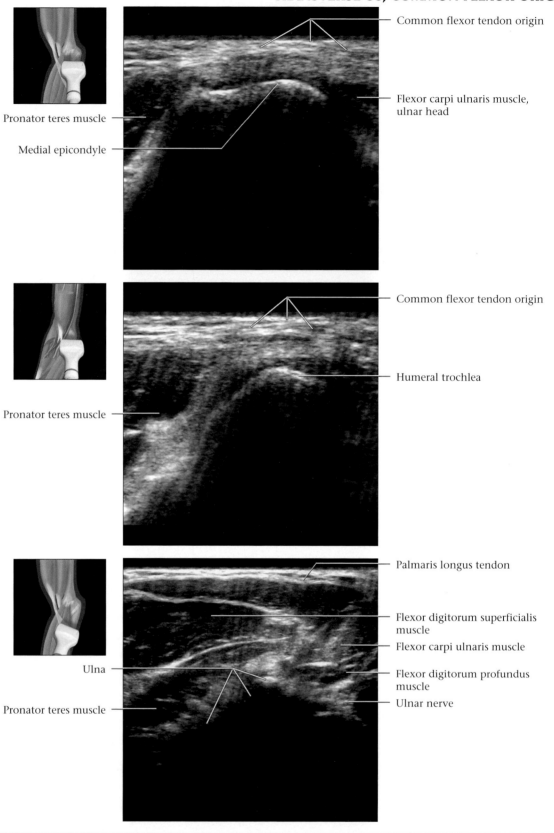

Common flexor tendon origin

Flexor carpi ulnaris muscle, ulnar head

Pronator teres muscle

Medial epicondyle

Common flexor tendon origin

Humeral trochlea

Pronator teres muscle

Palmaris longus tendon

Flexor digitorum superficialis muscle

Flexor carpi ulnaris muscle

Flexor digitorum profundus muscle

Ulnar nerve

Ulna

Pronator teres muscle

(Top) Transverse grayscale ultrasound at the common flexor tendon origin. Tendinosis of the common flexor tendon is termed "golfer's elbow", "medial epicondylitis". Yet most people who get this injury are involved in other sports particularly tennis. **(Middle)** Transverse grayscale ultrasound of the common flexor tendons just distal to the elbow. The different components of the common flexor tendons can be seen by following the tendon distally and proximally. **(Bottom)** Transverse grayscale ultrasound of the forearm more distal to the common flexor origin.

Upper Limb

VI

68

ELBOW

TRANSVERSE US, POSTERIOR ELBOW

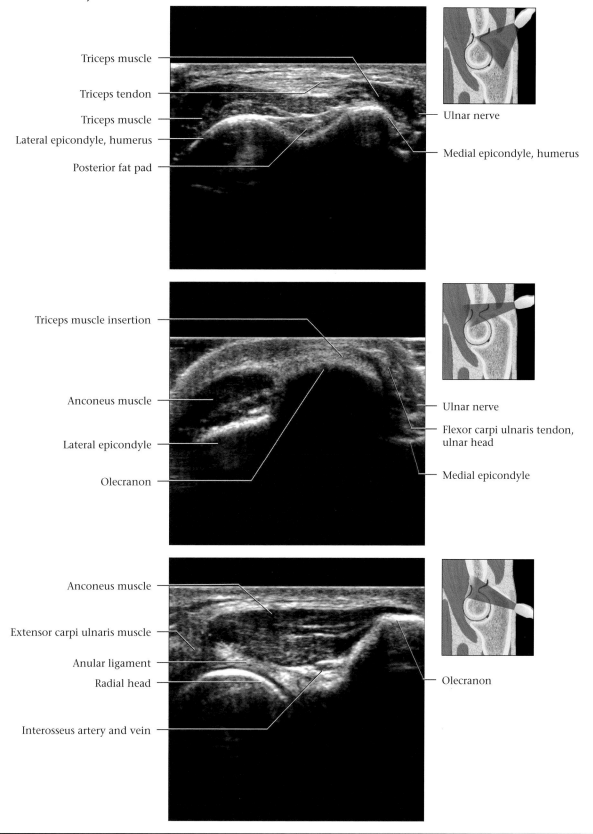

Triceps muscle
Triceps tendon
Triceps muscle
Lateral epicondyle, humerus
Posterior fat pad
Ulnar nerve
Medial epicondyle, humerus

Triceps muscle insertion
Anconeus muscle
Lateral epicondyle
Olecranon
Ulnar nerve
Flexor carpi ulnaris tendon, ulnar head
Medial epicondyle

Anconeus muscle
Extensor carpi ulnaris muscle
Anular ligament
Radial head
Interosseus artery and vein
Olecranon

(Top) Transverse grayscale ultrasound of the posterior elbow. There are three fat pads in the elbow. These are the anterior fat pad (radial and coronoid fossa) and posterior fat pad (olecranon fossa). The synovium extends from the articular surface of the humerus and lines these fossae, i.e. it lies deep to the fat pad in which the capsule encloses the fat pads. The fat pads therefore are intra-articular but extrasynovial. Fluid distension of the synovial cavity elevates the fat pads. (Middle) Transverse grayscale ultrasound of the elbow at the level of the olecranon. The anconeus is a small muscle on the posterior aspect of elbow that extends from the lateral epicondyle to the olecranon. (Bottom) Transverse grayscale ultrasound at the proximal radioulnar joint. The anular ligament is attached to the anterior and posterior margins of the radial notch of the ulna.

FOREARM

Imaging Anatomy

Flexors
- Deep flexor group
  - Flexor digitorum profundus (FDP)
    - Origin: Proximal ulna
    - Insertion: Index, middle, ring & little finger distal phalangeal bases
  - Flexor pollicis longus (FPL)
    - Origin: Radius, interosseous membrane, coronoid process
    - Insertion: Thumb distal phalangeal base
  - Pronator quadratus (PQ)
    - Origin: Medial distal volar ulna
    - Insertion: Lateral distal dorsal radius
- Superficial
  - Flexor carpi radialis (FCR)
    - Origin: Medial epicondyle/common flexor tendon
    - Insertion: 2nd MC base; slip to 3rd MC base
  - Palmaris longus (PL)
    - Origin: Medial epicondyle/common flexor tendon
    - Insertion: Volar distal flexor retinaculum and palmar aponeurosis
  - Flexor carpi ulnaris (FCU)
    - Origin: Medial epicondyle (humeral head) & medial proximal ulna (ulnar head)
    - Insertion: Pisiform
  - Flexor digitorum superficialis (FDS)
    - Origin: Medial epicondyle & ulnar coronoid process (humeroulnar head); volar proximal radius (radial head)
    - Insertion: Middle phalanges index, middle, ring & little fingers

Extensors
- Deep
  - Abductor pollicis longus (AbPL)
    - Origin: Dorsal lateral ulna, dorsal mid-radius
    - Insertion: 1st MC radial base
  - Extensor pollicis brevis (EPB)
    - Origin: Dorsal mid radius
    - Insertion: Thumb proximal phalangeal base
  - Extensor pollicis longus (EPL)
    - Origin: Dorsal mid-ulna; insertion: Thumb distal phalanx base
    - Variant: Fused with EPB
  - Extensor indicis (EI)
    - Origin: Dorsal mid ulna & interosseous membrane
    - Insertion: Extensor hood of index finger
- Superficial
  - Extensor carpi radialis longus (ECRL)
    - Origin: Lateral epicondyle/common extensor tendon
    - Insertion: Dorsal radial 2nd MC
  - Extensor carpi radialis brevis (ECRB)
    - Origin: Lateral epicondyle/common extensor tendon
    - Insertion: Dorsal radial 3rd MC
  - Extensor digitorum (ED)
    - Origin: Lateral epicondyle/common extensor tendon
    - Insertion: Middle & distal phalanges of index, middle, ring, little fingers
  - Extensor digiti minimi (EDM)
    - Origin: Lateral epicondyle/common extensor tendon
    - Insertion: Extensor hood of little finger proximal phalanx with slip to ring finger
  - Extensor carpi ulnaris (ECU)
    - Origin: Common extensor tendon & dorsal ulna
    - Insertion: Dorsal ulnar 5th MC base

Anomalous Muscles
- May present as a soft tissue mass; may create neural compression
- Accessory palmaris longus: Superficial to FD tendons, medial to FCR
- Extensor digitorum manus brevis: Arises from distal radius or dorsal radiocarpal ligament; inserts on 2nd MC
  - May be tender or present as mass
- Extensor carpi radialis intermedius: Arises from humerus or as accessory slip from ECRB or ECRL; inserts on 2nd &/or 3rd MC
- Extensor carpi radialis accessory: Arises from humerus or ECRL; inserts 1st MC, APB, or 1st dorsal interosseous

Anatomy-Based Imaging Issues

Imaging Pitfalls
- Many variations of flexor & extensor muscles & tendons
- Extensor pollicis brevis may be absent or fused with EPL
- Palmaris longus absent in 10%; short tendon with extended muscle belly may compress median nerve
- Multiple tendon slips can mimic longitudinal tendon tears (e.g., APL)
- Small amount of fluid common in tendon sheath (e.g., ECRB, ECRL, ECU)

Imaging Issues
- APL & EPB intersect ECRB & ECRL just proximal to extensor retinaculum; may impinge at musculotendinous intersection ("intersection syndrome")
- Sites of radial nerve entrapment in forearm
  - Posterior interosseous nerve within radial tunnel under arcade of Frohse
  - Posterior interosseous nerve between deep & superficial heads of supinator muscle
  - Superficial radial nerve between brachioradialis & ECRL in mid- to distal forearm
- Sites of ulnar nerve entrapment in forearm
  - Cubital tunnel
  - Beyond cubital tunnel it passes between the humeral and ulnar origins of flexor carpi ulnaris muscle
- Sites of medial nerve entrapment in forearm
  - Between heads of pronator teres

GRAPHIC, COMMON EXTENSOR TENDON

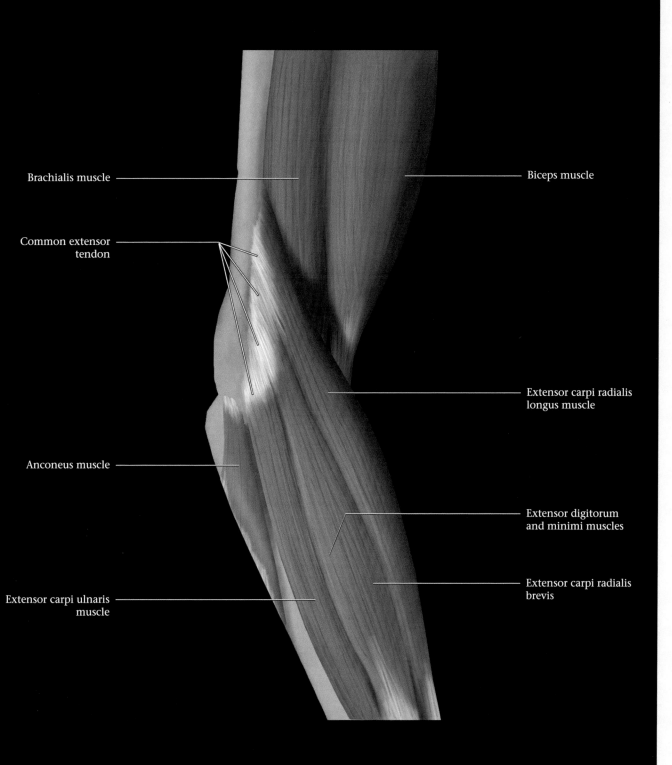

Brachialis muscle

Common extensor tendon

Anconeus muscle

Extensor carpi ulnaris muscle

Biceps muscle

Extensor carpi radialis longus muscle

Extensor digitorum and minimi muscles

Extensor carpi radialis brevis

Graphic of a side view of the lateral aspect of the elbow shows extensor-supinator group and its common extensor tendon, attaching to the lateral epicondyle and supracondylar aspect of the humerus. The common extensor tendon is comprised of the extensor carpi radialis brevis, extensor digitorum, extensor digiti minimi, and extensor carpi ulnaris.

FOREARM

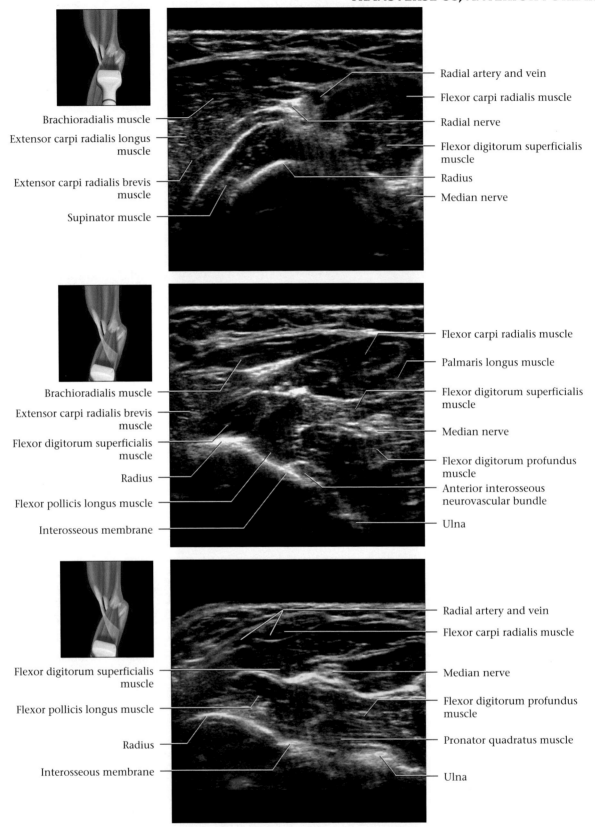

Brachioradialis muscle

Extensor carpi radialis longus muscle

Extensor carpi radialis brevis muscle

Supinator muscle

Radial artery and vein

Flexor carpi radialis muscle

Radial nerve

Flexor digitorum superficialis muscle

Radius

Median nerve

Brachioradialis muscle

Extensor carpi radialis brevis muscle

Flexor digitorum superficialis muscle

Radius

Flexor pollicis longus muscle

Interosseous membrane

Flexor carpi radialis muscle

Palmaris longus muscle

Flexor digitorum superficialis muscle

Median nerve

Flexor digitorum profundus muscle

Anterior interosseous neurovascular bundle

Ulna

Flexor digitorum superficialis muscle

Flexor pollicis longus muscle

Radius

Interosseous membrane

Radial artery and vein

Flexor carpi radialis muscle

Median nerve

Flexor digitorum profundus muscle

Pronator quadratus muscle

Ulna

(Top) Transverse grayscale ultrasound at the anterior aspect of the proximal third of the forearm. The anterior aspect of the forearm consists of five flexor muscles, three superficial and two deep. (Middle) Transverse grayscale ultrasound at the anterior aspect of the mid-forearm. The three superficial flexor muscles are, from ulnar to radial aspect, the flexor carpi ulnaris, the flexor digitorum superficialis and the flexor carpi radialis. The two deep flexor muscles are flexor digitorum profundus and flexor pollicis longus. (Bottom) Transverse grayscale ultrasound at the anterior aspect distal third of the forearm. The pronator quadratus is an easily recognized muscle that helps to pronate the forearm.

FOREARM

TRANSVERSE US, ANTEROMEDIAL FOREARM

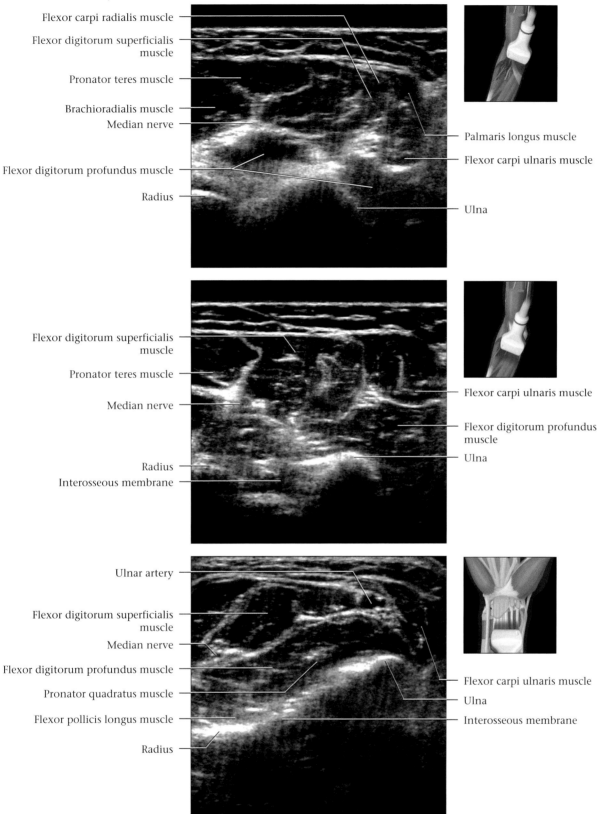

Flexor carpi radialis muscle
Flexor digitorum superficialis muscle
Pronator teres muscle
Brachioradialis muscle
Median nerve
Flexor digitorum profundus muscle
Radius

Palmaris longus muscle
Flexor carpi ulnaris muscle
Ulna

Flexor digitorum superficialis muscle
Pronator teres muscle
Median nerve
Radius
Interosseous membrane

Flexor carpi ulnaris muscle
Flexor digitorum profundus muscle
Ulna

Ulnar artery
Flexor digitorum superficialis muscle
Median nerve
Flexor digitorum profundus muscle
Pronator quadratus muscle
Flexor pollicis longus muscle
Radius

Flexor carpi ulnaris muscle
Ulna
Interosseous membrane

(Top) Transverse grayscale ultrasound at the anteromedial aspect of the proximal third of the forearm. The main flexors of the wrist are contained along the anterior and anteromedial aspect of the forearm. These are divided into two groups as superficial and deep. (Middle) Transverse grayscale ultrasound at the anteromedial aspect of the middle third of the forearm. The superficial group comprises the flexor carpi ulnaris, the flexor digitorum superficialis and the flexor carpi radialis. The deep group consists of the flexor digitorum profundus and the flexor pollicis longus. (Bottom) Transverse grayscale ultrasound at the antero-medial aspect of the distal third of the forearm. The ulnar nerve lies deep to the flexor carpi ulnaris, while the median nerve lies between the flexor digitorum superficialis and profundus.

TRANSVERSE US, ANTEROLATERAL FOREARM

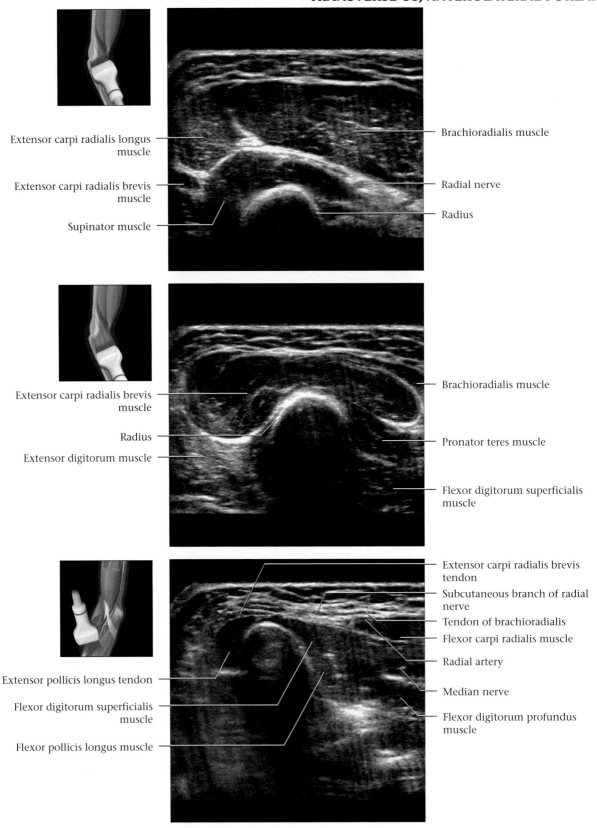

Extensor carpi radialis longus muscle

Extensor carpi radialis brevis muscle

Supinator muscle

Brachioradialis muscle

Radial nerve

Radius

Extensor carpi radialis brevis muscle

Radius

Extensor digitorum muscle

Brachioradialis muscle

Pronator teres muscle

Flexor digitorum superficialis muscle

Extensor carpi radialis brevis tendon

Subcutaneous branch of radial nerve

Tendon of brachioradialis

Flexor carpi radialis muscle

Radial artery

Median nerve

Flexor digitorum profundus muscle

Extensor pollicis longus tendon

Flexor digitorum superficialis muscle

Flexor pollicis longus muscle

(Top) Transverse grayscale ultrasound of the anterolateral proximal third of the forearm. The anterolateral aspect of the forearm comprises four extensor muscles running along the course of the radius. **(Middle)** Transverse grayscale ultrasound of the anterolateral aspect of the middle third of the forearm. The anterolateral group comprises the extensor carpi radialis brevis, the extensor carpi radialis longus, the brachioradialis and the pronator teres. **(Bottom)** Transverse grayscale ultrasound of the anterolateral aspect of the distal third of the forearm.

FOREARM

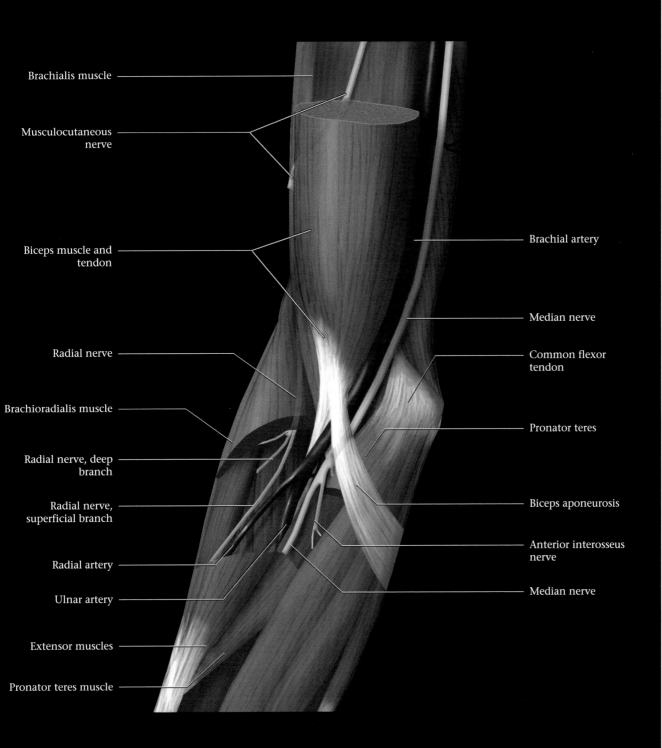

Brachialis muscle

Musculocutaneous nerve

Biceps muscle and tendon

Radial nerve

Brachioradialis muscle

Radial nerve, deep branch

Radial nerve, superficial branch

Radial artery

Ulnar artery

Extensor muscles

Pronator teres muscle

Brachial artery

Median nerve

Common flexor tendon

Pronator teres

Biceps aponeurosis

Anterior interosseus nerve

Median nerve

Graphic of the anterior view of the cubital fossa shows the median nerve and brachial artery passing underneath the biceps aponeurosis. The anterior interosseus nerve arises from the median nerve as the median nerve passes between the two heads of the pronator teres muscle. The radial nerve, deep to the brachioradialis muscle, is seen dividing into the superficial and deep branches.

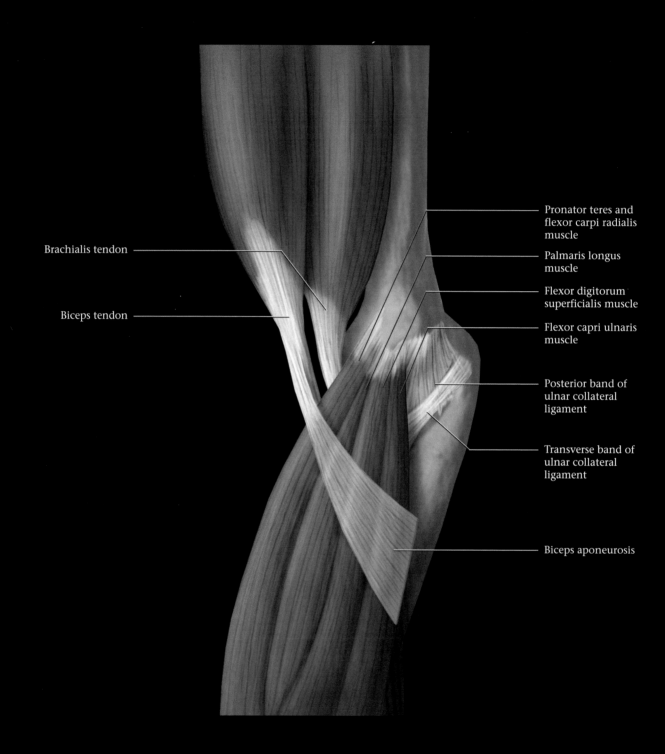

Brachialis tendon

Biceps tendon

Pronator teres and flexor carpi radialis muscle

Palmaris longus muscle

Flexor digitorum superficialis muscle

Flexor capri ulnaris muscle

Posterior band of ulnar collateral ligament

Transverse band of ulnar collateral ligament

Biceps aponeurosis

Graphic of the side view of the medial aspect of the elbow shows the flexor-pronator group and its common flexor tendon attaching to the medial epicondyle. The anterior band of the ulnar collateral ligament is deep to the common tendon. The biceps aponeurosis blends with the anterior aspect of the common flexor mass. The flexor digitorum profundus arises from the proximal humerus, posterior and deep to the flexor carpi ulnaris, and does not act on the elbow and is not part of the flexor-pronator group.

FOREARM

TRANSVERSE US, POSTERIOR ASPECT

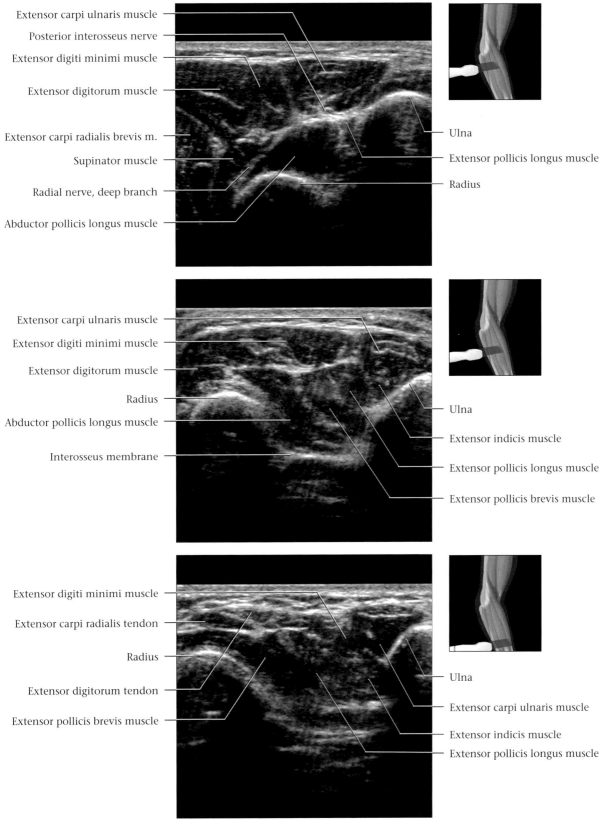

Extensor carpi ulnaris muscle
Posterior interosseus nerve
Extensor digiti minimi muscle
Extensor digitorum muscle
Extensor carpi radialis brevis m.
Supinator muscle
Radial nerve, deep branch
Abductor pollicis longus muscle

Ulna
Extensor pollicis longus muscle
Radius

Extensor carpi ulnaris muscle
Extensor digiti minimi muscle
Extensor digitorum muscle
Radius
Abductor pollicis longus muscle
Interosseus membrane

Ulna
Extensor indicis muscle
Extensor pollicis longus muscle
Extensor pollicis brevis muscle

Extensor digiti minimi muscle
Extensor carpi radialis tendon
Radius
Extensor digitorum tendon
Extensor pollicis brevis muscle

Ulna
Extensor carpi ulnaris muscle
Extensor indicis muscle
Extensor pollicis longus muscle

(Top) Transverse grayscale ultrasound shows the posterior aspect of the proximal third of the forearm. The posterior aspect of the forearm contains the extensor muscles. They are contained in two groups as superficial and deep groups. (Middle) Transverse grayscale ultrasound of the posterior aspect of the middle third of the forearm. The superficial group comprises (ulnar to radial), the extensor carpi ulnaris, the extensor digiti minimi and extensor digitorum. The deep group comprises the extensor pollicis longus, extensor pollicis brevis and the abductor pollicis longus. (Bottom) Transverse grayscale ultrasound shows the posterior aspect of the distal third of the forearm.

FOREARM VESSELS

Gross Anatomy

Arteries

- Brachial artery
  - Continuation of axillary artery
  - Located in cubital fossa, medial to biceps tendon & deep to biceps aponeurosis
  - Accompanies median nerve
  - Gives off two medial branches, which descend toward elbow joint on medial side of brachial artery → contribute to anterior & posterior anastomosis around elbow
  - Brachial artery divides into radial artery & ulnar artery in cubital fossa
- Radial artery
  - Medial to distal biceps tendon
  - Covered by brachioradialis muscle
  - Distally, leaves forearm & moves laterally crossing floor of anatomical snuffbox
  - Terminates in deep palmar arch of hand
  - Branches
    - Radial recurrent artery: Runs proximally along lateral side of elbow to form anastomosis with branches of deep brachial artery
    - Muscular branches to lateral side of forearm
    - Distal anastomotic branches: Palmar carpal arch, superficial palmar arch & dorsal carpal arch
- Ulnar artery
  - Proximally deep to pronator teres
  - Distally lies on flexor digitorum profundus & lies lateral to ulnar nerve
  - Anterior & posterior ulnar recurrent arteries form anastomosis around medial side of elbow with branches of brachial artery
  - Branches
    - Common interosseus artery: Arises in distal aspect of cubital fossa, 2 cm below origin of ulnar artery from brachial artery
    - Anterior interosseus artery: Runs distally on interosseus membrane & ends in dorsal carpal arch; reaches posterior compartment by means of perforating branches; terminates at wrist joint after piercing interosseus membrane; supplies deep muscles of forearm
    - Posterior interosseus artery: Enters posterior compartment proximal to interosseus membrane, between supinator & abductor pollicis longus & supplies posterior muscles
    - Muscular branches to medial side of forearm
    - Distal anastomotic branches: Palmar carpal arch, dorsal carpal arch

Veins

- Veins of upper limb are variable in number & position
  - In hand there are two sets of veins, deep & superficial
    - Deep veins follow arteries traveling as paired venae comitantes; radial, ulnar & brachial veins
  - Superficial veins of hand & forearm are drained by cephalic & basilic veins
- Cephalic vein
  - Begins on lateral aspect of wrist by draining blood from venous plexus on dorsum of hand
    - Ascends along lateral side of forearm & upper arm in superficial fascia
    - As vein drains cranially, it receives tributaries from anterior & posterior aspects of forearm
    - Cephalic vein lies laterally in superficial fascia of antecubital fossa & gives off median cubital vein
    - Median vein of forearm flows into medial cubital vein
- Basilic vein
  - Begins on medial side of wrist & drains medial part of venous plexus on dorsum of hand
  - Basilic vein passes upwards on medial side of forearm receiving anterior & posterior tributaries
  - Passes to anteromedial aspect of elbow where it receives median cubital vein

Anatomy-Based Imaging Issues

Imaging Recommendations

- Venous examination
  - Examination of upper limb veins is normally performed with patient supine & arm abducted to about 90°
  - Use of high frequency linear transducer (5-10 MHz) is recommended
    - Determination of compressibility & flow pattern is normally performed
    - Phasicity with respiration noted
  - Augmentation of flow is obtained by manual compression of forearm
  - Alternatively, augmentation can be achieved by asking patient to clench fist
- Arterial examination
  - In patients with possible arterial compression syndromes, arteries are examined in various degrees of abduction so that any compression may be accentuated
  - If angle of insonation is > 60°, Doppler and color sensitivity ↓
  - Keep Doppler gate in centre of lumen for peak flow velocity
  - Match color signal scale with flow velocity

Imaging Pitfalls

- Gold standard for assessment of accuracy of arterial Doppler ultrasound is usually arteriography

Clinical Implications

Clinical Importance

- Brachial artery in antecubital fossa may be used for arterial access for angiography
- High take-off of radial artery from brachial artery is a common anatomical variant
  - On arterial Doppler studies if either radial or ulnar artery is difficult to trace distally from elbow, then artery should be sought at wrist & followed proximally
- Hemodialysis arteriovenous fistulae are generally constructed by joining cephalic veins to radial artery at wrist

GRAPHIC, FOREARM ARTERIES

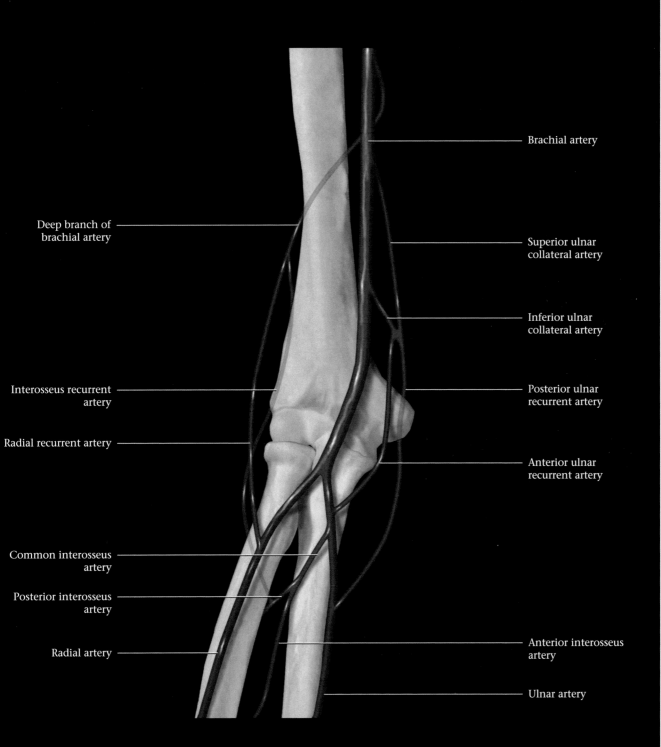

Deep branch of
brachial artery

Interosseus recurrent
artery

Radial recurrent artery

Common interosseus
artery

Posterior interosseus
artery

Radial artery

Brachial artery

Superior ulnar
collateral artery

Inferior ulnar
collateral artery

Posterior ulnar
recurrent artery

Anterior ulnar
recurrent artery

Anterior interosseus
artery

Ulnar artery

Graphic shows the brachial artery, the major artery of the arm. It divides into the radial and ulnar artery in the
proximal forearm.

FOREARM VESSELS

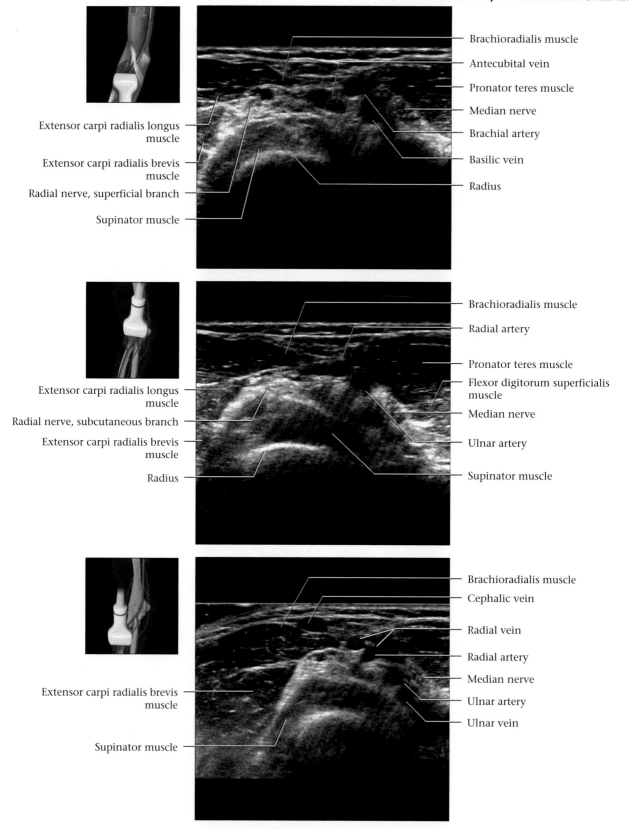

Top image labels:
- Extensor carpi radialis longus muscle
- Extensor carpi radialis brevis muscle
- Radial nerve, superficial branch
- Supinator muscle
- Brachioradialis muscle
- Antecubital vein
- Pronator teres muscle
- Median nerve
- Brachial artery
- Basilic vein
- Radius

Middle image labels:
- Extensor carpi radialis longus muscle
- Radial nerve, subcutaneous branch
- Extensor carpi radialis brevis muscle
- Radius
- Brachioradialis muscle
- Radial artery
- Pronator teres muscle
- Flexor digitorum superficialis muscle
- Median nerve
- Ulnar artery
- Supinator muscle

Bottom image labels:
- Extensor carpi radialis brevis muscle
- Supinator muscle
- Brachioradialis muscle
- Cephalic vein
- Radial vein
- Radial artery
- Median nerve
- Ulnar artery
- Ulnar vein

(Top) Transverse grayscale ultrasound of forearm vessels at the proximal forearm. The brachial artery divides into the radial and ulnar arteries in the proximal arm. The forearm veins are very variable in number and appearance. Both main veins should be assessed when investigating deep vein thrombosis. (Middle) Transverse grayscale ultrasound of radial vessels in the proximal forearm just distal to bifurcation of the brachial artery. (Bottom) Transverse grayscale ultrasound of radial vessels in the mid-forearm. The superficial branch of the radial nerve roughly follows the radial artery while the ulnar nerve closely follows the ulnar artery.

FOREARM VESSELS

TRANSVERSE US, RADIAL ARTERY

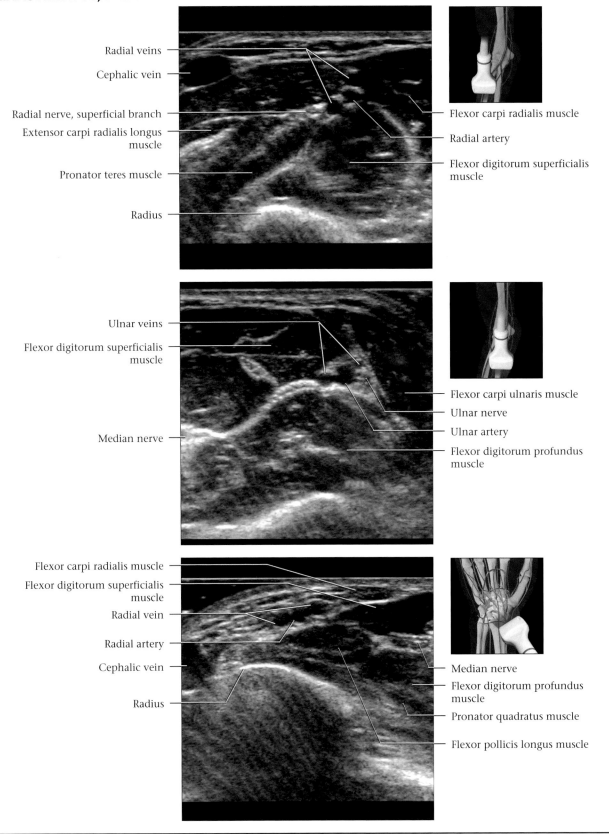

Radial veins

Cephalic vein

Radial nerve, superficial branch

Extensor carpi radialis longus muscle

Pronator teres muscle

Radius

Flexor carpi radialis muscle

Radial artery

Flexor digitorum superficialis muscle

Ulnar veins

Flexor digitorum superficialis muscle

Median nerve

Flexor carpi ulnaris muscle

Ulnar nerve

Ulnar artery

Flexor digitorum profundus muscle

Flexor carpi radialis muscle

Flexor digitorum superficialis muscle

Radial vein

Radial artery

Cephalic vein

Radius

Median nerve

Flexor digitorum profundus muscle

Pronator quadratus muscle

Flexor pollicis longus muscle

(Top) Transverse grayscale ultrasound of the radial artery mid-forearm. The radial artery serves as a landmark to divide the anterior (flexor) and posterior (extensor) compartments of the forearm. **(Middle)** Transverse grayscale ultrasound of the ulnar artery in mid-forearm. The ulnar artery is more variable in position than the radial artery. It may arise more proximal in the arm region. When the ulnar artery arises proximally, it often has an aberrant course and may lie superficial to the flexor muscles in the forearm. **(Bottom)** Transverse grayscale ultrasound of the radial artery in distal forearm. The radial artery is sometimes used instead of the long saphenous vein in coronary artery surgery. The caliber of the artery can be checked prior to surgery by ultrasound.

FOREARM VESSELS

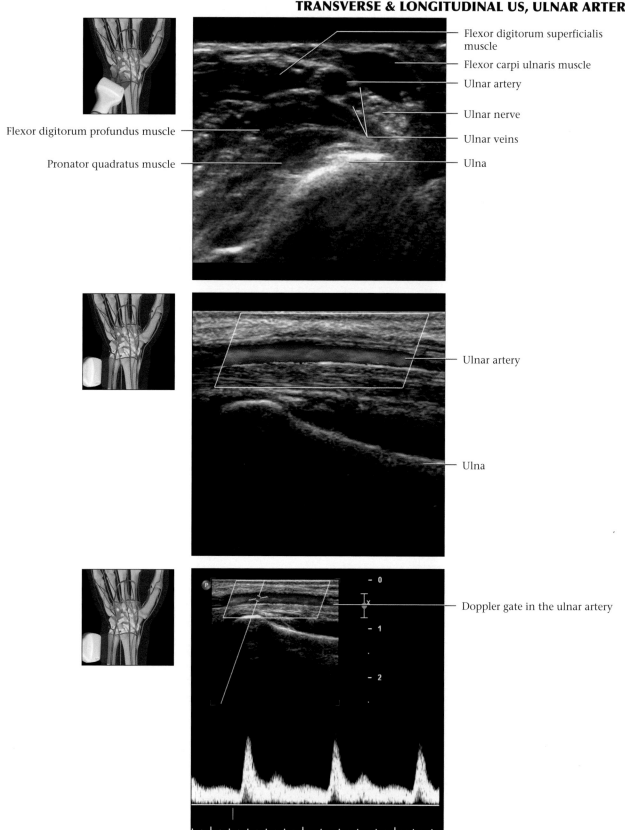

Flexor digitorum superficialis muscle

Flexor carpi ulnaris muscle

Ulnar artery

Ulnar nerve

Ulnar veins

Ulna

Flexor digitorum profundus muscle

Pronator quadratus muscle

Ulnar artery

Ulna

Doppler gate in the ulnar artery

(Top) Transverse grayscale ultrasound of the ulnar artery in the distal forearm. Allen's test is performed clinically to check dual arterial supply to the hand prior to radial artery cannulation or excision. (Middle) Longitudinal color Doppler ultrasound of the ulnar artery. Flow velocity and direction is denoted by the color signal. The normal diameter of the ulnar artery (1.9-2.2 mm) is measured near the wrist. (Bottom) Longitudinal spectral Doppler analysis of the ulnar artery. The spectral gate is placed in the middle of the arterial lumen. Normal uni-directional flow is present with a systolic peak and good diastolic flow. The peak systolic velocity (PSV) of the ulnar artery ranges between 40-90 cm/s while end-diastolic velocity ranges between 5-12 cm/s. Pulsatility index (PI) is variable ranging 3.9-5.0.

FOREARM VESSELS

ARTERIES AT DISTAL FOREARM AND HAND

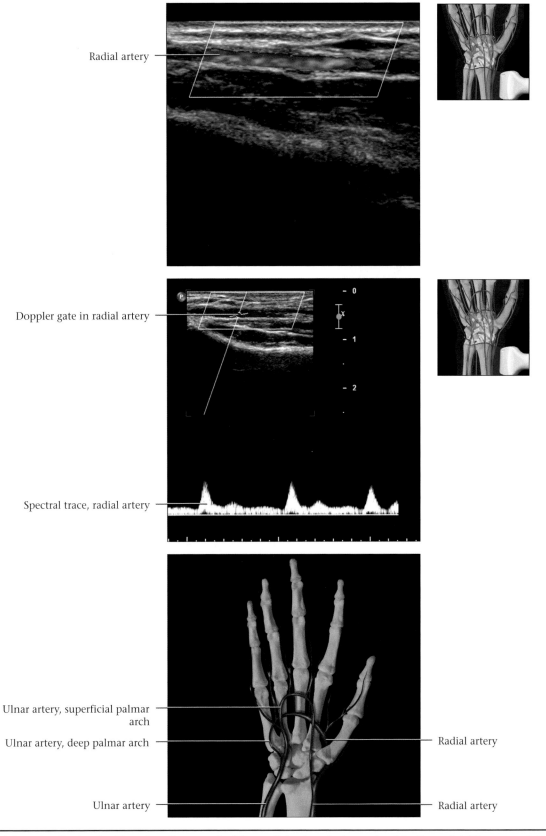

Radial artery

Doppler gate in radial artery

Spectral trace, radial artery

Ulnar artery, superficial palmar arch

Ulnar artery, deep palmar arch

Ulnar artery

Radial artery

Radial artery

Radial artery

(Top) Longitudinal color Doppler ultrasound of the radial artery just proximal to the wrist. The normal diameter of the radial artery just proximal to the wrist ranges 2.2-2.8 mm. (Middle) Spectral analysis of the radial artery just proximal to the wrist. Spectral analysis is best performed with the artery visualized longitudinally rather then transversely. The normal angle corrected peak systolic velocity (PSV) of the radial artery ranges from 40-90 cm/s, and the end diastolic velocity ranging 5-10 cm/s, pulsatility index (PI) is variable ranging 3.9-5.0. (Bottom) Graphic shows the distal aspect of the radial and ulnar artery in the forearm and their terminal course in the wrist and hand to form the superficial and deep palmar arterial arches.

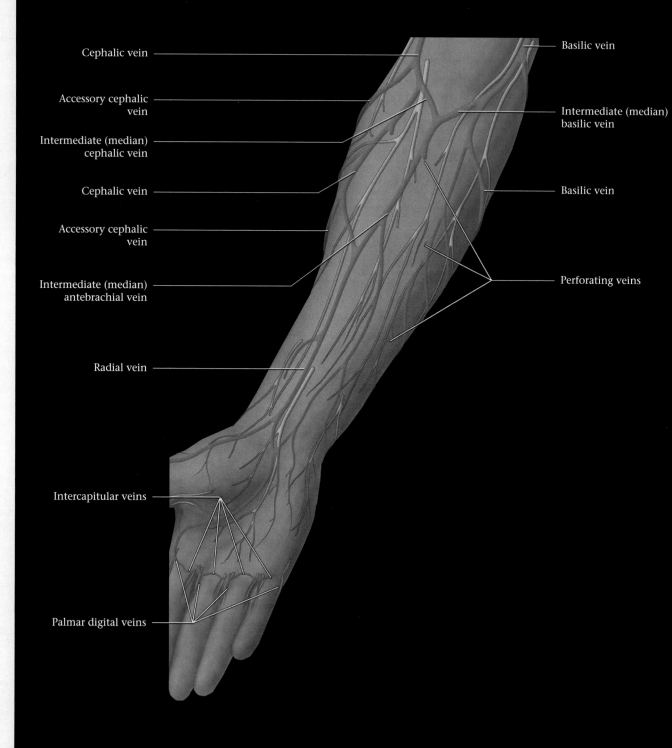

Cephalic vein

Accessory cephalic vein

Intermediate (median) cephalic vein

Cephalic vein

Accessory cephalic vein

Intermediate (median) antebrachial vein

Radial vein

Intercapitular veins

Palmar digital veins

Basilic vein

Intermediate (median) basilic vein

Basilic vein

Perforating veins

Graphic shows the superficial venous system of the forearm. The most important collecting vein of the forearm and arm is the cephalic vein. The cephalic vein proceeds from the radial margin of the dorsal venous rete of the hand, and follows a course diagonally above the radial margin of the forearm to the cubital fossa. From there, it continues in a stretched manner medially along the upper arm, 2-3 cm below the clavicle and into the axillary vein. It contains 6-10 valves. The ulnar and radial veins collect blood from the deep palmar arch and course along in pairs alongside the corresponding arteries. Blood is continuously shunted from these superficial veins in the subcutaneous tissue to deep veins via the perforating veins. Although the upper extremities also have many communicating veins, they have no clinical significance and are therefore not specifically named and located.

FOREARM VESSELS

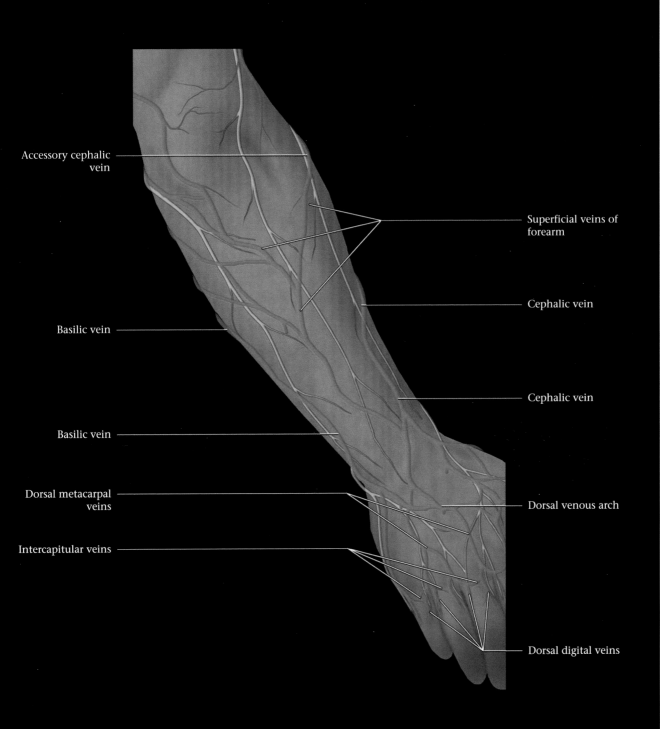

Accessory cephalic vein

Superficial veins of forearm

Cephalic vein

Basilic vein

Cephalic vein

Basilic vein

Dorsal metacarpal veins

Dorsal venous arch

Intercapitular veins

Dorsal digital veins

Graphic shows the posterior view of the superficial venous system of the forearm. The basilic vein starts from the ulnar margin of the dorsal venous plexus, and travels onwards to the bend of the elbow where it is joined by the cephalic vein. It contains 4-8 valves. There are two additional small branches that pass superficially on the volar side of the forearm, the median antebrachial vein and the median cubital vein, which flow into the cephalic vein and the basilic vein somewhat above the bend of the elbow. Although the upper extremities also have many communicating veins, they have no clinical significance and are therefore not specifically named and located.

WRIST

Gross Anatomy

Overview
- Wrist joint = articulation complex comprising distal radioulnar, radiocarpal, pisotriquetral, mid-carpal & carpometacarpal joints

Imaging Anatomy

Osseous Structures
- Distal radius: Lister tubercle on dorsal surface
- Distal ulna: Ulnar variance refers to length of ulnar head relative to distal radius; ulnar minus or ulnar plus
- Proximal carpal row: Scaphoid, lunate, triquetrum, pisiform
  - Scaphoid: Proximal & distal pole separated by waist
    - Tuberosity = volar prominence of distal pole
  - Lunate: Half-moon-shaped
  - Triquetrum: Triangular-shaped
  - Pisiform: Pea-shaped sesamoid-type bone to which flexor carpi ulnaris attaches & continues distally as pisohamate & pisometacarpal ligaments
- Distal carpal row: Trapezium, trapezoid, capitate, hamate
  - Trapezium: Saddle-shaped bone linking carpus & thumb
  - Trapezoid: Wedge-shaped bone
  - Capitate: Head (proximal), neck (mid portion) & body (bulky distal portion)
  - Hamate: Hook (hamulus) arises from palmar surface

Ligaments
- Extrinsic (on palmar or volar aspects of wrist) or intrinsic (between carpal bones)
- Major wrist stabilizers: Volar ligaments
- Extrinsic ligaments
  - Palmar: Radioscaphocapitate, radiolunotriquetral, radioscapholunate, ulnotriquetral, ulnolunate, scaphotriquetral
  - Dorsal: Scaphotriquetral, radiotriquetral, ulnotriquetral, radial collateral
- Intrinsic ligaments
  - Proximal interosseous: Scapholunate, lunotriquetral
  - Distal interosseous: Trapeziotrapezoid, trapeziocapitate, capitohamate

Muscles & Tendons
- **Flexors, deep**
  - Flexor digitorum profundus: Ulna → index, middle, ring & little finger distal phalangeal bases
  - Flexor pollicis longus: Radius, interosseous membrane & coronoid process ulna → distal phalangeal base thumb
- **Flexors, superficial**
  - Flexor carpi radialis: Medial epicondyle → 2nd metacarpal base
  - Palmaris longus: Medial epicondyle → palmar aponeurosis
  - Flexor carpi ulnaris: Medial epicondyle & medial olecranon/proximal ulna → pisiform
  - Flexor digitorum superficialis: Medial epicondyle & coronoid process of ulna & anterior radius → middle phalangeal bases digits 2-5
- **Extensors, deep**
  - Abductor pollicis longus: Ulna → radial aspect 1st metacarpal base
  - Extensor pollicis brevis: Radius → proximal phalangeal base thumb
  - Extensor pollicis longus: Mid-ulna → distal phalangeal base thumb
  - Extensor indicis: Mid-ulna → joins ulnar side of extensor digitorum tendon inserting into 2nd digit extensor hood
- **Extensors, superficial**
  - Extensor carpi radialis longus: Lateral supracondylar ridge of humerus → dorsal radial 2nd metacarpal base
  - Extensor carpi radialis brevis: Lateral humeral epicondyle → dorsal radial 3rd metacarpal base
  - Extensor digitorum: Lateral humeral epicondyle → distal phalangeal bases digits 2-5
  - Extensor digiti minimi: Lateral humeral epicondyle → extensor hood little finger
  - Extensor carpi ulnaris: Lateral humeral epicondyle → 5th metacarpal base

Retinacula
- **Flexor retinaculum**
  - Also called transverse carpal ligament: Attached to pisiform & hook of hamate, scaphoid & trapezium
- **Extensor retinaculum**
  - Attaches to ulnar styloid process, triquetrum & pisiform medially, crosses obliquely to attach to Lister tubercle & radial styloid process laterally
    - Sends septae to radius creating six compartments for extensor tendons
  - Compartment contents
    - 1) Abductor pollicis longus & extensor pollicis brevis (APL, EPB)
    - 2) Extensor carpi radialis longus & brevis (ECRL, ECRB)
    - 3) Extensor pollicis longus (EPL)
    - 4) Extensor digitorum & extensor indicis (ED, EI)
    - 5) Extensor digiti minimi (EDM)
    - 6) Extensor carpi ulnaris (ECU)

Anatomic Spaces
- **Carpal tunnel**
  - Margins: Carpal bones (dorsal margin); flexor retinaculum (volar margin); pisiform & hook of the hamate (ulnar margin), scaphoid & trapezium (radial margin), radiocarpal joint (proximal margin) & metacarpal base (distal margin)
    - Contents: Flexor digitorum superficialis, flexor digitorum profundus, flexor pollicis longus, median nerve
- **Guyon canal**
  - Margins: Fascial extension from flexor retinaculum, volar carpal ligament (volar margin), pisiform & flexor carpi ulnaris (ulnar margin), flexor retinaculum (radial & dorsal margins)
    - Contents: Ulnar artery & vein, ulnar nerve

WRIST

GRAPHICS, CARPAL BONES AND WRIST COMPARTMENTS

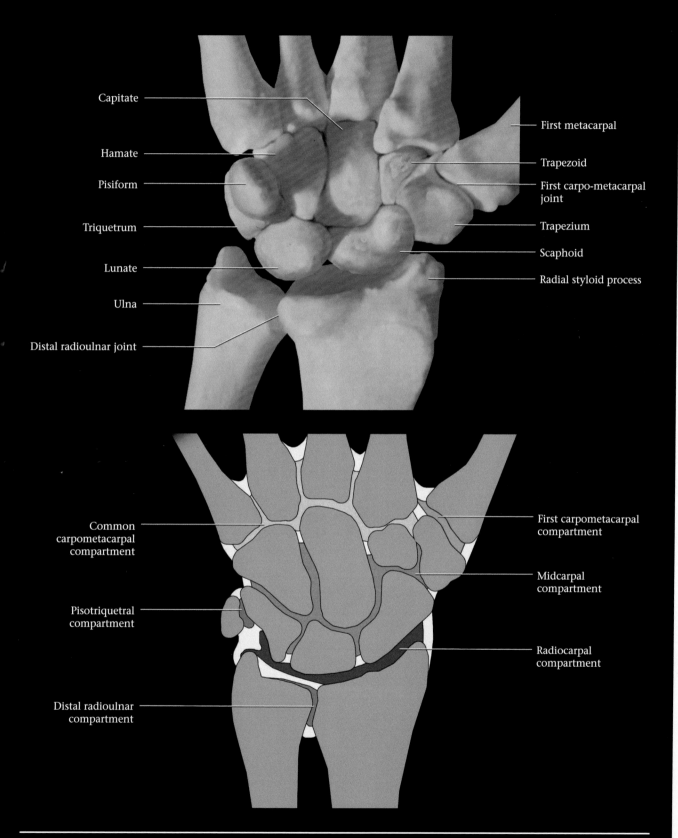

Capitate

Hamate

Pisiform

Triquetrum

Lunate

Ulna

Distal radioulnar joint

First metacarpal

Trapezoid

First carpo-metacarpal joint

Trapezium

Scaphoid

Radial styloid process

Common carpometacarpal compartment

Pisotriquetral compartment

Distal radioulnar compartment

First carpometacarpal compartment

Midcarpal compartment

Radiocarpal compartment

(Top) Graphic shows the bones of the wrist joint. (Bottom) Wrist compartments: Distal radioulnar, discretely separated by triangular fibrocartilage complex (TFCC). Radiocarpal, separated by proximal scapholunate and lunotriquetral ligaments as well as TFCC. Pisotriquetral, separated from radiocarpal in 20%. Midcarpal, separated by scapholunate and lunotriquetral ligaments, typically communicates with carpometacarpal joint. First carpometacarpal separated from common carpometacarpal by trapeziometacarpal ligament.

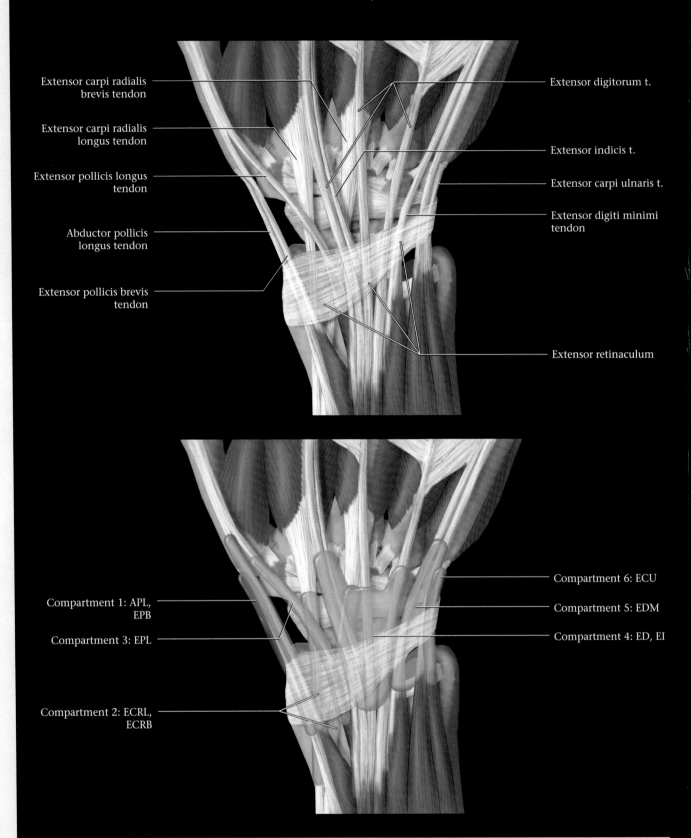

Extensor carpi radialis brevis tendon

Extensor carpi radialis longus tendon

Extensor pollicis longus tendon

Abductor pollicis longus tendon

Extensor pollicis brevis tendon

Extensor digitorum t.

Extensor indicis t.

Extensor carpi ulnaris t.

Extensor digiti minimi tendon

Extensor retinaculum

Compartment 1: APL, EPB

Compartment 3: EPL

Compartment 2: ECRL, ECRB

Compartment 6: ECU

Compartment 5: EDM

Compartment 4: ED, EI

(Top) Dorsal extensor tendons pass deep to extensor retinaculum, separated into six compartments by fibrous attachments of retinaculum to underlying bone. Compartment contents: #1-APL, EPB; #2-ECRL, ECRB; #3-EPL; #4-ED, EI; #5-EDM; #6-ECU. **(Bottom)** Separate tendon sheaths enclose dorsal extensor tendons in compartments 1-6 individually.

GRAPHICS, TENDONS: RELATIONS TO DORSAL & VOLAR WRIST

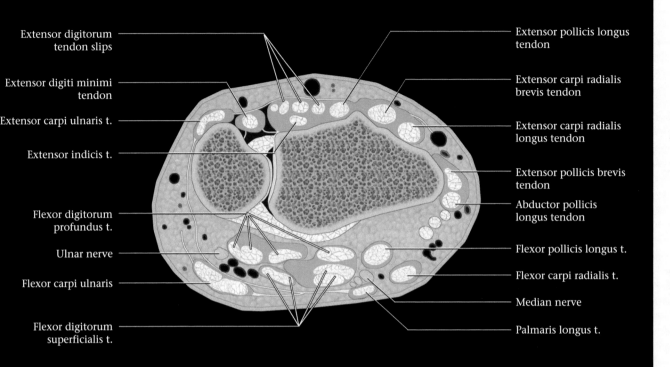

Extensor digitorum tendon slips — Extensor pollicis longus tendon

Extensor digiti minimi tendon — Extensor carpi radialis brevis tendon

Extensor carpi ulnaris t. — Extensor carpi radialis longus tendon

Extensor indicis t. — Extensor pollicis brevis tendon

Flexor digitorum profundus t. — Abductor pollicis longus tendon

Ulnar nerve — Flexor pollicis longus t.

Flexor carpi ulnaris — Flexor carpi radialis t.

Flexor digitorum superficialis t. — Median nerve

— Palmaris longus t.

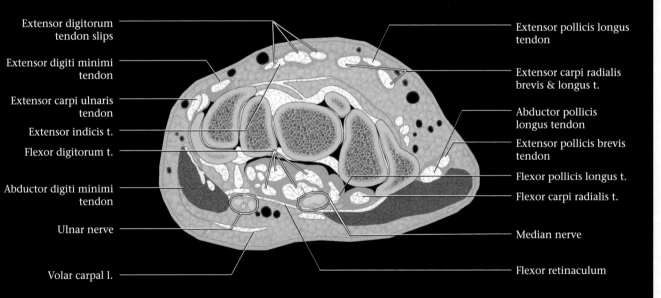

Extensor digitorum tendon slips — Extensor pollicis longus tendon

Extensor digiti minimi tendon — Extensor carpi radialis brevis & longus t.

Extensor carpi ulnaris tendon — Abductor pollicis longus tendon

Extensor indicis t. — Extensor pollicis brevis tendon

Flexor digitorum t. — Flexor pollicis longus t.

Abductor digiti minimi tendon — Flexor carpi radialis t.

Ulnar nerve — Median nerve

Volar carpal l. — Flexor retinaculum

(Top) Graphic representation of tendons in the proximal wrist. Extensor tendons are deep to the extensor retinaculum while flexor tendons are proximal to the flexor retinaculum at this level in the wrist. **(Bottom)** Mid carpal tunnel. Median nerve is slightly flattened as it passes deep to the flexor retinaculum & remains superficial to the flexor pollicis longus. Ulnar nerve, artery & veins lie lateral to the pisiform & may divide near the pisiform into deep & superficial branches.

TRANSVERSE US, RADIAL ASPECT

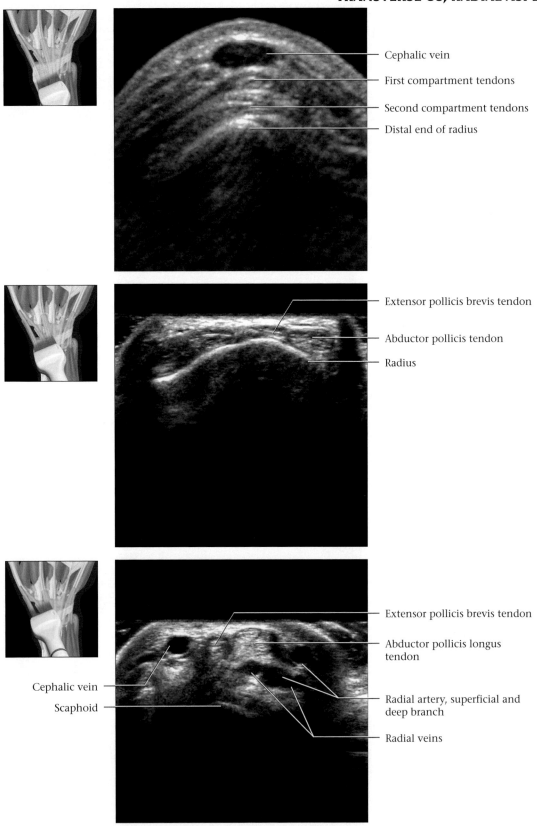

Cephalic vein

First compartment tendons

Second compartment tendons

Distal end of radius

Extensor pollicis brevis tendon

Abductor pollicis tendon

Radius

Extensor pollicis brevis tendon

Abductor pollicis longus tendon

Radial artery, superficial and deep branch

Radial veins

Cephalic vein

Scaphoid

(Top) Transverse grayscale US of the 1st extensor compartment proximal to the distal radius. 1st compartment comprises, EPB & larger APL. 1st compartment tendon runs obliquely over 2nd compartment tendons a few centimeters proximal to the wrist. Pain may occur at this intersection ("intersection syndrome"). **(Middle)** Transverse grayscale US of the 1st extensor compartment at the distal radius. EPB extends to the base of the proximal phalanx of the thumb, while APL inserts onto the base of the 1st metacarpal bone. They form the volar aspect of the anatomical snuff box. These tendons are swollen in patients with DeQuervain tenosynovitis. **(Bottom)** Transverse grayscale US of the 1st extensor compartment at the level of the scaphoid. Dorsal branch of the radial artery passes deep to the tendons of the 1st extensor compartment to enter the dorsum of the hand.

TRANSVERSE US, DORSAL WRIST

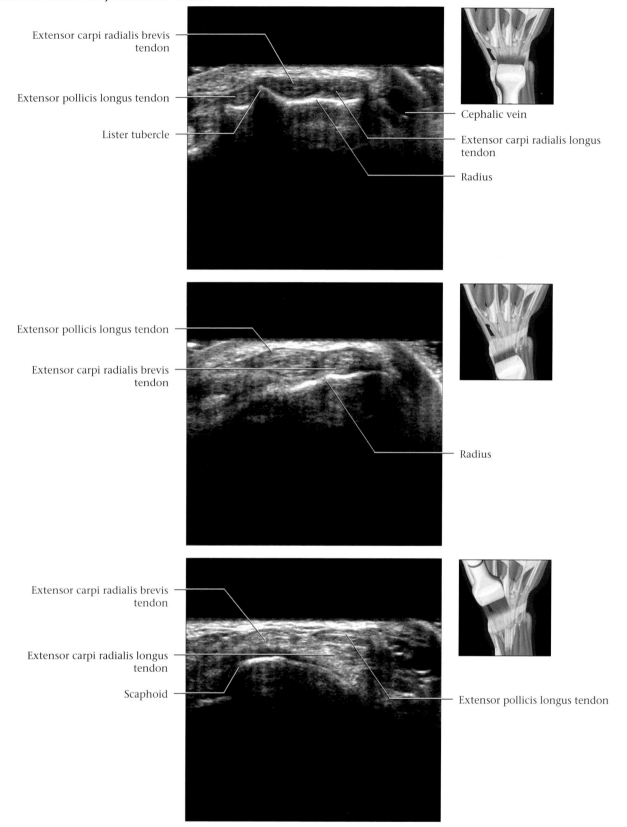

Extensor carpi radialis brevis tendon

Extensor pollicis longus tendon

Lister tubercle

Cephalic vein

Extensor carpi radialis longus tendon

Radius

Extensor pollicis longus tendon

Extensor carpi radialis brevis tendon

Radius

Extensor carpi radialis brevis tendon

Extensor carpi radialis longus tendon

Scaphoid

Extensor pollicis longus tendon

(Top) Transverse grayscale US of the 2nd & 3rd extensor compartment at the distal radius level. The 2nd extensor compartment comprises the ECRL and ECRB. ECRL inserts into the base of the index finger metacarpal while ECRB inserts into the middle finger metacarpal. The 2nd compartment is separated from the 3rd compartment, comprising the EPL, by Lister tubercle. **(Middle)** Transverse grayscale US of the 2nd and 3rd extensor compartments at the distal radius level. The second compartment forms the dorsal aspect of the anatomical snuff box. **(Bottom)** Transverse grayscale US of the 2nd extensor compartment at the scaphoid level. The EPL tendon hooks around Lister tubercle, and crosses superficial to the first compartment tendons as it runs towards its insertion on the base of the distal phalanx of the thumb. It is prone to rupture in inflammatory arthropathies and distal radial fractures.

TRANSVERSE US, EXTENSOR DIGITORUM

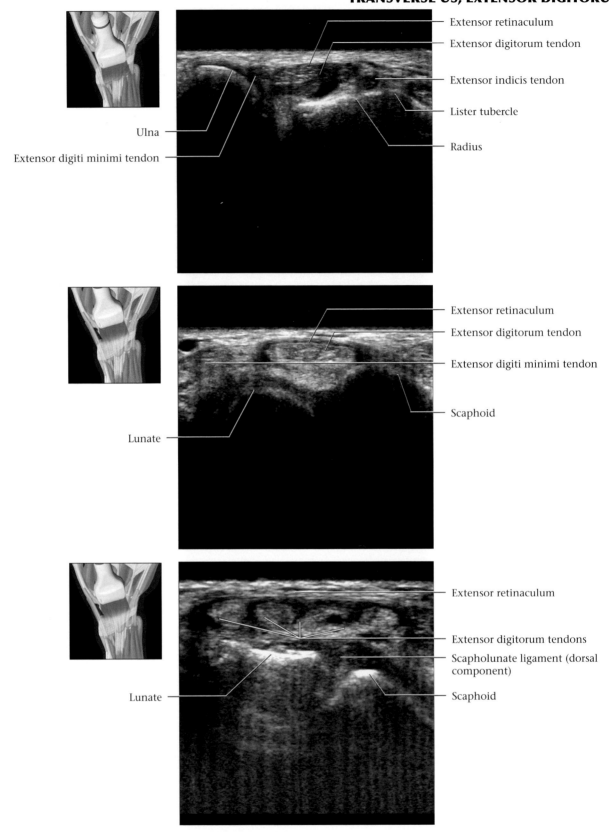

Extensor retinaculum

Extensor digitorum tendon

Extensor indicis tendon

Lister tubercle

Radius

Ulna

Extensor digiti minimi tendon

Extensor retinaculum

Extensor digitorum tendon

Extensor digiti minimi tendon

Scaphoid

Lunate

Extensor retinaculum

Extensor digitorum tendons

Scapholunate ligament (dorsal component)

Scaphoid

Lunate

(Top) Transverse grayscale ultrasound 4th extensor compartment at distal radius. The 4th extensor compartment comprises the four extensor digitorum tendons and the extensor indicis tendon which lies deep to the extensor digitorum tendons. The extensor digiti minimi has a separate compartment. (Middle) Transverse grayscale ultrasound fourth extensor compartment proximal carpal row. The extensor retinaculum is a thickened continuation of the antebrachial fascia. It is attached to the anterior aspect of distal radius, styloid process of ulna, triquetral and pisiform bones. (Bottom) Transverse grayscale ultrasound fourth extensor compartment proximal carpal row. The extensor retinaculum holds the extensor tendons in place. Because it is closely applied to the extensor tendons, with anisotropy, it may appear hypoechoic and be confused with tenosynovitis.

WRIST

TRANSVERSE US, EXTENSOR CARPI ULNARIS

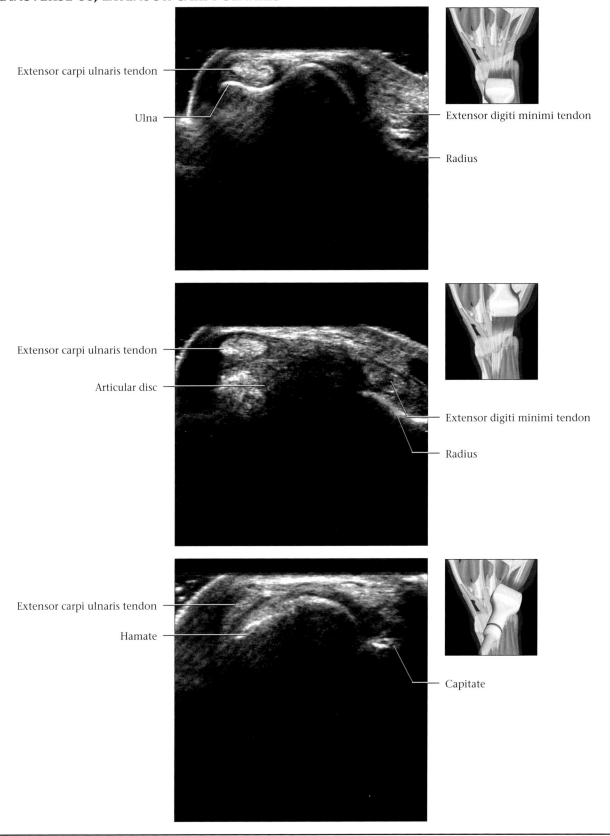

Extensor carpi ulnaris tendon

Ulna

Extensor digiti minimi tendon

Radius

Extensor carpi ulnaris tendon

Articular disc

Extensor digiti minimi tendon

Radius

Extensor carpi ulnaris tendon

Hamate

Capitate

(Top) Transverse grayscale ultrasound of the fifth and sixth extensor compartments. The fifth compartment contains the EDM. This tendon is joined by the ED tendon to the little finger just proximal to the MCP joint. The sixth compartment contains the ECU tendon which runs in a groove in the distal ulna. Its position in the groove will change with pronation and supination. (Middle) Transverse grayscale ultrasound of the fifth and sixth extensor compartments. The ECU tendon often has an midline irregular hypoechoic line within its substance close to insertion. This should not be mistaken for a longitudinal tear. (Bottom) Transverse grayscale ultrasound at insertion of the extensor carpi ulnaris. The ECU tendon widens as it passes the lunate bone on its way to insert onto the base of fifth metacarpal.

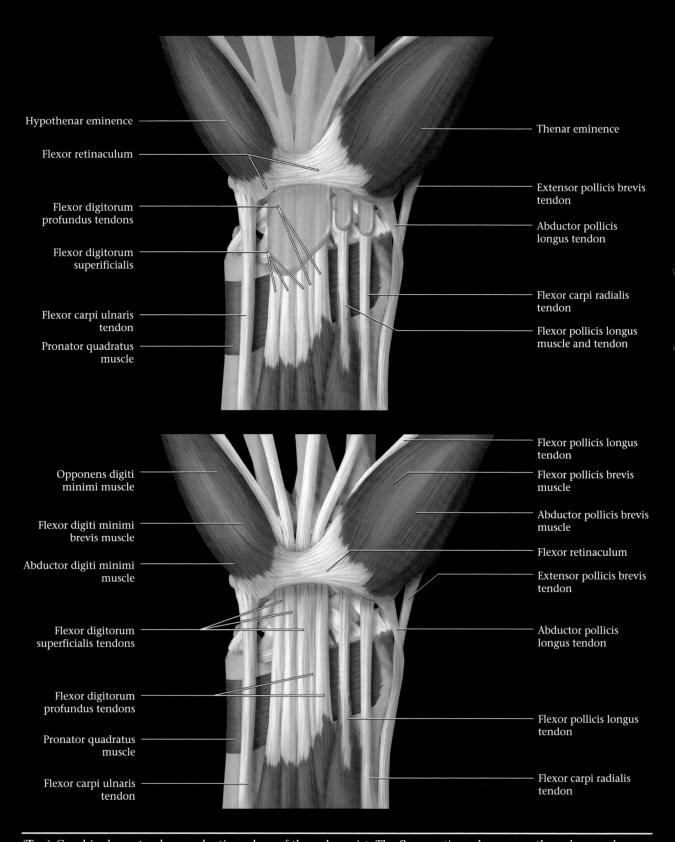

Hypothenar eminence

Flexor retinaculum

Flexor digitorum profundus tendons

Flexor digitorum superificialis

Flexor carpi ulnaris tendon

Pronator quadratus muscle

Thenar eminence

Extensor pollicis brevis tendon

Abductor pollicis longus tendon

Flexor carpi radialis tendon

Flexor pollicis longus muscle and tendon

Opponens digiti minimi muscle

Flexor digiti minimi brevis muscle

Abductor digiti minimi muscle

Flexor digitorum superficialis tendons

Flexor digitorum profundus tendons

Pronator quadratus muscle

Flexor carpi ulnaris tendon

Flexor pollicis longus tendon

Flexor pollicis brevis muscle

Abductor pollicis brevis muscle

Flexor retinaculum

Extensor pollicis brevis tendon

Abductor pollicis longus tendon

Flexor pollicis longus tendon

Flexor carpi radialis tendon

(Top) Graphic shows tendons and retinaculum of the volar wrist. The flexor retinaculum spans the palmar arch, attaching to the radial and ulnar styloid processes. The thenar eminence musculature includes abductor pollicis brevis, opponens pollicis, flexor pollicis brevis and adductor pollicis. The hypothenar musculature includes palmaris brevis, adductor digiti minimi, flexor digiti minimi brevis and opponens digiti minimi. **(Bottom)** Volar muscles and tendon are displayed with their relation to the flexor retinaculum. Note muscles of thenar and hypothenar eminences arise from the retinaculum itself. The flexor digitorum and flexor pollicis longus tendons pass deep to the retinaculum while the flexor carpi radialis is lateral but within fibers of the lateral retinaculum.

WRIST

TRANSVERSE US, VOLAR WRIST

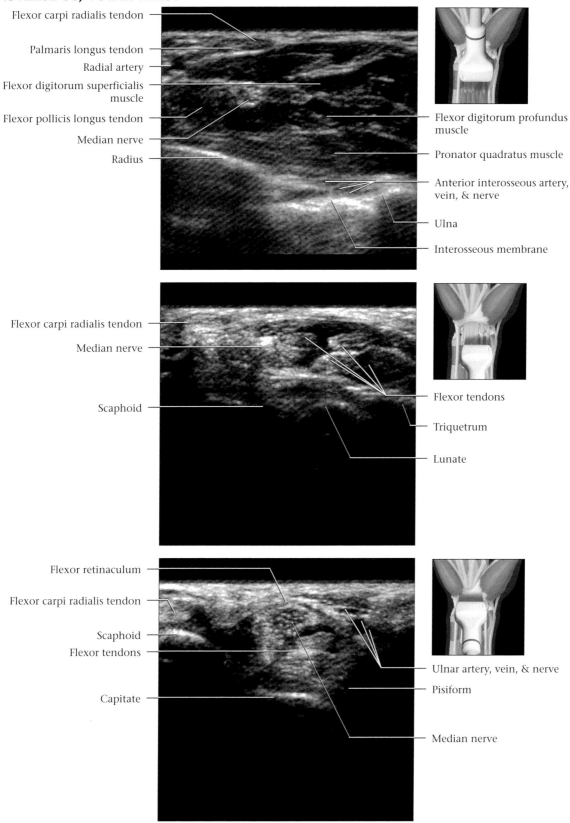

- Flexor carpi radialis tendon
- Palmaris longus tendon
- Radial artery
- Flexor digitorum superficialis muscle
- Flexor pollicis longus tendon
- Median nerve
- Radius
- Flexor digitorum profundus muscle
- Pronator quadratus muscle
- Anterior interosseous artery, vein, & nerve
- Ulna
- Interosseous membrane

- Flexor carpi radialis tendon
- Median nerve
- Scaphoid
- Flexor tendons
- Triquetrum
- Lunate

- Flexor retinaculum
- Flexor carpi radialis tendon
- Scaphoid
- Flexor tendons
- Capitate
- Ulnar artery, vein, & nerve
- Pisiform
- Median nerve

(Top) Transverse grayscale ultrasound of the volar aspect distal forearm just proximal to the wrist. In addition to the tendons which pass through the carpal tunnel, the flexor carpi ulnaris, flexor carpi radialis & palmaris longus tendons also traverse the wrist joint. (Middle) Transverse grayscale ultrasound of the volar aspect of the wrist just proximal to the carpal tunnel. The four tendons of FDS, four tendons of FDP & FPL tendon pass through the carpal tunnel. The median nerve dips deeply as it enters the carpal tunnel. (Bottom) Transverse grayscale ultrasound of the volar aspect of the wrist at the tunnel inlet. The inlet (and outlet) of the carpal tunnel can be best recognized by identifying the proximal & distal margins of the carpal tunnel. In evaluating carpal tunnel syndrome, the caliber of the nerve should be measured proximal to the tunnel, at the tunnel inlet & at the tunnel outlet.

WRIST

- Opponens pollicis muscle
- Ulnar artery
- Ulnar nerve & vein
- Flexor retinaculum
- Median nerve
- Flexor tendons
- Capitate
- Trapezium
- Abductor pollicis brevis muscle

- Abductor pollicis brevis muscle
- Flexor retinaculum
- Hook of hamate
- Median nerve
- Flexor tendons
- Capitate
- Opponens pollicis muscle
- Trapezium
- Base of 3rd metacarpal

- Abductor pollicis brevis muscle
- Ulnar artery
- Branch of median nerve
- Flexor tendons
- Adductor pollicis muscle
- Metacarpal of ring finger
- Metacarpal of third finger
- Flexor pollicis longus tendon
- Opponens pollicis muscle
- Flexor pollicis brevis muscle
- Metacarpal of index finger

(Top) Transverse grayscale ultrasound of the volar aspect at mid-carpal tunnel. The median nerve lies in the carpal tunnel just deep to the retinaculum in line with the ring finger. You may need to use anisotropy to clearly identify the margins of the median nerve separate from the adjacent flexor tendons. **(Middle)** Transverse grayscale ultrasound of the volar aspect of the wrist at the tunnel outlet. The tunnel outlet is considered to be the narrowest part of the carpal tunnel. **(Bottom)** Transverse grayscale ultrasound of the volar aspect of the wrist just beyond the tunnel outlet. The median nerve divides into its terminal branches just beyond the tunnel outlet.

WRIST

US, SCAPHOID

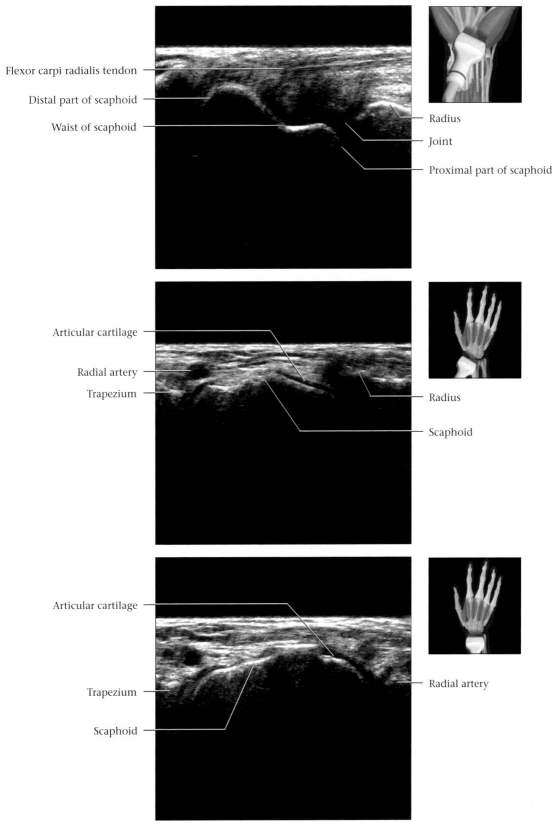

Flexor carpi radialis tendon

Distal part of scaphoid

Waist of scaphoid

Radius

Joint

Proximal part of scaphoid

Articular cartilage

Radial artery

Trapezium

Radius

Scaphoid

Articular cartilage

Trapezium

Scaphoid

Radial artery

(**Top**) Longitudinal grayscale ultrasound of the palmar aspect of the scaphoid bone. Ultrasound is a useful means of diagnosing a scaphoid fracture. Angulation of the transducer along the long axis of the scaphoid allows the palmar cortical outline to be appreciated. (**Middle**) Longitudinal grayscale ultrasound of the dorsal aspect of the scaphoid bone. There is often, particularly on the dorsal side, mild cortical irregularity of the scaphoid surface. The absence of surrounding edema, hematoma, periosteal thickening and cortical discontinuity allows one to differentiate this normal appearance from a fracture. (**Bottom**) Transverse grayscale ultrasound of the dorsal aspect of the scaphoid bone.

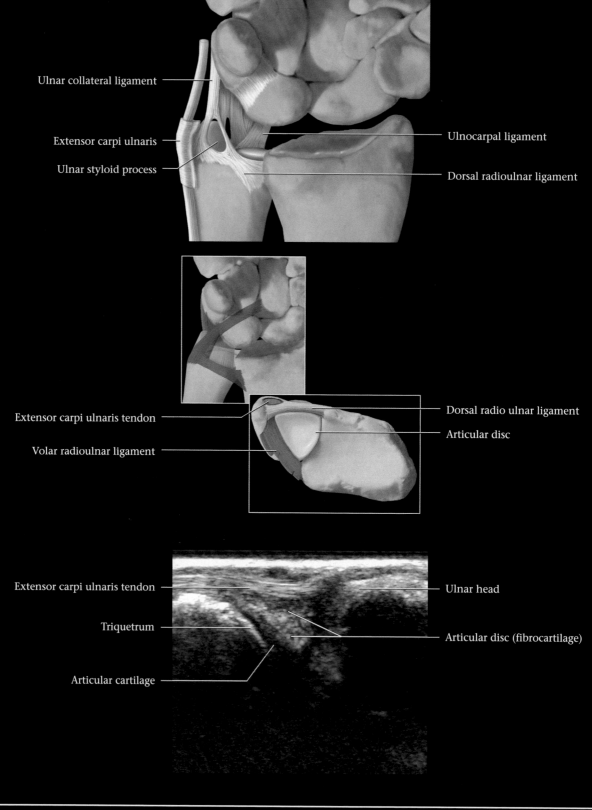

Ulnar collateral ligament

Extensor carpi ulnaris

Ulnar styloid process

Ulnocarpal ligament

Dorsal radioulnar ligament

Extensor carpi ulnaris tendon

Volar radioulnar ligament

Dorsal radio ulnar ligament

Articular disc

Extensor carpi ulnaris tendon

Triquetrum

Articular cartilage

Ulnar head

Articular disc (fibrocartilage)

(Top) Graphic shows supporting structures of TFCC. The ulno-carpal ligaments and the volar radioulnar ligament are on the volar side. At the ulnar border, there is the ulnar collateral ligament. On the dorsal surface there is the ECU tendon and its sub-sheath as well as the dorsal RUL. **(Middle)** Graphic depicting the axial view of the articular disc of TFCC. The articular disc is inseparable from supporting dorsal and volar radioulnar ligaments. The disc is widest at its radial attachment. Central tears are more common while peripheral tears have the capacity to heal, being better vascularized. **(Bottom)** Longitudinal grayscale ultrasound of the ulnar aspect of TFCC. The fibrocartilaginous articular disc is of different echotexture to hypoechoic hyaline cartilage. US is not sensitive at depicting TFCC tears.

GRAPHICS, VOLAR AND DORSAL LIGAMENTS

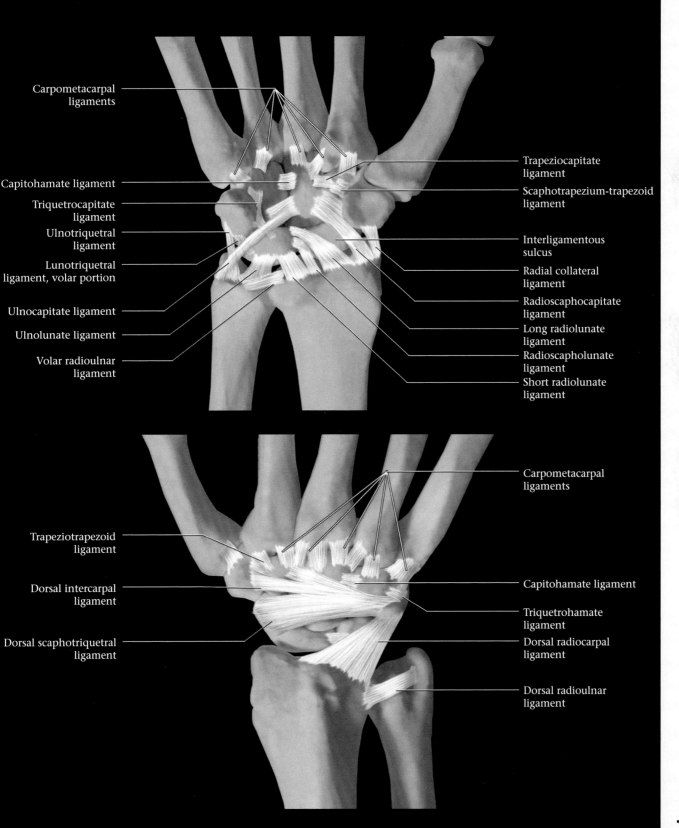

Carpometacarpal ligaments

Capitohamate ligament

Triquetrocapitate ligament

Ulnotriquetral ligament

Lunotriquetral ligament, volar portion

Ulnocapitate ligament

Ulnolunate ligament

Volar radioulnar ligament

Trapeziocapitate ligament

Scaphotrapezium-trapezoid ligament

Interligamentous sulcus

Radial collateral ligament

Radioscaphocapitate ligament

Long radiolunate ligament

Radioscapholunate ligament

Short radiolunate ligament

Trapeziotrapezoid ligament

Dorsal intercarpal ligament

Dorsal scaphotriquetral ligament

Carpometacarpal ligaments

Capitohamate ligament

Triquetrohamate ligament

Dorsal radiocarpal ligament

Dorsal radioulnar ligament

(Top) Graphic shows volar intrinsic and extrinsic ligaments. Extrinsic ligaments connect to the bones of the forearm (radius and ulna) and hand (metacarpals) and are often capsular. Intrinsic ligaments connect carpals to carpals. Note that the deltoid ligament, running parallel to the arcuate ligament, lies deep to these structures and is not shown here. **(Bottom)** Dorsal ligaments stabilize and restrict motion but are less critical to the stability of the wrist structures than volar ligaments.

HAND

Extrinsic Flexor Musculature: Digits 2 through 5

Flexor Digitorum Superficialis (FDS)
- Origin: Common flexor tendon origin (medial humeral epicondyle) & mid-radius
- Insertion: Volar plates proximal interphalangeal joints & bases of middle phalanges digits 2 → 5
- Innervation: Median nerve
- Superficialis tendons split level at bases of proximal phalanges, forming two tendon slips
  - Slips pass around flexor digitorum profundus tendon before inserting deep to this tendon
  - Forms "tunnel" for flexor digitorum profundus tendon
  - Just proximal to insertion, some fibers from each slip decussate to contralateral insertion
- Flexes metacarpophalangeal joints (aided by lumbricals & interossei) & proximal interphalangeal joints of digits 2 → 5

Flexor Digitorum Profundus (FDP)
- Origin: Proximal & mid-radius, as well as interosseus membrane
- Insertion: Volar plates, distal interphalangeal joints, & bases of distal phalanges of digits 2 → 5
- Innervation: Ulnar & median nerves
- Flexes distal interphalangeal joints & proximal interphalangeal, metacarpophalangeal (aided by lumbricals & interossei) joints of digits 2 → 5

Hypothenar Eminence
- Muscles: Abductor digiti minimi, flexor digiti minimi, opponens digiti minimi from superficial to deep
  - Origin: Abductor digiti minimi originates from pisiform
    - Flexor digiti minimi & opponens digiti minimi from flexor retinaculum & hook of hamate
  - Insertion: Abductor digiti minimi & flexor digiti minimi → combined insertion at ulnar aspect of base of proximal phalanx little finger
    - Opponens digiti minimi inserts to proximal two-thirds metacarpal shaft of little finger
  - Innervation: All by ulnar nerve
  - Actions are as their name implies

Adductor Pollicis Muscle
- Oblique (proximal) & transverse (distal) heads
- Origin: Capitate, trapezoid, 2nd & 3rd metacarpals
- Insertion: Ulnar aspect of base of proximal phalanx of thumb, interphalangeal joint, volar plate of thumb
  - Also contributes fibers to extensor hood of thumb which forms adductor aponeurosis
- Innervation: Ulnar nerve
- Actions: Adducts thumb toward 3rd digit & aids extension of interphalangeal joint
- Often grouped with thenar muscles though is distinct from them

- Separated from thenar muscles by fascial plane & innervated by ulnar rather than median nerve

Palmar Interossei
- Numbered 1-3 from radial to ulnar
- Origin: Mesial palmar diaphyses of 2nd, 4th, & 5th metacarpals
- Insertion: Mesial lateral bands & mesial aspect bases of proximal phalanges of same digit as origin
- Innervation: Ulnar nerve
- Actions: Adduct digits & assists lumbricals with flexion of metacarpophalangeal joints & extension of interphalangeal joints of digits 2, 4, & 5

Dorsal Interossei
- Numbered 1-4 from radial to ulnar
- Origin: Flexor digitorum profundus tendons just distal to carpal tunnel
- Insertion: Radial lateral bands of digits 2-5
- Innervation: Ulnar nerve
- Extends interphalangeal joints 2-5 and abducts digits 2-5

Tendon Sheaths
- Common flexor sheath (also known as ulnar bursa)
  - Contains flexor digitorum superficialis & profundus tendons
  - Begins just proximal to carpal tunnel
  - Ends just beyond carpal tunnel for digits 2 → 4
  - Encloses 5th digit flexor tendons over entire course to distal interphalangeal joint
- Common digital sheaths (digits 2 → 4)
  - Encloses flexor tendons from level of metacarpal necks to bases of distal phalanges
  - Common digital sheaths may connect to ulnar bursa in up to 10% of population
    - Potential route for spread of infection
- Flexor pollicis longus tendon sheath (also known as radial bursa)
  - Encloses flexor pollicis longus tendon from just proximal to carpal tunnel to tendon insertion at base of distal phalanx thumb
  - ± Communicates with ulnar bursa at level of carpal tunnel
    - Potential route for spread of infection

Extensor Expansion (or Extensor Hood)
- Expansions of extensor digitorum, extensor indicis, & extensor digiti minimi tendons on dorsum of fingers
  - Help prevent lateral translation
- Three bands of extensor expansion
  - Single wide middle band passes over dorsum of proximal phalanx & proximal half of middle phalanx
  - Two cord-like lateral bands extend from proximal phalanx to distal phalanx
    - Lumbricals, palmar & dorsal interossei insert into these lateral bands

HAND

GRAPHIC, PALMAR ASPECT

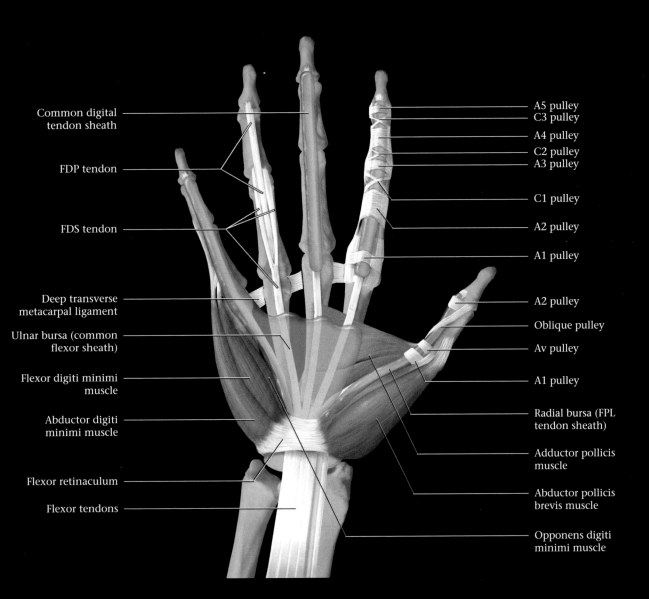

Common digital tendon sheath

FDP tendon

FDS tendon

Deep transverse metacarpal ligament

Ulnar bursa (common flexor sheath)

Flexor digiti minimi muscle

Abductor digiti minimi muscle

Flexor retinaculum

Flexor tendons

A5 pulley
C3 pulley
A4 pulley
C2 pulley
A3 pulley

C1 pulley

A2 pulley

A1 pulley

A2 pulley
Oblique pulley
Av pulley
A1 pulley

Radial bursa (FPL tendon sheath)

Adductor pollicis muscle

Abductor pollicis brevis muscle

Opponens digiti minimi muscle

Pulley system for the 3rd-5th digits is identical to that demonstrated for the 2nd digit. Common digital sheath of the 4th digit is removed to show the relationship of FDS & FDP tendons. Deep transverse metacarpal ligaments connect the volar plates (not shown) of digits 2-5. Although there is overlap of the radial & ulnar bursae in this image, these structures normally do not communicate. It is, however, important to know that the radial & ulnar bursae may communicate as a normal variation in a small percentage of the population. Similarly, any one or more of the common digital sheaths may communicate with the radial bursa in up to 10% of the normal population. These normal variant bursal communications are important as they can provide routes for more extensive spread of infection.

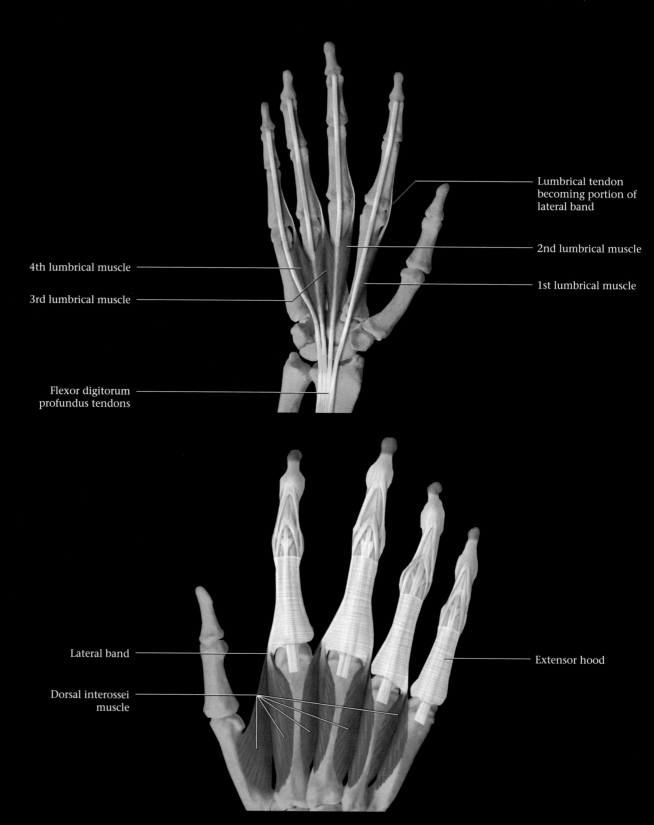

Lumbrical tendon becoming portion of lateral band

2nd lumbrical muscle

1st lumbrical muscle

4th lumbrical muscle

3rd lumbrical muscle

Flexor digitorum profundus tendons

Lateral band

Dorsal interossei muscle

Extensor hood

(Top) Lumbricals originate from the flexor digitorum profundus tendons as shown. Note how the 1st & 2nd lumbricals arise only from tendons to the 2nd & 3rd digits respectively (unipennate), whereas the 3rd & 4th lumbrical arise from the tendons to both the 3rd & 4th & the 4th & 5th digits respectively (bipennate). **(Bottom)** Graphic of the dorsal surface of the extensor mechanism of the hand and digits 2-5, demonstrates the complex relationship of the various fiber bands. As in imaging, distinction of individual fiber bands is often difficult and must be inferred by knowledge of where the structure "should" be with respect to more easily identifiable structures (such as bones and joints).

GRAPHIC, PALMAR INTEROSSEI

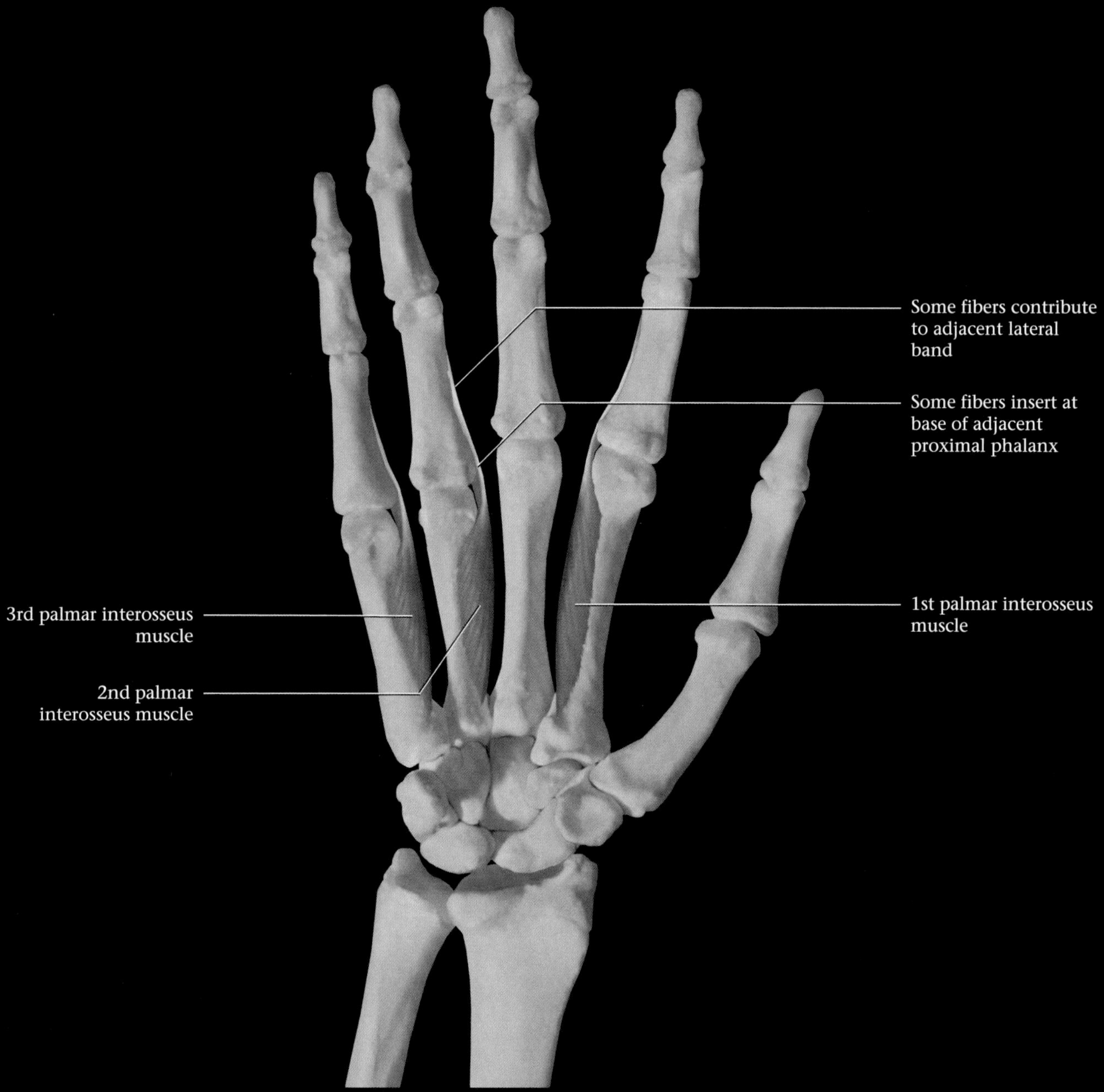

Some fibers contribute to adjacent lateral band

Some fibers insert at base of adjacent proximal phalanx

1st palmar interosseus muscle

3rd palmar interosseus muscle

2nd palmar interosseus muscle

Palmar interossei insert at both bases of adjacent proximal phalanges as well as adjacent lateral bands. The 2nd & 3rd palmar interossei contribute to the radial lateral bands of the 4th & 5th digits respectively, whereas the 1st palmar interosseus contributes to the ulnar lateral band of the 2nd digit.

HAND

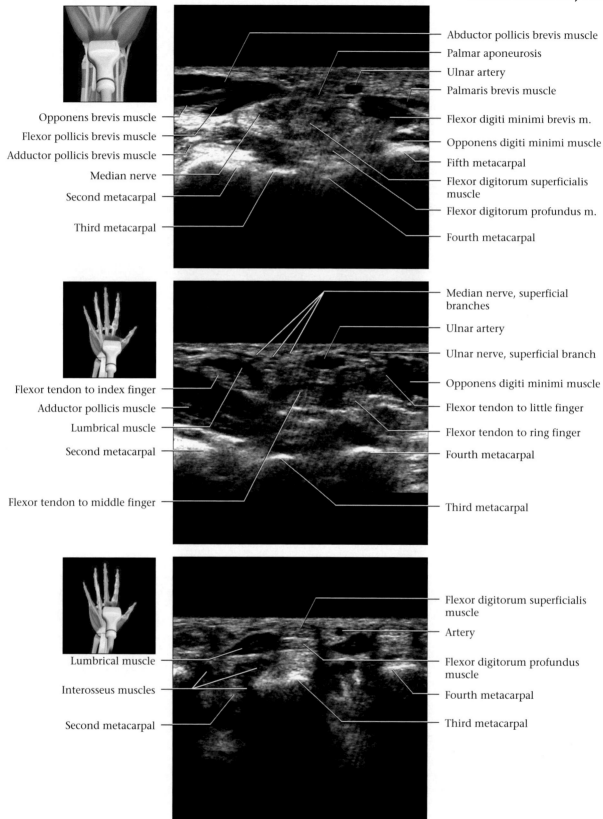

Opponens brevis muscle
Flexor pollicis brevis muscle
Adductor pollicis brevis muscle
Median nerve
Second metacarpal
Third metacarpal

Abductor pollicis brevis muscle
Palmar aponeurosis
Ulnar artery
Palmaris brevis muscle
Flexor digiti minimi brevis m.
Opponens digiti minimi muscle
Fifth metacarpal
Flexor digitorum superficialis muscle
Flexor digitorum profundus m.
Fourth metacarpal

Flexor tendon to index finger
Adductor pollicis muscle
Lumbrical muscle
Second metacarpal
Flexor tendon to middle finger

Median nerve, superficial branches
Ulnar artery
Ulnar nerve, superficial branch
Opponens digiti minimi muscle
Flexor tendon to little finger
Flexor tendon to ring finger
Fourth metacarpal
Third metacarpal

Lumbrical muscle
Interosseus muscles
Second metacarpal

Flexor digitorum superficialis muscle
Artery
Flexor digitorum profundus muscle
Fourth metacarpal
Third metacarpal

(Top) Transverse grayscale ultrasound at the proximal aspect of the palm. The palmar aponeurosis is thin and difficult to demonstrate in the mid to distal palm especially. (Middle) Transverse grayscale ultrasound of the mid portion of the palm. Beneath the aponeurosis lies the flexor tendons, the lumbrical muscles, the muscles of the thenar and hypothenar eminences and, most deeply, the interossei. There are three palmar interossei and four dorsal interossei muscles. (Bottom) Transverse grayscale ultrasound of the distal portion of the palm.

GRAPHIC, THENAR-HYPOTHENAR EMINENCE

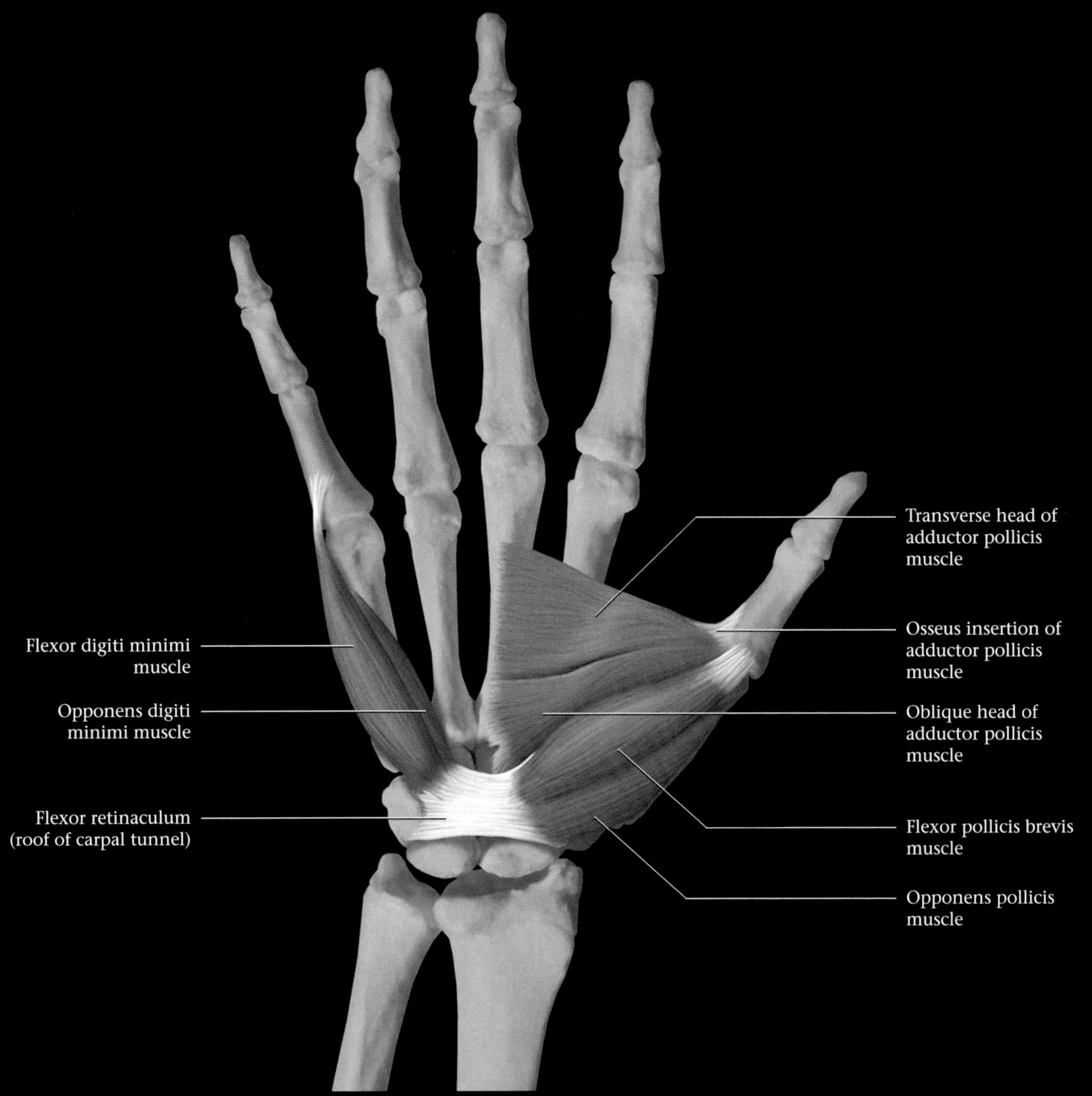

Flexor digiti minimi muscle

Opponens digiti minimi muscle

Flexor retinaculum (roof of carpal tunnel)

Transverse head of adductor pollicis muscle

Osseus insertion of adductor pollicis muscle

Oblique head of adductor pollicis muscle

Flexor pollicis brevis muscle

Opponens pollicis muscle

Graphic shows the thenar and hypothenar muscles of the hand. Strictly speaking, the adductor pollicis is not one of the thenar group of muscles since it has a separate fascia and separate nerve supply.

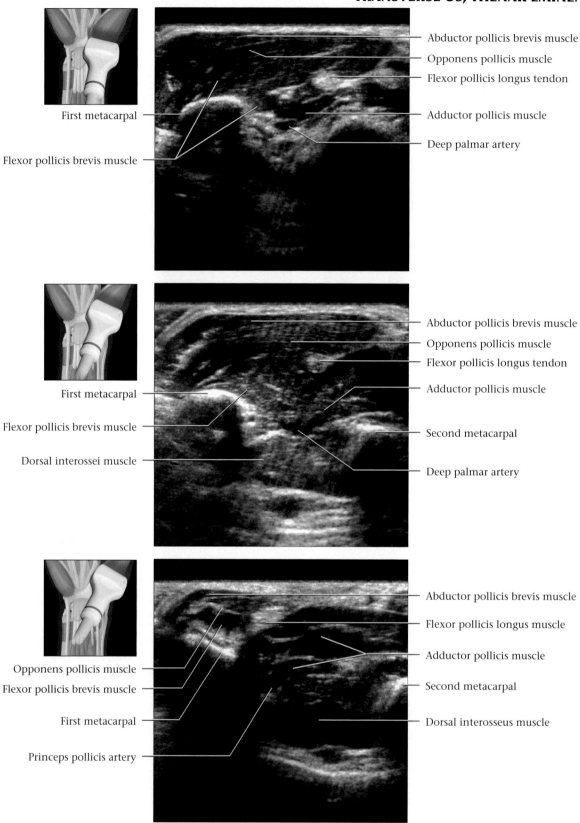

First metacarpal

Flexor pollicis brevis muscle

Abductor pollicis brevis muscle

Opponens pollicis muscle

Flexor pollicis longus tendon

Adductor pollicis muscle

Deep palmar artery

First metacarpal

Flexor pollicis brevis muscle

Dorsal interossei muscle

Abductor pollicis brevis muscle

Opponens pollicis muscle

Flexor pollicis longus tendon

Adductor pollicis muscle

Second metacarpal

Deep palmar artery

Opponens pollicis muscle

Flexor pollicis brevis muscle

First metacarpal

Princeps pollicis artery

Abductor pollicis brevis muscle

Flexor pollicis longus muscle

Adductor pollicis muscle

Second metacarpal

Dorsal interosseus muscle

(Top) Transverse grayscale ultrasound of the proximal aspect of the thenar eminence. The thenar eminence comprises four muscles: Abductor, opponens, flexor and adductor pollicis from above downwards. The adductor muscle is strictly speaking not part of the thenar eminence since it is separated by a fascial layer and has a separate innervation. **(Middle)** Transverse grayscale ultrasound of the mid-portion of the thenar eminence. The flexor pollicis longus tendon is easily recognized as an echogenic tendon alongside the flexor pollicis brevis, deep to the opponens pollicis and superficial to the adductor pollicis muscle. **(Bottom)** Transverse grayscale ultrasound of the distal portion of the thenar eminence.

HAND

LONGITUDINAL US, THENAR EMINENCE

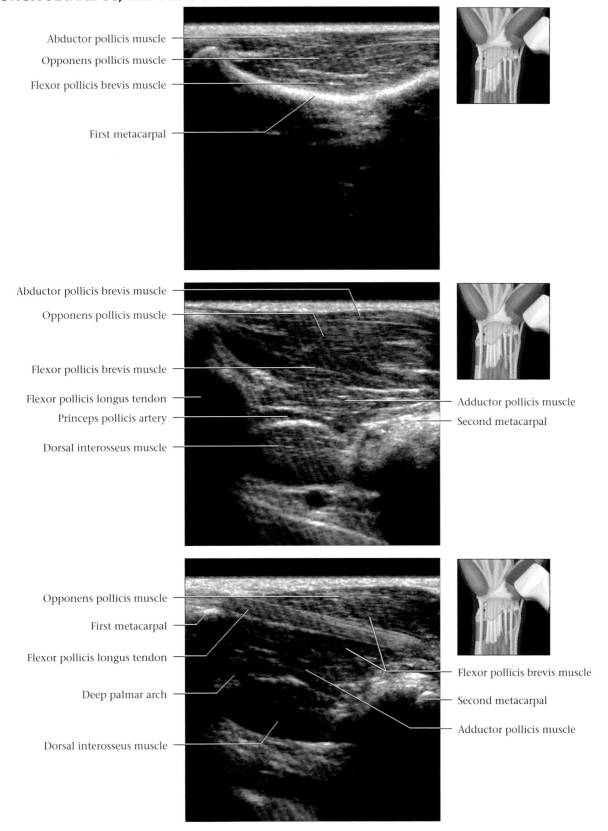

(Top) Longitudinal grayscale ultrasound of the proximal aspect of the thenar eminence. Use the mnemonic ABOF to remember the muscles of the thenar eminence. **(Middle)** Longitudinal grayscale ultrasound at mid-thenar eminence. The abductor pollicis brevis, opponens pollicis and flexor pollicis brevis (ABOF) lie superficial to deep in that order. **(Bottom)** Longitudinal grayscale ultrasound of the distal aspect of the thenar eminence. The flexor pollicis longus tendon passes through the more distal aspect of the thenar eminence.

HAND

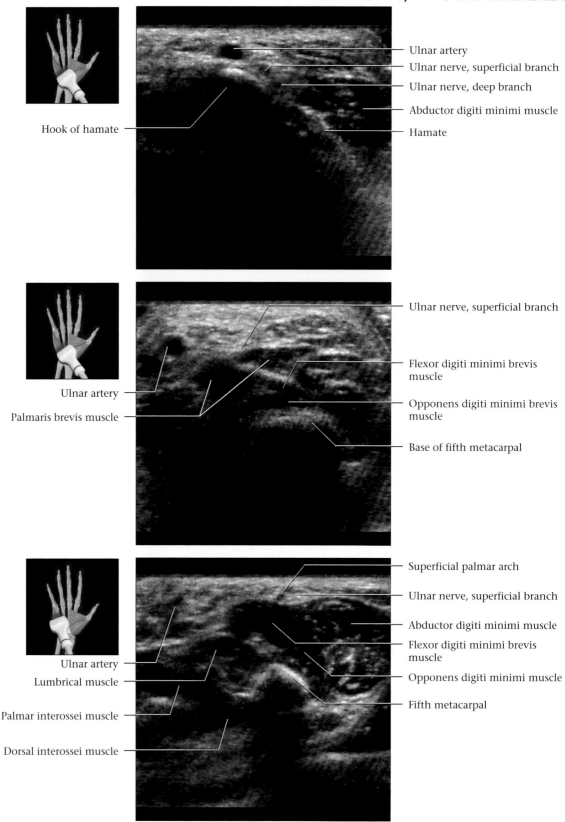

(Top) Transverse grayscale ultrasound of the proximal third of the hypothenar eminence. The hypothenar eminence along with the other muscles of the hand except for the thenar are supplied by the ulnar nerve. **(Middle)** Transverse grayscale ultrasound of the middle third of the hypothenar eminence. Hypothenar muscle atrophy can occur with injury to the deep branch of the ulnar nerve just distal to Guyon canal. **(Bottom)** Transverse grayscale ultrasound of the distal third of the hypothenar eminence. The order of muscles in the hypothenar eminence is different from the thenar eminence, with abductor digiti minimi, flexor digiti minimi and opponens digiti minimi from superficial to deep.

HAND

GRAPHIC, DORSAL ASPECT OF HAND

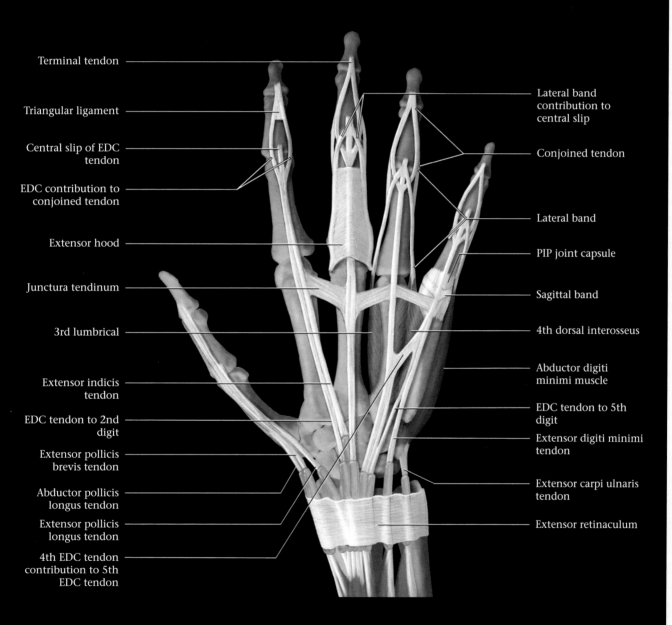

Terminal tendon

Triangular ligament

Central slip of EDC tendon

EDC contribution to conjoined tendon

Extensor hood

Junctura tendinum

3rd lumbrical

Extensor indicis tendon

EDC tendon to 2nd digit

Extensor pollicis brevis tendon

Abductor pollicis longus tendon

Extensor pollicis longus tendon

4th EDC tendon contribution to 5th EDC tendon

Lateral band contribution to central slip

Conjoined tendon

Lateral band

PIP joint capsule

Sagittal band

4th dorsal interosseus

Abductor digiti minimi muscle

EDC tendon to 5th digit

Extensor digiti minimi tendon

Extensor carpi ulnaris tendon

Extensor retinaculum

Extensor mechanism composite shows different components of the extensor mechanism on different digits. With the exception of the extensor indicis, extensor digiti minimi, abductor digiti minimi, & 4th EDC tendon contribution to the 5th EDC tendon, any structure on any of the 2nd-5th digits can be extrapolated to any & all of the other 2nd-5th digits. Note that the 2nd extensor retinaculum compartment & its contents (extensor carpi radialis longus & brevis tendons) are not included in this graphic. Although the abductor pollicis longus tendon travels in the 1st compartment of the extensor retinaculum, its insertion (not shown) is actually on the radial aspect of the volar surface of the base of the first metacarpal.

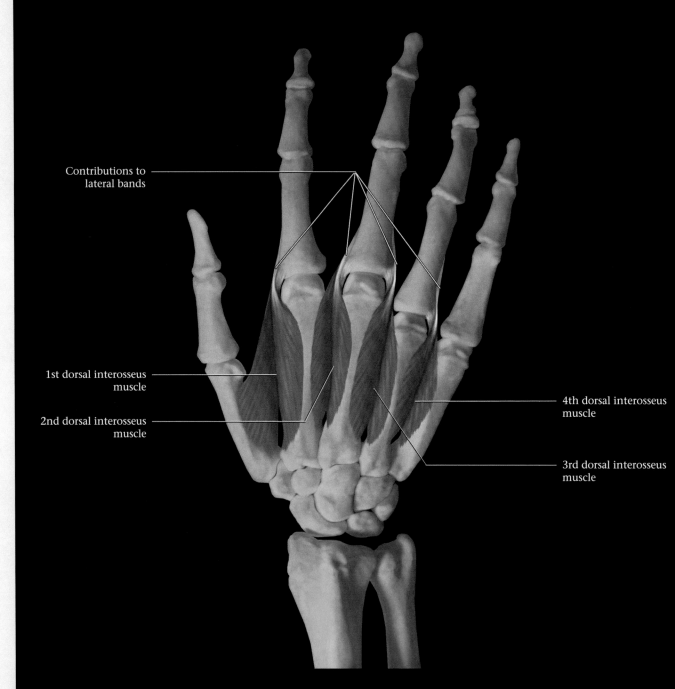

Contributions to lateral bands

1st dorsal interosseus muscle

2nd dorsal interosseus muscle

4th dorsal interosseus muscle

3rd dorsal interosseus muscle

Tendons of the dorsal interossei muscle (along with tendons of the palmar interossei & tendons of the lumbricals) help form lateral bands. Note how each interosseus only contributes fibers to the mesial-most adjacent lateral band. The dorsal interossei do not contribute any lateral band fibers to the 1st or 5th digits.

HAND

TRANSVERSE US, DORSUM HAND

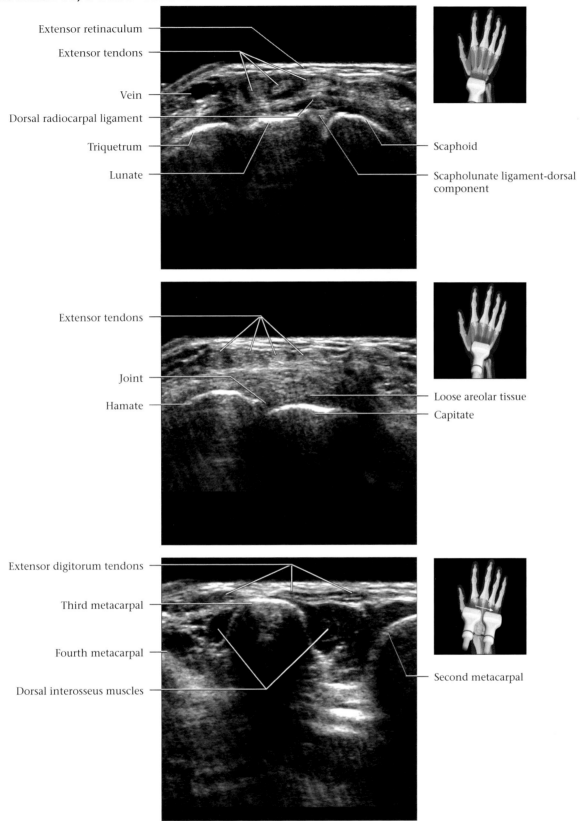

Extensor retinaculum

Extensor tendons

Vein

Dorsal radiocarpal ligament

Triquetrum

Lunate

Scaphoid

Scapholunate ligament-dorsal component

Extensor tendons

Joint

Hamate

Loose areolar tissue

Capitate

Extensor digitorum tendons

Third metacarpal

Fourth metacarpal

Dorsal interosseus muscles

Second metacarpal

(Top) Transverse grayscale ultrasound of the proximal aspect of the dorsum hand. The tissues on the dorsum hand are less tightly bound than the tissues on the palmar aspect of the hand and this part of the hand tends to swell much more with inflammatory or edematous processes. (Middle) Transverse grayscale ultrasound of the mid-aspect of the dorsum of hand. Loose areolar tissue separates the extensor tendons from the metacarpal bones. The extensor tendons do not have a complete tendon sheath from the level of the extensor retinaculum to the insertion. (Bottom) Transverse grayscale ultrasound of the distal-aspect of the dorsal hand. There are four dorsal interossei, one for each metacarpal interspace.

HAND VESSELS

Terminology

Abbreviations
- Abductor pollicis longus (AbPL)
- Extensor pollicis longus (EPL)
- Extensor pollicis brevis (EPB)
- Flexor retinaculum (FR)
- Flexor digiti minimi brevis (FDMB)
- Pronator quadratus (PQ)

Gross Anatomy

Arteries
- Radial artery
  - Terminal branch of brachial artery
  - Located superficial to pronator quadratus → continues dorsally around radial styloid process → passes deep to abductor pollicis longus & extensor pollicis brevis, across anatomic snuffbox & deep to extensor pollicis longus
  - Branches of radial artery
    - Superficial palmar branch continues distally superficial to flexor retinaculum through thenar eminence to anastomose with ulnar artery as superficial palmar arch
  - Deep palmar arch is continuation of radial artery in hand
    - Main radial artery continues dorsally at radial styloid across anatomic snuffbox deep to extensor pollicis brevis & abductor pollicis longus
    - Passes over dorsal aspect of scaphoid bone
    - Passes between heads of 1st dorsal interosseus muscle to enter palm → joins ulnar artery to form deep palmar arch
    - Deep palmar arch located at level of metacarpal bases 1 cm proximal to superficial palmar arch
    - Lies deep to long flexor tendons & superficial to interossei
    - Deep branch of ulnar nerve lies on convexity of deep palmar arch
    - Princeps pollicis artery, radial artery of index finger & palmar metacarpal arteries arise from deep palmar arch
- Ulnar artery
  - Terminal branch of brachial artery
  - Located superficial to pronator quadratus → runs between flexor carpi ulnaris & flexor digitorum superficialis tendons
  - Branches of ulnar artery
  - Common interosseus artery branches in forearm → anterior & posterior interosseus arteries
    - Anterior interosseus artery travels distally; at proximal pronator quadratus gives small branch which pierces membrane, enters dorsal forearm & anastomoses with posterior interosseus artery
    - Median artery (branch of anterior interosseus artery) arises in forearm & may persist accompanying median nerve into carpal tunnel contributing to superficial palmar arch
    - Posterior interosseus artery travels distally between deep & superficial extensors to anastomose with anterior interosseus artery
  - Superficial palmar arch is continuation of ulnar artery in hand
    - Located along line extended in arch across palm from thumb web space
    - Similar to metacarpal shaft level about 1 cm distal to deep palmar arch
    - Located deep to palmar aponeurosis but superficial to long flexor tendons & digital nerves
    - Common palmar digital arteries arise from superficial palmar arch
    - Run distally on surface of 2nd, 3rd & 4th lumbrical muscles
    - Near the MCP joints, each common palmar digital artery divides → two proper digital arteries
    - Run in subcutaneous fat of digits (lateral aspects)

Veins
- Dorsal venous network of hand + network formed by dorsal metacarpal veins
  - Found on dorsum of hand
  - Unite to form cephalic vein (radial side of wrist) & basilic vein (ulnar side of wrist)
    - Basilic and cephalic veins travel proximally in superficial tissues
    - Both veins unite at antecubital fossa via median cubital vein
    - Continues proximally as cephalic vein until it joins brachial vein in axilla to form axillary vein
  - Layout of superficial veins in hand and forearm is highly variable
- Causes of DVT in upper limb extremity are different from that of the lower limb
  - Related to IV cannulations, infusions, radiotherapy, effort induced thrombosis and malignant obstruction

Imaging Anatomy

Overview
- Extensive volar & dorsal anastomoses typically exist

Anatomy-Based Imaging Issues

Imaging Recommendations
- Assessment of caliber of small arteries of hand best performed by digital substraction angiography as they are close to the limit of resolution by ultrasound
  - For example, suspected Raynaud disease or Buerger disease

Imaging Pitfalls
- Vessel visualization on standard imaging is limited
  - Radial & ulnar artery: 2-3 mm; typically visualized
  - Vascular arches: 1 mm; inconsistently visualized
  - Multiple branches & anastomoses; < 1 mm; rarely visualized
- Entry points of nutrient vessels should not be mistaken for erosions
- If angle of insonation of ultrasound beam is at or near 90° to vessel, Doppler and color sensitivity will ↓
- Optimize gate size for small caliber arteries & position at center of arterial lumen to detect peak flow velocity

GRAPHICS

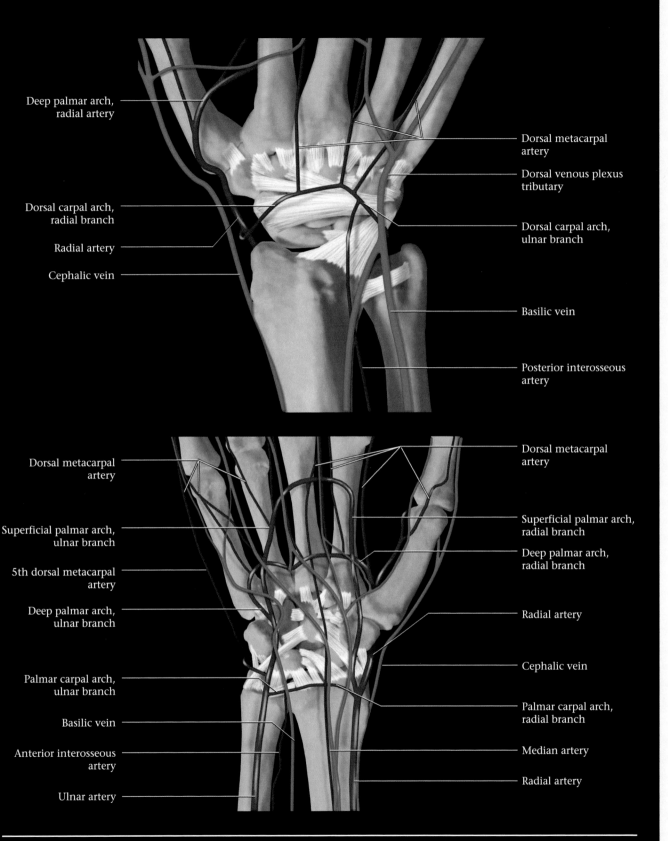

Deep palmar arch, radial artery

Dorsal metacarpal artery

Dorsal venous plexus tributary

Dorsal carpal arch, radial branch

Radial artery

Cephalic vein

Dorsal carpal arch, ulnar branch

Basilic vein

Posterior interosseous artery

Dorsal metacarpal artery

Dorsal metacarpal artery

Superficial palmar arch, ulnar branch

5th dorsal metacarpal artery

Deep palmar arch, ulnar branch

Palmar carpal arch, ulnar branch

Basilic vein

Anterior interosseous artery

Ulnar artery

Superficial palmar arch, radial branch

Deep palmar arch, radial branch

Radial artery

Cephalic vein

Palmar carpal arch, radial branch

Median artery

Radial artery

(Top) Vasculature of the dorsal wrist. The dorsal carpal arch supplies the distal radius, distal carpal row and lateral proximal carpal row. The venous plexus drains into two main venous systems, the cephalic and basilic, with multiple anastomotic communications. **(Bottom)** Vasculature of the volar wrist. Three major arterial arches are contributed to by the radial, ulnar and interosseous arteries: Palmar (volar) carpal, deep and superficial palmar arches. A dorsal venous plexus drains into the cephalic and basilic veins.

HAND VESSELS

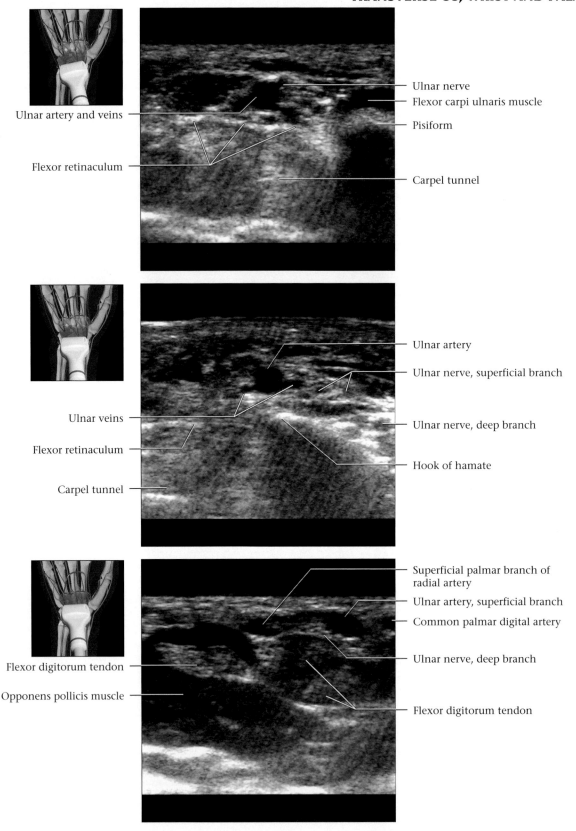

Ulnar artery and veins

Flexor retinaculum

Ulnar nerve
Flexor carpi ulnaris muscle
Pisiform

Carpel tunnel

Ulnar veins

Flexor retinaculum

Carpel tunnel

Ulnar artery

Ulnar nerve, superficial branch

Ulnar nerve, deep branch

Hook of hamate

Flexor digitorum tendon

Opponens pollicis muscle

Superficial palmar branch of radial artery

Ulnar artery, superficial branch
Common palmar digital artery

Ulnar nerve, deep branch

Flexor digitorum tendon

(Top) Transverse grayscale ultrasound of the ulnar artery at the level of the pisiform bone in the Guyon canal. The ulnar artery at the wrist lies on the radial side of the pisiform. Between the ulnar artery and the pisiform lies the ulnar nerve. The ulnar artery divides either within or just beyond the Guyon canal. (Middle) Transverse grayscale ultrasound of the ulnar artery at the level of the hook of hamate. Here it is prone to compression injury which may damage its walls leading to either thrombosis, occlusion or aneurysms. It is usually the superficial branch of the ulnar artery which is most prone to hypothenar hammer syndrome. (Bottom) Transverse grayscale ultrasound of the ulnar artery at the level of the mid palm. The superficial branch of the ulnar artery contributes to the superficial palmar arch.

HAND VESSELS

TRANSVERSE US, DORSAL ASPECT

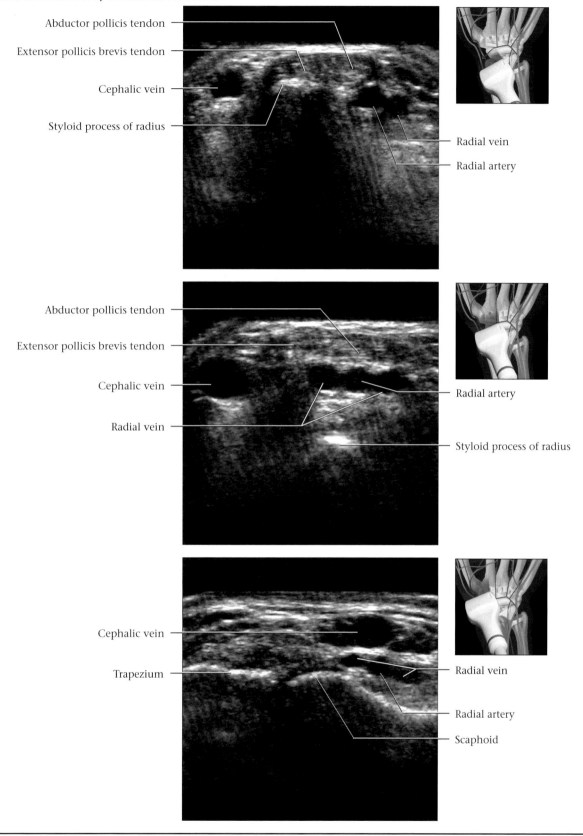

Abductor pollicis tendon

Extensor pollicis brevis tendon

Cephalic vein

Styloid process of radius

Radial vein

Radial artery

Abductor pollicis tendon

Extensor pollicis brevis tendon

Cephalic vein

Radial vein

Radial artery

Styloid process of radius

Cephalic vein

Trapezium

Radial vein

Radial artery

Scaphoid

(Top) Transverse grayscale US of the radial artery just proximal to the wrist. Radial artery runs in a superficial course parallel with the shaft of the radius in the distal forearm. At the wrist it lies alongside the 1st extensor compartment comprising abductor pollicis & extensor pollicis brevis tendons. (Middle) Transverse grayscale US of the radial artery at the wrist joint level. Radial artery runs deep to the 1st extensor compartment tendons. Just before it winds around the wrist it gives off the superficial palmar branch which helps form the superficial palmar arch. (Bottom) Transverse grayscale US of the radial artery at aspect dorsum of the hand. Deep branch of the radial artery runs on the dorsal surface of the scaphoid & trapezium bones, passes deep between the oblique & transverse heads of the adductor pollicis to enter the palm to form the deep palmar arch with the deep branch of the ulnar artery.

HAND VESSELS

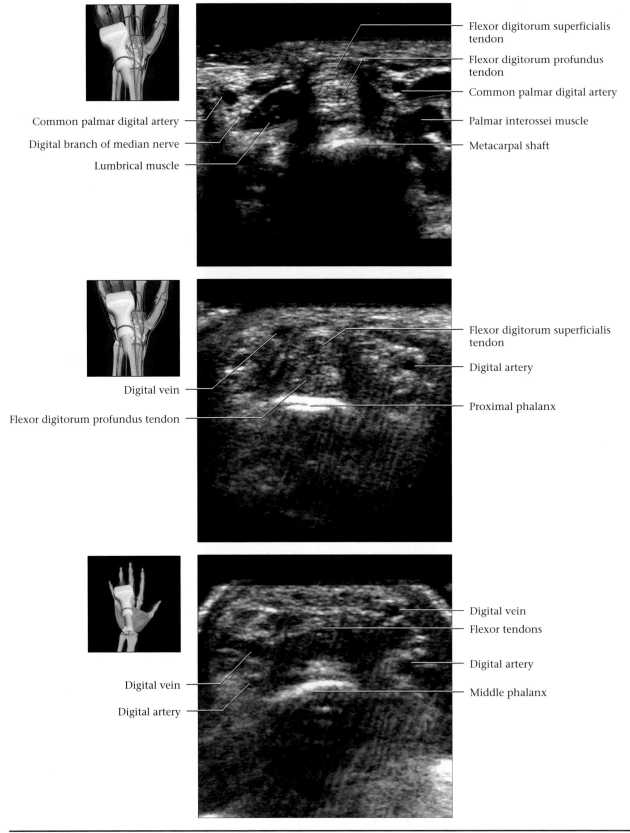

Flexor digitorum superficialis tendon

Flexor digitorum profundus tendon

Common palmar digital artery

Palmar interossei muscle

Metacarpal shaft

Common palmar digital artery

Digital branch of median nerve

Lumbrical muscle

Flexor digitorum superficialis tendon

Digital artery

Proximal phalanx

Digital vein

Flexor digitorum profundus tendon

Digital vein

Flexor tendons

Digital artery

Middle phalanx

Digital vein

Digital artery

(Top) Transverse grayscale US of the vessels of the mid-palm at the mid-metacarpal shaft level. The common palmar digital arteries arise from the superficial palmar arch and divide at the finger bases into proper digital arteries. Each finger has four (two volar, two dorsal) proper digital arteries. **(Middle)** Transverse grayscale US of the digital vessels at the proximal phalanx level. The palmar digital arteries lie dorsal to the digital nerves. The palmar digital arteries are usually bigger than the dorsal digital arteries. Ulno-palmar arteries are twice as big as the radiopalmar arteries (1.8 mm as opposed to 1.1 mm). PSV in hand arteries is variable, it ranges 30-70 cm/s. **(Bottom)** Transverse grayscale ultrasound of vessels at middle phalanx level. The veins of the fingers and the hand are variable in number and location. Dorsal veins are of variable size, ranging between 1.0-1.5 mm.

GRAPHICS

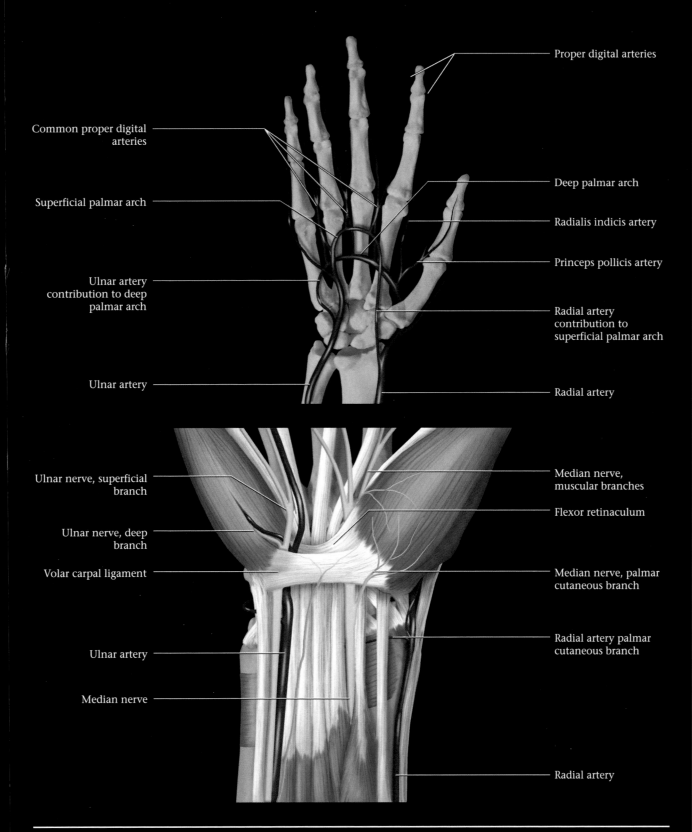

Proper digital arteries

Common proper digital arteries

Superficial palmar arch

Deep palmar arch

Radialis indicis artery

Princeps pollicis artery

Ulnar artery contribution to deep palmar arch

Radial artery contribution to superficial palmar arch

Ulnar artery

Radial artery

Ulnar nerve, superficial branch

Median nerve, muscular branches

Flexor retinaculum

Ulnar nerve, deep branch

Volar carpal ligament

Median nerve, palmar cutaneous branch

Radial artery palmar cutaneous branch

Ulnar artery

Median nerve

Radial artery

(Top) Graphic shows the hand arteries. After giving off its contribution to the superficial palmar arch, the radial artery travels around the radial aspect of the wrist to the dorsum of the hand where it travels in the anatomic snuffbox. It then dives into the 1st interspace between the heads of the 1st dorsal interosseus as well as between the transverse and oblique heads of the adductor pollicis before forming the deep palmar arch. **(Bottom)** Graphic shows the relationship of the nerves and arteries to the volar carpal ligament (superficial fibers of flexor retinaculum which form the roof of the Guyon canal) and flexor retinaculum (which forms the roof of the carpal tunnel). The ulnar nerve (and accompanying artery) pass deep to the volar ligament before branching into the deep and superficial branches.

THUMB

Terminology

Abbreviations
- Abductor pollicis brevis (AbPB)
- Extensor pollicis longus (EPL)
- Flexor digitorum superficialis (FDS)
- Flexor digitorum profundus (FDP)
- Flexor pollicis longus (FPL)
- Flexor pollicis brevis (FPB)
- Metacarpophalangeal joint (MCP joint)
- Opponens pollicis (OP)

Definitions
- Ulnar aspect - medial side
- Radial aspect - lateral side

Gross Anatomy

Muscles
- Thenar muscle
  - Comprises four muscles
    - Abductor pollicis brevis
    - Flexor pollicis brevis
    - Opponens pollicis
    - Adductor pollicis
  - Origin: All originate from flexor retinaculum & tubercle of trapezium
    - Abductor pollicis brevis also originates from tubercle of scaphoid
  - Insertion: AbPB, FPB share combined insertion at base of proximal phalanx radial aspect
    - OP inserts onto volar aspect 1st metacarpal
  - Adductor pollicis often grouped with thenar muscles but is distinct from them
    - AP is separated from thenar muscles by fascial plane & innervated by ulnar nerve rather than median nerve
- Extensor muscles
  - Extensor pollicis longus
    - Origin: Mid-ulna & interosseus membrane
    - Insertion: Dorsal aspect base of distal phalanx thumb
    - Extends both metacarpophalangeal & interphalangeal joints of thumb
  - Extensor pollicis brevis
    - Origin: Distal radius & interosseus membrane
    - Insertion: Dorsal aspect base of proximal phalanx of thumb
    - Extends MCP joint of thumb
- Flexor pollicis longus
  - Origin: Mid-radius & interosseus membrane
  - Insertion: Base of distal phalanx of thumb
  - Flexes metacarpophalangeal & interphalangeal joints of thumb
  - FPL tendon sheath (also known as radial bursa)
    - Encompasses FPL tendon from just proximal to carpal tunnel to its insertion (distal phalanx of thumb)
    - Radial bursa occasionally communicates with ulnar bursa (common flexor sheath) at level of carpal tunnel
- Extensor expansion
  - Formed by fibers from adductor pollicis ulnarly & abductor pollicis brevis radially
  - Aids extension of interphalangeal joint
  - Adductor pollicis contribution to extensor expansion is also known as adductor aponeurosis

Pulley
- A1 pulley: Level of metacarpophalangeal joint
- Av pulley: Variable in position & may be anywhere over proximal half of proximal phalanx
- Oblique pulley: Runs from ulnar aspect of proximal phalanx to radial aspect of distal phalanx
  - Crosses interphalangeal joint, so becomes lax in flexion
- A2 pulley: Level of interphalangeal joint
  - Clinically most important pulley of thumb

Imaging Anatomy

Overview
- On dorsal transverse imaging, extensor expansions seen as thin, regular, hypoechoic bands arising from edges of extensor tendon
- On palmar transverse imaging, annular pulleys seen as thin ring-shaped structures covering flexor tendons & inserting in palmar plate

Anatomy-Based Imaging Issues

Imaging Recommendations
- Thenar muscles can be identified reliably on ultrasound
  - All thenar muscles can be identified by placing transducer in orthograde position, parallel to direction of muscle fibers
- Extensor & flexor tendons of thumb bear similar ultrasound features to a normal tendon

Clinical Implications

Clinical Importance
- Radial bursa may communicate with ulnar bursa at level of carpal tunnel allowing spread of infection
- Ulnar collateral ligament of MCP joint of thumb is especially prone to tearing in forced abduction & extension
  - Referred to as gamekeeper's thumb or skier's thumb
  - If ulnar collateral ligament is torn, position of its proximal free end with respect to adductor aponeurosis is of importance
    - If proximal portion is displaced superficial to adductor aponeurosis, it is referred to as Stener lesion & surgery is usually required
    - Stener lesion = interposition of adductor aponeurosis between proximally retracted torn ulnar collateral ligament & distal portion
    - If proximal portion remains deep to adductor aponeurosis, conservative management may suffice
- First annular pulley believed to play a role in pathogenesis of trigger finger

GRAPHIC, DEEP DISSECTION OF HAND

Common digital tendon sheath

FDP tendon

FDS tendon

Deep transverse metacarpal ligament

Ulnar bursa (common flexor sheath)

Flexor digiti minimi muscle

Abductor digiti minimi muscle

Flexor retinaculum

Flexor tendons

A5 pulley
C3 pulley
A4 pulley
C2 pulley
A3 pulley

C1 pulley
A2 pulley

A1 pulley

A2 pulley

Oblique pulley

Av pulley

A1 pulley

Radial bursa (FPL tendon sheath)

Adductor pollicis muscle

Abductor pollicis brevis muscle

Opponens digiti minimi muscle

Graphic of pulley system for 3rd-5th digits is identical to that demonstrated for 2nd digit. Common digital sheath of 4th digit is removed to show relationship of FDS & FDP tendons. Deep transverse metacarpal ligaments connect volar plates (not shown) of digits 2-5. Although there is overlap of radial & ulnar bursae in this image, these structures normally do not communicate. It is, however, important to know that radial & ulnar bursae may communicate as a normal variation in a small percentage of population. Similarly, any one or more of common digital sheaths may communicate with radial bursa in up to 10% of normal population. These normal variant bursal communications are important as they can provide routes for more extensive spread of infection.

THUMB

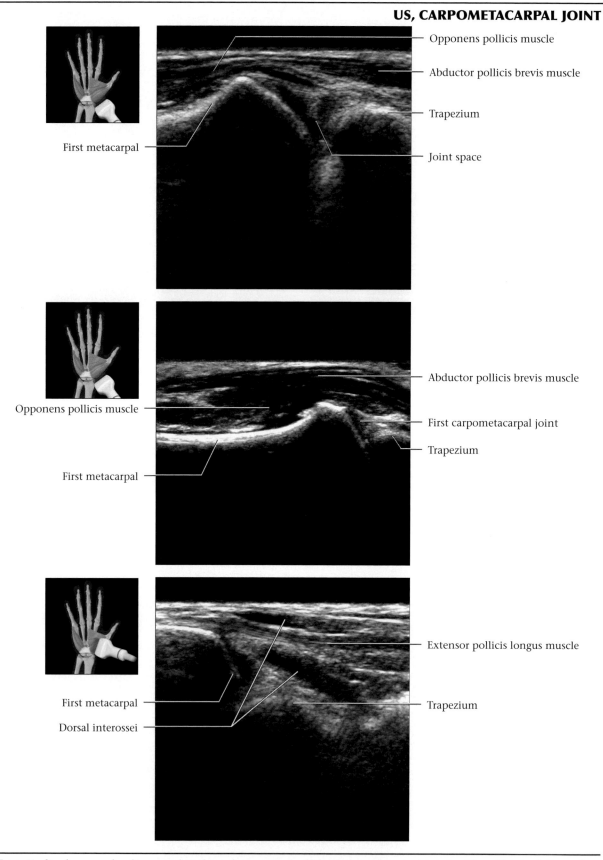

First metacarpal — Opponens pollicis muscle
Abductor pollicis brevis muscle
Trapezium
Joint space

Opponens pollicis muscle — Abductor pollicis brevis muscle
First metacarpal — First carpometacarpal joint
Trapezium

First metacarpal — Extensor pollicis longus muscle
Dorsal interossei — Trapezium

(**Top**) Longitudinal grayscale ultrasound at the palmar aspect of the carpometacarpal joint with radial deviation of thumb. The carpometacarpal joint of the thumb is by far the most mobile of the carpometacarpal joints. It is best viewed by radially deviating the thumb. (**Middle**) Longitudinal grayscale ultrasound at the palmar aspect of the carpometacarpal joint thumb. Because of its mobility, the carpometacarpal joint of the thumb is the only one of the carpometacarpal joints prone to osteoarthrosis. This gives rise to deep pain in the thenar eminence. (**Bottom**) Longitudinal grayscale ultrasound at the dorsal aspect of the carpometacarpal joint of thumb. The large dorsal component of the first metacarpal relative to the articulating surface on the trapezium leads to a normal step-off on the dorsal aspect of the joint.

THUMB

METACARPOPHALANGEAL JOINT

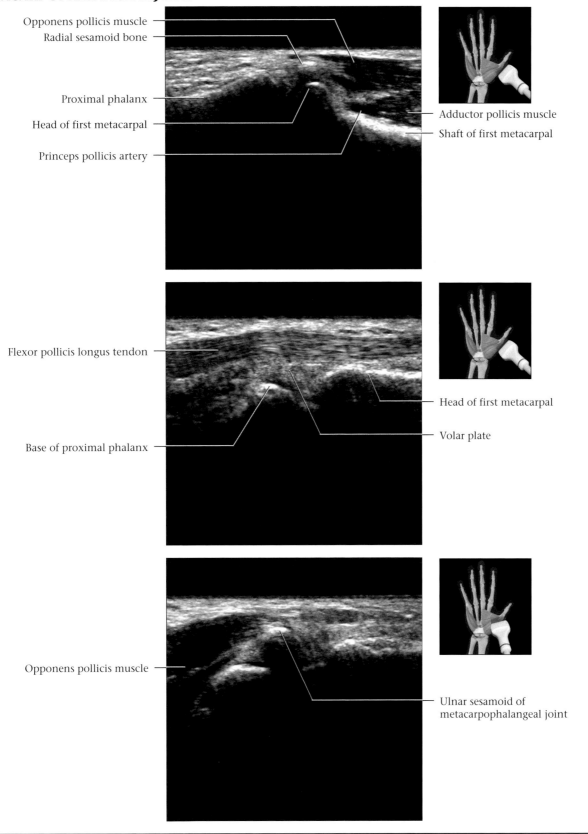

Opponens pollicis muscle

Radial sesamoid bone

Proximal phalanx

Head of first metacarpal

Princeps pollicis artery

Adductor pollicis muscle

Shaft of first metacarpal

Flexor pollicis longus tendon

Head of first metacarpal

Volar plate

Base of proximal phalanx

Opponens pollicis muscle

Ulnar sesamoid of metacarpophalangeal joint

(Top) Longitudinal grayscale ultrasound of metacarpo-phalangeal joint of thumb. Collateral ligament complex constitutes majority of lateral aspects of joint capsules of all metacarpophalangeal and interphalangeal joints. Ulnar collateral ligament of 1st metacarpophalangeal joint is especially prone to tearing in forced abduction and extension. Such an injury is commonly referred to as gamekeeper's thumb or skier's thumb. (Middle) Longitudinal grayscale ultrasound at metacarpophalangeal joint of thumb. Volar plate constitutes majority of volar aspect of joint capsule of metacarpophalangeal joint. Volar plate may be avulsed with forced extension. (Bottom) Transverse grayscale ultrasound of the first metacarpophalangeal joint. Metacarpal head is usually involved in erosions before adjacent proximal phalanx. Metacarpophalangeal joint is the location of initial erosions in inflammatory arthritis.

THUMB

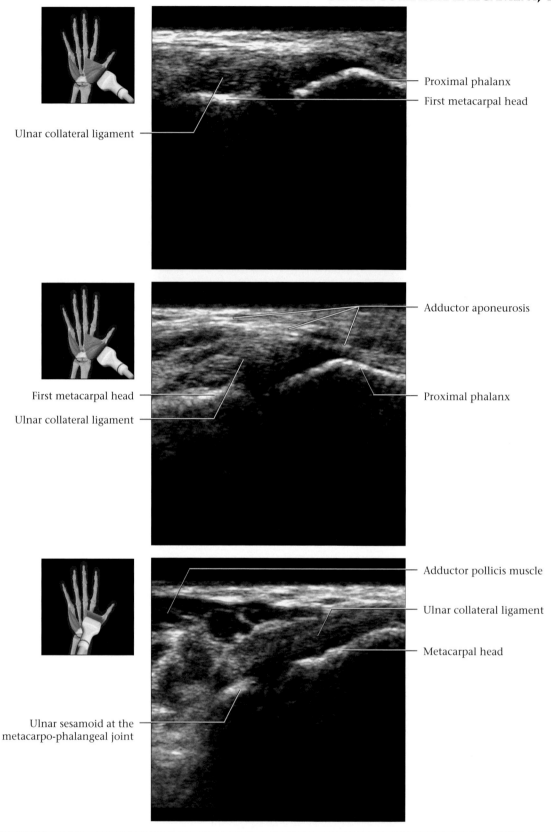

Proximal phalanx

First metacarpal head

Ulnar collateral ligament

Adductor aponeurosis

First metacarpal head

Ulnar collateral ligament

Proximal phalanx

Adductor pollicis muscle

Ulnar collateral ligament

Metacarpal head

Ulnar sesamoid at the metacarpo-phalangeal joint

(Top) Longitudinal grayscale ultrasound along the palmar aspect of ulnar collateral ligament of the thumb. The ulnar collateral ligament of the metacarpophalangeal joint is commonly injured by forced abduction of the thumb. Avulsion normally occurs at the distal i.e. proximal phalangeal attachment. **(Middle)** Longitudinal grayscale ultrasound of the ulnar collateral ligament at the mid portion. The adductor pollicis aponeurosis overlies the ulnar collateral ligament. The thin adductor aponeurosis is attached to the medial side of the proximal phalanx base and the ulnar sesamoid bone. If the torn ulnar collateral ligament displaces above the adductor aponeurosis (Stener lesion) this is an indication for operative repair. **(Bottom)** Transverse grayscale ultrasound at the metacarpophalangeal joint of thumb. This shows the normal thick ulnar collateral ligament in transverse section.

THUMB

TRANSVERSE US PALMAR ASPECT, THUMB

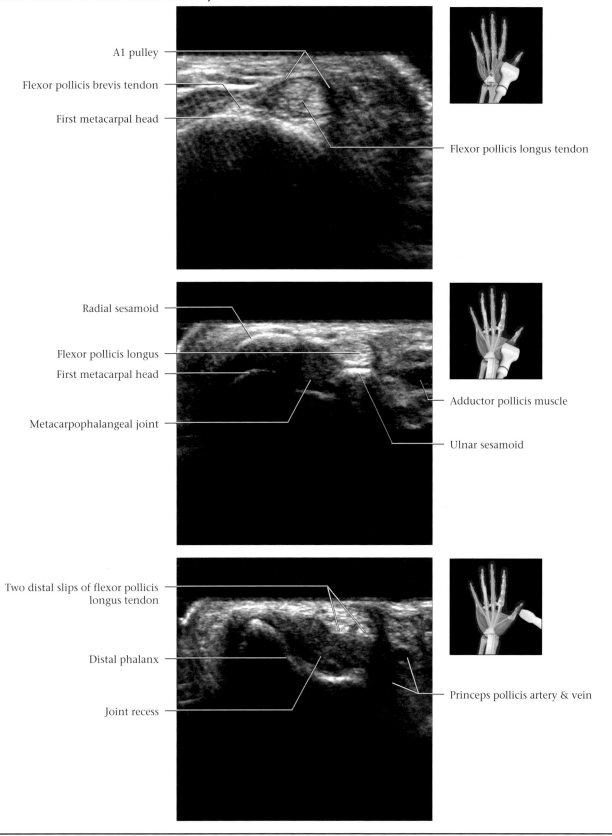

A1 pulley

Flexor pollicis brevis tendon

First metacarpal head

Flexor pollicis longus tendon

Radial sesamoid

Flexor pollicis longus

First metacarpal head

Metacarpophalangeal joint

Adductor pollicis muscle

Ulnar sesamoid

Two distal slips of flexor pollicis longus tendon

Distal phalanx

Joint recess

Princeps pollicis artery & vein

(Top) Transverse grayscale ultrasound along the flexor aspect of the thumb at the metacarpal head level. The flexor pollicis brevis inserts into the radial sesamoid and base of proximal phalanx. The flexor pollicis longus extends into the base of distal phalanx. (Middle) Transverse grayscale ultrasound along the flexor aspect of the thumb at the metacarpophalangeal joint level. The flexor pollicis longus tendon passes over the ulnar sesamoid bone of the metacarpophalangeal joint. (Bottom) Transverse grayscale ultrasound along the flexor aspect of the thumb at the interphalangeal joint level. The flexor pollicis longus tendon is held in position primarily by the A1 pulley at the metacarpophalangeal joint and the A2 pulley at the interphalangeal joint. The flexor pollicis longus tendon may divide into two slips at its insertion.

THUMB

Extensor pollicis longus tendon

First metacarpal

Joint recess

Proximal phalanx

Nail base

Distal phalanx

Extensor pollicis longus tendon

Proximal phalanx

Joint recess

Interphalangeal joint

Dorsal digital vessels

Extensor pollicis longus tendon

Dorsal digital vessels

Proximal phalanx

(Top) Longitudinal grayscale ultrasound along the extensor aspect of the thumb at the metacarpophalangeal joint level. The extensor pollicis longus tendon thins as it merges with the extensor expansion on the dorsum of the thumb. **(Middle)** Longitudinal grayscale ultrasound along the extensor aspect of the thumb at the interphalangeal joint level. The extensor pollicis longus tendon inserts into the distal phalanx. **(Bottom)** Transverse grayscale ultrasound along the extensor aspect of the thumb at the proximal phalanx level. The thin extensor expansion of the extensor pollicis longus is visible.

THUMB

TRANSVERSE US, THENAR EMINENCE

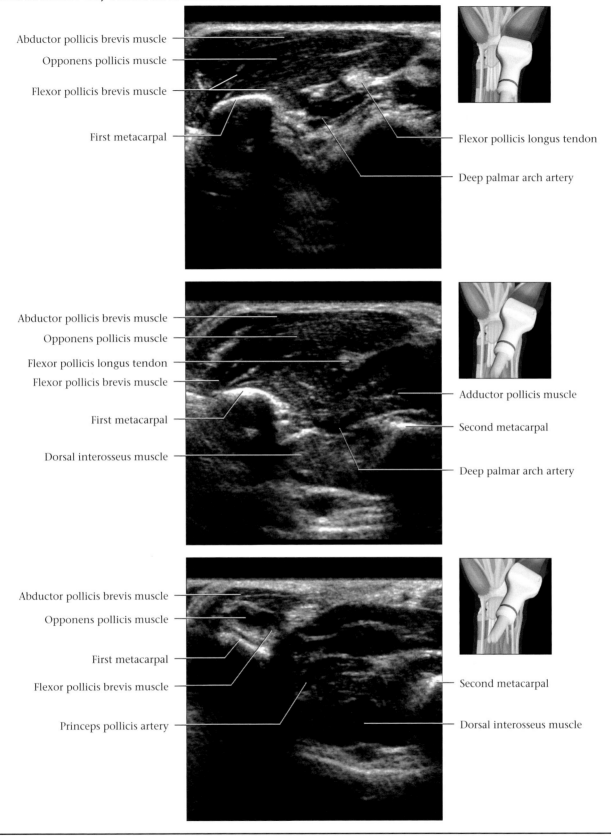

Abductor pollicis brevis muscle
Opponens pollicis muscle
Flexor pollicis brevis muscle
First metacarpal
Flexor pollicis longus tendon
Deep palmar arch artery

Abductor pollicis brevis muscle
Opponens pollicis muscle
Flexor pollicis longus tendon
Flexor pollicis brevis muscle
First metacarpal
Dorsal interosseus muscle
Adductor pollicis muscle
Second metacarpal
Deep palmar arch artery

Abductor pollicis brevis muscle
Opponens pollicis muscle
First metacarpal
Flexor pollicis brevis muscle
Princeps pollicis artery
Second metacarpal
Dorsal interosseus muscle

(Top) Transverse grayscale ultrasound along the proximal aspect of the thenar eminence. The thenar eminence comprises four muscles, the abductor, opponens, flexor and adductor pollicis from above downwards. The adductor muscle is, strictly speaking, not part of the thenar eminence since it is separated by a fascial layer and has a separate innervation. **(Middle)** Transverse grayscale ultrasound at the mid portion of thenar eminence. The flexor pollicis longus tendon is easily recognized as an echogenic tendon alongside the flexor pollicis brevis, deep to the opponens pollicis and superficial to the adductor pollicis muscle. **(Bottom)** Transverse grayscale ultrasound at the distal portion of the thenar eminence.

THUMB

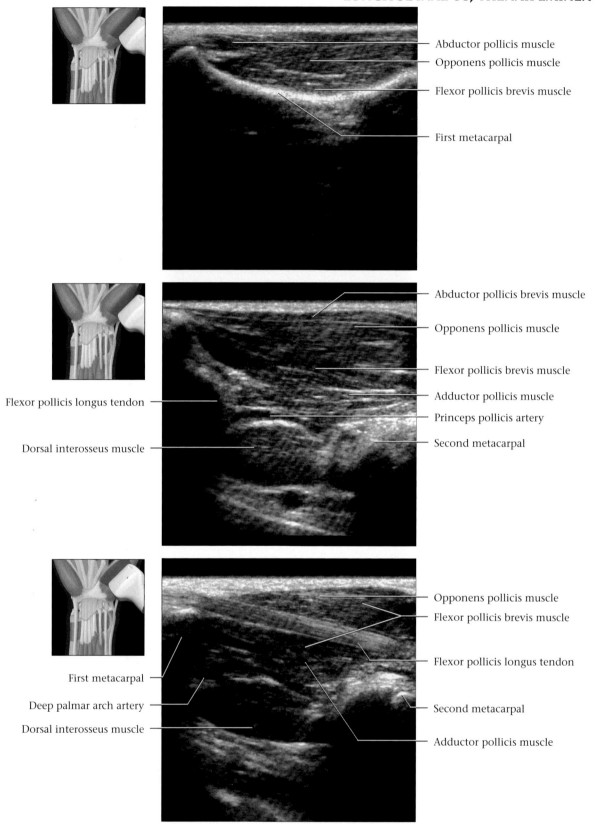

Top image labels:
- Abductor pollicis muscle
- Opponens pollicis muscle
- Flexor pollicis brevis muscle
- First metacarpal

Middle image labels:
- Abductor pollicis brevis muscle
- Opponens pollicis muscle
- Flexor pollicis brevis muscle
- Adductor pollicis muscle
- Princeps pollicis artery
- Second metacarpal
- Flexor pollicis longus tendon
- Dorsal interosseus muscle

Bottom image labels:
- Opponens pollicis muscle
- Flexor pollicis brevis muscle
- Flexor pollicis longus tendon
- Second metacarpal
- Adductor pollicis muscle
- First metacarpal
- Deep palmar arch artery
- Dorsal interosseus muscle

(Top) Longitudinal grayscale ultrasound along the the proximal aspect of thenar eminence. Use the mnemonic ABOF to remember the muscles of the thenar eminence. (Middle) Longitudinal grayscale ultrasound at the mid-thenar eminence. ABOF stands for abductor pollicis brevis, opponens pollicis and flexor pollicis brevis which lie superficial to deep in that order. Abductor pollicis brevis and flexor pollicis brevis share a combined insertion at the lateral base of the proximal phalanx of the 1st digit. (Bottom) Longitudinal grayscale ultrasound along the ulnar aspect of the thenar eminence. Although often grouped with the thenar muscles (by virtue of proximity), the adductor pollicis is distinct from them, as it is separated from the thenar muscles by a fascial plane, and innervated by ulnar nerve (as opposed to median nerve).

THUMB

STENER LESION

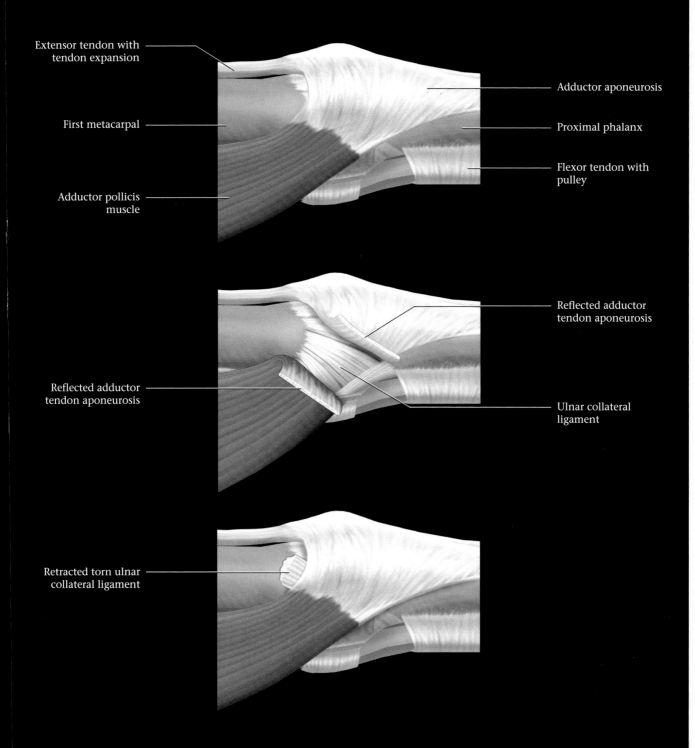

Extensor tendon with tendon expansion

First metacarpal

Adductor pollicis muscle

Adductor aponeurosis

Proximal phalanx

Flexor tendon with pulley

Reflected adductor tendon aponeurosis

Reflected adductor tendon aponeurosis

Ulnar collateral ligament

Retracted torn ulnar collateral ligament

Graphic shows the ulnar aspect of the metacarpophalangeal joint of thumb. On the top image, the adductor tendon aponeurosis attaches to the extensor expansion on the dorsum of the thumb. The middle image shows a reflected adductor aponeurosis with the ulnar collateral ligament beneath. When a complete tear of the ulnar collateral ligament occurs, shown in the bottom image, the proximal end of the ligament gets retracted back over the adductor aponeurosis. This is referred to as a "Stener lesion".

FINGERS

Terminology

Abbreviations
- Extensor digitorum communis (EDC)
- Extensor digiti minimi (EDM)
- Interphalangeal (IP) joint
- Metacarpophalangeal joint (MCP) joint

Gross Anatomy

Muscles
- Flexor aspect
  - Flexor digitorum superficialis (FDS)
    - Origin: Common flexor tendon origin & mid-radius
    - Insertion: Volar plates of proximal IP joints & bases of middle phalanges digits 2-5
    - Superficialis tendon is superficial to profundus tendon in palm until it divides at level of proximal third proximal phalanx
    - Two slips of superficialis tendon pass around profundus tendon & reunite deep to profundus tendon prior to insertion
    - Flexes both MCP joints, aided by lumbricals & interossei & proximal IP joints of digits 2-5
  - Flexor digitorum profundus (FDP)
    - Origin: Proximal & mid-radius & interosseus membrane
    - Profundus tendon passes through divided superficialis tendon to insert at base of distal phalanx
    - Insertion: Volar plates of distal IP joints & bases of distal phalanges digits 2-5
    - Flexes distal & proximal IP joints as well as MCP joints aided by lumbricals & interossei
- Palmar interossei
  - Denoted 1-3 from radial to ulnar
  - Origin: Mesial palmar diaphyses of 2nd, 4th & 5th metacarpals
  - Insertion: Mesial lateral bands & proximal phalanges bases of same digit as origin
  - Adducts digits & assists lumbricals with flexion MCP & extension IP joints digits 2, 4 & 5
- Extensor aspect
  - Extensor digitorum communis
    - Origin: Common extensor tendon origin (lateral humeral epicondyle)
    - Insertion: As central slip at bases of middle phalanges & proximal IP joint capsule
    - Separate EDC tendon to 5th digit tendon present in 50%
  - Extensor indicis
    - Origin: Posterior, distal ulna & interosseus membrane
    - Insertion: Blends with 2nd digit EDC tendon & extensor hood
  - Extensor digiti minimi
    - Origin: Common extensor tendon origin (lateral humeral epicondyle)
    - Insertion: Two tendons of EDM fuse with one another & with 5th digit EDC tendon prior to insertion at base of proximal phalanx 5th digit

- Lumbricals
  - Numbered 1-4 from radial to ulnar
  - Origin: Flexor digitorum profundus tendons, just distal to carpal tunnel
  - Insertion: Radial lateral bands of digits 2-5
    - Extend IP & flex MCP joints of digits 2-5
- Dorsal interossei
  - Numbered 1-4 from radial to ulnar
  - Origin: Dorsolateral metacarpal diaphyses
  - Insertion: Adjacent lateral bands of digits 2-4
    - Extend 2nd-5th IP joints & abduct digits 2-5

Tendon Pulley System
- Annular pulley
  - Retinacula that retain flexor tendons at 5 points = annular pulleys
  - Prevent tendon bowstringing during finger flexion
  - **Odd** numbered pulleys at **oval** parts (i.e. joints)
  - **Even** numbered pulleys at **elegant** waists (i.e. shafts)
  - A2 & A4 functionally most important
    - A1: MCP joint → base proximal phalanx
    - A2: Middle & distal thirds of proximal phalanx
    - A3: Proximal interphalangeal joint
    - A4: Mid-portion of middle phalanx
    - A5: Distal interphalangeal joint
  - Also cruciform pulleys, C1-C3
- Extensor expansion
  - Begins just proximal to MCP joints & terminates just proximal to proximal IP joint
  - Dorsal expansion of fibers oriented perpendicular to long axis of extensor tendons
  - Fibers of extensor expansion interdigitate with EDC tendons to prevent lateral translation

Tendon Sheaths
- 2nd-4th flexor synovial sheaths extends from metacarpal neck to bases of distal phalanges
- Encompasses the 5th digit flexor tendons over their entire course (to level of distal IP joint)

Anatomy-Based Imaging Issues

Imaging Approaches
- Extensor tendons in digits often seen best on longitudinal imaging
- Pulleys seen as focal hyperechoic thickening overlying tendon sheath, widening at base
  - Do not misdiagnose as tendon sheath thickening
  - A1 & A2 pulley can be depicted in most cases
  - Injury inferred by bowstringing of flexor tendons
  - Compare with normal fingers

Clinical Implications

Clinical Importance
- Digital sheaths may connect to ulnar bursa in up to 10% of population providing route for spread of infection from digits 2-4 to common flexor sheath & vice versa
- Pulley injury inferred by bowstringing of flexor tendons

FINGERS

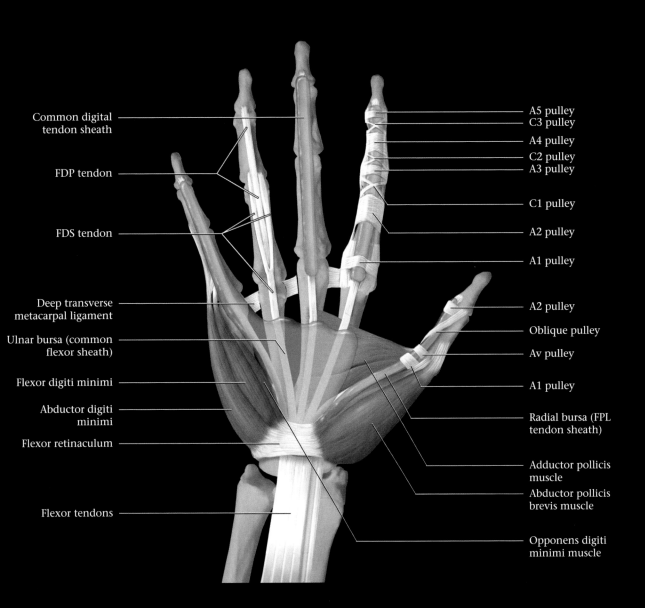

Common digital tendon sheath

FDP tendon

FDS tendon

Deep transverse metacarpal ligament

Ulnar bursa (common flexor sheath)

Flexor digiti minimi

Abductor digiti minimi

Flexor retinaculum

Flexor tendons

A5 pulley
C3 pulley
A4 pulley
C2 pulley
A3 pulley

C1 pulley

A2 pulley

A1 pulley

A2 pulley

Oblique pulley

Av pulley

A1 pulley

Radial bursa (FPL tendon sheath)

Adductor pollicis muscle

Abductor pollicis brevis muscle

Opponens digiti minimi muscle

Graphic of pulley system for the 3rd-5th digits is identical to that demonstrated for the 2nd digit. The common digital sheath of the 4th digit is removed to show the relationship of the FDS & FDP tendons. Deep transverse metacarpal ligaments connect the volar plates (not shown) of digits 2-5. Although there is overlap of the radial & ulnar bursae in this image, these structures normally do not communicate. It is, however, important to know that the radial & ulnar bursae may communicate as a normal variation in a small percentage of the population. Similarly, any one or more of the common digital sheaths may communicate with the radial bursa in up to 10% of the normal population. These normal variant bursal communications are important as they can provide routes for more extensive spread of infection.

FINGERS

Terminal tendon

Triangular ligament

Central slip of EDC tendon

EDC contribution to conjoined tendon

Extensor hood

Junctura tendinum

3rd lumbrical muscle

Extensor indicis tendon

EDC tendon to 2nd digit

Extensor pollicis brevis tendon

Abductor pollicis longus tendon

Extensor pollicis longus tendon

4th EDC tendon contribution to 5th EDC tendon

Lateral band contribution to central slip

Conjoined tendon

Lateral band

PIP joint capsule

Sagittal band

4th dorsal interosseus muscle

Abductor digiti minimi muscle

EDC tendon to 5th digit

Extensor digiti minimi tendon

Extensor carpi ulnaris tendon

Extensor retinaculum

Graphic of the hand and finger extensor mechanism composite shows different components of the extensor mechanism on different digits. With the exception of the extensor indicis, extensor digiti minimi, abductor digiti minimi, & 4th EDC tendon contribution to the 5th EDC tendon, any structure on any of the 2nd-5th digits can be extrapolated to any & all of the other 2nd-5th digits. Note that the 2nd extensor retinaculum compartment & its contents (extensor carpi radialis longus & brevis tendons) are not included in this graphic. Although the abductor pollicis longus tendon travels in the 1st compartment of the extensor retinaculum, its insertion (not shown) is actually on the radial aspect of the volar surface of the base of the first metacarpal.

FINGERS

PULLEY SYSTEM

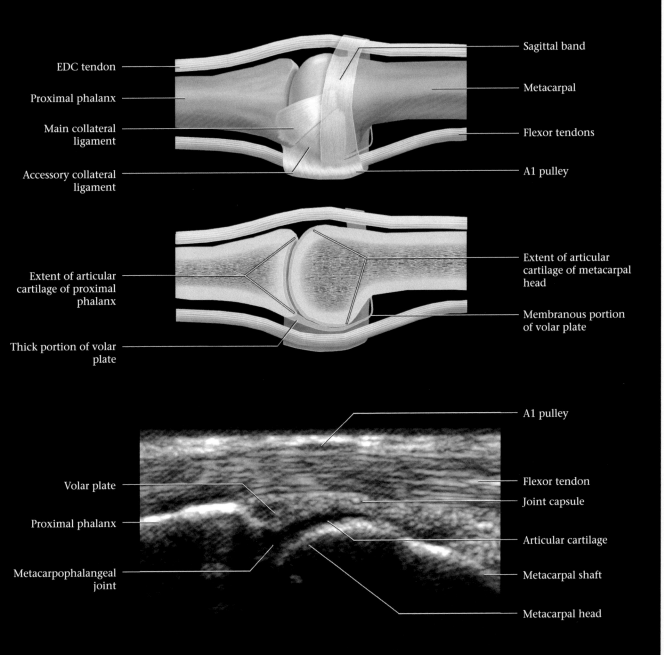

EDC tendon

Proximal phalanx

Main collateral
ligament

Accessory collateral
ligament

Sagittal band

Metacarpal

Flexor tendons

A1 pulley

Extent of articular
cartilage of proximal
phalanx

Thick portion of volar
plate

Extent of articular
cartilage of metacarpal
head

Membranous portion
of volar plate

A1 pulley

Volar plate

Proximal phalanx

Metacarpophalangeal
joint

Flexor tendon

Joint capsule

Articular cartilage

Metacarpal shaft

Metacarpal head

(Top) Surface & cut-section graphics of the MCP joint. The collateral ligament complex is composed of two separate fiber bands. The main collateral ligament inserts on the base of the adjacent phalanx. The accessory collateral ligament inserts on the volar plate. The volar plate is thick distally & thin & redundant proximally. With the exception of the sagittal band (present only at MCP joints), anatomy in this graphic is duplicated in all MCP & IP joints in the hand. (Bottom) Longitudinal grayscale ultrasound of the middle finger at the metacarpophalangeal joint.

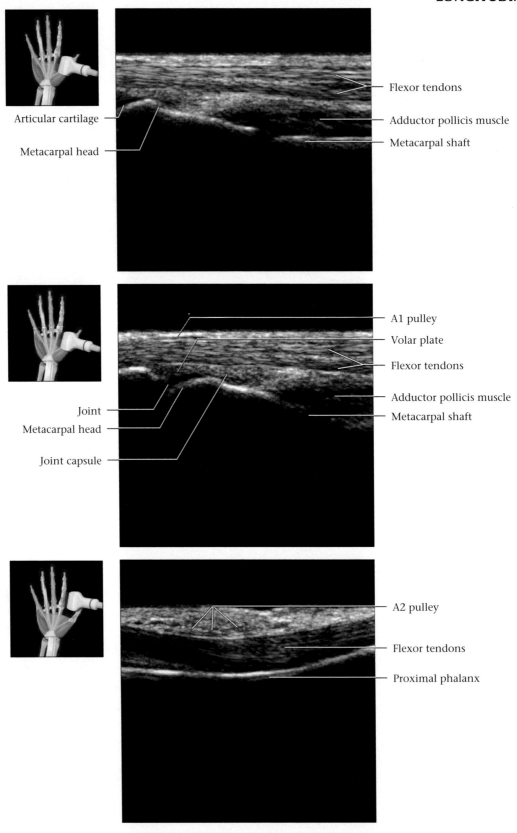

Articular cartilage

Metacarpal head

Flexor tendons

Adductor pollicis muscle

Metacarpal shaft

A1 pulley

Volar plate

Flexor tendons

Adductor pollicis muscle

Metacarpal shaft

Joint

Metacarpal head

Joint capsule

A2 pulley

Flexor tendons

Proximal phalanx

(Top) Longitudinal grayscale US of the finger at the metacarpal shaft level. From the base of the metacarpals (carpal tunnel outlet) to the neck of the metacarpals, the flexor tendons of the 2nd to 4th fingers (i.e. index, middle and ring fingers) are devoid of flexor tendon sheaths. A normal flexor tendon sheath cannot be clearly depicted on ultrasound and can only be seen when it is distended. Do not confuse the flexor tendon pulleys with tendon sheath thickening. **(Middle)** Longitudinal grayscale US of fingers at the metacarpophalangeal joint level. Metacarpophalangeal joints are narrowed dorsally & flare in the volar direction increasing contact with the proximal phalanx as the joint is flexed. Capsule of the metacarpophalangeal joint extends from the neck of the metacarpal to the base of proximal phalangeal joint. **(Bottom)** Longitudinal grayscale US of middle finger at proximal phalanx.

FINGERS

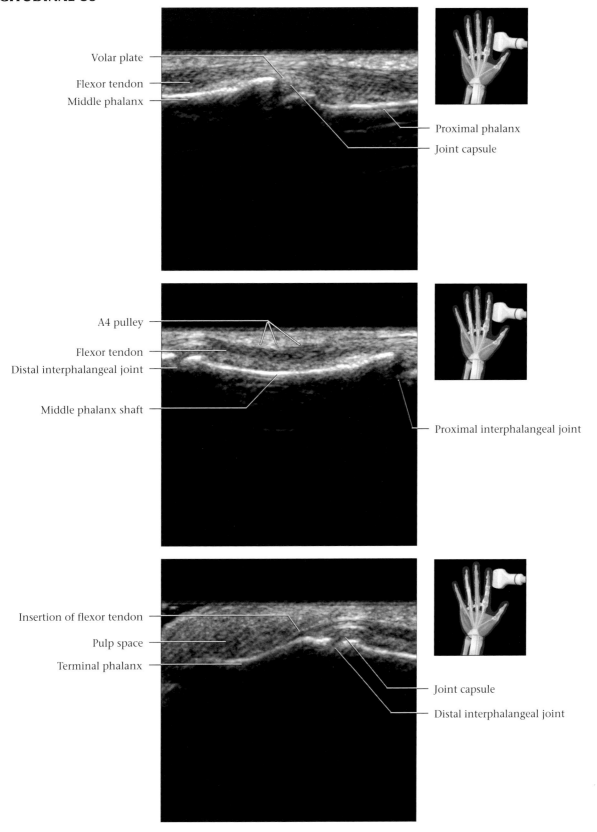

Volar plate

Flexor tendon

Middle phalanx

Proximal phalanx

Joint capsule

A4 pulley

Flexor tendon

Distal interphalangeal joint

Middle phalanx shaft

Proximal interphalangeal joint

Insertion of flexor tendon

Pulp space

Terminal phalanx

Joint capsule

Distal interphalangeal joint

(Top) Longitudinal grayscale US of the proximal IP joint of the middle finger. Volar plate is a fibrocartilaginous thickening on the volar aspect of the MCP joint & proximal IP joints. At the proximal IP joint it is attached to the base of the middle phalanx & has a thinner insertion to the distal end of the proximal phalanx. It may become avulsed during hyperextension injuries often associated with a small avulsion fracture. There is inability to fully extend & flex the joint, a condition which usually improves with time unless the joint is locked. **(Middle)** Longitudinal grayscale US of the middle finger at the middle phalanx. A4 pulley prevents bowstringing of flexor tendons at the middle phalanx. **(Bottom)** Longitudinal grayscale US at the distal IP joint middle finger. Avulsion of flexor tendons from the distal phalangeal joint base is usually accompanied by a small avulsion fracture.

FINGERS

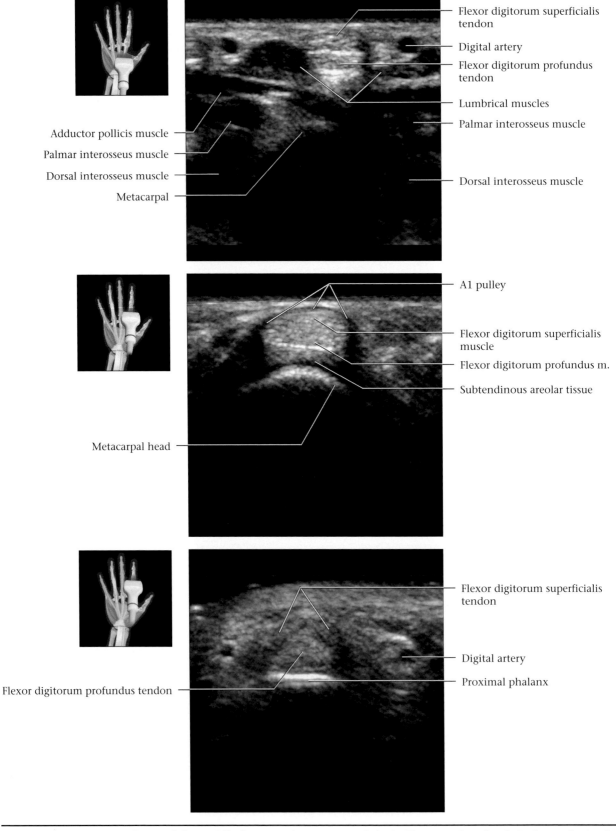

Flexor digitorum superficialis tendon

Digital artery

Flexor digitorum profundus tendon

Lumbrical muscles

Palmar interosseus muscle

Dorsal interosseus muscle

Adductor pollicis muscle

Palmar interosseus muscle

Dorsal interosseus muscle

Metacarpal

A1 pulley

Flexor digitorum superficialis muscle

Flexor digitorum profundus m.

Subtendinous areolar tissue

Metacarpal head

Flexor digitorum superficialis tendon

Digital artery

Proximal phalanx

Flexor digitorum profundus tendon

(Top) Transverse grayscale US of the middle finger at the metacarpal shaft. There are four lumbrical muscles in the hand. These are unusual muscles in that they do not originate from body but instead originate from the flexor digitorum tendons and insert into the extensor expansions. **(Middle)** Transverse grayscale US of the middle finger at the metacarpal head. This image from the A1 pulley level. The A1 pulley extends from the metacarpal head to the proximal phalanx base. It is seen as a thin hypoechoic to hyperechoic rim (depending on the beam angulation) around the flexor tendons. It broadens considerably at the base which cannot be clearly depicted. **(Bottom)** Transverse grayscale US of the middle finger at the proximal phalanx. The flexor digitorum superificialis tendon splits just proximal to the insertion, enabling the flexor digitorum profundus tendon to push through the gap.

FINGERS

A2 pulley

Flexor digitorum profundus tendon

Digital artery

Flexor digitorum superficialis tendon

Shaft of proximal phalanx

Flexor digitorum superficialis tendon

Flexor digitorum profundus tendon

Capsule

Head of proximal phalanx

Digital artery

Flexor digitorum superficialis tendon

Flexor digitorum profundus tendon

Digital artery

Proximal end of middle phalanx

(Top) Transverse grayscale ultrasound of the middle finger shaft of the proximal phalanx. Do not confuse the thickening of the A2 pulley with tendon sheath thickening. (Middle) Transverse grayscale ultrasound of the middle finger proximal phalangeal head region just distal to the A2 pulley. The small slips of the flexor digitorum superficialis tendon descend on either side of the flexor digitorum profundus tendon to insert onto the volar aspect of the base of the middle phalanx. (Bottom) Transverse grayscale ultrasound of the middle finger proximal end of the middle phalanx. The insertions of the slips of the flexor digitorum superficialis are small. As such, particularly in the presence of edema, it may be difficult to confirm isolated avulsion of one slip on ultrasound. In this situation the superficialis tendon will not be retracted.

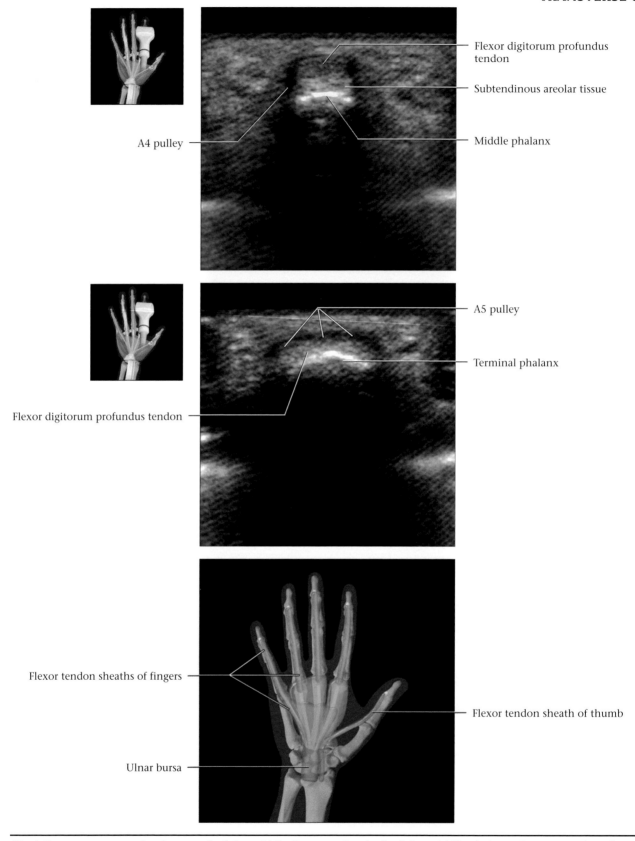

Flexor digitorum profundus tendon

Subtendinous areolar tissue

A4 pulley

Middle phalanx

A5 pulley

Terminal phalanx

Flexor digitorum profundus tendon

Flexor tendon sheaths of fingers

Flexor tendon sheath of thumb

Ulnar bursa

(Top) Transverse grayscale ultrasound of the middle finger at the shaft of the middle phalanx. Do not confuse the subtendinous connective tissue as part of the tendon. **(Middle)** Transverse grayscale ultrasound of the middle finger at the base of the distal phalanx. The flexor digitorum profundus tendon gains broad attachment to the base of the distal phalanx and is supported by the A5 pulley just proximal to the insertion. **(Bottom)** Graphic shows the tendon sheaths of the fingers. Digital sheaths may connect to the ulnar bursa in up to 10% of population providing a route for the spread of infection from digits 2-4 to the common flexor sheath & vice versa.

FINGERS

LONGITUDINAL US, EXTENSOR ASPECT

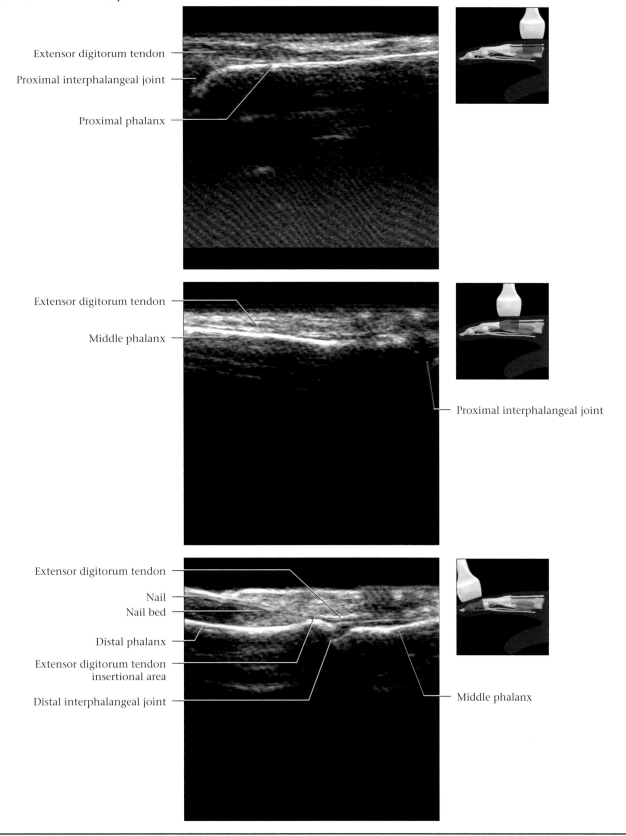

(Top) Longitudinal grayscale ultrasound of the dorsal aspect of the proximal phalanx. The extensor expansion on the dorsum of the fingers is thin and flat and does not have an enclosed synovial sheath. **(Middle)** Longitudinal grayscale ultrasound of the dorsal aspect of the middle phalanx. No pulleys are present on the extensor aspect of the fingers, the extensor expansion (or hood) being attached to the phalanges and the lateral bands. **(Bottom)** Longitudinal grayscale ultrasound of the dorsal aspect of the distal phalanx. The extensor digitorum is attached to the base of the distal phalanx. This is a common site of avulsion, often with a small avulsion fracture.

FINGERS

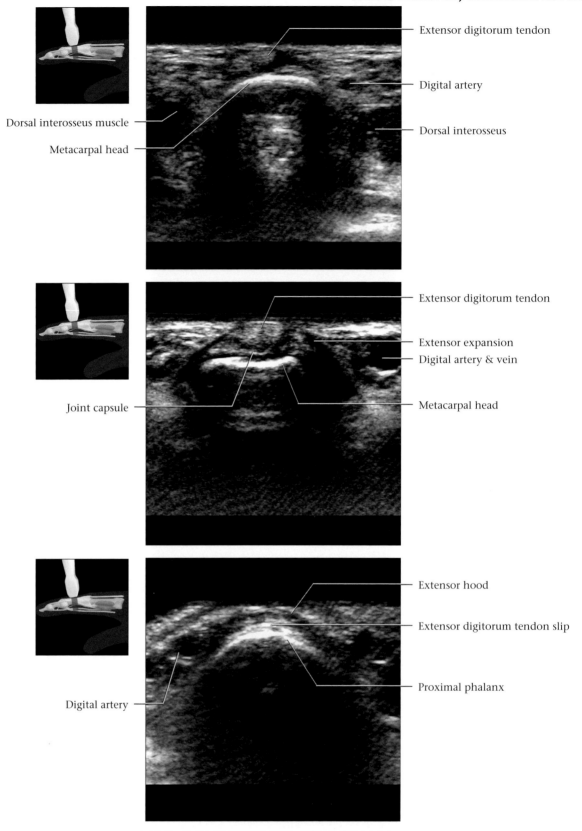

Top image labels:
- Extensor digitorum tendon
- Digital artery
- Dorsal interosseus
- Dorsal interosseus muscle
- Metacarpal head

Middle image labels:
- Extensor digitorum tendon
- Extensor expansion
- Digital artery & vein
- Metacarpal head
- Joint capsule

Bottom image labels:
- Extensor hood
- Extensor digitorum tendon slip
- Proximal phalanx
- Digital artery

(Top) Transverse grayscale ultrasound at the metacarpal head/neck region of the extensor aspect of the fingers. The extensor tendons of the hand do not have a complete synovial sheath. They are covered by thin paratenon. The tendons have an ovoid configuration. (Middle) Transverse grayscale ultrasound at the extensor aspect of the fingers at the metacarpal head region. At the proximal phalanx extending over the middle phalanx, the extensor tendons spread out and connect to the extensor expansion or hood. (Bottom) Transverse grayscale ultrasound of the extensor aspect of the fingers at the proximal phalanx level. With expansion of the extensor tendon it becomes very thin such that the normal tendon is difficult to illustrate on the dorsum of the fingers. If injured, it is usually more readily seen.

FINGERS

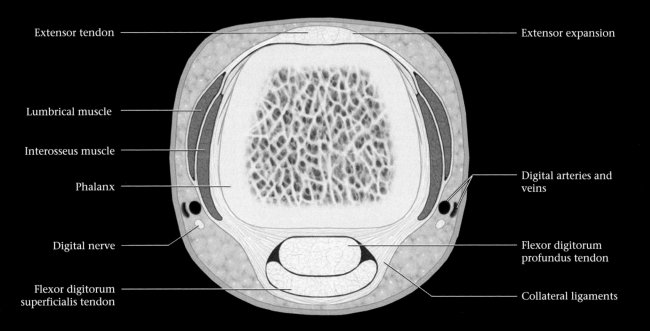

Extensor tendon · Extensor expansion · Lumbrical muscle · Interosseus muscle · Phalanx · Digital arteries and veins · Digital nerve · Flexor digitorum profundus tendon · Flexor digitorum superficialis tendon · Collateral ligaments

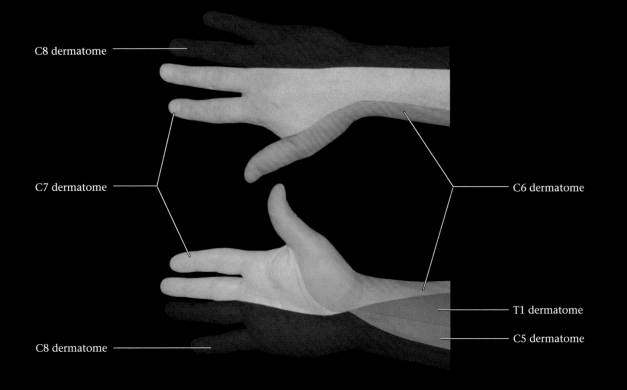

C8 dermatome · C7 dermatome · C6 dermatome · T1 dermatome · C5 dermatome · C8 dermatome

(Top) Graphic shows the transverse section of a finger depicting the relationships of the digital nerve, vessels, tendons to the phalanx. (Bottom) Dermatomes of hand and wrist correlated to corresponding cervical or thoracic nerves.

RADIAL NERVE

Terminology

Abbreviations
- Extensor digitorum (ED)
- Extensor carpi radialis brevis (ECRB)
- Extensor digiti minimi (EDM)
- Extensor carpi ulnaris (ECU)
- Extensor pollicis longus (EPL)
- Abductor pollicis longus (APL)
- Extensor indicis (EI)

Gross Anatomy

Arm
- Radial nerve is largest branch of posterior cord of brachial plexus
  - It receives contributions from cervical roots C5 → C8
  - Contains motor & sensory components that supply muscles of extensor compartments of arm, forearm & hand
- Lies between coracobrachialis & teres major muscles, & then between bellies of medial & lateral head of triceps
- Runs deep to triceps in spiral groove & then deep to brachioradialis
- Approximately 10 cm proximal to lateral epicondyle of humerus, radial nerve penetrates lateral intermuscular septum to enter anterior space of upper arm
- Just anterior to lateral epicondyle, nerve bifurcates into sensory (superficial branch of radial nerve) & motor (deep branch of radial nerve & posterior interosseous nerve) components

Forearm
- Branches of radial nerve
  - Divides at level of lateral epicondyle
  - Superficial
    - Purely sensory
    - Direct continuation of radial nerve
    - Courses distally, deep to brachioradialis, → posterior compartment distal forearm → dorsal wrist
    - Divides into lateral branch (supplies radial wrist & thumb skin) & medial branch (supplies mid & ulnar wrist skin)
    - Dorsal digital nerves supply ulnar thumb, index, middle & radial ring fingers
  - Deep
    - Purely motor
    - Enters supinator → exits distally → runs posteriorly as posterior interosseous nerve
    - Supplies ECRB, supinator, ED, EDM, ECU, EPL, APL & EL

Hand: Branches of Radial Nerve
- Not usually seen on routine imaging
- No motor innervation in hand
- Sensory: Dorsal surface from radiocarpal joint to just distal to proximal interphalangeal joints for digits 1-3 & radial 1/2 of 4th digit
  - Gives terminal branches to supply skin of lateral 2/3 of dorsum of wrist, hand & lateral 2 1/2 fingers

Anatomy-Based Imaging Issues

Imaging Recommendations
- Use high frequency ± 7.5 MHz transducer
- Radial nerve is best identified at lateral aspect distal arm where it runs deep to brachialis
  - Identified deep to triceps in spiral groove mid-humeral level
  - Or in proximal aspect arm medially
    - Lies just deep to brachial artery
- Assess shape, size, echotexture & integrity of nerve
  - Trace medium-sized branches by following their course as they branch from parent nerve
- Examination of nerves along transverse plane is preferable to longitudinal scanning because it allows following nerves continuously throughout limb

Imaging Approaches
- Ultrasound
  - Nerve echotexture
    - Transverse: Uniformly dispersed hypoechoic dots (nerve fascicles) separated by hyperechoic epineurium
    - Longitudinal: Parallel hypoechoic tracts of uniform caliber
    - Overall gain control & focus settings optimized for adequate visualization of nerve

Imaging Pitfalls
- Smaller nerves & nerve branches (1-2 mm) are difficult to identify & their location may only be inferred by adjacent vessels
- Anisotropy artifacts may affect scanning, especially in short axis; tilting transducer during scanning helps to achieve best view
- Structural compression is easier to appreciate than functional compression

Clinical Implications

Clinical Importance
- Sites of nerve entrapment of radial nerve
  - Lateral to long head of triceps due to fibrous arch
  - Spiral groove between medial and lateral heads of triceps muscle due to fibrous arch, fractures, tourniquet
  - Between brachialis and brachioradialis muscles at antecubital fossa due to muscle (body builders)
  - Posterior interosseous nerve by arcade of Frohse (superficial proximal margin of supinator) due to recurrent radial artery (leash of Henry) crossing just proximal to arcade
  - Posterior interosseous nerve between deep & superficial heads of supinator muscle (supinator syndrome)
  - Superficial radial nerve between brachioradialis and ECRL in mid to distal forearm (Wartenberg syndrome)

GRAPHICS

Posterior cord

Axillary nerve

Nerve to triceps muscle

Lower lateral cutaneous nerve of arm

Superficial terminal branch of radial nerve

Radial nerve

Nerve to anconeus

Supinator

Posterior interosseus nerve

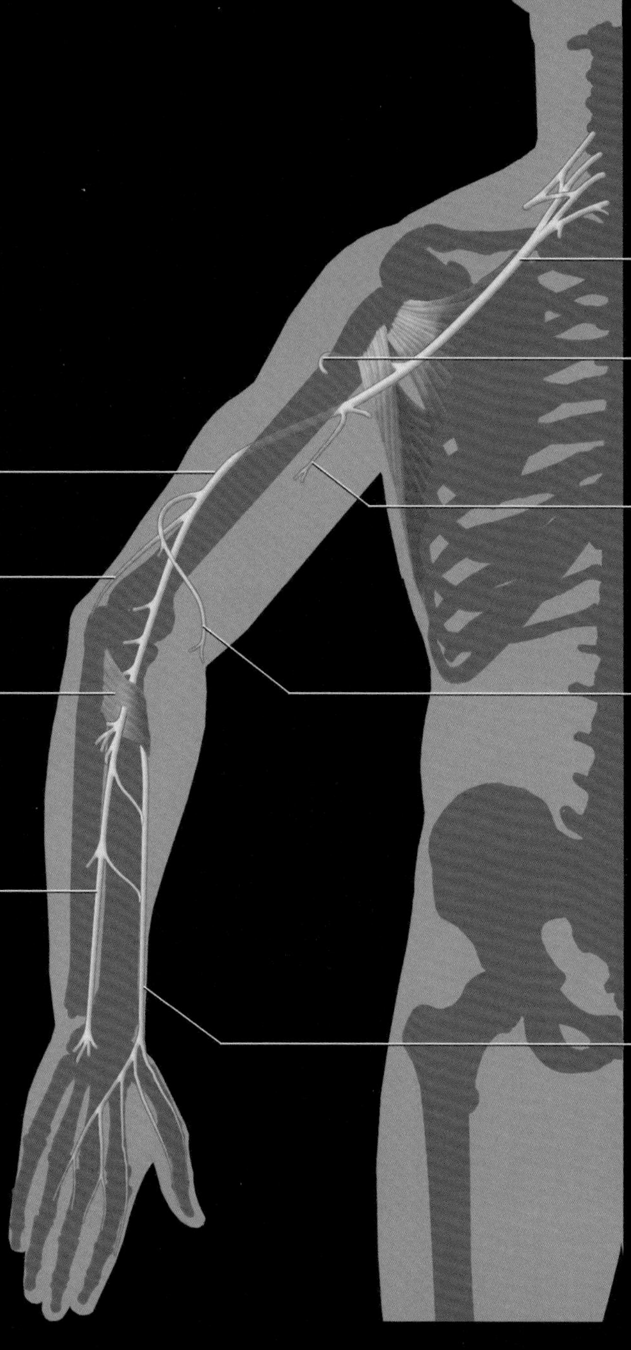

Graphic shows the course and distribution of the radial nerve. The radial nerve arises from the posterior cord of the brachial plexus (C5-8, T1). It spirals posterolaterally around the humerus with the deep brachial artery located anterolateral between the brachialis and the brachioradialis. It gives off the posterior cutaneous nerve of the forearm, which passes posterior to the lateral condyle and supplies the posterior forearm. It divides into deep and superficial branches at the lateral epicondyle. The deep branch is purely motor and it pierces the supinator muscle and winds around the lateral aspect of the radial neck. The superficial branch is purely sensory and is located in the anterolateral aspect of the forearm, superficial to the supinator and pronator teres muscles.

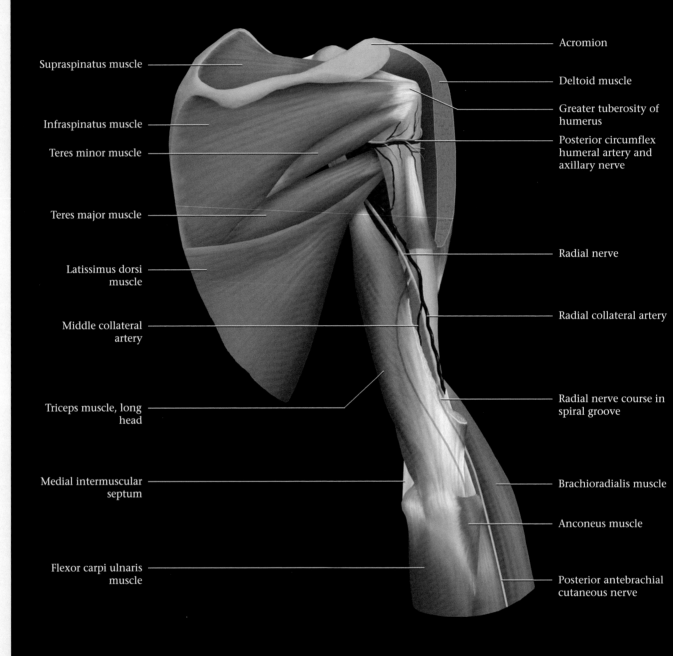

Supraspinatus muscle

Infraspinatus muscle

Teres minor muscle

Teres major muscle

Latissimus dorsi muscle

Middle collateral artery

Triceps muscle, long head

Medial intermuscular septum

Flexor carpi ulnaris muscle

Acromion

Deltoid muscle

Greater tuberosity of humerus

Posterior circumflex humeral artery and axillary nerve

Radial nerve

Radial collateral artery

Radial nerve course in spiral groove

Brachioradialis muscle

Anconeus muscle

Posterior antebrachial cutaneous nerve

Graphic shows the course of the radial nerve in the posterior aspect of the arm. The radial nerve spirals posterolaterally around the humerus with the deep brachial artery. It gives off the posterior cutaneous nerve of the forearm, which passes posterior to the lateral condyle and supplies the posterior forearm. It is located anterolaterally, between the brachialis and brachioradialis, where it supplies the triceps, anconeus, brachioradialis and the lateral portion of the brachialis.

RADIAL NERVE

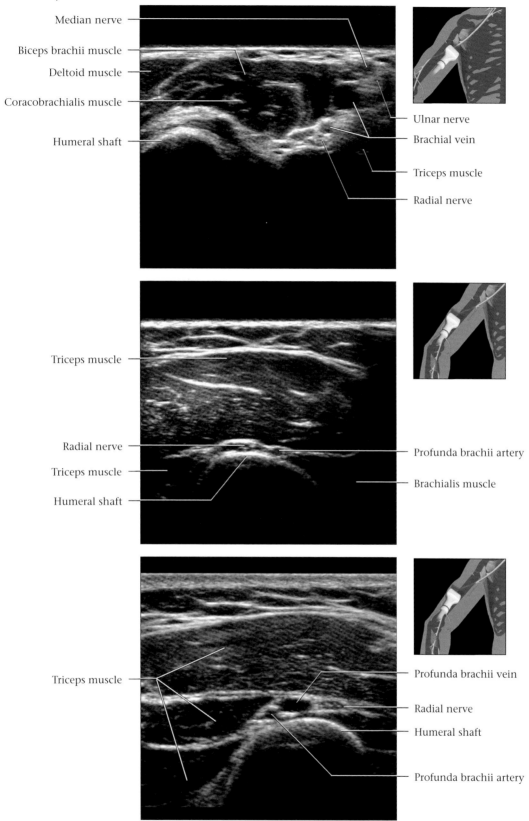

Median nerve

Biceps brachii muscle

Deltoid muscle

Coracobrachialis muscle

Humeral shaft

Ulnar nerve

Brachial vein

Triceps muscle

Radial nerve

Triceps muscle

Radial nerve

Triceps muscle

Humeral shaft

Profunda brachii artery

Brachialis muscle

Triceps muscle

Profunda brachii vein

Radial nerve

Humeral shaft

Profunda brachii artery

(Top) Transverse grayscale ultrasound section of the radial nerve in the proximal third of the arm. The radial nerve is a continuation of the posterior cord of the brachial plexus. It supplies the triceps and the supinator. In the proximal arm it lies deep to the brachial artery and vein. (Middle) Transverse grayscale ultrasound shows the radial nerve at the mid-third of the arm. The radial nerve may be injured as it passes around the posterior aspect of the mid to distal third of the humeral shaft. This injury may occur at the time of fracture, during fracture manipulation or fixation or as a result of post-operative fibrosis. (Bottom) Transverse grayscale ultrasound of the radial nerve at the mid-third of the arm (coned view). The radial nerve is accompanied in the spiral groove by the profunda brachii artery and vein.

RADIAL NERVE

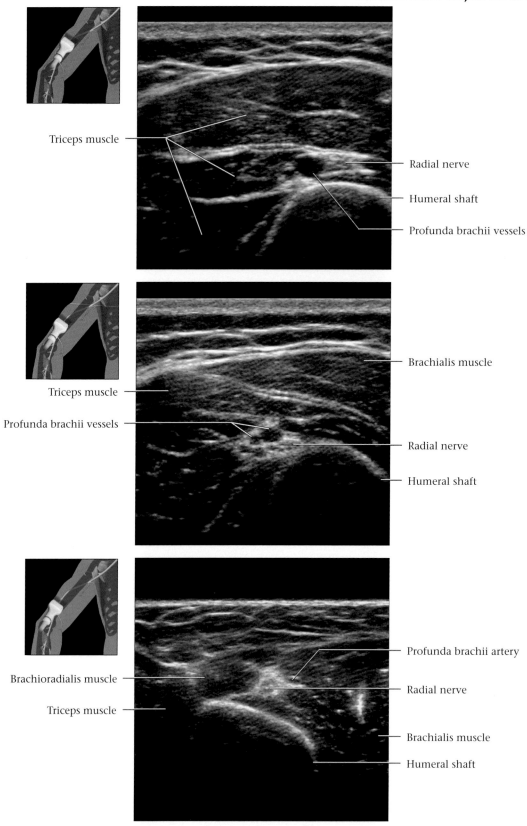

Triceps muscle

Radial nerve

Humeral shaft

Profunda brachii vessels

Brachialis muscle

Triceps muscle

Profunda brachii vessels

Radial nerve

Humeral shaft

Profunda brachii artery

Brachioradialis muscle

Radial nerve

Triceps muscle

Brachialis muscle

Humeral shaft

(Top) Transverse grayscale ultrasound of the radial nerve in the mid-part of the spiral groove (coned view). The surgeon must be aware of the site of the radial nerve when performing fixation of the humerus as the fixator screws or plate may potentially damage the radial nerve. (Middle) Transverse grayscale ultrasound of the radial nerve in the distal aspect of the spiral groove, mid-humerus. (Bottom) Transverse grayscale ultrasound of the radial nerve at the distal third of the arm. The radial nerve passes from the posterior to anterior compartment by piercing the lateral intermuscular septum. Compression of the radial nerve at the lateral intermuscular septum may occur. In very muscular individuals, the radial nerve may be compressed between the brachioradialis and brachialis muscles.

RADIAL NERVE

TRANSVERSE US, POSTERIOR FOREARM

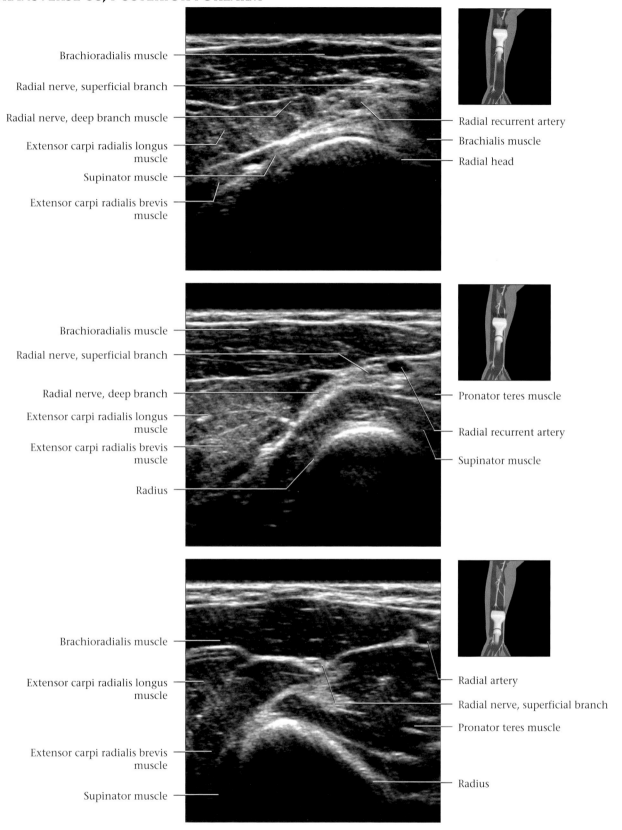

Brachioradialis muscle

Radial nerve, superficial branch

Radial nerve, deep branch muscle

Extensor carpi radialis longus muscle

Supinator muscle

Extensor carpi radialis brevis muscle

Radial recurrent artery

Brachialis muscle

Radial head

Brachioradialis muscle

Radial nerve, superficial branch

Radial nerve, deep branch

Extensor carpi radialis longus muscle

Extensor carpi radialis brevis muscle

Radius

Pronator teres muscle

Radial recurrent artery

Supinator muscle

Brachioradialis muscle

Extensor carpi radialis longus muscle

Extensor carpi radialis brevis muscle

Supinator muscle

Radial artery

Radial nerve, superficial branch

Pronator teres muscle

Radius

(Top) Transverse grayscale ultrasound shows the radial nerve course in the proximal forearm. The radial nerve passes in front of the lateral epicondyle. It can be readily identified deep to brachioradialis muscle. In the region of the radial head, it divides into superficial and deep branches. The radial nerve is prone to compression between the radial head and the supinator muscle (radial tunnel syndrome). (Middle) Transverse grayscale ultrasound of the radial nerve at the proximal forearm. The superficial branch of the radial nerve continues to descend in the forearm deep to the brachioradialis muscle. The deep branch pierces the supinator muscle, after which it is known as the posterior interosseus nerve. (Bottom) Transverse grayscale ultrasound of the radial nerve in the mid-forearm. The deep branch of the radial nerve may be compressed as it passes through the supinator muscle (arcade of Frohse).

RADIAL NERVE

Extensor digiti minimi muscle

Extensor digitorum muscle

Radial nerve deep branch

Extensor carpi radialis brevis muscle

Radial recurrent artery

Radius

Extensor pollicis longus muscle

Ulna

Brachioradialis muscle

Flexor digitorum superficialis muscle

Flexor digitorum profundus muscle

Radial nerve, superficial branch

Radial shaft

Extensor carpi radialis longus muscle

Interosseus membrane

Radial nerve, superficial branch

Extensor digiti minimi muscle

Extensor carpi ulnaris muscle

Extensor indicis muscle

Ulna

(Top) Transverse grayscale ultrasound of the deep branch of the radial nerve in the distal forearm. (Middle) Transverse grayscale ultrasound of the superficial branch of the radial nerve in the distal forearm. About 8 cm proximal to the radial styloid, the superficial branch of the radial nerve emerges from underneath the brachioradialis to lie between the brachioradialis and the extensor carpi radialis longus. It may be compressed in this location (Wartenberg syndrome). (Bottom) Transverse grayscale ultrasound of the superficial branch of the radial nerve in the forearm.

RADIAL NERVE

GRAPHICS

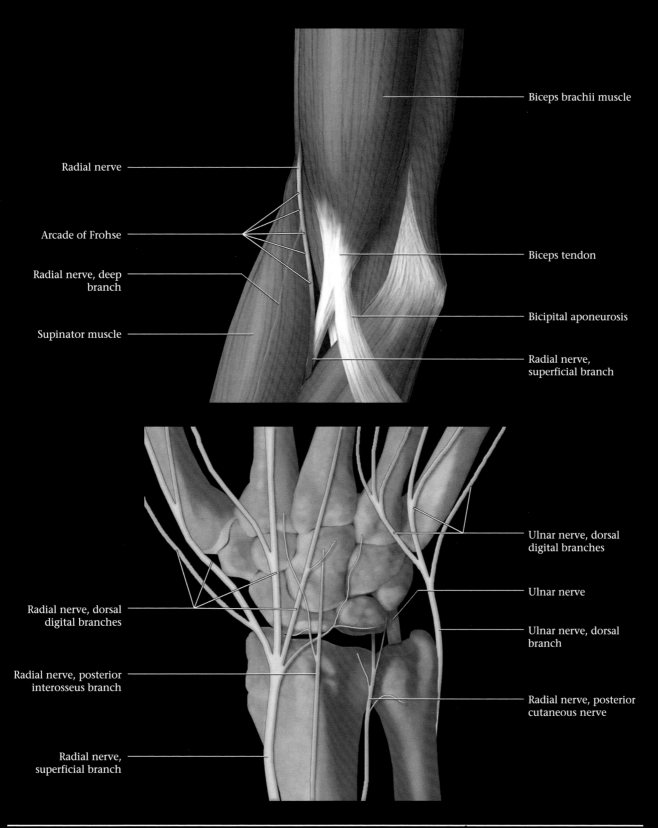

Radial nerve

Arcade of Frohse

Radial nerve, deep branch

Supinator muscle

Biceps brachii muscle

Biceps tendon

Bicipital aponeurosis

Radial nerve, superficial branch

Radial nerve, dorsal digital branches

Radial nerve, posterior interosseus branch

Radial nerve, superficial branch

Ulnar nerve, dorsal digital branches

Ulnar nerve

Ulnar nerve, dorsal branch

Radial nerve, posterior cutaneous nerve

(Top) Graphic shows the radial nerve course at the anterolateral aspect of the elbow. The deep branch of the radial nerve is prone for impingement at the superficial proximal margin of the supinator muscle (arcade of Frohse) resulting in posterior interosseus nerve syndrome. **(Bottom)** Graphic shows the nerves of the dorsal wrist. The radial nerve branches in the forearm with the superficial, posterior cutaneous and posterior interosseus branches serving the wrist and hand. The ulnar nerve provides branches to the dorsal and volar wrist.

MEDIAN NERVE

Terminology

Abbreviations
- Flexor digitorum profundus (FDP)
- Flexor digitorum superficialis (FDS)
- Flexor carpi ulnaris (FCU)
- Flexor pollicis longus (FPL)
- Pronator quadratus (PQ)
- Palmaris longus (PL)

Gross Anatomy

Arm: Median Nerve
- Arises from both medial & lateral cords of brachial plexus (C6-8, T1)
- Lies medial to brachial artery & vein
- Located deep to biceps aponeurosis in cubital fossa
- Gives articular branches to elbow joint
- Supplies pronator teres, pronator quadratus & flexors of anterior compartment forearm (except FCU, medial half of FDP which are supplied by ulnar nerve)

Forearm: Median Nerve and Branches
- Enters forearm by passing between heads of pronator teres, & located in forearm between FDP & FDS
  - Courses distally attached to deep surface of FDS by a fascial sheath
  - Anterior interosseus nerve
    - Arises from median nerve at level of pronator teres
    - Located in forearm anterior to interosseus membrane, between FPL & FDP
- At wrist, median nerve emerges from lateral side of FDS → becomes more superficial & runs deep to PL tendon towards carpal tunnel
  - Supplies FPL, PQ & lateral half of FDP

Wrist & Hand: Median Nerve and Branches
- Median nerve lies along axis of ring finger, i.e., to the ulnar side of midline
- Lies superficial to antebrachial fascia & palmaris longus before dipping deeply to enter carpal tunnel
- At distal radio-ulnar joint: Nerve is rounded; deep to PL, medial & superficial to FCR & FPL, lateral & superficial to FDS
- Carpal tunnel = fibro-osseous tunnel located immediately distal to volar wrist crease
  - Formed by carpal bones & flexor retinaculum (transverse carpal ligament)
  - Flexor retinaculum attaches pisiform, hook of hamate, scaphoid and trapezium
  - Nine structures pass through carpal tunnel
    - Four FDS tendons, four FDP tendons, FPL tendon & median nerve
    - Median nerve located superficially just deep to retinaculum
  - Narrowest part of carpal tunnel = tunnel outlet
- Branches
  - Motor to thenar & 1st & 2nd lumbrical muscles
  - Sensory to radial half of palm, radial 3½ digits
    - Palmar cutaneous branch arises proximal to carpal tunnel though variable
  - Median nerve divides just distal to carpal tunnel

Anatomy-Based Imaging Issues

Imaging Recommendations
- Examination of nerve in transverse plane is preferable to longitudinal scanning since it allows the nerve to be followed continuously throughout limb
- Use proximal & distal borders of retinaculum as markers of carpal tunnel

Imaging Approaches
- Ultrasound
  - Use high frequency ± 7.5 MHz transducer

Imaging Pitfalls
- Median nerve may be bifid
  - If quantifying size of nerve, both components should be measured & summated
- Angle transducer at right angle to nerve if possible as angulation will ↑ nerve caliber
  - May need to make use of anisotropy to best differentiate nerve from tendons in carpal tunnel
- Avoid too much transducer pressure as this will ↓ nerve caliber
- Median nerve may be difficult to see at tunnel outlet in subjects with thick palmar skin

Clinical Implications

Clinical Importance
- Normal cross-sectional area of median nerve ranges 3.9-9.0 mm²
  - Mean fascicular diameter ranges 0.3-0.5 mm
  - Nerve thickening and enlargement of the fascicles is considered if size changes beyond the above mentioned limits (e.g., > 10 mm² cross-sectional area and > 0.6 mm fascicular diameter in Charcot-Marie-Tooth disease)
- Sites of medial nerve compression
  - Deep to ligament of Struthers
    - Ligament between medial epicondyle & anomalous bony spur arising from distal humeral diaphysis (present in 1% population)
    - May compress median nerve or brachial artery or both
  - Between brachialis and bicipital aponeurosis
    - Bicipital aponeurosis = medial fascial expansion of biceps tendon that extends superficial to brachial artery & median nerve and merges with investing fascia forearm
  - Between heads of pronator teres
    - Either medial nerve or anterior interosseus nerve may be compressed
  - Carpal tunnel
    - Carpal tunnel syndrome = pain, paresthesia, numbness due to compression of nerve in carpal tunnel
    - Most common compressive neuropathy
    - Nerve swollen proximal to inlet ± at inlet ± at outlet ± distal to outlet
    - Should not use opposite side as comparative standard as subclinical compression common

GRAPHICS

Lateral cord of
brachial plexus

Musculocutaneous
nerve

Biceps brachii muscle

Pronator teres

Lateral cutaneous
nerve of forearm

Anterior interosseus
nerve

Nerves to thenar
muscles

Medial cord of
brachial plexus

Median nerve in arm

Lateral cutaneous
nerve of forearm

Bicipital aponeurosis

Median nerve in
forearm

Digital branches of
median nerve

Graphic shows the course and distribution of the median and musculocutaneous nerves. The median nerve arises
from the medial and lateral cords of the brachial plexus (C6-8, T1). It travels together with other nerves of the arm.
In the elbow it is located deep to the biceps aponeurosis, enters the forearm by passing between the heads of the
pronator teres, and located in the forearm between flexor digitorum superficialis and profundus muscles. The
musculocutaneous nerve arises from the lateral cord of brachial plexus (C5, 6, 7). It lies between the brachialis and
biceps brachii muscles and supplies both of them and then becomes superficial at the elbow, continuing laterally as
the lateral cutaneous nerve of the forearm which innervates the skin of the lateral side of the forearm.

MEDIAN NERVE

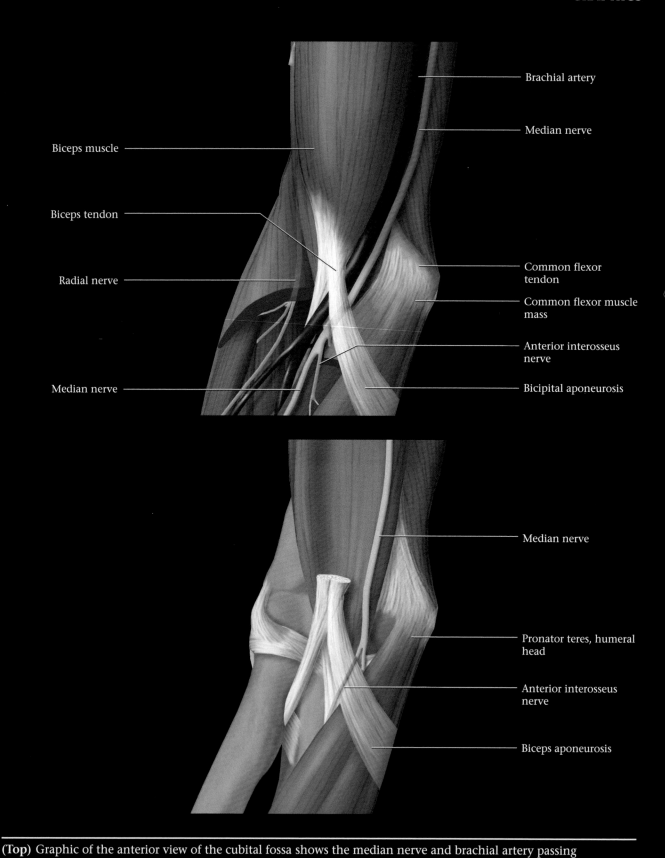

Brachial artery

Median nerve

Biceps muscle

Biceps tendon

Radial nerve

Common flexor tendon

Common flexor muscle mass

Anterior interosseus nerve

Median nerve

Bicipital aponeurosis

Median nerve

Pronator teres, humeral head

Anterior interosseus nerve

Biceps aponeurosis

(Top) Graphic of the anterior view of the cubital fossa shows the median nerve and brachial artery passing underneath the biceps aponeurosis. The anterior interosseus nerve arises from the median nerve as the median nerve passes between two heads of the pronator teres muscle. **(Bottom)** The median nerve may be entrapped between two heads of the pronator teres muscle or by the overlying biceps aponeurosis. The median nerve gives the articular branches to the elbow joint. It supplies the pronator teres, pronator quadratus, and flexors of the anterior compartment of the forearm (except the flexor carpi ulnaris and medial half of the flexor digitorum profundus which are supplied by the ulnar nerve).

MEDIAN NERVE

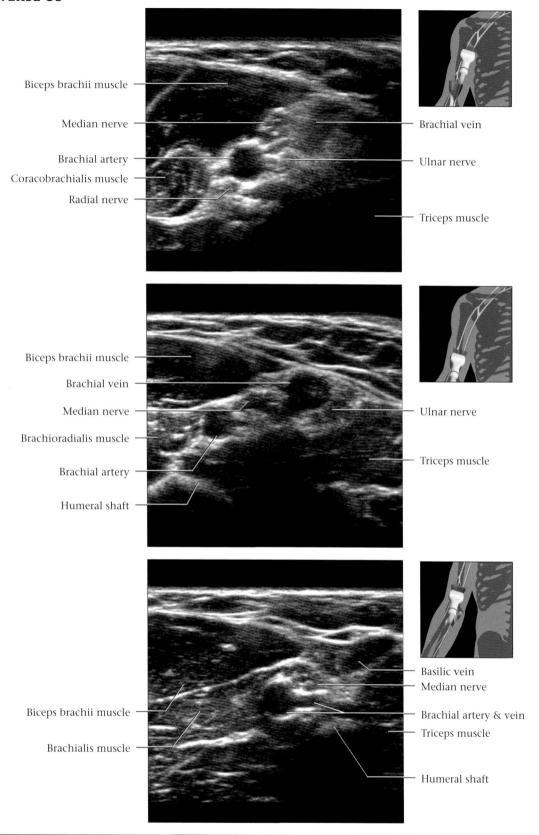

Biceps brachii muscle

Median nerve

Brachial artery
Coracobrachialis muscle
Radial nerve

Brachial vein

Ulnar nerve

Triceps muscle

Biceps brachii muscle

Brachial vein

Median nerve

Brachioradialis muscle

Brachial artery

Humeral shaft

Ulnar nerve

Triceps muscle

Basilic vein
Median nerve

Biceps brachii muscle

Brachialis muscle

Brachial artery & vein
Triceps muscle

Humeral shaft

(Top) Transverse grayscale ultrasound of the median nerve at the proximal arm. The median nerve arises from the lateral and medial cords of the brachial plexus. In the proximal arm it lies just lateral to the brachial vein and artery. **(Middle)** Transverse grayscale ultrasound section of the median nerve of the mid-arm. Little happens to the median nerve in the upper to mid-arm. It gives off no branches and is not prone to compression by normal structures. **(Bottom)** Transverse grayscale ultrasound of the median nerve distal arm. The median nerve passes over the brachial artery and vein from lateral to medial. There is occasionally a ligament (of Struther) in the distal arm (± bony spur) attached to the humerus about 5 cm proximal to the medial epicondyle. Pronator teres gains additional attachment from this ligament. The medial nerve may be compressed deep to this ligament.

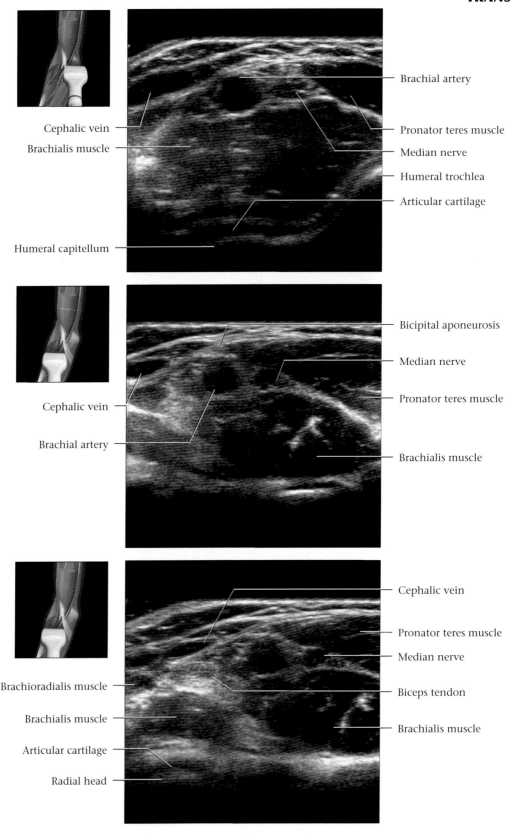

Brachial artery

Cephalic vein

Brachialis muscle

Pronator teres muscle

Median nerve

Humeral trochlea

Articular cartilage

Humeral capitellum

Bicipital aponeurosis

Median nerve

Cephalic vein

Brachial artery

Pronator teres muscle

Brachialis muscle

Cephalic vein

Pronator teres muscle

Median nerve

Brachioradialis muscle

Brachialis muscle

Biceps tendon

Articular cartilage

Brachialis muscle

Radial head

(Top) Transverse grayscale US of median nerve at the distal arm. Median nerve travels deep to the bicipital aponeurosis: A fascial aponeurosis (also known as lacertus fibrosis) arises from the biceps musculotendinous junction & inserts into the antebrachial fascia. The median nerve may be compressed deep to this fascia. **(Middle)** Transverse grayscale US of median nerve at the elbow region. **(Bottom)** Transverse grayscale US of median nerve at the proximal forearm. Median nerve is also prone to compression between two heads of pronator teres muscle (i.e. common flexor origin head & coronoid process head). Median nerve branches as it passes through these heads (giving rise to the anterior interosseus nerve) & may be compressed at this location (pronator teres syndrome). Pain in forearm or hand occurs with either prolonged forearm pronation or recurrent pronation & supination of forearm.

MEDIAN NERVE

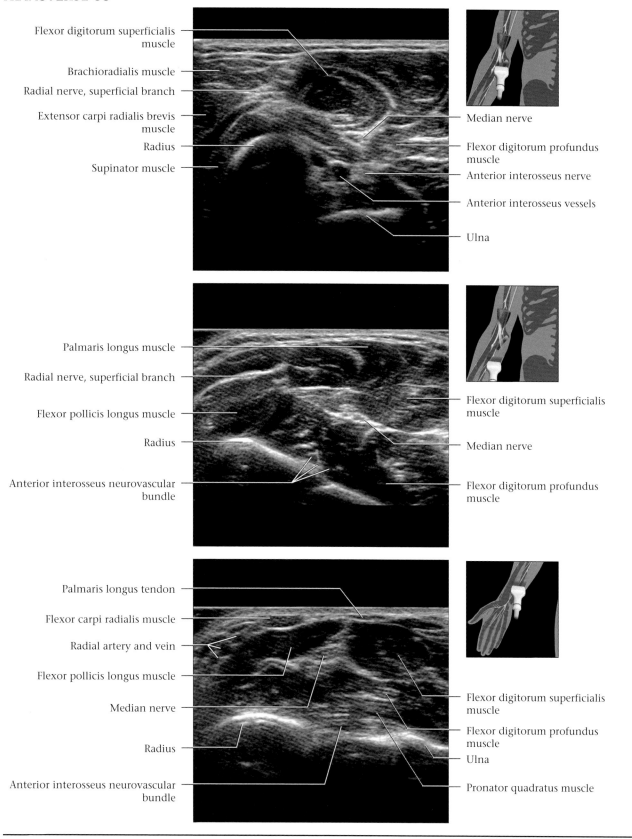

Flexor digitorum superficialis muscle

Brachioradialis muscle

Radial nerve, superficial branch

Extensor carpi radialis brevis muscle

Radius

Supinator muscle

Median nerve

Flexor digitorum profundus muscle

Anterior interosseus nerve

Anterior interosseus vessels

Ulna

Palmaris longus muscle

Radial nerve, superficial branch

Flexor pollicis longus muscle

Radius

Anterior interosseus neurovascular bundle

Flexor digitorum superficialis muscle

Median nerve

Flexor digitorum profundus muscle

Palmaris longus tendon

Flexor carpi radialis muscle

Radial artery and vein

Flexor pollicis longus muscle

Median nerve

Radius

Anterior interosseus neurovascular bundle

Flexor digitorum superficialis muscle

Flexor digitorum profundus muscle

Ulna

Pronator quadratus muscle

(Top) Transverse grayscale ultrasound of the median nerve proximal forearm. The anterior interosseus nerve supplies all the muscles of the anterior compartment of the forearm except the ulnar half of the flexor digitorum profundus muscle. It may be injured with fracture of the radial shaft. **(Middle)** Transverse grayscale ultrasound of the median nerve mid-forearm. The median nerve is clearly identified in the mid distal forearm as it travels between the flexor digitorum superficialis and profundus muscles. **(Bottom)** Transverse grayscale ultrasound of the median nerve distal forearm.

MEDIAN NERVE

Top image labels:
- Flexor carpi radialis tendon
- Palmaris longus tendon
- Flexor digitorum superficialis muscle
- Flexor carpi ulnaris muscle
- Median nerve
- Flexor digitorum profundus tendon
- Pronator quadratus muscle
- Radial artery and vein
- Flexor pollicis longus muscle

Middle image labels:
- Flexor carpi radialis tendon
- Palmaris longus tendon
- Flexor digitorum superficialis muscle
- Flexor carpi ulnaris muscle
- Flexor digitorum profundus muscle
- Pronator quadratus muscle
- Anterior interosseus neurovascular bundle
- Ulna
- Radial artery
- Flexor pollicis longus muscle
- Radius
- Median nerve

Bottom image labels:
- Flexor carpi radialis muscle
- Palmaris longus tendon
- Flexor digitorum superficialis muscle
- Median nerve
- Flexor digitorum profundus muscle
- Radius
- Radial artery and vein
- Flexor pollicis longus muscle

(Top) Transverse grayscale ultrasound of the median nerve in the distal forearm. **(Middle)** Transverse grayscale ultrasound of the median nerve just proximal to the wrist. The median nerve gives off the palmar cutaneous branch in the distal forearm. This branch innervates the skin on the palm of the hand. **(Bottom)** Transverse grayscale ultrasound of the median nerve just proximal to the carpal tunnel. Just proximal to the carpal tunnel, the median nerve ascends from a deeper position (between the flexor digitorum profundus and superficialis) to lie just deep to palmaris longus tendon. Enlargement of the median nerve in patients with carpal tunnel syndrome may present clinically as a mass-like lesion in this area. In suspected carpal tunnel syndrome the caliber of the nerve should be measured at this location.

MEDIAN NERVE

TRANSVERSE US, CARPAL TUNNEL

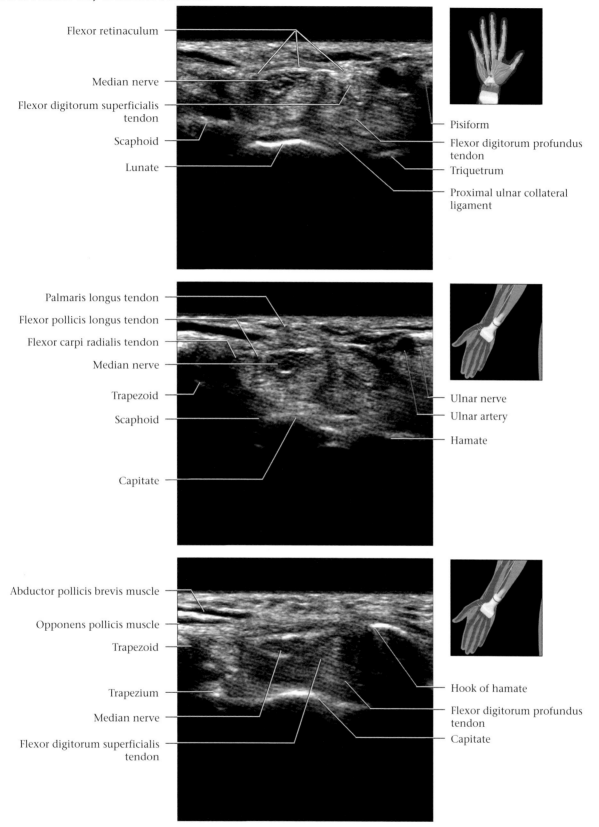

Top image labels:
- Flexor retinaculum
- Median nerve
- Flexor digitorum superficialis tendon
- Scaphoid
- Lunate
- Pisiform
- Flexor digitorum profundus tendon
- Triquetrum
- Proximal ulnar collateral ligament

Middle image labels:
- Palmaris longus tendon
- Flexor pollicis longus tendon
- Flexor carpi radialis tendon
- Median nerve
- Trapezoid
- Scaphoid
- Capitate
- Ulnar nerve
- Ulnar artery
- Hamate

Bottom image labels:
- Abductor pollicis brevis muscle
- Opponens pollicis muscle
- Trapezoid
- Trapezium
- Median nerve
- Flexor digitorum superficialis tendon
- Hook of hamate
- Flexor digitorum profundus tendon
- Capitate

(Top) Transverse grayscale ultrasound of the median nerve at the carpal tunnel inlet. The best way to identify the carpal tunnel is to identify the leading and trailing edges of the flexor retinaculum. The median nerve dips deep to the retinaculum. The cross-sectional area should be measured at this location in suspected carpal tunnel syndrome. (Middle) Transverse grayscale ultrasound of the median nerve at the mid-carpal tunnel. The median nerve lies just deep to the retinaculum. It is variable in shape and changes with flexor tendon movement. (Bottom) Transverse grayscale ultrasound of median nerve at carpal tunnel outlet. The cross sectional area of the median nerve should also be measured at this location in patients with suspected carpal tunnel syndrome. This is the narrowest part of the carpal tunnel.

MEDIAN NERVE

Opponens pollicis muscle

Abductor pollicis brevis muscle

Palmar aponeurosis

Ulnar artery

Opponens digiti minimi

Branches of median nerve

Flexor digitorum profundus tendon

Flexor digitorum superficialis tendon

Adductor pollicis muscle

Flexor pollicis brevis muscle

Flexor pollicis longus tendon

Flexor retinaculum

Median nerve

Flexor tendons

Radius

Lunate

Capitate

Flexor digitorum superficialis

Median nerve

Flexor digitorum profundus

(Top) Transverse grayscale ultrasound of the median nerve just beyond the carpal tunnel outlet. The median nerve fairly consistently divides into its digital branches just beyond the tunnel outlet. This makes it difficult to get consistent results for nerve caliber at this location. **(Middle)** Longitudinal grayscale ultrasound of the median nerve in the carpal tunnel. **(Bottom)** Longitudinal grayscale ultrasound of the median nerve in the distal forearm.

GRAPHICS, PALMAR NERVES

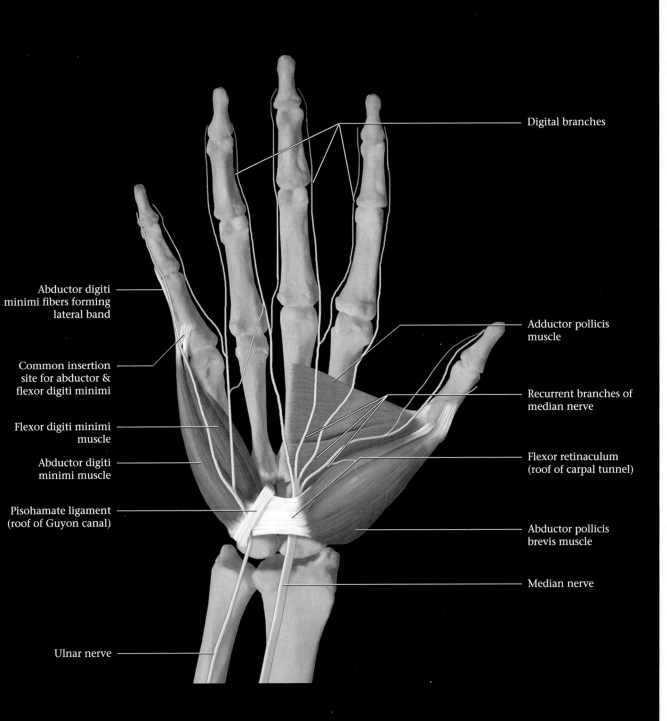

Digital branches

Abductor digiti minimi fibers forming lateral band

Common insertion site for abductor & flexor digiti minimi

Flexor digiti minimi muscle

Abductor digiti minimi muscle

Pisohamate ligament (roof of Guyon canal)

Ulnar nerve

Adductor pollicis muscle

Recurrent branches of median nerve

Flexor retinaculum (roof of carpal tunnel)

Abductor pollicis brevis muscle

Median nerve

The median nerve travels deep to the flexor retinaculum (within the carpal tunnel). The ulnar nerve travels superficial to the flexor retinaculum & deep to the pisohamate ligament (within the Guyon canal). Both are prone to compression syndromes within these fibroosseous tunnels. Motor supply of the median nerve is to the thenars (via recurrent branch) & 1st & 2nd lumbricals. The ulnar nerve motor supply is to all intrinsic muscles of the hand not supplied by the median nerve. Muscle atrophy should prompt an evaluation of the supplying nerve.

ULNAR NERVE

Terminology

Abbreviations
- Flexor carpi ulnaris (FCU)
- Flexor digitorum profundus (FDP)

Gross Anatomy

Arm: Ulnar Nerve
- Arises from medial cord of brachial plexus (C8, T1)
- Located posteromedially, deep to triceps muscles in distal arm
- Cubital tunnel: Fibro-osseous tunnel formed by medial epicondyle, olecranon & cubital retinaculum (Osborn fascia)
  - Cubital tunnel syndrome: Pain, weakness & numbness 4th & 5th fingers due to compression of ulnar nerve in cubital tunnel
- May sublux anterior to medial epicondyle in 15% normal elbows during flexion

Forearm: Ulnar Nerve and Branches
- Passes behind medial epicondyle, enters forearm between humeral & ulnar heads of FCU
- Courses distally between FCU & FDP
  - Supplies: FCU, medial half of FDP
- Palmar cutaneous branch: Arises mid-forearm & supplies skin on ulnar half of palm
- Dorsal cutaneous branch: Arises distal forearm & supplies skin on ulnar side of dorsum hand
- Distally, becomes superficial & passes into wrist superficial to flexor retinaculum

Hand: Ulnar Nerve and Branches
- In Guyon canal, ulnar nerve lies radial to pisiform & at ulnar & dorsal aspect of ulnar artery
- Enters Guyon canal; small triangular-shaped fibroosseous tunnel
  - Floor = flexor retinaculum; ulnar wall = pisiform & hook of hamate; roof = fascia continuous with flexor retinaculum (superficial palmar ligament)
  - Contains ulnar artery & ulnar nerve
  - Nerve lies between ulnar artery & pisiform or hook of hamate
  - At distal tunnel divides → superficial sensory branch & deep motor branch
    - Superficial branch
    - Sensory to ulnar side of palm, little finger & ulnar 1/2 of ring finger
    - Deep branch → medial to hook of hamate where prone to injury
    - Motor to hypothenar muscles, all interossei, 3rd & 4th lumbricals, & adductor pollicis

Anatomy-Based Imaging Issues

Imaging Recommendations
- Knowledge of nerve location & anatomic relationships is essential for sonographic identification

- Examination of nerves in transverse plane is preferable to longitudinal plane as it allows nerves to be followed continuously throughout limb

Imaging Approaches
- Ultrasound
  - Use of high frequency ± 7.5 MHz transducer
  - Nerve echogenicity
    - Transverse scan: Irregularly dispersed hypoechoic dots, due to nerve fascicles separated by hyperechoic epineurium
    - Longitudinal scan: Parallel hypoechoic tracts of uniform caliber
    - Gain control & focus settings should be optimized for adequate visualization

Imaging Pitfalls
- Smaller nerves & nerve branches (1-2 mm) are difficult to identify & their location may only be inferred by adjacent vessels
- Anisotropy artifacts may affect scanning, especially in short axis; tilting transducer during scanning helps to achieve best view
- Fixed structural causes of nerve compression are more easy to identify than functional structural compression
- Ulnar nerve normally swells to a mild degree in cubital tunnel though not as much as in cubital tunnel syndrome

Clinical Implications

Clinical Importance
- Direct sonographic visualization of nerves can reveal a focal abnormality or injury, differentiate from extraneural tumor, show extent of lesion & relationship to adjacent structures & vessels
- Ulnar nerve prone to compression in cubital tunnel, between humeral and ulnar origins of FCU & in Guyon canal
  - Cubital tunnel syndrome = compression of nerve in cubital tunnel
    - Mostly idiopathic without structural cause being found
    - Nerve swelling in Guyon canal
    - Measure nerve caliber proximal to, within & distal to cubital tunnel
    - Compare with opposite side
  - Guyon canal compression is often structural
    - Due to ganglion cyst at Guyon canal from pisotriquetral joint, fracture hook of hamate, nerve sheath tumor
    - Other causes are occupational neuritis, ulnar artery aneurysm, anomalous muscle, lipoma, laceration, or giant cell tumor of tendon sheath
- Dislocation of ulnar nerve over medial epicondyle can be observed on ultrasound during elbow flexion
  - ± Dislocation of medial triceps muscle belly
  - Repeated dislocation of ulnar nerve may lead to ulnar neuritis & functional impairment

ULNAR NERVE

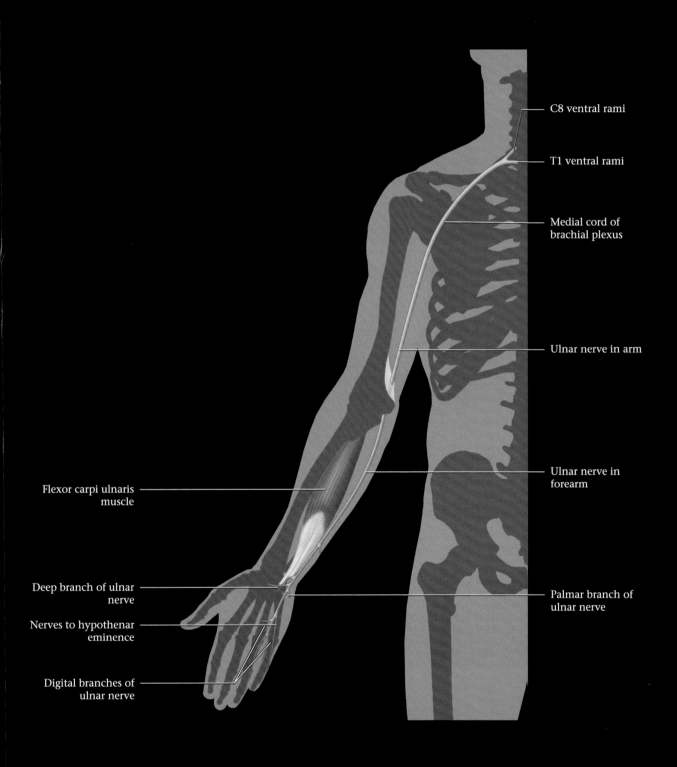

- C8 ventral rami
- T1 ventral rami
- Medial cord of brachial plexus
- Ulnar nerve in arm
- Ulnar nerve in forearm
- Palmar branch of ulnar nerve

- Flexor carpi ulnaris muscle
- Deep branch of ulnar nerve
- Nerves to hypothenar eminence
- Digital branches of ulnar nerve

Graphic shows the course of the ulnar nerve. The ulnar nerve arises from the medial cord of the brachial plexus (C8, T1). It is located posteromedially, deep to the triceps muscles in the distal arm, where it passes posterior to medial epicondyle in the cubital tunnel (cubital syndrome resultant due to compression of ulnar nerve in cubital tunnel). The ulnar nerve may sublux anterior to the medial epicondyle in about 15% of people, usually during flexion. It continues into the forearm by dividing into the superficial and deep heads of the flexor carpi ulnaris. The ulnar nerve supplies the flexor carpi ulnaris and medial half of the flexor digitorum profundus.

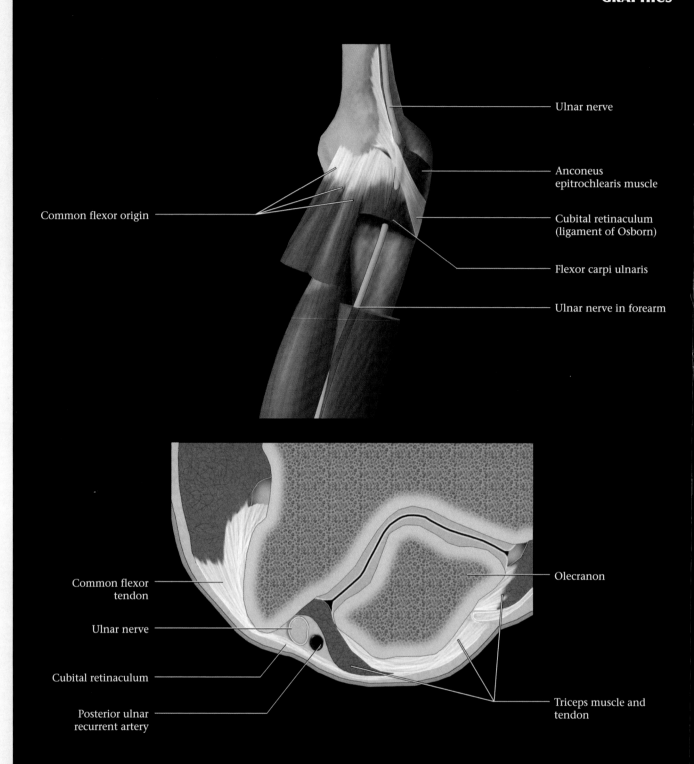

Ulnar nerve

Anconeus epitrochlearis muscle

Common flexor origin

Cubital retinaculum (ligament of Osborn)

Flexor carpi ulnaris

Ulnar nerve in forearm

Common flexor tendon

Olecranon

Ulnar nerve

Cubital retinaculum

Posterior ulnar recurrent artery

Triceps muscle and tendon

(Top) Medial graphic of the cubital tunnel. The anconeus epitrochlearis is an inconstant accessory muscle that is deep to the ulnar nerve and may compress the nerve against the cubital retinaculum. **(Bottom)** Axial graphic of the cubital tunnel. The ulnar nerve may be compressed within the cubital tunnel (cubital tunnel syndrome) by a mass, post-traumatic osseus deformity, or aneurysm of the recurrent ulnar artery. The ulnar nerve may also be subluxed out of the cubital tunnel by the adjacent medial head of the triceps.

ULNAR NERVE

TRANSVERSE US, ARM

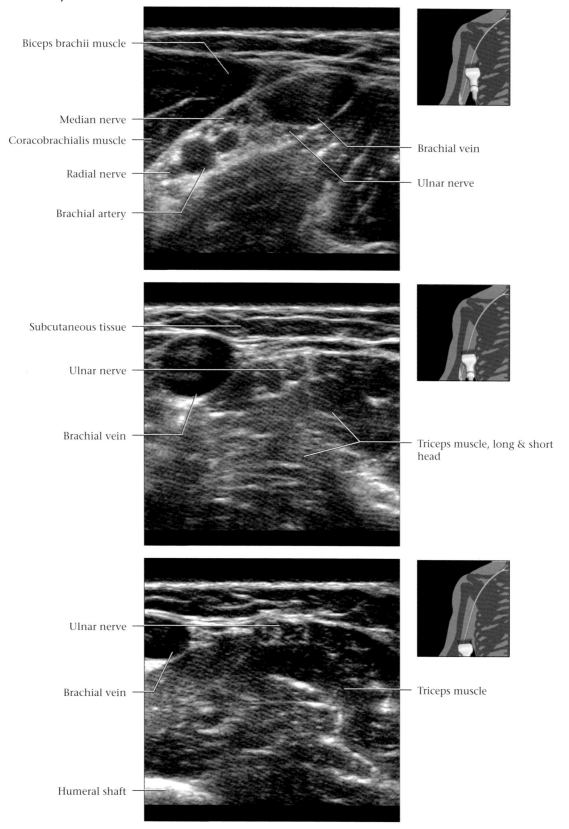

Biceps brachii muscle

Median nerve

Coracobrachialis muscle

Radial nerve

Brachial artery

Brachial vein

Ulnar nerve

Subcutaneous tissue

Ulnar nerve

Brachial vein

Triceps muscle, long & short head

Ulnar nerve

Brachial vein

Triceps muscle

Humeral shaft

(Top) Transverse grayscale ultrasound of the ulnar nerve at the proximal arm. The ulnar nerve arises from the medial cord of the brachial plexus and lies just medial to the brachial vein. (Middle) Transverse grayscale ultrasound of the ulnar nerve at the mid-arm. The ulnar nerve pierces the medial intermuscular septum in the mid-arm where it may be compressed. The ulnar nerve gives off no branch in the arm. (Bottom) Transverse grayscale ultrasound of the ulnar nerve in the distal arm. The ulnar nerve runs distally on the surface of the triceps muscle to reach the area between the olecranon and the medial epicondyle, i.e., the cubital tunnel.

ULNAR NERVE

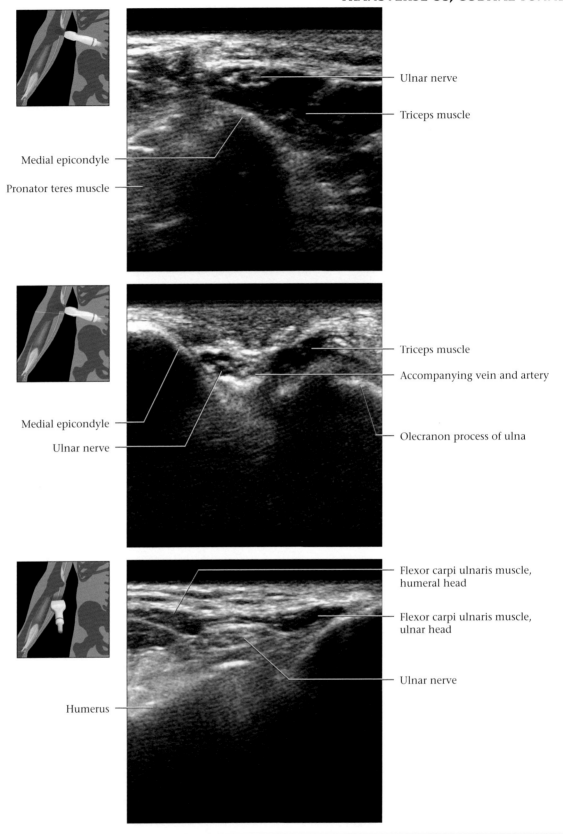

Ulnar nerve

Triceps muscle

Medial epicondyle

Pronator teres muscle

Triceps muscle

Accompanying vein and artery

Medial epicondyle

Ulnar nerve

Olecranon process of ulna

Flexor carpi ulnaris muscle, humeral head

Flexor carpi ulnaris muscle, ulnar head

Ulnar nerve

Humerus

(Top) Transverse grayscale US of the ulnar nerve just proximal to the cubital tunnel. The cubital tunnel is the most common site of ulnar neuropathy. Neuropathy may take the form of compression from the overlying retinaculum or fibrous bands, bony impingement & tumors, subluxation of ulnar nerve over the medial epicondyle or direct injury. (Middle) Transverse grayscale US of the ulnar nerve at the cubital tunnel. The cubital tunnel retinaculum (formed from an extension of investing fascia of the flexor carpi ulnaris & the ligament of Osborn) forms the roof of the cubital tunnel. The retinaculum is 4 mm wide & difficult to depict on ultrasound. Floor & wall of cubital tunnel are formed by containing bones, elbow capsule & medial collateral ligament. Ulnar nerve normally enlarges slightly within cubital tunnel. (Bottom) Transverse grayscale ultrasound of the ulnar nerve just beyond the cubital tunnel.

ULNAR NERVE

TRANSVERSE US, FOREARM

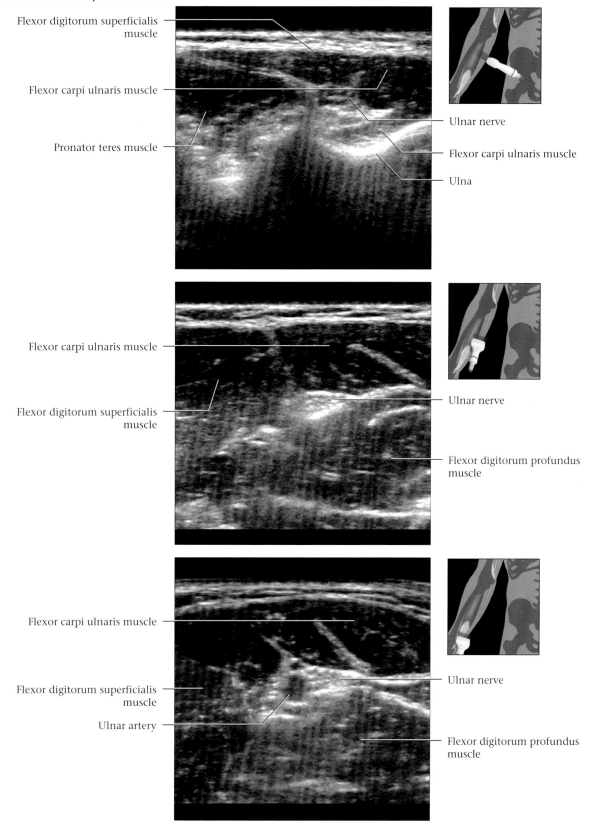

Flexor digitorum superficialis muscle

Flexor carpi ulnaris muscle

Pronator teres muscle

Ulnar nerve

Flexor carpi ulnaris muscle

Ulna

Flexor carpi ulnaris muscle

Flexor digitorum superficialis muscle

Ulnar nerve

Flexor digitorum profundus muscle

Flexor carpi ulnaris muscle

Flexor digitorum superficialis muscle

Ulnar artery

Ulnar nerve

Flexor digitorum profundus muscle

(Top) Transverse grayscale ultrasound the ulnar nerve just beyond the cubital tunnel, where the ulnar nerve passes between the two heads (humeral and ulnar) of the flexor carpi ulnaris tendon. This is a potential site of compression. **(Middle)** Transverse grayscale ultrasound of the ulnar nerve mid-forearm. The ulnar nerve pierces the intermuscular septum dividing the flexor and extensor compartments of the forearm to descend in the flexor compartment between flexor carpi ulnaris and flexor digitorum profundus muscles. **(Bottom)** Transverse grayscale ultrasound of the ulnar nerve distal forearm. The ulnar nerve is joined on its radial side by the ulnar artery in the distal forearm and the two structures travel to the wrist, deep to the flexor carpi ulnaris muscle.

ULNAR NERVE

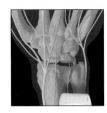

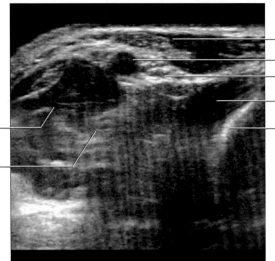

Flexor carpi ulnaris muscle

Ulnar artery

Ulnar nerve

Pronator quadratus muscle

Ulna

Flexor digitorum superficialis muscle

Flexor digitorum profundus muscle

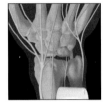

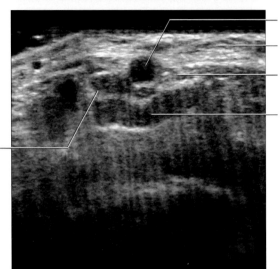

Ulnar artery

Flexor carpi ulnaris tendon

Ulnar nerve

Flexor digitorum profundus muscle

Flexor digitorum superficialis tendon

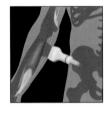

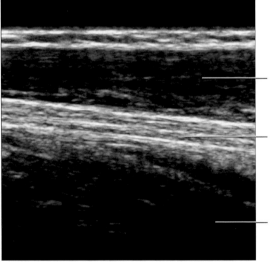

Flexor carpi ulnaris muscle

Ulnar nerve

Flexor digitorum profundus muscle

(Top) Transverse grayscale ultrasound on the ulnar nerve at the distal forearm. The ulnar nerve can be identified by first visualizing the ulnar artery and then identifying the nerve just ulnar to the artery. (Middle) Transverse grayscale ultrasound of the ulnar nerve just proximal to the wrist. At this location, the ulnar nerve is prone to injury from dog-bite, penetrating injury and non-accidental self injury. (Bottom) Longitudinal grayscale ultrasound of the ulnar nerve at the distal third of the forearm. Note the fibrillar pattern of the nerve with hypoechoic and hyperechoic pattern due to nerve fascicles separated by hyperechoic epineurium.

ULNAR NERVE

TRANSVERSE US, GUYON CANAL

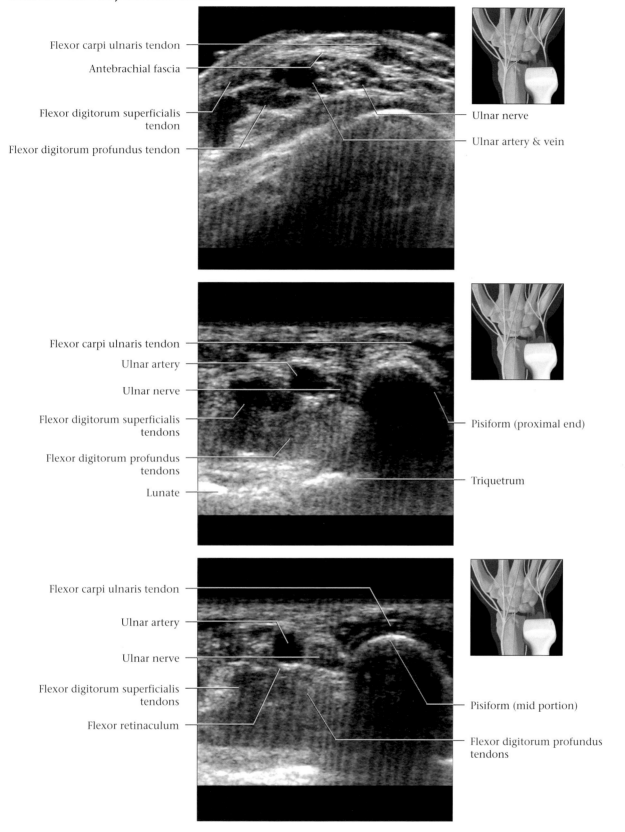

Flexor carpi ulnaris tendon
Antebrachial fascia
Flexor digitorum superficialis tendon
Flexor digitorum profundus tendon
Ulnar nerve
Ulnar artery & vein

Flexor carpi ulnaris tendon
Ulnar artery
Ulnar nerve
Flexor digitorum superficialis tendons
Flexor digitorum profundus tendons
Lunate
Pisiform (proximal end)
Triquetrum

Flexor carpi ulnaris tendon
Ulnar artery
Ulnar nerve
Flexor digitorum superficialis tendons
Flexor retinaculum
Pisiform (mid portion)
Flexor digitorum profundus tendons

(Top) Transverse grayscale ultrasound of the ulnar nerve just proximal to the Guyon canal. **(Middle)** Transverse grayscale ultrasound of the ulnar nerve at the proximal end of Guyon canal. Guyon canal is the second most common site of ulnar neuropathy. **(Bottom)** Transverse grayscale ultrasound of the ulnar nerve at the proximal end of Guyon canal. Ganglia arising from the pisiform-triquetral articulation are a common cause of ulnar nerve compression in the Guyon canal.

ULNAR NERVE

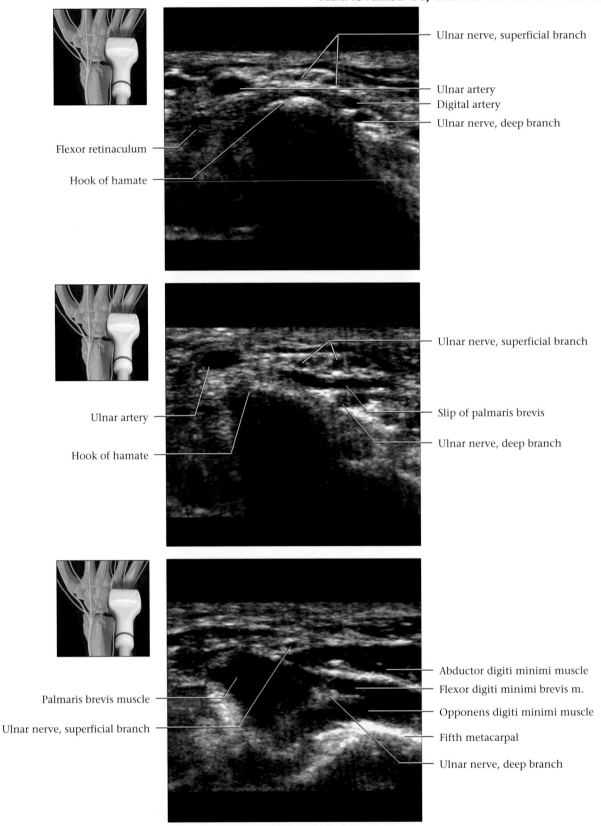

Top image labels:
- Ulnar nerve, superficial branch
- Ulnar artery
- Digital artery
- Ulnar nerve, deep branch
- Flexor retinaculum
- Hook of hamate

Middle image labels:
- Ulnar nerve, superficial branch
- Slip of palmaris brevis
- Ulnar nerve, deep branch
- Ulnar artery
- Hook of hamate

Bottom image labels:
- Abductor digiti minimi muscle
- Flexor digiti minimi brevis m.
- Opponens digiti minimi muscle
- Fifth metacarpal
- Ulnar nerve, deep branch
- Palmaris brevis muscle
- Ulnar nerve, superficial branch

(Top) Transverse grayscale ultrasound of the ulnar nerve at the distal end of Guyon canal, where the ulnar nerve divides into superficial and deep branches. These pass close to the top of (superficial branch) and side of (deep branch) the hook of hamate. (Middle) Transverse grayscale ultrasound of the ulnar nerve at the distal end of the hook of hamate level. Hook of hamate fractures (common in golfers, baseball players) and repeated blunt trauma (handle bar palsy) may injure the ulnar nerve as it passes by the hook of hamate. The ulnar artery can be injured at this location as well (hypothenar hammer syndrome). (Bottom) Transverse grayscale ultrasound of the ulnar nerve at the base of the hypothenar muscles. The superficial branch of the ulnar nerve stays superficial to supply the skin, while the deep branch stays deep to supply the hypothenar muscles & the 3rd & 4th lumbrical muscles.

ULNAR NERVE

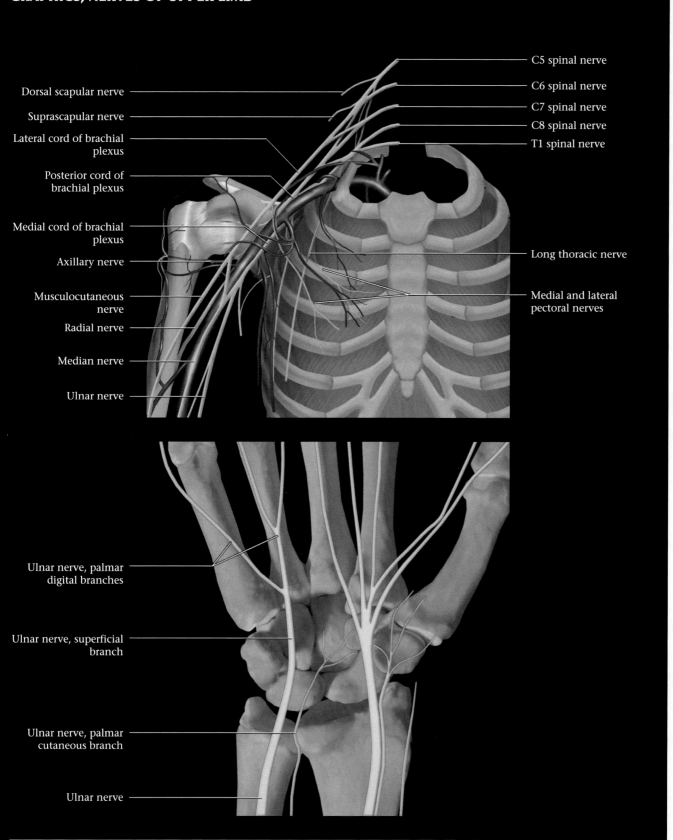

Dorsal scapular nerve

Suprascapular nerve

Lateral cord of brachial plexus

Posterior cord of brachial plexus

Medial cord of brachial plexus

Axillary nerve

Musculocutaneous nerve

Radial nerve

Median nerve

Ulnar nerve

C5 spinal nerve

C6 spinal nerve

C7 spinal nerve

C8 spinal nerve

T1 spinal nerve

Long thoracic nerve

Medial and lateral pectoral nerves

Ulnar nerve, palmar digital branches

Ulnar nerve, superficial branch

Ulnar nerve, palmar cutaneous branch

Ulnar nerve

(Top) Anterior graphic of the brachial plexus. **(Bottom)** Ulnar nerve serves the ulnar wrist and hand. A dorsal branch passes between the flexor carpi ulnaris and ulna to serve the dorsal ulnar wrist. Deep and superficial branches supply motor and sensory to the hypothenar eminence.

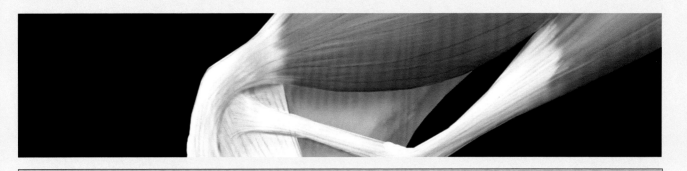

SECTION VII: Lower Limb

GROIN

Terminology

Abbreviations
- Artery (a.); anterior superior iliac spine (ASIS); insertion (I); ligament (l.); muscle (m.); origin (O); vein (v.)

Definitions
- Junctional region between thigh & trunk

Imaging Anatomy

Overview
- Incorporates lower abdominal wall, inguinal canal, femoral triangle & femoral adductor muscles

Osseous Anatomy
- Pubic bone
  - **Pubic tubercle:** Small protuberance, lateral border pubic crest
    - Attachment: Inguinal ligament
  - **Superior & inferior rami** extend from pubis
  - **Pecten:** Ridge, posterior aspect superior pubis
    - O of pectineus muscle
    - I of conjoint tendon (internal oblique and transverse abdominis)
  - **Pubic crest:** Superior surface, anterior aspect pubic body
    - O of rectus abdominis muscle
    - I of transversus abdominis & external oblique muscles
  - **Pubic symphysis:** Cartilaginous joint between pubic bodies
  - **Superior pubic ligament:** Laterally extends to pubic tubercles

Anterior Abdominal Wall
- Abdominal wall muscles
  - **Rectus abdominis:** Paired midline muscles
    - O: Superior pubic ramus, pubic crest
    - I: Xiphoid process, costal cartilages 5-7
  - **Linea alba:** Aponeurotic junction rectus femoris, transverse abdominis, internal & external oblique muscles
  - **External oblique:** Most superficial
    - O: Ribs 5-12
    - I: Pubic crest, anterior iliac crest, linea alba
    - Lower border of aponeurosis contributes to inguinal ligament
  - **Internal oblique:** Between external oblique, transversus abdominis
    - O: Lateral inguinal ligament, iliac crest, thoracolumbar fascia
    - I: Pecten (conjoined tendon), pubic crest, inferior aspect ribs 10-12, linea alba
    - Origin anterior to deep inguinal ring
    - Insertion lateral to rectus abdominis muscle, posterior & medial to superficial inguinal ring
    - Arches over inguinal canal forming roof
  - **Transversus abdominis:** Deepest
    - O: Iliac crest, posterior aspect of lateral inguinal ligament, thoracolumbar fascia

- I: Pubic crest, pecten (conjoined tendon), linea alba
- Remains posterior to inguinal canal

Inguinal Ligament
- Thickening inferior border external oblique aponeurosis
- Attachments: ASIS & pubic tubercle
- Separates lower extremity from pelvis
- Fascia lata attaches to inferior border
- **Subinguinal space:** Deep to inguinal ligament
  - Passageway for femoral vessels & nerve, iliopsoas muscle into femoral triangle
  - External iliac vessels become femoral vessels upon entering this space

Inguinal Canal
- Entrance: **Deep inguinal ring**
  - Located midinguinal ligament
  - Opening of evaginated transversalis fascia through which spermatic cord/round ligament pass
- Exit: **Superficial inguinal ring**
  - Division of external oblique aponeurosis lateral to pubic tubercle
- Contents: Ilioinguinal nerve; male - spermatic cord, female - round ligament; associated vessels
  - Covered by evaginated transversalis fascia

Femoral Triangle (see "Thigh" section)

Adductor Musculature
- **Adductor longus muscle:** Thin tendon arises from medial superior pubic ramus
  - Overlies origins of gracilis, adductor brevis & magnus muscles
- **Gracilis muscle:** Origin from anterior symphysis pubis & entire inferior pubic ramus
  - Origin medial to adductor brevis muscle, deep to adductor longus muscle

Clinical Notes
- Groin pain
  - Vague term attributable to multitude of causes
    - Internal derangements: Hip, symphysis pubis, abdominal wall muscles, adductor muscles
    - Stress fractures: Femur & pelvis

Anatomy-Based Imaging Issues

Imaging Recommendations
- Radiographs: For general assessment and for detecting fractures, bone destruction, enthesopathy (calcification/erosion)
- Ultrasound
  - Detecting masses: Hematoma, hernia, neoplasm etc.
  - Assessing vessels: Aneurysm, pseudoaneurysm, varicose veins etc.
- CT: Assess osseous & soft tissue integrity
- MR
  - High contrast resolution (especially for edema) helps with difficult diagnoses
  - Prone position may eliminate motion artifacts

GROIN

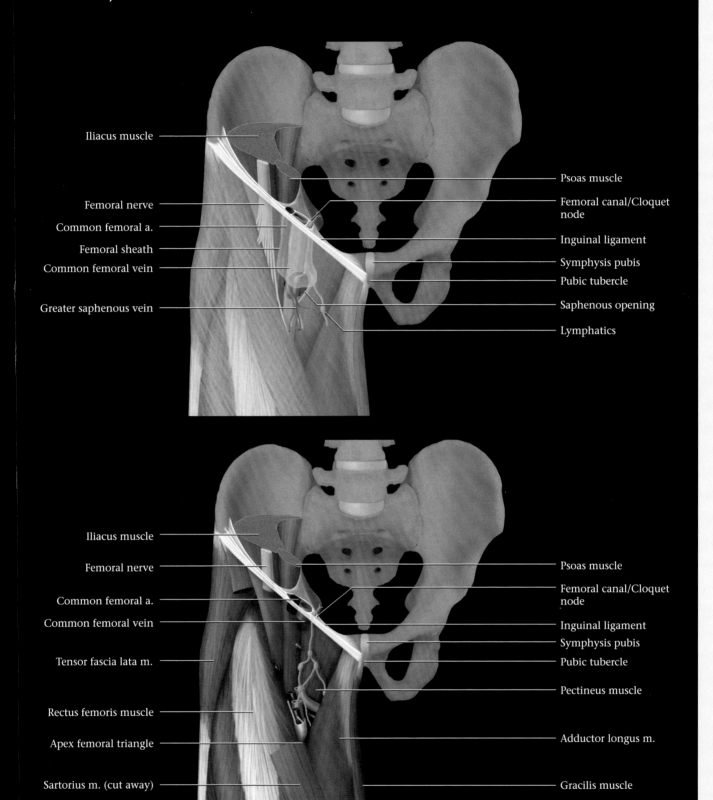

Iliacus muscle

Femoral nerve

Common femoral a.

Femoral sheath

Common femoral vein

Greater saphenous vein

Psoas muscle

Femoral canal/Cloquet node

Inguinal ligament

Symphysis pubis

Pubic tubercle

Saphenous opening

Lymphatics

Iliacus muscle

Femoral nerve

Common femoral a.

Common femoral vein

Tensor fascia lata m.

Rectus femoris muscle

Apex femoral triangle

Sartorius m. (cut away)

Psoas muscle

Femoral canal/Cloquet node

Inguinal ligament

Symphysis pubis

Pubic tubercle

Pectineus muscle

Adductor longus m.

Gracilis muscle

(Top) The contents of the femoral triangle from lateral to medial (NAVeL) are the femoral nerve, femoral artery & vein, and lymphatics. The nerve lies superficial to the iliopsoas muscle. The lateral border of the triangle is the sartorius muscle. The anterior wall is the inguinal ligament. The fascia lata encases the structures of the thigh. The femoral sheath is the fascial covering over the proximal vessels. At the cut away proximal boundary note the septa dividing the sheath into compartments. The femoral canal is the medial compartment. **(Bottom)** Femoral triangle after removal of the fascia lata, sartorius muscle and the vessels. The apex of the triangle is at the crossing of sartorius and adductor longus muscles. The pectineus, adductor longus and iliopsoas muscles form the floor of the triangle.

GRAPHICS, GROIN MUSCLES

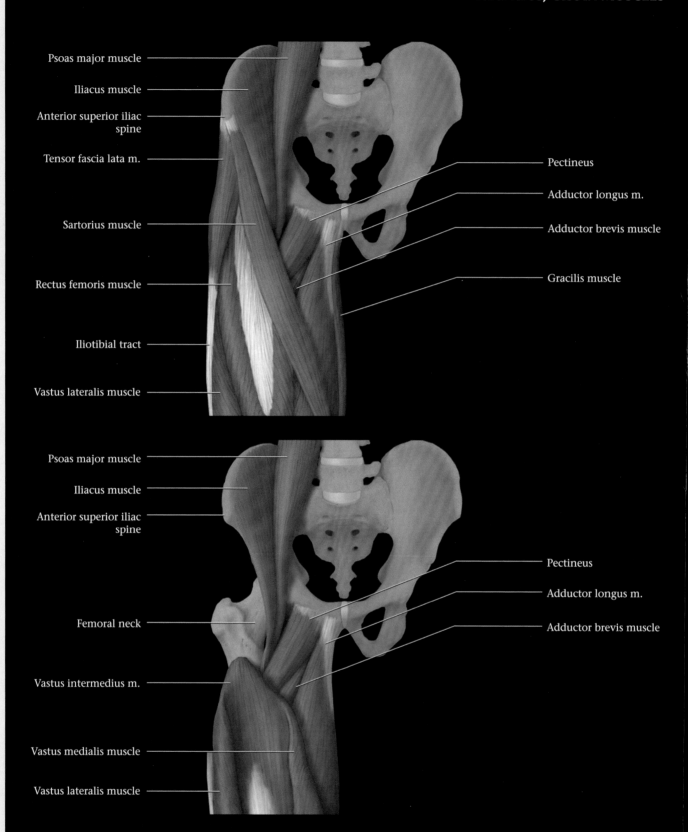

Psoas major muscle

Iliacus muscle

Anterior superior iliac spine

Tensor fascia lata m.

Sartorius muscle

Rectus femoris muscle

Iliotibial tract

Vastus lateralis muscle

Pectineus

Adductor longus m.

Adductor brevis muscle

Gracilis muscle

Psoas major muscle

Iliacus muscle

Anterior superior iliac spine

Femoral neck

Vastus intermedius m.

Vastus medialis muscle

Vastus lateralis muscle

Pectineus

Adductor longus m.

Adductor brevis muscle

(Top) Superficial muscles of the groin. The most lateral muscle is the sartorius & its oblique course is easily appreciated. The psoas major and iliacus muscle exit together from the pelvis over the pelvic brim to run inferiorly towards the lesser trochanter. On the medial side, the most medial muscle is the gracilis. The adductor brevis muscle is deep to the adductor longus and pectineus muscles. **(Bottom)** After removing the superficial layer of muscles, the floor of the femoral triangle is better appreciated. The iliopsoas muscle dives deeply to its trochanteric insertion. The adductors fan out laterally from their pubic origin and constitute the major medial component at a mid thigh level. The adductor magnus is in a deeper & more posterior position.

GROIN

GROIN OVERVIEW

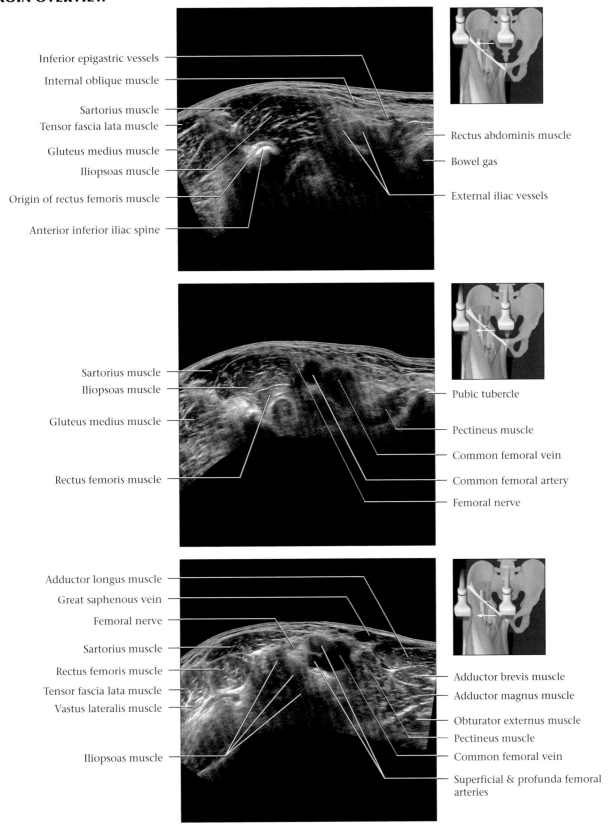

Top image labels (left):
- Inferior epigastric vessels
- Internal oblique muscle
- Sartorius muscle
- Tensor fascia lata muscle
- Gluteus medius muscle
- Iliopsoas muscle
- Origin of rectus femoris muscle
- Anterior inferior iliac spine

Top image labels (right):
- Rectus abdominis muscle
- Bowel gas
- External iliac vessels

Middle image labels (left):
- Sartorius muscle
- Iliopsoas muscle
- Gluteus medius muscle
- Rectus femoris muscle

Middle image labels (right):
- Pubic tubercle
- Pectineus muscle
- Common femoral vein
- Common femoral artery
- Femoral nerve

Bottom image labels (left):
- Adductor longus muscle
- Great saphenous vein
- Femoral nerve
- Sartorius muscle
- Rectus femoris muscle
- Tensor fascia lata muscle
- Vastus lateralis muscle
- Iliopsoas muscle

Bottom image labels (right):
- Adductor brevis muscle
- Adductor magnus muscle
- Obturator externus muscle
- Pectineus muscle
- Common femoral vein
- Superficial & profunda femoral arteries

(Top) Series of transverse panoramic scans of the groin. At this higher level, the lateral components of the groin include the sartorius and iliopsoas muscles, and at the medial boundary, the rectus abdominis muscle. At this level, where most structures are above the inguinal ligament, there is bowel (containing gas which produces shadowing artifact). At this level, vessels are named external iliac vessels. **(Middle)** At a lower level, through the pubic bone, the vessels have moved superficially after passing under the inguinal ligament and now become the common femoral vessels. Bowel is not normally present at this level; instead, pectineus muscle & superior pubic ramus form the floor. **(Bottom)** Further inferiorly, the adductor muscles become the major medial component. Femoral vessels divide into superficial & profunda branches.

GROIN

Rectus abdominis muscle
Transverse abdominis muscle

External oblique muscle
Adductor longus muscle
Adductor brevis muscle

Obturator externus muscle

Internal oblique muscle
Inguinal ligament
Adductor magnus muscle (ischiocondylar)
Gracilis muscle

Adductor magnus muscle (adductor)

Rectus sheath

Rectus abdominis muscle

Body of pubic bone

Pubic symphysis

Superior pubic ligament

Rectus abdominis muscle

Bowel gas with posterior shadow

Anterior surface of pubic bone

Superior surface of pubic bone

(Top) Anterior view of the anterior pelvis and the associated muscle attachments. A number of muscles take origin or insert onto the anterior aspect of the pelvis. These muscles aid in movement and stabilization of the trunk as well as movement and stabilization of the leg and form the medial components of the groin. (Middle) Transverse scan at the superior aspect of pubic symphysis. The superior pubic ligament runs horizontally across the symphysis, deep to rectus abdominis muscle origin. (Bottom) Sagittal image shows the lower rectus abdominis originating from the superior surface of pubic bone (pubic crest). Deep to the rectus abdominis muscle is the peritoneal cavity and bowel. Bowel gas produces posterior shadowing artifact, which obscures deeper structures.

Lower Limb

VII

6

GROIN

MEDIAL GROIN

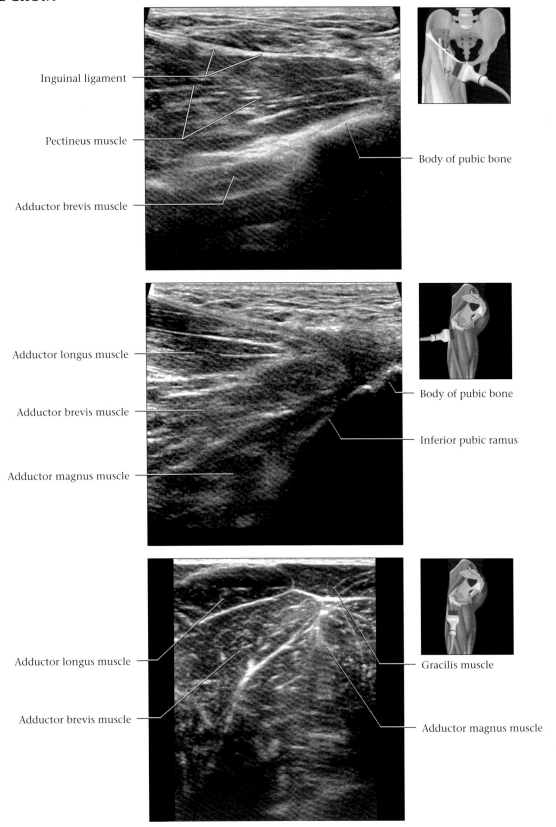

Inguinal ligament

Pectineus muscle

Adductor brevis muscle

Body of pubic bone

Adductor longus muscle

Adductor brevis muscle

Adductor magnus muscle

Body of pubic bone

Inferior pubic ramus

Adductor longus muscle

Adductor brevis muscle

Gracilis muscle

Adductor magnus muscle

(Top) Series of (oblique) transverse scans through adductor muscles. Superiorly, the pectineus muscle originates from pecten pubis & runs laterally (forming floor of femoral triangle) to insert on pectineal line of proximal femur. It runs superior & lateral to adductor longus muscle & is superficial to adductor brevis muscle. **(Middle)** Slightly inferiorly and scanning more obliquely, adductor longus, brevis & magnus can be seen originating from pubic body & inferior ramus. Scanning this region requires thigh abduction & balancing the transducer head on the bony landmark. From here, individual muscles can be traced inferolaterally. Note: Scout image is a graphic in this sagittal plane. **(Bottom)** Oblique transverse scan of adductors using a medial approach. Adductor longus & gracilis muscles form superficial layer, adductor brevis & magnus muscles run deeper. All muscles run inferolaterally to their femoral insertions.

GROIN

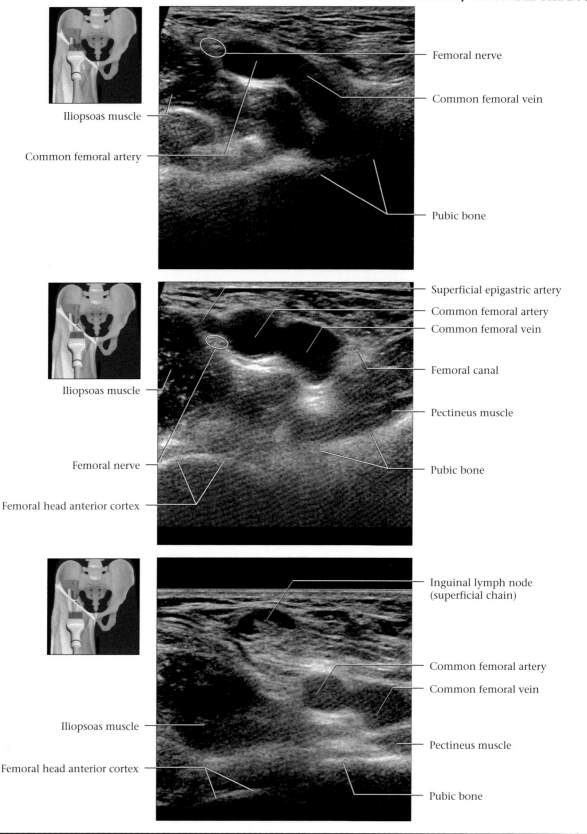

Iliopsoas muscle

Common femoral artery

— Femoral nerve

— Common femoral vein

— Pubic bone

Iliopsoas muscle

Femoral nerve

Femoral head anterior cortex

— Superficial epigastric artery
— Common femoral artery
— Common femoral vein

— Femoral canal

— Pectineus muscle

— Pubic bone

Iliopsoas muscle

Femoral head anterior cortex

— Inguinal lymph node (superficial chain)

— Common femoral artery

— Common femoral vein

— Pectineus muscle

— Pubic bone

(**Top**) Series of transverse scans through the femoral triangle. Above the inguinal ligament, the femoral nerve, artery & vein run medial to iliopsoas tendon. The pubic bone acts as a hard support for the iliopsoas and pectineus muscular floor. (**Middle**) Slightly inferiorly, below inguinal ligament, the femoral triangle commences. The mnemonic for the contents is NAVeL, standing for femoral Nerve, common femoral Artery, common femoral Vein & Lymph nodes (within femoral canal). The pectineus muscle forms the floor of femoral triangle. This floor is supported by the pubic bone & hip joint. (**Bottom**) In addition to lymph nodes in the femoral canal, lymph nodes are frequently seen superficially (the superficial inguinal chain) in the subcutaneous tissue.

GROIN

CENTRAL GROIN, FEMORAL TRIANGLE

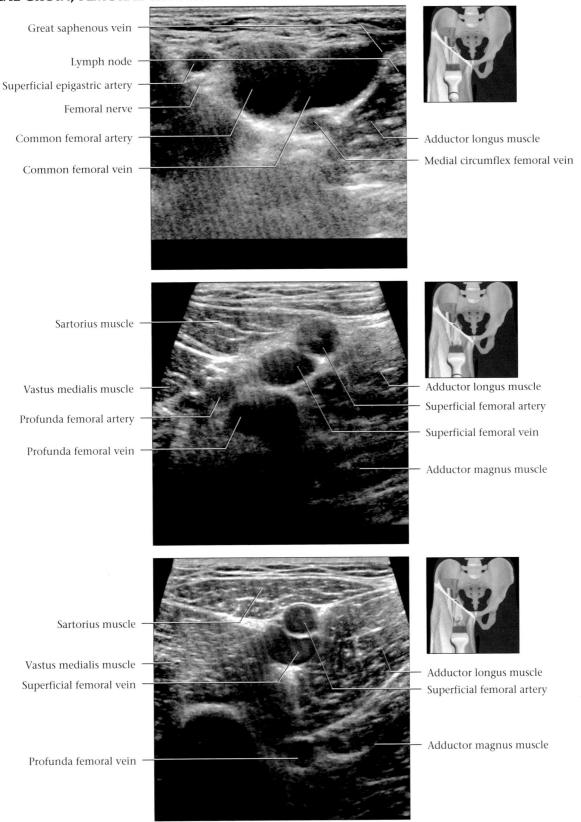

Great saphenous vein

Lymph node

Superficial epigastric artery

Femoral nerve

Common femoral artery

Common femoral vein

Adductor longus muscle

Medial circumflex femoral vein

Sartorius muscle

Vastus medialis muscle

Profunda femoral artery

Profunda femoral vein

Adductor longus muscle

Superficial femoral artery

Superficial femoral vein

Adductor magnus muscle

Sartorius muscle

Vastus medialis muscle

Superficial femoral vein

Profunda femoral vein

Adductor longus muscle

Superficial femoral artery

Adductor magnus muscle

(Top) Further inferiorly, & still within the femoral triangle, the great saphenous vein perforates the anterior wall of the femoral sheath to enter the femoral vein. Also, floor changes from pectineus to adductor longus muscle, with no bony support. **(Middle)** Transverse scan at the apex of the femoral triangle, defined as where the sartorius muscle becomes the roof of the femoral triangle. Just before exiting the femoral triangle, the femoral vessels divide into superficial and profunda branches. **(Bottom)** Transverse scan of the adductor canal. Distal to the femoral triangle, the superficial femoral vessels continue within a muscular conduit, the adductor canal. The groin muscles, the adductor longus and magnus muscles, form the medial wall and floor of this canal.

GROIN

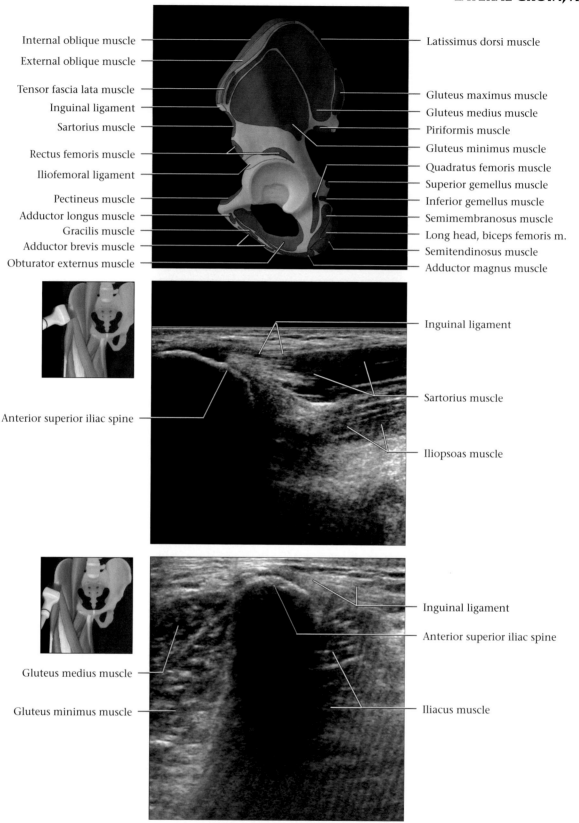

Top image labels (left):
- Internal oblique muscle
- External oblique muscle
- Tensor fascia lata muscle
- Inguinal ligament
- Sartorius muscle
- Rectus femoris muscle
- Iliofemoral ligament
- Pectineus muscle
- Adductor longus muscle
- Gracilis muscle
- Adductor brevis muscle
- Obturator externus muscle

Top image labels (right):
- Latissimus dorsi muscle
- Gluteus maximus muscle
- Gluteus medius muscle
- Piriformis muscle
- Gluteus minimus muscle
- Quadratus femoris muscle
- Superior gemellus muscle
- Inferior gemellus muscle
- Semimembranosus muscle
- Long head, biceps femoris m.
- Semitendinosus muscle
- Adductor magnus muscle

Middle image labels:
- Inguinal ligament
- Sartorius muscle
- Iliopsoas muscle
- Anterior superior iliac spine

Bottom image labels:
- Inguinal ligament
- Anterior superior iliac spine
- Gluteus medius muscle
- Gluteus minimus muscle
- Iliacus muscle

(Top) Muscle and ligament attachments to the external surface of the pelvis. Note the relatively small origin of the tendon of the adductor longus muscle. The adductor brevis muscle is just deep to the longus muscle. The origin of the gracilis muscle is lateral to the adductor brevis muscle. The adductor magnus muscle has a broad origin with its posterior fibers in close proximity to the hamstring tendon origins. **(Middle)** Oblique sagittal scan of ASIS shows origin of sartorius muscle (longest muscle in body). This slender muscle runs inferomedially over iliopsoas muscle, covers adductor canal & inserts at the proximal tibia as part of pes anserinus. **(Bottom)** Coronal scan of anterior superior iliac spine shows division of muscle groups by this bone. Gluteal muscles lie lateral & hip flexors medial. The inguinal ligament originates here & runs inferomedially to the pubic tubercle.

GROIN

ACROSS GROIN, INGUINAL LIGAMENT

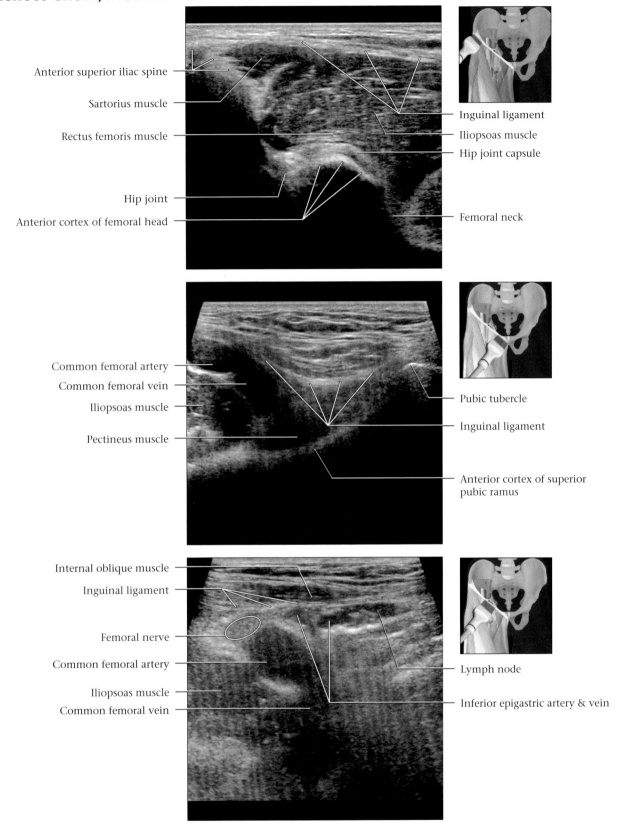

Top image labels:
- Anterior superior iliac spine
- Sartorius muscle
- Rectus femoris muscle
- Hip joint
- Anterior cortex of femoral head
- Inguinal ligament
- Iliopsoas muscle
- Hip joint capsule
- Femoral neck

Middle image labels:
- Common femoral artery
- Common femoral vein
- Iliopsoas muscle
- Pectineus muscle
- Pubic tubercle
- Inguinal ligament
- Anterior cortex of superior pubic ramus

Bottom image labels:
- Internal oblique muscle
- Inguinal ligament
- Femoral nerve
- Common femoral artery
- Iliopsoas muscle
- Common femoral vein
- Lymph node
- Inferior epigastric artery & vein

(**Top**) Oblique transverse scan of upper groin showing inguinal ligament attachment on ASIS, with the sartorius muscle originating immediately inferior to it. The inguinal ligament runs inferomedially and covers the iliopsoas muscle. (**Middle**) Oblique transverse scan along medial aspect of inguinal ligament. Medially, the inguinal ligament forms roof of femoral canal (covering the femoral vessels & nerve), it then runs over pectineus muscle to insert on the pubic tubercle. (**Bottom**) Superficially-focused oblique transverse scan over the upper femoral triangle shows the inguinal ligament forming its roof. Inferior epigastric vessels branch out from the femoral vessels and run superomedially. Clinically, the inferior epigastric vessels define the medial boundary of direct inguinal hernias. Inguinal hernias lateral to inferior epigastric vessels are considered indirect.

HIP

Imaging Anatomy

Overview
- Ball & socket joint with wide range of motion second only to glenohumeral joint

Acetabulum
- Formed by pubis, ilium, ischium
- Oriented anterior, inferior, lateral
- Covers > 50% femoral head
- **Anterior & posterior rims**: Osseous margins of acetabulum
- **Medial wall**: Quadrilateral plate ilium

Femoral Head
- 2/3 of sphere
- Covered by articular cartilage
  - Cartilage thickest superiorly
  - Cartilage thins at head/neck junction

Labrum
- Fibrocartilage lip deepening acetabular rim
- Joins transverse ligament at margins acetabular notch
- Thickest posterior & superior
- Widest anterior & superior
- Vascular supply: Branches obturator, superior & inferior gluteal arteries
  - Mainly capsular surface
- Shape
  - Triangular in 66-94%
    - Decreasing incidence with increasing age
  - Variants: Rounded/blunt or absent
  - Absent labra: Constellation absent anterior labrum & small remnant superiorly
    - In 10-14% asymptomatic individuals
- Function
  - Protect cartilage: Distributes forces by maintaining synovial fluid layer between articular surfaces
  - Prevents lateral translation femoral head
- Labral tear
  - Frequently has associated paralabral ganglion/cyst
  - Easier to detect in presence of joint effusion/arthrographic contrast

Joint Capsule
- 2 layers: Internal synovial; external fibrous (not usually separable on imaging)
  - External layer forms capsular ligaments
- Attachments
  - Acetabulum
    - Base of labrum anteriorly & posteriorly
    - Several millimeters above labrum superiorly
  - Femur
    - Anterior: Intertrochanteric line
    - Posterior: Proximal to intertrochanteric crest
    - Anterior attachment more lateral than posterior attachment
  - **Perilabral recess**: Between labrum & capsule
    - Smaller anterior & posterior
    - Larger superior

Vascular Supply
- Branches of medial & lateral circumflex femoral, deep division superior gluteal, inferior gluteal arteries, artery of ligamentum teres (branch of obturator artery)

Innervation
- Branches from nerve to rectus femoris, nerve to quadratus femoris, anterior division obturator nerve, accessory obturator nerve, superior gluteal nerve

Major Adjacent Structures
- **Greater trochanter**
  - I: Gluteus minimus & medius muscles
  - Separated from overlying iliotibial tract by thin trochanteric bursa (normally barely perceptible on imaging)
- **Lesser trochanter**
  - I: Iliopsoas muscle
- **Anterior inferior iliac spine**
  - O: Long head of rectus femoris muscle
- **Iliopsoas muscle**
  - Run inferomedially across anterior surface of hip joint
- **Femoral vessels**
  - Separated from hip joint by iliopsoas muscle

Neonatal Hip
- High success rate in treatment of developmental abnormalities demands early imaging diagnosis (with ultrasound)
- Established measurements of bony and cartilaginous components for comparison with normal reference
- Main measurements reflect depth of acetabulum and acetabular coverage of femoral head

Anatomy-Based Imaging Issues

Imaging Recommendations
- Radiographs for assessing osseous alignment
- Ultrasound for joint effusion & surrounding soft tissue
  - Also used for real-time guided procedures: Hip joint or abscess aspiration/biopsy; intra-articular contrast injection
  - Ideal in neonates for suspected developmental hip dysplasia
- MR-arthrography preferred to assess intra-articular structures

Imaging "Sweet Spots"
- Small joint effusions are best detected on ultrasound by a hypoechoic thickening/layer over anterior surface of femoral neck
  - Best site for aspirations/injections
- Para-labral ganglion cysts should alert to presence of labral tear

Imaging Pitfalls
- Synovial hypertrophy usually shows no evidence of vascularity on color Doppler scanning and is therefore difficult to distinguish from an effusion

GRAPHICS, AXIAL & SAGITTAL HIP SECTIONS

Femoral nerve

Iliopsoas bursa

Longitudinal capsular ligaments

Zona orbicularis

Greater trochanter

Femoral artery

Femoral vein

Anterior rim of acetabulum

Anterior column of acetabulum

Ligamentum teres

Medial wall of acetabulum

Posterior rim of acetabulum

Posterior column of acetabulum

Ischial spine

Internal pudendal a., v.

Anterior column of acetabulum

Anterior labrum

Femoral head

Ilium

Posterior column of acetabulum

Articular cartilage

Posterior labrum

Ischial tuberosity

(Top) Axial representation of the hip joint. The iliopsoas bursa is closely approximated to the joint anteriorly. The ligamentum teres is seen in profile as a flattened structure. The two layers of the external capsule are visible, the more superficial longitudinal fibers and deep circular fibers. **(Bottom)** Sagittal representation of the hip joint nicely demonstrates the inverted Y of the acetabulum. The ilium is the stem and the limbs are the anterior and posterior acetabular columns.

Lower Limb

VII

13

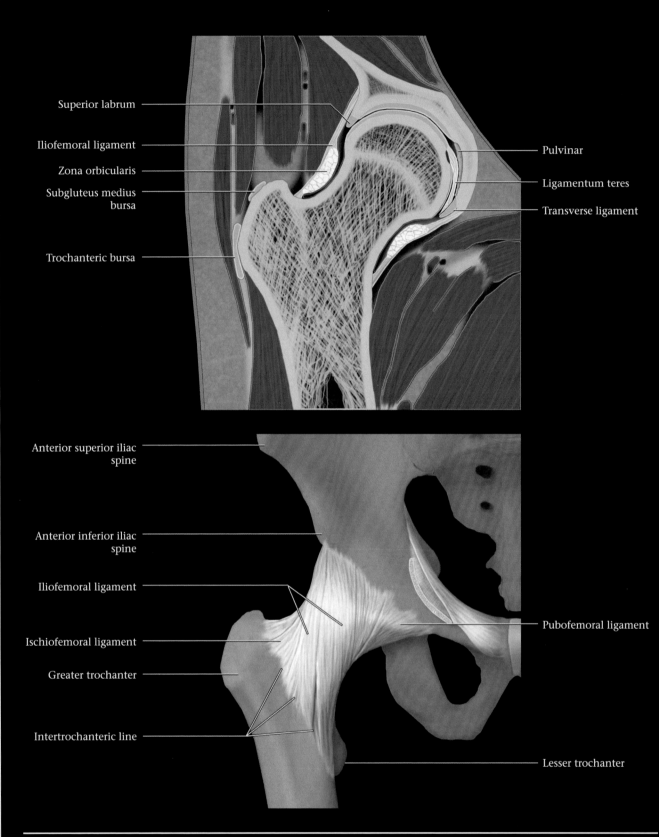

(Top) This coronal image demonstrates many of the important structures of the hip joint. The longitudinally oriented fibers of the ligaments of the external joint capsule and the deeper circularly oriented fibers of the zona orbicularis are visible. Note the long axis of the ligamentum teres and its insertion onto the transverse ligament. The pulvinar fills the acetabular fossa. **(Bottom)** Anterior ligaments. The longitudinal spiral of the iliofemoral and pubofemoral ligaments is well seen. Their attachments to the anterior inferior iliac spine and pubic aspect of the obturator foramen respectively are visible. The ischiofemoral ligament wraps over the superior aspect of the femoral neck to attach to the anterior femoral neck.

HIP OVERVIEW

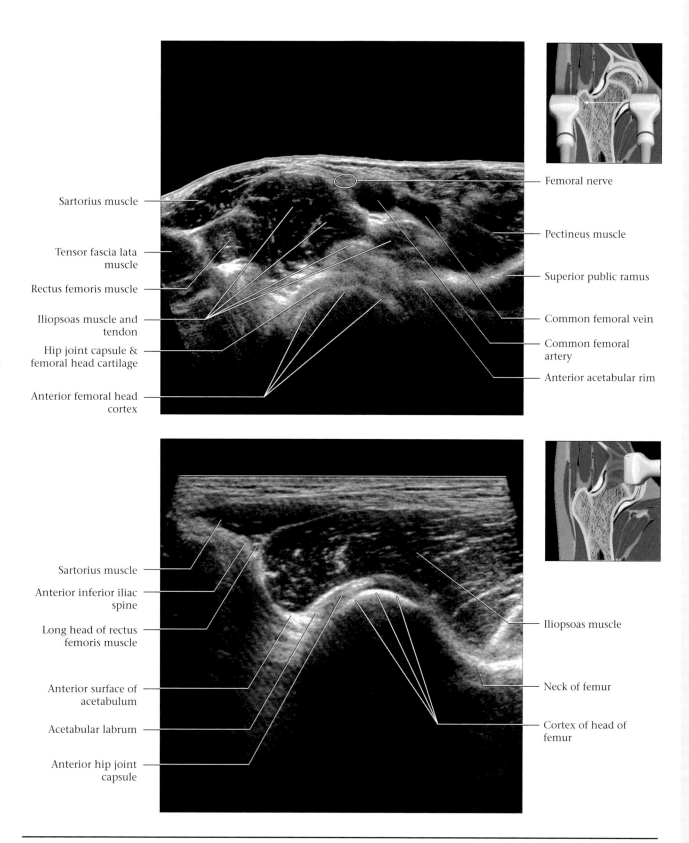

Sartorius muscle

Tensor fascia lata muscle

Rectus femoris muscle

Iliopsoas muscle and tendon

Hip joint capsule & femoral head cartilage

Anterior femoral head cortex

Femoral nerve

Pectineus muscle

Superior public ramus

Common femoral vein

Common femoral artery

Anterior acetabular rim

Sartorius muscle

Anterior inferior iliac spine

Long head of rectus femoris muscle

Anterior surface of acetabulum

Acetabular labrum

Anterior hip joint capsule

Iliopsoas muscle

Neck of femur

Cortex of head of femur

(Top) Transverse panoramic scan though femoral head. Medially & superiorly, femoral head is covered by bony acetabulum and not visible with ultrasound. Laterally, hip joint lies deep to the iliopsoas muscle & femoral triangle. Further laterally, hip joint is associated with gluteal muscles. **(Bottom)** Oblique sagittal scan of hip joint & anterior inferior iliac spine. Acetabular labrum, which is thickest and widest here, can be seen between acetabular rim & joint capsule. Small joint effusions are first detected not over the femoral head, but over the femoral neck as a hypoechoic layer. The femoral neck's relatively safe access makes it a suitable site for guided aspiration/injection.

ACETABULUM

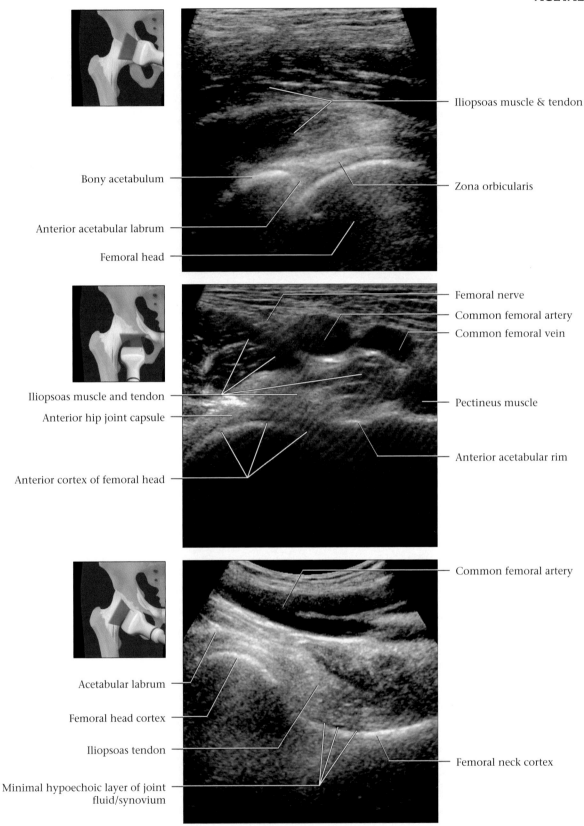

Iliopsoas muscle & tendon

Bony acetabulum

Zona orbicularis

Anterior acetabular labrum

Femoral head

Femoral nerve

Common femoral artery

Common femoral vein

Iliopsoas muscle and tendon

Anterior hip joint capsule

Pectineus muscle

Anterior cortex of femoral head

Anterior acetabular rim

Common femoral artery

Acetabular labrum

Femoral head cortex

Iliopsoas tendon

Femoral neck cortex

Minimal hypoechoic layer of joint fluid/synovium

(Top) Oblique sagittal scan along axis of femoral neck showing triangular cross-section of anterior acetabular labrum. Joint effusion/contrast tends to allow better delineation of its contour & lesions. **(Middle)** Transverse scan at level of hip joint. Anterior femoral cortex/cartilage, hip joint capsule & acetabular rim are well visualized. Contents of femoral triangle are separated from hip joint by iliopsoas muscle and tendon, which explains why paralabral cysts may tract along the iliopsoas muscle. **(Bottom)** Effusions are first detected not over the femoral head but over the femoral neck as an increase in the normally minimal hypoechoic layer of joint fluid and synovium. This is also the safest site for joint injections (intra-articular contrast or medication).

HIP

ILIOPSOAS INSERTION

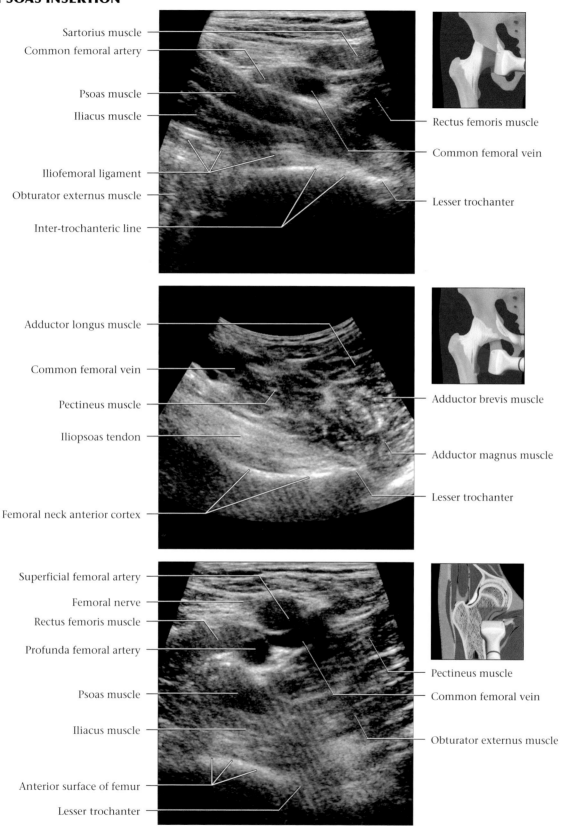

Top image labels:
- Sartorius muscle
- Common femoral artery
- Psoas muscle
- Iliacus muscle
- Iliofemoral ligament
- Obturator externus muscle
- Inter-trochanteric line
- Rectus femoris muscle
- Common femoral vein
- Lesser trochanter

Middle image labels:
- Adductor longus muscle
- Common femoral vein
- Pectineus muscle
- Iliopsoas tendon
- Femoral neck anterior cortex
- Adductor brevis muscle
- Adductor magnus muscle
- Lesser trochanter

Bottom image labels:
- Superficial femoral artery
- Femoral nerve
- Rectus femoris muscle
- Profunda femoral artery
- Psoas muscle
- Iliacus muscle
- Anterior surface of femur
- Lesser trochanter
- Pectineus muscle
- Common femoral vein
- Obturator externus muscle

(**Top**) Oblique sagittal scan along course of iliopsoas muscle. Resolution is reduced due to depth of structures, which may be partially improved by externally rotating hip to bring deep structures closer to surface. (**Middle**) Oblique sagittal scan slightly more distally than previous image. Insertion of iliopsoas tendon is onto lesser trochanter, which may be avulsed in injury. Notice the close relationship between these structures and the adductor compartment. (**Bottom**) Transverse scan of distal iliopsoas tendon just before insertion. A functional division is present between the hip flexor (iliopsoas) & hip adductors. This is also the apex level of femoral triangle where superficial & profunda vessels bifurcate.

HIP

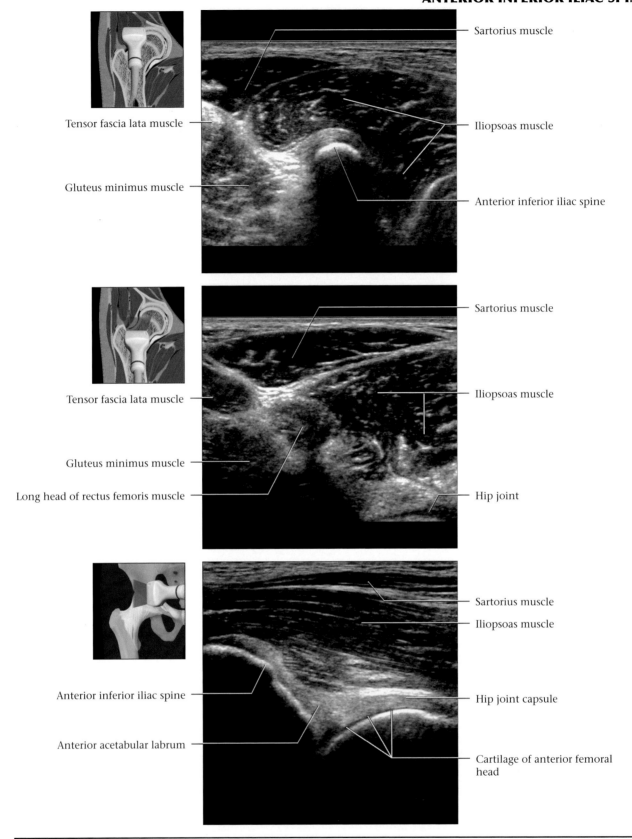

(Top) Transverse scan through anterior inferior iliac spine, origin of long head of rectus femoris muscle (part of quadriceps). Together with sartorius muscle, which originates from anterior superior iliac spine, & iliopsoas muscle, which originates from iliac fossa & lumbar transverse processes, they form hip flexors that cross the hip joint. (Middle) Transverse scan more inferior to previous image shows the long head of the rectus femoris muscle running deep to the sartorius muscle and lateral to the iliopsoas muscle. Note that the rectus muscle is the only quadriceps muscle that crosses the hip joint and thus acts as both hip flexor and knee extensor. (Bottom) Oblique scan along the sartorius muscle at hip joint level shows it to be roughly parallel with iliopsoas. The rectus femoris lies in a more lateral plane.

HIP

GREATER TROCHANTER

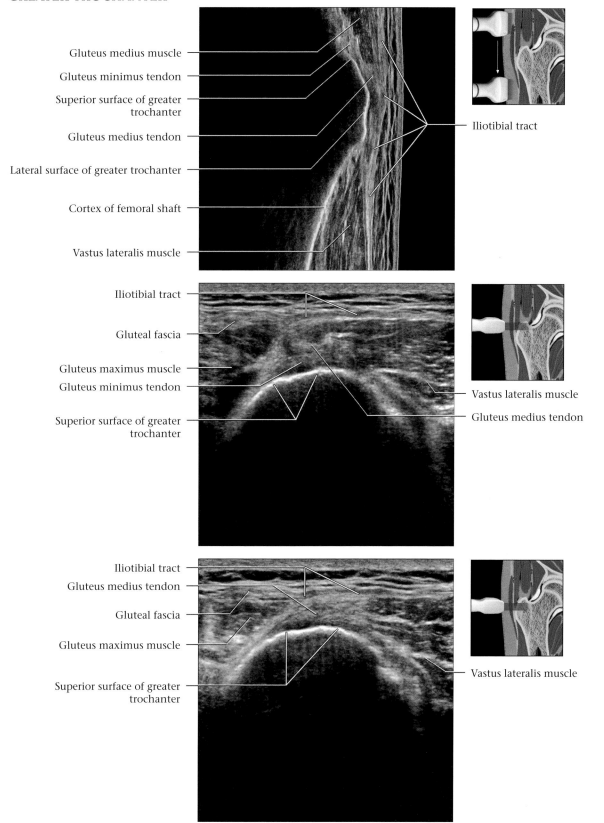

Gluteus medius muscle

Gluteus minimus tendon

Superior surface of greater trochanter

Gluteus medius tendon

Lateral surface of greater trochanter

Cortex of femoral shaft

Vastus lateralis muscle

Iliotibial tract

Iliotibial tract

Gluteal fascia

Gluteus maximus muscle

Gluteus minimus tendon

Superior surface of greater trochanter

Vastus lateralis muscle

Gluteus medius tendon

Iliotibial tract

Gluteus medius tendon

Gluteal fascia

Gluteus maximus muscle

Superior surface of greater trochanter

Vastus lateralis muscle

(Top) Coronal panoramic scan of the greater trochanter. The gluteus minimus & medius tendons insert on the superior and lateral surfaces of greater tuberosity. The iliotibial tract originates from the anterior aspect of iliac crest (as tensor fascia lata) and runs inferiorly passing superficial to the lateral surface of greater trochanter. **(Middle)** Transverse scan through the superior surface of the greater trochanter shows insertion of the gluteus minimus tendon. The gluteus medius tendon & iliotibial tract pass superficial to this. **(Bottom)** Transverse scan of the lateral surface of the greater trochanter shows the insertion of the gluteus medius tendon. The iliotibial tract is closest to the trochanter at this point and may be irritated resulting in formation of bursitis (trochanteric bursitis).

Gluteus medius
Unossified greater trochanter
Femoral shaft cortex
Femoral head

Gluteus minimus
Acetabular labrum
Acetabular roof
Part of tri-radiate cartilage

Gluteus medius
Unossified greater trochanter

Gluteus minimus
Acetabular roof
Femoral head
Part of tri-radiate cartilage

Gluteus medius

Gluteus minimus
Acetabular roof

Femoral head

Part of tri-radiate cartilage

(Top) Coronal scan of the hip of a one-month-old neonate with the hip in extension. The femoral head and the greater trochanter are purely cartilaginous. This allows ultrasound transmission and thus visualization of the acetabular fossa. **(Middle)** Coronal scan of the hip of a one-month-old neonate with the hip in flexion, which produces an axial section of the femoral head. The femoral head should appear round in this section. Both the femoral head and the greater trochanter are purely cartilaginous, allowing ultrasound transmission and thus better visualization of the depth of the acetabular fossa. **(Bottom)** Transverse scan of the femoral head with hip in extension shows also the central position of a normal femoral head on the tri-radiate cartilage (golf ball on a tee appearance).

HIP

PEDIATRIC HIP

Line c — Line a

Iliac cortex — Beta angle

Promontory — Alpha angle

Line b

Line a

Gluteus medius

Gluteus minimus

Acetabular labrum — Femoral shaft cortex

Acetabular roof — Ossification in femoral head

Part of tri-radiate cartilage

(Top) Using the standard image for a pediatric hip, 3 lines are drawn: (a) Along straight contour of iliac cortex; (b) from promontory along acetabular roof to describe the alpha angle; (c) from promontory to tip of labrum for beta angle. Normal ranges are: Alpha angle over 60 degrees and beta angle less than 55 degrees. Measurements outside of these ranges are suggestive of developmental hip dysplasia. **(Middle)** The proportion of femoral head within the acetabulum is calculated by dividing the depth (d) of femoral head below line a (see previous image) by the diameter of the femoral head (D). In normals, over 50% of the femoral head should be below line a. **(Bottom)** Coronal scan of the hip of a four-month-old with the hip in extension. The center of the femoral head has begun to ossify, showing up as an echogenic focus with posterior acoustic shadowing.

GLUTEAL MUSCLES

Terminology

Abbreviations
- Anterior superior iliac spine (ASIS)
- Artery (a.)
- Function (F)
- Insertion (I)
- Ligament (l.)
- Muscle (m.)
- Nerve supply (N)
- Origin (O)
- Vein (v.)

Imaging Anatomy

Gluteal Muscles
- Components: Gluteus maximus, gluteus medius, gluteus minimus, tensor fascia lata, piriformis, obturator internus & externus, superior & inferior gemellus, quadratus femoris
- Common functions: Hip abduction, external rotation
- **Inferior gemellus**
  - O: Ischial tuberosity
  - I: Piriformis fossa
  - N: Nerve to quadratus femoris muscle
  - F: Hip external rotation, weak abduction
- **Superior gemellus**
  - O: Ischial spine
  - I: Piriformis fossa
  - N: Nerve to obturator internus muscle
  - F: Hip external rotation, weak abduction
- **Gluteus maximus**
  - O: Posterior gluteal line (ilium), posterior sacrum & coccyx, sacrotuberous ligament
  - I: Iliotibial tract, gluteal tuberosity
  - N: Inferior gluteal
  - F: Hip extension, abduction and external rotation
- **Gluteus medius**
  - O: Between anterior & posterior gluteal lines (ilium)
  - I: Lateral & superoposterior facets greater trochanter
  - N: Superior gluteal
  - F: Hip abduction & internal rotation
- **Gluteus minimus**
  - O: External ilium between ant. & inf. gluteal lines
  - I: Anterior facet greater trochanter
  - N: Superior gluteal
  - F: Hip abduction & internal rotation
- **Obturator internus**
  - O: Internal surface obturator foramen & membrane
  - I: Piriformis fossa (joins with gemelli tendons)
  - N: L5, S1, S2
  - F: Hip external rotation, weak abduction
- **Obturator externus**
  - O: Edge of obturator foramen & obturator membrane
  - I: Posterior aspect of femur in trochanteric fossa
  - N: Obturator nerve
  - F: Lateral rotation of hip
- **Piriformis**
  - O: Anterior sacrum, sacrotuberous ligament
  - I: Greater trochanter (may fuse with obturator internus & gemellus muscles)
  - N: S1, S2
  - F: Hip external rotation, assists abduction
- **Tensor fascia lata**
  - O: External lip anterior iliac crest, external ASIS
  - I: Iliotibial tract
  - N: Superior gluteal
  - F: Hip flexion, abduction & weak internal rotation
- **Quadratus femoris**
  - O: Lateral ischial tuberosity
  - I: Quadrate line, intertrochanteric crest femur
  - N: L4, L5, S1
  - F: Strong hip external rotation

Rotator Cuff of Hip
- Gluteus medius & minimus tendons, trochanteric bursa, subgluteus medius & minimus bursa

Bursa
- Trochanteric
  - Greater trochanter & gluteus maximus muscle
- Ischiogluteal
  - Ischial tuberosity & gluteus maximus muscle
- Subgluteus medius
  - Greater trochanter & gluteus medius
- Subgluteus minimus
  - Greater trochanter & gluteus minimus muscle
- Gluteofemoral
  - Iliotibial tract & vastus lateralis muscle
- Obturator internus
  - Muscle & ischium
- Obturator externus
  - Synovial protrusion beneath inferior border

Piriformis Fossa
- Between posterior femoral neck & posterior medial surface of greater trochanter
- Insertion site for piriformis, superior & inferior gemelli, obturator internus

Ischial Tuberosity
- Covered by gluteus maximus muscle when hip extended, uncovered in hip flexion
- Origin of hamstrings and adductor magnus muscles

Sacroiliac Joint
- Anterior synovial joint
- Posterior syndesmosis: Tuberosities sacrum & ilium
- Function: Primarily weight transfer axial to appendicular skeleton
  - Limited gliding & rotation
- Widening anteriorly can occur without instability
- Posterior widening indicates instability
- **Sacroiliac ligaments**
  - **Interosseous sacroiliac:** Within syndesmotic joint
    - Between tuberosities ilium & sacrum
    - Oriented superiorly & laterally
    - Weight transferred to sacrum, sacrum displaced inferiorly, force transmitted to ligaments, ligaments pull ilii inward, compress sacrum & interlocking surfaces SI joints
    - Extremely strong
  - **Anterior sacroiliac:** Weak ligaments
    - Mainly anterior joint capsule

GLUTEAL MUSCLES

- ○ **Posterior sacroiliac:** Posterior fibers interosseous ligament
  - ■ **Short dorsal sacroiliac:** Horizontal; lateral sacral crest S1 & S2 to posterior iliac crest
  - ■ **Long dorsal sacroiliac:** Vertical oblique; posterior superior iliac spine to lateral sacral crest S3, S4

Posterior Sacroiliac Ligaments of Pelvis

- Primary stabilizers of pelvis
  - ○ Little contribution from anterior structures
- Resist rotational forces & vertical shear
- **Sacrotuberous:** Superior & inferior posterior iliac spines, sacrum & coccyx to ischial tuberosity
- **Sacrospinous:** Lateral sacrum & coccyx to ischial spine
- **Iliolumbar:** Tip L5 transverse process to iliac crest
- **Sacroiliac ligaments:** Interosseous, long & short dorsal

Greater Sciatic Foramen

- Greater sciatic notch converted to foramen by sacrospinous ligament
- Contents: Nerves, vessels, piriformis muscle
- Passageway from pelvis to thigh
  - ○ Structures identified as exiting pelvis above or below piriformis muscle
    - ■ Above: Superior gluteal artery, vein, nerve
    - ■ Below: Pudendal nerve, internal pudendal artery, vein, nerve to obturator internus, sciatic nerve, inferior gluteal artery, vein, nerve, posterior cutaneous nerve of thigh, nerve to quadratus femoris muscle
  - ○ Relationship of structures
    - ■ Most medial: Pudendal nerve
    - ■ Most lateral: Sciatic nerve
    - ■ Nerve to quadratus femoris muscle deep to sciatic nerve
- **Inferior gluteal artery**
  - ○ Larger terminal branch anterior division internal iliac artery
  - ○ Passes between S1 & S2 or S2 & S3
  - ○ Exits pelvis inferior to piriformis muscle
  - ○ Posteromedial to sciatic nerve
  - ○ Prenatally continuous with popliteal artery, remnant is artery to sciatic nerve
  - ○ S: Gluteus maximus, obturator internus, quadratus femoris, superior hamstrings muscles
  - ○ **Inferior gluteal vein** travels with artery, drains into internal iliac vein
- **Inferior gluteal nerve**
  - ○ Branch of sacral plexus
  - ○ Exits pelvis inferior to piriformis muscle
  - ○ Posterior to sciatic nerve
- **Superior gluteal artery**
  - ○ Continuation posterior division internal iliac artery
  - ○ Passes between lumbosacral trunk & S1
  - ○ Exits pelvis superior to piriformis muscle
  - ○ Superficial branch: S - gluteus maximus muscle
  - ○ Deep branch: S - gluteus medius & minimus, tensor fascia lata muscles
  - ○ **Superior gluteal vein** travels with artery, drains into internal iliac vein
- **Superior gluteal nerve**
  - ○ Branch of sacral plexus
  - ○ Exits pelvis superior to piriformis muscle

- **Sciatic nerve**
  - ○ Exits pelvis inferior to piriformis muscle
  - ○ Most lateral structure
- **Pudendal nerve & internal pudendal vessels**
  - ○ Exit inferior to piriformis muscle
  - ○ Nerve most medial structure
- **Nerve to obturator internus muscle**
  - ○ Exits pelvis inferior to piriformis muscle

Lesser Sciatic Foramen

- Lesser sciatic notch converted to foramen by intersection (crossing) sacrotuberous and sacrospinous ligaments
- Contents
  - ○ **Pudendal nerve & internal pudendal vessels**
    - ■ Pass over sacrospinous ligament
    - ■ Exit buttock, enter perineum
  - ○ **Obturator internus muscle**

Anatomy-Based Imaging Issues

Imaging Recommendations

- US
  - ○ Quick examination if patient can pin-point area of complaint
  - ○ Large area to be covered by ultrasound if symptoms non-specific
  - ○ Sensitivity could be increased by appreciating a disruption in the orientation of muscle fibers
  - ○ Anisotropy gives gluteal muscles varying echogenicity due to the different orientation of fibers
    - ■ This allows clear distinction between muscles
    - ■ Lesions may be better demonstrated/detected by scans along and across muscle fibers to make lesion more conspicuous
  - ○ Iliac crest, greater trochanter and ischial tuberosity are important bony landmarks for orientation
  - ○ Use of panoramic (extended field of view) images will help referring clinicians to understand the location of a lesion
    - ■ Panoramic images should be performed in standard anatomical planes to help interpretation
    - ■ Landmarks, especially osseous e.g., iliac crest, sacrum, ischial tuberosity, also help interpretation of a panoramic image
    - ■ Panoramic images do not provide accurate measurements
    - ■ Wide lesions are best assessed using dual screen/multiple contiguous images for a summated linear measurement
- MR
  - ○ Diagnose masses, anatomic anomalies, other causes of nerve compression
  - ○ Preferred modality for sacroiliitis
- CT
  - ○ Mainly used for assessing bone and joint (sacroiliac) abnormalities

Imaging Pitfalls

- Lower frequency transducers (5 MHz or below) should be used initially in an examination to exclude deep-seated lesions

GLUTEAL MUSCLES

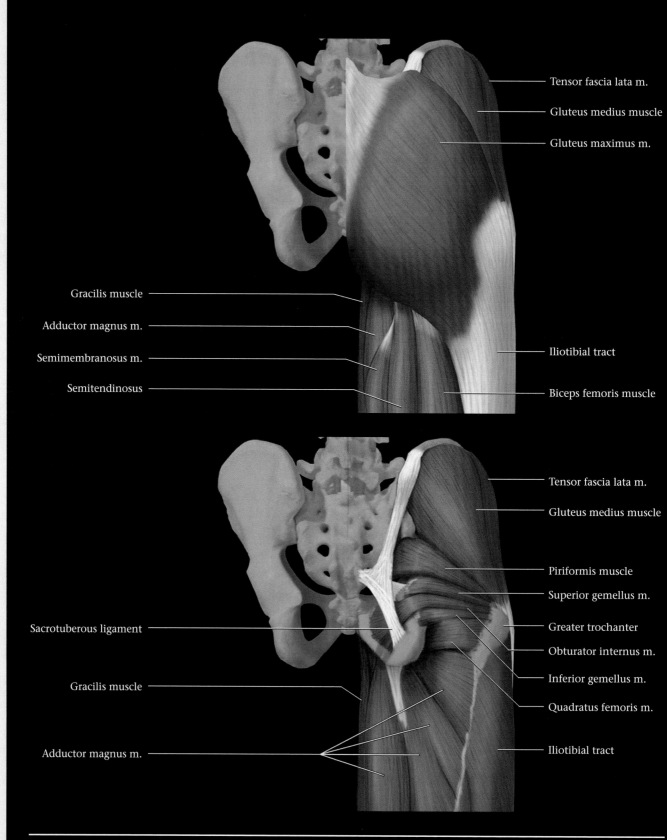

Tensor fascia lata m.

Gluteus medius muscle

Gluteus maximus m.

Gracilis muscle

Adductor magnus m.

Semimembranosus m.

Semitendinosus

Iliotibial tract

Biceps femoris muscle

Tensor fascia lata m.

Gluteus medius muscle

Piriformis muscle

Superior gemellus m.

Greater trochanter

Sacrotuberous ligament

Obturator internus m.

Inferior gemellus m.

Gracilis muscle

Quadratus femoris m.

Adductor magnus m.

Iliotibial tract

(Top) The gluteus muscles from anterior to posterior and deep to superficial are gluteus minimus, medius and maximus. These muscles form the bulk of the gluteal region. The gluteus maximus, in particular, covers most of the deep gluteal structures. **(Bottom)** After removing the gluteus maximus, the deep muscles are visible: Piriformis, superior gemellus, obturator internus, inferior gemellus, quadratus femoris. These all function as external rotators of the thigh. Note the piriformis muscle which exits via the greater sciatic foramen and the obturator internus muscle via the lesser sciatic foramen.

Lower Limb

VII

24

GLUTEAL MUSCLES

GRAPHIC, SCIATIC NERVE & OVERVIEW, GLUTEAL

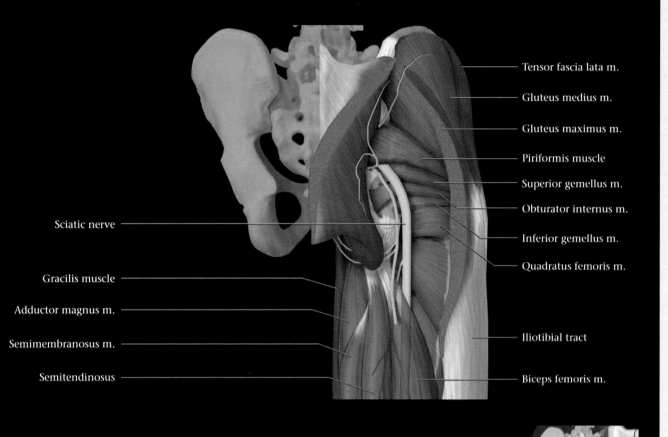

Tensor fascia lata m.

Gluteus medius m.

Gluteus maximus m.

Piriformis muscle

Superior gemellus m.

Obturator internus m.

Inferior gemellus m.

Quadratus femoris m.

Sciatic nerve

Gracilis muscle

Adductor magnus m.

Semimembranosus m.

Semitendinosus

Iliotibial tract

Biceps femoris m.

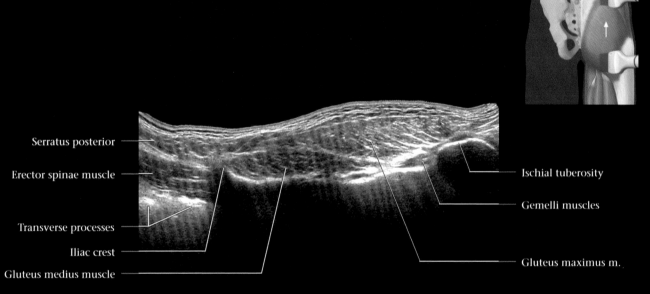

Serratus posterior

Erector spinae muscle

Transverse processes

Iliac crest

Gluteus medius muscle

Ischial tuberosity

Gemelli muscles

Gluteus maximus m.

(Top) The deep external rotators share an intimate relationship with the sciatic nerve, which emerges between the piriformis and superior gemellus muscles and then between gluteus maximus and the rest of the deep external rotators. Further inferiorly, the sciatic nerve runs covered by the biceps femoris muscle. **(Bottom)** Sagittal panoramic view of the medial aspect of the gluteal region. The iliac crest separates the back muscles from the glutei. At this level, the gluteus maximus muscle forms the main muscle bulk. Inferiorly, the gluteus maximus runs across the surface of the ischial tuberosity in this extended (hip joint) position. Coverage is lost (gluteus maximus moves superiorly) when the hip joint is flexed and the ischial tuberosity is exposed.

GLUTEAL MUSCLES

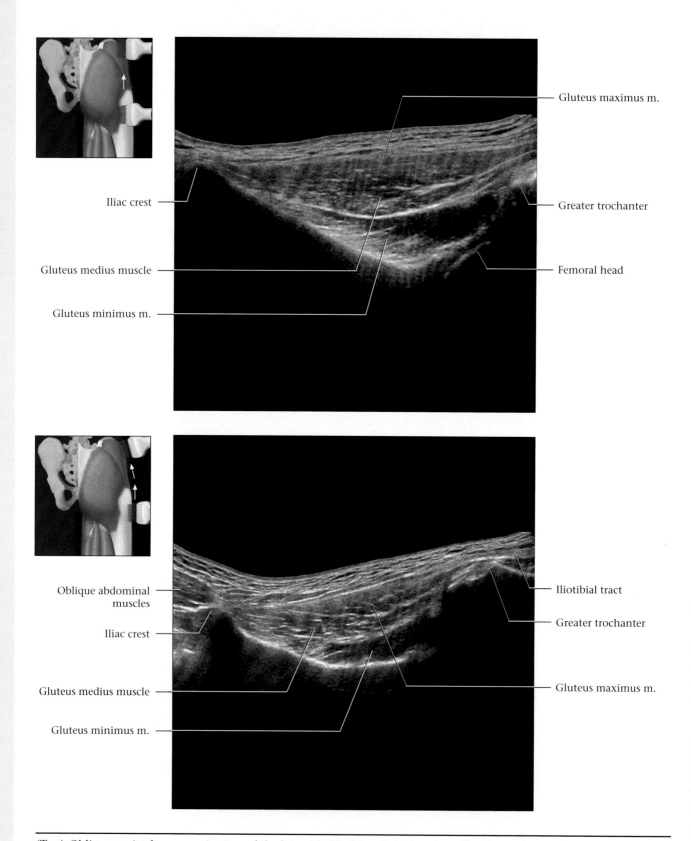

Gluteus maximus m.

Iliac crest

Greater trochanter

Gluteus medius muscle

Femoral head

Gluteus minimus m.

Oblique abdominal muscles

Iliotibial tract

Iliac crest

Greater trochanter

Gluteus medius muscle

Gluteus maximus m.

Gluteus minimus m.

(Top) Oblique sagittal panoramic view of the lateral half of the gluteal region. The close relationship between the gluteus minimus muscle and the posterior aspect of the hip joint can be appreciated here. In this region, all three gluteal muscles are present and can be distinguished by their different echogenicity. The gluteus maximus muscle fibers are running approximately horizontally along the scan plane and being most superficial, produce the highest echogenicity. The gluteus medius is running obliquely (lateral inferiorly) and thus shows short echogenic fibers. The gluteus minimus, after its iliac origin, runs obliquely in a sharp arc, plus being deepest, usually appears hypoechoic. **(Bottom)** Coronal panoramic view showing the gluteus medius and minimus muscles and their insertion on the greater trochanter. The iliotibial tract runs on the surface of the greater trochanter.

GLUTEAL MUSCLES

SAGITTAL GLUTEAL

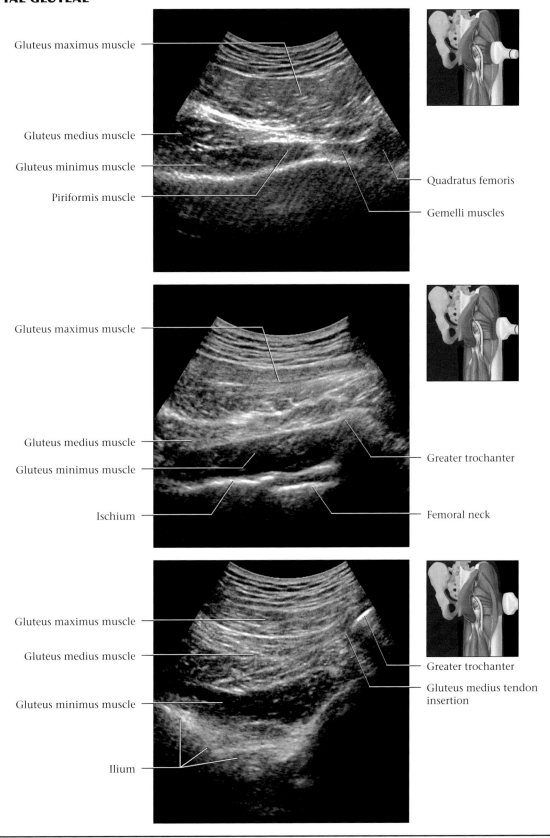

Gluteus maximus muscle

Gluteus medius muscle

Gluteus minimus muscle

Piriformis muscle

Quadratus femoris

Gemelli muscles

Gluteus maximus muscle

Gluteus medius muscle

Gluteus minimus muscle

Greater trochanter

Ischium

Femoral neck

Gluteus maximus muscle

Gluteus medius muscle

Greater trochanter

Gluteus medius tendon insertion

Gluteus minimus muscle

Ilium

(Top) Oblique sagittal scan in the lateral half of the gluteal region shows the three glutei and their relationship with the deeper, small external rotators: Piriformis, superior and inferior gemellus, and quadratus femoris muscles. **(Middle)** Further lateral, the femoral neck can be seen under the gluteus minimus. Again, the different echogenicity and echotexture of the three glutei can be appreciated. **(Bottom)** Further lateral, the gluteus medius tendon fibers insert onto the superior surface of the greater trochanter. The gluteus minimus tendon runs anteriorly under the gluteus medius to also insert on the lesser trochanter, but anterior to gluteus medius.

GLUTEAL MUSCLES

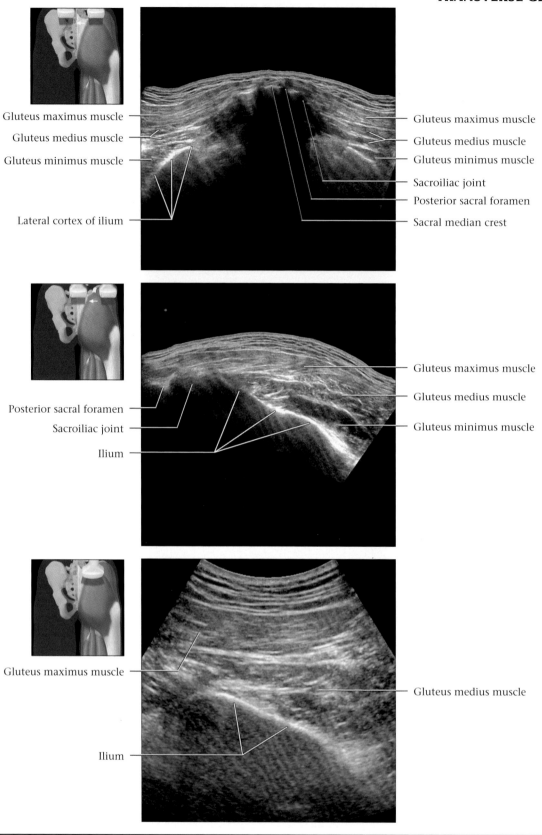

Gluteus maximus muscle

Gluteus medius muscle

Gluteus minimus muscle

Lateral cortex of ilium

Gluteus maximus muscle

Gluteus medius muscle

Gluteus minimus muscle

Sacroiliac joint

Posterior sacral foramen

Sacral median crest

Posterior sacral foramen

Sacroiliac joint

Ilium

Gluteus maximus muscle

Gluteus medius muscle

Gluteus minimus muscle

Gluteus maximus muscle

Gluteus medius muscle

Ilium

(Top) Transverse panoramic scan across the dorsal surface of the sacrum. This is the medial origin of the gluteus maximus muscle. Deep to this muscle, the gluteus medius and gluteus minimus muscles can be seen originating from the iliac surface. (Middle) Transverse panoramic view of the right gluteal region. The three gluteal muscles show their signature difference in echogenicity and echotexture even in the horizontal plane. (Bottom) Transverse focused view of the medial gluteal region shows the fiber orientation of the different muscles. Those of the gluteus maximus are longer as they run roughly horizontally, compared to those of the gluteus medius. This orderly fiber pattern is helpful in detecting intra- and inter-muscular lesions in the gluteal region (orderly fiber alignment tends to be disrupted in disease).

Lower Limb

VII

28

GLUTEAL MUSCLES

ISCHIAL REGION

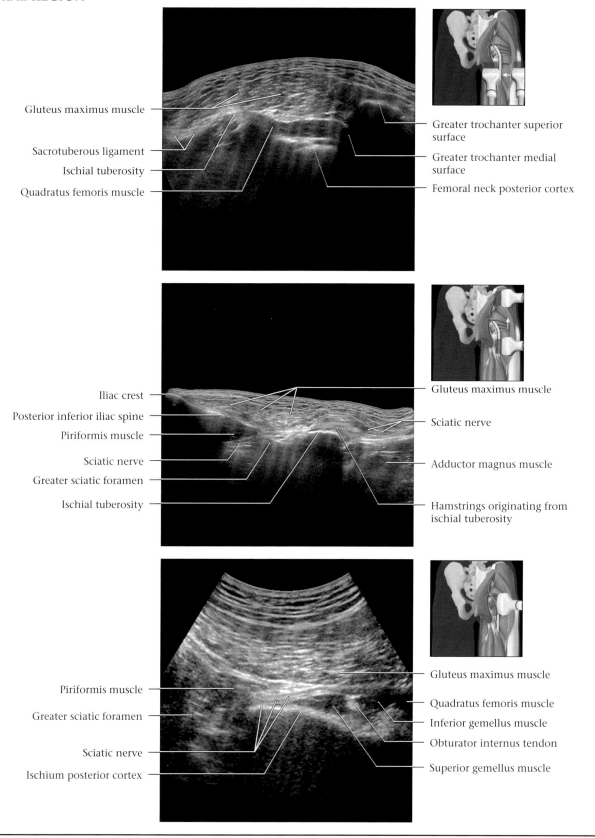

Gluteus maximus muscle

Sacrotuberous ligament

Ischial tuberosity

Quadratus femoris muscle

Greater trochanter superior surface

Greater trochanter medial surface

Femoral neck posterior cortex

Iliac crest

Posterior inferior iliac spine

Piriformis muscle

Sciatic nerve

Greater sciatic foramen

Ischial tuberosity

Gluteus maximus muscle

Sciatic nerve

Adductor magnus muscle

Hamstrings originating from ischial tuberosity

Piriformis muscle

Greater sciatic foramen

Sciatic nerve

Ischium posterior cortex

Gluteus maximus muscle

Quadratus femoris muscle

Inferior gemellus muscle

Obturator internus tendon

Superior gemellus muscle

(Top) Transverse panoramic view of the ischial region. The gluteus maximus forms most of the bulk at this lower gluteal level. Deep to this, small external rotators of the hip can be seen (in this scan the quadratus femoris muscle). (Middle) Sagittal panoramic scan from the lower iliac bone to below the ischial tuberosity. The greater sciatic foramen is demonstrated in this scan. The piriformis and sciatic nerve exit the pelvis via this foramen and run inferolaterally, the former to insert on the greater tuberosity and the latter inferiorly to supply the leg. (Bottom) Sagittal view of the greater sciatic foramen using the ischial tuberosity as a landmark. The sciatic nerve and its relationship with the small external rotators of the hip is shown here. The sciatic nerve emerges between the piriformis and superior gemellus muscles after exiting pelvis through the greater sciatic foramen.

GLUTEAL MUSCLES

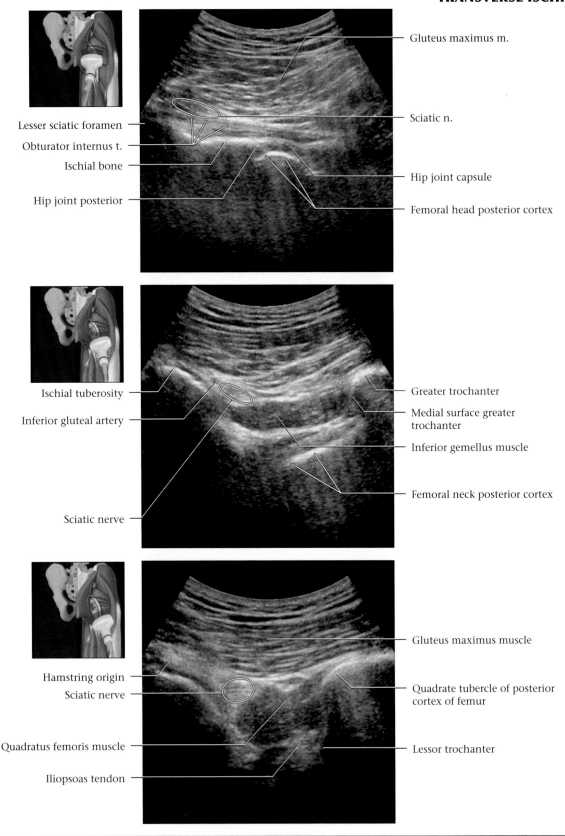

Gluteus maximus m.

Sciatic n.

Lesser sciatic foramen

Obturator internus t.

Ischial bone

Hip joint capsule

Hip joint posterior

Femoral head posterior cortex

Ischial tuberosity

Greater trochanter

Inferior gluteal artery

Medial surface greater trochanter

Inferior gemellus muscle

Femoral neck posterior cortex

Sciatic nerve

Gluteus maximus muscle

Hamstring origin

Sciatic nerve

Quadrate tubercle of posterior cortex of femur

Quadratus femoris muscle

Lessor trochanter

Iliopsoas tendon

(Top) Series of three transverse scans of inferomedial aspect of gluteal region. This image shows obturator internus tendon exiting lesser sciatic foramen, running laterally towards the lower aspect of hip joint. Sciatic nerve runs superficial to this tendon. (Middle) Slightly inferiorly, this image shows the inferior gemellus muscle arising from the ischial tuberosity, running laterally over the neck of the femur and inserting at the piriformis fossa on the medial surface of the greater trochanter. Sciatic nerve runs superficial to this muscle. (Bottom) Further inferiorly, this image shows the quadratus femoris muscle arising from the lateral border of the ischial tuberosity and running laterally to insert on the quadrate tubercle of the femur. The sciatic nerve also runs superficial to this tendon.

GLUTEAL MUSCLES

ISCHIAL TUBEROSITY

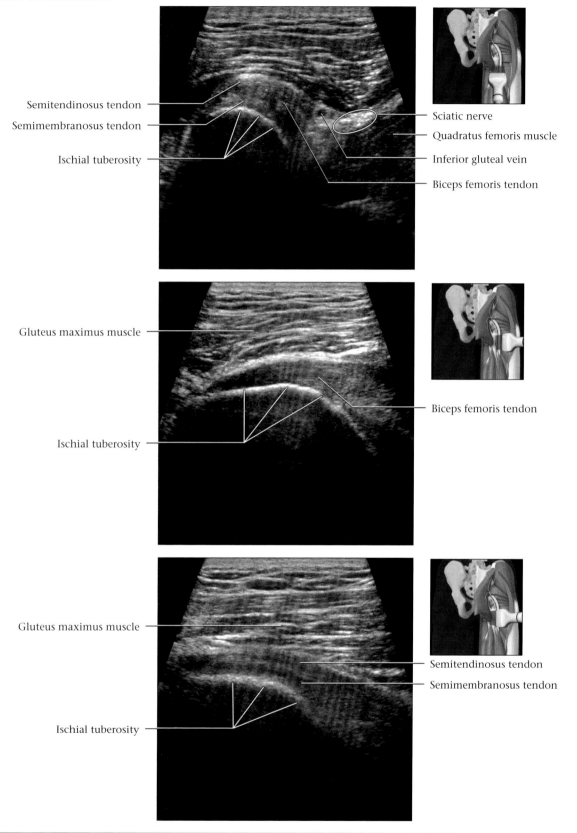

Semitendinosus tendon

Semimembranosus tendon

Ischial tuberosity

Sciatic nerve

Quadratus femoris muscle

Inferior gluteal vein

Biceps femoris tendon

Gluteus maximus muscle

Ischial tuberosity

Biceps femoris tendon

Gluteus maximus muscle

Semitendinosus tendon

Semimembranosus tendon

Ischial tuberosity

(Top) Transverse scan of the ischial tuberosity. The biceps femoris tendon originates lateral to semimembranosus & semitendinosus tendons. The sciatic nerve & inferior gluteal vessels run just lateral to the ischial tuberosity. Inflammation in this region (e.g., ischiogluteal bursitis) may cause irritation of the sciatic nerve. More importantly, aspiration or injection to treat the ischiogluteal bursitis should be performed with image guidance to avoid damaging the sciatic nerve. **(Middle)** Sagittal scan of the lateral aspect of the ischial tuberosity showing origin of the biceps femoris tendon. **(Bottom)** A sagittal scan more medially on the ischial tuberosity shows the insertion of the semitendinosus and semimembranosus tendons. The semitendinosus muscle originates & runs for most of its course on dorsal surface of semimembranosus.

THIG MUSCLES

Terminology

Abbreviations

- Anterior superior iliac spine (ASIS); artery (a.); function (F); insertion (I); ligament (l.); muscle (m.); nerve (n.); origin (O); vein (v.)

Imaging Anatomy

Compartment Anatomy

- **Compartmental anatomy is different from functional groupings below**
- Thigh divided into anterior, medial, and posterior compartments
  - **Anterior compartment**: Iliotibial tract, tensor fascia lata muscle, quadriceps muscles, sartorius muscle
  - **Medial compartment**: Gracilis muscle, adductor muscles
  - **Posterior compartment**: Hamstring muscles, short head of biceps femoris muscle, sciatic nerve
- Additional muscles at junction pelvis/thigh
  - Pectineus, iliopsoas, obturator externus, lateral femoral muscles
- Extensions from fascia lata divide compartments
  - Medial intermuscular septum: Anterior/medial
  - Lateral intermuscular septum: Anterior/lateral
  - Thin fascia separates medial, posterior compartments
- Clinical note: Compartment anatomy critical to tumor staging & biopsy planning
  - Cross compartment extension of tumor, contamination by biopsy requires change from limb salvage to amputation

Medial Femoral Muscles

- Anterior division: Adductor brevis & longus, gracilis muscles
- Posterior division: Adductor portion adductor magnus muscle
- Common function: Hip adduction; assist hip flexion, internal rotation (except obturator externus muscle)
- **Adductor brevis**
  - O: Inferior pubic ramus
  - I: Inferior 2/3 pectineal line, superior 1/2 medial lip linea aspera
- **Adductor longus**
  - O: Pubic body inferior to crest
  - I: Medial lip linea aspera
- **Adductor magnus**: Two separate muscles with different innervations & functions
  - Adductor portion
    - O: Ischiopubic ramus
    - I: Gluteal tuberosity, medial lip linea aspera, medial supracondylar line
  - Ischiocondylar portion: See "Posterior Femoral Muscles"
  - Adductor hiatus between 2 divisions of muscle in distal thigh
- **Gracilis**
  - O: Inferior pubic ramus, symphysis pubis
  - I: Medial proximal tibia (pes anserine)
  - F: Also assists knee flexion

- **Obturator externus**
  - O: External margins obturator foramen & membrane
  - I: Piriformis fossa
  - F: Hip external rotation only
- **Pectineus**
  - O: Superior pubic ramus, pecten
  - I: Pectineal line femur
  - Femoral nerve ± accessory obturator nerve
  - Unclear pre- or post-axial muscle

Anterior Femoral Muscles

- Common function: Knee extension (except sartorius muscle)
- **Rectus femoris**
  - O: Straight head - anterior inferior iliac spine, reflected head - groove above acetabulum
  - I: Superior patella, tibial tuberosity
  - F: Also hip flexion
  - Crosses 2 joints
- **Sartorius**: (Tailor's muscle)
  - O: ASIS, notch below
  - I: Proximal medial tibia (pes anserine)
  - F: Hip flexion, abduction, external rotation; knee flexion
  - Crosses 2 joints
  - Longest muscle in body
  - Separate fascial covering
- **Vastus lateralis**
  - O: Superior intertrochanteric line femur, anterior & inferior greater trochanter, gluteal tuberosity, lateral lip linea aspera, lateral intermuscular septum
  - I: Lateral tibial condyle (lateral patellar retinaculum) superolateral patella (quadriceps tendon)
  - Largest quadriceps muscle
- **Vastus medialis**
  - O: Entire medial lip linea aspera, inferior intertrochanteric line, medial intermuscular septum
  - I: Tendon rectus femoris muscle, superomedial patella (quadriceps tendon), medial condyle tibia (medial patellar retinaculum)
- **Vastus intermedius**
  - O: Anterior & lateral femoral shaft, inferior lateral lip linea aspera, lateral intermuscular septum
  - I: Blends along deep aspect rectus femoris, vastus medialis, vastus lateralis muscles
- **Quadriceps femoris**: Rectus femoris, vastus lateralis, vastus medialis, vastus intermedius muscles
  - Common tendon of insertion onto superior, lateral, medial patella

Posterior Femoral Muscles

- Common functions: Hip extension, knee flexion
- **Biceps femoris**
  - Long head: O - ischial tuberosity (inferior, medial)
    - Common tendon with semitendinosus muscle
  - Short head: O - lateral lip linea aspera femur, lateral supracondylar line, lateral intermuscular septum
    - Post-axial muscle
    - Not part of hamstring muscles
  - I: Fibular head, lateral condyle tibia
  - F: Also external rotation flexed knee
- **Semimembranosus**
  - O: Ischial tuberosity (superior, lateral)
  - I: Posterior medial condyle tibia, popliteal fascia

THIG MUSCLES

- Some fibers extend to form oblique popliteal ligament
  - F: Also internal rotation flexed knee
  - Membranous in upper thigh
- **Semitendinosus**
  - O: Ischial tuberosity (inferior, medial)
    - Common tendon long head biceps femoris muscle
  - I: Medial proximal tibia (pes anserine)
  - F: Also internal rotation flexed knee
  - Entirely tendinous in distal thigh
- **Ischiocondylar portion of adductor magnus**
  - O: Ischial tuberosity
  - I: Adductor tubercle
  - Medial-most aspect adductor magnus muscle
- **Hamstrings**: Long head biceps femoris, semimembranous, semitendinosus, ischiocondylar portion adductor magnus muscles
  - Does not include short head biceps femoris muscle
- **Pes anserine**
  - Common aponeurosis for insertion gracilis, semitendinosus, sartorius tendons
  - Pes anserine bursa between tendons & tibia

Lateral Femoral (Gluteal) Muscles
- Gluteal muscles (see "Gluteal Muscles" section)
- **Iliotibial tract/band**: Lateral thickening fascia lata
  - O: Tubercle iliac crest
  - I: Lateral condyle tibia
  - Insertion site tensor fascia lata muscle, portion of gluteus maximus muscle

Hip Flexors
- **Iliopsoas**: I - lesser trochanter
  - Iliacus
    - O: Iliac crest, iliac fossa, sacral ala, SI joint capsule
    - Femoral nerve
  - Psoas major
    - O: Lateral vertebral body & intervertebral discs T12-L5, all lumbar transverse processes
    - L1, L2, L3
  - Psoas minor
    - O: Lateral vertebral body T12, L1 & T12-L1 intervertebral disc
    - L1, L2
- Sartorius & pectineus

Femoral Triangle
- Anterior wall: Inguinal ligament
- Posterior wall: Adductor longus & pectineus muscles (medial), iliopsoas muscle (lateral)
- Medial border: Adductor longus muscle
- Lateral border: Sartorius muscle
- Apex: Crossing adductor longus & sartorius muscles
- Contents: Femoral nerve & branches, femoral vessels, lymph node (Cloquet node), femoral sheath
  - Structures lateral to medial at entrance: NAVeL
    - Nerve, Artery, Vein, Lymphatics
- Femoral artery/vein relationships
  - Entrance: Artery lateral
  - Apex: Artery anterior
- Femoral nerve branches within triangle
  - Saphenous nerve, & nerve to vastus medialis only branches to exit triangle

- **Femoral sheath**: Transversalis fascia covers vessels proximally
  - 3 compartments
    - Lateral: Artery
    - Middle: Vein
    - Medial: Lymph node (femoral canal)
- **Femoral canal**: Medial compartment femoral sheath
  - Anterior border: Inguinal ligament
  - Posterior border: Pubic bone
  - Medial border: Lacunar ligament
  - Lateral border: Femoral vein
  - Entrance: **Femoral ring**
    - Anterior border: Medial inguinal ligament
    - Posterior border: Superior pubic ramus
    - Medial border: Lacunar ligament
    - Lateral border: Septum between femoral canal & femoral vein
    - Open to peritoneal cavity
  - Contents: Lymphatic vessels & nodes (**Cloquet node**), fat, connective tissue
  - Clinical note: **Femoral hernia**
    - Lateral & inferior to pubic tubercle
    - Travels femoral ring to femoral canal to saphenous opening to subcutaneous tissue

Adductor (Subsartorial or Hunter) Canal
- Fascial passageway for vessels midthigh
  - Boundaries are fascial surfaces of adjacent muscles
- Anteromedial border: Sartorius muscle
- Anterolateral border: Vastus medialis muscle
- Posterior border: Adductor longus & magnus muscles
- Entrance: Apex femoral triangle
- Exit: Adductor hiatus
  - **Adductor hiatus**: Gap adductor magnus m. between adductor portion & ischiocondylar portion distal thigh
- Vessel passageway from thigh to popliteal fossa
- Contents: Femoral artery & vein, saphenous nerve
  - Nerve initially anterior to artery then medial
  - Artery anterior to vein
  - Descending geniculate artery arises in canal

Anatomy-Based Imaging Issues

Imaging Recommendations
- US
  - Highest combined spatial and contrast resolution of the different imaging modalities
    - Important for detecting and characterizing small lesions or fine anatomy e.g., small nerve sheath tumors, internal vascularity of lesions etc.
  - Real-time interrogation allows evaluation of muscle and tendon movement during dynamic maneuvers e.g., for snapping hips, nerve impingement etc.
  - Limited by depth of penetration
- CT
  - Best for evaluating osseous integrity
  - Soft tissue assessment inferior to US & MR
- MR
  - Highest contrast resolution when using fluid sensitive or contrast-enhanced sequences

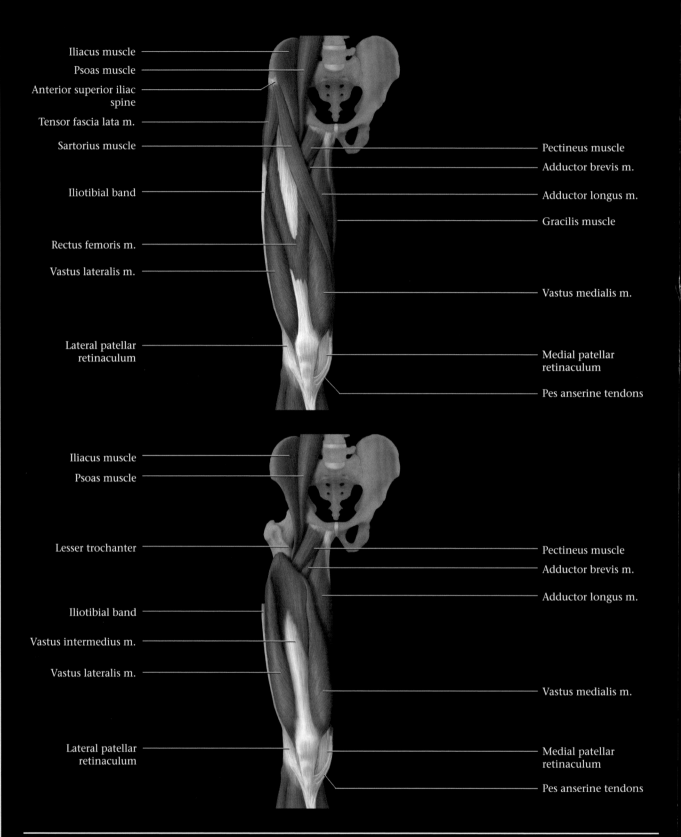

Iliacus muscle

Psoas muscle

Anterior superior iliac spine

Tensor fascia lata m.

Sartorius muscle

Iliotibial band

Rectus femoris m.

Vastus lateralis m.

Lateral patellar retinaculum

Pectineus muscle

Adductor brevis m.

Adductor longus m.

Gracilis muscle

Vastus medialis m.

Medial patellar retinaculum

Pes anserine tendons

Iliacus muscle

Psoas muscle

Lesser trochanter

Iliotibial band

Vastus intermedius m.

Vastus lateralis m.

Lateral patellar retinaculum

Pectineus muscle

Adductor brevis m.

Adductor longus m.

Vastus medialis m.

Medial patellar retinaculum

Pes anserine tendons

Lower Limb

VII

34

(Top) Superficial muscles of the anterior thigh. The oblique course of the sartorius muscle is easily appreciated. The adductor brevis muscle is deep to the adductor longus and pectineus muscles. The most medial muscle is the gracilis. The vastus lateralis and medialis muscles continue to their insertions as the lateral and medial patellar retinacula respectively. **(Bottom)** Deep muscles of the anterior thigh. The vastus intermedius muscle is deep to the rectus femoris muscle. The vastus intermedius muscle tendon blends with the rectus femoris tendon along its deep surface. The iliopsoas muscle dives deep after crossing over the pelvic brim. With removal of the sartorius muscle a little more of the adductor brevis muscle is visible. The pes anserine tendons, the gracilis, sartorius and semitendinosus, have a conjoined insertion onto the proximal medial tibia.

THIGH MUSCLES

OVERVIEW, ANTERIOR THIGH

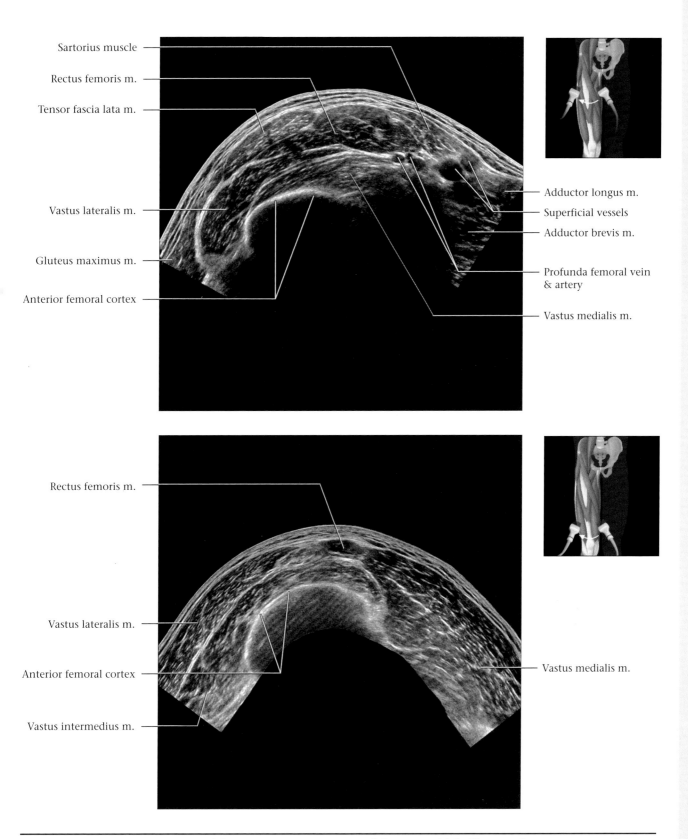

Sartorius muscle

Rectus femoris m.

Tensor fascia lata m.

Vastus lateralis m.

Gluteus maximus m.

Anterior femoral cortex

Adductor longus m.

Superficial vessels

Adductor brevis m.

Profunda femoral vein & artery

Vastus medialis m.

Rectus femoris m.

Vastus lateralis m.

Anterior femoral cortex

Vastus intermedius m.

Vastus medialis m.

(Top) Transverse panoramic view of the anterior compartment of the upper thigh. The anterior compartment is composed of the quadriceps muscle, tensor fascia lata/iliotibial tract and sartorius muscle. Medially, it is bordered by the femoral neurovascular bundle and adductor muscles. Laterally, it is bordered by the gluteal and hamstring muscles. **(Bottom)** In the lower thigh, the rectus femoris is much reduced in size and will continue inferiorly as the quadriceps tendon. The rest of the quadriceps continue as bulky muscles down to the suprapatellar level. They contribute directly to the quadriceps tendon. The major neurovascular bundle has moved to the posterior compartment and the only anterior compartment vessels are branches of the profunda femoral.

THIGH MUSCLES

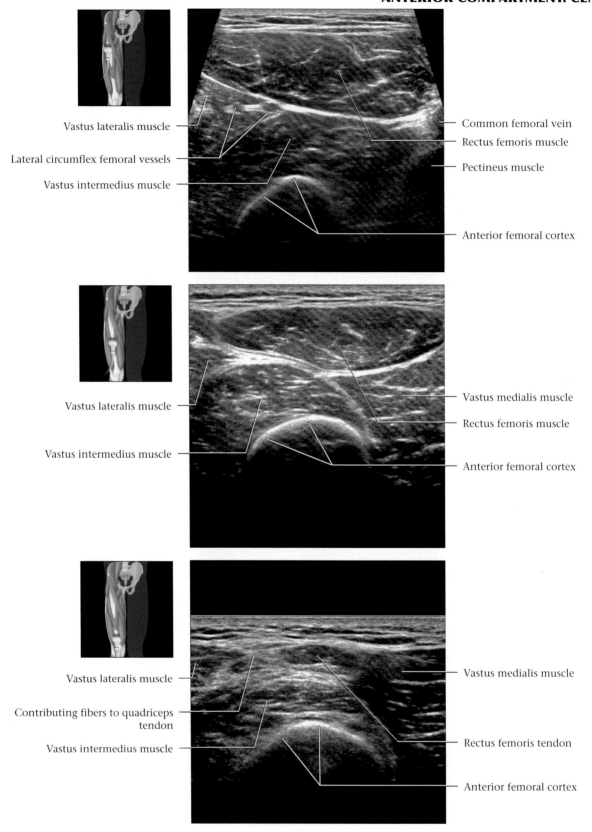

Vastus lateralis muscle

Lateral circumflex femoral vessels

Vastus intermedius muscle

Common femoral vein

Rectus femoris muscle

Pectineus muscle

Anterior femoral cortex

Vastus lateralis muscle

Vastus intermedius muscle

Vastus medialis muscle

Rectus femoris muscle

Anterior femoral cortex

Vastus lateralis muscle

Contributing fibers to quadriceps tendon

Vastus intermedius muscle

Vastus medialis muscle

Rectus femoris tendon

Anterior femoral cortex

(Top) Series of three transverse scans of the central part of the anterior compartment. At this proximal level, the dominant (in terms of bulk) quadriceps muscle is the rectus femoris muscle. It is easily identified by its central position; it is lateral to the femoral neurovascular bundle (the femoral triangle). The lateral circumflex artery is important because together with the medial circumflex, its posterior counterpart, they supply the head of the femur. (Middle) Transverse scan through the mid-thigh. The vastus medialis and intermedius have originated and at this level all four quadriceps muscles can be seen. (Bottom) Transverse scan of the distal thigh, above the level of the suprapatellar bursa. The rectus femoris has become a central tendon, which receives contributions from the vasti muscles.

THIGH MUSCLES

ANTERIOR COMPARTMENT: LATERAL

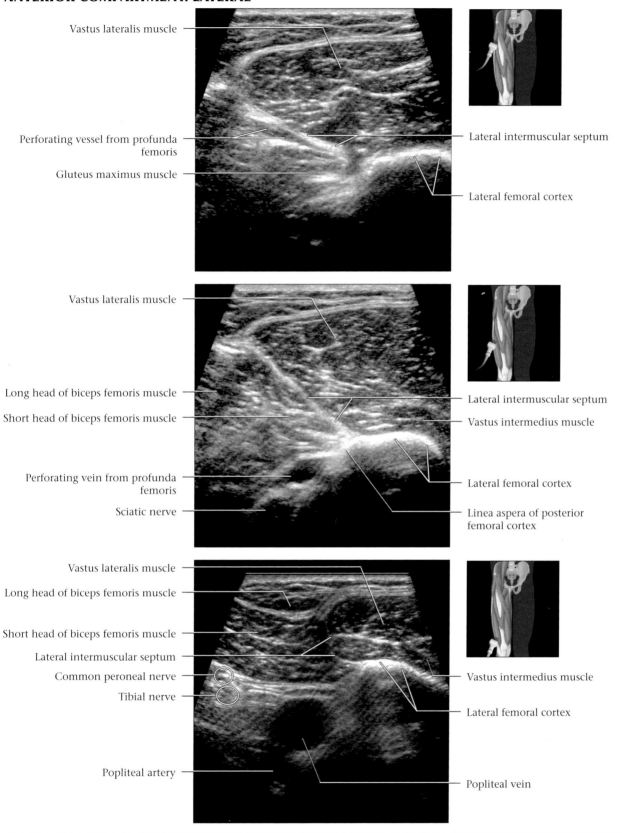

Vastus lateralis muscle

Perforating vessel from profunda femoris

Gluteus maximus muscle

Lateral intermuscular septum

Lateral femoral cortex

Vastus lateralis muscle

Long head of biceps femoris muscle

Short head of biceps femoris muscle

Perforating vein from profunda femoris

Sciatic nerve

Lateral intermuscular septum

Vastus intermedius muscle

Lateral femoral cortex

Linea aspera of posterior femoral cortex

Vastus lateralis muscle

Long head of biceps femoris muscle

Short head of biceps femoris muscle

Lateral intermuscular septum

Common peroneal nerve

Tibial nerve

Popliteal artery

Vastus intermedius muscle

Lateral femoral cortex

Popliteal vein

(Top) Series of transverse scans through lateral aspect of thigh. Proximally, the vastus lateralis muscle is dominant & borders with gluteus maximus muscle (which inserts onto the posterior surface of the femur). The lateral intermuscular septum separates anterior from posterior compartments laterally & also acts as conduit for vessels. **(Middle)** Further inferiorly, the vastus lateralis borders biceps femoris. The linea aspera is a distinct protrusion from the posterior femoral shaft where many muscles originate & insert, including the lateral intermuscular septum. On ultrasound, it is consistently seen and therefore serves as a useful bony landmark. **(Bottom)** At the superior popliteal level, the vastus lateralis muscle becomes less bulky (reverse occurs with the vastus intermedius muscle) as does the bordering long head of biceps muscle. The sciatic nerve divides into tibial and common peroneal branches.

THIGH MUSCLES

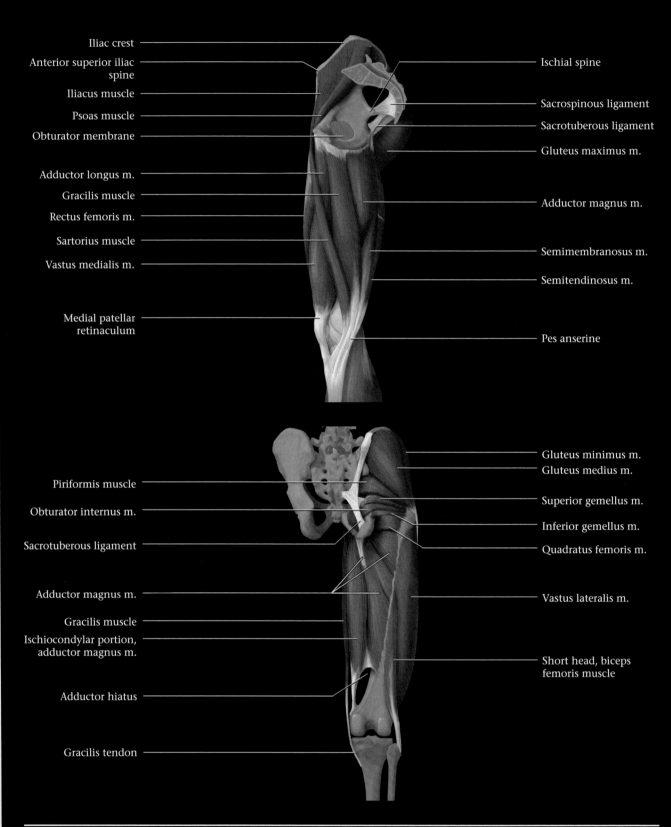

Iliac crest

Anterior superior iliac spine

Iliacus muscle

Psoas muscle

Obturator membrane

Adductor longus m.

Gracilis muscle

Rectus femoris m.

Sartorius muscle

Vastus medialis m.

Medial patellar retinaculum

Ischial spine

Sacrospinous ligament

Sacrotuberous ligament

Gluteus maximus m.

Adductor magnus m.

Semimembranosus m.

Semitendinosus m.

Pes anserine

Piriformis muscle

Obturator internus m.

Sacrotuberous ligament

Adductor magnus m.

Gracilis muscle

Ischiocondylar portion, adductor magnus m.

Adductor hiatus

Gracilis tendon

Gluteus minimus m.

Gluteus medius m.

Superior gemellus m.

Inferior gemellus m.

Quadratus femoris m.

Vastus lateralis m.

Short head, biceps femoris muscle

(Top) Medial muscles of the thigh. The gracilis muscle has a thin profile when viewed from the front, however when viewed from the side it is quite broad. The semimembranosus muscle runs along the deep surface of the semitendinous muscle and inserts onto the tibia posterior to the pes anserine tendons. Its insertion is hidden on this image. The iliopsoas muscle courses over the pelvic brim on its course to the lesser trochanter. **(Bottom)** Deep muscles of the posterior thigh. With removal of the hamstring muscles the expansive adductor magnus muscle is visible. The separation of its two heads in the distal thigh forms the adductor hiatus.

THIGH MUSCLES

OVERVIEW, MEDIAL THIGH

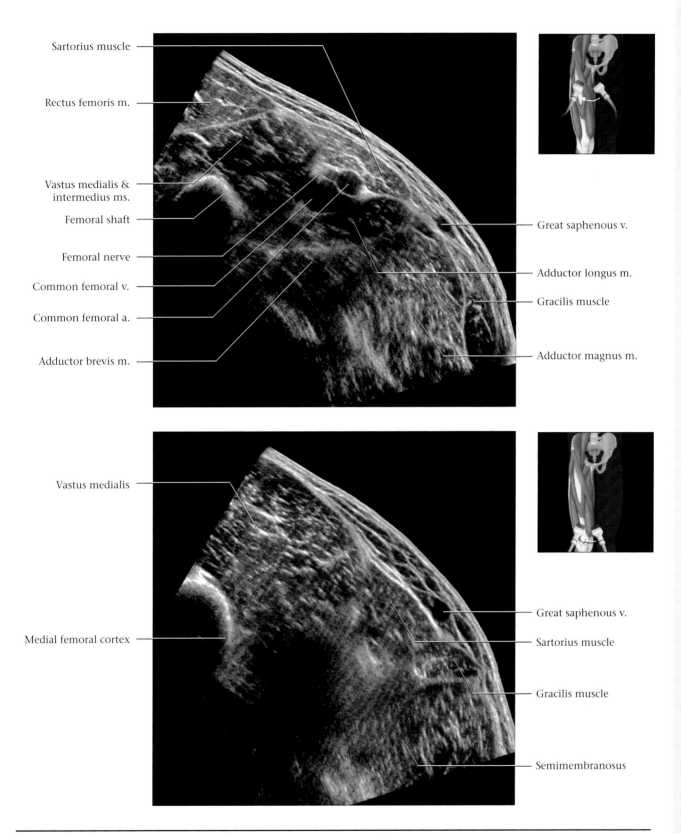

Sartorius muscle

Rectus femoris m.

Vastus medialis & intermedius ms.

Femoral shaft

Femoral nerve

Common femoral v.

Common femoral a.

Adductor brevis m.

Great saphenous v.

Adductor longus m.

Gracilis muscle

Adductor magnus m.

Vastus medialis

Medial femoral cortex

Great saphenous v.

Sartorius muscle

Gracilis muscle

Semimembranosus

(Top) Transverse panoramic view of the medial compartment at the upper thigh level. At this level, all three adductor muscles can be seen, together with the gracilis muscle. This compartment is bordered anteriorly by the femoral triangle, which continues inferiorly as the adductor canal. Posteriorly, the medial compartment is bordered by the semimembranosus muscle. (Bottom) Transverse panoramic scan of the medial aspect of the lower thigh. At this level, the adductor muscles have inserted superiorly, therefore, the medial compartment is much smaller and composed mainly of the gracilis muscle. The adductor hiatus, which is above this level, provides an entrance for the femoral vessels into the popliteal fossa.

THIGH MUSCLES

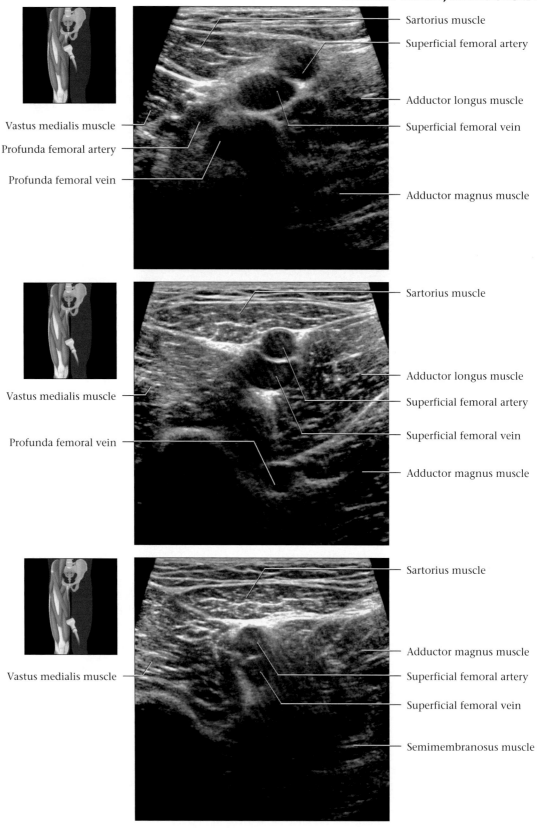

(Top) Transverse scan labels: Sartorius muscle, Superficial femoral artery, Adductor longus muscle, Superficial femoral vein, Adductor magnus muscle, Vastus medialis muscle, Profunda femoral artery, Profunda femoral vein

(Middle) Transverse scan labels: Sartorius muscle, Adductor longus muscle, Superficial femoral artery, Superficial femoral vein, Adductor magnus muscle, Vastus medialis muscle, Profunda femoral vein

(Bottom) Transverse scan labels: Sartorius muscle, Adductor magnus muscle, Superficial femoral artery, Superficial femoral vein, Semimembranosus muscle, Vastus medialis muscle

(Top) Transverse scan of the anterior part of the medial thigh. Above the adductor canal, the apex of the femoral triangle contains bifurcation of the common femoral vessels. The profunda will run deep to supply the thigh muscles and femur. The superficial femoral vessels continue into the adductor canal. (Middle) Transverse scan more inferiorly shows that the superficial femoral vessels are now under the cover of the sartorius muscle indicating that they are in the adductor canal. (Bottom) Transverse scan of the medial aspect of the mid-thigh. The common adductor canal continues medially and more deeply. At this level, the medial wall of the adductor canal changes from the adductor longus muscle to the adductor part of the adductor magnus muscle.

THIGH MUSCLES

MEDIAL THIGH

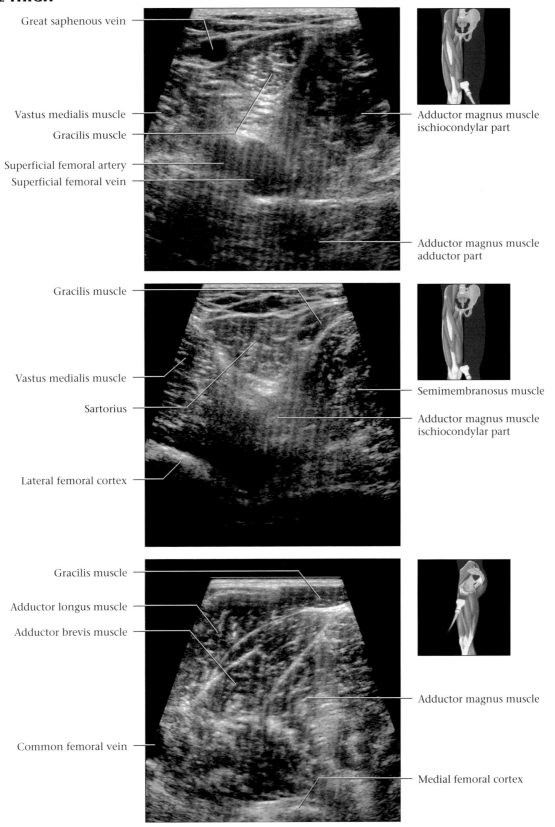

Great saphenous vein

Vastus medialis muscle

Gracilis muscle

Superficial femoral artery

Superficial femoral vein

Adductor magnus muscle ischiocondylar part

Adductor magnus muscle adductor part

Gracilis muscle

Vastus medialis muscle

Sartorius

Lateral femoral cortex

Semimembranosus muscle

Adductor magnus muscle ischiocondylar part

Gracilis muscle

Adductor longus muscle

Adductor brevis muscle

Common femoral vein

Adductor magnus muscle

Medial femoral cortex

(Top) Transverse scan using an anteromedial approach. At this level, the superficial femoral vessels enter the popliteal fossa via the adductor hiatus, which is a gap in the adductor magnus muscle, between the adductor and ischiocondylar parts before their insertions (on the medial supracondylar line and adductor tubercle respectively). (Middle) More inferiorly, only the gracilis muscle and the ischiocondylar part of the adductor magnus (acting like a hamstring) are left in the the medial compartment. This space is encroached on by the vastus medialis muscle anteriorly and semimembranosus muscle posteriorly. (Bottom) Using a medial approach (from the inner thigh), the deeper muscles can be demonstrated. The adductor longus and brevis muscle plus the gracilis muscle form an anterior division, while the bulky adductor magnus muscle forms the posterior division.

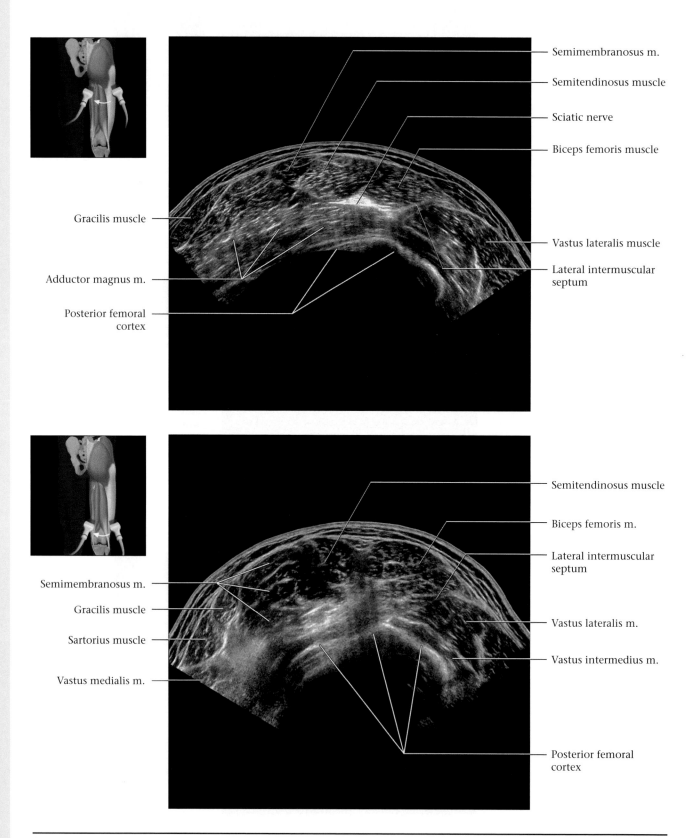

Semimembranosus m.

Semitendinosus muscle

Sciatic nerve

Biceps femoris muscle

Gracilis muscle

Vastus lateralis muscle

Lateral intermuscular septum

Adductor magnus m.

Posterior femoral cortex

Semitendinosus muscle

Biceps femoris m.

Lateral intermuscular septum

Semimembranosus m.

Gracilis muscle

Sartorius muscle

Vastus lateralis m.

Vastus intermedius m.

Vastus medialis m.

Posterior femoral cortex

(Top) Transverse panoramic scan of the posterior compartment at the upper-thigh level. At this level the hamstring muscles form a small proportion of the posterior muscle bulk, the main contributions come from adductors (the medial compartment) and vastus lateralis (the anterior compartment). The sciatic nerve runs under the cover of the biceps femoris muscle. **(Bottom)** Transverse panoramic scan of the posterior aspect of the distal thigh. At this more inferior level, the hamstrings form a much larger proportion of the posterior muscle bulk. In particular, the semimembranosus becomes the dominant muscle on posteromedial side as most of the adductors have inserted onto the femur above this level.

THIGH MUSCLES

POSTERIOR THIGH

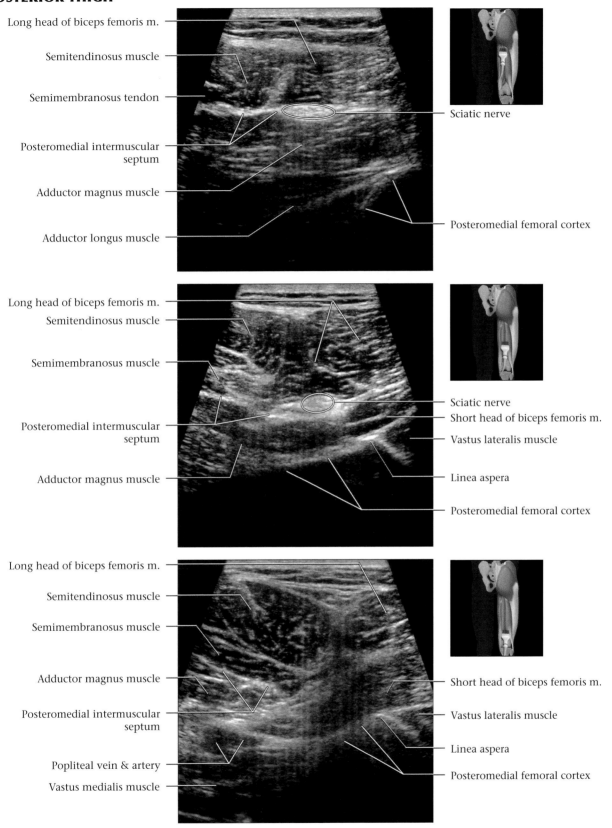

Long head of biceps femoris m.

Semitendinosus muscle

Semimembranosus tendon

Posteromedial intermuscular septum

Adductor magnus muscle

Adductor longus muscle

Sciatic nerve

Posteromedial femoral cortex

Long head of biceps femoris m.

Semitendinosus muscle

Semimembranosus muscle

Posteromedial intermuscular septum

Adductor magnus muscle

Sciatic nerve

Short head of biceps femoris m.

Vastus lateralis muscle

Linea aspera

Posteromedial femoral cortex

Long head of biceps femoris m.

Semitendinosus muscle

Semimembranosus muscle

Adductor magnus muscle

Posteromedial intermuscular septum

Popliteal vein & artery

Vastus medialis muscle

Short head of biceps femoris m.

Vastus lateralis muscle

Linea aspera

Posteromedial femoral cortex

(Top) Series of three transverse scans of the central portion of the posterior thigh. After their origin from the ischial tuberosity, the semitendinosus and semimembranosus muscles run on the medial side and the biceps femoris muscle runs on the lateral side. The sciatic nerve is under the cover of the biceps femoris for most of its way to the popliteal fossa. (Middle) At the mid-thigh level, the hamstrings are bulkier and the adductors smaller. The two groups are divided by the posteromedial intermuscular septum. (Bottom) Further inferiorly, the popliteal vessels enter via the adductor hiatus into the popliteal fossa. The superior aspect of the popliteal fossa is lined by the semimembranosus and semitendinosus muscle on the medial side and the biceps femoris laterally.

FEMORAL VESSELS AND NERVES

Terminology

Abbreviations
- Artery (a.)
- Ligament (l.)
- Muscle (m.)
- Nerve (n.)
- Vein (v.)
- Structure supplied by a nerve or vessel (S)

Imaging Anatomy

Femoral Vessels
- Enter thigh deep to inguinal ligament, midpoint between ASIS & symphysis pubis
  - Change from external iliac vessels to common femoral vessels
- Upper thigh: Vessels within femoral triangle
  - Enter: Artery lateral to vein
  - Exit: Artery anterior
- Mid thigh: Vessels within adductor canal
  - Enter: Artery anterior to vein
  - Exit: Artery anterior
- Distal thigh: Exit adductor canal via adductor hiatus, enter popliteal fossa
- **Common femoral artery branches**
  - **Superficial epigastric, superficial circumflex iliac, superficial external pudendal** arise anteriorly
  - **Deep external pudendal** arises medially
    - May branch from medial circumflex femoral
  - Divides into superficial & deep branches
  - **Superficial femoral artery**
    - Branch: **Descending genicular**
  - **Deep femoral (profunda femoris)**
    - Arises laterally in femoral triangle
    - Dives between pectineus & adductor longus ms.
    - Medial to femur, deep to adductor longus m.
    - Branches in femoral triangle: **Medial circumflex femoral** (main supply femoral head & neck), lateral circumflex femoral, muscular branches
    - Branches in adductor canal: 3 perforating branches, descending genicular
    - Terminal branch: 4th perforating artery
- **Femoral vein:** Travels with artery
  - Tributaries: Deep femoral, descending genicular, lateral circumflex femoral, medial circumflex femoral, deep external pudendal, greater saphenous veins
  - **Greater saphenous vein**
    - Longest vein in body
    - Toes to saphenous opening (fascia lata)
    - Tributaries: Accessory saphenous, superficial epigastric, superficial circumflex femoral, superficial external pudendal veins

Femoral Nerve
- Nerve contributions from L2, L3, L4, L5
- Largest branch lumbar plexus
- Exits plexus lower psoas muscle
- Travels in groove between psoas & iliacus muscles
- Exits pelvis beneath inguinal ligament, lateral to femoral vessels, enters femoral triangle
- Multiple branches in femoral triangle
  - Muscular branches: To pectineus, sartorius, rectus femoris, vastus lateralis, vastus medialis, vastus intermedius muscles
  - Cutaneous nerves: Anterior femoral cutaneous, saphenous
    - Saphenous n. exits triangle, enters adductor canal
  - Articular branches hip & knee

Sciatic Nerve
- Nerve contributions from: L4, L5, S1, S2, S3 levels
- Largest nerve in the body
- Two nerves in one sheath
  - Tibial n. (medial) & common peroneal n. (lateral)
  - Separate in popliteal fossa
- Course
  - Exits pelvis inferior to piriformis muscle
    - Anomalous relationship in 10%
  - Deep to gluteus maximus muscle, more inferiorly deep to biceps femoris muscle
    - Crosses over superior gemellus, obturator internus, inferior gemellus, quadratus femoris, adductor magnus muscles
    - Midway between ischial tuberosity and greater trochanter in the transverse plane
  - Runs deep to long head of biceps femoris muscle after exiting gluteal region
- Branches arising in thigh: Articular to hip, nerves to hamstring muscles
- Supply
  - In thigh: Biceps femoris, semitendinosus, semimembranosus, ischiocondylar portion of adductor magnus muscle
- **Tibial nerve:** Larger division of sciatic nerve
  - S: Posterior femoral muscles except short head biceps femoris muscle
- **Common peroneal nerve**
  - Oblique lateral course with biceps femoris muscle
  - S: Short head biceps femoris muscle

Anatomy-Based Imaging Issues

Imaging Recommendations
- Ultrasound is unique in that it assesses both morphology and functional response of vessels
  - Complete examination should include interrogation with color Doppler
  - In cases with stenosis, reflux or reverse flow, spectral Doppler helpful to demonstrate waveform and document flow velocity
  - Dynamic maneuvers, such as transducer compression, breath-holding, Valsalva, calf augmentation are helpful to assess patency of veins on color and spectral Doppler
  - Intravenous contrast is not necessary
- High spatial resolution makes ultrasound suitable for assessing superficial nerves
  - Disruption of parallel continuity of nerve bundles suggests pathology
  - Transducer angulation may need to be changed to avoid anisotropy

GRAPHICS, THIGH ARTERIES

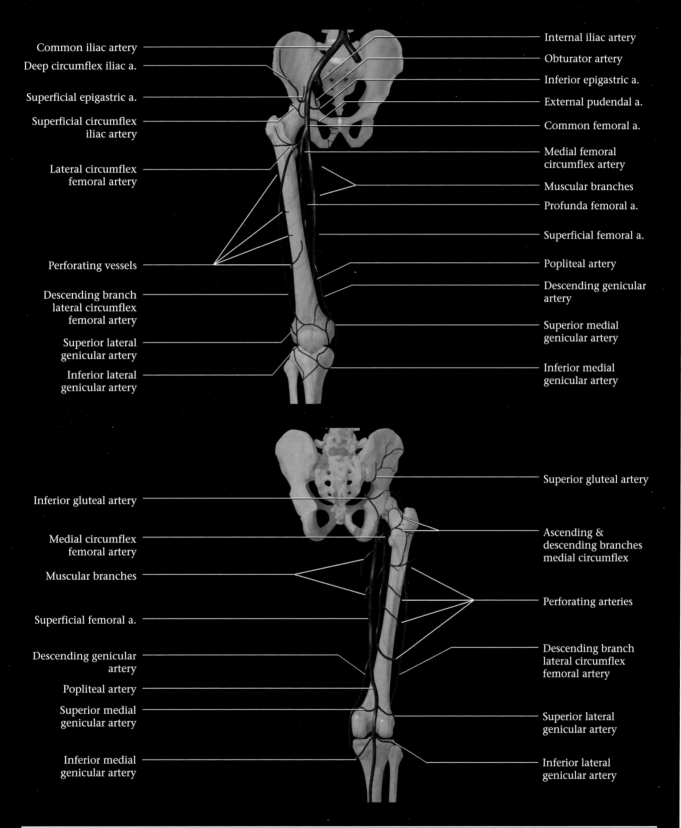

Common iliac artery

Deep circumflex iliac a.

Superficial epigastric a.

Superficial circumflex iliac artery

Lateral circumflex femoral artery

Perforating vessels

Descending branch lateral circumflex femoral artery

Superior lateral genicular artery

Inferior lateral genicular artery

Internal iliac artery

Obturator artery

Inferior epigastric a.

External pudendal a.

Common femoral a.

Medial femoral circumflex artery

Muscular branches

Profunda femoral a.

Superficial femoral a.

Popliteal artery

Descending genicular artery

Superior medial genicular artery

Inferior medial genicular artery

Inferior gluteal artery

Medial circumflex femoral artery

Muscular branches

Superficial femoral a.

Descending genicular artery

Popliteal artery

Superior medial genicular artery

Inferior medial genicular artery

Superior gluteal artery

Ascending & descending branches medial circumflex

Perforating arteries

Descending branch lateral circumflex femoral artery

Superior lateral genicular artery

Inferior lateral genicular artery

(Top) Anterior view of the external iliac, femoral and popliteal arteries and their branches. **(Bottom)** Posterior view of the femoral and popliteal arteries and the superior and inferior gluteal arteries of the greater sciatic notch.

FEMORAL VESSELS AND NERVES

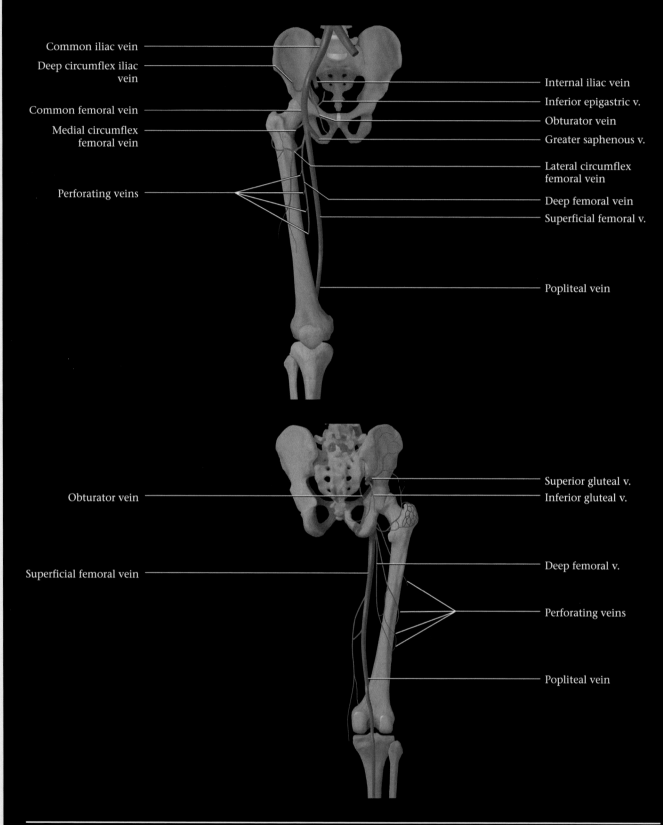

Common iliac vein
Deep circumflex iliac vein
Common femoral vein
Medial circumflex femoral vein
Perforating veins

Internal iliac vein
Inferior epigastric v.
Obturator vein
Greater saphenous v.
Lateral circumflex femoral vein
Deep femoral vein
Superficial femoral v.
Popliteal vein

Obturator vein
Superficial femoral vein

Superior gluteal v.
Inferior gluteal v.
Deep femoral v.
Perforating veins
Popliteal vein

(Top) Anterior view of the veins of the thigh. The veins typically follow the arterial tree. The main venous drainage is the superficial femoral vein which is actually a deep venous structure. Note the entrance of the greater saphenous vein into the femoral vein; it has no associated artery. **(Bottom)** Posterior view of the veins of the thigh and buttocks. The veins generally follow the arterial tree although more variability is seen within the venous system.

FEMORAL VESSELS AND NERVES

GRAPHICS, THIGH NERVES

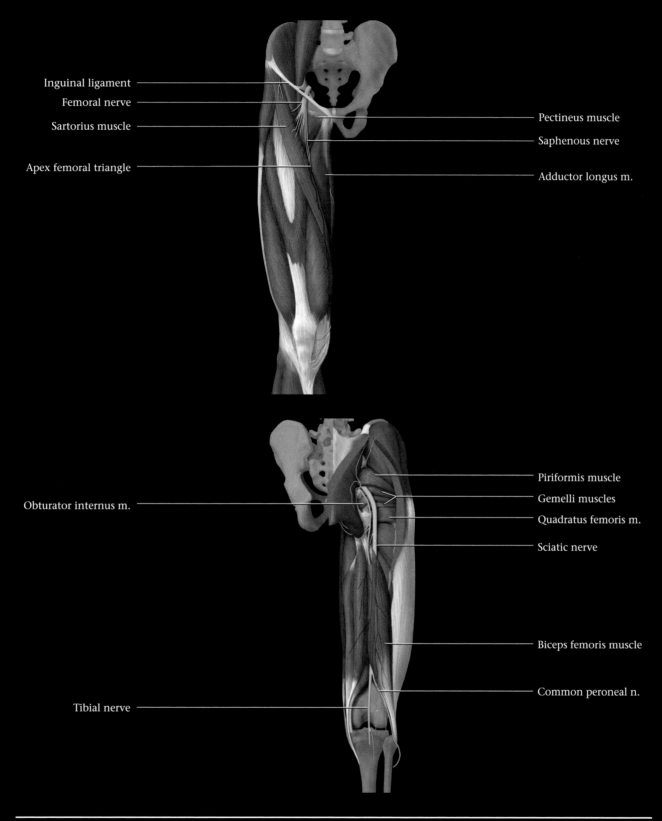

Inguinal ligament

Femoral nerve

Sartorius muscle

Apex femoral triangle

Pectineus muscle

Saphenous nerve

Adductor longus m.

Obturator internus m.

Piriformis muscle

Gemelli muscles

Quadratus femoris m.

Sciatic nerve

Biceps femoris muscle

Common peroneal n.

Tibial nerve

(Top) Femoral nerve. After emerging from the groove between the psoas and iliacus muscles the nerve passes under the inguinal ligament to enter the femoral triangle. It immediately branches into muscular, cutaneous, & articular nerves. The only nerve to pass through the femoral triangle into the adductor canal is the saphenous nerve.
(Bottom) Sciatic nerve. The sciatic nerve enters the lower extremity by passing under the inferior border of the piriformis muscle. The sciatic nerve passes posterior to the external rotator tendons and then courses deep to the biceps femoris muscle. It separates into the tibial and common peroneal nerves in the distal thigh. The tibial nerve bisects the popliteal fossa. The common peroneal nerve follows the biceps femoris muscle around the fibular head.

FEMORAL VESSELS AND NERVES

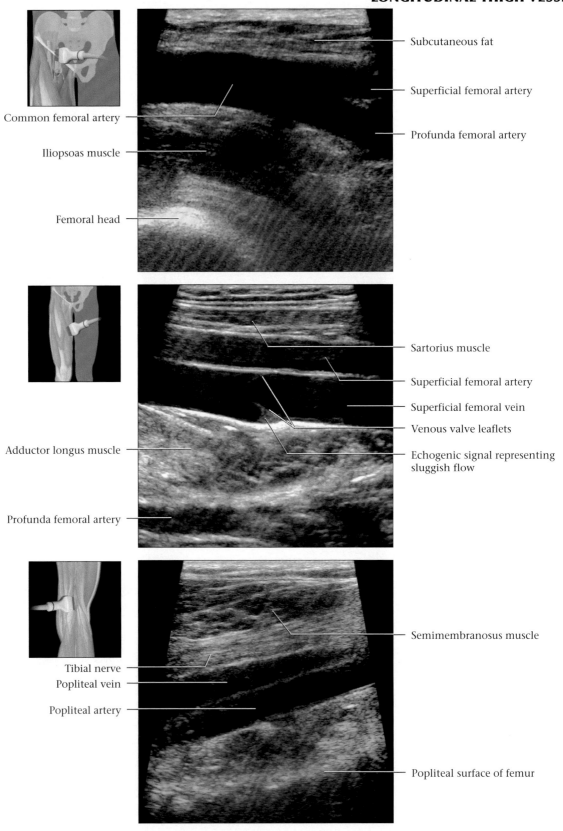

Common femoral artery

Iliopsoas muscle

Femoral head

Subcutaneous fat

Superficial femoral artery

Profunda femoral artery

Sartorius muscle

Superficial femoral artery

Superficial femoral vein

Venous valve leaflets

Echogenic signal representing sluggish flow

Adductor longus muscle

Profunda femoral artery

Tibial nerve

Popliteal vein

Popliteal artery

Semimembranosus muscle

Popliteal surface of femur

(Top) Sagittal scan of the common femoral artery and its bifurcation into the superficial femoral artery and the profunda femoral artery. The superficial femoral artery continues into the femoral triangle, adductor canal before ending at the adductor hiatus to become the popliteal artery. The profunda femoral artery supplies the muscles of the thigh. **(Middle)** Sagittal scan of the upper adductor canal. The superficial femoral vessels are covered by the sartorius muscle. The high spatial resolution of ultrasound allows venous valves and sluggish flow to be visualized (the latter as increased echogenicity). **(Bottom)** Sagittal scan of the popliteal vessels using a posterior approach. Note the reversed relationship between the vessels, the vein now lies more superficial than the artery.

Lower Limb

VII

48

FEMORAL VESSELS AND NERVES

TRANSVERSE THIGH VESSELS

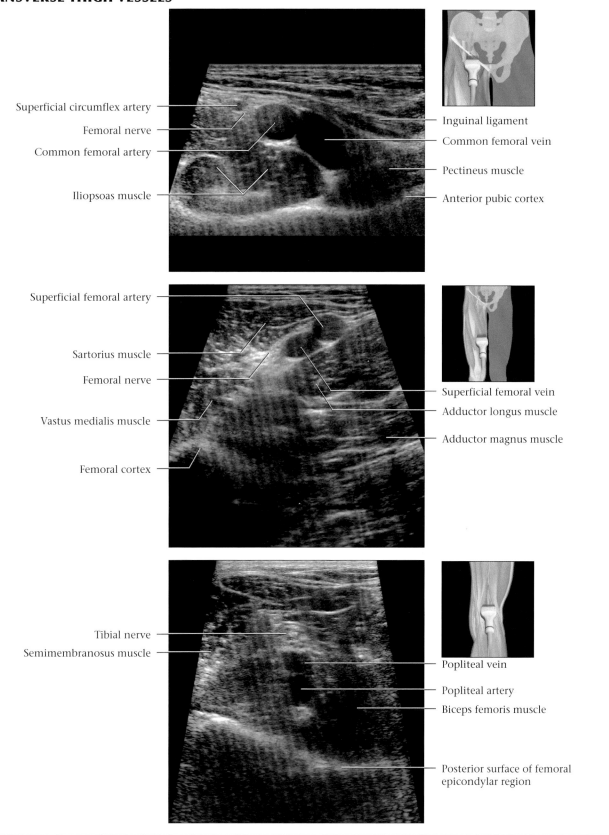

Superficial circumflex artery

Femoral nerve

Common femoral artery

Iliopsoas muscle

Inguinal ligament

Common femoral vein

Pectineus muscle

Anterior pubic cortex

Superficial femoral artery

Sartorius muscle

Femoral nerve

Vastus medialis muscle

Femoral cortex

Superficial femoral vein

Adductor longus muscle

Adductor magnus muscle

Tibial nerve

Semimembranosus muscle

Popliteal vein

Popliteal artery

Biceps femoris muscle

Posterior surface of femoral epicondylar region

(Top) Transverse scan of the common femoral vessels emerging from under the inguinal ligament. The femoral nerve lies lateral to the common femoral artery. The iliopsoas muscle and pectineus muscle form the floor. **(Middle)** Transverse scan of the lower aspect of the femoral triangle. The sartorius begins to cover the femoral vessels. The vastus medialis and the adductor longus muscles form the side walls. More inferiorly, the common femoral vessels bifurcate into the superficial and profunda branches. **(Bottom)** Transverse scan of the posterior thigh at the upper level of the popliteal fossa. After passing through the adductor hiatus, the superficial femoral vessels enter the popliteal fossa. The hamstring muscles form the side walls of this fossa.

FEMORAL VESSELS AND NERVES

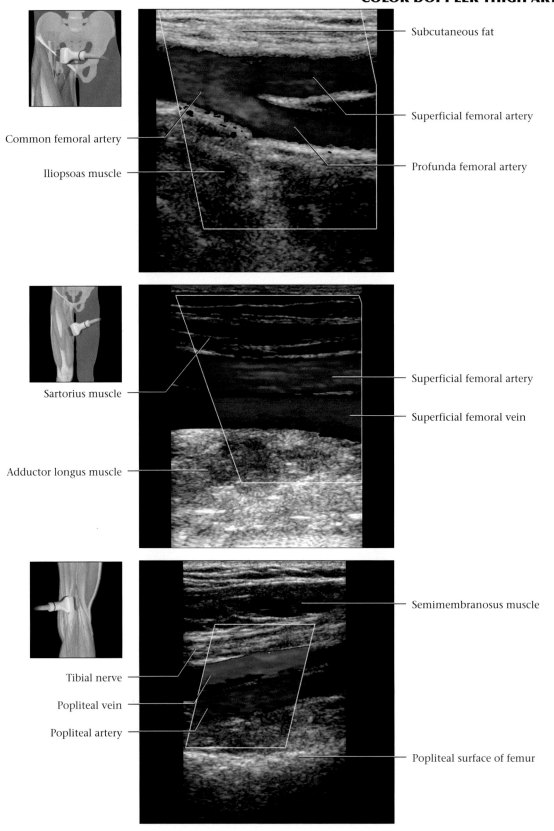

Subcutaneous fat

Common femoral artery

Iliopsoas muscle

Superficial femoral artery

Profunda femoral artery

Sartorius muscle

Adductor longus muscle

Superficial femoral artery

Superficial femoral vein

Tibial nerve

Popliteal vein

Popliteal artery

Semimembranosus muscle

Popliteal surface of femur

(Top) Sagittal color Doppler scan of the common femoral bifurcation. Color, representing flow, should fill the entire lumen with appropriate scan settings (as seen in this image). **(Middle)** Sagittal color Doppler scan of the superficial femoral vessels in the upper adductor canal. The color of flow is direction dependent (the Doppler effect) and here demonstrates the opposite direction of flow between the artery (red, away from the trunk) and vein (blue, toward the trunk). Again, the color should fill the entire lumen (red superficial to blue). **(Bottom)** Sagittal color Doppler scan of the popliteal vessels using a posterior approach. The change in relationship of the vessels, vein superficial to artery (blue superficial to red).

FEMORAL VESSELS AND NERVES

SPECTRAL DOPPLER THIGH ARTERIES

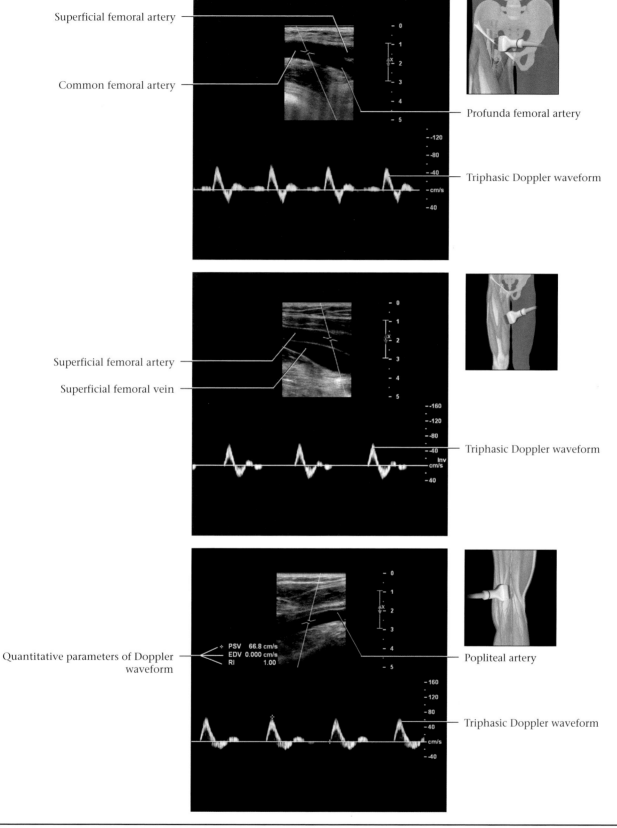

Superficial femoral artery

Common femoral artery

Profunda femoral artery

Triphasic Doppler waveform

Superficial femoral artery

Superficial femoral vein

Triphasic Doppler waveform

PSV   66.8 cm/s
EDV 0.000 cm/s
RI   1.00

Quantitative parameters of Doppler waveform

Popliteal artery

Triphasic Doppler waveform

(Top) Spectral Doppler trace at the common femoral artery. The typical waveform for an artery should be triphasic: Forward sharp upstroke of forward flow (systolic), then reverse flow (early diastolic) and finally slow forward flow (late diastolic), as seen in this trace. (Middle) Spectral Doppler spectral trace performed at the superficial femoral artery shows a similar waveform and slight decrease in the peak systolic flow. In general, as one moves further away from the heart, the peak velocity decreases. (Bottom) The typical arterial waveform is again seen in a spectral Doppler trace of the popliteal artery.

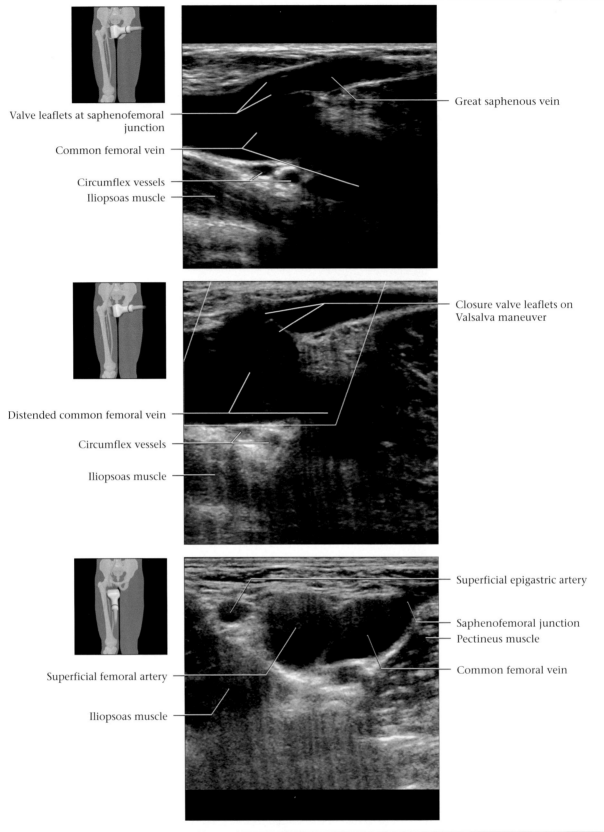

(Top) Valve leaflets at saphenofemoral junction — Great saphenous vein — Common femoral vein — Circumflex vessels — Iliopsoas muscle

(Middle) Closure valve leaflets on Valsalva maneuver — Distended common femoral vein — Circumflex vessels — Iliopsoas muscle

(Bottom) Superficial epigastric artery — Saphenofemoral junction — Pectineus muscle — Common femoral vein — Superficial femoral artery — Iliopsoas muscle

(Top) Sagittal scan at the confluence of the great saphenous vein with the common femoral vein. At this instance, the valve at the saphenofemoral junction is open to allow blood from the great saphenous vein to drain into the common femoral vein. **(Middle)** Sagittal color Doppler scan of the saphenofemoral junction during a Valsalva maneuver. The increased abdominal pressure is transmitted in the common femoral vein. This closes the valve at the saphenofemoral junction to prevent reflex into the great saphenous vein and also distends the common femoral vein (seen here as an increase in caliber). The lack of color flow across the valve indicates that the valve is competent. **(Bottom)** Transverse scan of the saphenofemoral junction. The great saphenous vein penetrates the femoral sheath to enter the common femoral vein.

FEMORAL VESSELS AND NERVES

DOPPLER SAPHENOUS VEIN

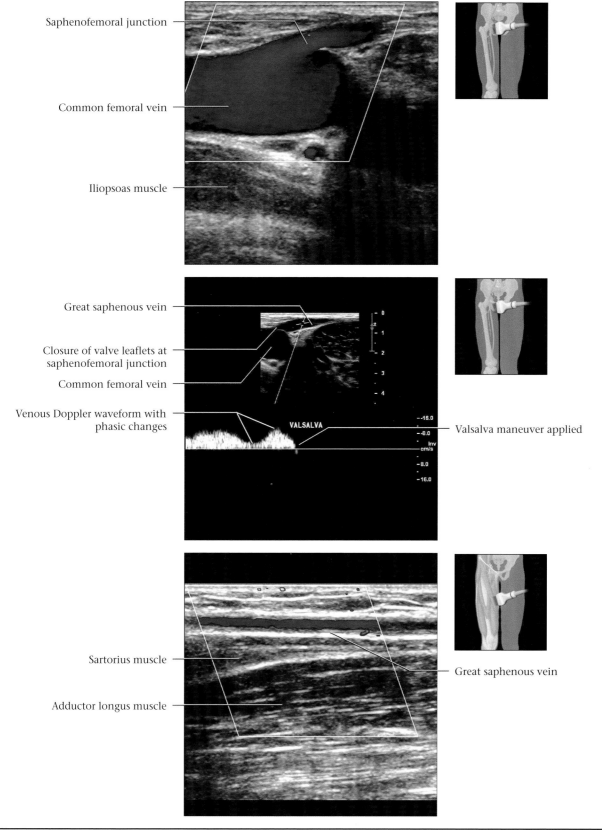

Saphenofemoral junction

Common femoral vein

Iliopsoas muscle

Great saphenous vein

Closure of valve leaflets at saphenofemoral junction

Common femoral vein

Venous Doppler waveform with phasic changes

Valsalva maneuver applied

Sartorius muscle

Adductor longus muscle

Great saphenous vein

(Top) Sagittal color Doppler scan of the saphenofemoral junction. The color flow in both the great saphenous vein and the common femoral vein is towards the trunk. (Middle) Spectral Doppler trace of the great saphenous vein before and during a Valsalva maneuver. The normal venous Doppler spectrum is biphasic due to respiratory variations. Applying a Valsalva maneuver, the valve closes abruptly at the saphenofemoral junction and stops flow in the great saphenous vein, which is seen as a zero flow velocity on the trace. (Bottom) Oblique coronal color Doppler scan of the great saphenous vein in the medial thigh shows blood flow towards the trunk (correct direction).

FEMORAL VESSELS AND NERVES

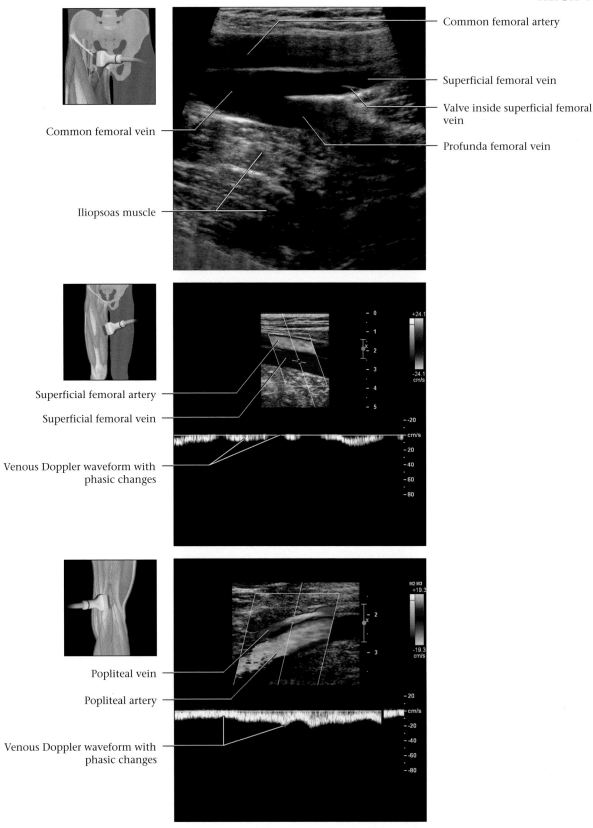

Common femoral artery

Superficial femoral vein

Valve inside superficial femoral vein

Profunda femoral vein

Common femoral vein

Iliopsoas muscle

Superficial femoral artery

Superficial femoral vein

Venous Doppler waveform with phasic changes

Popliteal vein

Popliteal artery

Venous Doppler waveform with phasic changes

(Top) Sagittal scan of the confluence of the common femoral vein. The common femoral vein is formed by its main tributaries, the superficial femoral vein and the profunda femoral vein (both accompanying the course of the arteries of the same name). (Middle) Spectral Doppler trace of the superficial femoral vein. The normal venous Doppler waveform is biphasic and varies with the phase of respiration. The flow velocity is also much slower than that in the artery. (Bottom) Spectral Doppler trace of the popliteal vein shows a similar venous waveform with respiratory phasic changes.

FEMORAL VESSELS AND NERVES

FEMORAL VEIN: COMPRESSION

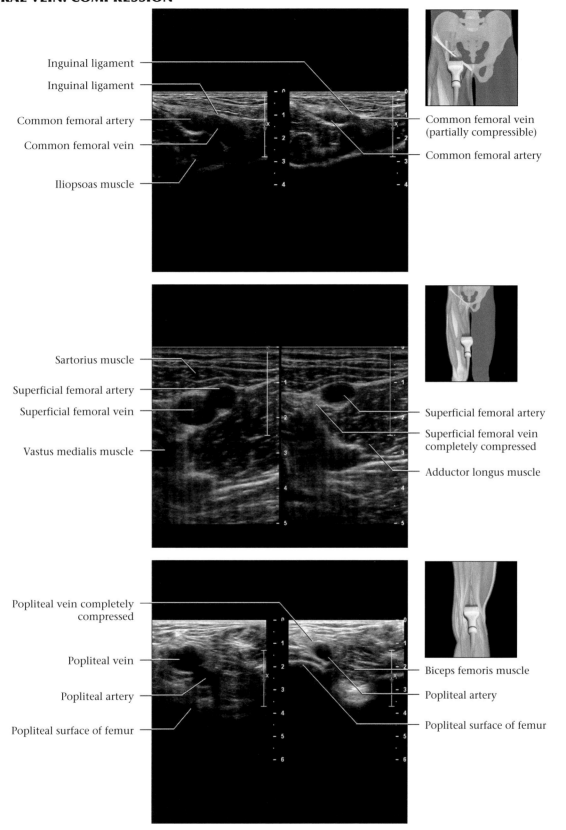

Inguinal ligament
Inguinal ligament
Common femoral artery
Common femoral vein
Iliopsoas muscle

Common femoral vein (partially compressible)
Common femoral artery

Sartorius muscle
Superficial femoral artery
Superficial femoral vein
Vastus medialis muscle

Superficial femoral artery
Superficial femoral vein completely compressed
Adductor longus muscle

Popliteal vein completely compressed
Popliteal vein
Popliteal artery
Popliteal surface of femur

Biceps femoris muscle
Popliteal artery
Popliteal surface of femur

(Top) Pre-/post-compression split screen transverse scan of the common femoral vessels. The left half image is obtained applying normal gentle transducer pressure, the right half scanned with firm compression. Patent veins are normally compressible with firm transducer pressure, with the exception demonstrated here due to the inguinal ligament. This is not a sign of venous thrombosis. **(Middle)** Pre-/post-compression split screen transverse scan in the adductor canal shows the normal compressible superficial femoral vein. With firm pressure, the superficial artery is distorted, but the lumen is not obliterated. **(Bottom)** Pre-/post-compression split screen transverse scan of the popliteal vessels show the same response: Obliterated venous lumen and distorted arterial lumen.

FEMORAL VESSELS AND NERVES

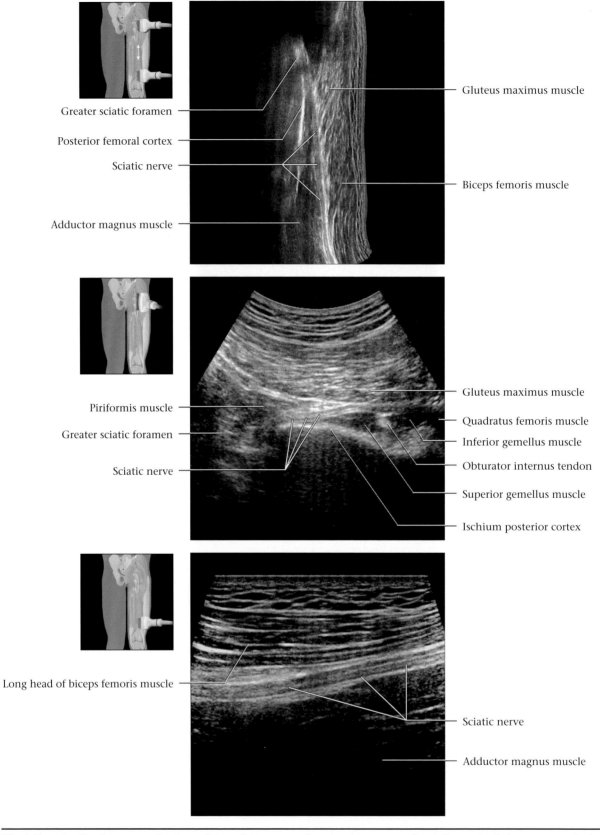

Greater sciatic foramen

Posterior femoral cortex

Sciatic nerve

Adductor magnus muscle

Gluteus maximus muscle

Biceps femoris muscle

Piriformis muscle

Greater sciatic foramen

Sciatic nerve

Gluteus maximus muscle

Quadratus femoris muscle

Inferior gemellus muscle

Obturator internus tendon

Superior gemellus muscle

Ischium posterior cortex

Long head of biceps femoris muscle

Sciatic nerve

Adductor magnus muscle

(Top) Longitudinal panoramic view of the sciatic nerve showing its course after it has exited the greater sciatic foramen. It runs distally deep to the gluteus maximus and then the biceps femoris to the popliteal fossa. **(Middle)** Sagittal scan of the greater sciatic foramen using the ischial tuberosity as a landmark. The sciatic nerve and its relationship with the small external rotators of the hip is shown here. The sciatic nerve emerges between the piriformis and superior gemellus muscles after the greater sciatic foramen. **(Bottom)** This longitudinal view of the sciatic nerve demonstrates the parallel and uniform hypoechoic tracts (representing nerve bundles). Any disruption of the uniformity or parallel course should be considered abnormal.

FEMORAL VESSELS AND NERVES

TRANSVERSE SCIATIC NERVE

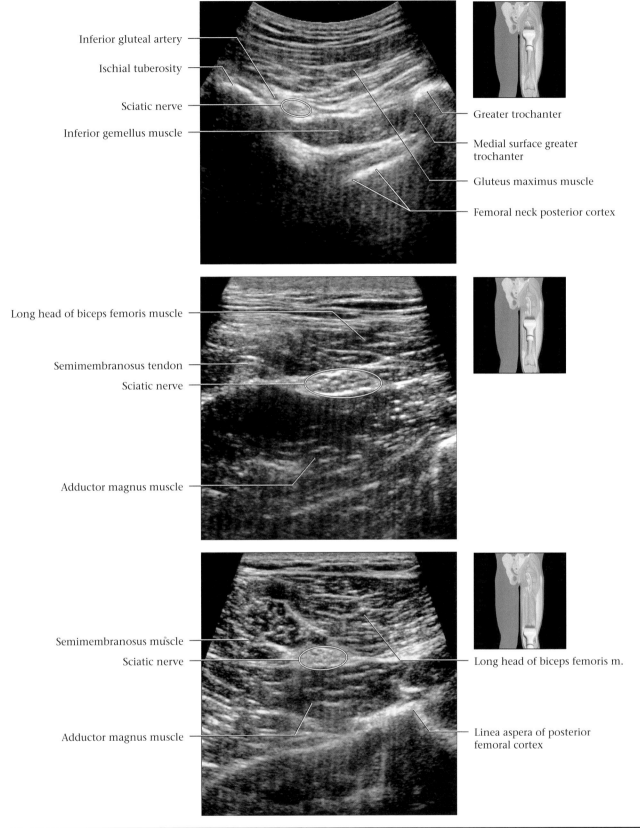

Inferior gluteal artery

Ischial tuberosity

Sciatic nerve

Inferior gemellus muscle

Greater trochanter

Medial surface greater trochanter

Gluteus maximus muscle

Femoral neck posterior cortex

Long head of biceps femoris muscle

Semimembranosus tendon

Sciatic nerve

Adductor magnus muscle

Semimembranosus muscle

Sciatic nerve

Adductor magnus muscle

Long head of biceps femoris m.

Linea aspera of posterior femoral cortex

(Top) Series of three transverse scans at different levels of the sciatic nerve. The sciatic nerve, after it has exited the greater sciatic foramen passes superficial to the small external rotators of the hip joint (obturator internus, superior and inferior gemelli and quadratus femoris). The inferior gluteal artery lies medial to the nerve. **(Middle)** At the upper-thigh level, the sciatic nerve is covered by the long head of biceps femoris muscle and is relatively superficial. The high spatial resolution of ultrasound allows individual nerve bundles to be identified as black dots in a bright matrix of epineurium. **(Bottom)** The same relationship with the long head of biceps femoris muscle continues inferiorly down the thigh until the sciatic nerve divides into the tibial and common femoral nerves.

KNEE

Terminology

Abbreviations
- Artery (a.); function (F); ligament (l.); medial collateral ligament (MCL); muscle (m.); tendon (t.); vein (v.)

Gross Anatomy

Overview
- Largest and most complex joint
  - Hinge joint throughout its greatest range of motion
  - Bones do not interlock; stability maintained by ligaments, tendons, capsule, and menisci
- **Motion** of knee and relationship of osseous structures
  - In full flexion
    - Posterior surfaces of femoral condyles articulate with posterior tibial condyles
    - Lateral facet of patella in contact with lateral femoral condyle
    - Supporting ligaments are not taut, and rotation of leg is allowed
  - During motion of extension
    - Patella slides upwards on femur, passing first on to its middle facet and then its lower facets
    - Femoral condyles roll forward on tibial condyles and menisci
    - Lateral femoral condyle shorter anteroposteriorly than medial and reaches full extension earlier
    - Medial femoral condyle continues to slide after lateral stops, and rotates slightly medially on tibia and medial meniscus ("screwing it home"), and tightens ACL, collateral ligaments, and posterior capsular ligaments, turning knee into a rigid pillar
  - Initiating flexion from fully extended knee
    - Requires slight medial rotation of tibia, produced by popliteus
    - "Unlocks" joint, allowing remainder of motion to take place
- **Muscles acting on knee joint**
  - **Extensors**: Four parts of quadriceps femoris
    - I: Patella
    - F: Acts together for hip flexion and knee extension
  - Rectus femoris
    - O: Anterior inferior iliac spine
  - Vastus medialis
    - O: Medial shaft of femur
  - Vastus intermedius
    - O: Anterior shaft of femur
  - Vastus lateralis
    - O: Lateral shaft of femur
  - **Flexors**
  - Biceps femoris
    - O: Ischial tuberosity
    - I: Fibular head and tibia
    - F: Crosses both hip and knee joints, extending hip and flexing knee
  - Sartorius
    - O: Anterior superior iliac spine
    - I: Anteromedial tibia
    - F: Flexes both hip and knee joints, rotating thigh laterally
  - Popliteus
    - O: Arises as tendon from popliteal groove at lateral femoral condyle
    - I: Posterior surface tibia
    - F: Flexes knee and medially rotates tibia at beginning of flexion
  - Gracilis
    - O: Pubis
    - I: Anteromedial tibia
    - F: Adducts thigh, flexes knee, and rotates flexed leg medially
  - Semitendinosus
    - O: Ischial tuberosity
    - I: Anteromedial tibia
    - F: Extends hip, flexes knee, medially rotates flexed leg
  - Semimembranosus
    - O: Ischial tuberosity
    - I: Posterior medial condyle tibia
    - F: Extends hip, flexes knee, medially rotates flexed knee

Imaging Anatomy

Osseous Anatomy
- **Distal femur**
  - Distal femoral metaphysis flares into medial and lateral epicondyles
  - Medial femoral condyle larger than lateral
  - Anteriorly, trochlear groove accommodates patella and is generally V-shaped
- **Proximal tibia**
  - Gerdy tubercle anterolateral just distal to joint
  - Tibial tubercle (apophysis) anterior and slightly lateral, several cm distal to joint
- **Proximal fibula**
  - Posterolateral relative to tibia
  - Fibular styloid process
- **Tibiofibular joint**
  - True synovial joint; subject to any arthritic process
  - Connects to knee joint in 20%
- **Patella**
  - Triangular sesamoid
  - Wider at base superiorly than at apex inferiorly
  - Non-articular outer surface may develop prominent enthesopathy where quadriceps tendon insertion blends into origin of inferior patellar tendon
  - Bipartite (multipartite) patella: Always upper outer quadrant; osseous fragments may not appear to "match", but cartilage is continuous over defect

Articular Capsule
- Highly complex, noncontiguous structure
- Contributions from multiple muscles, tendons, and ligaments

Extensor Mechanism
- **Quadriceps**
  - Composed of rectus femoris, vastus lateralis, medialis & intermedius muscles
  - Quadriceps tendon inserts on anterior surface of patella
  - Patellar tendon is mainly composed of rectus femoris fibers that course over patella

- o Patellar tendon runs from inferior pole of patellar to tibial tuberosity
- o Fibers of vastus lateralis and medialis contribute to lateral and medial retinacula, respectively

Fad Pads
- Suprapatellar: Anterior and posterior to the suprapatellar bursa
- Infrapatellar (Hoffa fat pad): Inferior to patella and between patellar ligament and anterior knee joint
- Posterior: Around the joint margin extending into the intercondylar region

Medial Supporting Structures
- Superficial (layer 1)
  - o Pes anserinus: Anteromedial tibial insertion
    - Sartorius embedded in crural fascia
    - Gracilis immediately deep to sartorius
    - Semitendinosus immediately deep to gracilis
- Middle (layer 2)
  - o Superficial medial collateral ligament (longitudinal and oblique components)
    - Origin medial epicondyle; runs slightly anteromedially to insert on tibia 5 cm distal to joint line
    - Anteriorly, longitudinal component fascia blends with layer 1
    - Posteriorly, oblique component blends with layer 3 as posterior oblique ligament
- Deep (layer 3)
  - o Capsular layers (sometimes termed deep fibers of MCL) at mid portion of knee
    - Meniscofemoral ligament: From outer superior aspect of body of meniscus to either superficial MCL or femur
    - Meniscotibial (coronary) ligament: From outer inferior aspect of body of meniscus to tibia just distal to joint line
  - o More posteriorly, superficial MCL blends with capsular layers MCL
  - o Posterior oblique ligament arises from superficial MCL
    - Blends with posteromedial meniscus
    - Receives fibers from semimembranosus tendon
    - Envelops posterior aspect femoral condyle, termed oblique popliteal ligament

Lateral Supporting Structures
- Superficial (layer 1)
  - o Iliotibial band anteriorly, inserting on Gerdy tubercle
  - o Superficial portion biceps femoris posterolaterally, inserting on fibular styloid
- Middle (layer 2)
  - o Quadriceps retinaculum anteriorly
  - o Posteriorly, two ligamentous thickenings which originate from lateral patella
    - Proximal one terminates at lateral intermuscular septum on femur
    - Distal one terminates at femoral insertion of posterolateral capsule and lateral head of gastrocnemius
- Deep (layer 3): Several thickenings in lateral part of capsule function as discrete structures

- o Lateral (fibular) collateral ligament originates from lateral femoral epicondyle, extends posterolaterally to insert on lateral fibular head
- o Arcuate ligament originates from styloid process fibular head, interdigitates with popliteus, and inserts into posterior capsule near oblique popliteal ligament
- o Several other small and inconstant structures located posterolaterally which are difficult to differentiate by imaging

Internal Structures
- **Menisci**
  - o Cushion, lubricate, and stabilize knee
  - o Fibrocartilage
  - o Only peripheral portion visualized by ultrasound
  - o Medial attached to capsule throughout extent
  - o Lateral attached to capsule at anterior horn and far posteriorly, but by fascicles to popliteus at body and posterior horn
- **Cruciate ligaments**
  - o Major stabilizing structures to anteroposterior motion
- The cruciate ligaments and the central portions of the menisci are not well visualized by ultrasound

Anatomy-Based Imaging Issues

Imaging Approaches
- US
  - o Ultrasound is good at assessing extracapsular structures and their abnormalities, but unable to satisfactorily interrogate the internal structures of the knee
  - o Given the size and complexity of this joint, an ultrasound examination needs to be compartmentalized to the area of complaint
    - e.g., posterior examination for popliteal mass, lateral examination for suspected iliotibial band syndrome etc.
  - o In an acutely inflamed joint, ultrasound is most effective as a screening tool for effusion, allowing image-guided aspiration at the same time
  - o Ultrasound is ideal for assessing extra-articular abnormalities e.g., tendinosis, ligament disruptions, bursitis, masses etc.
  - o For structures containing fibers e.g., ligaments and tendons, longitudinal scans tend to be more helpful both in confirming the course of the structure and assessing integrity
  - o For the above reason, during examination of the anterior knee, the knee should be flexed
    - Flexion tenses most of the tendinous and ligamentous structures and accentuates the straight course of its fibers

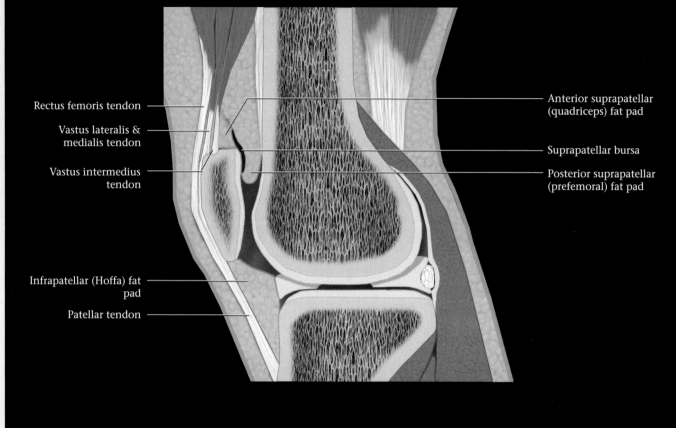

Rectus femoris tendon

Vastus lateralis & medialis tendon

Vastus intermedius tendon

Infrapatellar (Hoffa) fat pad

Patellar tendon

Anterior suprapatellar (quadriceps) fat pad

Suprapatellar bursa

Posterior suprapatellar (prefemoral) fat pad

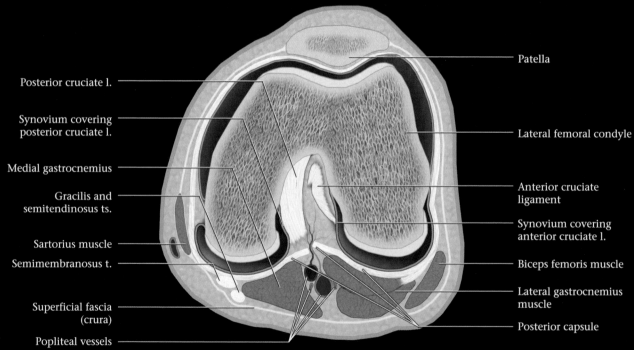

Posterior cruciate l.

Synovium covering posterior cruciate l.

Medial gastrocnemius

Gracilis and semitendinosus ts.

Sartorius muscle

Semimembranosus t.

Superficial fascia (crura)

Popliteal vessels

Patella

Lateral femoral condyle

Anterior cruciate ligament

Synovium covering anterior cruciate l.

Biceps femoris muscle

Lateral gastrocnemius muscle

Posterior capsule

(Top) Graphic shows trilaminar configuration of the quadriceps tendon. The superficial portion is rectus femoris, middle portion is the aponeurosis of vastus medialis and lateralis, and deep portion is vastus intermedius tendon. **(Bottom)** Graphic shows the relationships of the posterior capsule and overlying structures. The most superficial layer is the crural fascia, which envelops the sartorius and otherwise confines all the structures. The posterior capsule (white) is continuous with the synovium (pink) both posteromedially and posterolaterally. Superficial to the capsule are the plantaris and gastrocnemius muscles, hamstring muscle and tendons, plus the popliteal vessels.

EXTENSOR MECHANISM

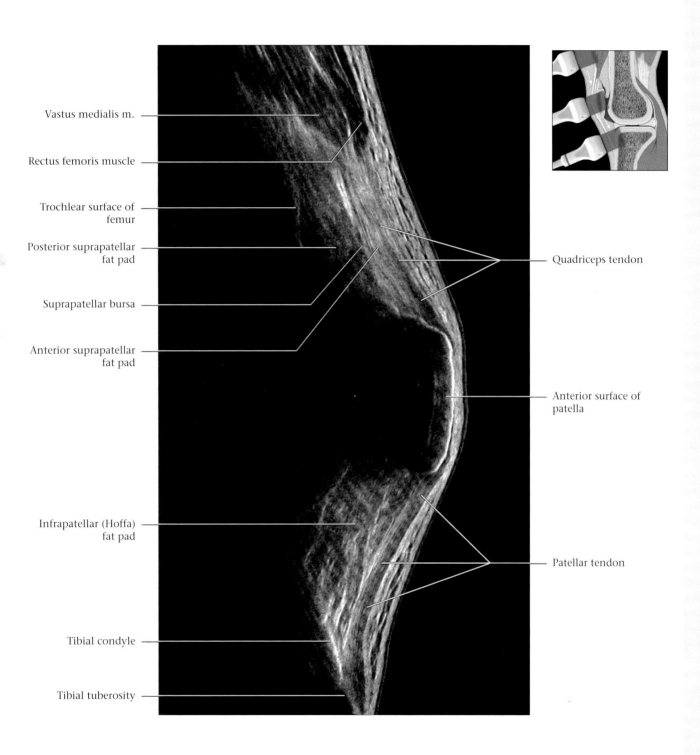

Vastus medialis m.

Rectus femoris muscle

Trochlear surface of femur

Posterior suprapatellar fat pad

Suprapatellar bursa

Anterior suprapatellar fat pad

Infrapatellar (Hoffa) fat pad

Tibial condyle

Tibial tuberosity

Quadriceps tendon

Anterior surface of patella

Patellar tendon

Sagittal panoramic scan of the anterior knee showing the main components of the extensor mechanism: Quadriceps muscle and tendon; patella; patellar tendon. The scan performed here is with the knee in extension. More focused views of individual components of the anterior knee can be performed with the knee in flexion (with a pillow to support the popliteal region). Flexion increases the tension of the extensor mechanism, thus straightening the tendons. This will help highlight abnormalities in terms of tendon alignment and continuity. However, the amount of suprapatellar fluid may be decreased (due to displacement) in flexion and assessment of the suprapatellar region in extension may be more sensitive in this respect.

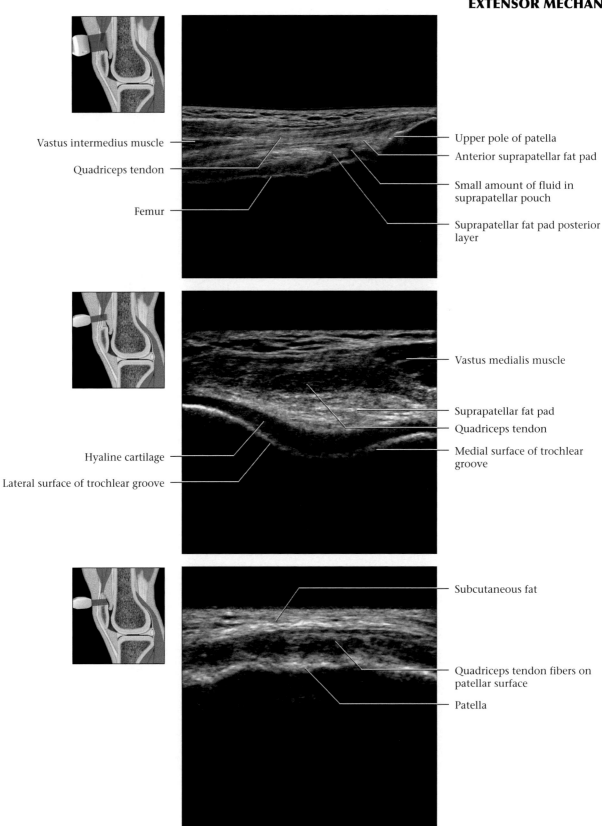

Vastus intermedius muscle

Quadriceps tendon

Femur

Upper pole of patella

Anterior suprapatellar fat pad

Small amount of fluid in suprapatellar pouch

Suprapatellar fat pad posterior layer

Vastus medialis muscle

Suprapatellar fat pad

Quadriceps tendon

Medial surface of trochlear groove

Hyaline cartilage

Lateral surface of trochlear groove

Subcutaneous fat

Quadriceps tendon fibers on patellar surface

Patella

(Top) Sagittal scan of the quadriceps tendon. The quadriceps tendon is the direct continuation of the rectus femoris with contributions medially and laterally from the vastus medialis and vastus lateralis respectively and posteriorly from vastus intermedius. The tendon inserts on the supero-anterior surface of the patella. In this scan, the supra-patellar pouch can be seen and normally contains a small amount of fluid (several millimeters thick). **(Middle)** Transverse scan of quadriceps tendon with the knee flexed. The central position of the quadriceps tendon can be appreciated here, receiving contributions from the vastus muscles. The articular cartilage of the trochlear groove can also be seen with the patella out of the way during flexion. **(Bottom)** Transverse scan of the anterior surface of the patella shows tendon fibers inserting or running on patellar surface.

KNEE

EXTENSOR MECHANISM

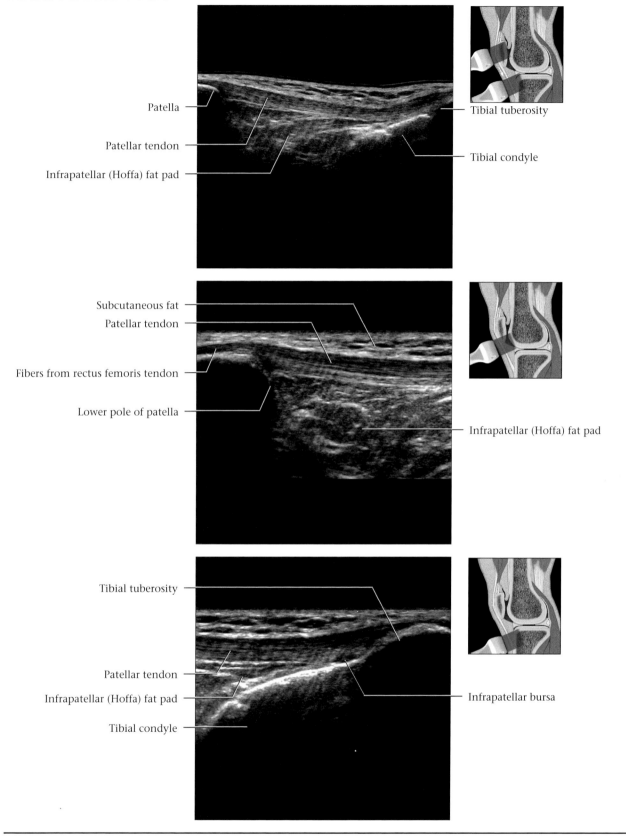

Patella

Patellar tendon

Infrapatellar (Hoffa) fat pad

Tibial tuberosity

Tibial condyle

Subcutaneous fat

Patellar tendon

Fibers from rectus femoris tendon

Lower pole of patella

Infrapatellar (Hoffa) fat pad

Tibial tuberosity

Patellar tendon

Infrapatellar (Hoffa) fat pad

Tibial condyle

Infrapatellar bursa

(Top) Sagittal panoramic view of the patellar tendon. Most of the fibers of the tendon are continuations of quadriceps tendon fibers. (Middle) Focused sagittal view of the apex of the patella, showing quadriceps fibers running on the anterior surface of the patella continuing distally as the patellar tendon. For this reason, many consider the patella a sesamoid bone. Also seen here are fibers originating from the apex of the patella itself. (Bottom) Focused sagittal scan of the tibial tuberosity. The distal fibers of the patellar tendon are separated from the anterior surface of the tibial condyle by the infrapatellar bursa. A small amount of fluid (2-3 mm thick) may be normally present in this bursa.

EXTENSOR MECHANISM

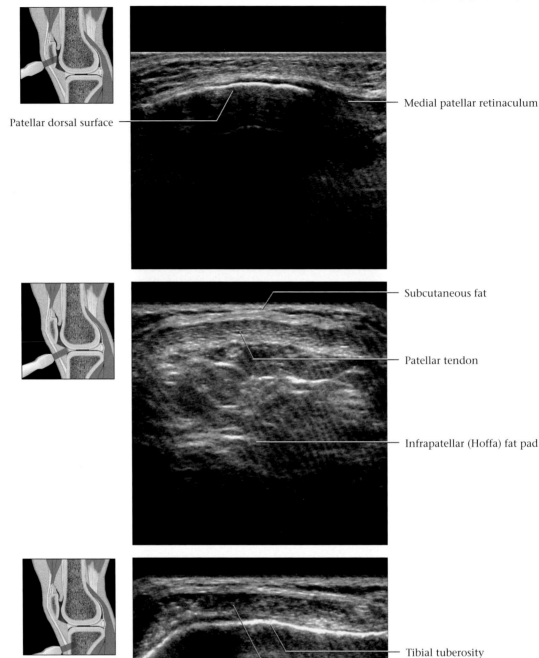

Patellar dorsal surface —

— Medial patellar retinaculum

— Subcutaneous fat

— Patellar tendon

— Infrapatellar (Hoffa) fat pad

— Tibial tuberosity

— Patellar tendon

(Top) Series of three transverse scans through the patellar tendon. Proximally, fibers from the quadriceps tendon continue over the anterior patellar surface to contribute to the patellar tendon. On both sides, fibers from the medial and lateral patellar retinaculum also insert onto the patella and blend with the patellar tendon fibers. (Middle) At the mid-substance of the patellar tendon, the tendon assumes a flattened appearance. The fibers within the tendon can be seen as tiny hyperechoic dots. A disruption to the uniformity of these dots or a change in thickness (focal or general) of the patellar tendon suggests tendinosis. (Bottom) More inferiorly, a transverse scan shows the patellar tendon inserting onto the tibial tuberosity. Note that throughout its course, the patellar tendon does not have a tendon sheath and therefore will not develop tenosynovitis.

KNEE

EXTENSOR MECHANISM

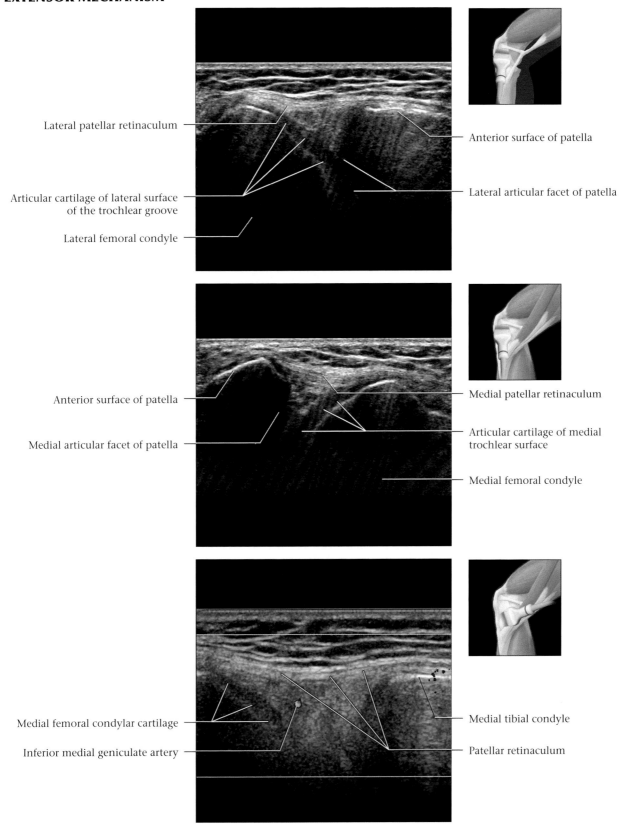

Lateral patellar retinaculum

Anterior surface of patella

Articular cartilage of lateral surface of the trochlear groove

Lateral articular facet of patella

Lateral femoral condyle

Anterior surface of patella

Medial patellar retinaculum

Medial articular facet of patella

Articular cartilage of medial trochlear surface

Medial femoral condyle

Medial femoral condylar cartilage

Medial tibial condyle

Inferior medial geniculate artery

Patellar retinaculum

(Top) Transverse scan at the medial margin of the patella shows the articulation between the lateral patella and the lateral surface of the trochlear groove. This articular plane is steeper (closer to sagittal) than the medial side for mechanical advantage. As a result of the obliquity of the course of the patellar tendon with respect to the tibial axis, the patella is prone to lateral dislocation or subluxation. The steeper lateral articular plane helps prevents this. (Middle) Transverse scan at the medial margin of the patella shows the articulation between the medial patella and the medial surface of the trochlear groove, showing patellar retinaculum as a thick structure. (Bottom) Sagittal color Doppler scan of the medial infrapatellar region shows the patellar retinaculum inserting onto the tibia. At this level the retinaculum has fanned out, becoming much thinner.

KNEE

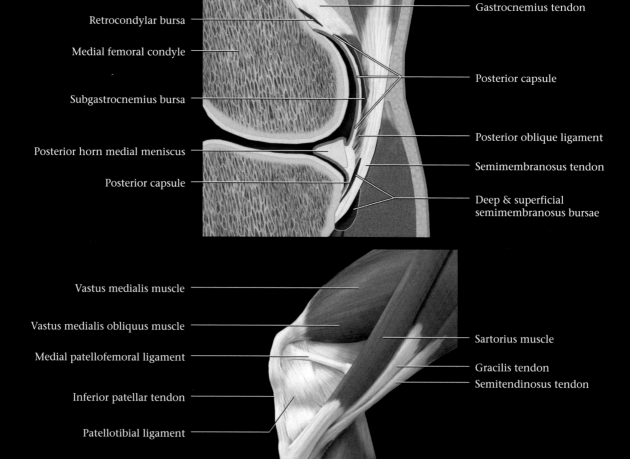

Posterior cruciate ligament

Medial femoral condyle

Meniscofemoral ligament
Superficial fibers medial collateral l.

Medial collateral bursa (variable)

Fat between superficial & deep
medial collateral fibers

Meniscotibial (coronary) ligament

Body medial meniscus

Semimembranosus muscle
Gastrocnemius tendon

Retrocondylar bursa

Medial femoral condyle

Subgastrocnemius bursa

Posterior capsule

Posterior horn medial meniscus

Posterior capsule

Posterior oblique ligament

Semimembranosus tendon

Deep & superficial
semimembranosus bursae

Vastus medialis muscle

Vastus medialis obliquus muscle

Medial patellofemoral ligament

Sartorius muscle

Gracilis tendon
Semitendinosus tendon

Inferior patellar tendon

Patellotibial ligament

(Top) Coronal graphic at mid joint, shows superficial fibers extending from adductor tubercle to approximately 5 cm below joint line. Deep fibers are shorter: Meniscotibial (coronary) ligament extends from meniscus to tibia adjacent to joint line & meniscofemoral ligament extends from meniscus to femur or superficial MCL. **(Middle)** Sagittal graphic of the far medial portion of posterior capsule. Superiorly the capsule attaches to cortex of posterior femoral condyle & fuses with fibers of medial gastrocnemius. **(Bottom)** Graphic shows the anteromedial attachment of pes anserinus tendons. Sartorius is most anterior & superficial. Gracilis inserts directly adjacent & deep to sartorius & semitendinosus inserts directly posterior & inferior to gracilis. These tendons & their crural fascia comprise the superficial layer of the medial capsuloligamentous complex.

KNEE

MEDIAL KNEE

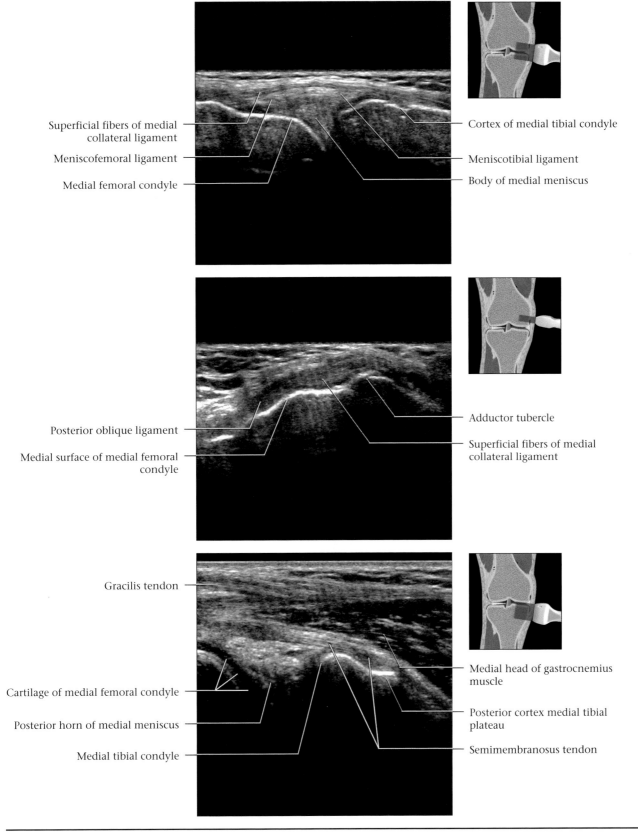

Superficial fibers of medial collateral ligament

Meniscofemoral ligament

Medial femoral condyle

Cortex of medial tibial condyle

Meniscotibial ligament

Body of medial meniscus

Posterior oblique ligament

Medial surface of medial femoral condyle

Adductor tubercle

Superficial fibers of medial collateral ligament

Gracilis tendon

Cartilage of medial femoral condyle

Posterior horn of medial meniscus

Medial tibial condyle

Medial head of gastrocnemius muscle

Posterior cortex medial tibial plateau

Semimembranosus tendon

(Top) Coronal scan of the medial joint line. The medial collateral ligament is composed of two layers: Superficial and deep. The superficial fibers run from the medial femoral epicondyle to the tibial condyle 5 cm below the joint line. The deep layer consists of the meniscofemoral (femoral condyle to body of meniscus) and meniscotibial (body of meniscus to tibia just distal to joint line). **(Middle)** Transverse scan of the medial epicondylar region. The superficial fibers of the medial collateral ligament arise adjacent to the adductor tubercle. The popliteal oblique ligament arises adjacent to this and runs posterior to the posterior joint capsule. **(Bottom)** Sagittal scan of the posteromedial joint line. The semimembranosus tendon inserts onto the posterior surface of the medial tibial condyle, just below the joint margin. Only the outer part of the meniscus is visible.

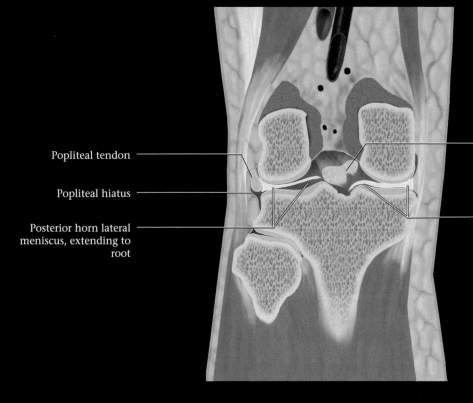

Popliteal tendon

Popliteal hiatus

Posterior horn lateral meniscus, extending to root

Posterior cruciate ligament

Posterior horn and root medial meniscus

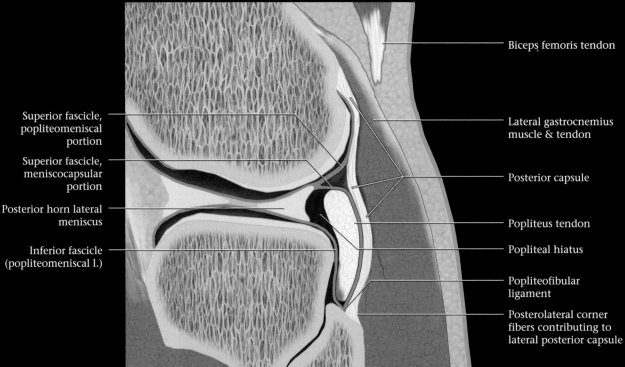

Superior fascicle, popliteomeniscal portion

Superior fascicle, meniscocapsular portion

Posterior horn lateral meniscus

Inferior fascicle (popliteomeniscal l.)

Biceps femoris tendon

Lateral gastrocnemius muscle & tendon

Posterior capsule

Popliteus tendon

Popliteal hiatus

Popliteofibular ligament

Posterolateral corner fibers contributing to lateral posterior capsule

(Top) Coronal graphic shows the roots of the posterior horns of both the medial and lateral menisci. The popliteal tendon is also seen coursing through the hiatus adjacent to the body/posterior horn of the lateral meniscus.
(Bottom) Sagittal graphic of lateral part of posterior capsule shows that it is intimately attached to lateral gastrocnemius muscle. The popliteus tendon is intra-articular but extrasynovial and is attached to capsule. Fibers from posterolateral corner and arcuate ligament originating from fibular head contribute to the lateral portion of the posterior capsule.

KNEE

LATERAL KNEE

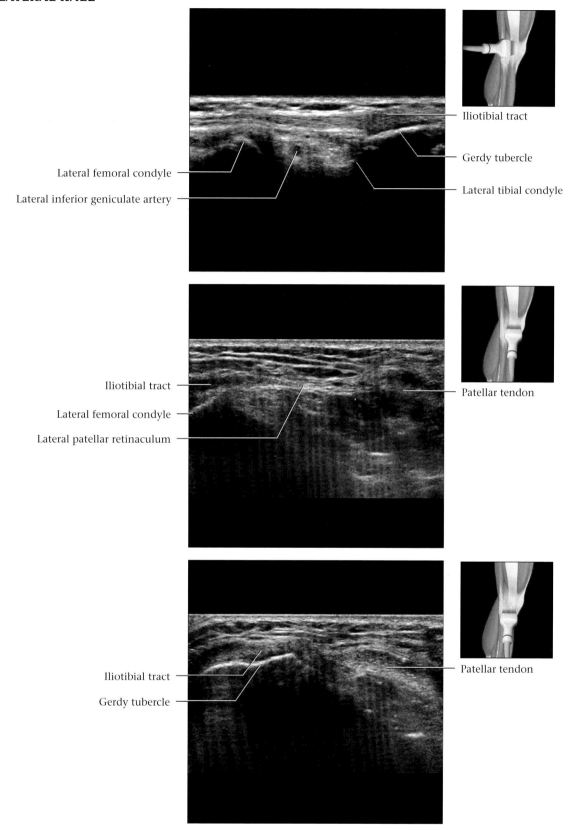

Iliotibial tract

Gerdy tubercle

Lateral tibial condyle

Lateral femoral condyle

Lateral inferior geniculate artery

Iliotibial tract

Lateral femoral condyle

Lateral patellar retinaculum

Patellar tendon

Iliotibial tract

Gerdy tubercle

Patellar tendon

(Top) Oblique sagittal scan of the lateral aspect of the joint line using Gerdy tubercle as a landmark. The iliotibial tract is shown here passing over the edge of the lateral femoral condyle (where it is liable to impingement (Iliotibial tract syndrome) before inserting on Gerdy tubercle on the anterior surface of the lateral tibial condyle. **(Middle)** Transverse scan of the anterolateral knee at the level of the femoral condyle shows that the iliotibial tract and the patellar tendon are connected by fibers of the lateral patellar retinaculum. **(Bottom)** More inferiorly, the two tendons have moved closer to each other. This transverse scan shows insertion of the iliotibial tract onto Gerdy tubercle. The patellar tendon is also approaching its tibial insertion.

KNEE

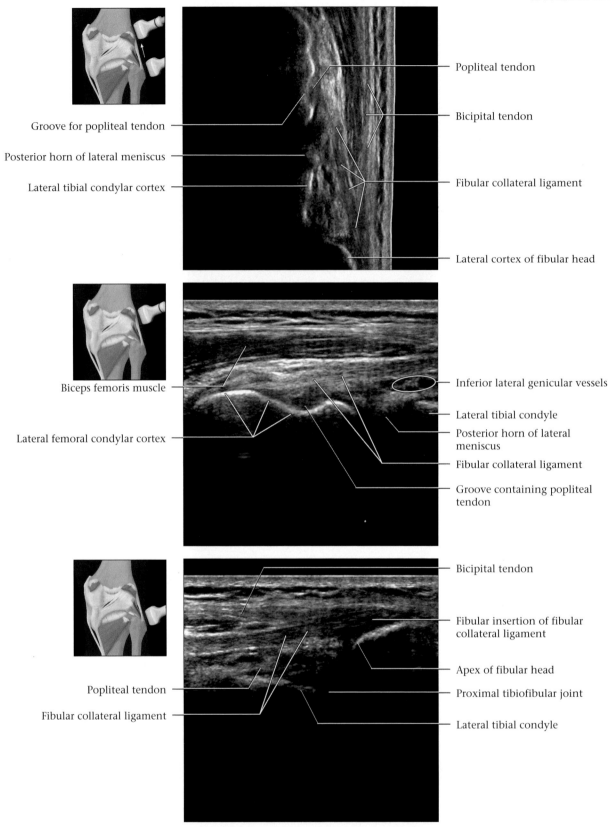

Groove for popliteal tendon

Posterior horn of lateral meniscus

Lateral tibial condylar cortex

Popliteal tendon

Bicipital tendon

Fibular collateral ligament

Lateral cortex of fibular head

Biceps femoris muscle

Lateral femoral condylar cortex

Inferior lateral genicular vessels

Lateral tibial condyle

Posterior horn of lateral meniscus

Fibular collateral ligament

Groove containing popliteal tendon

Bicipital tendon

Fibular insertion of fibular collateral ligament

Apex of fibular head

Proximal tibiofibular joint

Lateral tibial condyle

Popliteal tendon

Fibular collateral ligament

(Top) Coronal panoramic scan of the lateral collateral complex. The biceps femoris muscle is the dominant muscle on this side of the knee. It runs from the ischial tuberosity laterally and inferiorly to insert onto the lateral aspect of the head of the fibula. (Middle) Coronal scan of the lateral femoral condyle shows the insertion of the fibular collateral ligament. Just under this insertion is the groove for the popliteal tendon. The fibular collateral ligament is cord-like compared to the superficial component of the medial collateral ligament, which is a flatter strap. (Bottom) The fibular collateral ligament inserts onto the lateral wall of the head of the fibula. The tendon of biceps femoris inserts at and around the apex of the fibular head.

KNEE

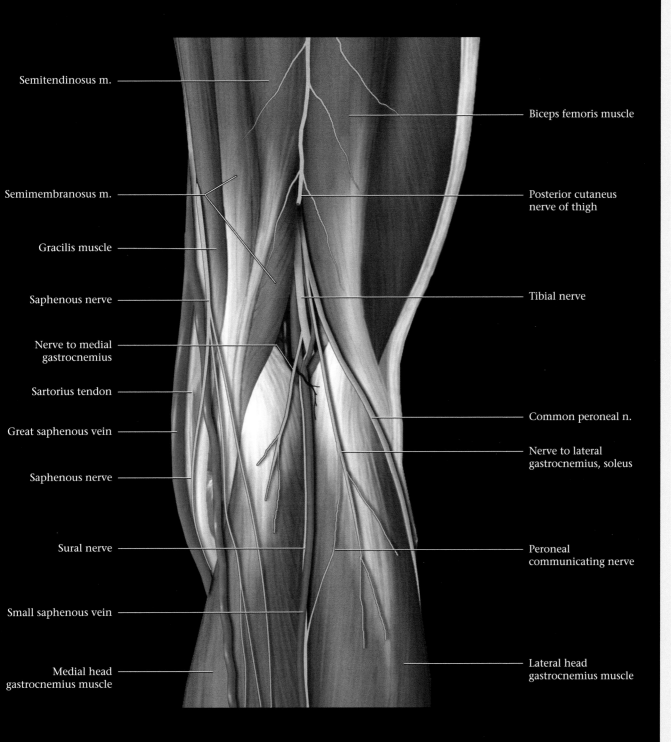

Semitendinosus m.

Biceps femoris muscle

Semimembranosus m.

Posterior cutaneus nerve of thigh

Gracilis muscle

Saphenous nerve

Tibial nerve

Nerve to medial gastrocnemius

Sartorius tendon

Great saphenous vein

Common peroneal n.

Nerve to lateral gastrocnemius, soleus

Saphenous nerve

Sural nerve

Peroneal communicating nerve

Small saphenous vein

Medial head gastrocnemius muscle

Lateral head gastrocnemius muscle

Graphic shows the superficial posterior muscles and nerves. The popliteal fossa is a diamond-shaped fossa bordered superiorly by the hamstring muscle and inferiorly by the head of the gastrocnemius muscle. Superiorly, the medial margin is represented by the semimembranosus & semitendinosus muscles; and laterally by the biceps femoris muscle. Inferiorly, the medial and lateral borders are the medial and lateral heads of the gastrocnemius muscle. This fossa contains the popliteal vessels, sciatic nerve and its branches. Note that the common peroneal nerve is part of the deeper nerve system, but travels more superficially, following the posterior biceps femoris muscle and tendon until it wraps around the fibular neck.

KNEE

Semitendinosus muscle

Biceps femoris muscle long head

Biceps femoris muscle short head

Gracilis muscle

Semimembranosus m.

Lateral head of gastrocnemius muscle

Plantaris muscle

Popliteal vein

Tibial nerve

Medial head of gastrocnemius muscle

Popliteal artery

(Top) Panoramic transverse scan of the posterior knee showing the upper popliteal fossa. At this level, the hamstring muscles form the superior boundaries (medial and lateral) of the popliteal fossa. The semimembranosus and semitendinosus muscles form the medial margin, while the biceps femoris muscle forms the lateral margin. **(Bottom)** Panoramic view of the posterior knee showing the lower aspect of the popliteal fossa. At this level the boundaries of the popliteal fossa are the heads of the gastrocnemius muscle, the lateral head of gastrocnemius being the lateral margin and the medial head the medial margin. The popliteal vessels are a continuation of the superficial femoral vessels after they have emerged through the adductor hiatus.

POSTERIOR KNEE

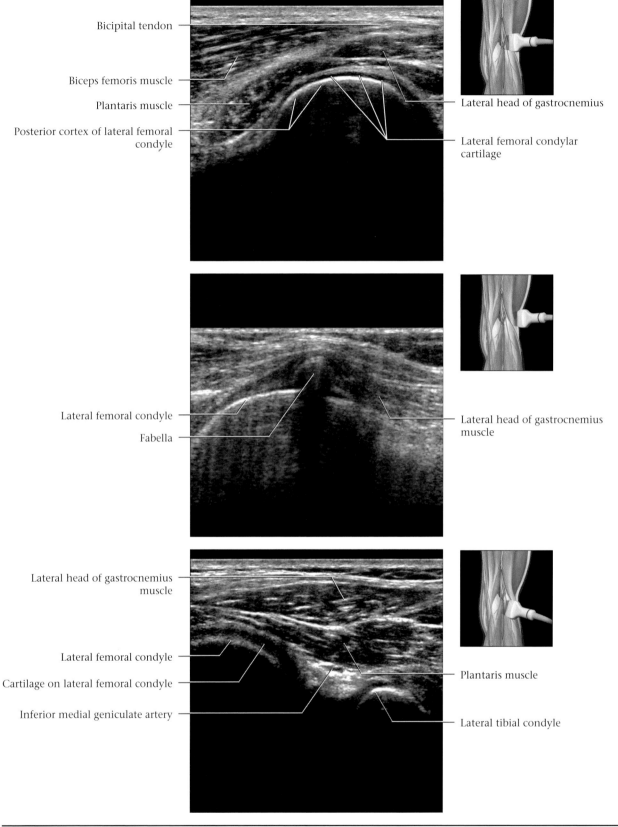

Top:
- Bicipital tendon
- Biceps femoris muscle
- Plantaris muscle
- Posterior cortex of lateral femoral condyle
- Lateral head of gastrocnemius
- Lateral femoral condylar cartilage

Middle:
- Lateral femoral condyle
- Fabella
- Lateral head of gastrocnemius muscle

Bottom:
- Lateral head of gastrocnemius muscle
- Lateral femoral condyle
- Cartilage on lateral femoral condyle
- Inferior medial geniculate artery
- Plantaris muscle
- Lateral tibial condyle

(Top) Sagittal scan of the lateral femoral condyle. The plantaris muscle originates slightly more superior and medial to the lateral head of gastrocnemius. The plantaris runs inferomedially across the thigh to lie on the medial side of the Achilles tendon. More superficially, the bicipital tendon runs laterally towards its fibular head insertion. (Middle) A more lateral sagittal view shows the sesamoid bone within the lateral head of gastrocnemius muscle, the fabella. (Bottom) A more inferior oblique scan shows both the plantaris and lateral heads of the gastrocnemius muscle running over the posterior surface of the knee joint. Further distally, the plantaris muscle becomes a thin tendon and is difficult to discern until it reaches the medial side of the Achilles tendon in the distal calf.

KNEE

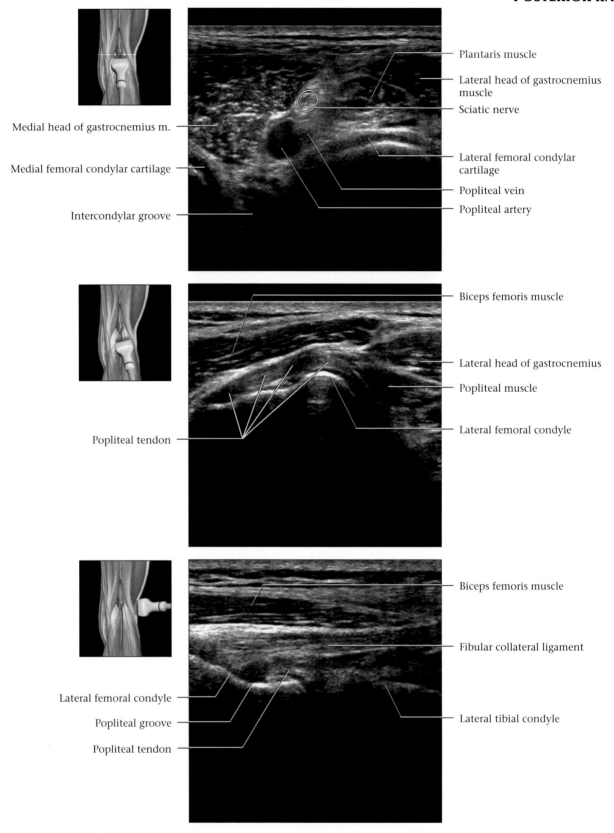

(Top) Transverse scan of the posterolateral aspect of the knee joint at the level of the inferior popliteal fossa. The sciatic nerve is the largest nerve in the body. In cross-section, nerve fibrils are seen as hypoechoic dots separated by hyperechoic perineurium. **(Middle)** Scanning more laterally and inferiorly, the popliteal muscle and its tendon can be demonstrated. The popliteal tendon originates from the proximal posterior tibial surface and runs superolaterally under the lateral head of the gastrocnemius muscle to insert onto the lateral cortex of the lateral femoral condyle. **(Bottom)** Coronal scan showing the popliteal groove on the lateral femoral condyle and the popliteal tendon entering this groove as its heads towards its insertion.

KNEE

POSTERIOR KNEE

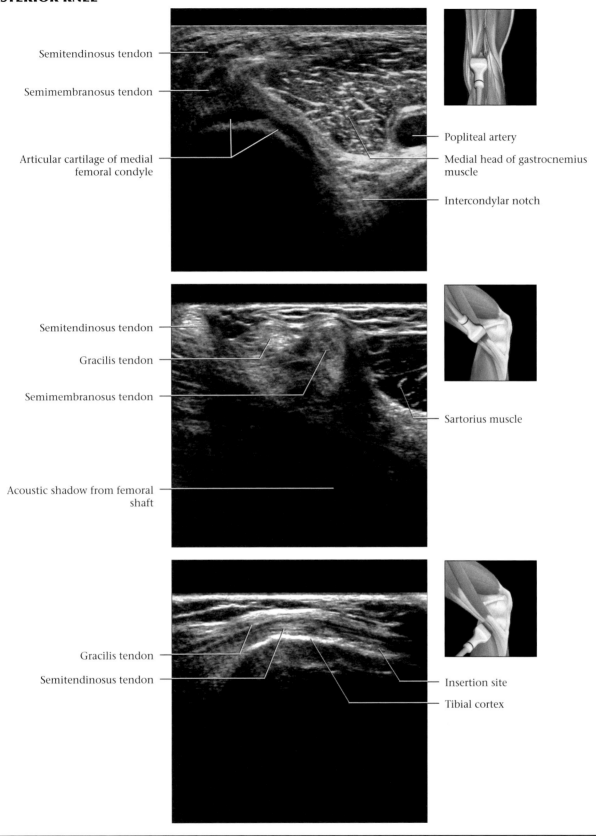

Semitendinosus tendon

Semimembranosus tendon

Articular cartilage of medial femoral condyle

Popliteal artery

Medial head of gastrocnemius muscle

Intercondylar notch

Semitendinosus tendon

Gracilis tendon

Semimembranosus tendon

Acoustic shadow from femoral shaft

Sartorius muscle

Gracilis tendon

Semitendinosus tendon

Insertion site

Tibial cortex

(Top) Transverse scan of the posteromedial knee at the level of the femoral condyles. The semimembranosus tendon can be seen running medial to the medial head of gastrocnemius muscle and deep to the semitendinosus tendon. The semimembranosus tendon will continue inferiorly to its posterior tibial insertion whereas the semitendinosus will be joined by others to insert on the anteromedial surface of the tibia. (Middle) More superiorly, transverse scan of the posteromedial aspect of the supracondylar region shows the medial tendons and muscles. Three of these, the sartorius, gracilis, and semitendinosus will continue together inferiorly and insert adjacent to each other as the pes anserine on the medial aspect of the proximal tibial shaft. (Bottom) Oblique transverse scan along the course of the pes anserine tendons showing their insertion on the medial tibial cortex.

LEG MUSCLES

Terminology

Abbreviations

- Artery = a.; ligament = l.; muscle = m.; vein = v.

Gross Anatomy

Osseous Anatomy

- **Tibia**
  - Proximal tibiofibular joint
    - Head of fibula and lateral condyle tibia joined by fibrous capsule
    - May communicate with knee joint
    - Posterolaterally located
    - Synovial; at risk for any articular process
  - Anterolateral tibia: Origin of anterior muscles of leg
  - Anterior border (shin): Sharp ridge running from tibial tuberosity proximally to anterior margin of medial malleolus
  - Medial tibial surface
    - Wide and flat
    - Proximally, covered by pes anserinus
    - Remainder is subcutaneous
  - Medial border of tibia: Saphenous nerve and great saphenous vein run along it
  - Posterior tibia: Origin of deep posterior muscles of leg
  - Lateral border of tibia: Ridge for attachment of interosseous membrane
  - Medial malleolus: 2 colliculi, anterior longer than posterior
  - Distal tibiofibular joint
    - Fibula articulates with tibia at fibular notch; joined by interosseous ligament
    - Strengthened by anterior and posterior tibiofibular ligaments
    - Posterolaterally located
- **Fibula**
  - Anterior fibula
    - Origin of lateral muscles of leg
  - Medial fibula
    - Origin of deep posterior muscles of leg
  - Posterolateral fibula
    - Origin of posterior muscles of leg
  - Lateral malleolus: 1 cm longer than medial malleolus

Interosseous Membrane

- Stretches across interval between tibia and fibula
- Greatly extends surface for origin of muscles
- Strong, oblique fibers run downwards and laterally from tibia to fibula
- In upper part, below lateral condyle of tibia, there is an opening for passage of anterior tibial vessels
- Distally, an opening allows passage of perforating branch of peroneal artery
- Tibialis posterior and flexor hallucis longus take partial origin from the back of membrane
- Tibialis anterior, long extensors of toes, and peroneus tertius take partial origin from front of membrane

Muscles of Leg

- Compartments separated by deep fascia, which give partial origin to several muscles
- **Posterior compartment: Superficial muscles**
  - **Gastrocnemius**
    - Origin: Medial from posterior femoral metaphysis; lateral from posterior edge of lateral epicondyle
    - Heads separated from posterior capsule by a bursa
    - 2 heads unite to form main bulk of muscle
    - Join in a thin aponeurotic tendon near mid leg
    - Joins soleus aponeurosis to form Achilles tendon; concave in cross section; musculotendinous junction 5 cm above calcaneal insertion
    - Nerve supply: Tibial nerve
    - Action: Plantar flexor of ankle and flexor of knee
  - **Plantaris**
    - Origin: Superior and medial to lateral head of gastrocnemius origin, as well as from oblique popliteal ligament
    - Continues deep to lateral head gastrocnemius
    - Myotendinous junction at level of origin of soleus (muscle is 5-10 cm long)
    - Tendon then lies between medial head gastrocnemius and soleus
    - Follows medial side of Achilles to insert either anteromedially on Achilles or on calcaneus
    - Plantaris absent 7-10%
    - Nerve supply: Tibial nerve
    - Action: Acts with gastrocnemius
  - **Soleus**
    - Origin: Extensive, from back of fibular head and upper 1/3 of posterior surface of shaft of fibula, from soleal line and middle 1/3 of medial border of tibia, and from tendinous arch joining these across the popliteal vessels
    - Flat, thick, powerful muscle ends in strong tendon
    - Joins with tendon of gastrocnemius to form Achilles tendon
    - Nerve supply: Tibial nerve
    - Action: Stabilizes ankle in standing, plantarflexes ankle
    - Accessory soleus: Rare variant, arises from anterior surface of soleus or from fibula and soleal line of tibia; inserts into Achilles or onto calcaneus anteromedially to Achilles; presents as mass
- **Posterior compartment: Deep muscles**
  - **Popliteus**
    - Origin: Tendon from popliteal groove of lateral femoral condyle
    - Passes through popliteal hiatus posteriorly and medially, pierces posterior capsule of knee
    - M. fibers directed medially & downwards to insert on posterior surface of tibia above soleal line
    - Nerve supply: Tibial nerve
    - Action: Flexes knee and medially rotates tibia with respect to femur at onset of flexion (unlocking extension "screwing home" mechanism)
  - **Tibialis posterior**
    - Origin: Interosseous membrane and adjoining parts of posterior surfaces of tibia and fibula
    - Superior end bifid; anterior tibial vessels pass forward between the 2 attachments

- Distally it inclines medially, under flexor digitorum longus
- Grooves and curves around medial malleolus
- Nerve supply: Tibial nerve
- Action: Plantarflexes and inverts foot
○ **Flexor digitorum longus**
  - Origin: Posterior surface of tibia, below popliteus, and medial to the vertical ridge
  - Crosses superficial to distal part of tibialis posterior
  - Tendon grooves lower end of tibia lateral to that of the tibialis posterior, passes around medial malleolus to foot
  - Nerve supply: Tibial nerve
  - Action: Flexes interphalangeal and metatarsophalangeal joints of lateral 4 toes; plantarflexes and inverts foot
○ **Flexor hallucis longus**
  - Origin: Posterior surface of fibula, below origin of soleus
  - Passes medially, descends down posterior to mid tibia
  - Associated with os trigonum posterior to talus
  - Tendon occupies deep groove on posterior surface of talus, passes around medial malleolus, under sustentaculum tali, to great toe
  - Nerve supply: Tibial nerves
  - Action: Flexes the interphalangeal and metatarsophalangeal joints of great toe; plantarflexes foot
- **Lateral compartment**
  ○ Peroneals separated from extensors by anterior intermuscular septum and from posterior muscles by posterior septum
  ○ **Peroneus longus**
    - Origin upper 2/3 lateral surface of fibula and intermuscular septa and adjacent muscular fascia
    - Becomes tendinous a few cm above lateral malleolus
    - Curves forward behind lateral malleolus, posterior to peroneus brevis
    - Nerve supply: Superficial peroneal
    - Action: Everts foot and secondarily plantarflexes foot
  ○ **Peroneus brevis**
    - Origin lower 2/3 lateral surface of fibula and intermuscular septa and adjacent muscular fascia
    - Muscle is medial to peroneus longus at origin but overlaps peroneus longus in middle 1/3
    - Tendon curves forward behind lateral malleolus, in front of peroneus longus tendon
    - Nerve supply: Superficial peroneal
    - Action: Everts foot and secondarily plantarflexes foot
  ○ Synovial sheath for peroneals begins 5 cm above tip of lateral malleolus and envelops both tendons; divides into 2 sheaths at level of calcaneus
  ○ **Peroneus quartus**: Accessory muscle with prevalence of 10%; originates from distal leg, frequently from peroneal muscles, with variable insertion sites at foot; at level of malleolus, located medial or posterior to both peroneal tendons

○ **Peroneus digiti minimi**: Accessory with prevalence of 15-36%; extends from peroneus brevis muscle around medial malleolus to foot; tiny tendinous slip
- **Anterior compartment**
  ○ **Tibialis anterior**
    - Origin: Upper half of lateral surface of tibia and interosseous membrane
    - Tendon originates in distal 1/3; passes deep to retinaculum
    - Nerve supply: Deep peroneal and recurrent genicular
    - Action: Dorsiflexor and invertor of foot
  ○ **Extensor digitorum longus**
    - Origin: From upper 3/4 anterior surface fibula
    - Descends behind extensor retinacula to ankle
    - Nerve supply: Deep peroneal
    - Action: Extends interphalangeal and metatarsophalangeal joints of lateral 4 toes, dorsiflexes foot
  ○ **Peroneus tertius**
    - Small, not always present
    - Origin: Continuous with extensor digitorum longus, arising from distal 1/4 of anterior surface of fibula and interosseous membrane
    - Inserts into dorsal surface base 5th metatarsal
    - Nerve supply: Deep peroneal
    - Action: Dorsiflexes ankle and everts foot
  ○ **Extensor hallucis**
    - Thin muscle hidden between tibialis anterior and extensor digitorum longus
    - Origin: Middle 2/4 of anterior surface of fibula and interosseous membrane
    - Tendon passes deep to retinacula to great toe
    - Nerve supply: Deep peroneal
    - Action: Extends phalanges of great toe and dorsiflexes foot

Anatomy-Based Imaging Issues

Imaging Recommendations
- US
  ○ Owing to its smaller size, compared to the thigh (less depth to penetrate), the leg muscles and vessels are well-demonstrated by ultrasound throughout their course
  ○ The relationship of different structures in the posterior compartment tend to change along their course. If in doubt, start from the ankle level and trace structures proximally

Imaging "Sweet Spots"
- The deep structures of the posterior compartment, such as the peroneal vessels and the tibialis posterior muscle, may be be difficult to visualize in very muscular patients.
  ○ The structures can be interrogated by scanning from anterior through the anterior compartment and the gap between the tibia and fibula

Lower Limb

VII

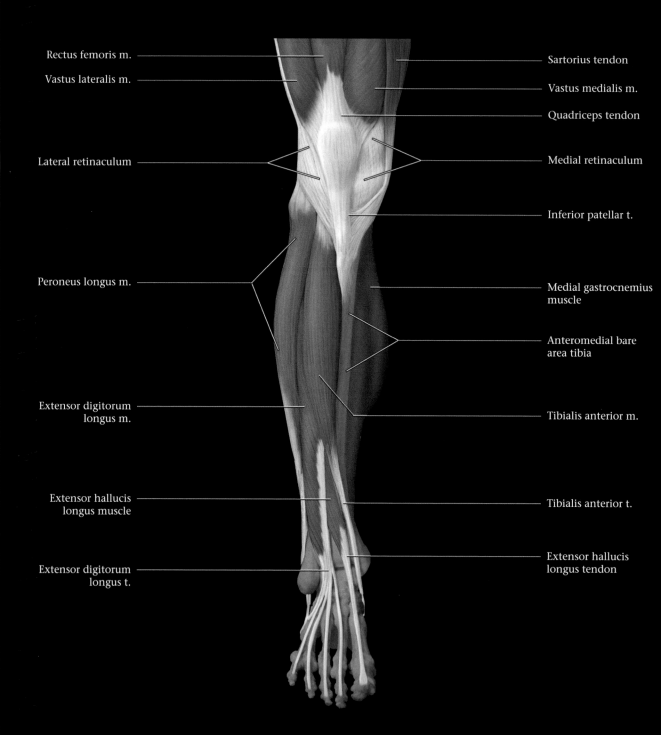

Rectus femoris m.

Vastus lateralis m.

Lateral retinaculum

Peroneus longus m.

Extensor digitorum
longus m.

Extensor hallucis
longus muscle

Extensor digitorum
longus t.

Sartorius tendon

Vastus medialis m.

Quadriceps tendon

Medial retinaculum

Inferior patellar t.

Medial gastrocnemius
muscle

Anteromedial bare
area tibia

Tibialis anterior m.

Tibialis anterior t.

Extensor hallucis
longus tendon

Graphic of anterior leg muscles. Note that nearly the entire anteromedial tibia is bare of muscle; it is thus poorly vascularized, resulting in slow fracture healing. The tibialis anterior has an extensive origin from both tibia and interosseous membrane and is the most substantial muscle of the anterior compartment. The extensor digitorum longus originates from the fibula. The extensor hallucis longus originates between the two, from the fibula and the interosseous membrane. These three muscles retain the same orientation as they become tendinous anterior to the ankle. The mnemonic "Tom, Harry, & Dick" applies to the tendon order, from medial to lateral (tibialis anterior, extensor hallucis longus, extensor digitorum).

LEG MUSCLES

PANORAMIC ANTEROLATERAL LEG

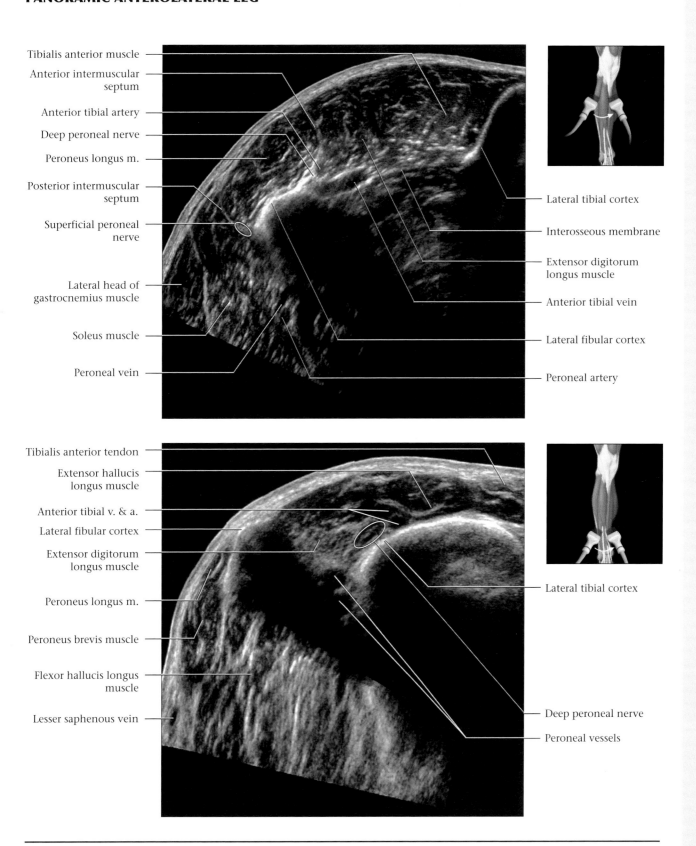

Tibialis anterior muscle
Anterior intermuscular septum
Anterior tibial artery
Deep peroneal nerve
Peroneus longus m.
Posterior intermuscular septum
Superficial peroneal nerve
Lateral head of gastrocnemius muscle
Soleus muscle
Peroneal vein

Lateral tibial cortex
Interosseous membrane
Extensor digitorum longus muscle
Anterior tibial vein
Lateral fibular cortex
Peroneal artery

Tibialis anterior tendon
Extensor hallucis longus muscle
Anterior tibial v. & a.
Lateral fibular cortex
Extensor digitorum longus muscle
Peroneus longus m.
Peroneus brevis muscle
Flexor hallucis longus muscle
Lesser saphenous vein

Lateral tibial cortex

Deep peroneal nerve
Peroneal vessels

(Top) Transverse panoramic view of the anterior and lateral compartments of the upper leg. The crural compartments are divided by the tibia, and the two intermuscular septae (anterior and posterior) into the anterior (extensor), lateral (peroneal) and posterior (flexor) compartments. The intermuscular septum separates the anterior from the posterior compartments. **(Bottom)** Transverse panoramic view of the anterior and lateral compartments of the inferior leg. All muscles are smaller in caliber compared to that seen superiorly. An interosseous gap is still present between the the tibia and fibula but ultrasound interrogation through this gap is no longer possible and the interosseous membrane cannot be demonstrated.

LEG MUSCLES

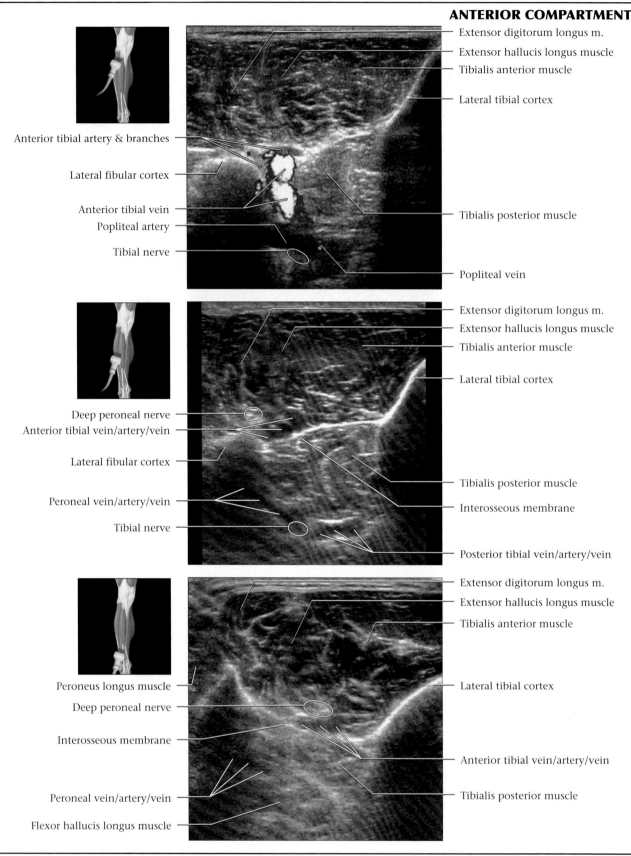

ANTERIOR COMPARTMENT

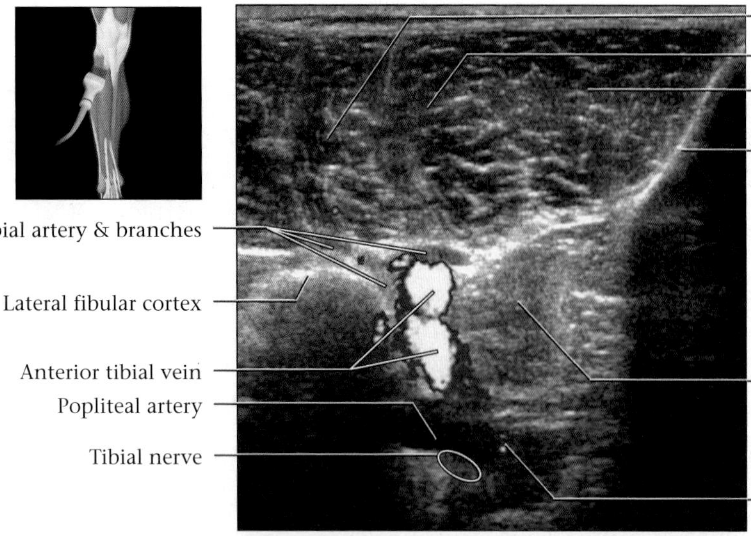

Extensor digitorum longus m.
Extensor hallucis longus muscle
Tibialis anterior muscle
Lateral tibial cortex
Anterior tibial artery & branches
Lateral fibular cortex
Anterior tibial vein
Popliteal artery
Tibial nerve
Tibialis posterior muscle
Popliteal vein

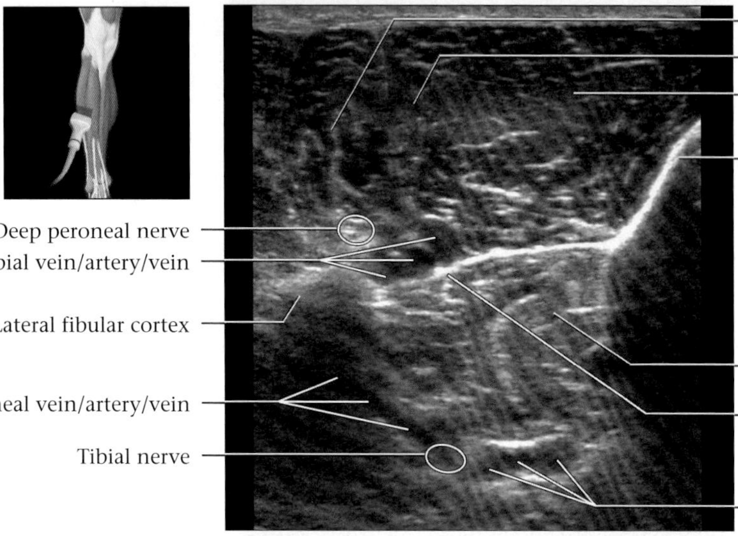

Extensor digitorum longus m.
Extensor hallucis longus muscle
Tibialis anterior muscle
Lateral tibial cortex
Deep peroneal nerve
Anterior tibial vein/artery/vein
Lateral fibular cortex
Peroneal vein/artery/vein
Tibial nerve
Tibialis posterior muscle
Interosseous membrane
Posterior tibial vein/artery/vein

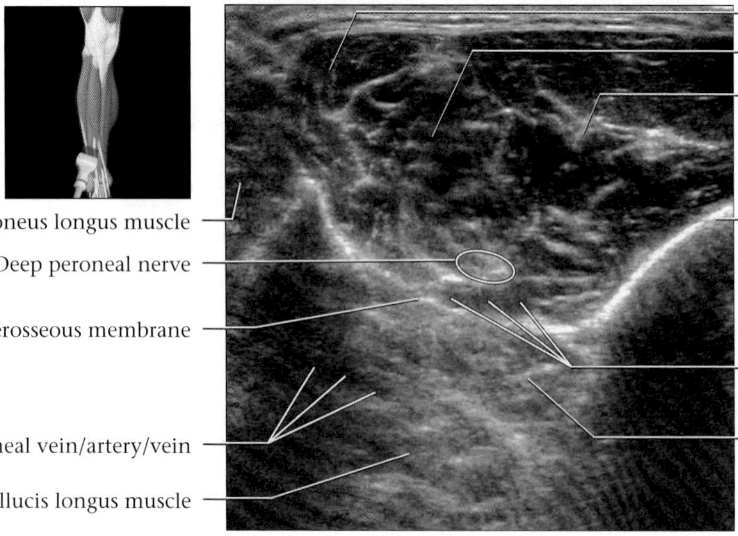

Extensor digitorum longus m.
Extensor hallucis longus muscle
Tibialis anterior muscle
Peroneus longus muscle
Lateral tibial cortex
Deep peroneal nerve
Interosseous membrane
Anterior tibial vein/artery/vein
Peroneal vein/artery/vein
Tibialis posterior muscle
Flexor hallucis longus muscle

(Top) Transverse color Doppler scan of the anterior compartment at the upper leg level slightly below the proximal tibiofibular joint. At this level, which is above the superior margin of the interosseous membrane, the anterior tibial artery and vein, which are branches of the popliteal artery and vein, run anteriorly to supply the anterior compartment. **(Middle)** Transverse scan of the anterior compartment at a slightly lower level. The tibialis anterior, extensor hallucis longus and extensor digitorum longus muscles form the muscular component of this compartment. The deep peroneal nerve has penetrated from laterally to supply this compartment. The anterior tibial vessels run on the surface of the interosseous membrane. **(Bottom)** Transverse scan more inferiorly shows a decrease in size of the extensor muscles and gradual migration of nerve and vessels more medially and superficially.

LEG MUSCLES

ANTERIOR COMPARTMENT

Tibialis anterior muscle

Tibialis posterior muscle

Anterior tibial vein

Anterior tibial artery

Soleus muscle

Anterior tibial artery

Tibialis anterior muscle/tendon/muscle

Tibialis posterior muscle

Interosseous membrane

Peroneal vein

Soleus muscle

Tibialis posterior muscle

Tibialis anterior muscle

Peroneal artery and vein

Soleus muscle

(Top) Sagittal scan of the anterior compartment at the upper leg level. The anterior tibial vessels pass above the superior margin of the interosseous membrane to enter the anterior compartment and supply the extensor muscles. (Middle) Sagittal scan of the anterior and posterior compartments at the mid-leg level, shows that the interosseous gap between the tibia and fibula can be used as a window to interrogate the deep posterior structures. (Bottom) Sagittal scan of the anterior compartment at a lower level. Within the posterior compartment the peroneal vessels run anteriorly, and just below the inferior margin of the interosseous membrane.

LEG MUSCLES

Soleus muscle
Peroneus longus muscle
Extensor digitorum longus m.
Deep peroneal nerve
Anterior tibial vein/artery/vein
Tibialis anterior muscle
Interosseous membrane
Tibialis posterior muscle
Posterior tibial cortex

Superficial peroneal nerve
Peroneal vein/artery/vein
Tibial nerve
Lateral fibular cortex

Soleus muscle
Peroneus longus muscle
Peroneus brevis muscle
Anterior intermuscular septum
Extensor digitorum longus m.
Anterior tibial vein/artery/vein
Tibialis anterior muscle
Interosseous membrane
Lateral tibial cortex

Posterior intermuscular septum
Lateral fibular cortex

Sural nerve
Short saphenous vein
Peroneus longus tendon
Lateral fibular cortex
Peroneal artery
Peroneal vein

Peroneus brevis muscle
Flexor hallucis longus muscle

(Top) Transverse scan of the lateral compartment at a high level. At this level, only the peroneus longus muscle has originated and is the only muscle occupying this compartment. The superficial peroneal nerve lies on its posterior surface. The deep peroneal nerve has already entered the anterior compartment after curving around the fibular neck (above this scan level). (Middle) Transverse scan at the mid-leg level shows that the peroneus brevis muscle has now originated and resides anterior and deep to the peroneus longus muscle. More inferiorly, the peroneus longus muscle will become smaller and turn into a tendon while the peroneus brevis will still have muscle fibers down to the level of the ankle joint. (Bottom) Transverse scan at the level of the lateral malleolus. The peroneal tendons will run posterior to the lateral malleolus and curve around its tip to run towards the lateral foot.

LEG MUSCLES

LATERAL COMPARTMENT

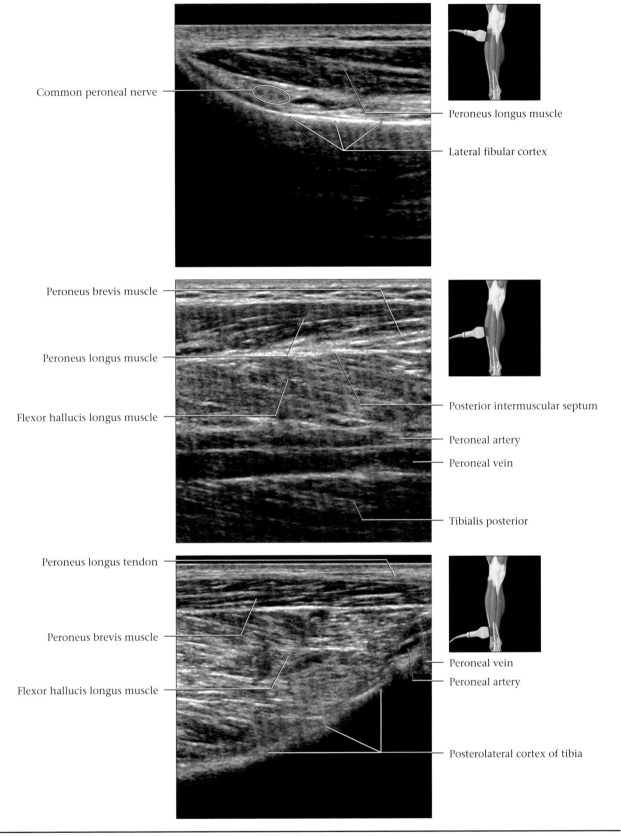

Common peroneal nerve

Peroneus longus muscle

Lateral fibular cortex

Peroneus brevis muscle

Peroneus longus muscle

Flexor hallucis longus muscle

Posterior intermuscular septum

Peroneal artery

Peroneal vein

Tibialis posterior

Peroneus longus tendon

Peroneus brevis muscle

Flexor hallucis longus muscle

Peroneal vein

Peroneal artery

Posterolateral cortex of tibia

(Top) Coronal scan of the lateral compartment at the level of the fibular neck. The common peroneal nerve runs together with the biceps femoris tendon, then curves anteriorly around the neck of fibula to enter the lateral and then the anterior compartments. (Middle) Coronal scan of the lateral compartment at the mid-leg level shows the transition between the peroneus longus and peroneus brevis muscles. These are separated from the posterior compartment by the posterior intermuscular septum. (Bottom) Coronal scan further inferiorly shows that the peroneus longus muscle is now only a tendon, compared to the muscular peroneus brevis. Similarly in the posterior compartment, the flexor hallucis longus muscle is the only muscle at this level as the others have also become tendons.

LEG MUSCLES

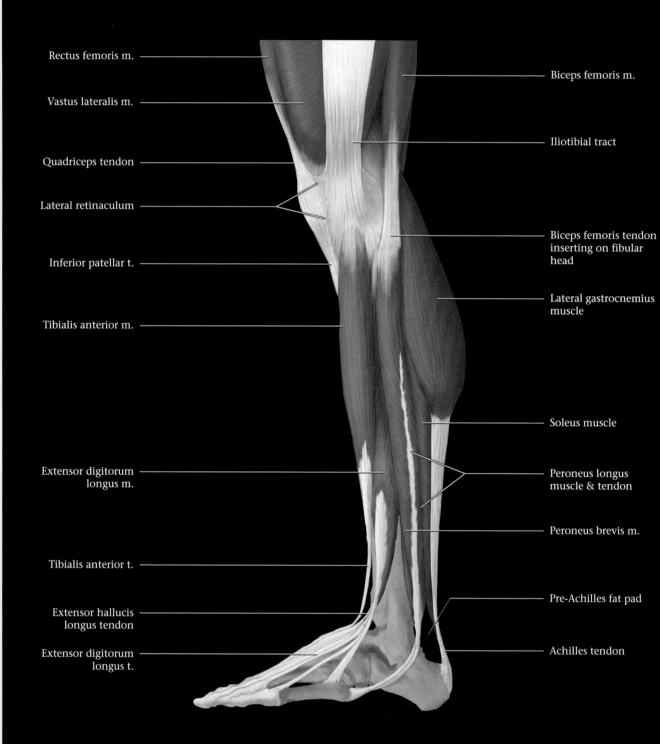

Rectus femoris m.

Vastus lateralis m.

Quadriceps tendon

Lateral retinaculum

Inferior patellar t.

Tibialis anterior m.

Extensor digitorum longus m.

Tibialis anterior t.

Extensor hallucis longus tendon

Extensor digitorum longus t.

Biceps femoris m.

Iliotibial tract

Biceps femoris tendon inserting on fibular head

Lateral gastrocnemius muscle

Soleus muscle

Peroneus longus muscle & tendon

Peroneus brevis m.

Pre-Achilles fat pad

Achilles tendon

Graphic of the lateral leg, showing the anterior compartment (extensors), lateral compartment (peroneals), and superficial muscles of the posterior compartment.

LEG MUSCLES

POSTERIOR LEG

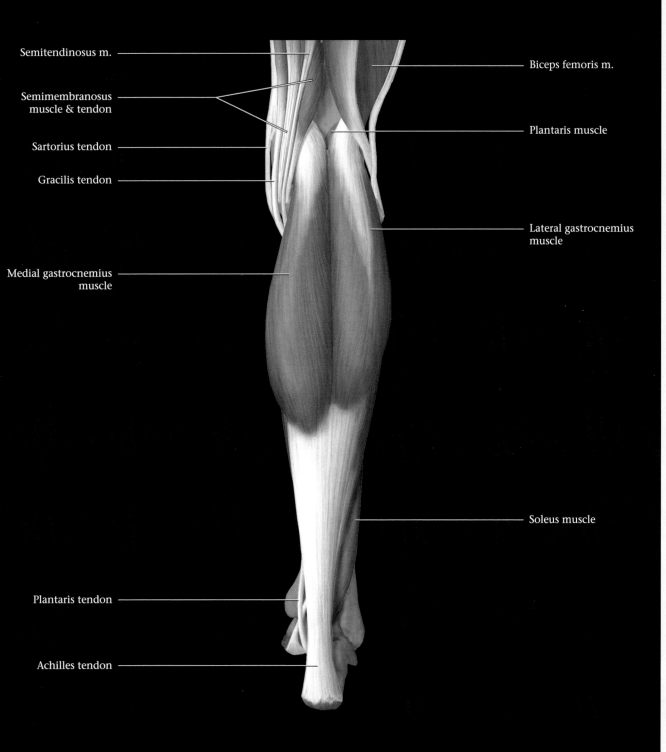

Semitendinosus m.

Semimembranosus muscle & tendon

Sartorius tendon

Gracilis tendon

Medial gastrocnemius muscle

Plantaris tendon

Achilles tendon

Biceps femoris m.

Plantaris muscle

Lateral gastrocnemius muscle

Soleus muscle

Posterior view of superficial muscles and tendons of the leg. The gastrocnemius muscles are bulky in the proximal half of the leg and taper to an aponeurosis which blends with the soleus more distally to become the Achilles tendon. The plantaris muscle is superficial only at its origin from the lateral femoral metaphysis, just medial to the origin of the lateral head of gastrocnemius. The muscle extends only a few centimeters before becoming tendinous, extending distally between the soleus and medial gastrocnemius; eventually, the plantaris tendon merges with the medial side of Achilles or inserts on the calcaneus medial to the Achilles insertion.

LEG MUSCLES

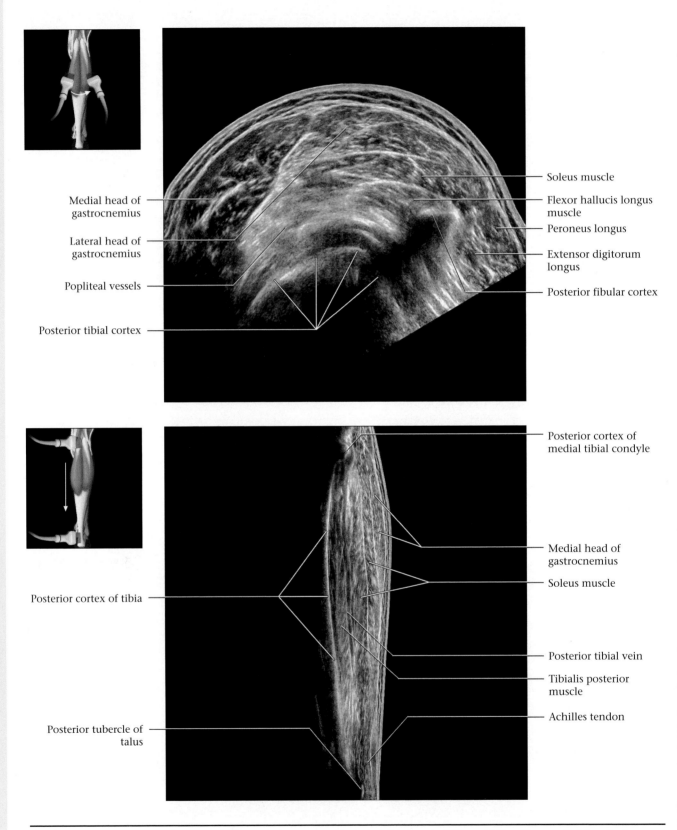

Medial head of gastrocnemius

Lateral head of gastrocnemius

Popliteal vessels

Posterior tibial cortex

Soleus muscle

Flexor hallucis longus muscle

Peroneus longus

Extensor digitorum longus

Posterior fibular cortex

Posterior cortex of medial tibial condyle

Medial head of gastrocnemius

Soleus muscle

Posterior tibial vein

Tibialis posterior muscle

Achilles tendon

Posterior cortex of tibia

Posterior tubercle of talus

(Top) Transverse panoramic scan of the posterior compartment at the level of the mid-leg. The medial head of gastrocnemius muscle is larger than the lateral throughout its course. From this mid-calf level downwards, the soleus will assume relatively more bulk as the gastrocnemius turns tendinous. **(Bottom)** Sagittal panoramic scan of the posterior compartment. The gastrocnemius is muscular down to approximately the level of the mid-calf. Below this level, it forms the Achilles tendon, receiving contributions from the soleus muscle. For the deep layer, the tibialis posterior muscle lies on the surface of the tibial shaft and interosseous membrane.

LEG MUSCLES

TRANSVERSE POSTERIOR LEG

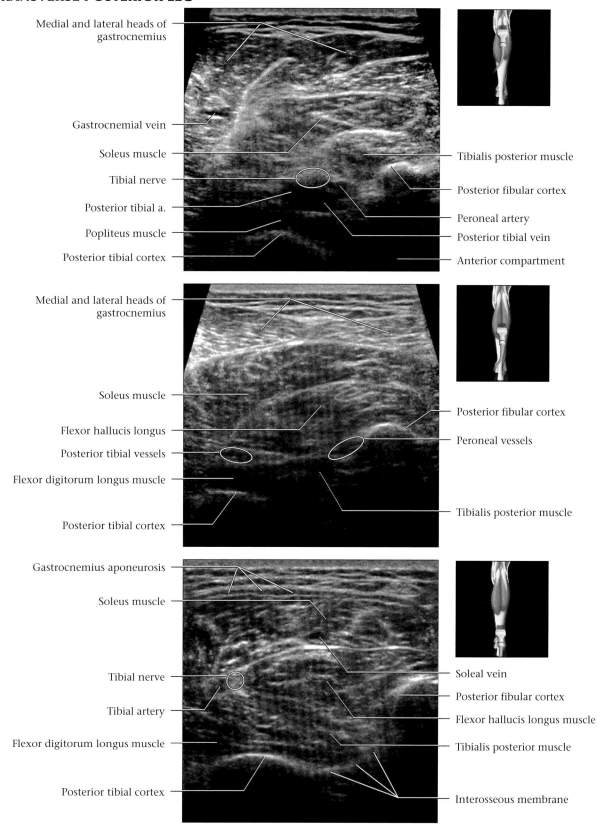

Medial and lateral heads of gastrocnemius

Gastrocnemial vein

Soleus muscle

Tibial nerve

Posterior tibial a.

Popliteus muscle

Posterior tibial cortex

Tibialis posterior muscle

Posterior fibular cortex

Peroneal artery

Posterior tibial vein

Anterior compartment

Medial and lateral heads of gastrocnemius

Soleus muscle

Flexor hallucis longus

Posterior tibial vessels

Flexor digitorum longus muscle

Posterior tibial cortex

Posterior fibular cortex

Peroneal vessels

Tibialis posterior muscle

Gastrocnemius aponeurosis

Soleus muscle

Tibial nerve

Tibial artery

Flexor digitorum longus muscle

Posterior tibial cortex

Soleal vein

Posterior fibular cortex

Flexor hallucis longus muscle

Tibialis posterior muscle

Interosseous membrane

(Top) Transverse scan through the posterior compartment at the upper-calf level. For this compartment, the superficial layer consists of the gastrocnemius, plantaris and soleus muscles. The deep layer consists of the popliteus, tibialis posterior, flexor digitorum longus and flexor hallucis longus muscles. **(Middle)** Transverse scan at the mid-calf level. The tibial vessels have bifurcated into their peroneal and posterior tibial branches, which delineates a separation between the tibialis posterior and flexor digitorum longus from the rest of the calf muscles. Given the thickness of the gastrocnemius and soleus muscle, these deep muscles may be better seen using the anterior compartment as a window. **(Bottom)** Further inferiorly, the gastrocnemius has become a thin aponeurosis and together with the tendon from the soleus muscle will form the Achilles tendon.

LEG VESSELS

Terminology

Abbreviations
- Artery (a.)
- Ligament (l.)
- Muscle (m.)
- Nerve (n.)
- Vein (v.)

Gross Anatomy

Vessels of Leg
- **Popliteal artery**
  - Begins as the continuation of the superficial femoral artery after it has passed through the adductor hiatus (inferior end of adductor canal)
  - Runs through the fat of the popliteal fossa
  - Relations
    - Deep to artery: Femoral shaft, knee joint capsule, popliteus fascia
    - Superficial to artery: Semimembranosus muscle and gastrocnemius muscle
  - Ends at distal border of popliteus in two branches: Anterior tibial artery and tibioperoneal trunk
- **Anterior tibial artery**
  - Smaller of the 2 terminal branches of popliteal artery
  - Origin in back of leg, at distal border of popliteus muscle
  - Passes through upper part of interosseous membrane
  - Straight course down front of leg to become dorsalis pedis artery
  - Runs on the anterior surface of the interosseous membrane, deep to the extensor muscles
  - Muscular branches along length
  - Malleolar branches ramify over malleoli; lateral one anastomoses with perforating branch of peroneal artery
- **Posterior tibial artery**
  - Larger of the 2 terminal branches of popliteal artery
  - Main blood supply to foot
  - Passes downwards and slightly medially along with tibial nerve to end in space between medial malleolus and calcaneus
  - Within the calf, the artery runs just deep to the transverse intermuscular septum
  - Divides into lateral and medial plantar arteries in the tarsal tunnel behind the medial malleolus
  - Branches
    - Circumflex fibular (may arise from anterior tibial), runs laterally around neck of fibula
    - Nutrient artery to tibia
    - Muscular branches
- **Peroneal artery**
  - Largest branch of posterior tibial artery
  - Runs obliquely downwards and laterally beneath soleus to fibula
  - It descends deep to flexor hallucis longus
- **Popliteal vein**
  - Paired venae comitantes of anterior and posterior tibial arteries join to form popliteal vein

  - Also receives the small saphenous vein in the popliteal fossa
  - Usually begins at the inferior border of the popliteus muscle
  - Crosses from the medial to the lateral side of the popliteal artery as it runs in the popliteal fossa, aside from always being superficial to the popliteal artery
  - Ends at adductor hiatus by becoming the superficial femoral vein
- **Great saphenous vein**
  - Begins at medial border of foot
  - Ascends in front of medial malleolus
  - Passes obliquely upwards and backwards across medial surface of distal 1/3 of tibia
  - Passes vertically upward along medial border of tibia to posterior part of medial side of knee
- **Small saphenous vein**
  - Extends behind lateral malleolus, ascends lateral to Achilles tendon
  - At midline of calf in lower popliteal region, pierces popliteal fascia and terminates in popliteal vein

Anatomy-Based Imaging Issues

Imaging Recommendations
- Ultrasound
  - Examination of the lower limb vessels requires the use of morphological and functional techniques
    - Morphology: Documentation of areas of stenosis or occlusion, sites of venous valves, aberrant branches, aneurysm formation, etc.
    - Functional: Combination of color and spectral Doppler examination
  - Veins require the use of dynamic maneuvers
    - Valsalva: To increase abdominal pressure and accentuate reverse flow and incompetent venous valves
    - Augmentation: To increase venous return (to demonstrate venous flow and patency) by manually squeezing the calf or by gently moving the toes
    - Compression: To demonstrate the absence of thrombus by using transducer pressure to cause complete luminal occlusion
  - Arteries require the use of spectral Doppler scanning to show their phasicity; normal scan is triphasic
    - Sharp forward flow upstroke (systolic phase)
    - Small reverse flow (early diastolic phase)
    - Final smaller forward flow (late diastolic phase)

Imaging Pitfalls
- Augmentation is frequently required to demonstrate flow in the deep calf veins (which normally show no color Doppler flow)

LEG VESSELS

GRAPHICS ANTERIOR AND POSTERIOR LEG VESSELS

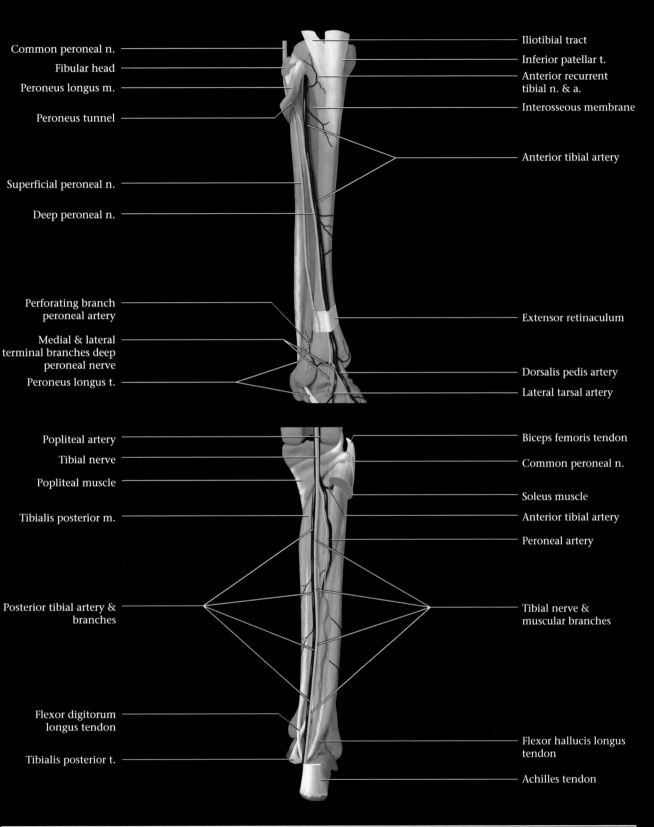

Common peroneal n.

Fibular head

Peroneus longus m.

Peroneus tunnel

Superficial peroneal n.

Deep peroneal n.

Perforating branch peroneal artery

Medial & lateral terminal branches deep peroneal nerve

Peroneus longus t.

Iliotibial tract

Inferior patellar t.

Anterior recurrent tibial n. & a.

Interosseous membrane

Anterior tibial artery

Extensor retinaculum

Dorsalis pedis artery

Lateral tarsal artery

Popliteal artery

Tibial nerve

Popliteal muscle

Tibialis posterior m.

Posterior tibial artery & branches

Flexor digitorum longus tendon

Tibialis posterior t.

Biceps femoris tendon

Common peroneal n.

Soleus muscle

Anterior tibial artery

Peroneal artery

Tibial nerve & muscular branches

Flexor hallucis longus tendon

Achilles tendon

(Top) Graphic of anterior leg shows anterior tibial artery perforating the interosseous septum proximally and descending along this membrane down the front of leg to terminate as dorsalis pedis. Distally one sees a perforating branch of the peroneal artery, which in a variant situation may provide the major blood supply to the dorsum of the foot. (Bottom) The popliteal artery ends at the distal border of popliteus in two branches: 1) Anterior tibial artery passes through a slit in tibialis posterior muscle and the interosseous membrane to the anterior compartment, and 2) posterior tibial artery passes downwards and slightly medially adjacent to tibial nerve to end in space between medial malleolus and calcaneus. The largest branch of the posterior tibial artery is the peroneal, which runs obliquely downwards and laterally beneath the soleus to the fibula.

LEG VESSELS

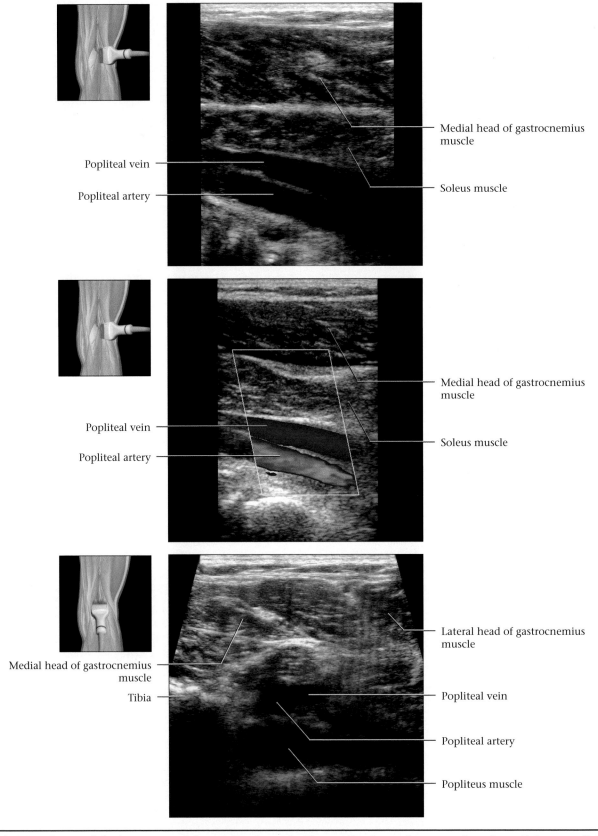

Popliteal vein

Popliteal artery

Medial head of gastrocnemius muscle

Soleus muscle

Popliteal vein

Popliteal artery

Medial head of gastrocnemius muscle

Soleus muscle

Medial head of gastrocnemius muscle

Tibia

Lateral head of gastrocnemius muscle

Popliteal vein

Popliteal artery

Popliteus muscle

(Top) Sagittal scan of the lower part of the popliteal vessels. The popliteal vessels are continuations of the superficial femoral vessels after they have exited the adductor canal through the adductor hiatus. The popliteal vein lies superficial to the popliteal artery, a reverse of the relationship between the superficial femoral vein and artery. The popliteal vessels pass inferolaterally through the fat of the popliteal fossa. (Middle) Sagittal color Doppler scan of the popliteal vessels shows complete color filling of the lumina (excluding luminal thrombus) and normal flow direction: Towards the trunk (blue) for the vein; and away from the trunk (red) for the artery. (Bottom) Transverse scan of the lower part of the popliteal vessels. The popliteal vein runs superficial to the popliteal artery and usually bifurcates at the inferior margin of the popliteus muscle.

LEG VESSELS

POPLITEAL VESSEL BIFURCATION

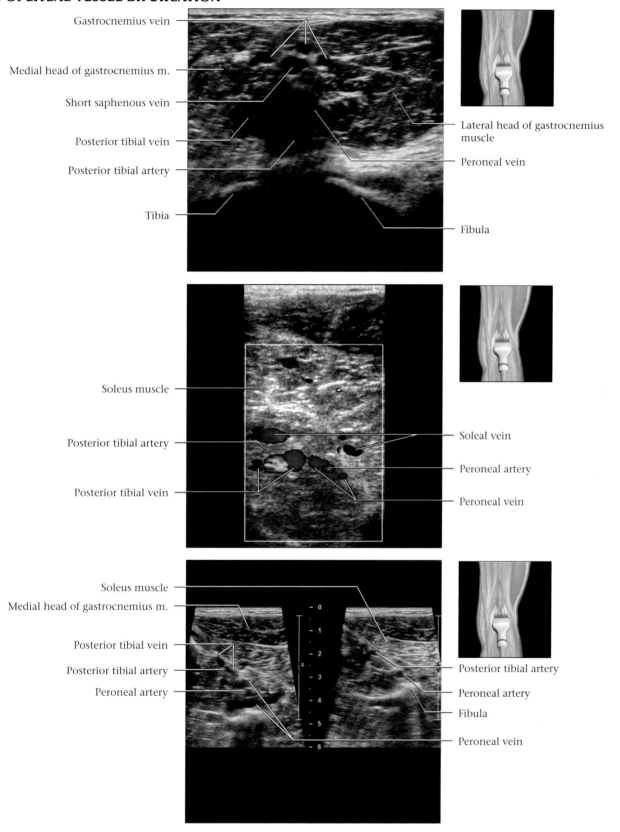

Gastrocnemius vein

Medial head of gastrocnemius m.

Short saphenous vein

Posterior tibial vein

Posterior tibial artery

Tibia

Lateral head of gastrocnemius muscle

Peroneal vein

Fibula

Soleus muscle

Posterior tibial artery

Posterior tibial vein

Soleal vein

Peroneal artery

Peroneal vein

Soleus muscle

Medial head of gastrocnemius m.

Posterior tibial vein

Posterior tibial artery

Peroneal artery

Posterior tibial artery

Peroneal artery

Fibula

Peroneal vein

(Top) Transverse scan below the bifurcation of the popliteal artery. The popliteal artery bifurcates into the anterior and posterior tibial arteries. The posterior tibial artery is the larger of the two terminal branches of the popliteal artery and passes inferiorly for a short distance before giving out its largest branch, the peroneal artery. (Middle) Transverse color Doppler scan showing the posterior compartment vessels of the proximal calf. Color flow highlights the paired venae comitantes nature of the posterior tibial and peroneal veins, lying on both sides of the corresponding artery. (Bottom) Transverse scan at the mid-proximal calf scanning from the medial side. The lumina of the peroneal and tibial veins can be compressed by firm transducer pressure (right half image) indicating the lack of thrombus.

LEG VESSELS

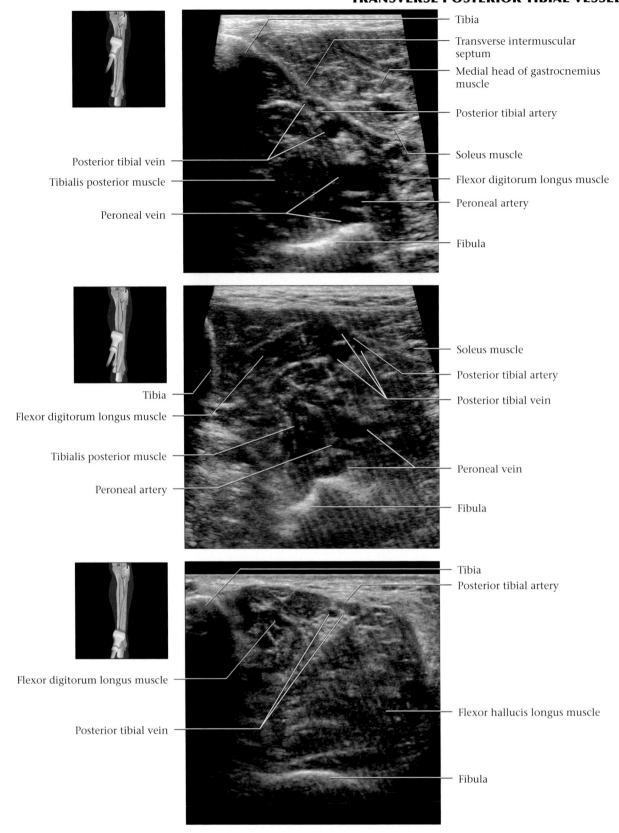

Top image labels:
- Tibia
- Transverse intermuscular septum
- Medial head of gastrocnemius muscle
- Posterior tibial artery
- Soleus muscle
- Flexor digitorum longus muscle
- Peroneal artery
- Fibula
- Posterior tibial vein
- Tibialis posterior muscle
- Peroneal vein

Middle image labels:
- Soleus muscle
- Posterior tibial artery
- Posterior tibial vein
- Peroneal vein
- Fibula
- Tibia
- Flexor digitorum longus muscle
- Tibialis posterior muscle
- Peroneal artery

Bottom image labels:
- Tibia
- Posterior tibial artery
- Flexor hallucis longus muscle
- Fibula
- Flexor digitorum longus muscle
- Posterior tibial vein

(Top) Series of three transverse scans of the posterior tibial vessels using a medial scanning approach. Superiorly, the posterior tibial vessels give off their main branch, the common peroneal vessels. The posterior tibial artery lies just deep to the transverse intermuscular septum while the peroneal arteries are deep to the flexor digitorum muscle. **(Middle)** At the mid-calf level, the posterior tibial vessels no longer line up side by side (three in a line). Anatomical variations occur, as seen here with three posterior tibial veins accompanying one artery. The peroneal vessels continue their deeper course, running on the surface of the tibialis posterior, which separates them from the anterior leg compartment. **(Bottom)** Further inferiorly, the posterior tibial vessels emerge superficially as they prepare to enter the tarsal tunnel behind the medial malleolus.

LEG VESSELS

LONGITUDINAL POSTERIOR TIBIAL VESSELS

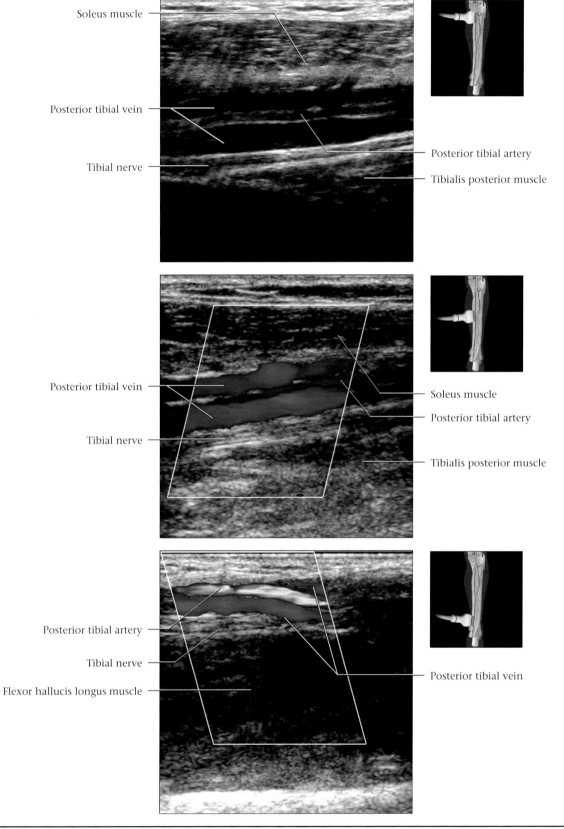

(Top) Oblique coronal scan of the posterior tibial vessels using a medial approach. The posterior tibial artery is accompanied by paired venae comitantes (posterior tibial veins) and the tibial nerve. They run deep to the transverse intermuscular septum of the leg. **(Middle)** Color Doppler scan of the posterior tibial vessels. Notice the marked difference in caliber between the artery and the veins, all of which show normal, complete color filling and normal direction of flow. **(Bottom)** Further inferiorly, oblique coronal scan of the lower-calf shows the distal part of the posterior tibial vessels running superficial to the flexor hallucis muscle and getting ready to curve under the medial malleolus. The posterior tibial vessels and tibial nerve run in the tarsal tunnel together with the flexors of the foot.

LEG VESSELS

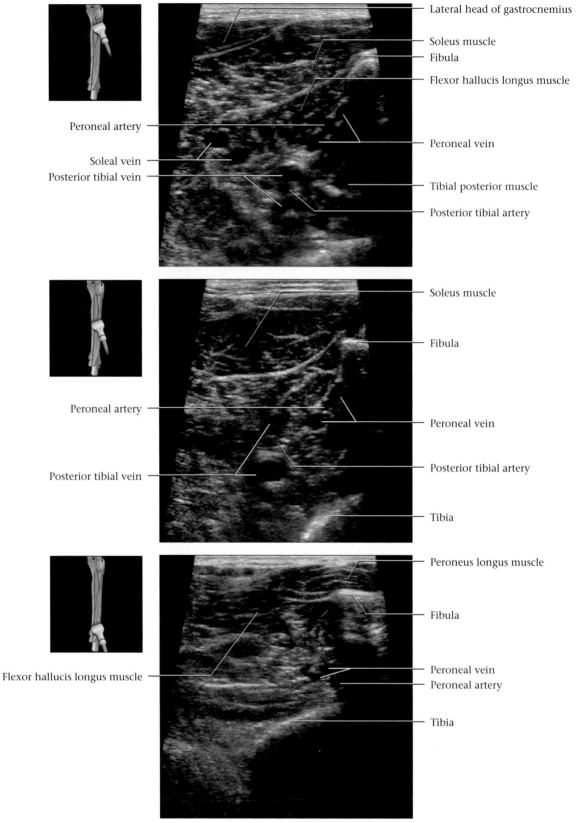

Lateral head of gastrocnemius

Soleus muscle

Fibula

Flexor hallucis longus muscle

Peroneal artery

Peroneal vein

Soleal vein

Posterior tibial vein

Tibial posterior muscle

Posterior tibial artery

Soleus muscle

Fibula

Peroneal artery

Peroneal vein

Posterior tibial artery

Posterior tibial vein

Tibia

Peroneus longus muscle

Fibula

Flexor hallucis longus muscle

Peroneal vein

Peroneal artery

Tibia

(Top) Series of three transverse scans of the calf using a lateral scanning approach. The peroneal vessels are branches of the posterior tibial. They run obliquely towards the fibula and then run along the medial surface of the fibula distally, sandwiched between the flexor hallucis longus muscle and tibialis posterior muscle. **(Middle)** More inferiorly, the relationship between the peroneal vessels and the fibula and flexor muscles remain the same. Nutrient vessels branch out to supply the fibula and the adjacent muscles. **(Bottom)** Most inferiorly, the peroneal artery passes anteriorly to pierce the interosseous membrane to enter into the anterior compartment and runs over the dorsum of the foot.

LONGITUDINAL PERONEAL VESSELS

Lateral head of gastrocnemius m.

Soleus muscle

Peroneal vein

Peroneal artery

Tibialis posterior muscle

Soleus muscle

Flexor hallucis longus muscle

Peroneal vein

Peroneal artery

Tibialis posterior muscle

Soleus muscle

Flexor hallucis longus muscle

Peroneal vein

Peroneal artery

Tibialis posterior muscle

(Top) Oblique coronal scan of the peroneal vessels using a lateral approach. The peroneal artery, like the posterior tibial, is also accompanied by venae comitantes (peroneal veins). The difference is that there is no peroneal nerve to accompany the vessels. The peroneal nerve runs in the lateral leg compartment after curving around the neck of fibula. (Middle) More inferiorly, oblique coronal scan shows the peroneus vessels lie deep to the flexor hallucis longus and soleus muscles, while running superficial to the tibialis posterior muscle. (Bottom) Further inferiorly, the peroneal vessels are much smaller in caliber after giving out many branches. They arch anteriorly toward the interosseous membrane.

LEG VESSELS

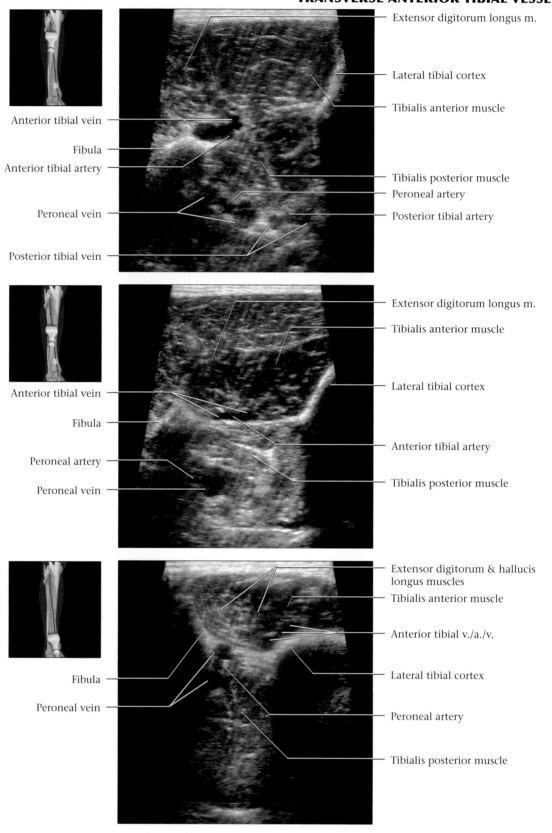

Top image labels:
- Anterior tibial vein
- Fibula
- Anterior tibial artery
- Peroneal vein
- Posterior tibial vein
- Extensor digitorum longus m.
- Lateral tibial cortex
- Tibialis anterior muscle
- Tibialis posterior muscle
- Peroneal artery
- Posterior tibial artery

Middle image labels:
- Anterior tibial vein
- Fibula
- Peroneal artery
- Peroneal vein
- Extensor digitorum longus m.
- Tibialis anterior muscle
- Lateral tibial cortex
- Anterior tibial artery
- Tibialis posterior muscle

Bottom image labels:
- Fibula
- Peroneal vein
- Extensor digitorum & hallucis longus muscles
- Tibialis anterior muscle
- Anterior tibial v./a./v.
- Lateral tibial cortex
- Peroneal artery
- Tibialis posterior muscle

(Top) Series of three transverse scans of the anterior tibial vessels using an anterior scanning approach. The anterior tibial vessels are the smaller terminal branches of the popliteal vessels (smaller compared to the posterior tibial vessels at the bifurcation). After its origin, the anterior tibial vessels run anterior through the interosseous membrane & then passes inferiorly on the anterior surface of this membrane. (Middle) At mid-leg level, the anterior tibial vessels continue to run in a deep position on the surface of the interosseous membrane. Through the window between the tibia & fibula, the peroneal vessels & tibialis posterior muscle are seen. (Bottom) In the most distal part of the leg, the anterior tibial vessels move medially to lie on the surface of the tibia. At this level the peroneal vessels run anteriorly to penetrate the interosseous membrane.

LEG VESSELS

LONGITUDINAL ANTERIOR TIBIAL VESSELS

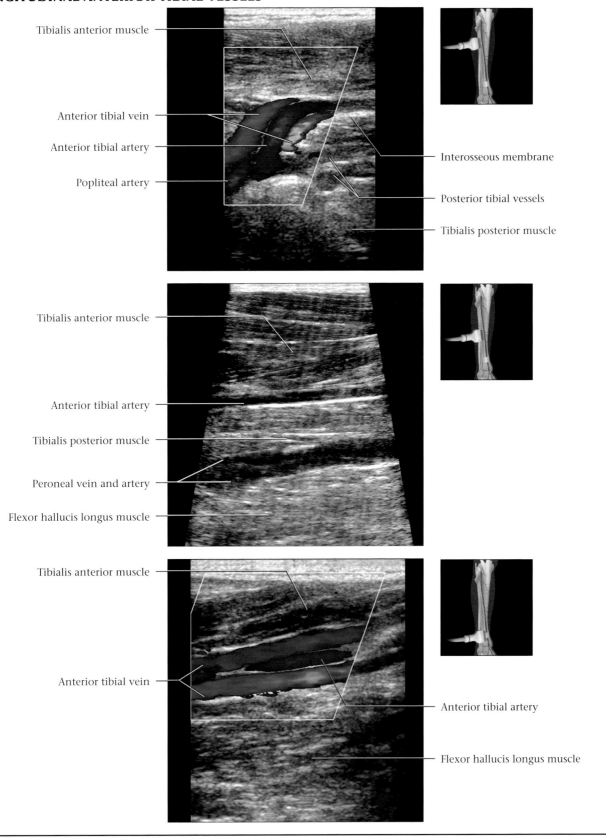

Tibialis anterior muscle

Anterior tibial vein

Anterior tibial artery

Popliteal artery

Interosseous membrane

Posterior tibial vessels

Tibialis posterior muscle

Tibialis anterior muscle

Anterior tibial artery

Tibialis posterior muscle

Peroneal vein and artery

Flexor hallucis longus muscle

Tibialis anterior muscle

Anterior tibial vein

Anterior tibial artery

Flexor hallucis longus muscle

(Top) Oblique sagittal color Doppler scan of the anterior tibial vessels as they bifurcate from the popliteal vessels. The anterior tibial vessels run anteriorly to penetrate the interosseous membrane into the anterior compartment. (Middle) Sagittal scan of the anterior tibial artery in the mid-leg level. The anterior tibial artery runs deep within the anterior compartment and on the surface of the interosseous membrane, being covered by the tibialis anterior muscle. (Bottom) Sagittal color Doppler scan of the lower aspect of the anterior tibial vessels. The vessels begin to run more superficially and in the foot the anterior tibial artery continues as the dorsalis pedis artery.

LEG VESSELS

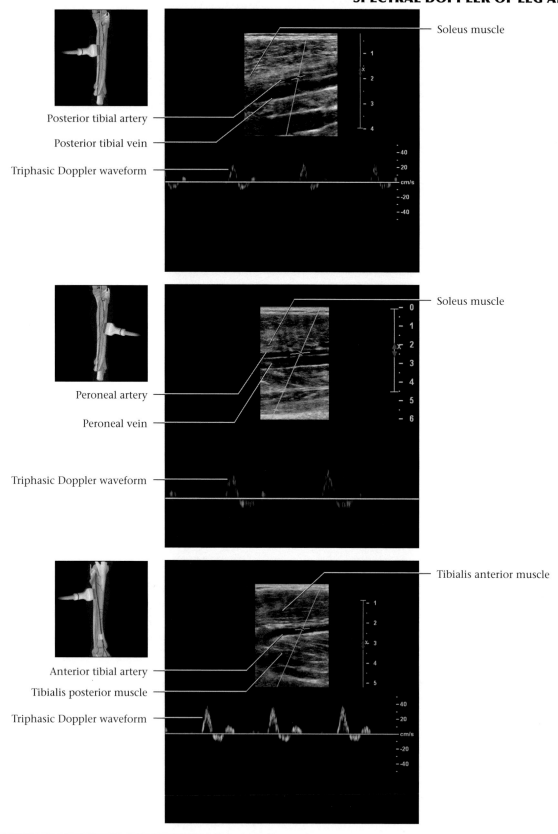

Soleus muscle

Posterior tibial artery

Posterior tibial vein

Triphasic Doppler waveform

Soleus muscle

Peroneal artery

Peroneal vein

Triphasic Doppler waveform

Tibialis anterior muscle

Anterior tibial artery

Tibialis posterior muscle

Triphasic Doppler waveform

(Top) Spectral Doppler scan of the posterior tibial artery demonstrates the typical triphasic pattern seen in normal arteries. Loss of the reverse flow in the diastolic phase is termed a biphasic pattern and is suggestive of stenosis proximal to the point of interrogation. With proximal stenosis, the peak flow velocity is also decreased. **(Middle)** Similarly, the peroneal artery shows a triphasic waveform on spectral Doppler. **(Bottom)** Oblique coronal spectral Doppler scan of the anterior tibial artery in the upper calf level also shows a normal triphasic pattern. Abnormal increase in reverse flow (negative flow in early diastolic phase) suggests increased distal resistance from stenosis.

LEG VESSELS

SPECTRAL DOPPLER OF LEG VEINS

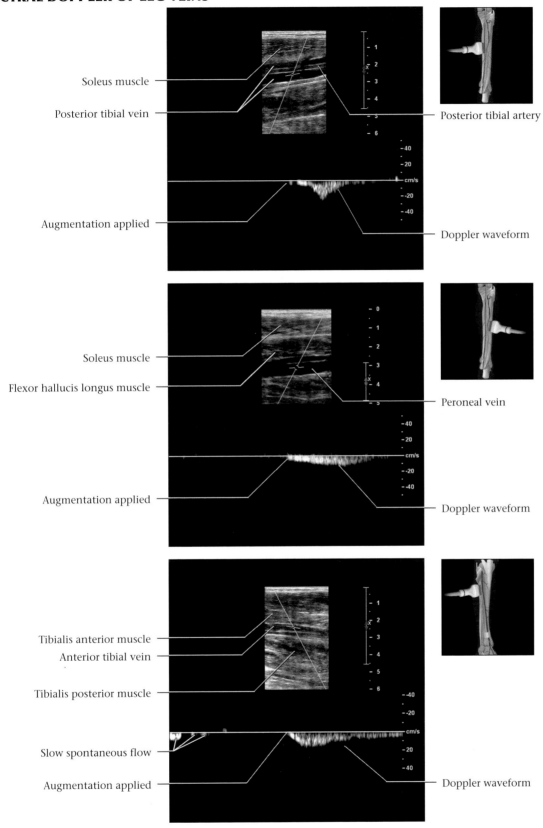

Soleus muscle

Posterior tibial vein

Augmentation applied

Posterior tibial artery

Doppler waveform

Soleus muscle

Flexor hallucis longus muscle

Augmentation applied

Peroneal vein

Doppler waveform

Tibialis anterior muscle

Anterior tibial vein

Tibialis posterior muscle

Slow spontaneous flow

Augmentation applied

Doppler waveform

(Top) Oblique coronal spectral Doppler scan of the posterior tibial vein shows absence of spontaneous flow at rest (left half of the spectral trace). After augmentation (squeezing calf muscles distal to transducer), a surge of blood flow towards the trunk (negative values) can be demonstrated and indicates luminal patency. **(Middle)** Oblique coronal spectral Doppler scan of the peroneal vein before and after augmentation shows a similar sudden surge of blood flow. **(Bottom)** Oblique coronal spectral Doppler scan of the anterior tibial vein demonstrates slow spontaneous flow at rest. After augmentation, a sustained surge of flow is demonstrated.

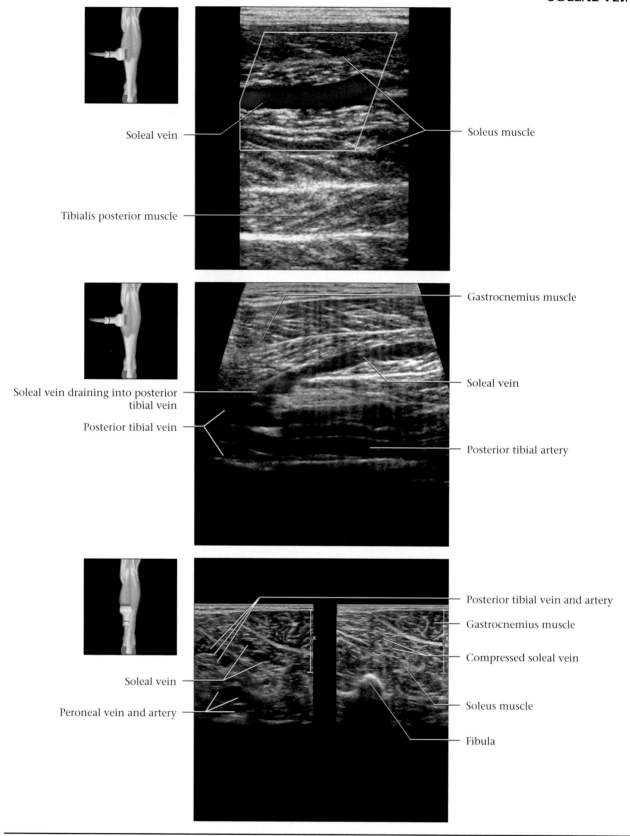

Soleal vein — Soleus muscle

Tibialis posterior muscle

Gastrocnemius muscle

Soleal vein draining into posterior tibial vein

Soleal vein

Posterior tibial vein

Posterior tibial artery

Posterior tibial vein and artery

Gastrocnemius muscle

Compressed soleal vein

Soleal vein

Soleus muscle

Peroneal vein and artery

Fibula

(Top) Oblique sagittal color Doppler scan of the posterior compartment in the mid-calf level. The soleal vein shows complete color filling of its lumen indicating the absence of thrombus. Soleal veins are the most common veins to develop thrombosis and should be assessed when scanning for deep venous thrombosis. (Middle) Oblique sagittal scan of the posterior compartment showing the soleal vein running proximally and joining the posterior tibial vein. This pathway allows a soleal vein thrombus to extend into the posterior tibial vein and propagate proximally. (Bottom) Dual transverse images of the posterior compartment using a medial approach, before (left side image) and during firm transducer compression (right-sided image). The soleal veins are completely compressed by transducer pressure indicating an absence of thrombus.

LEG VESSELS

GASTROCNEMIUS VEINS

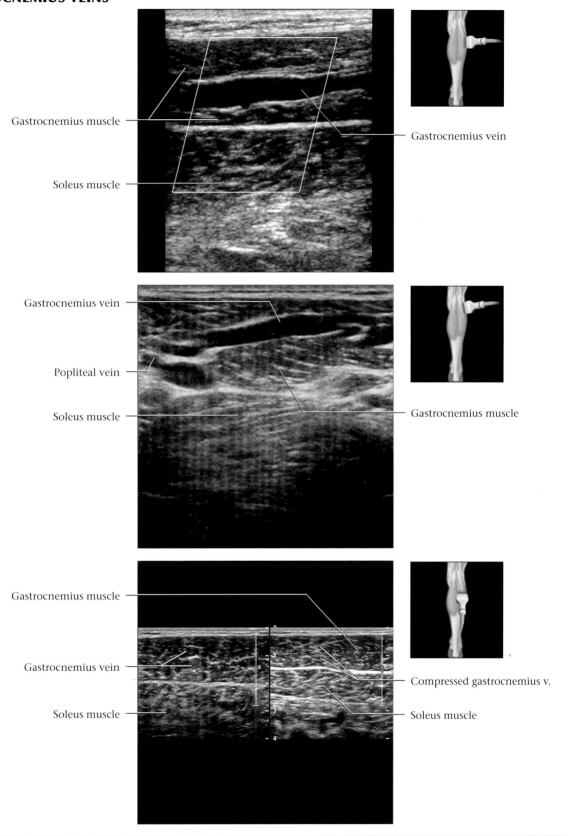

Gastrocnemius muscle

Soleus muscle

Gastrocnemius vein

Gastrocnemius vein

Popliteal vein

Soleus muscle

Gastrocnemius muscle

Gastrocnemius muscle

Gastrocnemius vein

Soleus muscle

Compressed gastrocnemius v.

Soleus muscle

(Top) Oblique sagittal color Doppler scan of the posterior leg compartment. The gastrocnemius vein shows complete color filling indicating absence of thrombus. The gastrocnemius veins are the second most common site for venous thrombosis. (Middle) Oblique sagittal scan of the posterior compartment of the upper-calf shows the gastrocnemius vein joining the popliteal vein, allowing a gastrocnemius vein thrombus to extend proximally to the popliteal vein. (Bottom) Dual transverse images of gastrocnemius veins before (left-side image) and during compression (right-side image). The gastrocnemius veins are completely compressed during compression indicating an absence of thrombus. Compression is regarded as the most reliable technique to rule out venous thrombosis.

LEG VESSELS

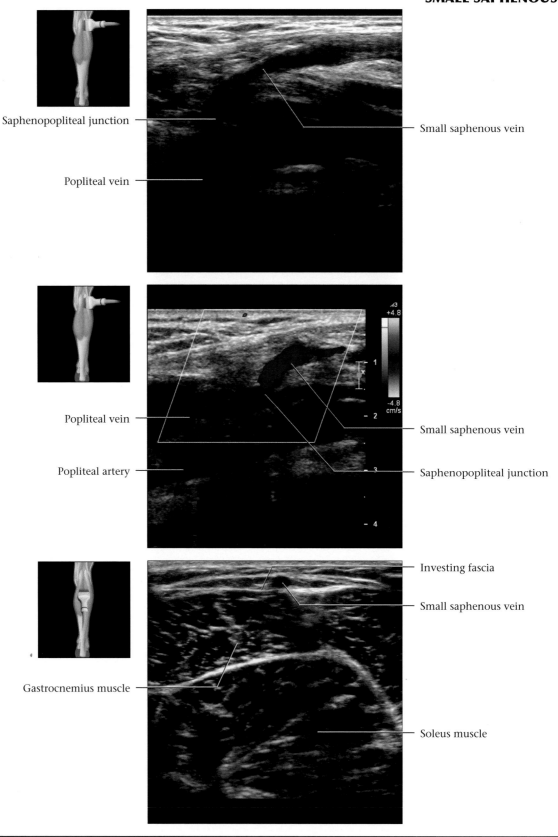

Saphenopopliteal junction — Small saphenous vein

Popliteal vein

Popliteal vein — Small saphenous vein

Popliteal artery — Saphenopopliteal junction

Investing fascia

Small saphenous vein

Gastrocnemius muscle

Soleus muscle

(Top) Sagittal scan of central popliteal fossa. The small saphenous vein running from the lateral surface of the calf turns medially, penetrates the popliteal fascia to drain into popliteal vein. Varicose veins arise as a result of reflux and stasis due to incompetent valves. Varicose veins on the lateral side of the calf suggest an incompetent small saphenous system. **(Middle)** Sagittal color Doppler scan of the central popliteal fossa with augmentation. Flow towards the popliteal vein (red) is demonstrated at the saphenopopliteal junction. Reverse flow into the small saphenous vein, would suggest valvular incompetence. **(Bottom)** Transverse scan of the posterior surface of the upper-calf. The small saphenous vein is sandwiched between two layers of investing fascia. Minimal probe pressure is required to avoid inadvertent compression of the small saphenous vein.

LEG VESSELS

GREAT SAPHENOUS VEINS

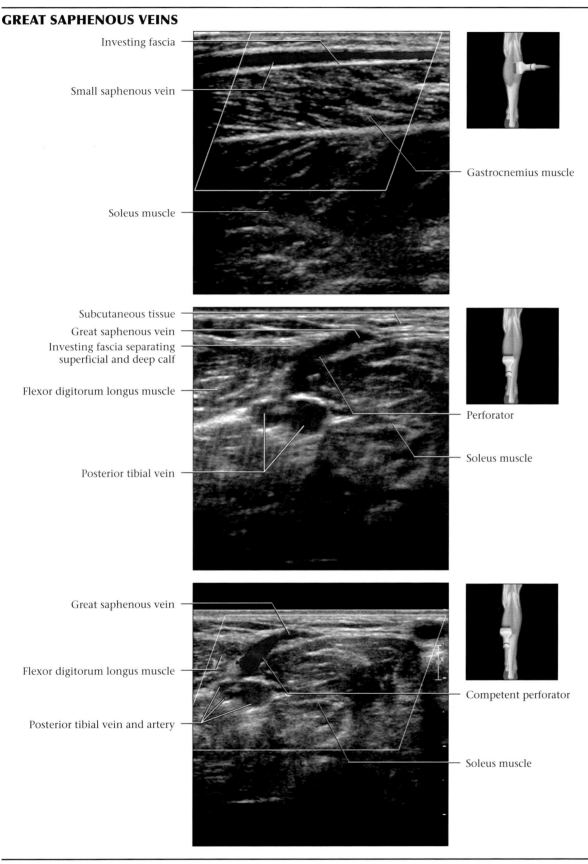

(Top) Sagittal color Doppler scan of upper mid-calf with augmentation. The complete filling of venous lumen of the small saphenous vein is demonstrated, indicating the absence of a superficial vein thrombus. If flow towards trunk is demonstrated, valvular incompetence can be excluded. **(Middle)** Transverse scan of the medial aspect of the lower third of the calf. A perforator arising from the great saphenous vein is seen penetrating through the investing fascia to join the posterior tibial vein. **(Bottom)** Transverse color Doppler scan of the medial aspect of the lower third of the calf. With augmentation, color filling of the perforator lumen is demonstrated in the perforator between the great saphenous vein and the posterior tibial vein, indicating patency of vessel. If flow towards the posterior tibial vein can be documented on Doppler study, incompetence can be excluded.

LEG NERVES

Terminology

Abbreviations
- Artery = a.
- Ligament = l.
- Muscle = m.
- Nerve = n.
- Vein = v.

Gross Anatomy

Nerves of Leg
- Sciatic nerve is actually two nerves (common peroneal and tibial) bound together
- **Common peroneal**
  - Smaller of 2 terminal divisions of sciatic nerve
  - Arises from dorsal divisions of sacral plexus (L4, L5, S1, S2)
  - Separates from tibial nerve mid thigh, at the superior angle of the popliteal fossa, runs downwards laterally along medial border of biceps femoris muscle and tendon
  - Leaves popliteal fossa by crossing plantaris and lateral head of gastrocnemius, passes posterior and superficial to head of fibula
  - Curves anteriorly over the posterior aspect of the head of fibula
  - Winds around the lateral surface of the fibular neck
  - This location at fibular head/neck puts peroneal nerve at risk in multiple clinical situations
    - Fibular neck fracture may result in foot drop
    - Total knee replacement in a patient (who had been in chronic valgus) may damage this nerve as a result of the knee realignment (correction of valgus deformity)
  - Ends between lateral side of neck of fibula and peroneus longus by dividing into 2 terminal branches
  - **Deep peroneal nerve**: One of 2 terminal branches
    - Arises on lateral side of neck of fibula, under peroneus longus
    - Pierces anterior intermuscular septum & extensor digitorum longus to enter anterior compartment
    - Extends down to ankle between tibialis anterior and long extensors
    - Near ankle, crossed by extensor hallucis and passes to ankle midway between malleoli
    - Muscular branches to anterior compartment and articular branch to ankle joint
    - Medial terminal branch to dorsum of foot
    - Lateral terminal branch to lateral dorsum of ankle
  - **Superficial peroneal nerve**: 2nd of 2 terminal branches of the common peroneal nerve
    - Descends in substance of peroneus longus until it reaches peroneus brevis
    - Passes obliquely over anterior border of brevis and descends in groove between peroneus brevis and extensor digitorum longus
    - In distal 1/3 of leg, pierces deep fascia and divides into medial and lateral branches to foot
- **Tibial nerve**
  - Arises from ventral surface of sacral plexus
  - Runs roughly along the central axis of the popliteal fossa
  - Descends under fascial septum which separates deep and superficial posterior muscle compartments
  - In upper 2/3, lies on fascia of tibialis posterior and on flexor digitorum longus
  - In lower 1/3, located midway between Achilles tendon and medial border of tibia
  - Crosses posterior surfaces of tibia and ankle joint
  - Posterior tibial vessels run with it, crossing in front of it from lateral to medial side
  - At ankle, under flexor retinaculum, divides into lateral and medial plantar nerves
- **Saphenous nerve**
  - Longest branch of femoral nerve, arising 2 cm below inguinal ligament and descending via adductor canal
  - Passes posterior to sartorius, descends posteromedial to knee where it pierces the deep fascia
  - In leg, accompanies great saphenous vein
- **Sural nerve**
  - Arises in popliteal fossa from tibial nerve
  - Descends between 2 heads of gastrocnemius
  - Pierces deep fascia midway between knee and ankle
  - Accompanies small saphenous vein to lateral border of foot

Anatomy-Based Imaging Issues

Imaging Approaches
- Ultrasound
  - Use high frequency transducers to assess nerves
  - Neural signature on ultrasound
    - Short axis: Uniformly dispersed hypoechoic dots (nerve fascicles) separated by hyperechoic epineurium
    - Long axis: Parallel hypoechoic tracts of uniform caliber
    - Overall gain control and focus settings may have to be optimized for ultrasound to demonstrate the nerve well
    - Anisotropy artifact may affect scanning, especially in the short axis; tilting the transducer during scanning helps achieve the best view
    - Distortion of this uniform appearance suggests pathology
  - Trace medium size nerves by following their course as they branch from their parent
  - Small (1-2 mm) nerves are difficult to identify and their location may only be inferred by the adjacent vessels
- MR
  - Also suffers from inability to detect small nerves
  - Use of superficial small field of view coils may improve resolution

LEG NERVES

ANTERIOR AND POSTERIOR LEG NERVES

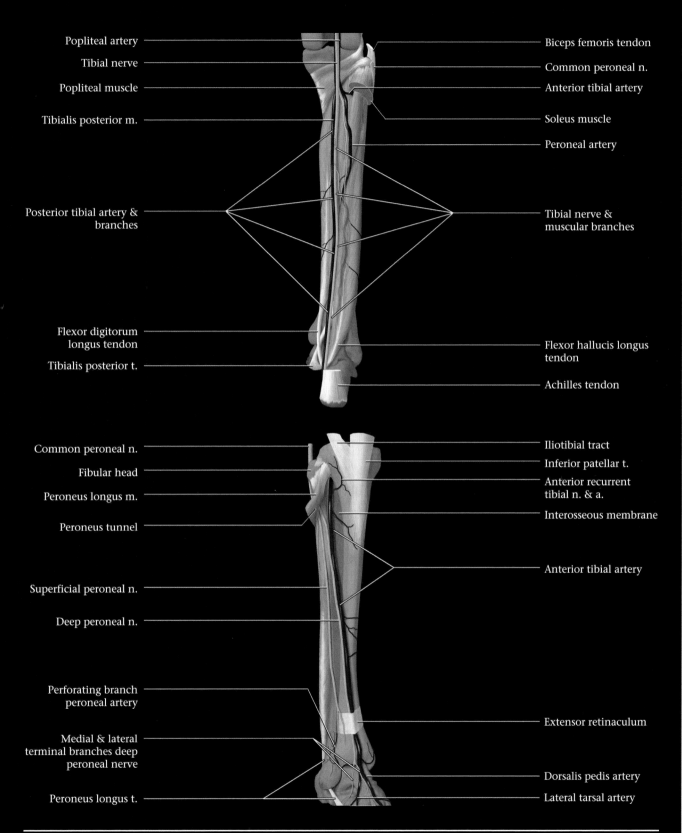

Popliteal artery

Tibial nerve

Popliteal muscle

Tibialis posterior m.

Posterior tibial artery & branches

Flexor digitorum longus tendon

Tibialis posterior t.

Biceps femoris tendon

Common peroneal n.

Anterior tibial artery

Soleus muscle

Peroneal artery

Tibial nerve & muscular branches

Flexor hallucis longus tendon

Achilles tendon

Common peroneal n.

Fibular head

Peroneus longus m.

Peroneus tunnel

Superficial peroneal n.

Deep peroneal n.

Perforating branch peroneal artery

Medial & lateral terminal branches deep peroneal nerve

Peroneus longus t.

Iliotibial tract

Inferior patellar t.

Anterior recurrent tibial n. & a.

Interosseous membrane

Anterior tibial artery

Extensor retinaculum

Dorsalis pedis artery

Lateral tarsal artery

(Top) Graphic of posterior leg nerves & arteries. The sciatic nerve divides into common peroneal & tibial branches. The common peroneal nerve then follows the biceps femoris around the lateral fibular neck. The tibial nerve descends between the deep and superficial posterior leg muscles, paralleling the posterior tibial artery. (Bottom) Graphic of the anterior leg shows the common peroneal nerve extending through the peroneal tunnel (between the peroneus longus tendon and the fibular neck), branching into deep and superficial components. Both have muscular branches along their length; deep peroneal nerve parallels the anterior tibial artery and terminates in the medial & lateral branches to the dorsum of the foot and ankle, respectively.

TIBIAL NERVE

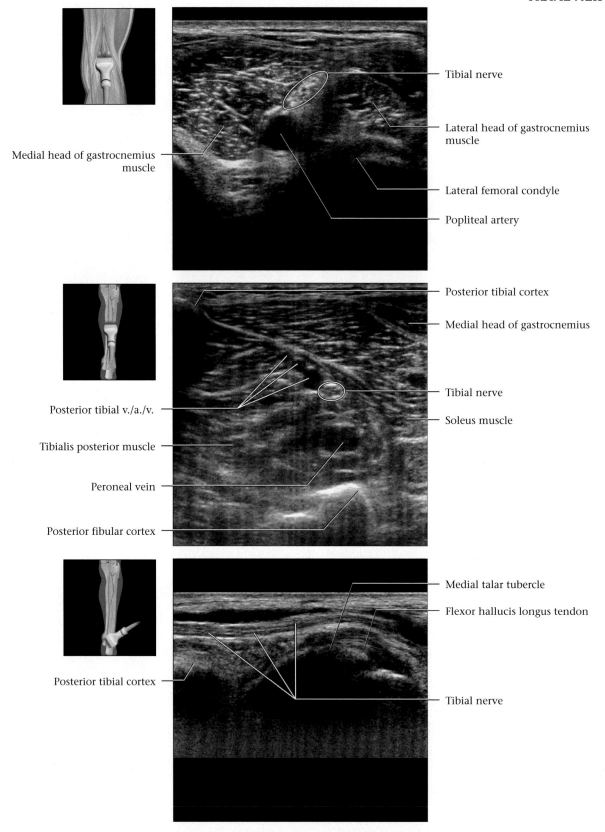

Tibial nerve

Lateral head of gastrocnemius muscle

Medial head of gastrocnemius muscle

Lateral femoral condyle

Popliteal artery

Posterior tibial cortex

Medial head of gastrocnemius

Posterior tibial v./a./v.

Tibial nerve

Tibialis posterior muscle

Soleus muscle

Peroneal vein

Posterior fibular cortex

Medial talar tubercle

Flexor hallucis longus tendon

Posterior tibial cortex

Tibial nerve

(Top) Transverse scan of the lower aspect of the popliteal fossa. The tibial nerve demonstrates the typical neural signature of small black dots within a bright matrix. It lies superficial to the popliteal artery. (Middle) Further inferiorly, at the level of the mid-calf, the tibial nerve is deep to the soleus muscle and lies lateral to the posterior tibial vessels. Notice that even at this depth, the neural signature is still visible. (Bottom) Sagittal scan of the posterior aspect of the medial ankle. The longitudinal neural signature of the tibial nerve is well-shown here with parallel hypoechoic tracts which are roughly uniform in size. Contrast this to the more densely packed appearance of tendons.

LEG NERVES

PERONEAL NERVE

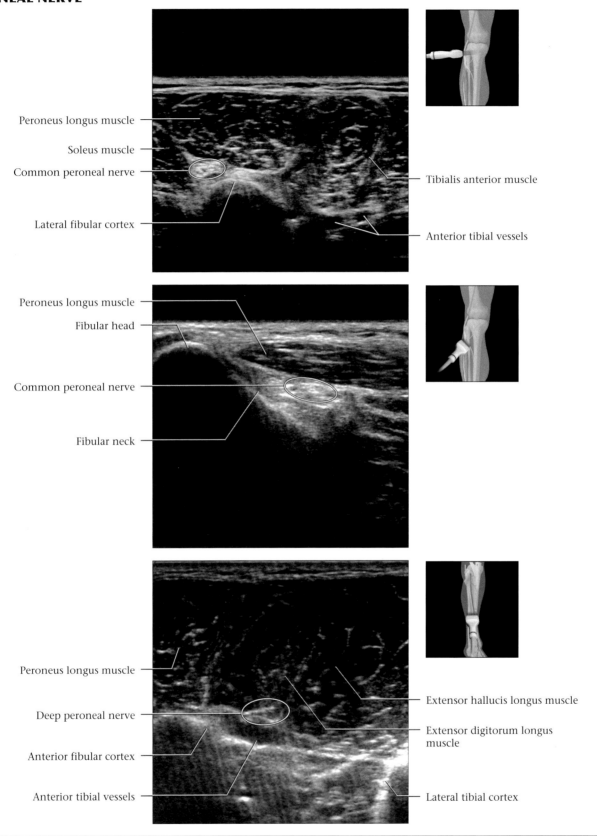

Peroneus longus muscle

Soleus muscle

Common peroneal nerve

Lateral fibular cortex

Tibialis anterior muscle

Anterior tibial vessels

Peroneus longus muscle

Fibular head

Common peroneal nerve

Fibular neck

Peroneus longus muscle

Deep peroneal nerve

Anterior fibular cortex

Anterior tibial vessels

Extensor hallucis longus muscle

Extensor digitorum longus muscle

Lateral tibial cortex

(Top) Transverse scan of the head of fibula showing the common peroneal nerve running along the posteromedial aspect of the peroneus longus muscle. Superior to this, the nerve is covered by the biceps femoris. **(Middle)** Coronal scan of the fibular neck shows the common peroneal nerve passing deep to the peroneus longus muscle. The nerve will then enter the anterior compartment. **(Bottom)** Transverse scan of the anterior compartment at the mid-leg level. The deep peroneal nerve runs anterior to the anterior tibial vessels deep in this compartment.

ANKLE

Terminology

Abbreviations
- Artery (a.); ligament (l.); muscle (m.); tendon (t.); vein (v.)

Gross Anatomy

Osseous Anatomy
- **Ankle (talocrural) joint**
  - Tibia, fibula & talus form synovial joint
  - Supported by lateral & medial collateral ligaments
  - Mainly uniaxial hinge joint, dorsiflexion, plantar flexion, also dynamic shift of axis of rotation during dorsi & plantar flexion
- **Distal tibiofibular joint**
  - Fibrous joint
  - Supported by syndesmotic ligaments
  - Synovial recess from ankle joint extends into joint
  - May have articular cartilage far distally
  - Minimal stretch ("give") during dorsiflexion: Allows increase in malleolar gap & slight fibular lateral rotation

Ligaments
- 3 sets bind ankle: Distal tibiofibular syndesmotic complex, lateral collateral & deltoid ligaments
- **4 tibiofibular syndesmotic ligaments**
  - **Anterior & posterior tibiofibular ligaments**
    - Extend obliquely between anterior & posterior tibial & fibular tubercles respectively
    - Distal anterior tibiofibular ligament: Bassett ligament
  - **Inferior transverse ligament**: Distal part of posterior tibiofibular ligament
  - **Interosseous ligament**: Distal thickening of syndesmotic membrane
- **3 lateral collateral ligaments**
  - **Anterior talofibular ligament**
    - Originates 1 cm proximal to lateral malleolar tip, inserts on talar neck
    - Stabilizes talus against anterior displacement, internal rotation & inversion
    - Weakest, first to tear
  - **Calcaneofibular ligament**
    - Originates from lateral malleolar tip, inserts on calcaneal trochlear eminence
    - Deep to peroneal tendons
    - Lateral restraint of subtalar joint, often tears with anterior talofibular ligament
  - **Posterior talofibular ligament**
    - Extends from lateral malleolar fossa to lateral talar tubercle
    - Strongest, rarely tears
- **Deltoid ligament (medial collateral ligament)**
  - Fan-shaped, originates from anterior, apex & posterior medial malleolus, inserts on talus, sustentaculum tali, spring ligament & navicular
  - Deep: Posterior & anterior tibiotalar bands
  - Superficial: Tibiocalcaneal, tibiospring, tibionavicular & posterior tibiotalar (variable) bands

- **Spring ligament (plantar calcaneonavicular ligament)**
  - Binds calcaneus to navicular, 3 components
  - Superomedial - **origin**: Sustentaculum tali, **insertion**: Superomedial navicular, tibiospring band of deltoid
  - Medioplantar oblique - **origin**: Calcaneal coronoid fossa, **insertion**: Plantar navicular
  - Inferoplantar longitudinal - **origin**: Coronoid fossa, **insertion**: Navicular beak

Retinacula
- Focal thickening of deep fascia
- Prevents bowstringing, binds tendons down
- **Superior extensor retinaculum**
  - A few cm above ankle joint
  - Attaches to anterior fibula laterally, tibia medially
  - Proximally continues with fascia cruris
  - Distally attaches to inferior extensor retinaculum
  - Binds down anterior compartment muscles
- **Inferior extensor retinaculum**
  - At ankle joint, Y-shaped, stem laterally, proximal & distal bands medially
  - Stem attaches laterally to upper calcaneus
    - Loops around extensor tendons
    - Roots extend into sinus tarsi
  - Proximal medial band has deep & superficial layers, loop around extensor hallus longus tendon & occasionally tibialis anterior tendon
  - Distal medial band superficial to extensor hallucis longus & tibialis anterior tendons
    - Attaches to plantar aponeurosis
  - Dorsalis pedis vessels, deep peroneal nerve: Deep to all layers of inferior extensor retinaculum
- **Flexor retinaculum**
  - Attaches to medial malleolus
  - Proximally continuous with deep fascia of leg
  - Distally continuous with plantar aponeurosis
  - Abductor hallucis partly attached to it
  - Binds deep flexor tendons to tibial & calcaneal grooves
  - Lateral border of tarsal tunnel
- **Superior peroneal retinaculum**
  - Origin: Lateral malleolus, insertions vary, most commonly to deep fascia of leg & calcaneus
  - Binds peroneal tendons into retrofibular groove
- **Inferior peroneal retinaculum**
  - Continuous with inferior extensor retinaculum
  - Inserts on lateral calcaneus, peroneal tubercle (trochlea)
  - Binds peroneus brevis, peroneus longus tendons to calcaneus

Tendons
- Muscles discussed in greater detail in leg module
- **Anterior (extensor) compartment**
  - **Tibialis anterior tendon**
    - Most medial & largest tendon in anterior compartment
    - Inserts on medial cuneiform, base of 1st metatarsal
    - Dorsiflexes ankle, inverts foot, tightens plantar aponeurosis
    - Supports medial longitudinal arch during walking

ANKLE

- **Extensor hallucis longus tendon**
  - Inserts on dorsal base of 1st distal phalanx
  - Extends 1st phalanges, dorsiflexes foot
- **Extensor digitorum longus tendon**
  - Divides into four slips on dorsum of foot
  - Slips receive tendinous contributions from extensor digitorum brevis, lumbricals & interosseous muscles
  - Each slip divides into 3: Central one inserts on dorsal base of middle phalanx & 2 collateral ones which reunite & insert on bases of 2nd-5th distal phalanges
  - Dorsiflexes ankle, extends toes, tightens plantar aponeurosis
- **Peroneus tertius tendon**
  - Typically part of extensor digitorum longus tendon
  - Inserts on dorsal base of 5th metatarsal
- **Lateral compartment**
  - **Peroneus longus tendon**
    - Posterolateral to peroneus brevis tendon in retrofibular groove, deep to superior peroneal retinaculum
    - Proximally has common tendon sheath with peroneus brevis
    - Second tendon sheath at sole of foot
    - Descends behind peroneal tubercle, deep to inferior peroneal retinaculum
    - Curves under cuboid deep to long plantar ligament
    - Inserts on plantar base of 1st metatarsal, medial cuneiform
    - Plantarflexes ankle, everts foot, supports longitudinal & transverse arches during walking
    - Os peroneum always present, ossified in about 20% of individuals
  - **Peroneus brevis tendon**
    - Anteromedial to peroneus longus tendon in retrofibular groove, deep to superior peroneal retinaculum
    - Descends anterior to peroneal tubercle of calcaneus, deep to inferior peroneal retinaculum
    - Inserts into base of 5th metatarsal
    - Everts foot, limits foot inversion
- **Superficial posterior compartment**
  - **Achilles tendon**
    - Largest & strongest tendon in body
    - Conjoined tendon of medial & lateral gastrocnemius & soleus muscles
    - Approximately 15 cm long
    - Lacks tendon sheath, enclosed by paratenon
    - Inserts on posterior calcaneal tuberosity
    - Retrocalcaneal bursa between distal tendon & calcaneal tuberosity
    - Main plantarflexor of ankle, foot
- **Plantaris tendon**
  - Vestigial, slender tendon, medial to Achilles tendon
  - Inserts on or medial to Achilles tendon
- **Deep posterior (flexor) compartment**
  - **Tibialis posterior tendon**
    - Crosses flexor digitorum longus tendon above ankle joint to become most posteromedial tendon
    - Shares tibial groove with flexor digitorum longus tendon
    - Inserts on navicular tuberosity, cuneiforms, sustentaculum tali, bases of 2nd-4th metatarsals
    - Main invertor of foot, aids in plantar flexion
    - Supports medial longitudinal arch
  - **Flexor digitorum longus tendon**
    - Lateral to tibialis posterior tendon in tibial groove
    - Crosses flexor hallucis longus tendon at knot of Henry (where there is also an exchange of tendon fibers at this crossing of two tendons)
    - Divides into 4 slips which give origin to lumbricals
    - Slips pass through openings in corresponding tendons of flexor digitorum brevis
    - Slips insert on bases of 2nd-5th distal phalanges
    - Flexes distal phalanges, assists in plantar flexion of ankle
    - When foot on ground: Maintains pads of toes on ground
    - When foot off ground: Plantar flexes 2nd-5th phalanges, aids in maintaining longitudinal arches
  - **Flexor hallucis longus tendon**
    - Passes 3 fibro-osseous tunnels: 1) between medial & lateral talar tubercles, 2) under sustentaculum tali, 3) between 1st medial & lateral sesamoids
    - Crosses & sends slip to flexor digitorum longus at knot of Henry
    - Inserts on base of 1st distal phalanx
    - When foot on ground: Maintains pad of 1st toe on ground
    - When foot off ground: Plantar flexes 1st phalanges, aids in maintaining medial longitudinal arch
    - Weak plantar flexor of ankle
    - Innervated by tibial nerve

Anatomy-Based Imaging Issues

Imaging Recommendations
- **Ultrasound**
  - Use ultrasound to assess tendon and ligamentous abnormalities aside from masses around the ankle joint
  - Ligaments and tendons need to be assessed in both long and short axis
  - Since most structures run obliquely and tendons make acute turns around the joint, a clear understanding of their relationships and associated bony landmarks is helpful
- **Computed tomography**
  - Best for bony anatomy
  - Superior to MR for detecting small avulsion fragments
- **MR of ankle & hindfoot**
  - Axials optimal for ankle tendons, ligaments
  - Coronals useful for bones, cartilage, ankle and sinus tarsi ligaments
  - Sagittals optimal for Achilles tendon, bones, cartilage, sinus tarsi ligaments

ANKLE

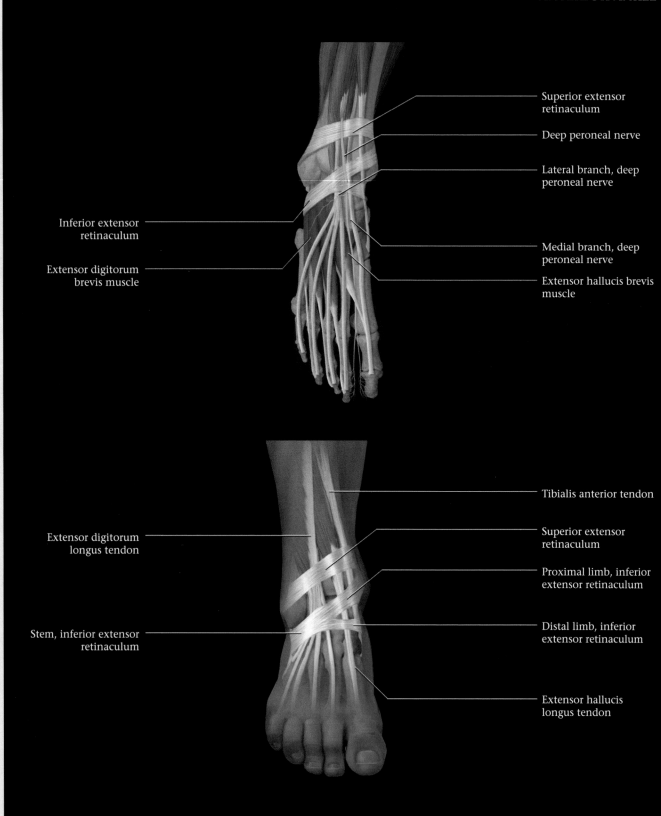

Superior extensor retinaculum

Deep peroneal nerve

Lateral branch, deep peroneal nerve

Inferior extensor retinaculum

Extensor digitorum brevis muscle

Medial branch, deep peroneal nerve

Extensor hallucis brevis muscle

Extensor digitorum longus tendon

Stem, inferior extensor retinaculum

Tibialis anterior tendon

Superior extensor retinaculum

Proximal limb, inferior extensor retinaculum

Distal limb, inferior extensor retinaculum

Extensor hallucis longus tendon

(Top) The deep peroneal nerve travels deep to extensor retinacula, in anterior tarsal tunnel, & gives a lateral motor branch to extensor digitorum brevis muscle. The medial branch continues dorsal to talonavicular joint, middle cuneiform & in between 1st & 2nd metatarsal to provide mostly sensory but some motor supply to 1st web space. **(Bottom)** Anterior view. The peroneus tertius and tibialis anterior tendon insert proximally, on the base of the 5th metatarsal and on the medial cuneiform and 1st metatarsal respectively. The rest of the extensor tendons continue distally toward their insertion sites on the digits. The extensor tendons are held in place by the superior and inferior extensor retinacula.

ANKLE

ANTERIOR ANKLE

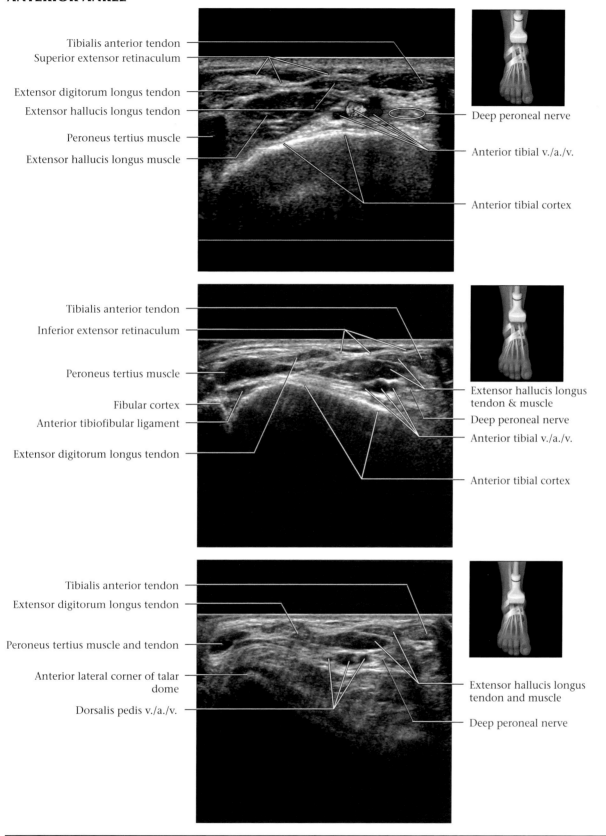

Top image labels (left):
- Tibialis anterior tendon
- Superior extensor retinaculum
- Extensor digitorum longus tendon
- Extensor hallucis longus tendon
- Peroneus tertius muscle
- Extensor hallucis longus muscle

Top image labels (right):
- Deep peroneal nerve
- Anterior tibial v./a./v.
- Anterior tibial cortex

Middle image labels (left):
- Tibialis anterior tendon
- Inferior extensor retinaculum
- Peroneus tertius muscle
- Fibular cortex
- Anterior tibiofibular ligament
- Extensor digitorum longus tendon

Middle image labels (right):
- Extensor hallucis longus tendon & muscle
- Deep peroneal nerve
- Anterior tibial v./a./v.
- Anterior tibial cortex

Bottom image labels (left):
- Tibialis anterior tendon
- Extensor digitorum longus tendon
- Peroneus tertius muscle and tendon
- Anterior lateral corner of talar dome
- Dorsalis pedis v./a./v.

Bottom image labels (right):
- Extensor hallucis longus tendon and muscle
- Deep peroneal nerve

(Top) Anterior transverse color Doppler scan above level of the ankle joint. The basic relationship of the main structures of the anterior ankle hold true here and down through the ankle joint. From medial to lateral the structures are: Tibialis anterior, extensor Hallucis longus; nerve AND vessels; extensor Digitorum longus (mnemonic: Tom Harry AND Dick). **(Middle)** Transverse scan of the ankle joint at the level of the anterior talofibular ligament. The anterior talofibular ligament, like most ankle ligaments runs an oblique course and thus may appear irregular or interrupted on a straight axial scan. This can be corrected by scanning obliquely along the long axis of the ligament. **(Bottom)** Transverse scan more inferiorly shows the asymmetrical soft tissue thickness anterior to the talus (thicker medially) due to different orientation axes of talus and foot.

ANKLE

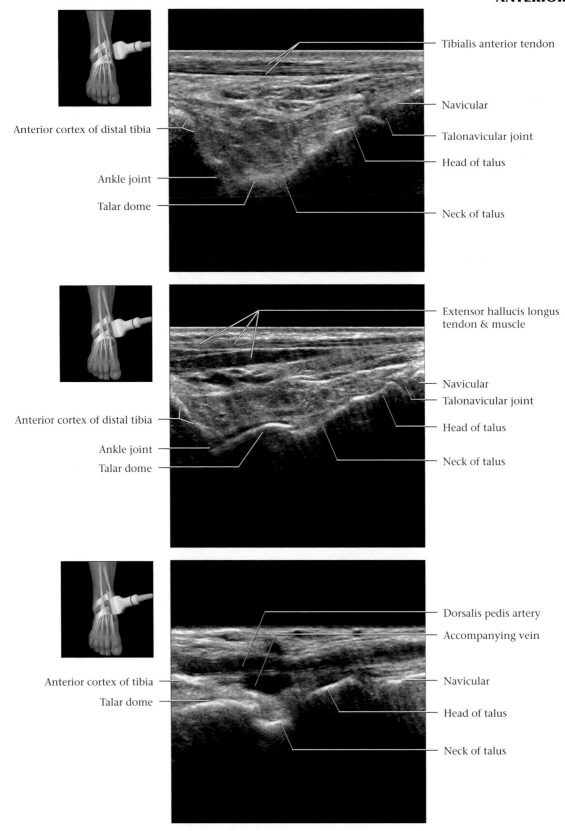

Tibialis anterior tendon

Navicular

Talonavicular joint

Head of talus

Neck of talus

Anterior cortex of distal tibia

Ankle joint

Talar dome

Extensor hallucis longus tendon & muscle

Navicular

Talonavicular joint

Head of talus

Neck of talus

Anterior cortex of distal tibia

Ankle joint

Talar dome

Dorsalis pedis artery

Accompanying vein

Navicular

Head of talus

Neck of talus

Anterior cortex of tibia

Talar dome

(Top) Longitudinal scan of the lateral aspect of the ankle showing the course of the tibialis anterior tendon. A thin hypoechoic synovial layer can be seen enveloping the tendon. (Middle) Slightly more laterally, sagittal scan shows the extensor hallucis longus tendon and muscle, the latter distinguishing it from the tibialis anterior tendon. (Bottom) Further laterally, the dorsalis pedis artery and the accompanying vein(s) come into view. At this point, the subcutaneous tissue is thinnest, a result of the transverse arch of the midfoot with apex roughly coinciding with the site of this artery. This creates a shallow bony backing for palpating the artery.

ANKLE

MEDIAL ANKLE

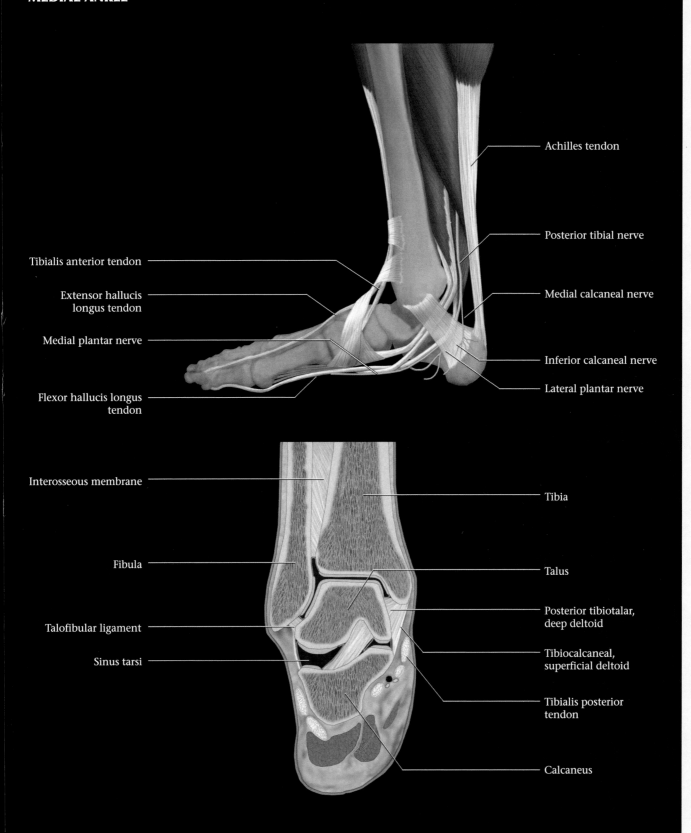

- Achilles tendon
- Posterior tibial nerve
- Medial calcaneal nerve
- Inferior calcaneal nerve
- Lateral plantar nerve

- Tibialis anterior tendon
- Extensor hallucis longus tendon
- Medial plantar nerve
- Flexor hallucis longus tendon

- Interosseous membrane
- Fibula
- Talofibular ligament
- Sinus tarsi

- Tibia
- Talus
- Posterior tibiotalar, deep deltoid
- Tibiocalcaneal, superficial deltoid
- Tibialis posterior tendon
- Calcaneus

(Top) Tarsal tunnel. The tunnel accommodates the posterior tibial neurovascular bundle. The medial calcaneal nerve supplies skin of medial heel. The medial plantar nerve supplies flexor hallucis brevis, abductor hallucis, flexor digitorum brevis and 1st lumbrical. It carries sensation from medial 2/3 of plantar foot. The lateral plantar nerve supplies all other plantar muscles including 2nd-4th lumbricals and all interossei, plus sensation from lateral 1/3 of mid & forefoot. **(Bottom)** Drawing of the ankle ligaments. On the medial side, the medial malleolus is connected via the deep and superficial deltoid ligaments to the medial tarsal bones. The tibialis posterior tendon passes over the deltoid ligament as it curves below the medial malleolus.

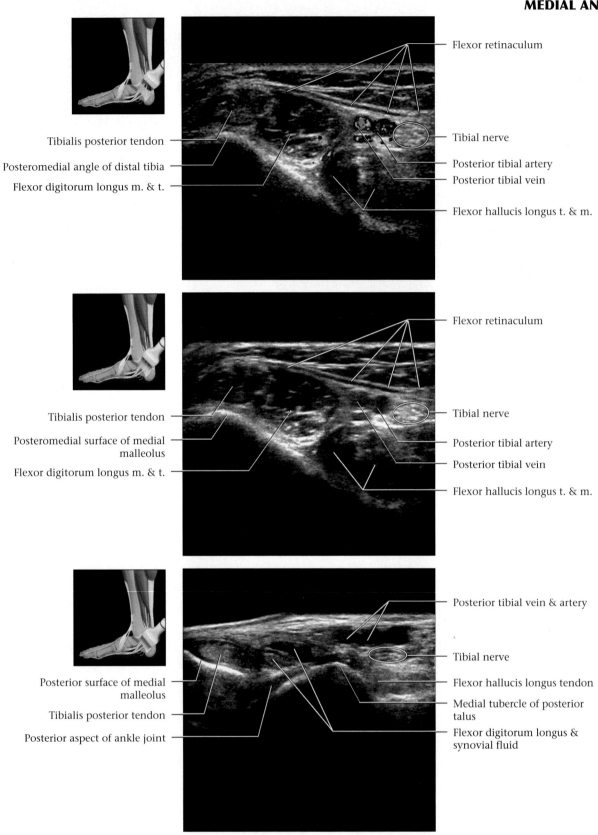

Flexor retinaculum

Tibial nerve

Posterior tibial artery
Posterior tibial vein

Flexor hallucis longus t. & m.

Tibialis posterior tendon

Posteromedial angle of distal tibia

Flexor digitorum longus m. & t.

Flexor retinaculum

Tibial nerve

Posterior tibial artery

Posterior tibial vein

Flexor hallucis longus t. & m.

Tibialis posterior tendon

Posteromedial surface of medial malleolus

Flexor digitorum longus m. & t.

Posterior tibial vein & artery

Tibial nerve

Flexor hallucis longus tendon

Medial tubercle of posterior talus

Flexor digitorum longus & synovial fluid

Posterior surface of medial malleolus

Tibialis posterior tendon

Posterior aspect of ankle joint

(Top) Transverse color Doppler scan of the posterior aspect of the distal tibia just above the medial malleolus. This area is held down by the flexor retinaculum and termed the tarsal tunnel. Within this tunnel are: Tibialis posterior, flexor Digitorum longus, vessels AND nerve, flexor Hallucis longus (mnemonic: Tom Dick AND Harry). **(Middle)** Corresponding grayscale transverse scan just above the medial malleolus. Image is less grainy without simultaneous color Doppler interrogation, and the nerve fibers (hypoechoic dots) give the typical neural signature. **(Bottom)** At the level of the talus, the tibial nerve moves anteriorly to run deep to the posterior tibial vessels and superficial to the flexor hallucis longus tendon. The flexor hallucis tendon runs in a groove on the posterior surface of the talus.

ANKLE

MEDIAL ANKLE

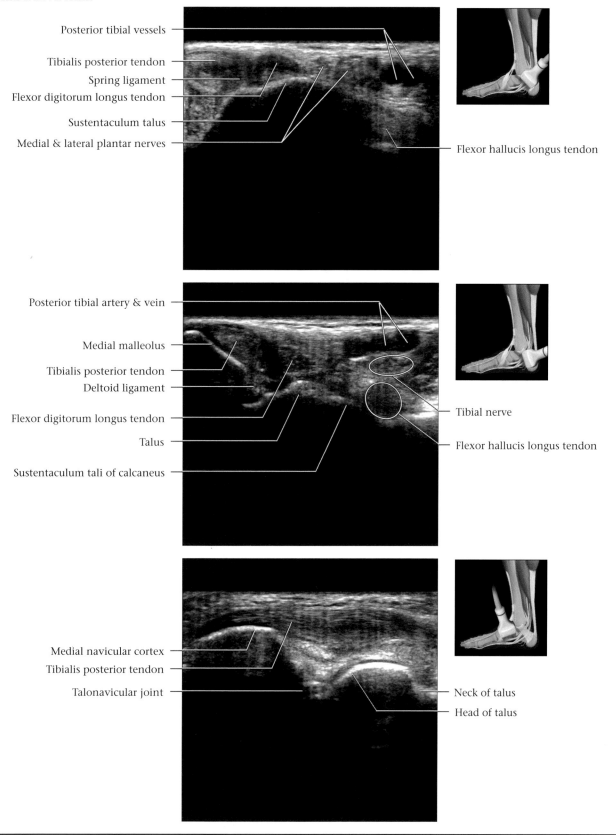

Posterior tibial vessels

Tibialis posterior tendon

Spring ligament

Flexor digitorum longus tendon

Sustentaculum talus

Medial & lateral plantar nerves

Flexor hallucis longus tendon

Posterior tibial artery & vein

Medial malleolus

Tibialis posterior tendon

Deltoid ligament

Flexor digitorum longus tendon

Talus

Sustentaculum tali of calcaneus

Tibial nerve

Flexor hallucis longus tendon

Medial navicular cortex

Tibialis posterior tendon

Talonavicular joint

Neck of talus

Head of talus

(**Top**) More inferiorly, oblique transverse scan through the sustentaculum tali of calcaneus shows that the mnemonic still holds (tibialis anterior anteriorly and flexor hallucis longus posteriorly). The flexor hallucis longus tendon now runs in a groove behind the sustentaculum tali. (**Middle**) Coronal scan of the tarsal tunnel. All structures within the tunnel curve around the medial malleolus to run forward to the midfoot. The tibialis posterior tendon runs on the surface of the deltoid ligament, flexor digitorum longus on the talus and flexor hallucis longus on the calcaneus under the sustentaculum tali. (**Bottom**) Transverse image showing the long axis of the tibialis posterior tendon inserting onto the medial pole of navicular. This insertion is sometimes complicated by an accessory navicular bone which may take on different shapes.

ANKLE

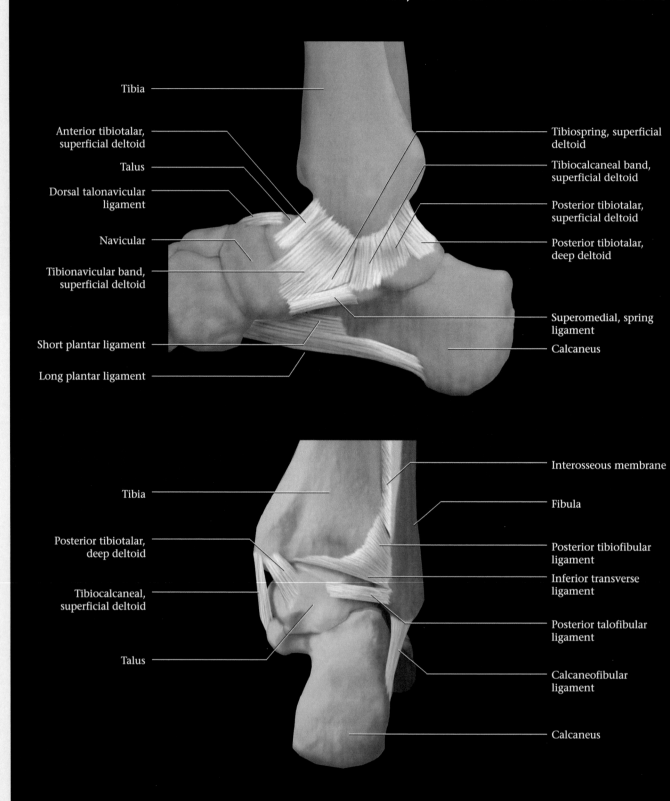

Tibia

Anterior tibiotalar, superficial deltoid

Talus

Dorsal talonavicular ligament

Navicular

Tibionavicular band, superficial deltoid

Short plantar ligament

Long plantar ligament

Tibiospring, superficial deltoid

Tibiocalcaneal band, superficial deltoid

Posterior tibiotalar, superficial deltoid

Posterior tibiotalar, deep deltoid

Superomedial, spring ligament

Calcaneus

Tibia

Posterior tibiotalar, deep deltoid

Tibiocalcaneal, superficial deltoid

Talus

Interosseous membrane

Fibula

Posterior tibiofibular ligament

Inferior transverse ligament

Posterior talofibular ligament

Calcaneofibular ligament

Calcaneus

(Top) Medial view of the ankle. The deltoid ligament is the major supporter of the ankle. It has many variable components but a commonly accepted division includes the deep anterior & posterior tibiotalar & superficial anterior & posterior tibiotalar, tibiocalcaneal, tibiospring & tibionavicular bands. Note that the superficial deltoid is band-like and distinction between its various components relies on the sites of insertion. **(Bottom)** Posterior view of the ankle. The tibiofibular ligaments are obliquely oriented and their fibular origin is above the fibular fossa. The inferior transverse ligament, which is the inferior aspect of the posterior tibiofibular ligament, extends distal to the tibial posterior surface.

ANKLE

DELTOID LIGAMENT

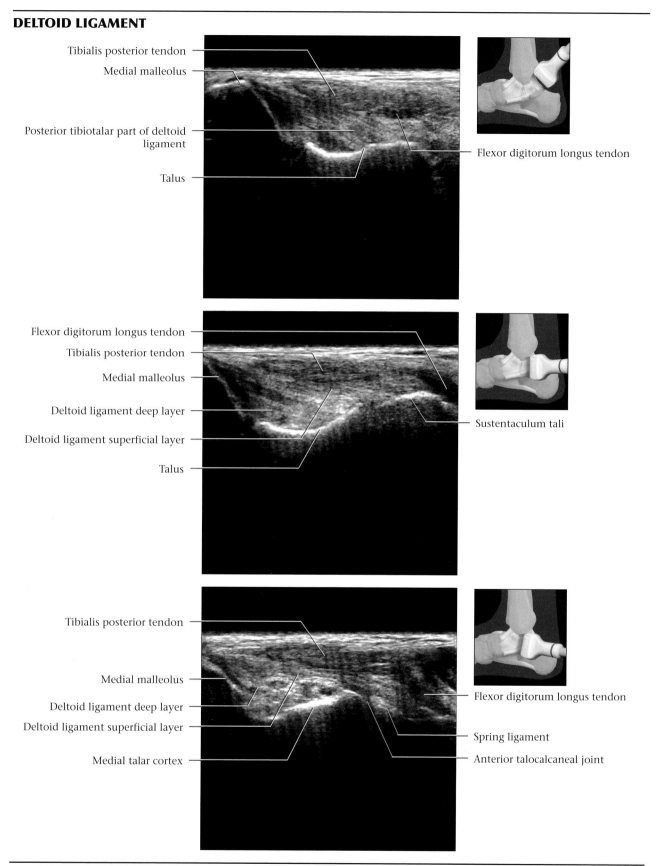

(Top) Coronal image through the posterior (posterior tibiotalar) portion of deltoid ligament, which runs from the medial malleolus to the talus. The tibialis posterior and flexor digitorum longus tendons run superficial to this ligament. **(Middle)** Coronal image through a more anterior portion of the deltoid ligament: The superficial layer (tibiocalcaneal) runs from the malleolus to the sustentaculum tali, the deep component (posterior tibiotalar) to the talus. **(Bottom)** Coronal image through the mid portion of the deltoid ligament: The superficial layer (tibiospring) runs from malleolus to the spring ligament, the deep component to the talus.

DELTOID LIGAMENT

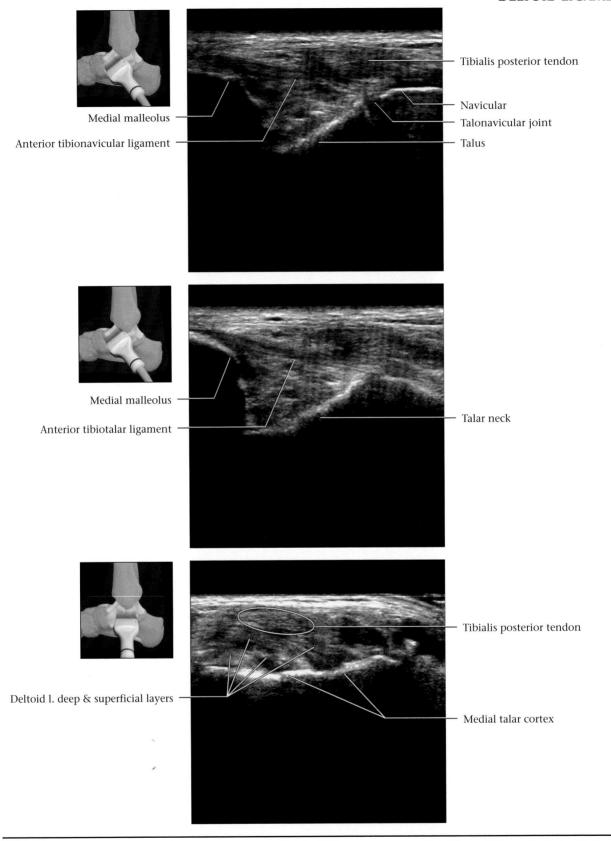

Medial malleolus

Anterior tibionavicular ligament

Tibialis posterior tendon

Navicular

Talonavicular joint

Talus

Medial malleolus

Anterior tibiotalar ligament

Talar neck

Deltoid l. deep & superficial layers

Tibialis posterior tendon

Medial talar cortex

(Top) Coronal image through the anterior portion of deltoid ligament, a superficial layer (talonavicular) which runs from the malleolus to the navicular. **(Middle)** Oblique sagittal image through the most anterior portion of the deltoid ligament, fibers (anterior tibiotalar) run from the malleolus to the talar neck. From front to back these superficial and deep components of the deltoid create a strong restraint against ankle eversion. **(Bottom)** Transverse scan through medial wall of talus, shows deep and superficial components of deltoid ligament. The tibialis posterior tendon runs superficial to this ligament.

ANKLE

LATERAL ANKLE

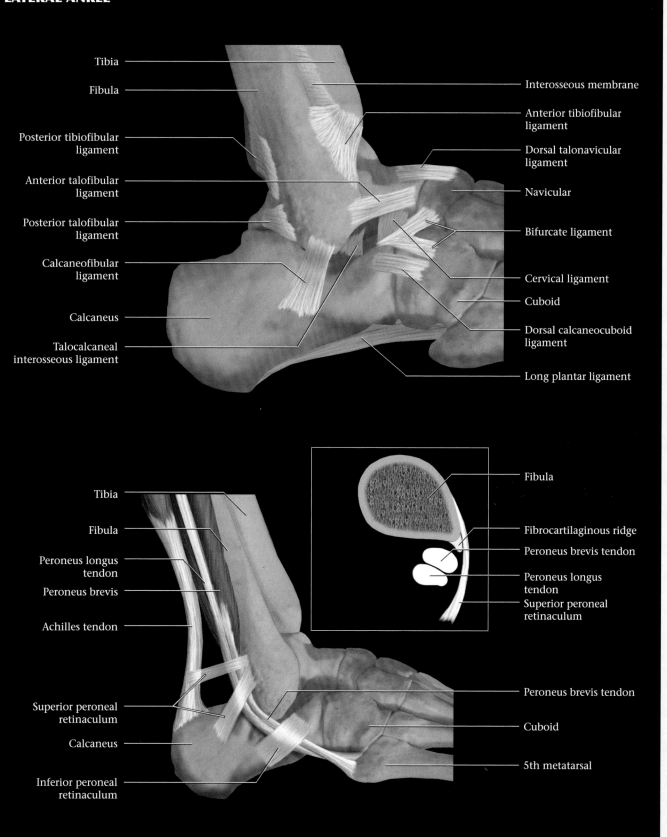

Tibia

Fibula

Posterior tibiofibular ligament

Anterior talofibular ligament

Posterior talofibular ligament

Calcaneofibular ligament

Calcaneus

Talocalcaneal interosseous ligament

Interosseous membrane

Anterior tibiofibular ligament

Dorsal talonavicular ligament

Navicular

Bifurcate ligament

Cervical ligament

Cuboid

Dorsal calcaneocuboid ligament

Long plantar ligament

Tibia

Fibula

Peroneus longus tendon

Peroneus brevis

Achilles tendon

Superior peroneal retinaculum

Calcaneus

Inferior peroneal retinaculum

Fibula

Fibrocartilaginous ridge

Peroneus brevis tendon

Peroneus longus tendon

Superior peroneal retinaculum

Peroneus brevis tendon

Cuboid

5th metatarsal

(Top) Lateral view of the ankle. Two groups of lateral ligaments support the ankle: 1) the syndesmotic ligaments, including the anterior tibiofibular, posterior tibiofibular & syndesmotic ligaments, and 2) the lateral collateral ligaments including the anterior talofibular, posterior talofibular & calcaneofibular ligaments. Other ligaments that bind the lateral hindfoot include the talocalcaneal interosseous ligament and cervical ligament in the sinus tarsi. Note the bifurcate ligament which extends from the calcaneus to the navicular and cuboid. (Bottom) Peroneal retinacula. The superior peroneal retinaculum holds the peroneal tendons in the retrofibular groove. The retinaculum has variable insertions but typically inserts on deep fascia of leg & on the calcaneus. The inferior peroneal retinaculum holds the peroneal tendons against calcaneus.

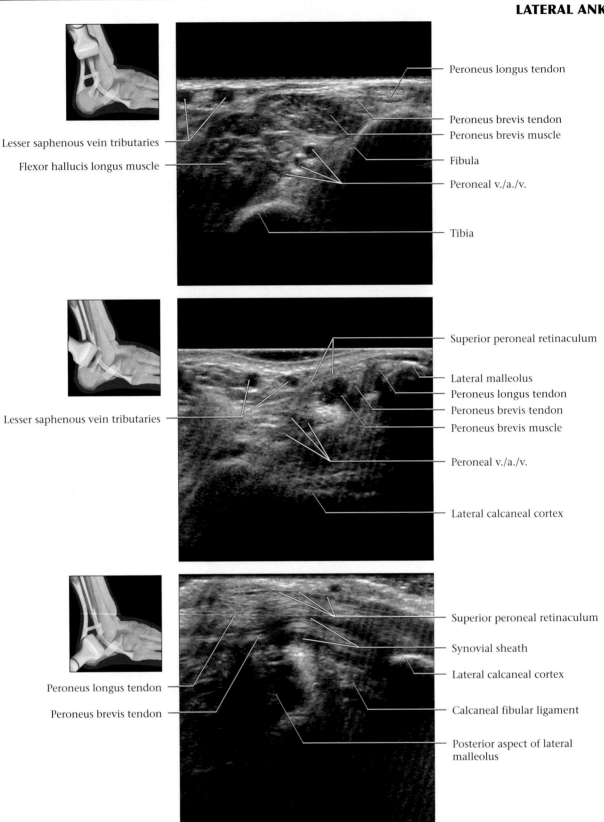

Peroneus longus tendon

Peroneus brevis tendon
Peroneus brevis muscle

Fibula

Peroneal v./a./v.

Tibia

Lesser saphenous vein tributaries

Flexor hallucis longus muscle

Superior peroneal retinaculum

Lateral malleolus
Peroneus longus tendon
Peroneus brevis tendon
Peroneus brevis muscle

Peroneal v./a./v.

Lateral calcaneal cortex

Lesser saphenous vein tributaries

Superior peroneal retinaculum

Synovial sheath

Lateral calcaneal cortex

Calcaneal fibular ligament

Posterior aspect of lateral malleolus

Peroneus longus tendon

Peroneus brevis tendon

(Top) Transverse scan of the posterior aspect of the distal fibula showing the distal peroneal muscles. The peroneus longus tendon runs anterior to the peroneus brevis. The latter is easily identified by its muscle component, which continues to just above the tip of the lateral malleolus. (Middle) Transverse scan at the level just above the tip of the lateral malleolus. The peroneal tendons are now held down by the superior peroneal retinaculum, which prevents tendon subluxation (bowstringing). There is still a residual component of the peroneus brevis muscle. (Bottom) Oblique coronal scan of the posterior aspect of the lateral malleolus shows the longitudinal course lof the peroneal tendons. Both tendons run inferior onto the lateral surface of the calcaneus, passing over the calcaneal fibular ligament on the way.

ANKLE

LATERAL ANKLE

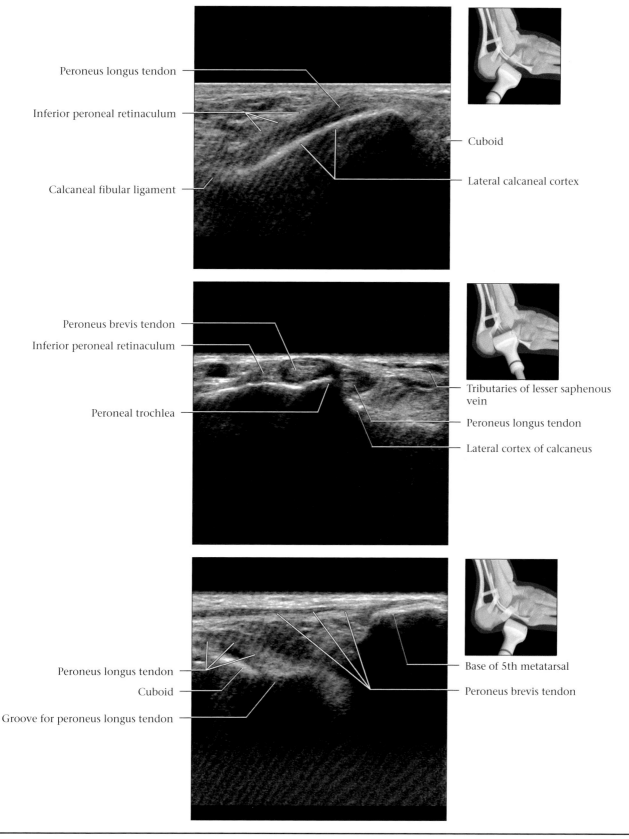

Peroneus longus tendon

Inferior peroneal retinaculum

Calcaneal fibular ligament

Cuboid

Lateral calcaneal cortex

Peroneus brevis tendon

Inferior peroneal retinaculum

Peroneal trochlea

Tributaries of lesser saphenous vein

Peroneus longus tendon

Lateral cortex of calcaneus

Peroneus longus tendon

Cuboid

Groove for peroneus longus tendon

Base of 5th metatarsal

Peroneus brevis tendon

(Top) Oblique transverse scan of the lateral aspect of the calcaneus along the course of the peroneus longus tendon. Close to the anterior end of the calcaneus, the peroneus longus turns medially and inferiorly to enter the plantar region. (Middle) Coronal scan of the lateral surface of the calcaneus shows the peroneal tendons held down by the inferior peroneal retinaculum but partially separated by peroneal trochlea, a protuberance on the lateral calcaneal cortex. The peroneus brevis tendon lies more superior than peroneus longus tendon at this level. (Bottom) Transverse scan of the lateral aspect of the foot showing insertion of the peroneus brevis tendon onto the base of fifth metatarsal bone. Also shown here is the peroneus longus tendon turning inferiorly on the surface of the cuboid to enter the plantar aspect, into a groove solely for this tendon.

Lateral malleolus

Anterior talofibular ligament

Ankle joint recess with fluid

Extensor digitorum brevis muscle

Neck of talus

Lateral malleolus

Peroneus longus tendon

Peroneus brevis tendon

Calcaneofibular ligament

Lesser saphenous vein

Lateral calcaneal cortex

Lateral malleolus posterior cortex

Peroneus longus tendon

Peroneus brevis tendon

Flexor hallucis longus muscle

Lateral tubercle of talus

Posterior talofibular ligament

Posterior recess of ankle joint

(Top) Oblique transverse scan of the lateral ankle along the course of the anterior talofibular ligament. An ankle joint recess exists deep to this ligament making it a good area to look for small effusions. The lateral fibers of the extensor digitorum brevis muscle run on the surface of this ligament. (Middle) Oblique coronal scan along the long axis of the calcaneofibular ligament. The peroneal tendons can be seen curving under the lateral malleolus and running partly on the surface of this ligament. (Bottom) Transverse scan of the posterior aspect of the lateral malleolus shows the posterior talofibular ligament. Deep to this ligament is the posterior recess of the ankle joint.

ANKLE

POSTERIOR ANKLE PANORAMA

Flexor hallucis longus muscle

Tibia

Posterior margin of talar dome

Lateral tubercle of talus

Recess from posterior subtalar joint

Soleus muscle

Inferior extent of soleal musculo-tendinous junction

Achilles tendon

Middle facet of posterior calcaneus

Achilles tendon insertion

Sagittal panoramic view of the posterior ankle. The dominant structure in the posterior ankle is the Achilles tendon, the largest tendon in the body. This runs craniocaudally just under the skin and is well-demonstrated by ultrasound. The ankle should be in dorsiflexion to tighten this tendon during examination so that the organization of its fibers and its continuity can be assessed. More superiorly, its contributing muscles, the soleus and gastrocnemius can be traced. Deep to this is the deep layer of the posterior compartment, and at the ankle level, predominantly the flexor hallucis longus muscle. Finally, the posterior cortices of the ankle bones can be seen.

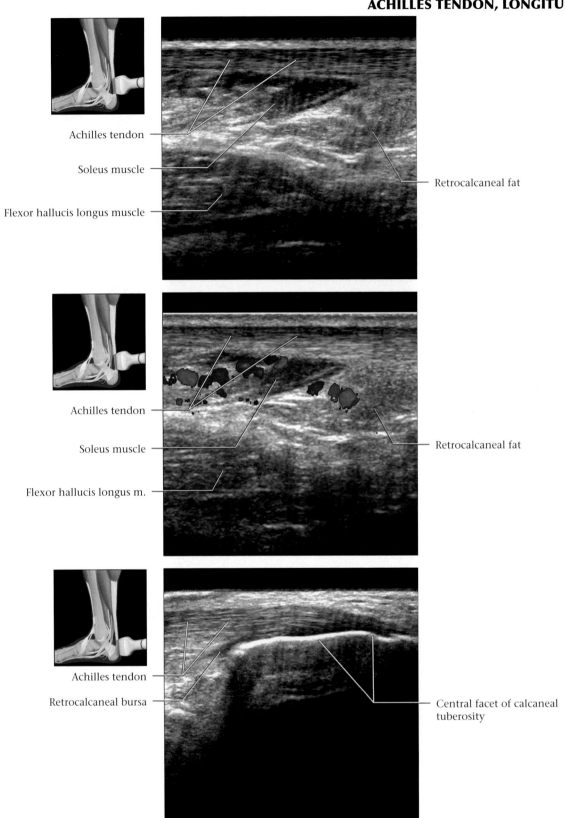

Achilles tendon

Soleus muscle

Flexor hallucis longus muscle

Retrocalcaneal fat

Achilles tendon

Soleus muscle

Flexor hallucis longus m.

Retrocalcaneal fat

Achilles tendon

Retrocalcaneal bursa

Central facet of calcaneal tuberosity

(Top) Sagittal scan of the lower posterior leg showing the musculotendinous junction between the soleus muscle and the Achilles tendon. These structures join at an angle with a crisp border. A disruption of this sharp transition (usually due to hemorrhage and rupture of inserting muscle fibers) is suggestive of injury to the musculotendinous junction. (Middle) Color Doppler scan of the same region showing the rich blood supply to this region and the cause for extensive bruising in tendon damage at this site. (Bottom) Sagittal scan more distally shows the insertion of Achilles tendon onto the middle facet of the posterior calcaneal surface. The retrocalcaneal bursa separates the Achilles tendon from the superior facet of the posterior calcaneal surface. This bursa usually contains a tiny amount of fluid detectable on ultrasound.

ANKLE

ACHILLES TENDON, AXIAL

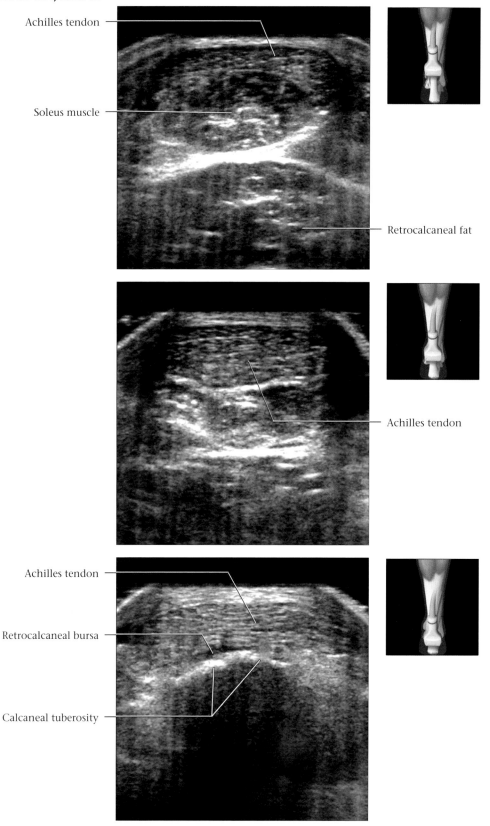

Achilles tendon

Soleus muscle

Retrocalcaneal fat

Achilles tendon

Achilles tendon

Retrocalcaneal bursa

Calcaneal tuberosity

(Top) Series of transverse scans through the Achilles tendon. At a superior level, the soleus muscle can be seen deep to the Achilles tendon. The Achilles tendon begins superiorly as a continuation of the gastrocnemius aponeurosis, which then joins with the soleus tendon to form the Achilles tendon. At the level of this scan, the tendon is crescent shaped to accommodate the soleus muscle. (Middle) Transverse scan of the Achilles tendon at its midportion. The tendon now assumes an oval shape. The fibrils within the tendon produce a coarsely dotted appearance. Focal hypoechogenicity or change in shape of this tendon should suggest tear/rupture or tendinosis. (Bottom) At a lower level before its insertion onto the calcaneal tuberosity, the Achilles tendon becomes flattened. A small amount of fluid is frequently seen in the retrocalcaneal bursa deep to the tendon.

TARSUS

Terminology

Abbreviations
- Artery (a.)
- Ligament (l.)
- Muscle (m.)
- Nerve (n.)
- Vein (v.)

Definitions
- **Three major divisions**
  - **Hindfoot**: Calcaneus and talus
  - **Midfoot**: Navicular, cuneiforms, and cuboid
  - **Forefoot**: Metatarsals and phalanges
- **Two columns**
  - **Medial column**: Talus, navicular, cuneiforms 1-3, digits 1-3
  - **Lateral column**: Calcaneus, cuboid, digits 4 and 5
- Some authors use 2 columns in hind and midfoot as above, but divide forefoot into 3 columns
  - Medial column: 1st toe
  - Middle column: 2nd-4th toes
  - Lateral column: 5th toe

Imaging Anatomy

Overview
- Alignment of foot can only be assessed on weight-bearing radiographs

Arches of Foot
- Foot is arched from posterior to anterior, and from medial to lateral
- **Transverse arch of foot**
  - Cuneiform bones form keystone of arch due to triangular shape
  - Major supporting structures of transverse arch
    - Spring ligament
    - Lisfranc ligament and intermetatarsal ligaments
    - Intertarsal ligaments
- **Longitudinal arch of foot**
  - From posterior process calcaneus to metatarsal heads
  - Medial side is higher than lateral
  - Apex of arch is at navicular and cuneiforms
  - Metatarsals slant downward from apex of arch to metatarsophalangeal (MTP) joint
    - This is called inclination angle
    - Inclination angle decreases from 20° at 1st to 5° at 5th metatarsal
  - Major supporting structures of longitudinal arch
    - Plantar fascia
    - Long and short plantar ligaments
    - Spring ligament
    - Posterior tibial tendon, peroneus longus tendon
- **Radiographic assessment of normal longitudinal arch**
  - Evaluate talometatarsal alignment
    - Normal: Axis of talus continues along axis of 1st metatarsal
    - Pes planus: Axis of talus points below axis of 1st metacarpal, due to the flattened arch
    - Pes cavus: Axis of talus points above axis of 1st metacarpal, due to the exaggerated arch

Distribution of Weight-Bearing
- 50% of weight borne on subtalar joint and calcaneus
- Remainder transmitted via arch anteriorly to metatarsophalangeal joints, greatest weight on 1st toe

Bony Anatomy
- **Cuboid bone**
  - Roughly cuboidal shape
  - 1 ossification center: Ossifies between 9th fetal month and 6 months age
  - Articulates with calcaneus, navicular, 3rd cuneiform, 4th and 5th metatarsals, rarely head of talus
    - Dorsal ligaments (calcaneocuboid, cubonavicular, cuneocuboid, cubometatarsal) strengthen each of these articulations
    - Short and long plantar ligaments attach to plantar surface
  - Sulcus at lateral margin, under which passes peroneus longus tendon
  - 5th metatarsal base extends beyond lateral margin
- **Navicular bone**
  - Curved shape, concave proximally and convex distally
  - 1 ossification center: Ossifies in 3rd year of life
  - Articulates with talus, cuboid, cuneiforms
    - Dorsal ligaments strengthen each of these articulations
    - Single facet proximally for articulation with head of talus
    - 3 facets distally for cuneiform articulations
    - 1 facet laterally for articulation with cuboid
    - Connected to anterior process of calcaneus by bifurcate ligament
    - Connected to sustentaculum tali by spring ligament
  - Large median eminence for attachment of posterior tibial tendon is located more plantar than main body of navicular
- **Cuneiform bones**
  - Wedge-shaped, with base of wedge at dorsal surface of 2nd and 3rd cuneiforms, dorsomedial surface 1st cuneiform
  - In combination, form arch
  - 1st cuneiform (medial cuneiform)
    - Articulates with navicular, 2nd cuneiform, 1st metatarsal
    - 1 or 2 ossifications centers: Ossify in 2nd year of life
  - 2nd cuneiform (middle or intermediate cuneiform)
    - Articulates with navicular, 1st and 3rd cuneiforms, 2nd metatarsal
    - Smallest of cuneiforms
    - 1 ossification center: Ossifies in 3rd year of life
  - 3rd cuneiform (lateral cuneiform)
    - Articulates with navicular, 2nd cuneiform, cuboid, 3rd metatarsal
- **Metatarsal bones**
  - 2 ossifications centers: Shaft ossifies in 9th prenatal week, epiphysis in 3rd-4th years of life
    - 1st metatarsal has epiphysis at proximal end, others at distal end

- 2nd-5th metatarsals have articulations at bases with adjacent metatarsals
- 1st metatarsal
  - Largest of metatarsals
  - Articulates with 1st cuneiform, 1st proximal phalanx, sesamoids of metatarsal head
  - Variable articulation with 2nd metatarsal base
- 2nd-3rd metatarsals
  - Articulate with respective cuneiforms and proximal phalanges
  - 2nd metatarsal base recessed relative to 1st and usually 3rd
- 4th-5th metatarsals
  - Articulate with cuboid and respective proximal phalanges
  - Styloid process of 5th metatarsal extends lateral to cuboid
- **Phalanges**
  - 1st toe is biphalangeal, other toes are triphalangeal
  - 5th toe sometimes has failure of segmentation of middle and distal phalanges
  - 2 ossification centers: Shaft ossifies 9th-15th prenatal weeks, epiphysis 2nd-8th years

Musculature

- **Plantar muscles**: 4 muscle layers, numbered from superficial to deep
  - 1st layer: Abductor hallucis, flexor digitorum brevis, abductor digiti minimi
  - 2nd layer: Quadratus plantae (flexor accessorius), flexor digitorum and hallucis longus ts., lumbricals
  - 3rd layer: Flexor hallucis brevis, adductor hallucis, flexor digiti minimi brevis, tibialis posterior t.
  - 4th layer: Plantar interossei (3), dorsal interossei (4)
  - Peroneus longus t. courses across all layers, from superficial plantar laterally to deep plantar medially
- **Dorsal muscles**: 2 muscle layers
  - Superficial layer: Tibialis anterior t., extensor hallucis longus t., extensor digitorum longus t., peroneus tertius t.
  - Deep layer: Extensor hallucis brevis, extensor digitorum brevis
  - In forefoot, long and short extensors run side by side in single layer

Compartments

- **4 plantar compartments** divided by fascial layers
  - Lateral and medial intermuscular septae determine major compartment divisions
- **Medial plantar compartment**
  - Contains abductor hallucis, flexor hallucis longus, and flexor hallucis brevis ts.
- **Central plantar compartment**
  - Superficial subcompartment: Contains flexor digitorum brevis, distal portion of flexor digitorum longus ts.
  - Intermediary subcompartment: Contains proximal plantar portion of flexor digitorum longus t., quadratus plantae, lumbricals
  - Deep subcompartment: Limited to forefoot, contains adductor hallucis
- **Lateral plantar compartment**
  - Contains abductor and flexor digiti minimi
- **Interosseous compartment**
  - Contains plantar and dorsal interosseous muscles
- **Dorsal compartment**
  - Superficial layer: Extrinsic extensor tendons
  - Deep layer: Intrinsic extensor muscles

Major Ligaments

- Plantar fascia (aponeurosis): 3 portions extend from tuberosity of calcaneus to transverse metatarsal ligaments of toes
  - Medial band: Thin structure superficial to abductor hallucis muscle
  - Central band: Thick, strong structure superficial to flexor digitorum brevis
    - Divides into separate bands to each toe; these are linked by transverse bands
    - Distally sends septae superficially into subcutaneous fat and deep to MTP joints
  - Lateral band: Thin structure superficial to abductor digiti minimi
  - Medial and lateral bands sometimes terminate at level of mid metatarsals
- Long plantar ligament: Originates calcaneal tuberosity, inserts cuboid and bases 2nd-4th metatarsals
  - Forms retinaculum for peroneus longus tendon as it courses medially on plantar aspect of foot
- Short plantar (plantar calcaneocuboid) ligament: Deep to long ligament, inserts more proximally on cuboid
- Plantar calcaneocuboid (spring) ligament: Originates sustentaculum tali, inserts plantar aspect navicular
- Bifurcate ligament: Originates anterior process of calcaneus dorsally, inserts navicular and cuboid
- Lisfranc ligament: Originates 1st cuneiform, inserts base 2nd metatarsal
- Intermetatarsal ligaments: Dorsal and plantar ligaments between 2nd-5th metatarsal bases
- Transverse metatarsal ligaments: Superficial and deep ligaments between metatarsal heads

Nerves

- **Tibial nerve** divides into medial and lateral plantar branches at level of tarsal tunnel
  - **Medial plantar nerve**
    - Between 1st and 2nd muscle layers, accompanies medial plantar artery
    - Motor branches: Abductor hallucis, flexor digitorum and hallucis brevis, 1st lumbrical
    - Plantar digital nerves to 1st-3rd toes, medial aspect 4th toe
  - **Lateral plantar nerve**: Has deep and superficial divisions
    - Motor branches: Flexor digiti minimi brevis, lumbricals, interossei, adductor hallucis
    - Superficial lateral plantar nerve: Between 1st and 2nd muscle layers
    - Plantar digital nerves to 5th toe, lateral aspect 4th toe
    - Deep lateral plantar nerve: Between 3rd and 4th muscle layers; accompanies lateral plantar artery
- **Deep peroneal nerve**: Extends along dorsum of foot, between tibialis anterior and extensor hallucis longus
  - Motor branch: Extensor digitorum brevis
- **Superficial peroneal nerve**: Divides into medial and lateral branches at dorsum of foot
  - Sensory branches to dorsal foot

- **Sural nerve:** Lateral, superficial branch of tibial nerve
  - Extends along lateral margin of foot
  - Sensory branches to lateral foot

Arteries

- Posterior tibial artery divides into medial and lateral plantar arteries at level of tarsal tunnel
  - Plantar arteries accompany medial and deep lateral plantar nerves
- Peroneal artery accompanies superficial peroneal nerve down anterolateral aspect ankle
  - May join or replace posterior tibial artery
- Anterior tibial artery continues into foot as dorsalis pedis artery, deep to extensor retinaculum
  - Divides into multiple branches in midfoot, forming arcade

Bursae

- Extensor digitorum brevis: Between muscle and 2nd cuneiform and metatarsal bases
- Extensor hallucis longus: Between tendon and 1st cuneiform and metatarsal bases
- Abductor digiti minimi: Between muscle and tuberosity of 5th metatarsal
- Metatarsophalangeal joints: Dorsally; between metatarsal heads; and medial to 1st metatarsal head

Anatomy-Based Imaging Issues

Imaging Recommendations

- Radiographs
  - Weight-bearing when possible
  - Standard views: Anteroposterior (dorsoplantar), lateral, oblique
- US
  - Offers highest spatial resolution for muscle and tendons
  - Particularly useful given limited depth of most soft tissue structures in foot
  - As a result of transverse arch of foot, interrogation should be performed separately for medial and lateral sides for best visualization
  - Due to complex soft tissue anatomy, panoramic (extended field of view) images provide better depiction of location and extent of a lesion and course of different structures
  - Dorsal foot structures tend to be very superficial and thin (tendons) or compressible (vessels)
    - To better visualize these structures, minimal compression and a thick layer of coupling gel may help
- CT
  - Multidetector 1 mm images with sagittal and coronal reformations
  - Three dimension reconstructions often useful for analyzing relationship between bones and bone fragments
- MR
  - Better images obtained when field of view limited to area of concern, not entire foot
  - Demonstration of bone marrow edema aside from soft tissue lesions

Imaging "Sweet Spots"

- Tendon movement can be easily demonstrated with ultrasound by moving the bone it inserts onto
  - This helps with confirming tendon location and also with establishing tendon integrity
- Tarsal ligaments are usually seen as hypoechoic thickenings on cortices and between bones
  - Orientation of transducer along long axis makes ligament stand out and easier to identify

Imaging Pitfalls

- Alignment can only be reliably assessed on weight-bearing radiographs

Clinical Implications

Foot Motion

- **Supination:** Elevation of medial arch of foot
  - Combination of inversion and adduction
- **Pronation:** Depression of medial arch of foot
  - Combination of eversion and abduction
- Complex motions at multiple joints
  - Chopart (calcaneocuboid and talonavicular) joint
    - These 2 joints move together on an oblique axis to produce compound motions
    - Pronation-abduction-extension to supination-adduction-flexion
  - Tarsometatarsal joints
    - Dorsiflexion and plantar flexion
    - 2nd and 3rd tarsometatarsal joints relatively immobile
    - Slight abduction of 1st tarsometatarsal joint
  - Metatarsophalangeal joints
    - Dorsiflexion and plantar flexion
    - Abduction and adduction at 1st metatarsophalangeal joint

Alignment

- Normal weight-bearing and gait depend on normal foot alignment
- Evaluated initially with anteroposterior and lateral weight-bearing radiographs

Malalignment

- Forefoot adductus: Medial angulation of metatarsals from axis of hindfoot
- Forefoot varus: Inversion of metatarsals resulting in shift of weight-bearing to 5th metatarsal from 1st metatarsal
- Metatarsus primus varus: Medial deviation of 1st metatarsal axis relative to 2nd
- Hallux valgus (hallux abductus): Lateral deviation of 1st proximal phalanx relative to axis of 1st metatarsal
  - Valgus refers to an angular deformity in vertical plane, where apex points medially
  - Abductus refers to an angular deformity in horizontal plane, where apex points medially
  - Hallux valgus is a misnomer, but it remains the term commonly used for hallux abductus

DORSAL FOOT

Superior extensor retinaculum

Deep peroneal nerve

Lateral branch, deep peroneal nerve

Medial branch, deep peroneal nerve

Extensor hallucis brevis muscle

Inferior extensor retinaculum

Extensor digitorum brevis muscle

Bifurcate ligament

Dorsal talonavicular ligament

Dorsal tarsometatarsal ligaments

Dorsal Lisfranc ligament

Cuneiform-cuboid ligament

Dorsal intermetatarsal ligaments

Transverse metatarsal ligaments

(Top) The deep peroneal nerve travels deep to the extensor retinacula, in the anterior tarsal tunnel, & gives a lateral motor branch to the extensor digitorum brevis muscle. The medial branch continues dorsal to the talonavicular joint, middle cuneiform & in between 1st & 2nd metatarsal to provide mostly sensory but some motor supply to 1st web space. **(Bottom)** Graphic of the dorsal ligaments shows dense ligaments between the tarsal bones, and between tarsals and metatarsals. Ligaments are generally named for the bones they bridge. Exceptions are the bifurcate ligament, which extends from the anterior process calcaneus to the cuboid and the navicular, and the dorsal Lisfranc ligament, from the 1st cuneiform to the 2nd metatarsal.

Lower Limb

VII

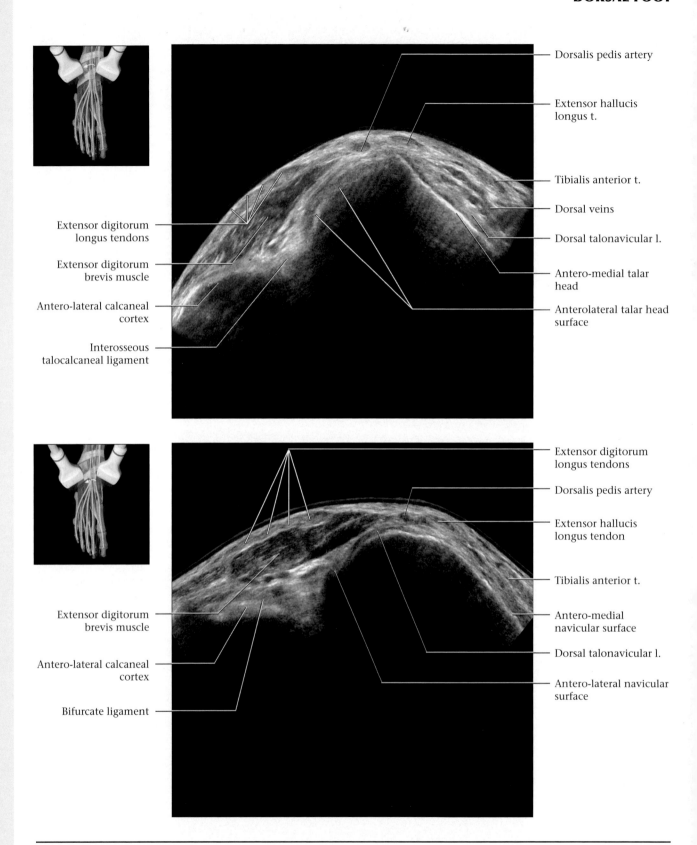

Dorsalis pedis artery

Extensor hallucis longus t.

Tibialis anterior t.

Dorsal veins

Dorsal talonavicular l.

Antero-medial talar head

Anterolateral talar head surface

Extensor digitorum longus tendons

Extensor digitorum brevis muscle

Antero-lateral calcaneal cortex

Interosseous talocalcaneal ligament

Extensor digitorum longus tendons

Dorsalis pedis artery

Extensor hallucis longus tendon

Tibialis anterior t.

Antero-medial navicular surface

Dorsal talonavicular l.

Antero-lateral navicular surface

Extensor digitorum brevis muscle

Antero-lateral calcaneal cortex

Bifurcate ligament

(Top) Coronal panoramic scan of the dorsal foot at the talo-calcaneus level. The foot can be divided into two columns: The medial column (talus, navicular & cuneiforms) & lateral column (calcaneus & cuboid) form antero-medial & antero-lateral surfaces of transverse mid-foot arch. The dorsalis pedis artery runs at the apex of this arch. **(Bottom)** Coronal panoramic scan of the dorsal foot through the navicular-calcaneal level. The transverse arch of the dorsal foot creates two surfaces: Anteromedial and anterolateral, over which extensor tendons and small muscles lie. More focal examination of these structures requires scanning along each surface separately. Panoramic scans give an overview of anatomy. However, high resolution of the site of interest provides more details and both should be performed as complementary techniques.

TARSUS

DORSAL FOOT

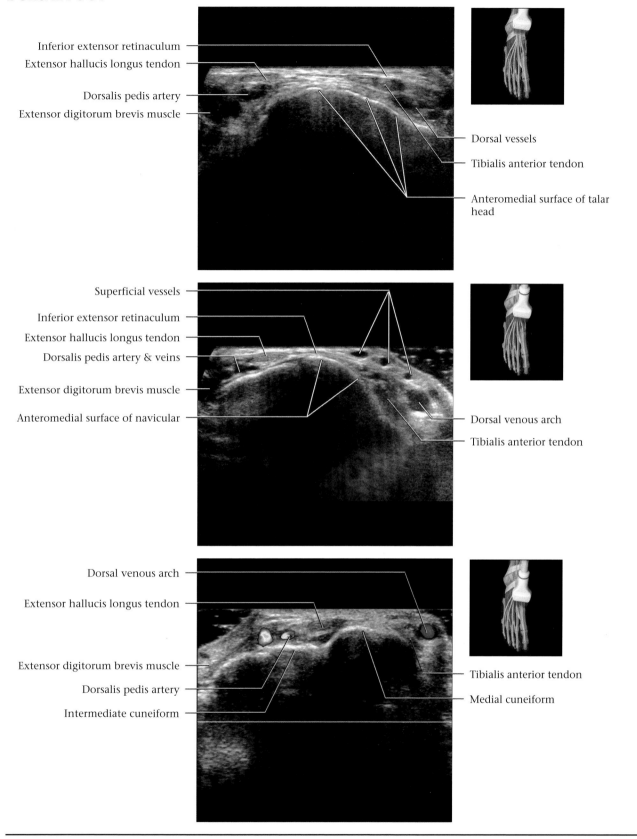

Inferior extensor retinaculum
Extensor hallucis longus tendon
Dorsalis pedis artery
Extensor digitorum brevis muscle

Dorsal vessels
Tibialis anterior tendon
Anteromedial surface of talar head

Superficial vessels
Inferior extensor retinaculum
Extensor hallucis longus tendon
Dorsalis pedis artery & veins
Extensor digitorum brevis muscle
Anteromedial surface of navicular

Dorsal venous arch
Tibialis anterior tendon

Dorsal venous arch
Extensor hallucis longus tendon
Extensor digitorum brevis muscle
Dorsalis pedis artery
Intermediate cuneiform

Tibialis anterior tendon
Medial cuneiform

(Top) Series of three coronal scans of the dorsal medial surface of the foot. At this most proximal level, the talus is the underlying bone. The extensor hallucis can be seen partially covering the dorsalis pedis artery. More medially, the tibialis anterior tendon can be found. (Middle) At a mid-tarsal level, this coronal scan shows the anteromedial surface of the navicular. The tibialis anterior tendon begins to turn acutely medially to curve around to the medial edge of the foot, eventually inserting on the medial cuneiform. As seen here, the use of light pressure and copious amounts of gel will allow visualization of small superficial veins, which are numerous on the dorsum of the foot. (Bottom) Coronal color Doppler scan at the level of the cuneiforms. The intimate relationship between the dorsalis pedis artery and the extensor hallucis longus tendon continues.

TARSUS

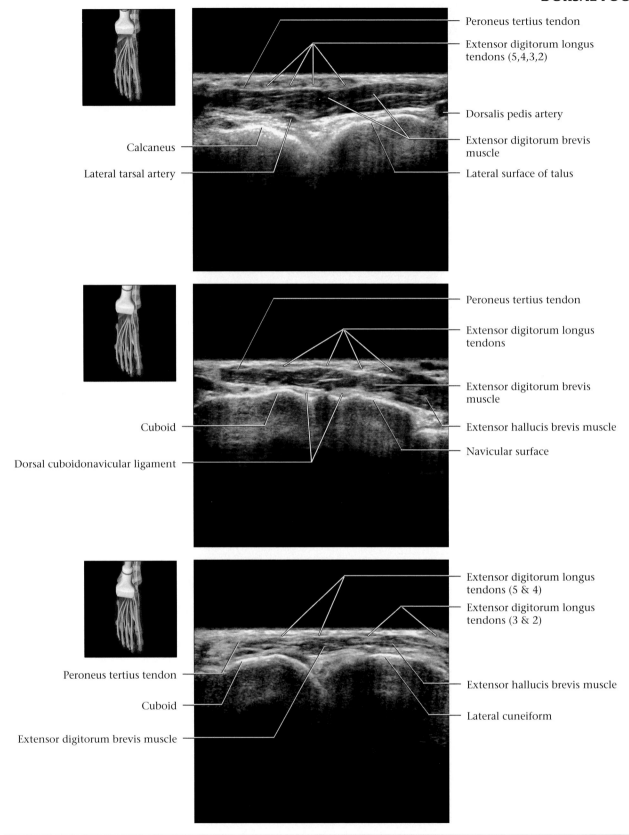

Top image labels:
- Peroneus tertius tendon
- Extensor digitorum longus tendons (5,4,3,2)
- Dorsalis pedis artery
- Extensor digitorum brevis muscle
- Lateral surface of talus
- Calcaneus
- Lateral tarsal artery

Middle image labels:
- Peroneus tertius tendon
- Extensor digitorum longus tendons
- Extensor digitorum brevis muscle
- Extensor hallucis brevis muscle
- Navicular surface
- Cuboid
- Dorsal cuboidonavicular ligament

Bottom image labels:
- Extensor digitorum longus tendons (5 & 4)
- Extensor digitorum longus tendons (3 & 2)
- Extensor hallucis brevis muscle
- Lateral cuneiform
- Peroneus tertius tendon
- Cuboid
- Extensor digitorum brevis muscle

(Top) Series of three coronal scans over the dorsal lateral surface of the tarsus. At this proximal level, the lateral surface of the calcaneus and the talus are the underlying bones. The extensor digitorum longus tendons are close to each other and share a common synovial sheath. The extensor digitorum brevis muscle lies deep to the longus tendons. The lateral tarsal artery runs deeper and is a branch of the dorsalis pedis artery. **(Middle)** At the level of the mid-tarsus, the extensor digitorum longus tendons for individual toes begin to spread out and also flatten (the latter making them just discernible on ultrasound). At this level, the extensor hallucis brevis muscle can also be seen. **(Bottom)** At a more distal level, the extensor digitorum brevis muscle and the extensor hallucis brevis muscle are much thinner and will turn into tendons distally.

TARSUS

DORSAL FOOT

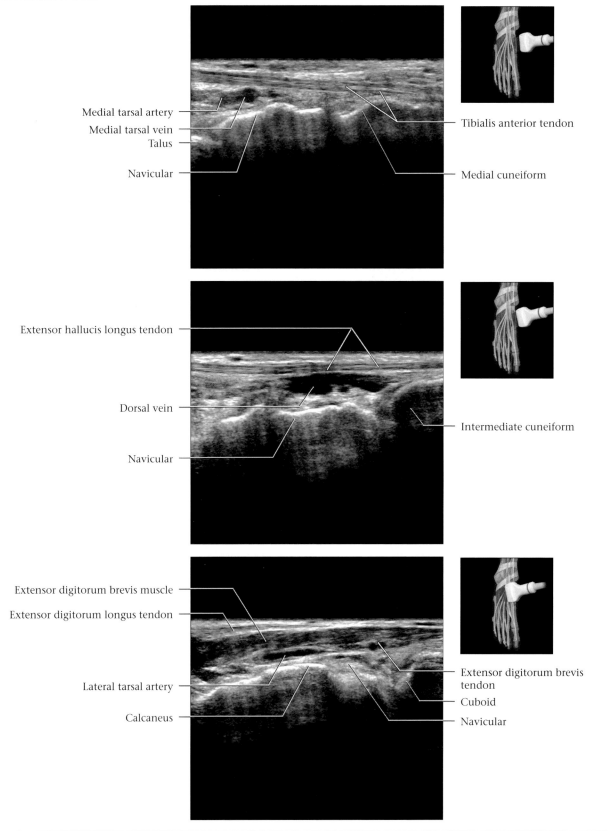

Medial tarsal artery — Talus — Medial tarsal vein — Navicular — Tibialis anterior tendon — Medial cuneiform

Extensor hallucis longus tendon — Dorsal vein — Navicular — Intermediate cuneiform

Extensor digitorum brevis muscle — Extensor digitorum longus tendon — Lateral tarsal artery — Calcaneus — Extensor digitorum brevis tendon — Cuboid — Navicular

(Top) Series of sagittal scans through the tarsus. Medially, the tibialis anterior is seen running over the medial tarsal vessels (branch of dorsalis pedis) to insert on the medial and inferior surfaces of the base of the medial cuneiform. (Middle) Slightly laterally, the extensor hallucis longus tendon runs towards the big toe, passing over the intermediate cuneiform bone. (Bottom) More laterally, the extensor digitorum longus tendon and the extensor digitorum brevis muscle come into view. They lie on the surface of the calcaneus with the lateral tarsal artery coursing between the muscle and bone. The gradual tapering of the extensor digitorum brevis muscle distally can be appreciated here.

PLANTAR MUSCLES SUPERFICIAL LAYERS

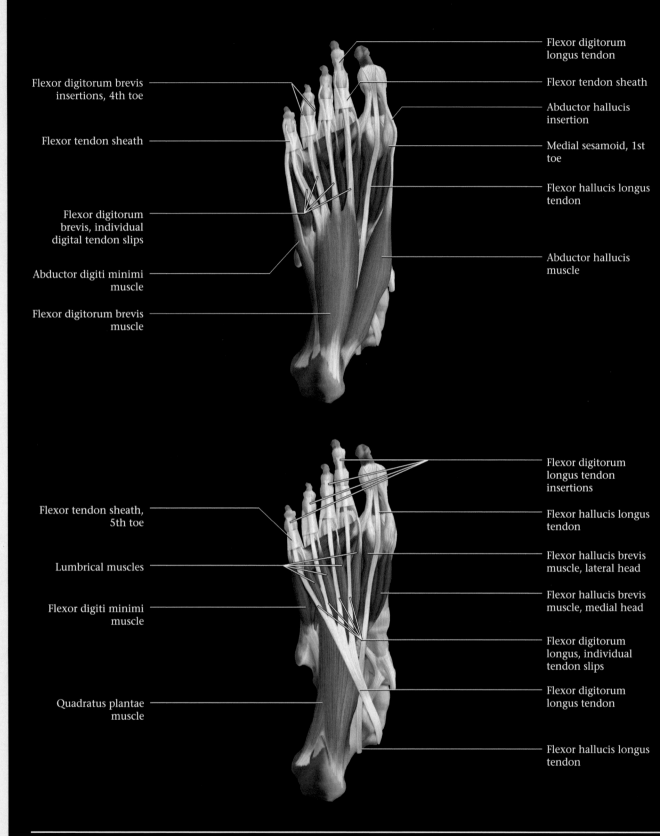

Flexor digitorum brevis insertions, 4th toe

Flexor tendon sheath

Flexor digitorum brevis, individual digital tendon slips

Abductor digiti minimi muscle

Flexor digitorum brevis muscle

Flexor digitorum longus tendon

Flexor tendon sheath

Abductor hallucis insertion

Medial sesamoid, 1st toe

Flexor hallucis longus tendon

Abductor hallucis muscle

Flexor tendon sheath, 5th toe

Lumbrical muscles

Flexor digiti minimi muscle

Quadratus plantae muscle

Flexor digitorum longus tendon insertions

Flexor hallucis longus tendon

Flexor hallucis brevis muscle, lateral head

Flexor hallucis brevis muscle, medial head

Flexor digitorum longus, individual tendon slips

Flexor digitorum longus tendon

Flexor hallucis longus tendon

(Top) Graphic shows the superficial layer of the plantar foot muscles: Abductor digiti minimi, flexor digitorum brevis, and abductor hallucis. The deep muscles are partially visible deep to the superficial layer. The flexor digitorum brevis tendons split in each digit (4th digit labeled), tatching at lateral aspects of the middle phalangeal bases. The flexor tendon sheaths hold the flexor mechanism in close proximity to the phalanges. **(Bottom)** Graphic shows the 2nd layer of plantar muscles. The interesting arrangement of interactions between flexors is well seen: Quadratus plantae inserting on flexor digitorum longus tendon, and lumbricals arising from individual flexor digitorum longus tendon slips. In the toes, the flexor tendons are contained with fibrous tendon sheaths.

TARSUS

PLANTAR FOOT MUSCLES DEEP LAYERS

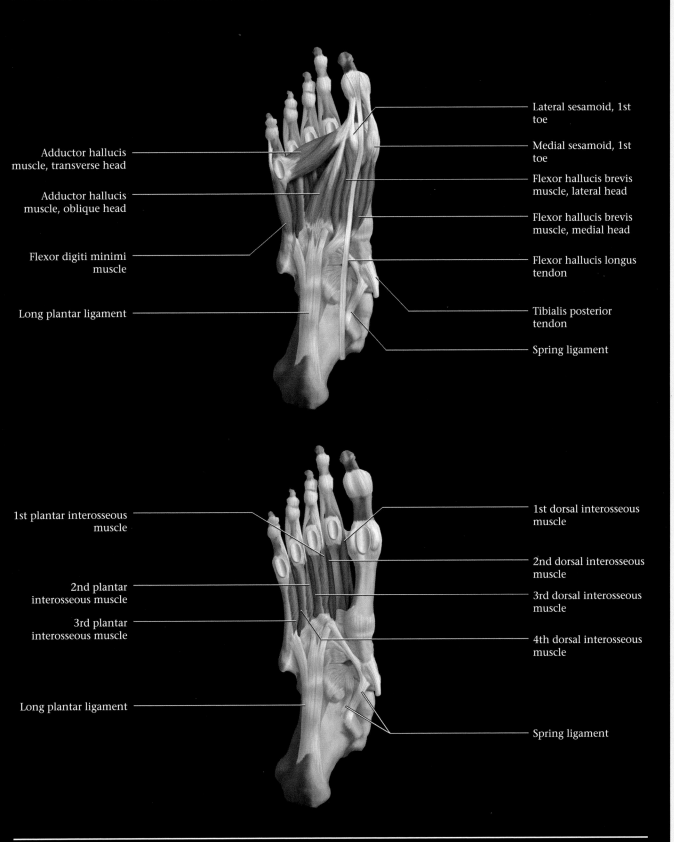

Adductor hallucis muscle, transverse head

Adductor hallucis muscle, oblique head

Flexor digiti minimi muscle

Long plantar ligament

Lateral sesamoid, 1st toe

Medial sesamoid, 1st toe

Flexor hallucis brevis muscle, lateral head

Flexor hallucis brevis muscle, medial head

Flexor hallucis longus tendon

Tibialis posterior tendon

Spring ligament

1st plantar interosseous muscle

2nd plantar interosseous muscle

3rd plantar interosseous muscle

Long plantar ligament

1st dorsal interosseous muscle

2nd dorsal interosseous muscle

3rd dorsal interosseous muscle

4th dorsal interosseous muscle

Spring ligament

(Top) Graphic shows 3rd layer of plantar muscles. This layer contains the flexor hallucis brevis and flexor digiti minimi, as well as the adductor hallucis muscle. The oblique head of the adductor hallucis is thick and broad, whereas the transverse head is thin. **(Bottom)** Graphic shows the 4th layer of plantar muscles, the interosseous muscles. There are 4 dorsal interossei. They have bipennate origins from 2 adjacent metatarsals. There are 3 plantar interossei. The 1st plantar interosseous muscle originates from the medial side of the 3rd metatarsal, and inserts on the medial side of the 3rd proximal phalanx. The 2nd and 3rd plantar interossei originate on the medial sides of the 4th and 5th metatarsals, respectively, and insert on the medial side of the corresponding proximal phalanx.

TARSUS

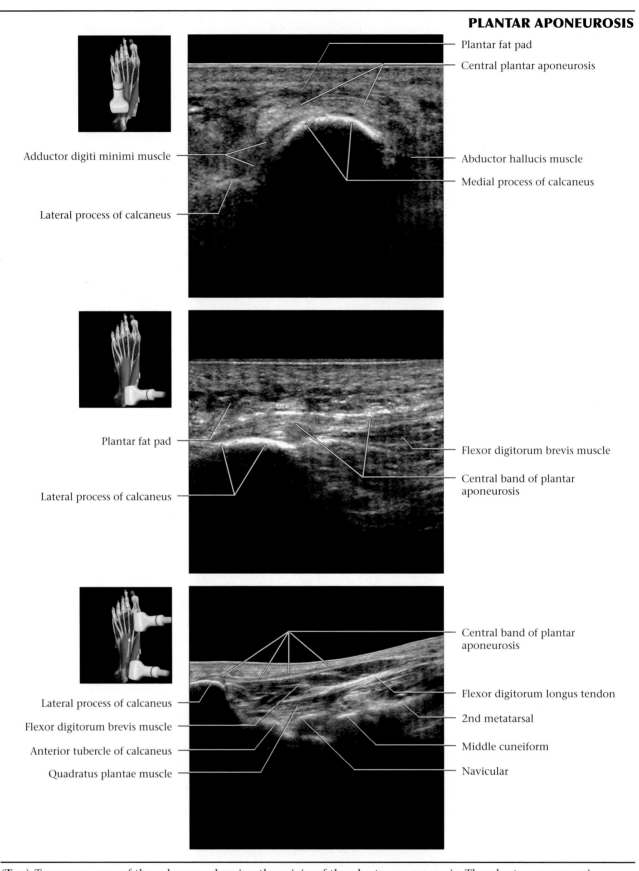

(Top) Transverse scan of the calcaneus showing the origin of the plantar aponeurosis. The plantar aponeurosis consists of three parts: Strong, thick central band over the flexor digitorum brevis muscle; lateral band over the abductor digiti muscle; thin band over the abductor hallucis muscle. **(Middle)** Sagittal scan of the origin of the central band of the plantar aponeurosis. This arises from the medial process of the calcaneus and runs anteriorly deep to the plantar subcutaneous fat. **(Bottom)** Sagittal panoramic scan of central band of plantar aponeurosis. The central is the thickest and most easily identified component of the plantar aponeurosis. Deep to this are the flexor digitorum brevis and quadratus plantae muscles which form the bulk of the central tarsal plantar compartment.

TARSUS

SAGITTAL FOOT OVERVIEW

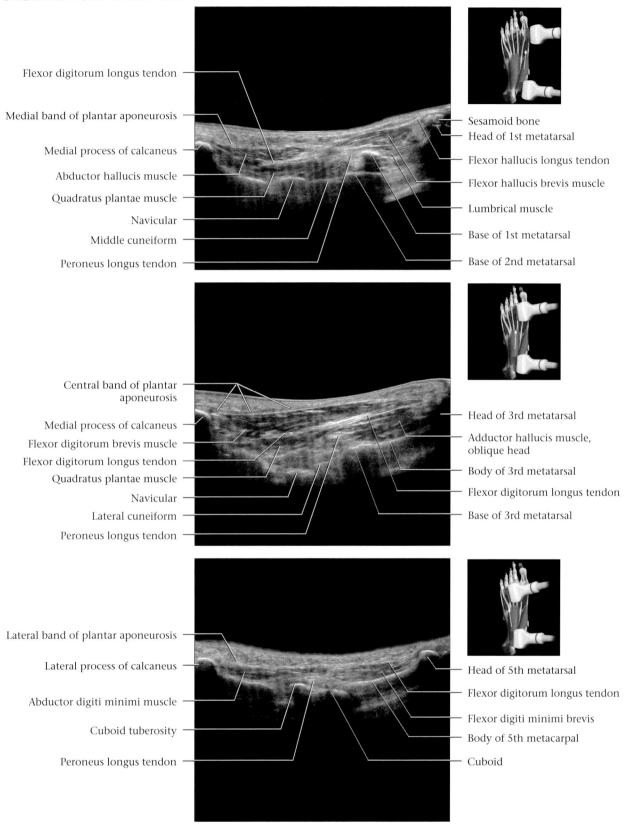

Flexor digitorum longus tendon

Medial band of plantar aponeurosis

Medial process of calcaneus

Abductor hallucis muscle

Quadratus plantae muscle

Navicular

Middle cuneiform

Peroneus longus tendon

Sesamoid bone

Head of 1st metatarsal

Flexor hallucis longus tendon

Flexor hallucis brevis muscle

Lumbrical muscle

Base of 1st metatarsal

Base of 2nd metatarsal

Central band of plantar aponeurosis

Medial process of calcaneus

Flexor digitorum brevis muscle

Flexor digitorum longus tendon

Quadratus plantae muscle

Navicular

Lateral cuneiform

Peroneus longus tendon

Head of 3rd metatarsal

Adductor hallucis muscle, oblique head

Body of 3rd metatarsal

Flexor digitorum longus tendon

Base of 3rd metatarsal

Lateral band of plantar aponeurosis

Lateral process of calcaneus

Abductor digiti minimi muscle

Cuboid tuberosity

Peroneus longus tendon

Head of 5th metatarsal

Flexor digitorum longus tendon

Flexor digiti minimi brevis

Body of 5th metacarpal

Cuboid

(Top) Series of three panoramic sagittal scans through the plantar aspect of the foot. This first scan shows the content of the medial compartment: The abductor hallucis muscle, flexor hallucis longus tendon, and flexor hallucis brevis muscle; together with smaller structures. (Middle) In the central plantar compartment, the contents can be divided into layers. Superficially, there are the flexor digitorum brevis muscle, and the flexor digitorum longus tendon. Deep to this layer are the quadratus plantae muscle, oblique head of the adductor hallucis muscle and the lumbricals. (Bottom) A scan through the lateral compartment, which contains the abductor digiti minimi muscle and the flexor digiti minimi muscle.

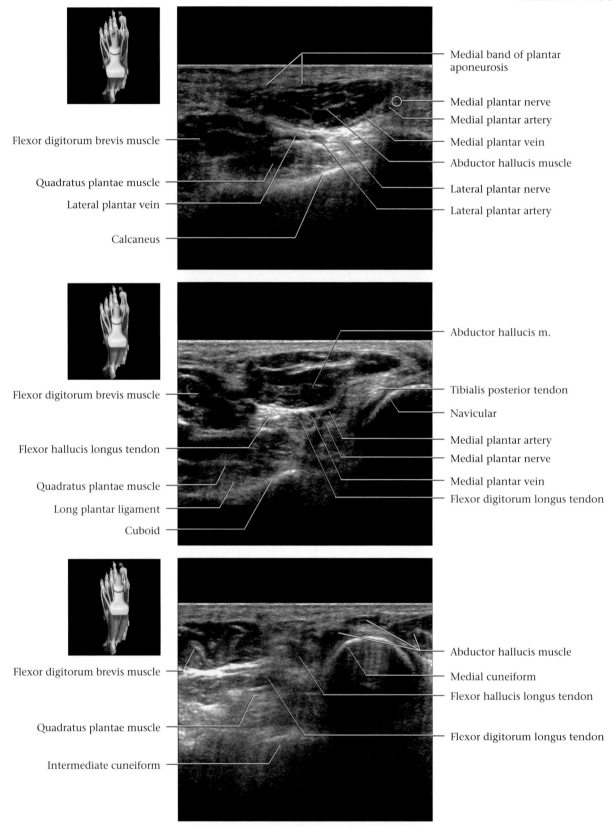

Top image labels:

- Medial band of plantar aponeurosis
- Medial plantar nerve
- Medial plantar artery
- Medial plantar vein
- Abductor hallucis muscle
- Lateral plantar nerve
- Lateral plantar artery
- Flexor digitorum brevis muscle
- Quadratus plantae muscle
- Lateral plantar vein
- Calcaneus

Middle image labels:

- Abductor hallucis m.
- Tibialis posterior tendon
- Navicular
- Medial plantar artery
- Medial plantar nerve
- Medial plantar vein
- Flexor digitorum longus tendon
- Flexor digitorum brevis muscle
- Flexor hallucis longus tendon
- Quadratus plantae muscle
- Long plantar ligament
- Cuboid

Bottom image labels:

- Abductor hallucis muscle
- Medial cuneiform
- Flexor hallucis longus tendon
- Flexor digitorum longus tendon
- Flexor digitorum brevis muscle
- Quadratus plantae muscle
- Intermediate cuneiform

(Top) Series of three coronal scans through the medial half of the plantar aspect of the foot. At this proximal level, the two main muscles (flexor digitorum brevis and quadratus plantae) of the central compartment can be seen lying superficial to the calcaneus. The medial compartment muscle (abductor hallucis) can also be seen medially. **(Middle)** At the level of the mid-tarsus, the knot of Henry can be seen. This is where tendons of the flexor digitorum longus & flexor hallucis longus tendons cross and exchange fibers. The medial plantar neurovascular bundle lies in close proximity to this. **(Bottom)** More distally, the flexor hallucis longus and digitorum longus tendons separate and head towards their respective insertions.

TARSUS

LATERAL TARSUS

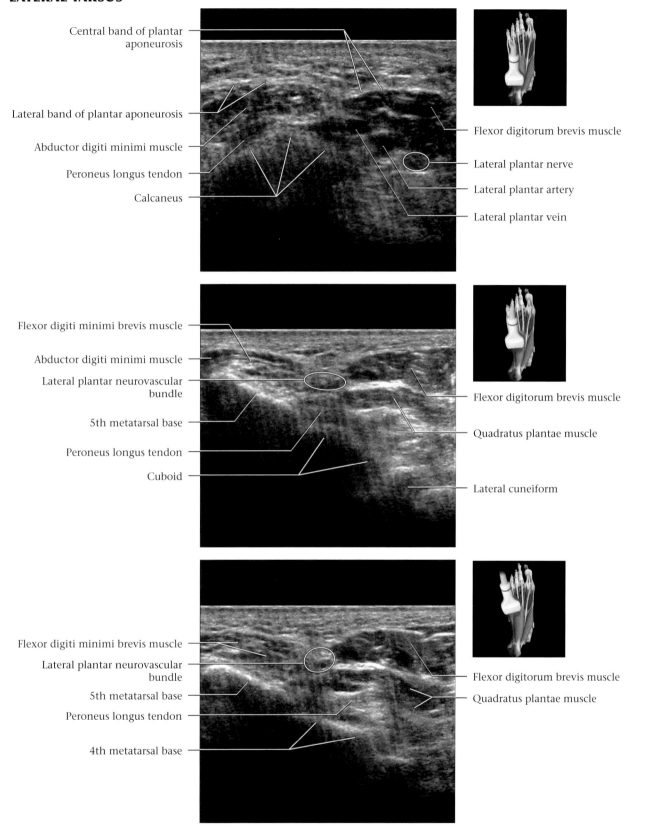

Central band of plantar aponeurosis

Lateral band of plantar aponeurosis

Abductor digiti minimi muscle

Peroneus longus tendon

Calcaneus

Flexor digitorum brevis muscle

Lateral plantar nerve

Lateral plantar artery

Lateral plantar vein

Flexor digiti minimi brevis muscle

Abductor digiti minimi muscle

Lateral plantar neurovascular bundle

5th metatarsal base

Peroneus longus tendon

Cuboid

Flexor digitorum brevis muscle

Quadratus plantae muscle

Lateral cuneiform

Flexor digiti minimi brevis muscle

Lateral plantar neurovascular bundle

5th metatarsal base

Peroneus longus tendon

4th metatarsal base

Flexor digitorum brevis muscle

Quadratus plantae muscle

(Top) Series of three coronal scans through the lateral half of the plantar aspect of the foot. The lateral compartment (abductor digiti minimi) and half of the central compartment can be seen here separated by the lateral plantar neurovascular bundle. The calcaneus forms the bony support of all structures at this level. (Middle) At the level of the mid-tarsus, the separation between the lateral and the central compartment by the neurovascular bundle continues. Within the lateral compartment, the abductor digiti minimi muscle moves laterally, to give way to the other component of the lateral compartment, the flexor digiti minimi brevis muscle. (Bottom) Most distally, the abductor digiti minimi muscle runs on the lateral border and only the flexor digiti minimi brevis muscle is seen on the plantar aspect of the foot.

FOOT VESSELS

Imaging Anatomy

Arteries

- **Dorsalis pedis artery**
  - Dorsal artery of foot
  - Direct continuation of anterior tibial artery, changing name at ankle joint
  - Course and relations
    - Crosses superficial to talocrural articular capsule, talus, navicular and intermediate cuneiform bones
    - Passes deep to inferior extensor retinaculum and distally, extensor hallucis brevis
    - Lies lateral to extensor hallucis longus tendon
    - Passes to proximal end of intermetatarsal space and curves deeply to enter sole between heads of first dorsal interosseous muscle
    - Forms part of plantar arch
  - Main branches
    - Medial and lateral tarsal arteries: Arise at the level of the navicular
    - Lateral tarsal artery runs under extensor digitorum brevis
    - Two or three medial tarsal arteries run on the medial surface of the tarsus
  - Lateral tarsal artery runs under extensor digitorum brevis; two or three medial tarsal arteries run on the medial surface of the tarsus
  - Arcuate artery: Arises at medial cuneiform level and runs laterally over metatarsal bases, deep to extensor tendons; gives off branches to the metatarsals and toes
  - First dorsal metatarsal artery: Arises just before dorsalis pedis dives deep into the sole
- **Posterior tibial artery**
  - Continuation of the calf vessel by the same name, a branch of the popliteal artery
  - Runs in the tarsal tunnel behind and below the medial malleolus accompanied by the tibial nerve
  - Divides into its terminal branches in the tarsal tunnel, the medial and plantar arteries
  - Medial plantar artery: runs in medial aspect of foot medial to medial plantar nerve
    - Then deep to abductor hallucis and flexor digitorum brevis muscles
  - Lateral plantar artery: Runs in lateral aspect of foot lateral to the lateral plantar nerve
    - Then deep to the abductor hallucis muscle and distally between the flexor digitorum brevis and quadratus plantae muscles
    - Distally runs between flexor digitorum brevis and abductor digiti minimi; between base of first and second metatarsals, finally joins dorsalis pedis to form the plantar arch
- **Plantar arch**
  - An arterial arch at level of metatarsals
  - Formed by dorsalis pedis and lateral plantar arteries
  - Gives off branches to metatarsals and toes
- **Peroneal artery**
  - Accompanies superficial peroneal nerve down anterolateral aspect of ankle and sends off a perforating branch that joins a communicating branch from anterior tibial artery
  - May join or replace posterior tibial artery

Veins

- Superficial veins
  - Great saphenous vein
    - Arises from medial part of dorsal venous arch of foot
    - Runs subcutaneously over muscles and tendons to pass anterior to medial malleolus
    - Passes superiorly on medial aspect of calf and thigh to join common femoral vein at femoral triangle
  - Small saphenous vein
    - Arises from lateral part of dorsal venous arch
    - Runs subcutaneously over muscles and tendons to pass posterior to lateral malleolus
    - Passes superiorly on lateral and posterior side of calf to join popliteal vein in popliteal fossa
- Deep veins
  - Plantar venous arch: Receives venous drainage from dorsal and plantar aspects of toes and metatarsals
  - Medial and lateral plantar veins: Arise from plantar venous arch to accompany same named arteries
  - Communication exists with great and small saphenous veins
  - Medial and lateral plantar veins form posterior tibial veins in tarsal tunnel and run proximally to calf, accompanying posterior tibial artery

Anatomy-Based Imaging Issues

Imaging Recommendations

- US
  - Provides greatest amount of information on vasculature of foot of the different imaging modalities available
  - Morphology and functional status of vessels can be assessed
  - Color Doppler scans allow assessment for vessel occlusion and thrombosis
  - Spectral Doppler scans allow quantitative and semiquantitative documentation of flow velocity, resistance, waveform etc.
  - Augmentation of foot veins usually only requires small degrees of flexion/extension of toes to produce enough venous flow for detection (unlike need to squeeze muscles in calf)

Imaging Pitfalls

- Superficial veins are easily compressed even with lightest transducer pressure
  - A thick layer of coupling gel helps act as a spacer between the transducer and skin to minimize pressure and allows better visualization of vessels

FOOT VESSELS

DORSAL AND PLANTAR ARTERIES AND NERVES

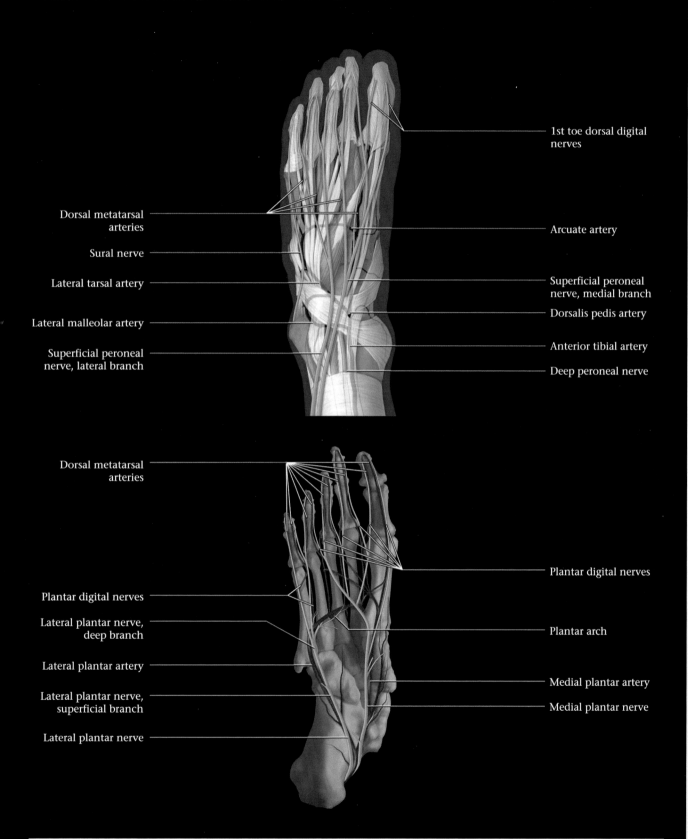

Dorsal metatarsal arteries

Sural nerve

Lateral tarsal artery

Lateral malleolar artery

Superficial peroneal nerve, lateral branch

1st toe dorsal digital nerves

Arcuate artery

Superficial peroneal nerve, medial branch

Dorsalis pedis artery

Anterior tibial artery

Deep peroneal nerve

Dorsal metatarsal arteries

Plantar digital nerves

Lateral plantar nerve, deep branch

Lateral plantar artery

Lateral plantar nerve, superficial branch

Lateral plantar nerve

Plantar digital nerves

Plantar arch

Medial plantar artery

Medial plantar nerve

(Top) Graphic of arteries and nerves at dorsal aspect of the foot. The deep peroneal nerve accompanies the anterior tibial artery. The superficial peroneal nerve divides into medial and lateral branches in distal 3rd of leg. Anterior tibial artery is called dorsalis pedis in foot. It terminates in arcuate artery, which communicates with plantar arterial arch, and in digital vessels. **(Bottom)** Graphic of arteries and nerve at the plantar aspect of the foot. The posterior tibial nerve and artery divide into medial and lateral plantar branches. These divide further into digital branches to the medial and lateral aspects of each toe. The plantar arch sends vessels dorsally as well as to the plantar aspect of the toes.

FOOT VESSELS

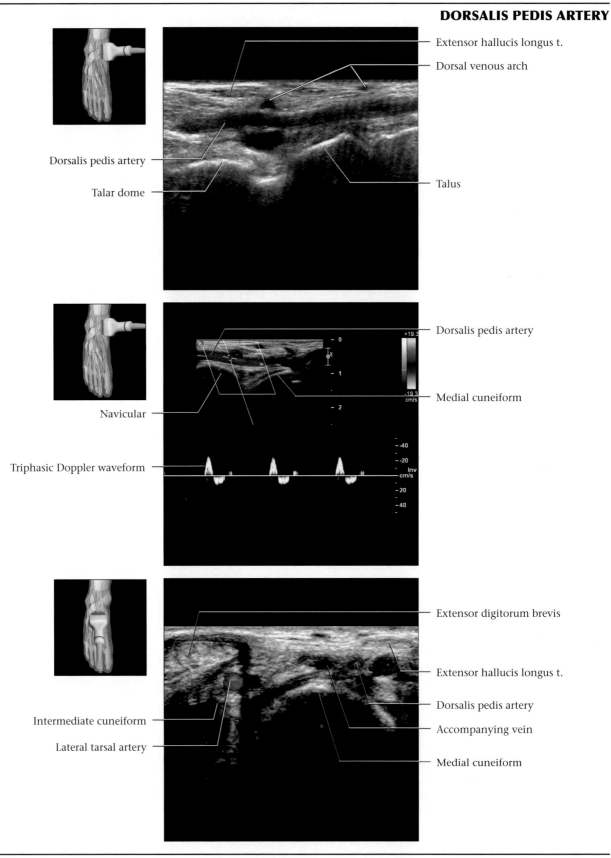

(Top) Sagittal scan of the dorsum of the foot. The dorsalis pedis artery runs at the anterior aspect of the transverse arch formed by the tarsal bones. It is a continuation of the anterior tibial artery and runs lateral to the extensor hallucis longus tendon. **(Middle)** Sagittal spectral Doppler scan of the dorsalis pedis artery shows the typical triphasic artery flow. **(Bottom)** Coronal color Doppler scan of the dorsum of the foot at the level of the cuneiform. The dorsalis pedis artery gives rise to medial and lateral tarsal arteries at the level of the navicular. The dorsalis pedis artery remains lateral to the extensor hallucis longus tendon even at this distal level.

Labels (Top): Extensor hallucis longus t.; Dorsal venous arch; Dorsalis pedis artery; Talar dome; Talus

Labels (Middle): Dorsalis pedis artery; Medial cuneiform; Navicular; Triphasic Doppler waveform

Labels (Bottom): Extensor digitorum brevis; Extensor hallucis longus t.; Dorsalis pedis artery; Accompanying vein; Medial cuneiform; Intermediate cuneiform; Lateral tarsal artery

FOOT VESSELS

METATARSAL & DIGITAL ARTERIES

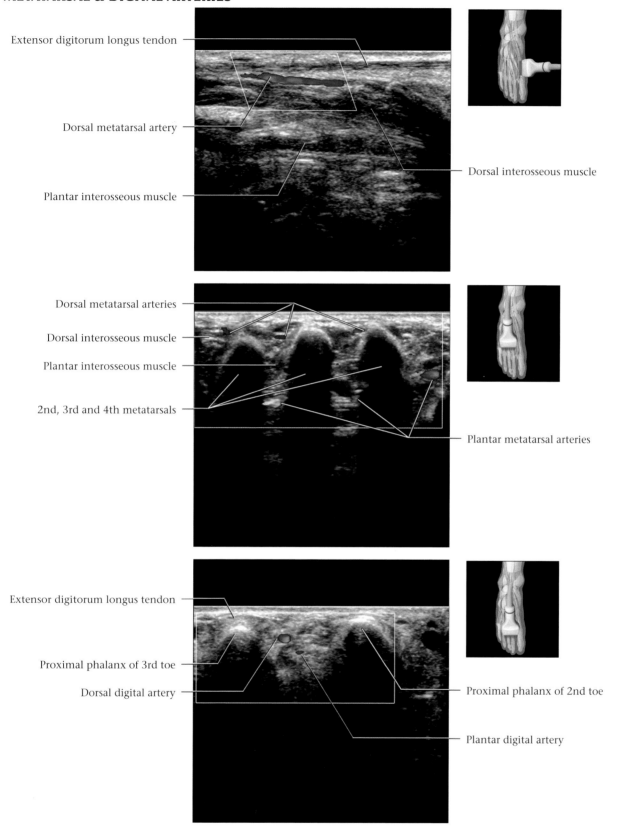

Extensor digitorum longus tendon

Dorsal metatarsal artery

Plantar interosseous muscle

Dorsal interosseous muscle

Dorsal metatarsal arteries

Dorsal interosseous muscle

Plantar interosseous muscle

2nd, 3rd and 4th metatarsals

Plantar metatarsal arteries

Extensor digitorum longus tendon

Proximal phalanx of 3rd toe

Dorsal digital artery

Proximal phalanx of 2nd toe

Plantar digital artery

(Top) Sagittal color Doppler of the second interosseous space. The arcuate artery gives rise to dorsal metatarsal arteries which run in the interosseous spaces to supply the metatarsals and toes. The two layers of interosseous muscles can be appreciated here. (Middle) Transverse color Doppler scan of the metatarsal bodies. Both the dorsal and plantar interosseous muscles can be seen between the bones. The dorsal and plantar metatarsal arteries are also demonstrable by the use of color Doppler. The plantar metatarsal arteries arise from the plantar arch. (Bottom) Coronal color Doppler scan of the second web space. The dorsal and plantar metatarsal arteries continue distally as the digital arteries, which will divide further to run on the sides of the phalanges.

FOOT VESSELS

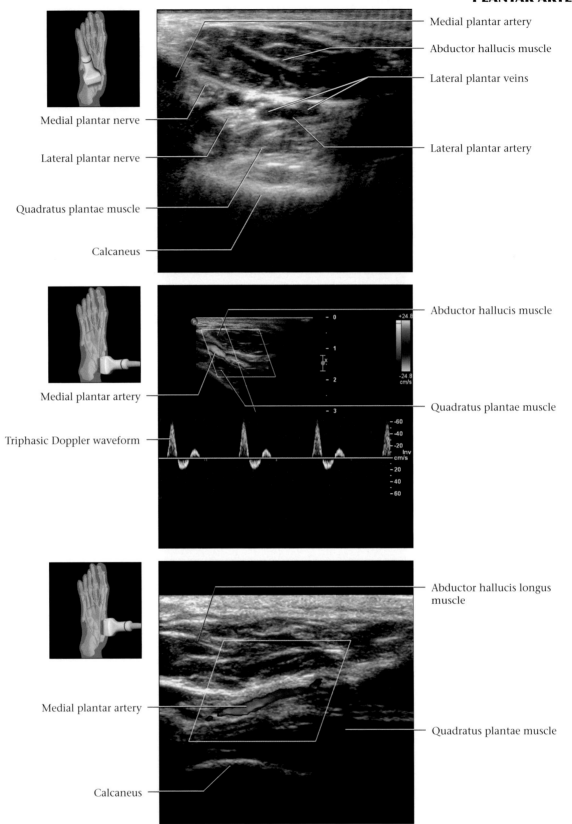

Top image labels:
- Medial plantar artery
- Abductor hallucis muscle
- Lateral plantar veins
- Lateral plantar artery
- Medial plantar nerve
- Lateral plantar nerve
- Quadratus plantae muscle
- Calcaneus

Middle image labels:
- Abductor hallucis muscle
- Medial plantar artery
- Quadratus plantae muscle
- Triphasic Doppler waveform

Bottom image labels:
- Abductor hallucis longus muscle
- Medial plantar artery
- Quadratus plantae muscle
- Calcaneus

(Top) Coronal scan of the medial plantar compartment. The tibial nerve has divided into the medial and lateral plantar nerves and similarly the posterior tibial vessels have divided into medial and lateral plantar vessels. Note that this is a scan of the left foot and the lateral side is on the right of the image. **(Middle)** Spectral Doppler scan of the medial plantar artery showing a typical triphasic arterial waveform. **(Bottom)** Oblique sagittal color Doppler scan of the medial compartment shows the medial plantar artery running between the abductor hallucis muscle and the quadratus plantae muscle.

FOOT VESSELS

PLANTAR ARTERIES

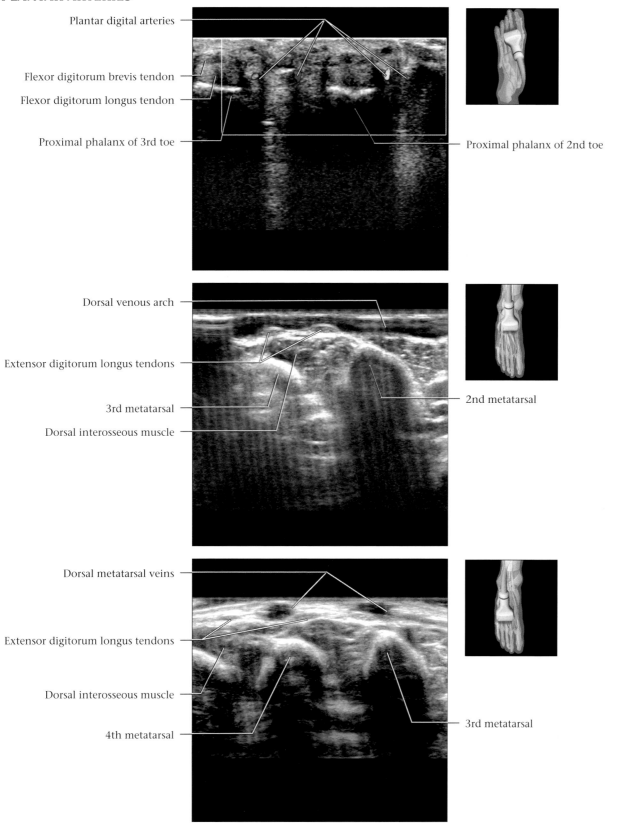

Plantar digital arteries

Flexor digitorum brevis tendon

Flexor digitorum longus tendon

Proximal phalanx of 3rd toe

Proximal phalanx of 2nd toe

Dorsal venous arch

Extensor digitorum longus tendons

3rd metatarsal

Dorsal interosseous muscle

2nd metatarsal

Dorsal metatarsal veins

Extensor digitorum longus tendons

Dorsal interosseous muscle

4th metatarsal

3rd metatarsal

(Top) Coronal color Doppler scan of the plantar aspect of the toes. The digital arteries can be seen on both sides of the phalanges as they travel more distally. **(Middle)** Coronal scan of the dorsum of the foot at the metatarsal level. Minimal pressure was used during this scan to prevent compression of the superficial (subcutaneous) veins. Here, the transversely running dorsal venous arch is demonstrated. The extensor tendons and the interossei run deep to this arch. **(Bottom)** More distally, a coronal scan of the dorsum of the foot shows the tributaries of the dorsal venous arch, the dorsal metatarsal veins.

METATARSALS AND TOES

Imaging Anatomy

Overview
- In normal weight-bearing stance, all of the metatarsal heads are at same level, and all are weight-bearing
  - Metatarsophalangeal (MTP) joints are slightly extended in standing position
- Each metatarsophalangeal joint is a separate synovial cavity

Metatarsal Bones
- 1st metatarsal
  - Largest metatarsal
  - Articulates with 1st cuneiform, 1st proximal phalanx, sesamoids
  - Medially receives attachments from the tibialis anterior tendon, plantar side receives peroneus longus tendon
  - Origin of medial head of first dorsal interosseous muscle on its lateral surface
- Second to fourth metatarsals
  - Gradually smaller and shorter moving laterally
  - Receive the interosseous muscle on the medial and lateral sides
- Fifth metatarsal
  - Insertion of peroneus tertius & brevis

Phalanges
- Distal phalanx is insertion site for: Tendons from flexor and extensor digitorum longus
- Middle phalanx is insertion site for tendons from flexor and extensor digitorum brevis
- Second to fourth proximal phalanges are the attachments of interosseous muscles on both sides and lumbricals on the medial side

1st Metatarsophalangeal Joint
- Dorsiflexion of toe important in push-off phase of gait
- Metatarsal head has 2 concave facets at plantar surface, 1 for each sesamoid, separated by ridge (crista)
- Distal articular surface of metatarsal head may be flat, rounded, or have a central prominence
- Base of proximal phalanx has concave contour
- **Sesamoids**
  - Either sesamoid may be unipartite or bipartite
  - Medial sesamoid in medial head flexor hallucis brevis and abductor hallucis
  - Lateral sesamoid in lateral head flexor hallucis brevis and adductor hallucis and deep metatarsal ligament
  - Medial and lateral sesamoids joined by intersesamoid ligament
    - Intersesamoid ligament is floor of canal in which runs flexor hallucis longus tendon
  - Both are embedded in plantar plate of joint
  - **Sesamophalangeal apparatus**
    - Sesamoids fixed in position relative to 1st proximal phalanx, move relative to 1st metatarsal
    - Therefore displaced laterally in hallux valgus
- **Plantar plate**
  - Fibrocartilaginous plantar capsular thickening extending from metatarsal neck to base proximal phalanx
  - Incorporates sesamoids

Lateral Metatarsophalangeal Joints
- Convex metatarsal head articular surface articulates with concave articular surface of proximal phalangeal base
- Plantar aspect of metatarsal head has rounded contour
- Dorsal aspect of metatarsal head is smaller than plantar aspect
  - Has concave or notched contour along medial and lateral margins
- Sesamoids variably present, most commonly at 5th toe
- **Phalangeal apparatus** is combination of plantar plate and proximal phalanx
- **Plantar plate**
  - Fibrocartilaginous plantar capsular thickening extending from metatarsal neck to base proximal phalanx
  - Attached to deep transverse metatarsal ligament, plantar fascia and flexor tendon sheath, medial and lateral collateral ligaments
  - Instability may mimic Morton neuroma

Anatomy-Based Imaging Issues

Imaging Recommendations
- Ultrasound
  - Good for assessing tendon integrity and joint alignment
    - Tendon integrity recognized by morphology (continuity of tendon and densely packed appearance of tendon fibers) and by behavior during passive movement
    - Joints can also be assessed dynamically during flexion and extension
  - Limited use in assessing for global bony alignment

Clinical Implications

Clinical Importance
- Instability of MTP joints results in pain and deformity of forefoot

Stability of 1st MTP Joint
- Collateral ligaments
- Flexor and extensor hallucis brevis muscles
- Flexor and extensor hallucis longus have a smaller contribution to stability

Stability of Lateral MTP Joints
- Collateral ligaments
- Plantar plate
  - Rupture of plantar plate results in dorsal subluxation of MTP joint and hammer toe deformity

Short 1st Metatarsal (Morton Foot)
- Normal variant but increases stress on 2nd metatarsal
- Predisposes to osteonecrosis of 2nd metatarsal head (Freiberg infraction)

METATARSALS AND TOES

FIRST METATARSAL HEAD SECTION AND TOES

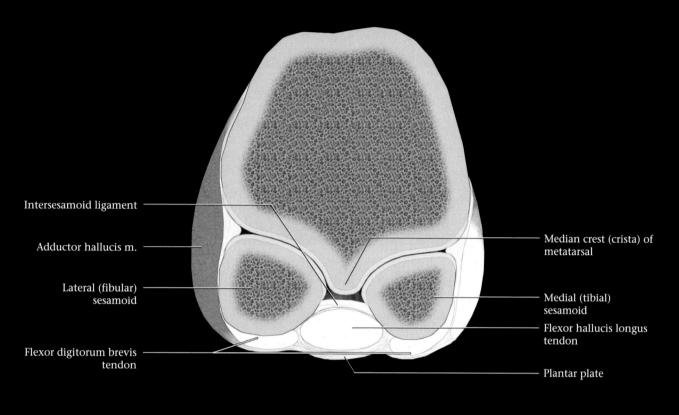

Intersesamoid ligament

Adductor hallucis m.

Lateral (fibular) sesamoid

Flexor digitorum brevis tendon

Median crest (crista) of metatarsal

Medial (tibial) sesamoid

Flexor hallucis longus tendon

Plantar plate

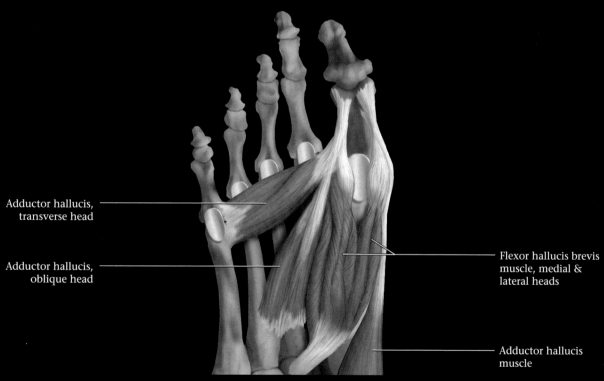

Adductor hallucis, transverse head

Adductor hallucis, oblique head

Flexor hallucis brevis muscle, medial & lateral heads

Adductor hallucis muscle

(Top) Coronal graphic shows sesamoids positioned at the plantar surface of the 1st metatarsal head, separated by the median crest of metatarsal. The sesamoids are united by the intersesamoid ligament. The intersesamoid ligament forms the floor of the groove between the sesamoids, and the flexor hallucis longus tendon runs along this groove. **(Bottom)** Axial graphic shows muscle attachments to sesamoids of 1st metatarsophalangeal joint. Abductor hallucis and medial head of flexor hallucis brevis attach to medial sesamoid. Lateral head of flexor hallucis brevis and adductor hallucis attach to lateral sesamoid.

METATARSALS AND TOES

Extensor digitorum brevis ts. for 2nd & 3rd metatarsals

Extensor hallucis brevis tendon

Extensor hallucis longus t.

5th metatarsal

Dorsal interossei muscles

1st metatarsal

Dorsal venous arch

Medial cuneiform

Base of metatarsal

Extensor hallucis longus t.

Shaft of metatarsal

Dorsal venous arch

Extensor hallucis longus tendon

Shaft of 1st metatarsal

Head of 1st metatarsal

Neck of 1st metatarsal

(Top) Coronal panoramic scan of the dorsal surface of the bodies of the metatarsals. The dorsal interosseous muscles lie between the bodies of the metatarsals. Their action is to abduct the toes. The plantar interosseous muscles act to adduct the toes. The extensor digitorum longus and extensor hallucis longus tendons receive assistance from their brevis tendons which are deeper and approach from a lateral aspect. **(Middle)** Sagittal scan of the dorsum of the big toe at the level of the tarsometatarsal joint. The extensor hallucis longus tendon is in close proximity to the bones around the joint. Note the densely packed and parallel echogenic tendon fibers. **(Bottom)** Sagittal scan of the head of the 1st metatarsal. The extensor hallucis longus tendon is separated from the neck and most of the body of the metatarsal by fat.

METATARSALS AND TOES

PLANTAR METATARSAL

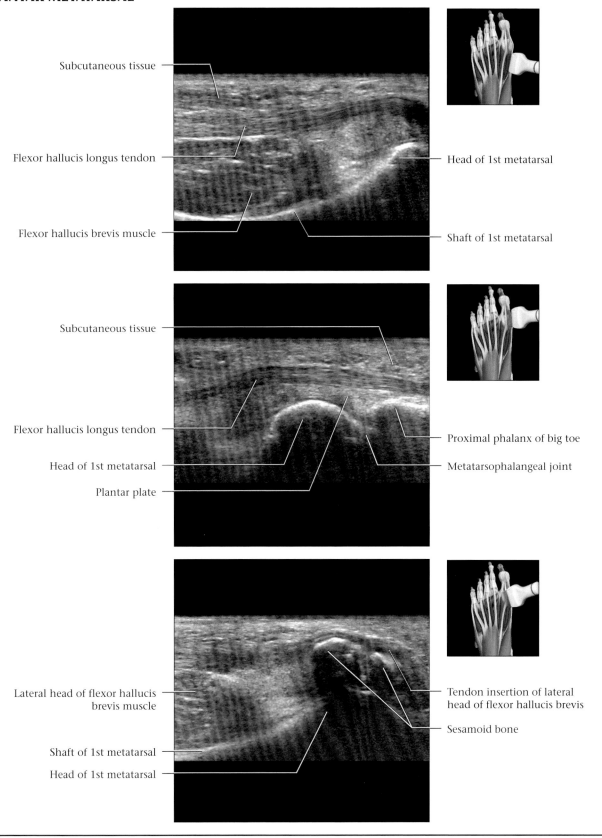

Subcutaneous tissue

Flexor hallucis longus tendon

Flexor hallucis brevis muscle

Head of 1st metatarsal

Shaft of 1st metatarsal

Subcutaneous tissue

Flexor hallucis longus tendon

Head of 1st metatarsal

Plantar plate

Proximal phalanx of big toe

Metatarsophalangeal joint

Lateral head of flexor hallucis brevis muscle

Shaft of 1st metatarsal

Head of 1st metatarsal

Tendon insertion of lateral head of flexor hallucis brevis

Sesamoid bone

(**Top**) Sagittal scan of the plantar aspect of the head of the 1st metatarsal. The flexor hallucis longus muscle originates in the calf, while the brevis muscle arises from the cuboid and lateral cuneiform bones and tendon of the tibialis posterior. (**Middle**) Sagittal scan of the center of the 1st metatarsophalangeal joint. The flexor hallucis longus tendon passes over the plantar plate of this joint to reach its insertion at the distal phalanx. (**Bottom**) Oblique sagittal scan of the first metatarsophalangeal joint, just lateral to the center. The flexor hallucis brevis tendons insert on to both sides of the base of the proximal phalanx via two tendons. Each tendon contains a sesamoid bone. Sesamoid bones may be bipartite as seen here, especially for the medial sesamoid.

METATARSALS AND TOES

Flexor hallucis longus tendon

Flexor digitorum brevis muscle

Abductor hallucis muscle

Base of 1st metatarsal

Flexor hallucis brevis muscle

Bases of 2nd, 3rd and 4th metatarsals

Flexor digitorum longus tendons

3rd metatarsal base

Flexor digitorum brevis tendons

2nd metatarsal base

Common plantar digital artery

Flexor hallucis longus tendon

Medial slip of flexor hallucis brevis tendon

Sesamoid bone in medial head of flexor hallucis brevis tendon

2nd metatarsal

Sesamoid bone in lateral head of flexor hallucis brevis tendon

Head of 1st metatarsal, partially obscured by sesamoid

(Top) Transverse scan of plantar aspect of the bases of the medial metatarsals. The abductor hallucis muscle is superficial to the first and second metatarsals. The base of the first metatarsal is uniquely large compared to the rest of the metatarsals and is easily identifiable. The flexor hallucis longus tendon runs superficial to the brevis muscle. (Middle) Transverse scan of the plantar surface of the base of the second and third metatarsals. The base of the metatarsals form an arch with plantar concavity. The flexor digitorum longus tendons run centrally on the plantar surfaces of the metatarsals. (Bottom) Transverse scan of the plantar surface of the first metatarsal. The flexor hallucis longus runs between the two sesamoid bones on the plantar aspect of the first metatarsal. The sesamoids adhere to the medial and lateral heads of the flexor hallucis brevis tendons.

METATARSALS AND TOES

TOE, PLANTAR AND DORSUM

Superficial veins

Flexor hallucis longus tendon

Proximal phalanx

Head of 1st metatarsal

Metatarsal-phalangeal joint

Flexor digitorum longus and brevis tendons

Insertion of flexor digitorum longus tendon

Proximal phalanx

Distal phalanx

Middle phalanx

Distal interphalangeal joint

Nail

Coupling gel as acoustic window

Extensor digitorum longus tendon

Nail bed

Proximal phalanx of big toe

Superficial veins

Distal phalanx of big toe

(Top) Sagittal scan of the plantar surface of the first tarsometatarsal joint. The flexor hallucis tendon runs close to the plantar surface of the phalanges and inserts at the base of the distal phalanx. (Middle) Sagittal scan of the plantar surface of the second toe. The flexor digitorum longus tendon inserts centrally at the base of the distal phalanx. The flexor digitorum brevis inserts on the sides of the base of the middle phalanx. Passive flexion of only the distal interphalangeal joint allows isolated evaluation of the tendon's movement (and integrity) of the flexor digitorum longus tendon. (Bottom) Sagittal color Doppler scan of the dorsal surface of the distal phalanx of the big toe. The extensor digitorum longus tendon inserts on the dorsal surface of the base of the distal phalanx. The nail bed has a rich vascular supply as demonstrated by the color flow.

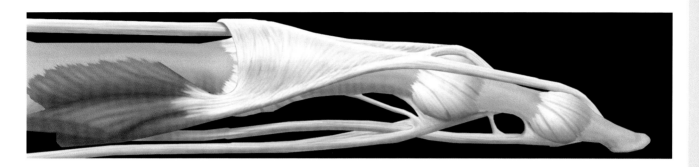

INDEX

INDEX

INDEX

INDEX

INDEX

INDEX

INDEX

INDEX

INDEX

INDEX

INDEX

INDEX

INDEX

INDEX

Index

INDEX

INDEX

INDEX

INDEX

INDEX

INDEX

INDEX

INDEX

INDEX

P

INDEX

INDEX

INDEX

INDEX

INDEX

INDEX

INDEX

INDEX

INDEX

INDEX

INDEX